Pedia[illegible] Pulmonology

Author
American Academy of Pediatrics Section on Pediatric Pulmonology

Editor in Chief
Michael J. Light, MD, FAAP

Associate Editors
Carol J. Blaisdell, MD, FAAP
Douglas N. Homnick, MD, FAAP
Michael S. Schechter, MD, FAAP
Miles M. Wienberger, MD, FAAP

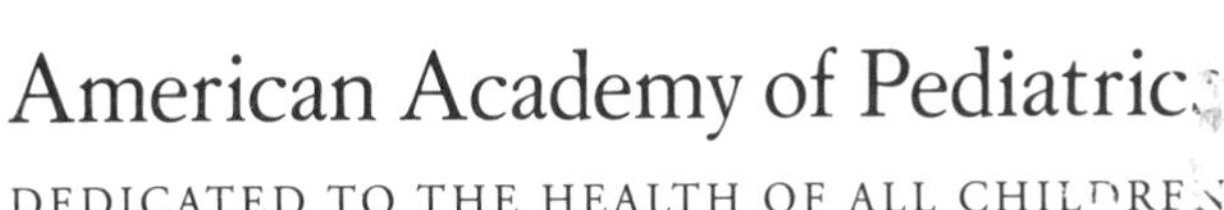

American Academy of Pediatrics Department of Marketing and Publications Staff

Maureen DeRosa, MPA, Director, Department of Marketing and Publications

Mark Grimes, Director, Division of Product Development

Martha Cook, MS, Senior Product Development Editor

Carrie Peters, Editorial Assistant

Sandi King, MS, Director, Division of Publishing and Production Services

Kate Larson, Manager, Editorial Services

Theresa Wiener, Manager, Publications Production and Manufacturing

Linda Diamond, Manager, Art Direction and Production

Kevin Tuley, Director, Division of Sales and Marketing

Linda Smessaert, Manager, Publication and Program Marketing

Library of Congress Control Number: 2010906482
ISBN: 978-1-58110-492-9
MA0562

The recommendations in this publication do not indicate an exclusive course of treatment or serve as a standard of medical care. Variations, taking into account individual circumstances, may be appropriate.

The mention of product names in this publication is for informational purposes only and does not imply endorsement by the American Academy of Pediatrics.

Every effort has been made to ensure that the drug selection and dosage set forth in this text are in accordance with the current recommendations and practice at the time of publication. It is the responsibility of the health care provider to check the package insert of each drug for any change in indications and dosage and for added warnings and precautions.

The publishers have made every effort to trace the copyright holders for borrowed material. If they have inadvertently overlooked any, they will be pleased to make the necessary arrangements at the first opportunity.

3-227/0511

1 2 3 4 5 6 7 8 9 10

Editorial Board

American Academy of Pediatrics Reviewers

John Curran, MD, FAAP,
Board of Directors

Committee on Drugs

Richmond Center

Committee on Bioethics

Committee on Genetics

Committee on Hospital Care

Committee on Infectious Diseases

Committee on Nutrition

Council on Environmental Health

Section on Allergy and Immunology

Section on Cardiology and Cardiac Surgery

Section on Clinical Pharmacology and Therapeutics

Section on Endocrinology

Section on Epidemiology

Section on Gastroenterology, Hepatology & Nutrition

Section on Hematology/Oncology

Section on Home Care

Section on Infectious Diseases

Section on Radiology

Section on Rheumatology

Contributors

Julian L. Allen, MD
Professor of Pediatrics
University of Pennsylvania School of Medicine
Chief, Division of Pulmonary Medicine and Cystic Fibrosis Center
The Children's Hospital of Philadelphia
Philadelphia, Pennsylvania

Molly K. Ball, MD
Fellow, Neonatal-Perinatal Medicine
Northwestern University
Chicago, Illinois

Suzanne E. Beck, MD
Associate Professor of Clinical Pediatrics
The Children's Hospital of Philadelphia
Philadelphia, Pennsylvania

Renee Benson, MD
Pediatric Pulmonology Fellow
Children's Hospital & Research Center Oakland
Oakland, California

Ariel Berlinski, MD, FAAP
Associate Professor
Pediatric Pulmonology Section, Department of Pediatrics
University of Arkansas for Medical Sciences, College of Medicine
Director, Aerosol Research Laboratory at ACHRI
Little Rock, Arkansas

Ellen K. Bowser, MD
Associate in Pediatrics
University of Florida College of Medicine
Pediatric Pulmonary Division
Gainesville, Florida

John S. Bradley, MD, FAAP
Professor of Clinical Pediatrics
Chief, Division of Infectious Diseases, Department of Pediatrics
University of California, San Diego
School of Medicine
Director, Division of Infectious Diseases
Rady Children's Hospital San Diego
San Diego, California

Lee J. Brooks, MD
Attending Physician
Division of Pulmonary and Sleep Medicine
The Children's Hospital of Philadelphia
Philadelphia, Pennsylvania

Robyn T. Cohen, MD, MPH
Assistant Professor of Pediatrics
Drexel University College of Medicine
Section of Pulmonology and Allergy
St Christopher's Hospital for Children
Philadelphia, Pennsylvania

John L. Colombo, MD, FAAP
Director, Pediatric Pulmonology and NE Cystic Fibrosis Center
University of Nebraska Medical Center
Clinical Service Chief, Children's Hospital Medical Center and University of Nebraska Medical Center, Pediatric Pulmonology
Omaha, Nebraska

Carol Conrad, MD
Associate Professor of Pediatrics
Director, Pediatric Lung and Heart-Lung Transplant Program
Stanford University
Palo Alto, California

Robin R. Deterding, MD
Professor of Pediatrics
University of Colorado
The Children's Hospital Denver
Aurora, Colorado

Mark F. Dovey, MD
Associate Professor of Pediatrics
Drexel University College of Medicine
Chief, Section of Pulmonology and Allergy
St Christopher's Hospital for Children
Philadelphia, Pennsylvania

Martin B. Draznin, MD, FAAP
Director, Pediatric Endocrine Sub Specialty Clinics
Associate Program Director, Pediatrics
Michigan State University Kalamazoo Center for Medical Studies
Professor, Pediatrics and Human Development
Michigan State University College of Human Medicine
Kalamazoo, Michigan

Harold J. Farber, MD, MSPH, FAAP
Associate Professor of Pediatrics, Section of Pulmonology
Baylor College of Medicine
Texas Children's Hospital
Houston, Texas

Elizabeth K. Fiorino, MD, FAAP
Assistant Professor of Pediatrics
Division of Pediatric Pulmonology
New York University School of Medicine
New York, New York

Edward W. Fong, MD
Pediatric Pulmonologist
Bay Area Pediatric Pulmonary Medical Corporation
Children's Hospital & Research Center at Oakland
California Pacific Medical Center
Oakland, California

Alexandra Freeman, MD
Staff Clinician
Laboratory of Clinical Infectious Diseases
NIAID/NIH
Bethesda, Maryland

David Geller, MD
Nemours Children's Clinic
Associate Clinical Professor, Pediatrics
Florida State University and
University of Central Florida Schools of Medicine
Orlando, Florida

Samuel B. Goldfarb, MD
Assistant Professor of Clinical Pediatrics
University of Pennsylvania
Philadelphia, Pennsylvania

Karen A. Hardy, MD, FAAP
Director, Pediatric Pulmonary, BAPP, CHRCO and CPMC
Associate Clinical Scientist, CHORI
Clinical Professor, University of California, San Francisco
San Francisco, California

Christopher E. Harris, MD, FAAP
Director, Pediatric Pulmonary Medicine
Cedars-Sinai Medical Center
Associate Clinical Professor
David Geffen School of Medicine
University of California-Los Angeles
Los Angeles, California

Leslie Hendeles, PharmD
Professor, Pharmacotherapy and Translational Research
Professor of Pediatrics
University of Florida
Gainesville, Florida

Michael Henrickson, MD, MPH, FAAP
Clinical Director, Division of Rheumatology
Cincinnati Children's Hospital Medical Center
Associate Professor
University of Cincinnati College of Medicine
Cincinnati, Ohio

H. William Kelly, PharmD
Professor Emeritus of Pediatrics and Pharmacy
Department of Pediatrics, School of Medicine
University of New Mexico Health Sciences Center
Professor Emeritus of Pediatrics
Department of Pediatrics
Pediatrics/Pulmonary
Albuquerque, New Mexico

Katharine Kevill, MD, FAAP
Assistant Professor
Division of Pediatric Pulmonary Medicine
Duke University School of Medicine
Durham, North Carolina

T. Bernard Kinane, MD
Associate Professor of Pediatrics
Chief of Pediatric Pulmonology
Massachusetts General Hospital for Children
Harvard Medical School
Boston, Massachusetts

Richard M. Kravitz, MD, FAAP
Associate Professor of Pediatrics
Duke University Medical Center
Durham, NC

Nandini Madan, MD
Attending Cardiologist
St. Christopher's Hospital for Children
Assistant Professor of Pediatrics
Drexel University
Philadelphia, Pennsylvania

Oscar Henry Mayer, MD
Clinical Assistant Professor of Pediatrics
The Children's Hospital of Philadelphia
University of Pennsylvania School of Medicine
Philadelphia, Pennsylvania

Susanna B. McColley, MD, FAAP
Head, Division of Pulmonary Medicine
Children's Memorial Hospital
Associate Professor of Pediatrics
Northwestern University Feinberg School of Medicine
Chicago, Illinois

Peter H. Michelson, MD, MS
Associate Professor of Pediatrics
Washington University School of Medicine
St. Louis, Missouri

Manisha Newaskar, MBBS
Pediatric Pulmonologist
Children's Hospital and Research Center at Oakland
Oakland, California

Brian P. O'Sullivan, MD, FAAP
Professor of Pediatrics
UMass Memorial Medical Center
University of Massachusetts Medical School
Worcester, Massachusetts

Julieta M. Oneto, MD
Pediatric Radiologist
Palm Beach Radiology Professionals
Atlantis, Florida

Kenneth N. Olivier, MD, MPH
Staff Clinician
Laboratory of Clinical Infectious Diseases
NIAID/NIH
Bethesda, Maryland

Sebnem Ozdogan, MD
Pediatric Pulmonary Fellow
Children's Hospital and Research Center at Oakland
Oakland, California

Howard B. Panitch, MD
Professor of Pediatrics
University of Pennsylvania School of Medicine
Director of Clinical Programs
Division of Pulmonary Medicine
The Children's Hospital of Philadelphia
Philadelphia, PA

Theresa D. Pattugalan, MD, FAAP
Department of Pediatrics
Albert Einstein Medical Center
Philadelphia, Pennsylvania

Madhuri Penugonda, MD
Pediatric Pulmonology Fellow
Emory University
Atlanta, Georgia

Adrienne Prestridge, MD
Attending Physician, Pulmonary Medicine
Associate Director, Cystic Fibrosis Center
Director, Pulmonary Function Lab
Director, Pediatric Pulmonary Fellowship
Children's Memorial Hospital
Chicago, Illinois

Patricia M. Quigley, MD
Assistant Medical Director
Director of Pulmonary Medicine
Mount Washington Pediatric Hospital
Assistant Professor of Pediatrics
Johns Hopkins University School of Medicine
Baltimore, Maryland

Keyvan Rafei, MD, MBA
Chief, Division of Pediatric Pulmonology
Division of Pediatric Pulmonology
University of Rochester
Rochester, New York

Clement L. Ren, MD, FAAP
Associate Professor of Pediatrics
Chief, Division of Pediatric Pulmonology
Division of Pediatric Pulmonology
University of Rochester
Rochester, New York

Ricardo Restrepo, MD
Pediatric Radiology Fellowship Program Director
Radiology Department
Miami Children's Hospital
Miami, Florida

David P.L. Sachs, MD
Director, Palo Alto Center for Pulmonary Disease Prevention
Attending Physician, Pulmonary and Critical Care Medicine
Stanford University Hospital
Palo Alto, California

Paul H. Sammut, MD, FAAP
Associate Professor of Pediatrics
University of Nebraska Medical Center
Omaha, NE

James W. Schroeder Jr, MD, FACS, FAAP
Division of Pediatric Otolaryngology
Children's Memorial Hospital
Assistant Professor
Department of Otolaryngology Head and Neck Surgery
Feinberg School of Medicine
Northwestern University
Chicago, Illinois

Daniel J. Schidlow, MD, FAAP
Professor and Chair, Department of Pediatrics
Senior Associate Dean
Drexel University College of Medicine
Physician in Chief
St. Christopher's Hospital for Children
Philadelphia, PA

John Schuen, MD
Chief, Pediatric Pulmonary & Sleep Medicine Division
Helen DeVos Children's Hospital
Associate Professor of Pediatrics & Human Development
Michigan State University College of Human Medicine
A Diplomate of the American Board of Pediatrics in
General Pediatrics, Pediatric Pulmonary & Sleep Medicine
Grand Rapids, Michigan

Girish D. Sharma, MD, FAAP
Associate Professor of Pediatrics
Director, Section of Pediatric, Pulmonology and Rush Cystic Fibrosis Center
Rush University Medical Center
Chicago, Illinois

Eli J. Sills, MD, FAAP
The Permanente Medical Group
Oakland, California

Dawn M. Simon, MD, FAAP
Assistant Professor of Pediatrics
Emory University
Atlanta, Georgia

Marianna M. Sockrider, MD, DrPH, FAAP
Associate Professor
Pediatric Pulmonology
Chief of Pediatric Pulmonary Clinics
Texas Children's Hospital
Houston, Texas

Jonathan Steinfeld, MD
Assistant Professor of Pediatrics
Drexel University School of Medicine
Section of Pulmonology
St. Christopher's Hospital for Children
Philadelphia, Pennsylvania

Paul C. Stillwell, MD, FAAP
Senior Instructor
Department of Pediatrics
University of Colorado-Denver
The Children's Hospital Denver
Aurora, Colorado

Robert Strunk, MD
Professor of Pediatrics
Washington University School of Medicine
St. Louis, Missouri

Danna Tauber, MD, MPH
Attending Physician, Section of Pulmonology
Medical Director, Sleep Disorders Center
St. Christopher's Hospital for Children
Assistant Professor of Pediatrics
Drexel University College of Medicine
Philadelphia, Pennsylvania

Karen Kay Thompson, MD
Pediatrician
Helen Devos Children's Hospital
Pediatric Pulmonary and Sleep Medicine
Grand Rapids, Michigan

Karen Z. Voter, MD, FAAP
Associate Professor of Pediatrics
University of Rochester School of Medicine and Dentistry
Rochester, New York

Mary H. Wagner, MD
Associate Professor
Department of Pediatrics
University of Florida
Gainesville, Florida

Pnina Weiss, MD, FAAP
Assistant Professor, Yale University School of Medicine
Director, Subspecialty Resident Education
Medical Director, Pediatric Pulmonology Function Laboratory
Associate Director, Pediatric Pulmonology Fellowship
New Haven, CT

Eric Zee, MD
Pediatric Pulmonologist
Bay Area Pediatric Pulmonary Medical Corporation
Children's Hospital & Research Center at Oakland
California Pacific Medical Center
San Francisco, California

Table of Contents

Foundation

Anatomical Disorders

Upper Airway Infections

19 Pneumonia 391

Noninfectious Pulmonary Disorders

Genetic Disorders

Lung Disease Associated With Systemic Disorders

44 Pulmonary Complications of Immunologic Disorders 857

45 Pulmonary Complications of Neuromuscular Disorders 875

Treating and Managing Pulmonary Disease

Preface

We proudly present the first edition of *Pediatric Pulmonology,* written by members of the Section on Pediatric Pulmonology of the American Academy of Pediatrics (AAP). This handbook was written primarily for primary care providers who look after children with acute and chronic respiratory problems. However, we expect that specialists who are not pulmonologists will find it useful and that pediatric pulmonologists may occasionally find it an accessible and reliable tool as well. The dominant color throughout the book is blue, which is intentional, so that it may become known as the "Blue Book." Credit needs to be given to Dr Bettina Hilman (the 2011 recipient of the Edward L. Kendig Jr Award for lifetime achievement in pediatric pulmonology), who approached Michael Light when he was chair of the Section on Pediatric Pulmonology and suggested that a "blue book of pediatric pulmonology for the general pediatrician" be written. A few years later, this is the product of her suggestion.

In designing the first edition of this handbook, we attempted to provide a broad-based reference that is as evidence-based as possible. However, for most respiratory conditions in pediatrics there is a paucity of strong evidence to support clinical practice, so reliance still rests to a large degree on experience, anecdote, and extrapolation from adult literature. The guidance to the authors who submitted the chapters was broad. The authors were asked to provide a pragmatic and practical approach to the various subjects that pediatricians need to know about the respiratory care of children. The first 2 chapters introduce the topics of anatomy and physiology. Subsequent chapters include clinical approaches that cover the major topics of pediatric pulmonology from a practical clinical angle. These chapters contain information and recommendations from recognized authorities in the field but, except where they quote formal evidence-based guidelines, should be regarded as earnest opinions but not absolute authority. It is likely that others in the field may disagree with some of the descriptions and recommendations. We expect that this first edition of the Blue Book will undergo extensive change and improvement over time—consider the Piagetian metaphor of accommodation and assimilation or the quality improvement model of Plan-Do-Study-Act cycles—and we welcome input from specialists and generalists alike regarding future editions.

The bulk of the heavy lifting for this book was borne by its editor, Michael Light, and the Section on Pediatric Pulmonology is indebted to him for his time and efforts. Dr Light has accepted a position in the Department of Integrated Medical Education with the Ross University School of Medicine, on the Caribbean island of Dominica. Of course, it was Martha Cook, our staff manager from the AAP, who supported Dr Light while he was doing that heavy lifting. The assistant editors, all current members of the section executive committee, volunteered hours of their time in dedication to this task, and we owe a tremendous debt of gratitude to all of the authors of individual chapters who tolerated our picky criticisms and occasionally heavy-handed rewrites of their contributions. Finally, we thank the AAP for its support of this work, and for its efforts in support of the health of all children.

Michael S. Schechter, MD

Michael J. Light, MD

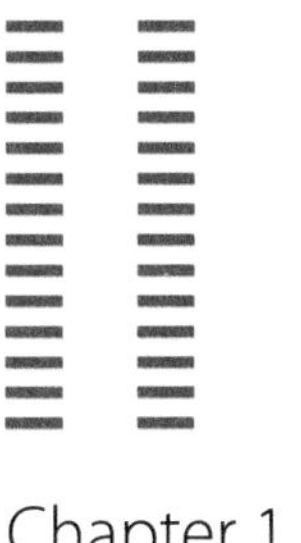

Chapter 1

Anatomy of the Lung

Michael J. Light, MD

Introduction

Knowledge of the development of the lungs helps us to understand congenital pulmonary anomalies. The lungs develop with the ultimate goal of sustaining life after delivery of the newborn. To sustain life, oxygen from the atmosphere is breathed into the lungs and carbon dioxide is excreted. Oxygen provides the fuel to allow the human body to function. Here we describe the gross anatomy of the lung, rather than microscopic anatomy.

Embryology of the Lungs

The 3 laws of development of the lungs according to Reid are as follows:

1. The bronchial tree is developed by the 16th week of intrauterine life.
2. Alveoli develop after birth, increasing in number until 5 to 8 years of age and increasing in size until growth of the chest wall finishes with adulthood.
3. The pre-acinar vessels (arteries and veins) follow the development of the airways; development of the intra-acinar vessels follows that of the alveoli. Muscularization of the intra-acinar arteries does not keep pace with the appearance of new arteries.[1]

There are 5 phases or periods of lung development (Figure 1-1). Before 3 weeks of gestation a pouch arises from the primitive foregut, at which time the embryo is 3 mm in length. This period constitutes the embryonic phase. The lung bud divides into right and left, which will become the right and left lungs. By the end of the embryonic period there will be 5 additional branches, which are the major bronchi, and the lung buds will have elongated into primary lung sacs. Developmental anomalies at this stage will result in anomalies of the major airways, including atresia (closed or undeveloped) and tracheoesophageal fistula.

The glandular period (also called pseudoglandular) starts at the end of the 5th week and continues to the 16th week as the conducting airways are formed by dichotomous branching. It is called pseudoglandular because the airways are blind tubes lined by columnar or cuboidal epithelium. The terminal bronchioles are formed and primitive acinar (terminal airway) structures are developing. If there is a diaphragmatic hernia there is the potential for a reduction in the number of branches formed on the side of the hernia, with resultant hypoplastic lung.

The canalicular period is from the 17th week until the 24th week. During this period the terminal bronchioles will have divided to produce a number of respiratory bronchioles, and the capillary bed is forming so that toward the end of this stage gas exchange can occur and potentially life can be sustained, even though the alveoli have not yet formed.

The airways from the trachea to the 19th generation are the conducting airways and the gas-exchanging units are from the 20th to 27th generation and are the terminal respiratory units. From the major bronchi at the 8th generation to the 20th are the non-respiratory bronchioles, and the respiratory bronchioles are from 20th to 23rd generation (Figure 1-1).

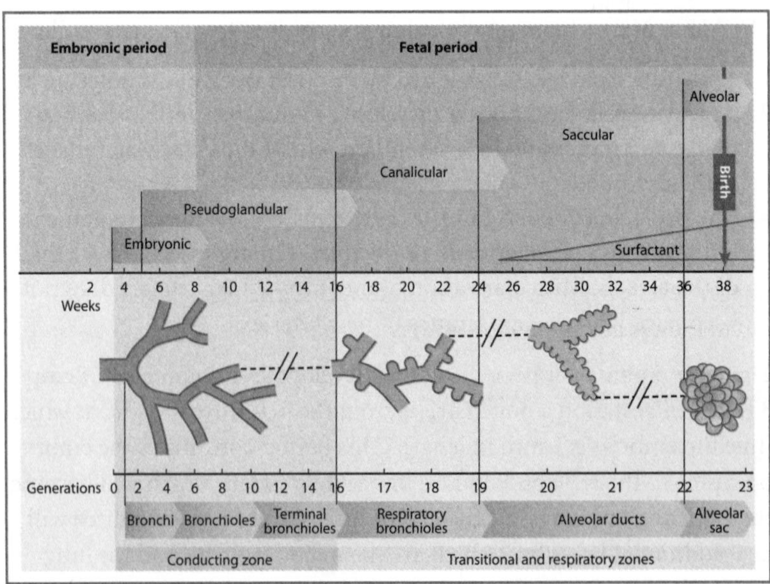

Figure 1-1. The 5 phases of embryonic development, which are approximate and overlapping.

The saccular period extends from the end of the canalicular phase until birth and overlaps with the alveolar period, which extends to 5 to 8 years of age. The terminal respiratory unit comprises the respiratory bronchiole and the alveolar ducts, including the alveoli, and the unit is also known as the acinus. Alveoli are lined by type I (95%) and type II pneumocytes. Type II pneumocytes are cuboidal and synthesize surfactant and divide during repair. Eventually most of them flatten out to form type I pneumocytes, which are supportive. The primitive airways, prior to delivery, contain lung fluid, which drains into the amniotic fluid.

In the postnatal period, alveoli continue to develop until 5 to 8 years of age and enlarge through adolescence. The term infant has between 20 to 50 million alveoli at birth, and this number increases to about 300 million at age 8 years. The alveolar surface area is approximately 2.8 square meters at birth, 32 square meters at 8 years of age, and 75 square meters at adulthood. This last number is often equated to the size of a tennis court.

Blood Supply

During the embryonic and glandular periods, the development of the pulmonary arteries parallels that of the branching airways. During this same period the bronchial vessels are close to the pulmonary vessels. The bronchial arteries supply blood for the nutrition of the lung; they are derived from the thoracic aorta or from the upper aortic intercostal arteries. The conducting airways receive their blood supply from the bronchial vessels, and the terminal respiratory units receive their blood from the pulmonary vessels. The pulmonary veins form from the capillary network and join together to form the 4 main pulmonary veins, which drain oxygenated blood into the left atrium. The pulmonary artery pressures are high at birth and fall, in response to the higher oxygen levels, over the next days and weeks. The bronchial arterial circulation is at systemic pressures.

Pulmonary Lymphatics

The lymphatics draining from the lung comprise lymph ducts, lymph nodes, and the thoracic duct. At birth the pulmonary lymphatics are vital to the removal of lung liquid. There are 2 lymphatic networks: the pleural network and the parenchymal network. Most drainage is toward the hilum and, because of the valves in the lymph channels, the flow moves in one direction. Fully formed lymph nodes are not seen until birth and develop further in infancy. The main right lymphatic ducts follow the right side of the trachea, joining the venous system at the junction of the right jugular and subclavian veins. On the left side the veins follow the trachea and empty into the thoracic duct, which drains into the veins on the left side of the neck. Pulmonary lymphatic drainage is complex and is very variable from individual to individual.

Nerve Supply

The nerve supply of the lungs is from branches of the thoracic sympathetic ganglia and the vagus nerve. The upper 3 to 5 branches of the sympathetic ganglia supply the lungs and the lower supply the intercostal nerves. Almost all of the afferent (sensory) pathways are through the vagus nerve. Figure 1-2 shows the efferent or motor component. The efferent fibers control the caliber of the conducting airways, the activity of bronchial glands, and the state (constricted or dilated) of the pulmonary vessels. The parietal pleura is richly innervated with pain fibers. The visceral pleura has no pain fibers. The phrenic nerves supply the diaphragm, originating from the third to fifth cervical roots (Figure 1-2).

Gross Anatomy of the Lung

The lungs are within the thoracic cavity, separated by the heart and mediastinum (Figures 1-3 and 1-4). The airways terminate in the acinus where gas exchange occurs. The whole lung is sponge-like and pink in the early years, gradually becoming grayer with age. The apex extends into the root of the neck, and the base is concave resting on the convexity of the diaphragm. The right lung has 3 lobes and 2 fissures, the left lung has 2 lobes and one fissure (Figure 1-5). The lobes of the lung are further divided into segments, and these are shown diagrammatically in Figures 1-6 and 1-7.

The lungs are covered by the visceral pleura (also called pulmonary pleura), and this membrane extends into the fissures. The parietal pleura lines the inner surface of the thoracic cavity, and the visceral and parietal pleurae join at the root of the lung (hilum). There is an expandable space between the 2 layers that contains a small amount of fluid.

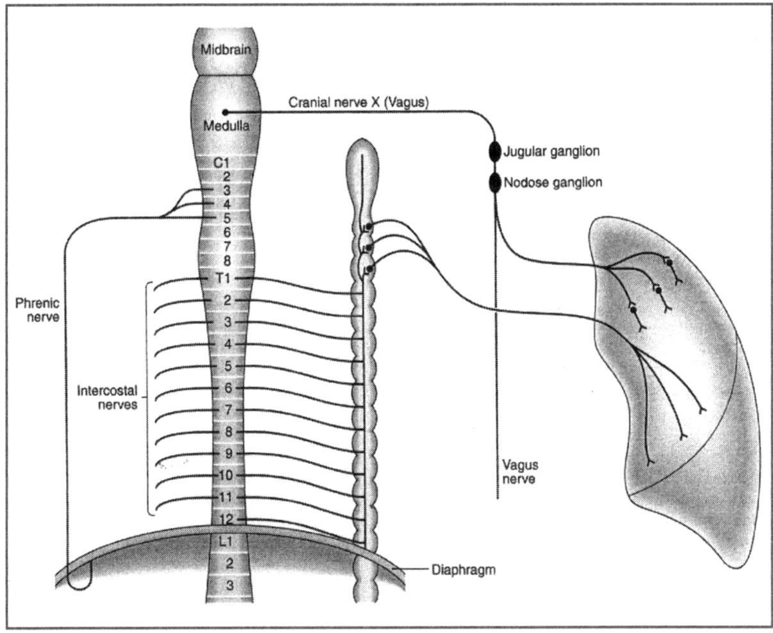

Figure 1-2. Efferent nervous system of the lungs. Innervation of the diaphragm, intercostal muscles, and lungs. The efferent (motor) systems are shown. The afferent (sensory) system is mainly in the vagus nerves.

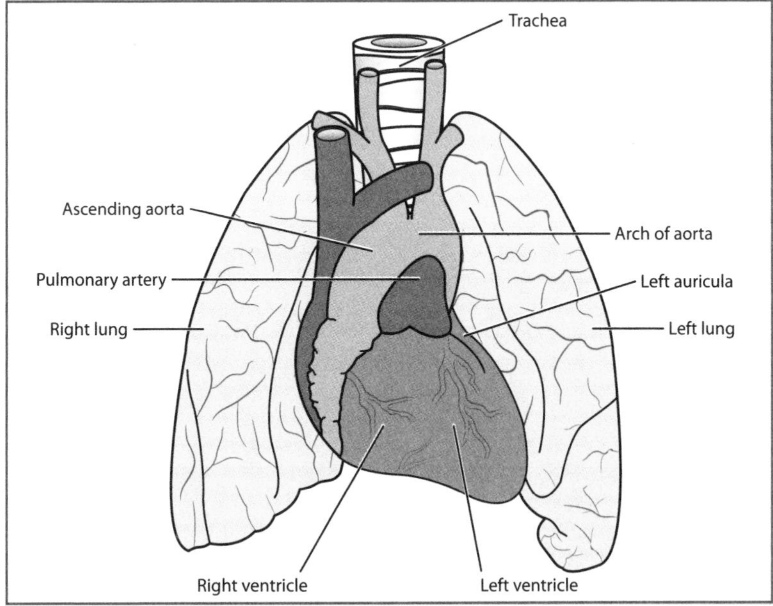

Figure 1-3 . Front view of the lungs and heart (anterior borders of the lungs retracted).

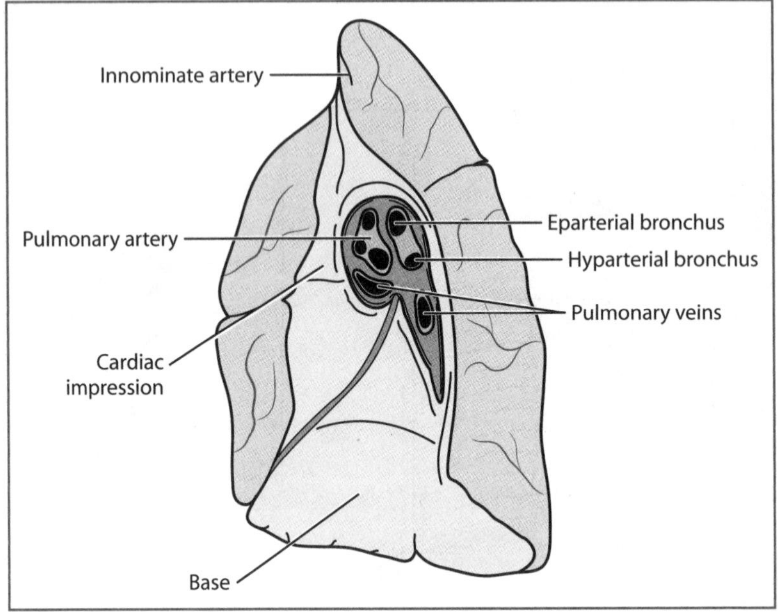

Figure 1-4. Mediastinal surface of the right lung.

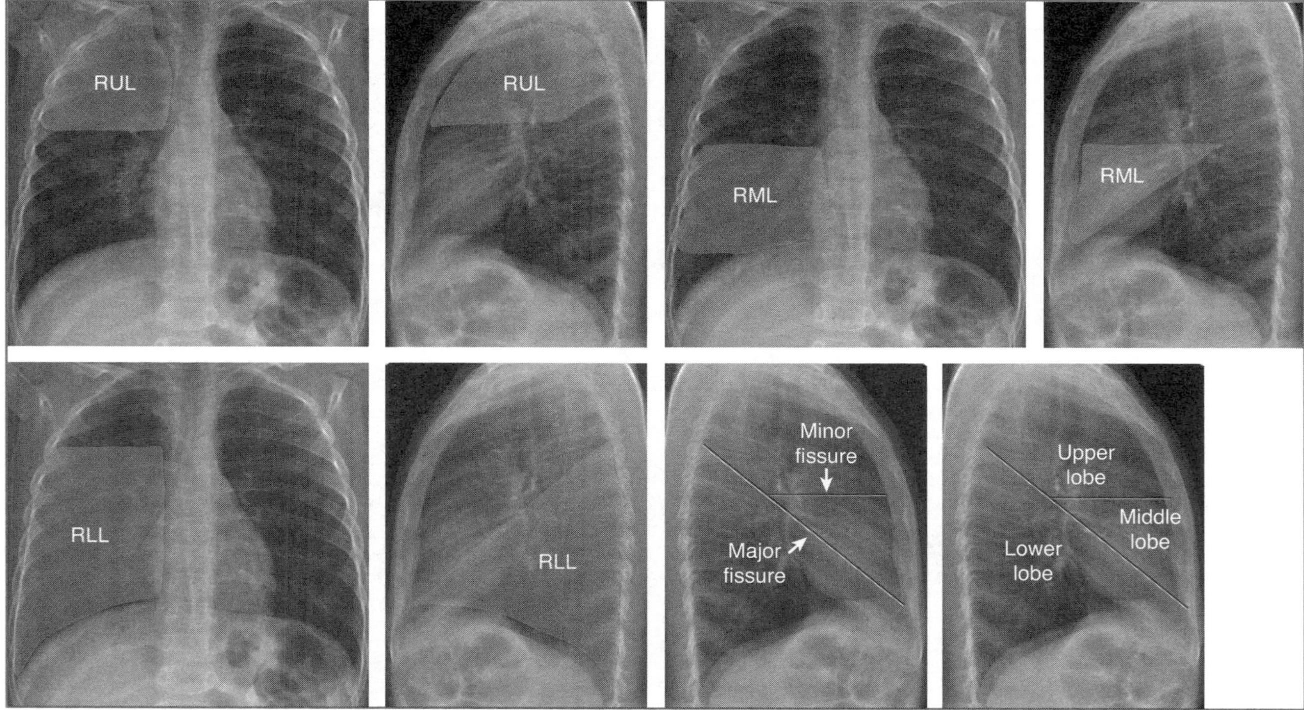

Figure 1-5A. Chest radiograph with overlying lobes and fissures. Right lung. (http://www.wikiradiography.com/page/Lung+Anatomy)

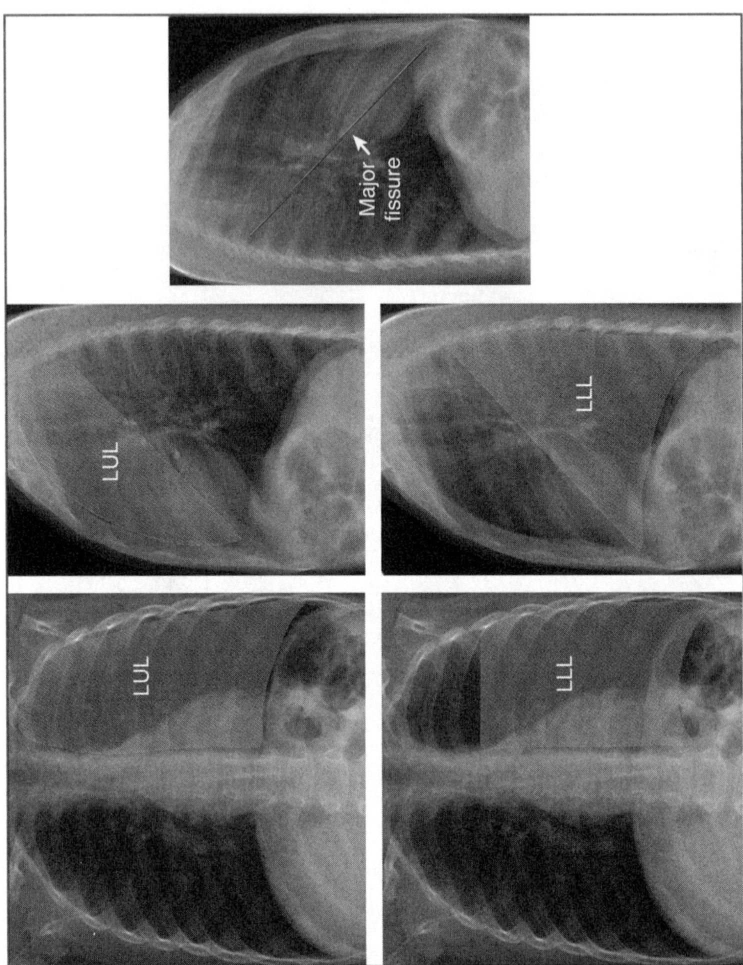

Figure 1-5B . Chest radiograph with overlying lobes and fissures. Left lung.

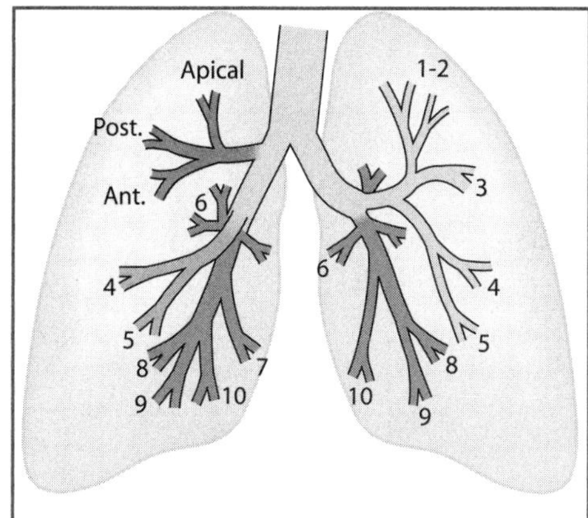

Figure 1-6A. Upper lobe, anterior view.

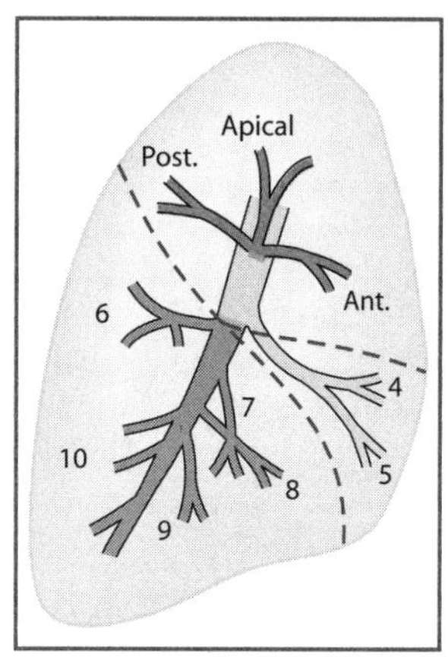

Figure 1-6B. Right upper lobe, lateral view.

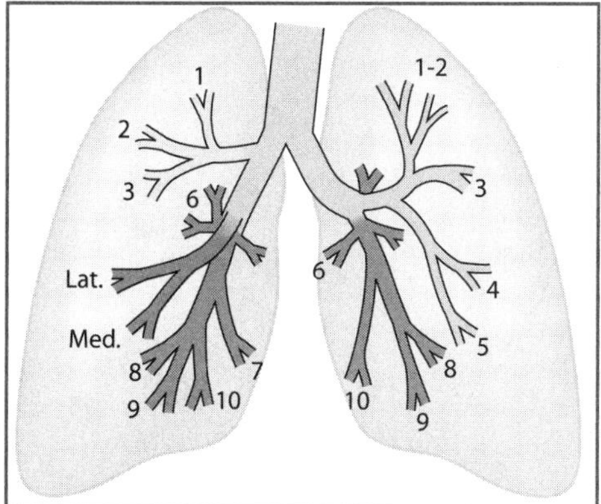

Figure 1-6C. Right middle lobe, anterior view.

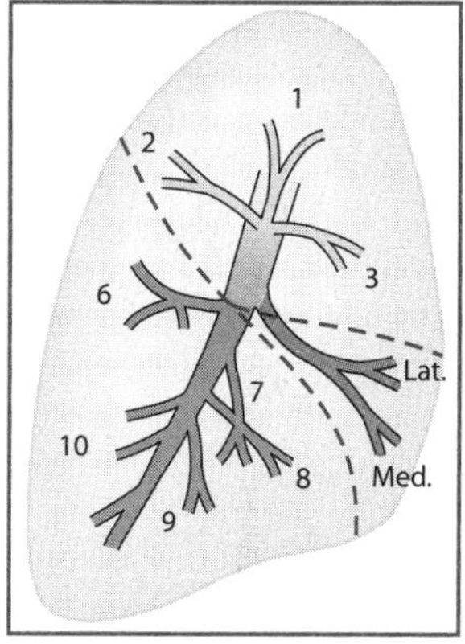

Figure 1-6D. Right middle lobe, lateral view.

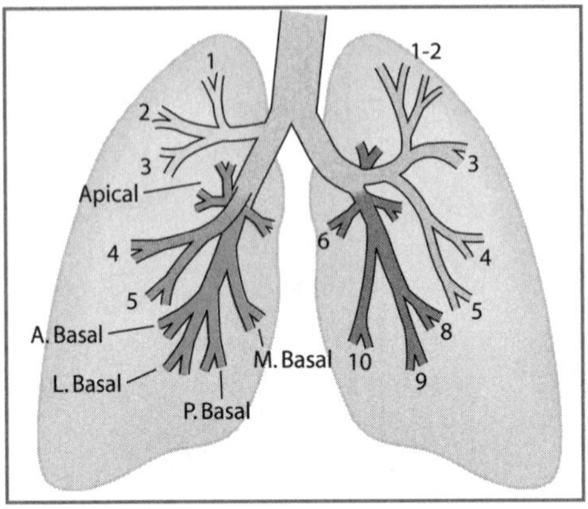

Figure 1-6E. Right lower lobe, anterior view.

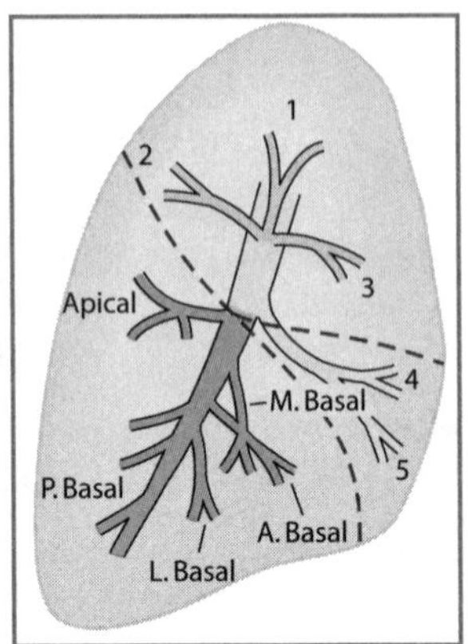

Figure 1-6F. Right lower lobe, lateral view.

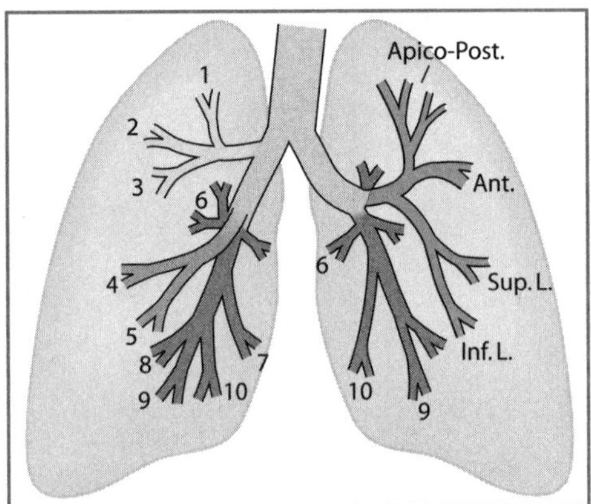

Figure 1-7A. Left upper lobe (includes lingula), anterior view.

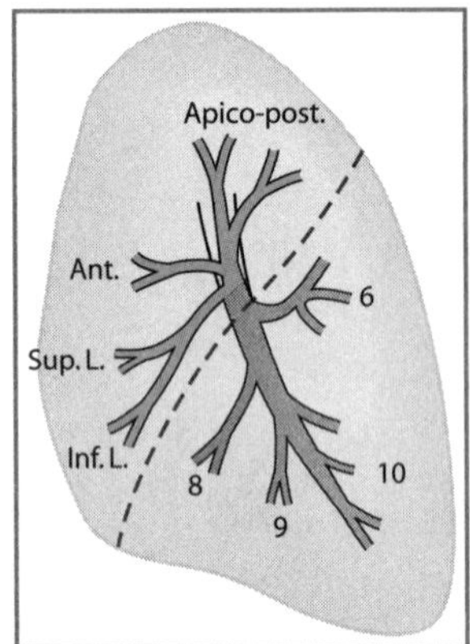

Figure 1-7B. Left upper lobe (includes lingula), lateral view.

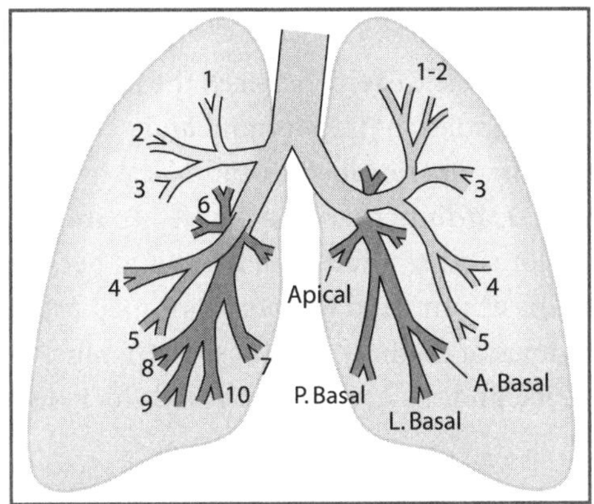

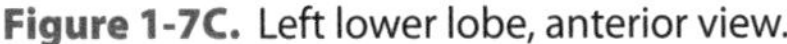

Figure 1-7C. Left lower lobe, anterior view.

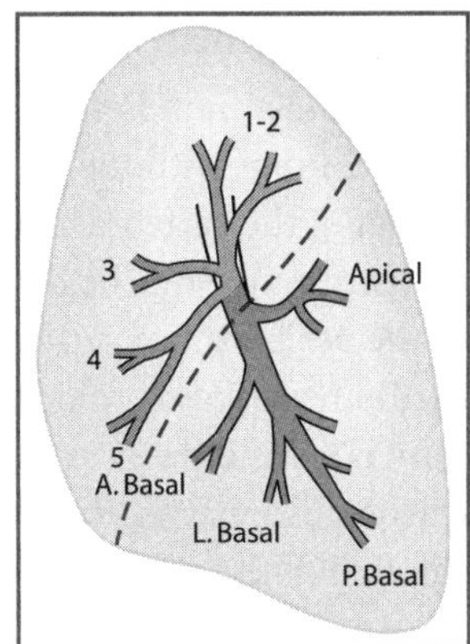

Figure 1-7D. Left lower lobe, lateral view.

Mediastinum

The mediastinum lies within the thoracic cavity between the pleurae of the 2 lungs with the anterior boundary of the sternum and posterior border of the vertebral column. The superior mediastinum is above the pericardium, while below the pericardium there are 3 parts. In front of the pericardium is the anterior mediastinum, the heart and pericardium are in the middle mediastinum, and the posterior mediastinum is behind the heart. The superior mediastinum has the thymus, trachea, esophagus, thoracic duct, and the upper great vessels including the arch of the aorta (Figure 1-3).

The hila of the lungs are where the structures of the lung enter from the mediastinum. The usual level of the hilum is anteriorly the third to fourth costal cartilage and posteriorly the fifth to seventh thoracic vertebrae.

Intercostal Muscles and Diaphragm

The muscles of respiration are the intercostals and the diaphragm. The anatomy of the diaphragm is shown in Figure 1-8. The right diaphragm overlies the liver and is higher than the left diaphragm, which overlies the stomach and spleen. The 3 major openings are the inferior vena cava at thoracic vertebral level (T) 12, esophagus (T10), and aorta

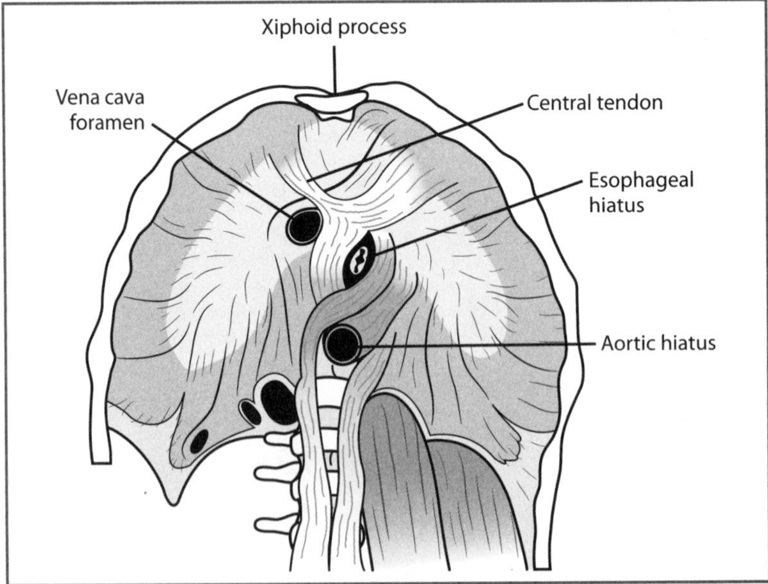

Figure 1-8. View of the diaphragm from below showing the important openings.

(T12). The opening of the anterior diaphragm is the foramen of Morgagni and of the posterior diaphragm is the foramen of Bochdalek. These 2 foramina are the sites of diaphragmatic hernia, with the Bochdalek hernia being the most common and known as the posterolateral diaphragmatic hernia, mostly (80%–85%) on the left.

It is important to understand the surface anatomy of the lungs, and this is shown in the Figure 1-9. Knowing the area of the lung below the surface while percussing and auscultating the lungs is important in localizing the pathology. The diaphragm is attached to the lower costal margin and the leaves are dome-shaped. With inspiration, the diaphragm flattens and the lower border of the lungs correspondingly descend. This will result in a different level of the lower lung border, which changes by several centimeters during deep breathing.

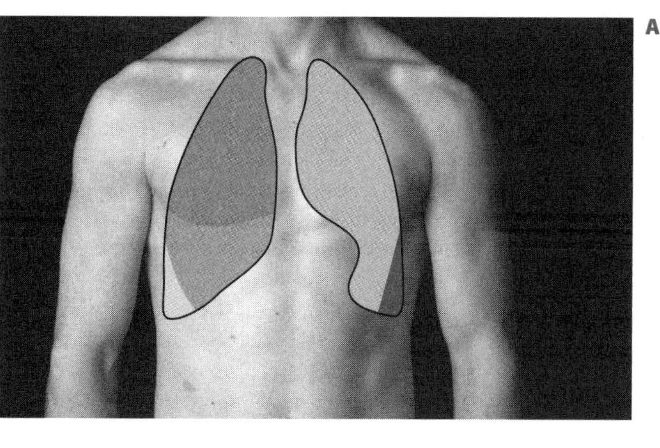

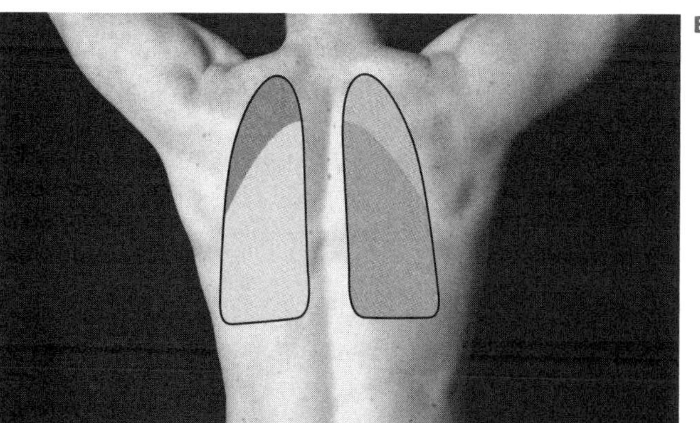

Figure 1-9A–B. Note that the lung images on the surface of the chest wall indicate the lobes and lungs at full inspiration. With tidal breathing and full expiration the images will be smaller and much smaller, respectively.

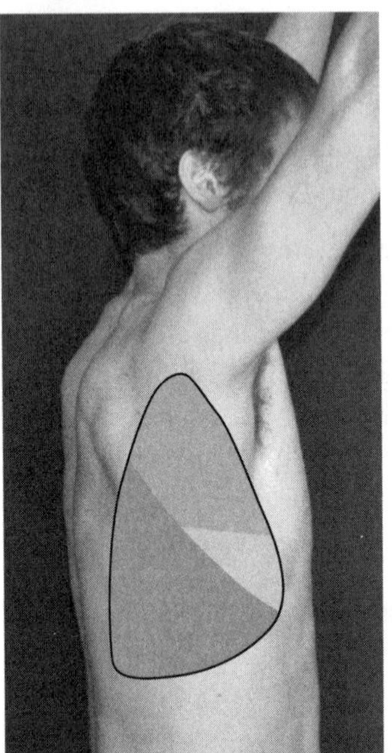

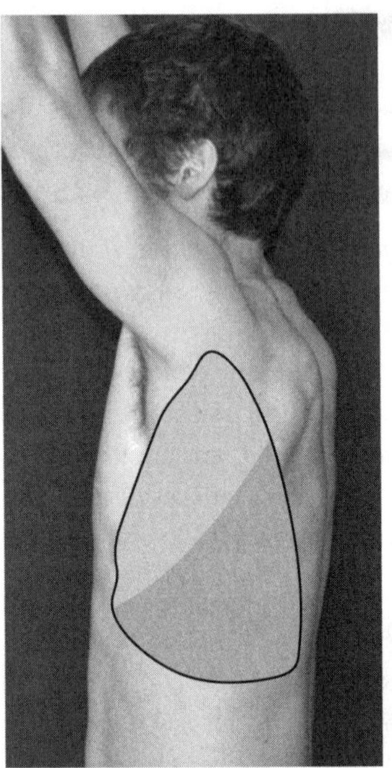

Figure 1-9C–D. Note that the lung images on the surface of the chest wall indicate the lobes and lungs at full inspiration. With tidal breathing and full expiration the images will be smaller and much smaller, respectively.

Key Points

- Lung development occurs in 5 stages. Extrauterine life can be sustained at 20 to 22 weeks of gestation.
- The airways branch from the trachea. The first 19 branches are the conduction airways and the 20th to 27th branches are the gas-exchanging units.
- It is important to know the surface position of lung anatomy to aid in localizing pathology of the lung.

Reference

1. Hislop A, Reid L. Growth and development of the respiratory system. In: Davis JA, Dopping J, eds. *Scientific Foundations of Pediatrics*. London: Heineman; 1974:214–254

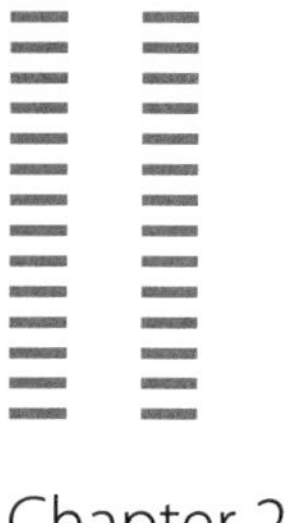

Chapter 2

Pulmonary Physiology

Pnina Weiss, MD

Introduction

The function of the respiratory system is to provide oxygen to arterial blood to nourish the body's tissues and to remove carbon dioxide from the returning venous blood. Gas exchange takes place at the level of the alveoli surrounded by a network of thin capillaries. Oxygen and carbon dioxide move between the air and blood by a process of diffusion. Air is brought to the alveoli by branching bronchi and bronchioles. The muscles of respiration act as a pump to move air in and out of the lungs. Elastic properties of the lung and chest wall and airway resistance affect the work and efficiency of the system. Disease processes that alter these relationships can lead to respiratory failure that is defined as failure of the lungs to oxygenate and ventilate adequately.

Gas Exchange

The tensions or pressures of dissolved oxygen or carbon dioxide in the blood are designated as Po_2 and Pco_2 (individual partial pressures of the gases), respectively. Table 2-1 shows the partial pressures of gases in

Table 2-1. Partial Pressure of Gases in the Atmosphere and the Lung

	Air (mm Hg)	Humidified Air (mm Hg)	Alveoli (mm Hg)
Oxygen	159	149	104
Carbon dioxide	0.3	0.3	40
Nitrogen	600.6	564	569
Water vapor	0	47	47

Adapted with permission from Levitzky M. *Pulmonary Physiology.* 4th ed. New York: McGraw-Hill, Inc; 1995:74–75.

the atmosphere and the lung. Dry atmospheric air is composed primarily of nitrogen. Oxygen constitutes 20.93% of the atmosphere; there is a minimal amount of carbon dioxide.[1]

Dry atmospheric air is humidified as it travels down the airways into the lungs. The Po_2 in the alveoli is determined by the balance between the amount that flows in and the amount that is removed by the pulmonary capillaries. It will be decreased if barometric pressure is low (ie, high altitude), if there is no fresh supply of air (ie, atelectasis), or if Pco_2 is elevated (ie, hypoventilation).

As gas moves in and out of the alveolus, blood flows through the pulmonary capillary vessels, which provide a large surface for gas exchange. Figure 2-1 depicts how gas exchange occurs in the alveolus. The driving force for gas exchange is the difference in pressures of Po_2 and Pco_2 between the venous blood and alveoli. Under normal conditions, the gases equilibrate fully and the Po_2 and Pco_2 of pulmonary capillary blood equals that of the alveoli.[2]

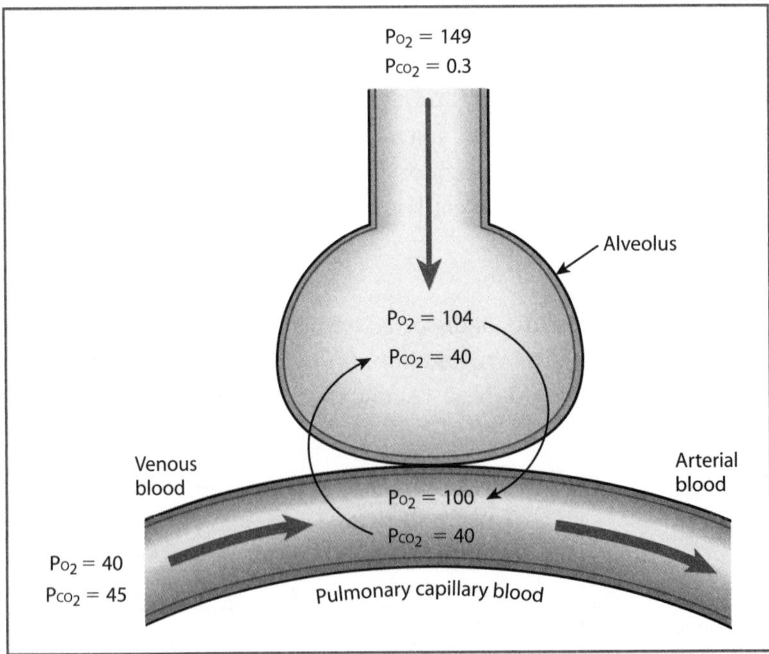

Figure 2-1. Gas exchange in the alveolus (values in mm Hg). Oxygen and carbon dioxide diffuse across the alveolar-capillary membrane. There is little carbon dioxide in the atmosphere. The Po_2 in the alveolus is high and oxygen diffuses into the capillary blood. Pco_2 is high in the venous blood and carbon dioxide diffuses into the alveolus.

Oxygen Consumption and Carbon Dioxide Production

The total amount of oxygen that is taken up by the body in 1 minute is called the *oxygen consumption* ($\dot{V}o_2$) and the amount of carbon dioxide produced is the carbon dioxide production ($\dot{V}co_2$). Oxygen consumption and carbon dioxide production are increased with exercise. The ratio between the two is known as the *respiratory quotient* and is usually 0.8. The respiratory quotient rises (ie, more carbon dioxide is produced for each molecule of oxygen consumed) on a high carbohydrate diet. For patients in respiratory failure, low carbohydrate and high lipid formulas are suggested in order to decrease the respiratory quotient and decrease carbon dioxide production.[3]

Ventilation

The process of ventilation brings air in and out of the lungs. During inspiration, the size of the thoracic cavity increases and air moves into the lungs. The fresh air is carried through conducting airways to the alveoli, which are responsible for gas exchange.

Alveolar and Dead Space Ventilation

The volume of a breath is known as the *tidal volume.*[2] However, only part of the breath is used for gas exchange. Only the air that reaches the alveolus is involved in gas exchange; this is known as *alveolar volume* and is shown in Figure 2-2. The conducting airways are not involved in gas exchange and the volume of air in them is known as dead space. About 30% of each breath ends up in *dead space.*[4] In some disease processes, the dead space volume increases and less air is available in each breath for gas exchange.

Total ventilation is the total volume of fresh air that reaches the lung each minute. It is determined by the volume of each breath, multiplied by the number of breaths per minute. The relationship between tidal volume, respiratory rate, and total ventilation is shown in Figure 2-3. If a child has a tidal volume of 100 mL and is breathing 15 breaths/min, then the total ventilation is 1,500 mL/min. *Alveolar ventilation* is the total volume of air *that reaches the alveoli* and is available for gas exchange each minute. Thus, if a disease process decreases the respiratory rate and/or the volume of each breath or increases the dead space, it will decrease the effective ventilation. Total ventilation is easy to quantify since tidal volume is easily measured; alveolar ventilation is more difficult since dead space is more difficult to measure.

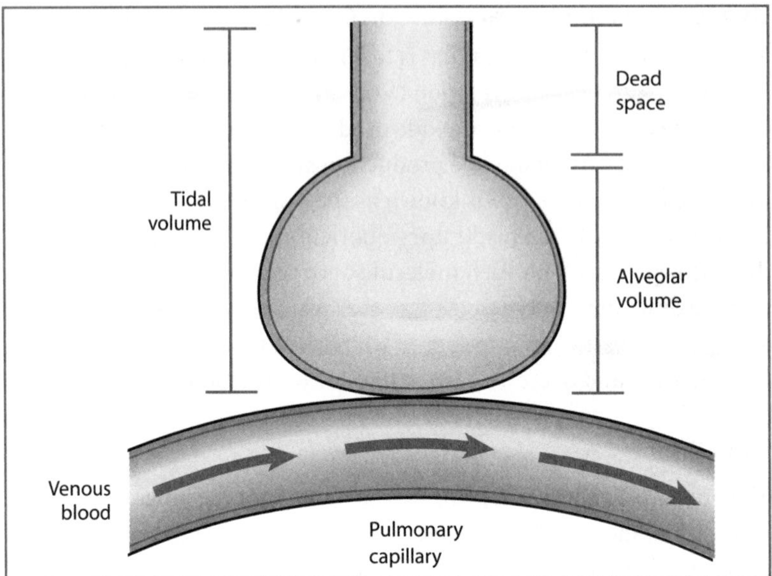

Figure 2-2. The relationship of tidal volume to dead space and alveolar volume. In each breath (tidal volume), some of the air goes into the alveoli (alveolar volume) and is available for gas exchange. The rest remains in the conducting airways and is known as dead space.

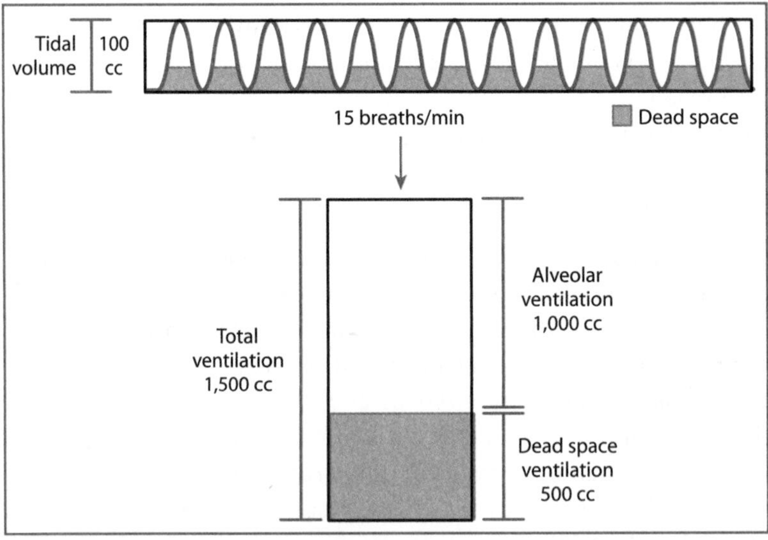

Figure 2-3. Components of total ventilation: tidal volume, respiratory rate, alveolar ventilation, and dead space ventilation. Total ventilation is determined by the volume of each breath multiplied by the number of breaths per minute. In this diagram, dead space is one-third of total volume.

Relationship of Ventilation to Arterial P_{CO_2}

The removal of carbon dioxide from the blood depends on alveolar ventilation. If alveolar ventilation increases, then the elimination of carbon dioxide increases and its concentration in the arterial blood decreases.[1] This relationship is shown in Figure 2-4. If alveolar ventilation decreases, then the elimination of carbon dioxide decreases and it accumulates in the arterial blood. There is a direct relationship between the alveolar ventilation and the arterial carbon dioxide concentration: If alveolar ventilation doubles, the arterial carbon dioxide concentration is halved. If the alveolar ventilation decreases by 50%, then the arterial carbon dioxide concentration doubles.

The effect of changes in respiratory rate, tidal volume, and dead space on ventilation and arterial carbon dioxide level are depicted in Table 2-2. Decreased alveolar ventilation with an increase in

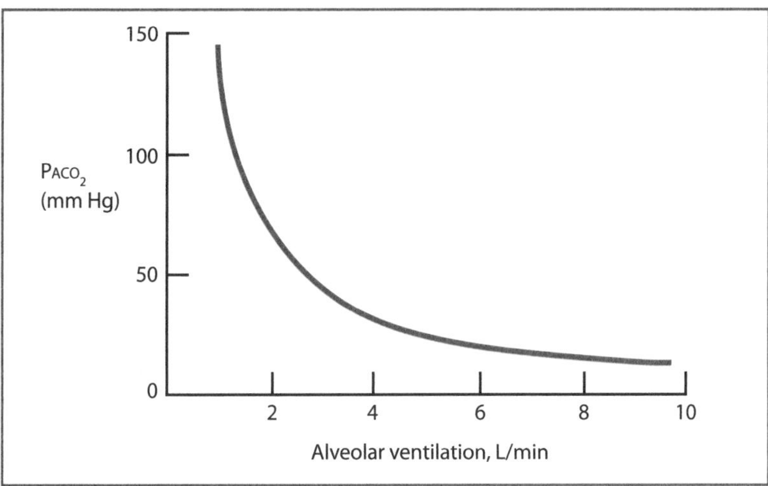

Figure 2-4. The relationship between ventilation and carbon dioxide levels in the lung. Increases in alveolar ventilation will decrease carbon dioxide levels; conversely, decreases in ventilation will increase carbon dioxide levels. P_{ACO_2} is the partial pressure of carbon dioxide in the alveolus. (Adapted from Lumb AB. *Nunn's Applied Respiratory Physiology.* 5th ed. Edinburgh: Butterworth Heinemann; 2000, with permission.)

Table 2-2. Effect of Respiratory Rate, Tidal Volume, and Dead Space on Total Ventilation and Arterial Carbon Dioxide Level

Respiratory Rate (breaths/min)	Tidal Volume	Dead Space	Total Ventilation	Arterial Pco_2	Causes
↓	↔	↔	↓	↑	Medications, alcohol, central nervous system infections, seizures, apnea
↔	↓	↔	↓	↑	Chest wall trauma, neuromuscular weakness, lung disease
↔	↔	↑	↔	↑	Acute respiratory distress syndrome, scoliosis, pulmonary embolus
↑	↔	↔	↑	↓	Metabolic acidosis, salicylate overdose, anxiety, pain
↔	↑	↔	↑	↓	Metabolic acidosis, salicylate overdose, anxiety, pain
↔	↔	↓	↔	↓	Mechanical ventilation, deep breathing

Decreases in respiratory rate and tidal volume decrease total ventilation and increase arterial carbon dioxide tension. Increases in respiratory rate and tidal volume increase total ventilation and decrease arterial carbon dioxide tension. Changes in dead space do not affect total ventilation; they will, however, affect alveolar ventilation and carbon dioxide levels.

arterial carbon dioxide tension (PCO_2) can be caused by a wide variety of factors. A decrease in respiratory rate or tidal volume can result from drugs such as opiates, benzodiazepines, or alcohol; central nervous system infection; trauma; seizures; or sepsis. Premature infants can have cessation of breathing, or apnea of prematurity. In congenital central hypoventilation syndrome, children have a decreased central drive to breathe and, consequently, hypoventilation. In children with obstructive sleep apnea, there is a relative decrease in their tidal volume because they can't get an effective breath in. Chest wall trauma or deformity, neuromuscular weakness, and lung disease can also decrease the tidal volume and impair ventilation. Disease processes, such as acute respiratory distress syndrome, scoliosis, pulmonary embolus, or general anesthesia, can increase the dead space and thus impair the proportion of effective ventilation.

Increased alveolar ventilation results in a decrease in PCO_2. Causes for increasing respiratory rate and tidal volume are depicted in Table 2-2. The most common etiologies include metabolic acidosis, salicylate ingestion, anxiety, central nervous system disorders, and pain. There are also some instances in which the dead space can be decreased.

Regulation of Arterial PCO_2

The arterial carbon dioxide concentration reflects a balance between carbon dioxide production and elimination. More carbon dioxide is produced when the metabolic rate is increased. Fever or increased muscle activity (shivering, seizures) produce more carbon dioxide and can produce elevations in arterial carbon dioxide levels unless ventilation is increased.

Ventilation is controlled by sensors called *chemoreceptors* that are located in the brain and the carotid bodies, which lie at the bifurcation of the carotid arteries. These receptors sense changes in arterial carbon dioxide concentration. They respond by activating effectors that alter ventilation to keep arterial carbon dioxide concentration normal.

Acid-Base Status

Carbon dioxide is transported in the blood in 3 forms: dissolved, bicarbonate, and combined with proteins such as carbamino compounds. In arterial blood, most of it is carried as bicarbonate (90%).[5]

$$CO_2 + H_2O \underset{}{\overset{\text{Carbonic Anhydrase}}{\leftrightarrows}} H_2CO_3 \leftrightarrows H^+ + HCO_3^-$$

Carbon dioxide and water are converted to carbonic acid by the enzyme carbonic anhydrase in red blood cells. Carbonic acid spontaneously dissociates into hydrogen ions (acid) and bicarbonate.

The pH of the blood depends on the relationship of bicarbonate and carbon dioxide. As the arterial P_{CO_2} increases, the pH decreases, which is known as *respiratory acidosis.* As the arterial P_{CO_2} decreases, the pH increases, which is known as *respiratory alkalosis.*

While the lungs regulate the concentration of carbon dioxide, the kidneys control the bicarbonate concentration. In response to a respiratory acidosis, the kidneys will compensate over 3 to 5 days by conserving bicarbonate and will create a secondary *metabolic alkalosis.* Table 2-3 provides a list of primary acid-base disorders and their secondary compensation. In contrast, in response to a respiratory alkalosis, the kidneys will eliminate excess bicarbonate and create a secondary *metabolic acidosis* in compensation. It is possible to determine the primary acid-base disorder and the compensation by plotting the values on a nomogram.[6] An example of this nomogram is shown in Figure 2-5.

In general, for acute respiratory acidosis an increase in P_{CO_2} of 10 mm Hg will decrease the pH by 0.08 and the bicarbonate by 1 meq/L. In chronic respiratory acidosis, after renal compensation, the bicarbonate will increase by a total of 4 meq/L for each 10 mm rise in P_{CO_2}. In acute and chronic respiratory alkalosis, similar changes in the opposite direction occur. Remembering the relationship between change in P_{CO_2} and pH can be useful in determining whether a patient has a compensated, partially compensated, or uncompensated respiratory acidosis. For example, a patient with a severe acute asthma exacerbation may present to the emergency department with a pH of 7.24, a P_{CO_2}

Table 2-3. Primary Acid-Base Disorders and Compensation

	Carbon Dioxide Level	pH	Bicarbonate
Acute respiratory acidosis	⬆	↓	↑
Chronic respiratory acidosis	⬆	↓	↑
Acute respiratory alkalosis	⬇	↑	↓
Chronic respiratory alkalosis	⬇	↑	↓
Metabolic acidosis	↓	↓	⬇
Metabolic alkalosis	↑	↑	⬆

[a]The primary event is shown in bold arrows; the secondary effects are listed. The length of the arrows is proportional to the magnitude of the change. For example, in acute respiratory acidosis, the primary event is an elevation in arterial Pco_2. There is a concomitant decrease in pH and a very small increase in bicarbonate. In chronic respiratory acidosis, there is renal compensation and bicarbonate increases. As a result, the Pco_2 is still elevated, but the pH is not as dramatically decreased as in acute respiratory acidosis.

of 60 mm Hg, and a bicarbonate of 22 meq/L, which represents an acute uncompensated respiratory acidosis. If his ventilation does not improve, over the course of 2 to 3 days his kidneys would start to compensate and a follow-up blood gas may have a pH of 7.30, Pco_2 of 60 mm Hg, and a bicarbonate of 25 meq/L, which reflects partial compensation. In contrast, an infant with bronchopulmonary dysplasia who has chronic respiratory failure may have a blood gas with a pH of 7.35, Pco_2 of 60 mm Hg, and a bicarbonate of 28 meq/L, which represents a compensated respiratory acidosis.

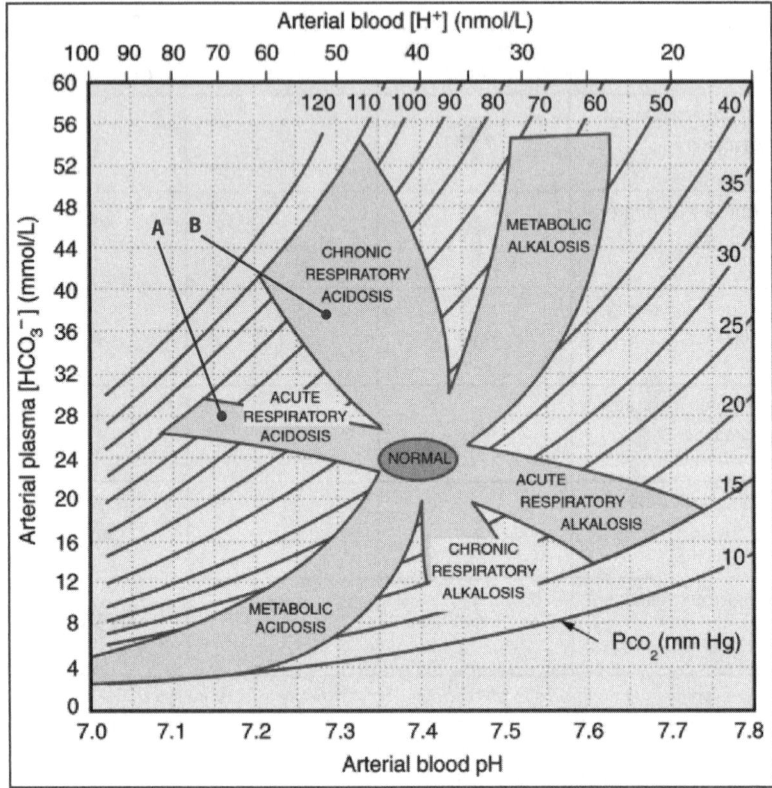

Figure 2-5. Nomogram of acid-base abnormalities. From this nomogram, the primary acid-base abnormality can be determined. **A.** Patient A has a pH 7.18, Pco_2 of 80 mm Hg, and HCO^-_3 of 26 mmol/L. It is consistent with an acute respiratory acidosis. **B.** Patient B has a Pco_2 of 80 mm Hg and a pH 7.3, with a HCO^-_3 of 37 mmol/L, which is consistent with chronic respiratory acidosis. (Adapted from DuBose TD. Disorders of acid-base balance. In: Brenner BM, ed. *Brenner and Rector's The Kidney.* Philadelphia, PA: Saunders Elsevier; 2007, with permission from Elsevier.)

Oxygenation

Oxygen reaches the alveoli through the conducting airways, where it diffuses across the very thin membrane to the capillary blood. Under normal instances, oxygen composes approximately 21% of air. The amount of oxygen in the alveolus is determined by the presence of other gases such as carbon dioxide, a supply of fresh air, and changes in barometric pressure. The Po_2 decreases when the Pco_2 increases. The Po_2 depends on a fresh flow of air; if there is no airflow, such as in cases of mucus plugging, atelectasis, or apnea, then the Po_2 in the alveolus decreases. In addition, the Po_2 depends on the atmospheric pressure. At high altitudes, the atmospheric pressure is lower and there is less oxygen available, which accounts for the development of hypoxemia, or low arterial oxygen level, at Mount Everest or when flying.

Oxygen is primarily bound to hemoglobin in the red blood cell; a small amount is dissolved in plasma. A red blood cell takes about three-quarters of a second to transverse the pulmonary capillary bed; under normal conditions, it takes about one-quarter of a second for oxygen to be fully transferred to the red blood cell.[2] If the capillary membrane is thickened, then transfer may take longer and make not be complete by the end of its transit time. This may be aggravated by exercise; as the blood moves more quickly through the lungs, it may not have adequate time to become fully saturated.[7]

Mechanisms of Hypoxemia

The primary processes that contribute to hypoxemia (abnormally low oxygen in the arterial blood) are hypoventilation, diffusion impairment, shunt, ventilation/perfusion ($\dot{V}/\dot{Q}$) mismatch, and low venous blood saturation.[8] These processes are depicted in Figure 2-6. In addition, as was mentioned in the prior section, hypoxemia may result from low inspired Po_2. This may occur at high altitudes or in the laboratory under experimental conditions.

Hypoventilation

If ventilation is inadequate, the Pco_2 in the alveoli rises and the Po_2 falls. Inadequate ventilation may be caused by depressed respiratory drive (medications, sepsis, brain trauma), damage to the chest wall, or weakness of the respiratory muscles.

The relationship between the rise in arterial carbon dioxide and fall in oxygen tension can be seen from the alveolar gas equation:

$$P_{AO_2} = P_{IO_2} - Pa_{CO_2}/R$$

where P_{AO_2} is the alveolar Po_2, P_{IO_2} is the inspired Po_2, Pa_{CO_2} is the arterial Pco_2, and R is the respiratory exchange ratio of carbon dioxide and oxygen, which is estimated to be 0.8 for the whole lung. So roughly every increase in alveolar Pco_2 of 10 mm Hg would decrease the Po_2 by 12.5 mm Hg. For example, if a child without lung disease with a resting Pco_2 of 40 mm Hg and Po_2 of 100 mm Hg has an episode of apnea and his Pco_2 rises to 80 mm Hg, his Po_2 will fall to 50 mm Hg.

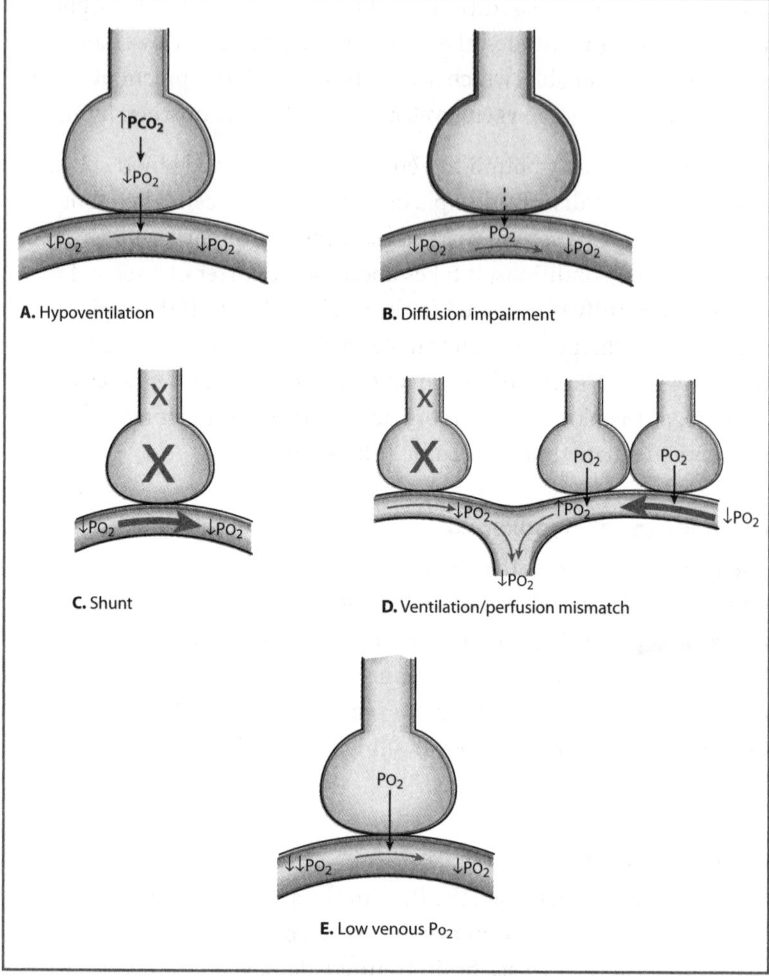

Figure 2-6. Causes of hypoxemia. **A.** Hypoventilation: Ventilation is decreased and there is an increase in Pco_2. Consequently, the Po_2 in the alveolus decreases. **B.** Diffusion impairment: Diffusion across the alveolar-capillary membrane to the hemoglobin in the red blood cells is decreased. **C.** Shunt: Pulmonary venous blood bypasses the lung without being oxygenated. This may occur in congenital cardiac disease or arteriovenous malformation where there is a right-to-left shunt. **D.** Ventilation/perfusion mismatch: Some areas of the lung are nonfunctional and poorly oxygenate the venous blood. There is mixing of blood from functioning alveolar units. **E.** Low venous Po_2: The Po_2 in the venous blood may be abnormally low because of anemia, fever, or decreased cardiac output. In the presence of lung disease, shunt, or exercise, it may not be fully oxygenated as it completes its course through the lung.

Diffusion

Problems with diffusion can be seen in pediatric patients. Diffusion of a gas through tissues depends on the cross-sectional area, the partial pressure difference across and the thickness of the tissue, and inherent characteristics of the gas (its solubility and molecular weight). Diffusion can be impaired if the surface area of the lung is decreased (such as in a lobectomy or emphysema) or the capillary basement membrane is thickened (such as in pulmonary edema or interstitial fibrosis). Problems with diffusion can be detected by using a surrogate marker, carbon monoxide, and testing the diffusing capacity of the lung for carbon monoxide (DLCO). The DLCO may be low in the conditions noted above and also with reduced thoracic blood volume or reduced hemoglobin.

Neonates, particularly premature infants, have a decrease in their diffusion capacity relative to adults. They have a decrease in surface area, because they do not have complete alveolarization when they are born. In bronchopulmonary dysplasia, a chronic lung disease of infancy, there may be arrested alveolarization, which also results in a decrease in surface area.[9] In addition, in premature infants, there is a greater distance between the capillary and alveolus, which impairs diffusion because the gas needs to travel over a larger distance.

Shunt

Shunt occurs when deoxygenated blood bypasses the lungs and goes directly into the arterial circulation. Small shunts exist under normal physiological conditions. Deoxygenated blood from the bronchial arteries drains directly into the pulmonary veins and the coronary veins drain directly into the left ventricle through the thebesian veins. In some circumstances, there can be an abnormal connection between the veins and arteries (arteriovenous malformation). In addition, a right to left shunt can occur with congenital heart disease (pulmonary atresia with ventriculoseptal defect, pulmonary hypertension with an atrial septal defect or patent foramen ovale). The amount of blood going through the shunt can be calculated from the following equation:

$$\frac{\dot{Q}_S}{\dot{Q}_T} = \frac{Cc'_{O_2} - Ca_{O_2}}{Cc'_{O_2} - C\bar{v}_{O_2}}$$

Where $\dot{Q}s/\dot{Q}T$ is the fraction of blood going through the shunt, $Cc'o_2$ is the pulmonary capillary oxygen content, Cao_2 is the arterial oxygen content, and $C\bar{v}o_2$ is the mixed venous oxygen content. Shunt fractions can also be calculated from nomograms (Figure 2-7).

A shunt will result in decreased oxygen concentration but does not usually produce elevated arterial carbon dioxide levels. The chemoreceptors normally sense the elevation of arterial carbon dioxide and respond by increasing ventilation.

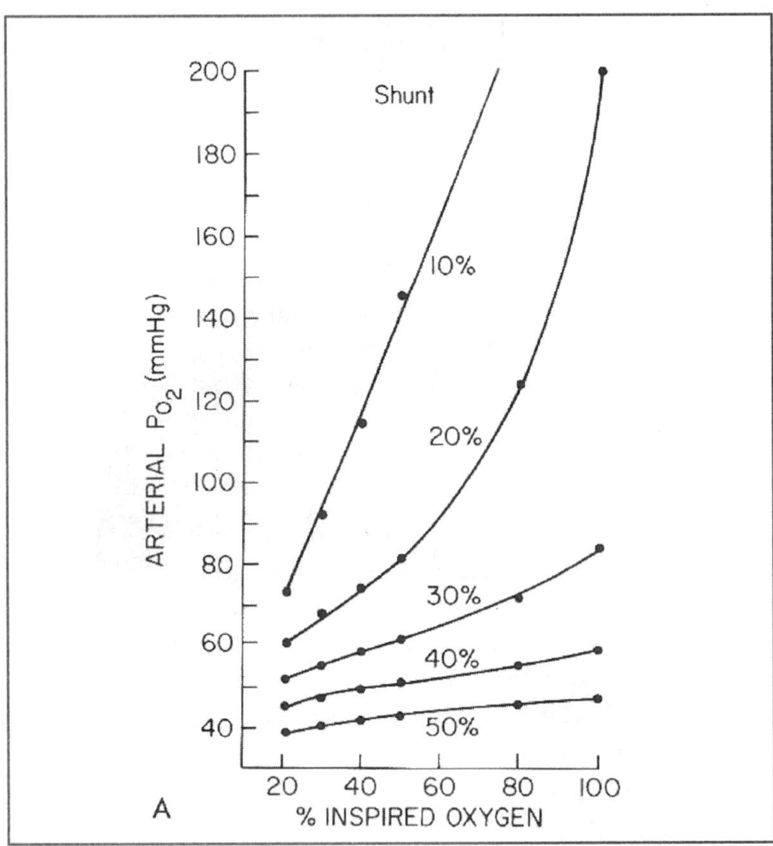

Figure 2-7. Effect of changing inspired oxygen concentration on arterial Po_2 in lungs with shunts of varying degrees from 10% to 50%. In larger shunts, administering supplemental oxygen has little effect on arterial Po_2. Addition of 100% oxygen has little effect on arterial Po_2 when the shunt is greater than 30%. (From Dantzker DR. Gas exchange in the adult respiratory distress syndrome. *Clin Chest Med.* 1982;3:57–67, with permission from Elsevier.)

$\dot{V}/\dot{Q}$ Mismatch

This is one of the most difficult of the causes to understand. If blood flow and ventilation are not matched in areas of the lung, then inadequate gas exchange occurs. If an area of the lung is perfused but not ventilated, as in the case of pneumonia or atelectasis (lung collapse), then it acts like a small shunt. Deoxygenated blood goes through the nonfunctional lung without being oxygenated. It then mixes with blood from other areas of the lung that are oxygenated.

A shunt can be distinguished from $\dot{V}/\dot{Q}$ mismatch by the hyperoxia test. In the case of the latter, addition of 100% oxygen will increase the arterial oxygen saturation. However, if a true shunt exists, the supplemental oxygen will raise the arterial saturation by only a small amount (<5%).

Low Venous Oxygen Content

The normal Po_2 of venous blood is 45 mm Hg and has a saturation of 75%. If the venous blood has an unusually low Po_2 then the blood may not be fully oxygenated by the time it finishes its course through the pulmonary capillaries. A low venous Po_2 may result when the body extracts more oxygen from the blood than usual, such as in anemia, fever, and low cardiac output. Normally the lung can compensate for the abnormally low venous Po_2. However, it may not if there is another superimposed problem such as $\dot{V}/\dot{Q}$ mismatch, shunt, diffusion impairment, or exercise.

Oxygen Transport

Oxygen is primarily carried in the blood bound to hemoglobin; a very small amount is dissolved in plasma. The total amount that is carried by the blood is called the *oxygen content.* The maximum amount of oxygen that can be combined with hemoglobin is called the *oxygen capacity.* One gram of hemoglobin can combine with 1.34 mL of oxygen.[2] The oxygen capacity for a normal child with a hemoglobin of 14 g/100 mL is 19.5 mL oxygen/100 mL blood.

The *oxygen saturation* is the percentage of binding sites of hemoglobin that have oxygen attached. The normal oxygen saturation is 98% for arterial blood and 75% for venous blood. In general, oxygen saturation increases as the Po_2 of the blood increases. The dissociation curve for oxygen is “S”-shaped and is shown in Figure 2-8. Between an oxygen tension of 20 and 75 mm Hg, there is a sharp, linear rise in oxygen saturation. After that, large rises in arterial Po_2 cause small rises in oxygen saturation. The P_{50} is the oxygen tension at which 50% of the hemoglobin is saturated.

Factors That Alter the Affinity of Hemoglobin for Oxygen

Many factors can affect the affinity of hemoglobin for oxygen. Acidosis, hypercarbia, and hyperthermia can decrease the affinity of hemoglobin for oxygen. The result is a shift in the oxygen dissociation curve to the right, which is shown in Figure 2-9. As a result, the hemoglobin is less saturated at a given oxygen tension. The converse is true: Alkalosis, hypocarbia, and hypothermia shift the oxygen dissociation curve

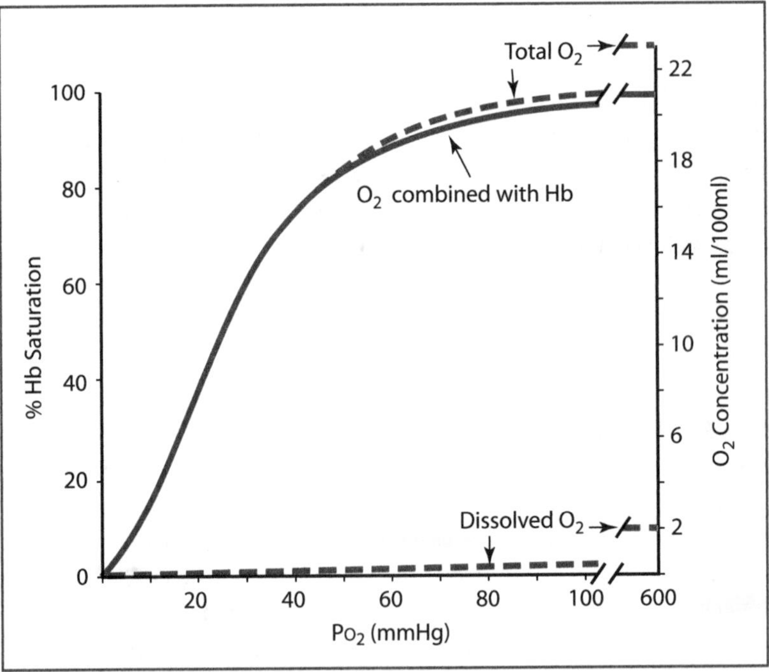

Figure 2-8. Oxygen dissociation curve. The oxygen dissociation curve is shown for pH 7.4, Pco_2 40 mm Hg, 37°C, and hemoglobin concentration 15 g/100 mL. There is a very small amount of oxygen dissolved in the blood; the bulk is combined with hemoglobin. The P_{50} is the Po_2 at which 50% of the hemoglobin sites are saturated. (Adapted from West JB. *Respiratory Physiology: The Essentials.* 8th ed. Baltimore, MD: Lippincott Williams & Wilkins; 2008, with permission from Wolters Kluwer Health.)

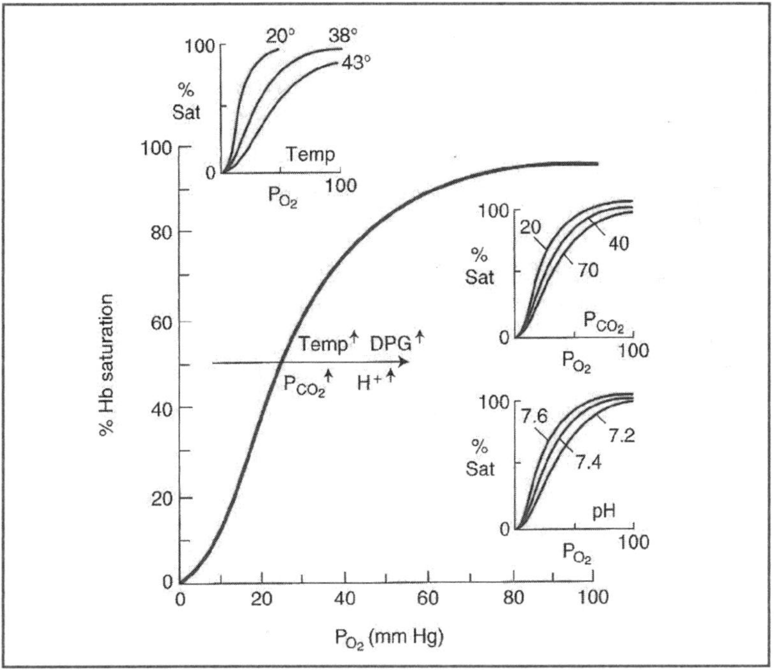

Figure 2-9. Factors that change the oxygen dissociation curve. Many factors can shift the oxygen dissociation curve to the right and cause oxygen to bind less avidly to hemoglobin: increased temperature, acidosis, hypercarbia, and increased 2,3 diphosphoglycerate. Conversely, decreased temperature, alkalosis, and low CO_2 levels shift the curve to the left; thus oxygen binds more avidly to the hemoglobin. The effect of the latter is decreased delivery to the tissues. (Adapted from West JB. *Respiratory Physiology: The Essentials.* 8th ed. Baltimore, MD: Lippincott Williams & Wilkins; 2008, with permission from Wolters Kluwer Health.)

to the left and the hemoglobin has a higher saturation at a given oxygen tension.

Another common reason for altered oxygen affinity is alterations in the hemoglobin itself. The hemoglobin of patients with sickle cell disease has less affinity for hemoglobin than those with normal hemoglobin. Thus patients with sickle cell may have a lower oxygen saturation in room air.[10,11] In contrast, fetal hemoglobin or red blood cells, which have been stored in a blood bank, have a higher affinity for oxygen. The cause of the latter is a decreased amount of 2,3 diphosphoglycerate (2,3 DPG).[12] The saturation of oxygen can also be lower because it is bound by other molecules, such as in carbon monoxide poisoning or methemoglobinemia.

Decreases in oxygen capacity and, consequently, impaired oxygen delivery to tissues can be caused by a decrease in oxygen saturation or anemia. As previously described, decreases in oxygen saturation can be caused by decreases in arterial oxygen concentration (pneumonia, atelectasis, lung disease, high altitude), affinity of hemoglobin for oxygen, or if sites are bound by other molecules.

Assessment of Oxygenation and Ventilation

It is extremely difficult to assess the adequacy of oxygenation and ventilation by physical examination. The most specific sign of impaired oxygenation is cyanosis, which can usually be detected at an oxyhemoglobin saturation of 80%.[13] However, it may be difficult to assess in children with anemia or dark-colored skin. Other associated signs are tachypnea, tachycardia, confusion, motor incoordination, and agitation (the latter are late signs). Impaired ventilation is even more difficult to determine. Certainly, when a patient is apneic or has an extremely low respiratory rate, an impairment of ventilation is likely. Tidal volume is difficult to determine from examination of chest excursion; dead space cannot be assessed.[14] Other late signs of impaired ventilation are hypotension, flushed skin, diaphoresis, tachycardia, and lethargy.

Noninvasive Monitoring of Oxygen and Carbon Dioxide

Both oxygenation and ventilation can be assessed noninvasively. Pulse oximetry is the most common way to assess oxygenation and is based on the principle that oxyhemoblobin and reduced hemoglobin have different light absorption spectra. Oxyhemoglobin detects arterial pulsations and measures the arterial oxygen saturation. It has a few problems: It is insensitive to changes at high arterial Po_2 (because of the shape of the oxygen dissociation curve) and inaccurate at low arterial oxygen saturation (Sao_2). There is also a delay in response to changes in Sao_2, particularly when it is placed on an extremity. In addition, a number of factors can give spurious results; these factors are listed in Box 2-1.[15,16]

End-tidal carbon dioxide monitoring (capnography) can be used to assess ventilation.[17] The carbon dioxide in exhaled air is measured by infrared light absorption or mass spectrometry. A representative capnograph is shown in Figure 2-10. In normal healthy individuals, the carbon dioxide in the exhaled air will be slightly less than the arterial

P_{CO_2}. Larger differences may occur in disease states where there is more dead space, such as in anesthetized patients or with pulmonary embolism.[18]

Box 2-1. Causes of Inaccuracies in Pulse Oximetry

- Carboxyhemoglobin
- Methemoglobin
- High-intensity ambient light
- Impaired perfusion
- Nail polish and artificial nails
- Intravenous dyes
  - Methylene blue
  - Indigo carmine
  - Indocyanine green

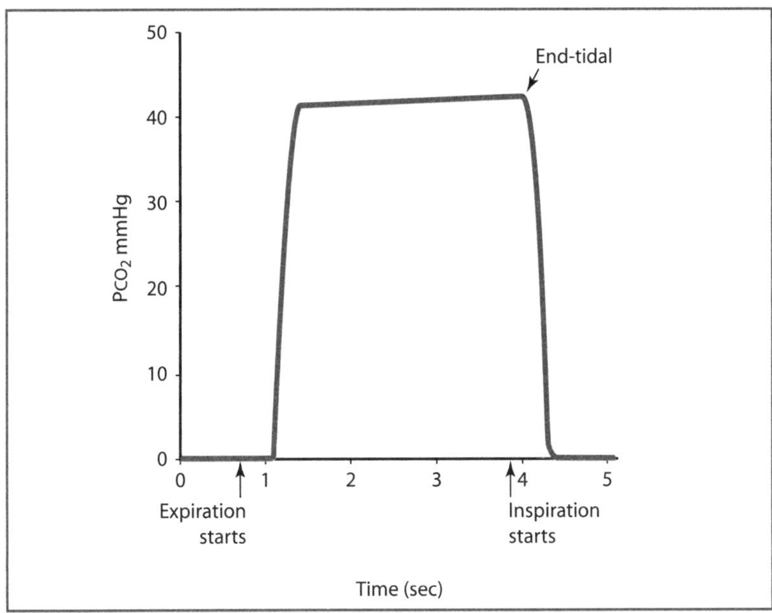

Figure 2-10. Normal capnograph. Carbon dioxide is measured in the exhaled air. The beginning of the breath is filled with dead space volume. At the end of the breath, the end-tidal P_{CO_2} reflects alveolar P_{CO_2}. It is a noninvasive way of monitoring arterial P_{CO_2}. (From Levitzky M. *Pulmonary Physiology.* 4th ed. New York: McGraw-Hill, Inc; 1995:73, with permission.)

Arterial Blood Gas Analysis

The gold standard for assessing both oxygenation and ventilation is arterial blood gas analysis.[19] The actual value of measured arterial Po_2 is important. However, in patients with hypoventilation or on supplemental oxygen, it is also useful to compare it to what it should ideally be. The difference between the predicted arterial Po_2 (calculated from the alveolar Po_2: P_{AO_2}) and what is measured is known as the *alveolar-arterial (A-a) gradient;* it is usually less than 10 mm Hg.[20] The P_{AO_2} can be calculated from the alveolar gas equation:

$$P_{AO_2} = P_{IO_2} - Paco_2/R$$

$$\text{since } P_{IO_2} = F_{IO_2}\,(Patm - P_{H_2O})$$

$$P_{AO_2} = F_{IO_2}\,(Patm - P_{H_2O}) - Paco_2/R$$

where P_{AO_2} is the alveolar Po_2, P_{IO_2} is the inspired Po_2, $Paco_2$ is the arterial Pco_2, and R is the respiratory exchange ratio of carbon dioxide and oxygen (which is estimated to be 0.8 for the whole lung). F_{IO_2} is the percentage of oxygen, Patm is atmospheric pressure (760 mm Hg at sea level), and P_{H_2O} is water vapor pressure (47 mm Hg at 37°C). So, for example, a patient breathing 40% oxygen with an arterial Pco_2 of 35 mm Hg has a Po_2 of 100 mm Hg. However, based on the equation, he/she should have an arterial Po_2 of 240 mm Hg at sea level. The A-a gradient is extremely elevated at 140 mm Hg. There are other ways to assess impairment of oxygenation using the P_{AO_2}[21] (Table 2-4).

The adequacy of ventilation can be assessed with an arterial blood gas; there is an inverse correlation between ventilation and the arterial Pco_2. However, the number must be assessed in the context of the clinical picture. For example, an asthmatic patient who is in severe distress with a respiratory rate of 60 breaths/min has a Pco_2 of 40 mm Hg.

Table 2-4. Measures of Impairment in Oxygenation

Oxygen	Normal Values (mm Hg)
$P_{AO_2} - Pao_2$	<10
Pao_2 / P_{AO_2}	1
Pao_2 / F_{IO_2}	500

The severity of an impairment in oxygenation can be assessed by comparing the ideal or alveolar Po_2 (P_{AO_2}) to the actual arterial Po_2 (Pao_2).

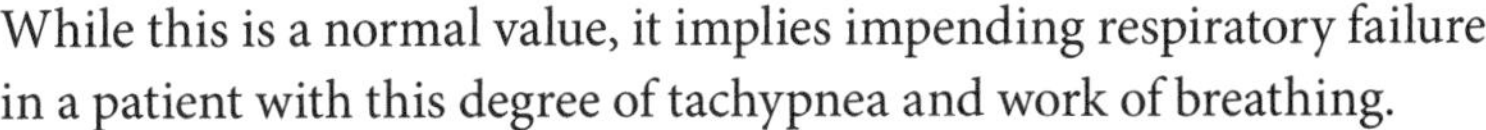

While this is a normal value, it implies impending respiratory failure in a patient with this degree of tachypnea and work of breathing.

Arterial blood gases are invasive, painful, and sometimes technically difficult. Surrogate measures are obtained either by using a venous or capillary blood sample. In the latter, a finger or toe is pierced with a lancet and the blood collected. Neither measure is useful for assessing arterial oxygenation, since they're mixed with venous blood. Since venous blood has a higher Pco_2, both will overestimate the true arterial Pco_2 (and give the worst-case scenario). In cases of cardiac arrest, the discrepancy between the 2 values widens.[22]

Mechanics of Breathing

The muscles of respiration act like a pump to move air in and out of the lungs. The efficiency of the pump is determined by the elastic properties of the chest wall and lungs and the resistance of the airways. Disease processes can alter these relationships and lead to respiratory failure.

Muscles of Breathing

The muscles of inspiration are depicted in Figure 2-11. The diaphragm is the primary muscle of inspiration. It is a dome-shaped muscle and is responsible for two-thirds of the air that enters the lungs during quiet breathing. When it contracts, it forces the abdominal contents down and widens the rib cage. When it is paralyzed, as in the case of phrenic nerve or cervical spine injury, it moves up instead of down during inspiration. Other muscles of inspiration are the external intercostal muscles and other "accessory muscles," such as the scalene and sternocleidomastoid muscles.

In normal quiet breathing, expiration is passive; the recoil of the lungs forces the air out. However, in active breathing, such as with exercise, coughing, singing, or in lower airway obstruction, expiratory muscles are recruited.[1] The muscles of expiration are the abdominal and internal intercostal muscles. Neuromuscular disease, abdominal muscle weakness, or postoperative abdominal pain may impair cough, leading to a decreased ability to clear secretions.

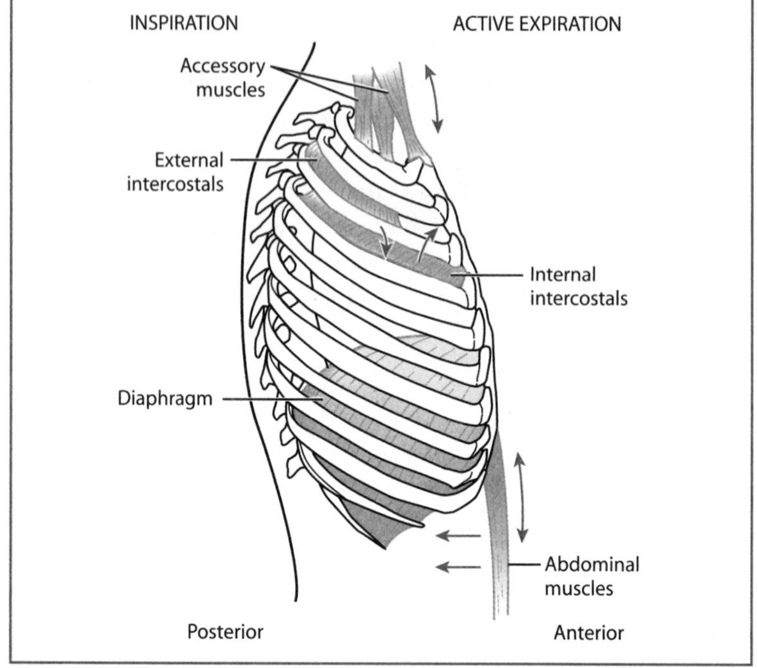

Figure 2-11. Muscles of breathing. The inspiratory muscles are the diaphragm, external intercostals, and accessory muscles such as the sternocleidomastoid and scalene. Expiration with quiet breathing is passive. Active expiration requires the use of the abdominal and internal intercostal muscles.

Elastic Properties of the Lung and Chest Wall

It is the interaction of the lungs and chest wall that determines the effectiveness of the "pump." The lungs and individual alveoli act like balloons. Pressure is required to inflate the lungs; without it they would tend to collapse. At low volumes it is difficult to overcome the elastic forces and to inflate the lung; high pressures are required. At medium volumes, less pressure is required to inflate them. At high volumes, it is again more difficult and higher pressures are required. The ease by which the lungs can be stretched is known as compliance. Reduced lung compliance can be seen in conditions such as fibrosis, pulmonary edema, or acute respiratory distress syndrome. Increased lung compliance is seen in emphysema and aging. One of the important functions of surfactant, a phospholipid produced by the lung, is to increase lung compliance by reducing the surface tension of alveoli. Consequently, in premature infants where there is a developmental decrease in surfactant production, there is a decrease in lung compliance and the development of neonatal respiratory distress syndrome.

The chest wall has elastic properties and its own compliance. Its inherent tendency is to expand, which counterbalances the tendency of the lungs to collapse. The relationship between the forces of the chest wall and lung volume are shown in Figure 2-12. The resting lung volume (functional residual capacity, FRC) represents the equilibrium between the 2 forces (Figure 2-12A). Lung volumes will be smaller if the compliance of either chest wall (Figure 2-12B) or the lung (Figure 2-12C) is decreased.

Airway Resistance

Resistance is the force that opposes the forward motion of the airflow. Approximately 25% to 40% of the total resistance to airflow is located in the upper airway: nose and mouth passages and larynx.[1,5] The airways and lung tissue provide the remainder of the resistance.

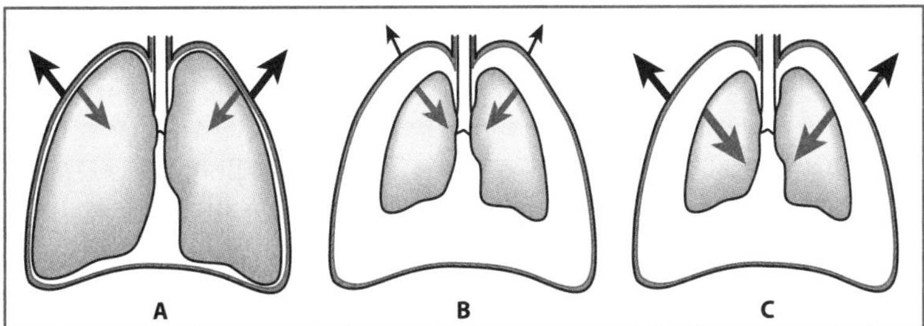

Figure 2-12. Interactions of the chest wall and lung in diseased states. **A.** In the normal lung, the outward recoil of the chest wall balances the inward recoil of the lung. The final volume of the lung depends on the equilibrium betweenthe two. **B.** If the chest wall becomes less compliant and more stiff, there is less outward force to balance out the inward recoil of the lungs. The result is a smaller lung volume. Examples: obesity, neuromuscular weakness, trauma to or defects in the chest wall. **C.** If the lungs become less compliant, they overcome the outward force of the chest wall and have a smaller resting volume. Examples: pulmonary edema, interstitial fibrosis, acute respiratory distress syndrome.

Air flows through the airways as if they were tubes. In some areas, the flow is very orderly and is known as *laminar flow.* In some places, such as in narrowed or branch points, it is disorganized and is known as *turbulent flow.* In laminar flow, resistance is directly proportional to the radius[4] of the airways. Consequently, if the radius of an airway is narrowed by half, the resistance increases by 16-fold. In the airway of an infant or child, which is already narrow relative to an adult's, small changes in caliber produce large changes in the degree of obstruction. Turbulent flow depends on gas density. Thus gases with a low density, such as helium, are administered to decrease resistance in patients with airway obstruction.[23]

Work of Breathing

The work involved in breathing is proportional to the tidal volume and the change in pressure that is required to move the air. The work of breathing increases when the compliance of the chest wall and lung is decreased; it requires more negative pressure to breathe. In addition, it increases with increased airway resistance, such as with asthma or upper airway obstruction. Infants and young children are at a mechanical disadvantage; their respiratory system works less efficiently than an adult's. Their chest walls are more compliant and their diaphragms are flatter and more likely to fatigue, which predisposes them to respiratory failure.

Assessment of Lung Mechanics

An alteration in lung mechanics is often described as *respiratory distress.* Decreases in lung and chest wall compliance are usually heralded by tachypnea. Increased effort of breathing is manifest by recruitment of accessory muscles, such as the sternocleidomastoid or scalene muscles. Retractions, bowing in of muscle and soft tissue of the chest wall with inspiration, indicate that high pressures are generated in order to move air through the airways. They can be seen subcostal, intercostal, and in the suprasternal notch. The higher the retractions, the more severe the respiratory distress. Nasal flaring is an attempt to decrease the resistance of breathing by decreasing the resistance of the nasal passages.

Airflow, lung volumes, and airway resistance can be measured by pulmonary function testing and will be further described in Chapter 6, Pulmonary Function Testing.

Key Points

Gas Exchange

- The Po_2 in the alveoli is determined by the balance between the amount that flows in and the amount that is removed by the pulmonary capillaries.
- The total amount of oxygen that is taken up by the body in 1 minute is called the *oxygen consumption* ($\dot{V}o_2$) and the amount of carbon dioxide produced is the *carbon dioxide production* ($\dot{V}co_2$).

Ventilation

- The volume of a breath is known as the *tidal volume.*
- The conducting airways are not involved in gas exchange, and the volume of air in them is known as dead space.
- *Total ventilation* is the total volume of fresh air that reaches the lung each minute.
- *Alveolar ventilation* is the total volume of air that reaches the alveoli and is available for gas exchange each minute.
- The removal of carbon dioxide from the blood depends on alveolar ventilation.
  - If alveolar ventilation increases, then the elimination of carbon dioxide increases and its concentration in the arterial blood decreases.
  - If alveolar ventilation decreases, then the elimination of carbon dioxide decreases and it accumulates in the arterial blood.
- Increases in arterial Pco_2 can be caused by decreased tidal volume, decreased respiratory rate, increased dead space, or increased carbon dioxide production.
- Most of the carbon dioxide in the blood is transported as bicarbonate.
- In respiratory acidosis, the arterial Pco_2 increases and the pH decreases
- In respiratory alkalosis, the arterial Pco_2 decreases and the pH increases.
- The kidneys compensate for a primary respiratory acidosis or alkalosis by conserving and losing bicarbonate, respectively.

Key Points (continued)

Oxygenation

- The amount of oxygen that is in the alveoli will decrease if barometric pressure is low (eg, high altitude), if there is no fresh supply of air (eg, atelectasis), or if Pco_2 is elevated (eg, hypoventilation).
- Under normal conditions, the red cells have enough time to become fully saturated as they pass through the pulmonary capillary circulation; however, this may not be true in exercise.
- Hypoxemia, or low arterial Po_2, may be caused by hypoventilation, diffusion impairment, shunt, ventilation/perfusion mismatch, and abnormally low venous blood saturation.
- Oxygen is primarily carried in the blood bound to hemoglobin; a very small amount is dissolved in plasma.
- *Oxygen saturation* is the percentage of binding sites of hemoglobin that have oxygen attached.
- The P_{50} is the oxygen tension at which 50% of the hemoglobin is saturated.
- The affinity of hemoglobin for oxygen can by altered by changes in blood pH, Pco_2, temperature, and 2,3 DPG levels.
- Arterial oxygen saturation can be assessed noninvasively using pulse oximetry.
- Arterial Pco_2 can be assessed noninvasively by end-tidal CO_2 monitoring.
- Arterial blood gas analysis is the gold standard for assessing Po_2 and Pco_2.
- The degree of impairment in oxygenation can be assessed by calculating the A-a gradient.

Key Points (continued)

Mechanics of Breathing

- The diaphragm is the primary muscle of inspiration.
- In quiet breathing, expiration is passive; in active breathing, expiratory muscles such as the abdominal muscles are used.
- The ease by which the lungs can be stretched is known as *compliance*.
  - Reduced lung compliance can be seen in conditions such as fibrosis, pulmonary edema, or acute respiratory distress syndrome.
  - Increased lung compliance is seen in emphysema and in aging.
- The resting lung volume (FRC) represents the balance between the tendency of the lungs to collapse and the chest wall to recoil outward.
- Resistance is the force that opposes the forward motion of the airflow.
- Approximately 25% to 40% of the total resistance to airflow is located in the upper airway: nose and mouth passages and larynx.
- In laminar airflow, resistance is directly proportional to the radius^4 of the airways. Therefore, small changes in the airway caliber produce large changes in resistance.
- The work of breathing increases when the compliance of the chest wall or lung is decreased or airway resistance is increased.
- Infants and young children are at higher risk of respiratory failure because their chest walls are more compliant and their diaphragms are flatter and more prone to fatigue.

References

1. Levitzky M. *Pulmonary Physiology.* 4th ed. New York, NY: McGraw-Hill, Inc; 1995:12–54, 73–80, 130–186
2. West JB. *Respiratory Physiology: The Essentials.* 8th ed. Baltimore, MD: Lippincott Williams & Wilkins; 2008:13–34, 55–122, 126–129
3. Angelillo VA, Bedi S, Durfee D, Dahl J, Patterson AJ, O'Donohue WJ Jr. Effects of low and high carbohydrate feedings in ambulatory patients with chronic obstructive pulmonary disease and chronic hypercapnia. *Ann Intern Med.* 1985;103:883–885
4. Kerr AA. Dead space ventilation in normal children and children with obstructive airways disease. *Thorax.* 1976;31:63–69
5. Lumb AB. *Nunn's Applied Respiratory Physiology.* 6th ed. Philadelphia, PA: Elsevier Limited; 2006:25–54, 76–91, 148–155, 189–200
6. DuBose TD. Disorders of acid-base balance. In: Brenner BM, ed. *Brenner and Rector's The Kidney.* Philadelphia, PA: Saunders Elsevier; 2007:505–520
7. Presson RG Jr, Graham JA, Hanger CC, et al. Distribution of pulmonary capillary red blood cell transit times. *J Appl Physiol.* 1995;79:382–388
8. Dantzker DR. Pulmonary gas exchange. In: Dantzker D, ed. *Cardiopulmonary Critical Care.* Orlando, FL: Grune &Stratton, Inc; 1986:25–46
9. Bancalari E, Claure N, Sosenko IR. Bronchopulmonary dysplasia: changes in pathogenesis, epidemiology and definition. *Semin Neonatol.* 2003;8:63–71
10. Needleman JP, Setty BN, Varlotta L, Dampier C, Allen JL. Measurement of hemoglobin saturation by oxygen in children and adolescents with sickle cell disease. *Pediatr Pulmonol.* 1999;28:423–428
11. Rackoff WR, Kunkel N, Silber JH, Asakura T, Ohene-Frempong K. Pulse oximetry and factors associated with hemoglobin oxygen desaturation in children with sickle cell disease. *Blood.* 1993;81:3422–3427
12. Watkins GM, Rabelo A, Pizak LF, Sheldon GF. The left shifted oxyhemoglobin curve in sepsis: a preventable defect. *Ann Surg.* 1974;180:213–220
13. Comroe JH Jr, Botelho S. The unreliability of cyanosis in the recognition of arterial anoxemia. *Am J Med Sci.* 1947;124:1–6
14. Mithoefer JC, Bossman OG, Thibeault DW, Mead GD. The clinical estimation of alveolar ventilation. *Am Rev Respir Dis.* 1968;98:868–871
15. Brockway J, Hay WW Jr. Prediction of arterial partial pressure of oxygen with pulse oxygen saturation measurements. *J Pediatr.* 1998;133:63–66
16. Brown M, Vender J. Noninvasive oxygen monitoring. In: Vender J, ed. *Intensive Care Monitoring.* Philadelphia, PA: WB Saunders; 1988:493–509
17. Stock MC. Noninvasive carbon dioxide monitoring. In: Vender J, ed. *Intensive Care Monitoring.* Philadelphia, PA: WB Saunders; 1988:511–526
18. Nunn JF, Hill DW. Respiratory dead space and arterial to end-tidal carbon dioxide tension difference in anesthetized man. *J Appl Physiol.* 1960;15:383–389

19. Shapiro BA. Arterial blood gas monitoring. In: Vender J, ed. *Intensive Care Monitoring.* Philadelphia, PA: WB Saunders; 1988:479–492
20. Filley GF, Gregoire F, Wright GW. Alveolar and arterial oxygen tensions and the significance of the alveolar-arterial oxygen tension difference in normal men. *J Clin Invest.* 1954;33:517–529
21. Covelli HD, Nessan VJ, Tuttle WK III. Oxygen derived variables in acute respiratory failure. *Crit Care Med.* 1983;11:646–649
22. Adrogue HJ, Rashad MN, Gorin AB, Yacoub J, Madias NE. Assessing acid-base status in circulatory failure. Differences between arterial and central venous blood. *N Engl J Med.* 1989;320:1312–1316
23. Gupta VK, Cheifetz IM. Heliox administration in the pediatric intensive care unit: an evidence-based review. *Pediatr Crit Care Med.* 2005;6:204–211

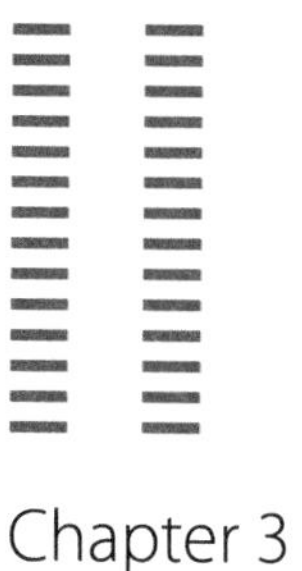

Chapter 3

Applied Pulmonary Physiology

Michael J. Light, MD
Douglas N. Homnick, MD, MPH

Exercise Physiology

Understanding exercise physiology in children is important because of the increasing popularity of young children participating in competitive sports.

The energy to power skeletal muscle depends on ATP. Combined with water, hydrolysis splits one of the phosphate groups, which results in formation of ADP. To replenish the limited stores of ATP, phosphorylation adds a phosphate group to ADP. If phosphorylation occurs in the presence of oxygen the reaction is aerobic metabolism, and in the absence of oxygen the reaction is anaerobic metabolism.

The ventilatory response to exercise results from increased demand for oxygen and excretion of carbon dioxide (CO_2). Exercise results in an almost immediate increase in oxygen consumption and without oxygen stores in the body, the carotid chemoreceptors register hypoxemia. This simplistic understanding is inadequate because ventilation appears to increase before there is hypoxemia and is probably driven by a neural response. Hypoxemia results in higher minute ventilation, which is the tidal volume (the volume of air inspired and expired during a passive breath) multiplied by the number of breaths per minute (frequency). Both tidal volume and frequency increase in response to increased metabolic demands. There is also an increase in blood flow to the lungs and an increase in lung diffusion capacity, which is a measure of the transport of oxygen passing from the alveolus across the alveolar-capillary membrane into the pulmonary circulation. The frequency increases from the resting 12 to 15 breaths/min to 45 to 70 breaths/min depending on age. The tidal volume increases to levels that may reach

50% to 60% of the vital capacity, which is the largest active breath than can be inspired and expired. As the degree of exercise increases there is a linear increase in tidal volume that reaches a maximum, and increased minute ventilation then results from increase in the frequency of breathing.

The cardiac responses are increased heart rate and stroke volume, which increases cardiac output. Resting heart rate averages 60 to 80 beats/min and increases in direct proportion to the degree of exercise to a maximum that is approximately 220 minus the age in years. Stroke volume also increases with exercise intensity, and training can increase this volume significantly.

The point at which the oxygen consumption does not rise with increasing exercise intensity is $\dot{V}O_2max$. It is also known as maximal oxygen uptake or aerobic capacity, and it is expressed as milliliters of oxygen per kilogram of body weight per minute. The expression relative to weight or body surface area is useful in comparing with other children (and adults of different sizes).

There is a great deal of variety in $\dot{V}O_2max$ and genetics plays a major role in these differences.[1] Responders make significant improvement and nonresponders make little or no progress to the same training program. Maximal ventilation increases to some extent with training, but at submaximal levels of exercise ventilation is consistently lower after training.[2] In children, both aerobic and anaerobic work capacity increase with training as measured by increase in $\dot{V}O_2max$ and decreased lactate production for a given workload.[3]

High-Altitude Illness

Ascending to high altitude results in hypoxia because the partial pressure of oxygen of inspired air decreases the higher the ascent. High altitude is considered to be over 1,500 m. Mild altitude elevation is considered to be over 1,500 m (4,900 ft), moderate 2,000 to 3,500 m (6,600–11,500 ft), very high 3,500 to 5,500 m (11,500–18,000 ft), and extreme high altitude is over 5,500 m (18,000 ft). Table 3-1 shows the approximate alveolar oxygen, the oxygen concentration at the level of the gas exchange portion of the lung, at different altitudes. The physiological effect of the reduced inspired oxygen depends principally on the rate of ascent and to a lesser extent on the medical history of the individual.

Table 3-1. Altitude and Oxygen Tensions

Altitude	Meters	(Feet)	Approximate Alveolar Oxygen Tension (mm Hg)
Sea level	0		100
Mild elevation	>1,500–2,000	(4,900–6,600)	80
Moderate	2,000–3,500	(6,600–11,500)	60
Very high	3,500–5,500	(11,500–18,000)	40
Extreme	>5,500	(>18,000)	<40

Acclimatization

The percentage (fraction) of oxygen in inspired air remains approximately 21% (0.21) but on ascent the partial pressure of oxygen decreases with the decrease in barometric pressure. The response to hypoxia depends on the magnitude of reduction and the rate of the change. Adaptation to hypoxia is known as acclimatization. The physiological response to hypoxia occurs immediately and also over time. The immediate response is an increase in minute ventilation when the carotid body registers the hypoxemia. As alveolar ventilation increases there is resultant decrease in partial pressure of CO_2, which causes a mild respiratory alkalosis and a reduction in the degree of hyperventilation. Over time, renal compensation for the respiratory alkalosis causes excretion of bicarbonate, which normalizes the pH. This ventilatory acclimatization takes place over 3 to 4 days (see Chapter 2). Ascent to altitude also results in circulatory changes to improve oxygen delivery to the tissues. There is increased sympathetic nerve activity, which increases the heart rate. Hypoxia causes pulmonary vasoconstriction and an increase in cerebral blood flow.

The first few nights of sleep at high altitude are associated with more frequent arousals, headache, and disturbed sleep that tends to improve over time.

Hemoconcentration results from reduction in plasma volume as a result of fluid shifts and diuresis, which improves oxygen-carrying capacity of the blood. Over time, weeks and months, there is increased red cell production. Dwellers at high altitude who develop polycythemia have a blunted response to hypoxia, and chronic hypoxia typically results in pulmonary hypertension. Individuals who are susceptible to high-altitude sickness, particularly the severe forms, should ascend to altitude more slowly as the recurrence risk is high.

Acute Mountain Sickness

The Lake Louise Consensus Group[4] defined acute mountain sickness (AMS) as the presence of headache in an unacclimatized person who has recently ascended to an altitude above 2,500 m. In addition there should be one or more symptoms, including anorexia, nausea, vomiting, insomnia, dizziness, lassitude, or fatigue. Onset of symptoms tends to be 6 to 10 hours after ascent but can be as early as 1 hour. Children are at risk for AMS, but not necessarily more so than adults.

High-Altitude Cerebral Edema

High-altitude cerebral edema (HACE) may be associated with AMS or high-altitude pulmonary edema. The major symptoms are ataxia and altered consciousness. High-altitude cerebral edema is essentially the severe form of AMS. The cerebral edema may cause papilledema or retinal hemorrhage and even cranial nerve palsy. Drowsiness is followed by stupor. Death may occur from brain stem herniation.

High-Altitude Pulmonary Edema

High-altitude pulmonary edema (HAPE) is a noncardiogenic pulmonary edema. As noted previously, hypoxia causes pulmonary vasoconstriction, and pulmonary hypertension results. The combination of increased pressure and hypoxia-related increased capillary permeability leads to leakage of fluid in the lungs. The risk of HAPE appears to be genetically determined in some individuals who are more susceptible, and in research studies a difference in the amiloride-sensitive sodium channel has been demonstrated.[5] In addition, the presence of preexisting pulmonary hypertension prior to the ascent exaggerates the effect of hypoxia. The risk of HAPE is increased by exercise because of the increased cardiac output and oxygen deficit.

Reentry HAPE occurs when persons who live at high altitude leave for a time and then return. Children are more susceptible than adults. Symptoms develop as rapidly as 24 hours after returning. It is diagnosed and managed the same as HAPE.

High-altitude pulmonary edema usually occurs 2 to 4 days after the ascent and tends to be worse at night. The primary symptom is cough with progressive dyspnea. It may be associated with central nervous system (CNS) symptoms, especially drowsiness. The chest radiograph

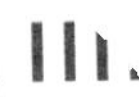

shows unilateral or bilateral patchy infiltrates. The heart siz(normal.

It is important to recognize HAPE because it has the potential to be life-threatening within a few hours. The Lake Louise Consensus definition of HAPE[4] is summarized in Box 3-1.

Box 3-1 Lake Louise Consensus Definition of High-Altitude Pulmonary Edema

At least 2 of the following symptoms and at least 2 of the following signs are necessary for diagnosis.

Symptoms

Weakness or decreased exercise ability
Cough
Dyspnea at rest
Chest tightness or congestion

Signs

Rales or wheezing in at least one lung field
Central cyanosis or arterial oxygen desaturation relative to altitude
Tachycardia
Tachypnea

It is important to be aware that fever may be present, and so a diagnosis of pneumonia may be incorrectly considered. The cough and decreased exercise ability are the early warning symptoms, and only late in the illness does production of frothy blood-stained sputum occur. Fifty percent of people with HAPE have AMS, and 14% have HACE.

Chronic Mountain Sickness

Chronic mountain sickness (CMS) occurs with persons born at high altitude as well as lowlanders who spend a prolonged period at high altitude. The condition has also been termed *chronic mountain polycythemia.* The symptoms are related to the polycythemia and include headache, dizziness, lethargy, difficulty sleeping, and impaired mentation and memory. The disorder is incompletely understood because actual hematocrit levels tend to be higher than expected considering the oxygen saturation. In addition there is hypoventilation and blunted hypoxic ventilatory response. Pulmonary hypertension may develop. The first consideration is to descend to a lower altitude, but this may not be practical. The management of CMS is lowering the red cell volume by phlebotomy. Low-flow oxygen may be beneficial.

Management of High-Altitude Illness

The first treatments of AMS are oxygen at 4 L/min and descent to a lower altitude. Symptoms of AMS may improve with a descent as small as 500 to 1,000 m. Reduction of symptoms can be achieved with acetazolamide, effective within 24 hours. Dexamethasone is equivalently effective, with a response within about 12 hours. The headache associated with AMS responds well to ibuprofen. Acetazolamide is also used as a preventive treatment, especially in those with prior history of AMS or HAPE. It is not used in the treatment of HAPE. Table 3-2 presents medical therapies for high-altitude sickness, but caution is necessary for children because data are limited.

Early diagnosis of HAPE is essential because it is the cause of most deaths from high-altitude illness. It is important not to exacerbate hypoxia during the descent by additional exertion. If high-dose supplemental oxygen does not improve the oxygen saturation to over 90% within 5 minutes, descent to a lower altitude or hyperbaric chamber may be lifesaving. Nifedipine is indicated if oxygen is not available or descent is not possible. Inhaled β-agonists have been shown to increase clearance of fluid from the alveolar space and may be helpful in the prevention and management of HAPE. Lasix is not indicated because the blood volume is already contracted.

Table 3-2. Therapy for High-Altitude Illness

Agent	Indication	Dose	Duration
Oxygen	All	2–4 L/min to keep oxygen saturation >90%	
Acetazolamide	Prevent AMS (adult)	125–250 mg	Twice a day for 24 hours before ascent and then first 2 days at altitude
	Treat pediatric AMS	5 mg/kg/day	2 or 3 times a day
Dexamethasone	Prevent AMS	8 mg per day	2 or 3 times a day
	Treat AMS	4 mg	Every 6 hours
	Treat HACE	8 mg initial then 4 mg oral, IM, or IV	Every 6 hours
	Pediatric AMS or HACE	0.15 mg/kg oral, IM, or IV	Every 6 hours

Abbreviations: AMS, acute mountain sickness; HACE, high-altitude cerebral edema; IM, intramuscular; IV, intravenous.

Simulated descent in a hyperbaric chamber has the same effect as descent to a lower altitude. Portable hyperbaric chambers are used by adventure and climbing groups. The chambers are coated fabric bags that are sealed and manually inflated to 105 to 220 mm Hg above ambient atmospheric pressure.

Underwater Medicine

Shallow Water Blackout

Hyperventilation before diving lowers CO_2, which reduces the stimulus to breathe. This prolongs the breath-holding time, but it can be dangerous. This occurs when free diving because as the diver descends, alveolar partial pressure of oxygen (Po_2) and partial pressure of carbon dioxide (Pco_2) increase but the CO_2 is so soluble that it diffuses into the tissues. Partial pressure of oxygen rises artificially, prolonging the breath-holding time, and then when the diver ascends the Po_2 falls dramatically so that unconsciousness may occur before reaching the surface. The risk is increased because of simultaneous hypocapnic vasoconstriction of the cerebral vessels. This combination is thought to explain many of the accidents that occur in swimming pools. Advice to parents should include telling their child not to hyperventilate before swimming underwater.

Thoracic Squeeze

This condition results during breath-hold diving, also known as free diving. Taking a full breath and free diving to 33 ft would cause the lungs to be half of their original size. At 66 ft they would be one-third, and at 99 ft they would be one-fourth. The air within the lungs is compressed during descent, and it is possible to compress to a volume smaller than the residual volume of the lungs. The chest wall will not be able to be compressed further, and the squeeze results in blood being forced into the alveoli because of the negative pressure within the lungs. The result is wheezing and hemoptysis. Free divers attempt to improve their ability to dive to deeper levels by "packing" or "stacking," which consists of glossopharyngeal breathing whereby the tongue and pharynx force air into the lung to exceed total lung capacity.

Scuba Diving

The effect of underwater pressure on gases is described by Boyle's law, which states that as the pressure of a gas increases, the volume decreases proportionately. By going from the surface (1 atmosphere) to 10 m (33 ft), which is 2 atmospheres and is the greatest change in pressure, the volume of air within the lungs is halved. Charles' law states that if the pressure is constant, the volume of gas alters with temperature, expanding with heating and contracting with cooling. This means that when a scuba tank is filled it will have less air if it is filled at a high temperature and later cools versus a tank that is filled at a low temperature. Charles' law is important when nitrogen in the tissues is expelled as gas in the lungs. If someone is close to the bends (see below) and the diver is warmed, there will be increased risk of the bends. If a scuba tank is left in a hot car it is more at risk for bursting (temperature rises, volume constant and pressure increases). Also important is Dalton's law, which states that in a mixture of gases the total gas pressure is equal to the sum of the individual pressures. This implies that as air is compressed into the scuba tank the percentages of each gas will remain the same. Many of the complications of diving are related to Henry's law, which states that the amount of gas that dissolves in a liquid is a function of the partial pressure of the gas and how easily the liquid absorbs gas. As a result, when a diver is at great depths the amount of nitrogen absorbed into blood and tissues is increased because of the increased pressure. This explains in part why the risk of decompression sickness is greater at depths of 100 ft than 30 ft.

Oxygen toxicity may occur if a diver descends below 200 ft, producing CNS effects including tremor and seizure, nausea, and tunnel vision. These effects may be seen at lower depths if the diver is using Nitrox, a blend of oxygen and nitrogen. Nitrox 1 has 32% oxygen, Nitrox 2 has 36%, and some divers use 40%. The advantage of Nitrox is that there is less risk of nitrogen narcosis and decompression sickness because the percentage of nitrogen decreases as the oxygen percentage increases.

Scuba is an acronym for self-contained underwater breathing apparatus, and the sport of scuba diving is very popular. There are limits of lower age set by the 2 major certifying agencies in North America. The Professional Association of Diving Instructors (PADI) requires that the child be 10 or older to take the certification course. Students younger than 15 will receive the PADI Junior Open Water Diver certification. It can then be upgraded to PADI Open Water Diver certification on reaching age 15. The National Association of Underwater Instructors' minimum age for certification is 12 years.

Pulmonary Complications of Scuba

Nitrogen Narcosis

The symptoms of nitrogen narcosis include euphoria, difficulty concentrating, and poor judgment. Because it happens at depths around 100 ft, this can be a dangerous situation for the diver. It is called "rapture of the deep" because the symptoms are similar to the effects of alcohol. It resolves very quickly during the ascent.

Decompression Sickness (DCS)

During descent, nitrogen under pressure is absorbed into tissues throughout the body. The amount is increased in fatty tissues and in those with good blood flow and less in other tissues, such as cartilage and tendons. During ascent the nitrogen is released again, and with slow ascent the nitrogen travels to the lung and is exhaled. If the ascent is too rapid the nitrogen forms bubbles in the blood that can block circulation in blood vessels. This produces the symptoms, commonly known as the bends, which result from blockage in the small veins of joints, especially the elbow, knee, and shoulder joints.

Type I DCS is the non-neurogenic form, which causes itching, rashes, joint pains, fatigue, and vertigo. The more severe form of DCS is Type II, when the bubbles interfere with the cerebral and spinal circulation resulting in weakness, paralysis, and behavioral changes. Decompression sickness occurs within a short time after the dive. Thalmann[6] reported 42% within 1 hour, 60% within 3 hours, and 98% within 24 hours, so that later symptoms are unlikely to be due to DCS.

Preventing DCS

Good diving practice is the most important way to prevent DCS, although there are differences in age, body size, and shape, as well as degree of fitness, which may make certain individuals more susceptible. Dive tables indicate how much time can be spent at a certain depth, and dive computers are helpful to define these depths, particularly if multiple dives are attempted. The rate of ascent is very important, and decompression stops should be routine, including a stop at half of the maximum dive and a safety stop at 15 ft. It is recommended that 24 hours elapse after diving before flying.

Treating DCS

Mild symptoms of DCS can be treated with oxygen (100%), fluids, aspirin, and rest. More severe forms require immediate recompression in a hyperbaric chamber. The recompression dissolves the bubbles, which can then be gradually eliminated by slow decompression.

Barotrauma

As every diver is aware, breath-holding during ascent is extremely dangerous. Air in the lung expands, especially in the last 10 m, and if unable to escape can produce an arterial gas embolism, pneumothorax, pneumomediastinum, or subcutaneous emphysema. These complications are more likely to occur if there is air trapping, such as occurs with asthma, pneumonia, or cystic fibrosis (see Diving and Asthma below). Arterial gas embolism is the most serious complication, whereby the alveolar sacs rupture and air enters the pulmonary capillary circulation. Bubbles travel to the left ventricle and then into the systemic circulation. The bubbles form an embolus with ischemia distal to the obstruction. Immediate recompression is necessary to reduce the size of the bubble that is causing the obstruction.

Carbon Monoxide (CO) Poisoning in Divers

The usual cause of excess CO in the breathing supply is proximity of the compressor intake to the exhaust of an internal combustion engine. The CO molecules displace oxygen from hemoglobin, which does not become apparent until at depth or during ascent. Symptoms of headache, confusion, and tunnel vision may result and the diver may lose consciousness because of hypoxia. On the surface of the water, the characteristic cherry red appearance of the skin may be noted. Smokers are at greater risk because of already elevated CO levels in the blood. This is treated with oxygen and may require recompression in the hyperbaric chamber (see discussion of CO poisoning under Inhalation Injury on page 57).

An important resource for divers is Divers Alert Network or DAN, which has a 24-hour consultative service to assist with diagnosis and treatment, and referral for hyperbaric treatment (see Resources).

Diving and Asthma

Not uncommonly parents and patients will inquire about the safety of underwater sports for their child with asthma. Unfortunately, there are no definitive data with which to make a specific recommendation for an individual child or youth. It has been suggested that several factors occurring naturally in the course of undertaking scuba diving can put individuals with increased airway hyperresponsiveness at risk of acute asthma. These include the inspiration of cold and dry gas, increased airway resistance, increased inspired partial pressure of oxygen, possible gas contamination with allergens and irritants, saltwater aspiration, and extreme exertion.[7]

A recent systematic review of the literature, covering 15 studies of safety of asthma in scuba diving, concluded that, although there is a sizeable subpopulation of divers who have asthma, aside from isolated case reports there was no rigorous epidemiological evidence for an increased relative risk of pulmonary barotrauma.[8] A large review by the DAN of DCS (1,213 cases) failed to demonstrate an increased risk of injury to asthmatic divers.[9] However, a subsequent survey by the same authors of 279 divers participating in 56,334 dives with active asthma (using medications at the time of study) revealed a slightly increased risk of DCS.[10] Much of the data from these studies rely on self-reporting of symptoms and are inherently flawed. Safety is of prime concern when counseling young divers with asthma.

The question as to whether a child with asthma should be permitted to become certified to dive and whether they are fit to dive at a specific time because of their asthma may be guided by the information in Box 3-2.

Box 3-2. Guidance for Young Divers With Asthma

1. Currently accepted (National Heart, Lung, and Blood Institute Expert Panel Report 3) guidelines for asthma should be followed in order to achieve optimal asthma control under all conditions in all seasons. (See Chapter 12.)
2. Diving should be avoided when actively wheezing, for a minimum of 2 weeks following wheezing, and within 48 hours of using a rescue inhaler (short-acting β-agonist).[8,11]
3. Diving is absolutely contraindicated in persons subject to spontaneous pneumothorax (eg, previous pneumothorax).[12]
4. Patients with moderate to severe persistent asthma should not dive.[11]
5. Airway function must be normal as demonstrated on standard pulmonary function tests, including the absence of demonstrable airway obstruction and air trapping.[13]

With conflicting data as to the increased risk of pulmonary barotraumas and DCS in asthmatic divers, it is ultimately up to the physician, parent, and patient regarding the decision to participate as a result of an informed, shared decision.

Near-Drowning

Drowning is the result of submersion or immersion in liquid resulting in various outcomes, including death, or survival, with or without morbidity. Near-drowning is the description if death is not the outcome. Various categories have been described, including dry drowning, wherein water has not entered the lungs; freshwater drowning, when freshwater enters the lungs; and saltwater drowning, when saltwater enters the lungs. Drowning is the third most common cause of accidental death in 1- to 4-year-olds and second most common in 5- to 15-year-olds.

The composition of the body usually allows an individual to float in water with about 3% by weight above the surface. If a breath is taken, then more of the body can be above water, conversely on deep expiration the body will sink somewhat. This is one of the reasons that shouting when a person is drowning may cause that person to sink. In addition, restrictive lung disease will reduce buoyancy.

An important factor relating to near-drowning includes the temperature of the water. Immersion in cold water results in hypothermia, which may have the potential to prolong survival. The mammalian dive reflex results from immersion of the face in cold water. This dive reflex leads to an immediate response with reduced physiological functioning of various body systems, including respiratory, cardiac, and nervous systems, entering a state of near suspended animation.

The sequence of events in a drowning accident is usually immersion followed by a sharp inspiration, initially resulting in a spasm of the larynx preventing water from entering the lungs. Hypoxia leads to unconsciousness, with subsequent laryngeal relaxation allowing water to enter the lungs. The major contribution to mortality and morbidity is the degree and duration of hypoxia with resultant cerebral injury. The pulmonary effects are from aspiration. Saltwater aspiration draws fluid into the alveoli and washes out surfactant. Freshwater aspiration also disrupts surfactant because it is hypo-osmolar relative to plasma.

The reduction in surfactant results in atelectasis and injury to the alveolar-capillary membrane and ventilation/perfusion ($\dot{V}/\dot{Q}$) mismatching resulting in hypoxemia (see Chapter 2). Acute respiratory distress syndrome is an important complication of both forms of near-drowning.

The cause of the near-drowning needs to be evaluated because other injuries may be present including traumatic (intentional, or perhaps unintentional, head injury), seizures, syncope, or cardiac disease. Hypoglycemia or alcohol intoxication may also have been involved. Pneumonia complicates the recovery from near-drowning, especially when the submersion is in stagnant or polluted water and the organisms responsible for infection may be unusual, including *Burkholderia pseudomallei, Chromobacterium violaceum, Aeromonas,* and *Pseudallescheria boydii,* as well as the more expected *Escherichia coli, Streptococcus pneumoniae,* and *Haemophilus influenzae.*

Inhalation Injury

Inhalation of Products of Combustion

Inhalation injury most commonly occurs during the inhalation of smoke containing chemicals and particulates and/or steam from fires, but also may occur with the inhalation of oils or corrosive chemicals. Pulmonary injuries from products of combustion will be considered first and are common, with fires and burns being the fourth most common cause of unintentional injury-related death in the United States.[14] The injury is caused by both chemical and thermal exposures, with most of the thermal injury occurring in the upper airway. The exception to this is steam, which can carry thermal injury to the lower airways due to its large heat capacity. Chemical injury can result from incomplete products of combustion and release of various substances that may combine with water vapor to form corrosive substances. These include compounds, such as nitrous oxide and sulfur dioxide forming nitric and sulfuric acids.

Bronchoscopic evaluation, especially of children and youth with facial burns, can reveal the extent and level of the thermal injury and may also provide a means to clear debris from the airway and enhance ventilation and oxygenation. The pathologic lesions encountered include bronchial erythema with vascular engorgement, edema, and epithelial necrosis, with formation of obstructing bronchial casts composed of sooty debris, exudated fibrin, and other circulatory derived products including inflammatory cells. Superinfection may eventually affect both the damaged airways and lung.

In the lung, small airway damage may occur directly or as a result of the effects of hypoxemia and hypotension. Edema of the interstitium, alveoli, and alveolar vessels are found and acute pulmonary edema often ensues due to increased vascular permeability. Atelectasis from both obstruction of small airways and loss of pulmonary surfactant may complicate $\dot{V}/\dot{Q}$ mismatching, leading to significant hypoxemia. Patients who die from their acute injury show a severe necrotizing bronchitis and bronchiolitis, intra-alveolar hemorrhage, hyaline membrane formation, and massive pulmonary edema.[15] Stridor from upper airway edema and increased airway hyperreactivity with reflex bronchoconstriction increase airway resistance, significantly increasing work of breathing.

Asphyxiants are chemicals generated during combustion that can displace oxygen and lead to absolute or relative hypoxemia. Carbon monoxide is the most common gas resulting from incomplete combustion of carbon-containing materials such as wood. It is responsible for 50% of fire-related fatalities and should be an immediate concern for caregivers of burn victims. Carbon monoxide combines with great affinity to hemoglobin (approximately 250 times the affinity of oxygen), forming carboxyhemoglobin (COHb), and leads to severely reduced tissue oxygenation.

With prolonged exposure it impairs mitochondrial function, reducing the production of ATP, and binds to myoglobin, impairing muscle function. It is important to understand that oxygen content of the blood is reduced but the Po_2 on a blood gas will not reflect this. Nor will pulse oximetry be accurate, as it measures both saturated normal hemoglobin and COHb. Co-oximetry can distinguish between the two. The CO level measured in blood can indicate the severity of exposure with expected associated symptoms as outlined in Table 3-3.

Table 3-3. Signs and Symptoms Associated With Carbon Monoxide Intoxication

Carboxyhemoglobin Level (%)	Signs and Symptoms
Mild (<20%)	Headache, slight dyspnea, decreased visual acuity, dyscoordination, slowed thinking
Moderate (20%–40%)	Irritability, nausea, decreased vision, impaired judgment, rapid fatigue
Severe (>40%)	Confusion, hallucination, ataxia, coma
Critical (>60%)	Death

Treatment is directed at CO intoxication, airway management, and respiratory support. Carbon monoxide intoxication is treated with high-flow oxygen to attain inspired concentrations near 100%. The role and risks and benefits of hyperbaric oxygen (where available) are unclear in children, although some authors have advocated it for severe exposures.[16]

Significant airway injury may require endotracheal intubation and mechanical ventilation with positive end-expiratory pressure (PEEP) to reduce pulmonary edema from vascular leak. Awake and cooperative patients with lesser pulmonary involvement and few facial burns may benefit from noninvasive ventilation with continuous positive airway pressure devices. Attention to fluid management and antibiotics as needed for superinfection is important. Corticosteroids should be used only for conditions where benefit is proven, such as asthma.[16] Corticosteroids have not been shown to alter morbidity or mortality in smoke inhalation injury.[17] The long-term prognosis after thermal, chemical, and smoke inhalation injury is guarded. Inhalation injury limits exercise endurance and leads to reduced lung function at between 3 and 8 years post-injury.[17,18]

Acute Aspiration of Hydrocarbons

Lung injury from aspiration of hydrocarbons occurs most commonly during accidental ingestion in children. The most commonly ingested and aspirated substances include household cleaning products, solvents, and fuels.[15] Gasoline and kerosene, particularly when kept in nonstandard and non-approved containers, cause a large percentage of these injuries.

Besides systemic toxicity, the most serious effect of hydrocarbon aspiration is pneumonitis, which is the leading cause of death. Similar to thermal injury, necrotizing bronchitis, bronchiolitis, alveolitis, atelectasis, interstitial inflammation, hemorrhage, pulmonary edema, necrotizing bronchopneumonia, and hyaline membrane formation all occur to a variable extent and are responsible for the clinical and laboratory findings. These include retractions, cough, grunting, tachypnea, and fever. With severe ingestion or aspiration, hemoptysis and pulmonary edema develop, and death may occur from respiratory failure. Initial radiographs may be normal immediately after the aspiration but usually show infiltrates and atelectasis by 2 hours. As necrotic obstruction of airways with secondary atelectasis occurs, ventilation/perfusion mismatching occurs, leading to hypoxemia, increased work of breathing, and possible respiratory failure. Treatment of symptomatic children and youth includes supplemental oxygen with increasing degrees of respiratory support, including noninvasive ventilation with continuous positive airway pressure and mechanical ventilation with PEEP as required. Gastric lavage should be avoided, as this may lead to further aspiration. Antimicrobial therapy is rarely needed, and corticosteroids have shown no benefit in this type of aspiration.[19] Like inhalation injury, prognosis is guarded. Small airway obstruction with residual air trapping can be found years after aspiration.

Effect of Pregnancy on Pulmonary Function

When the uterus expands, the diaphragm is displaced as much as 4 cm higher in the thoracic cavity. The function of the diaphragm remains normal. The thoracic cavity expands at its lower level by increasing circumference. The major physiological effect on pulmonary function is reduction in the functional residual capacity by about 20% during the latter half of pregnancy. This results from reduction in both expiratory reserve volume and residual volume. The changes in vital capacity tend to be small, and the forced expired volume in 1 second is essentially unchanged.

The minute volume increases by nearly 50% at term as a result of increased tidal volume with respiratory rates that do not increase. This effect is thought to be related to increased levels of progesterone. The change in minute volume is associated with a corresponding decrease in arterial P_{CO_2}, which tends to be about 30 mm Hg at term, and an increase in arterial P_{O_2} because of reduced alveolar CO_2 levels.

Key Points

- The definitive treatment of AMS, HACE, and HAPE is descent to lower altitude.
- Individuals may be particularly susceptible to AMS, HACE, and HAPE and can experience recurrence on ascent to altitude.
- Chronic mountain sickness is treated with low-flow oxygen and phlebotomy.
- Shallow water blackout can occur with hyperventilation before swimming and diving, and children and youth should be warned against this practice.
- Qualified diving instruction and good diving practice help prevent decompression sickness.
- Scuba diving is contraindicated in patients with moderate to severe persistent asthma and in those with unstable mild asthma with abnormal pulmonary function, or those who have wheezed in the last 2 weeks. See Box 3-2.
- Corticosteroids are of no proven benefit in inhalation injury.
- Gastric lavage is contraindicated in hydrocarbon aspiration.
- Compensatory increase in minute volume avoids hypoxemia in pregnancy as a consequence of reduction in functional residual capacity.

Resources

Exercise Physiology and Related Exercise Resources

The American Academy of Pediatrics Council on Sports Medicine and Fitness has a number of policy statements that address important issues, which can be viewed at www.aap.org/sections/sportsmedicine/PolicyStatements.cfm.

Diving Resources

Professional Association of Diving Instructors: www.padi.com/scuba/
National Association of Underwater Instructors: www.naui.org/
Divers Alert Network: www.diversalertnetwork.org/

References

1. Bouchard C, Dionne FT, Simoneau JA, Boulay MR. Genetics of aerobic and anaerobic performances. *Exerc Sport Sci Rev.* 1992;20:27–58
2. Homnick DN. Chest and pulmonary conditions. In: Patel DR et al, eds. *Pediatric Practice-Sports Medicine.* New York, NY: McGraw-Hill Medical; 2009:119–131
3. Sjodin B, Svedenhag J. Oxygen uptake during running as related to body mass in circumpubertal boys: a longitudinal study. *Eur J Appl Physiol Occup Physiol.* 1992;65(2):150–157
4. The Lake Louise consensus on the definition and quantification of altitude illness. In: Sutton JR, Coates G, Houston CS, eds. *Hypoxia and Mountain Medicine.* Burlington, VT: Queen City Printers; 1992
5. Sartori C, Duplain H, Lepori M, et al. High altitude impairs nasal transepithelial sodium transport in HAPE-prone subjects. *Eur Respir J.* 2004;23:916–920
6. Thalmann ED. *Phase II Testing of Decompression Algorithms for Use in the US Navy Underwater Decompression Computer.* Panama City, FL: Navy Experimental Diving Unit; 1984:1–84
7. Cirillo I, Vizzaccaro A, Crimi E. Airway reactivity and diving in healthy and atopic subjects. *Med Sci Sports Exerc.* 2003;35(9):1493–1498
8. Koehle M, Loyd-Smith R, McKenzie D, Taunton J. Asthma and recreational diving—a systematic review. *Sports Med.* 2003;33(2):109–116
9. Corson KS, Dovenbarger JA, Moon RE, Hodder S, Bennett PB. Risk assessment of asthma for decompression illness (abstract). *Undersea Biomed Res.* 1991;18S:16–17
10. Corson KS, Moon RE, Nealen M, Dovenbarger JA, Bennett PB. A survey of diving asthmatics (abstract). *Undersea Biomed Res.* 1992;19S:18–19
11. Tetzlaff K, Muth CM, Waldhauser LK. A review of asthma and scuba diving. *J Asthma.* 2002;39(7):566–577
12. Melamed Y, Shupak A, Bitterman H. Medical problems associated with underwater diving. *Undersea Hyperb Med.* 1999;326(1):30–35
13. Davies MJ, Fisher LH, Chegani S, Craig TJ. Asthma and the diver. *Clin Rev Allergy Clin Immunol.* 2005;29:131–138
14. American Academy of Pediatrics Committee on Injury and Poison Prevention. Reducing the number of deaths and injuries from residential fires. *Pediatrics.* 2000;105:1355–1357
15. Lee A, Bye MR, Mellins RB. Lung injury from hydrocarbon aspiration and smoke inhalation. In: Chernick et al, eds. *Kendig's Disorders of the Respiratory Tract in Children.* Philadelphia, PA: WB Saunders; 2006:653–660
16. Ruddy RM. Smoke inhalation injury. *Pediatr Clin North Am.* 1994;41:317–336
17. Lee AS, Mellins RB. Lung injury from smoke inhalation. *Pediatr Respir Rev.* 2006;7:123–128

18. Micak R, Desai MH, Robinson E, Nichols R, Herdon DN. Lung function following thermal injury in children—an 8-year follow up. *Burns.* 1998;24(3):213–216
19. Steele RW, Conklin RH, Mark HM. Corticosteroids and antibiotics for the treatment of fulminant hydrocarbon aspiration. *JAMA.* 1972;219:1434–1437

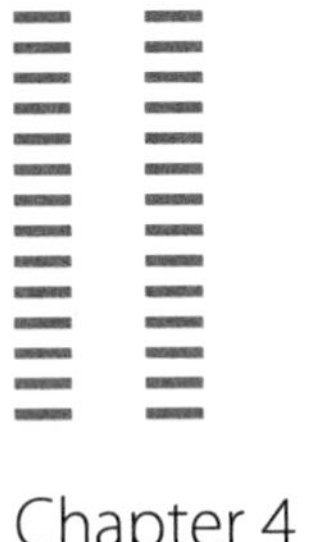

Chapter 4

Taking the Pulmonary History

Douglas N. Homnick, MD, MPH
Christopher Harris, MD

Pulmonary History

When evaluating children with respiratory complaints, it is crucial to obtain a complete and thorough, system-directed history. This history should be considered a supplement to the general pediatric history, a guide to which can be found in several comprehensive texts.[1,2] The pulmonary history is an information gathering process; sensitivity is key to the formation of a good therapeutic relationship. Parents and other care providers are often under great stress, especially when dealing with a chronic illness. Multiple people may care for the patient and, with appropriate parental or guardian consent, attention should be placed on getting information from grandparents, teachers, and others in the child's life so that a clear picture is obtained of the symptom complex. Sensitivity must also be shown to cultural aspects of the child and family. This may include the nuances of language that trained translators can provide. Finally, ingrained beliefs about conditions are often present and may influence how a parent or care provider is able to understand and trust the information given. For instance, parents may not believe that their active child has asthma because of a long-held idea that asthma causes children to be sickly and inactive. Assurance that persons with asthma may be Olympic-class athletes helps dispel this idea.

History of Present Illness

As in the general pediatric history of present illness, determining *onset* (gradual or acute), *duration* (chronic = >3 weeks), *recurrent* (periods of wellness alternating with periods of illness) or *persistent,* and *trigger factors* (eg, viral upper respiratory infection) are essential, all obtained in chronological fashion. Since the lungs are in constant contact with the external environment, the *environmental history* is particularly important. Indoor (environmental tobacco smoke [ETS], woodstoves, pets, stuffed animals in the bedroom, etc) and outdoor exposures (animals, cold air, industrial pollutants, etc) must be carefully sought. Environmental tobacco smoke exposures will adversely affect children's lung health. Parents and other caregivers should be questioned about tobacco use with a strong recommendation to quit using, a brief intervention or, at minimum, removing all secondhand smoke from a child's environment (eg, not smoking in the house or car, sitting in nonsmoking areas of restaurants, avoiding family gatherings where smoke cannot be avoided, or asking family members to smoke away from the child). Teen smoking is a growing problem and all teens and preteens, starting in middle school years, should be questioned about primary smoking. Additional environmental inquiry should include the age of the home; type of construction; and sources of heating, cooling, and ventilation.

Family History

Family history of respiratory illness is also very important because many diseases manifesting in childhood have a genetic basis. Various conditions result in pulmonary abnormalities. The Mendelian defects are single gene defects that may include autosomal dominant, recessive, X-linked dominant, and X-linked recessive. Additionally there are chromosome and multifactorial disorders that may result in pulmonary abnormalities. Some examples are shown in Box 4-1. If there appears to be a genetic basis for disease, an extended family tree may be useful.

Medical History

The neonatal history may also indicate a reason for persistent or recurrent respiratory disease, especially in infancy, although even teens may manifest chronic airway obstruction as a result of neonatal disease such as post-infant respiratory distress syndrome (IRDS) or chronic lung disease/bronchopulmonary dysplasia (BPD). Precise details of the antenatal history and clinical course after delivery are key to providing rational and appropriate care. Attention should be paid to birth weight and gestational age, both of which are known antecedents to neonatal

Box 4-1. Genetic or Chromosome Defects That Result in Pulmonary Disorders

Dominant
- Marfan syndrome
- Neurofibromatosis 1
- Achondroplasia
- Familial pulmonary fibrosis

Recessive
- Cystic fibrosis
- Primary ciliary dyskinesia
- Sickle cell disease
- Mucopolysaccharidoses
- Spinal muscular atrophy

X-linked
- Dominant
  - Rett syndrome
- Recessive
  - Duchenne muscular dystrophy
  - Hemophilia

Chromosome
- Down syndrome
- Other trisomy

Other (multifactorial)
- Cleft lip and palate
- Asthma
- Allergic rhinitis
- Gastroesophageal reflux
- Autoimmune disorders
- Diabetes type 1
- Heart disease
- Interstitial lung disease

lung disease. The pregnancy history should also include maternal use of tobacco and other substances. Other important points include maternal complications during pregnancy, such as pregnancy-induced hypertension or diabetes mellitus. Also, problems at the time of delivery are relevant because they may immediately place the infant at risk for lung disease and injury. For instance, a prolonged labor increases the risk for fetal distress and the antenatal passage of meconium. With sufficient stress, aspiration may occur, which can be associated with significant lung injury and pulmonary hypertension. Additionally, details of treatment in the intensive care nursery aid in understanding how severely the child's lungs may have been affected by both antenatal factors and postnatal treatment. Certainly the child born with transient tachypnea of the newborn and a 12-hour intubation is very different from the 500-g child born at 26 weeks' gestation who was intubated and mechanically ventilated for weeks. Finally, the total length of oxygen therapy can provide information regarding the degree of lung injury.

Surgical History

Surgical procedures relevant to the respiratory tract, including cardiac, gastric, esophageal, otolaryngologic, orthopedic, and urologic/nephrologic procedures, may be a clue to persistent respiratory problems. For example, a repair of a tracheoesophageal fistula may leave significant residual airway problems in the form of localized tracheomalacia.

Tympanostomy (ear tubes) or tonsillectomy and adenoidectomy may not be declared without prompting the parent or caretaker.

A history of contact with the medical system and the use of medical resources can give valuable information about the severity, chronicity, and control of a respiratory condition. For example, hospitalizations and emergency department (ED) visits provide important information about the patient's history.

Quality health care includes efficient use of resources and limiting unnecessary repeat studies. Many times, a few precisely directed calls will yield valuable information regarding previous studies and investigations that can be summarized quickly. This will often obviate the need for repeating some studies, allowing further diagnostic testing to be streamlined, lowering cost, and lessening the burden of health care visits for the family. In some cases, however, repeat studies are necessary. For example, if a sweat chloride test for cystic fibrosis (CF) is not done per Cystic Fibrosis Foundation standards by experienced personnel (most often found in a CF care center), the results may be suspect and the test should be repeated.

The past response to various therapeutic trials is also helpful information for the health care provider. For example, if a child with chronic cough fails to respond to oral antibiotics but responds well after a several day course of corticosteroid, then a diagnosis of asthma is supported. Alternatively, if the patient responds well to oral antibiotics, then conditions such as chronic sinusitis, cystic fibrosis, bronchiectasis, or possible aspirated foreign body are more likely. Medication delivery information is also critical because a lack of response to therapy may be caused by an inadequate delivery of medication. For example, it is appropriate to inquire whether nebulized medications were given by blow-by rather than with a properly fitted mask. Further, was there an attempt to give a metered-dose inhaler to a small child who lacks the skill to use it?

Social History

Additional social history will supplement the environmental history. For example, an appropriate social history should determine whether a child spends time in 2 different households. Exposure to ETS in one home may make asthma control difficult, and education of both caregivers is essential. Other questions to ask include the following: Who is caring for the child or youth? Is there an adult in the home who can supervise administration of medication and provide for early medical intervention when symptoms exacerbate? Is the child receiving treatments as prescribed or are there adherence issues evident from medical or pharmacy refill records? Does the family keep follow-up appointments? Are there financial barriers that prevent adherence to a therapeutic regimen or that may promote ED use rather than primary or subspecialty follow-up care? Is there a history of a psychiatric disorder in a parent or guardian or in the child or youth that may affect adherence to therapeutic recommendations? Are there educational or language barriers that prevent the family from reading and understanding educational and instructional information regarding illness treatment and prevention? A medical social worker can help sort through possible barriers to quality care and help families obtain the resources necessary to deal with the respiratory condition with minimal stress.

As in the general pediatric history, *immunization* and specific *medication allergy history* are important to record. The child with chronic respiratory disease is at particular risk from influenza and complicating *Streptococcus pneumoniae* infection and, if no contraindication, will benefit from the pneumococcal vaccine and yearly influenza vaccination as are recommended by the Centers for Disease Control and Prevention and American Academy of Pediatrics. Occasionally, travel may expose a patient to an infectious agent that is not common in a local area. Certain fungal agents have a particular propensity for a geographic region, and it is helpful to know about a patient's travel history. Foreign travel can increase risk for *Mycobacterium tuberculosis* exposure with varying degrees of susceptibility to antimicrobials.

Copies of previous medical records, including radiographic studies, will help avoid unnecessary tests, confirm response or lack thereof to medication or other therapeutic trials, and confirm the severity and frequency of symptoms and chronicity of a condition. A list of elements of the pediatric pulmonary history is found in Box 4-2.

Review of Systems

A complete review of systems is always necessary for the thorough evaluation of a new patient. The review of systems relevant to the respiratory tract is listed in Box 4-3. Important information not otherwise gleaned in the history of present illness may become evident here and may shed light on the current situation.

Box 4-2. Elements of the Pediatric Pulmonary History

Present Illness

Onset
Duration
Recurrence
Persistence
Triggers

Medical History

Birth history
Immunizations
Allergy
Hospitalizations and emergency department (ED) visits
Response to therapeutic interventions
Imaging and laboratories

Family History

Allergy/allergic rhinitis, bronchitis, asthma, cystic fibrosis, sinus problems, pneumonia, tuberculosis, inflammatory bowel disease, childhood cancer, HIV/immune problems, eczema, congenital heart disease, juvenile onset diabetes mellitus, early onset emphysema, liver disease

Environmental History

Smoke and other toxic exposures
- Primary and secondhand environmental tobacco smoke exposure
- Woodstoves
- Industrial and household aerosols
- Dust, mold, construction dust, and debris
- Other toxins

Allergen exposure
- Age and condition of the house and the child's bedroom
- Stuffed toys
- Pets
- Heat source, humidifiers, air filters
- Other environments including a second household and child care
- Attempts at allergy reduction

Travel

Social History

Family dynamics
- Who is the caregiver?
- Is the child supervised in taking medications?
- Educational and reading level
- Language barriers

Financial support

- Can the family afford medications?
- Are follow-up visits avoided because of finances (eg, co-pays or lack of transportation)?
- ED use because of financial hardship

Box 4-3. Review of Systems Relevant to the Respiratory Tract

Constitutional
Fever, weight loss, night sweats, fatigue, pain

Skin
Eczema, other rashes, urticaria

Head, Eyes, Ears, Nose, Throat
Sinusitis, otitis media, congestion

Respiratory
Cough, wheeze, stridor, shortness of breath, chest discomfort or pain, hemoptysis, sputum production, chest tightness, symptoms with exercise, pneumonia diagnosis

Cardiovascular
Congenital heart disease, hypertension, syncope, previous surgery

Gastrointestinal
Stool volume and consistency, constipation, diarrhea, regurgitation or gastroesophageal reflux disease, choking or gagging with feedings, food intolerance, hematochezia

Genital/Urinary
Urinary anomalies, poly- or oligohydramnios, renal disease, recurrent infection

Neurologic
Known neuromuscular disease, known developmental disabilities, choking or gagging, stridor

Musculoskeletal
Scoliosis, chest wall deformity, previous chest wall surgery, muscle weakness, joint pain or swelling, chest wall pain or discomfort

Allergy/Immunology
Wheezing or known asthma, chronic cough, chronic congestion, itching and sneezing, recurrent infection, HIV or other exposures, skin or serum testing

Blood Disorders
Sickle cell disease, coagulopathies, bleeding, cancer, other blood dyscrasias, transfusion history

Endocrine
Diabetes, thyroid, parathyroid disease, growth

Common Symptoms Related to the Pulmonary System

Common symptoms that the pediatrician will encounter include cough, wheezing and stridor, chest pain, dyspnea (shortness of breath), and cyanosis. The causes of these symptoms often vary by age of the child, although considerable overlap may occur. Details on the various causes presented here can be found in the specific diseases discussed in other chapters and in other pediatric pulmonary texts.[3]

Cough

Coughing arises from an irritation of the airways where receptors are concentrated at airway bifurcations. It occurs in a phased sequence involving a deep inspiration, closure of the glottis and relaxation of the diaphragm along with contraction of muscles of expiration, and sudden opening of the glottis with forceful expired airflow. Cough can be classified as acute or chronic depending on duration; continued symptoms beyond 3 weeks are termed chronic.

Cough during infancy most commonly accompanies infection, usually viral, and is productive of thin, white mucus resolving over about 10 days. Croup syndrome produces a brassy, seal-like cough following an upper airway infection. Exposure to irritants such as ETS and woodstoves may produce acute cough in infants. Chronic cough in infants requires a more extensive and comprehensive evaluation. Causes include CF, less common infections *(Bordetella pertussis, Chlamydia, Mycoplasma),* aspiration due to developmental disabilities or traumatic birth injury (suck-swallow dyscoordination, recurrent laryngeal nerve injury, complications of neonatal intubation), gastroesophageal reflux disease (GERD), the sequela of neonatal lung injury (BPD), and congenital lung malformations (bronchogenic cyst, congenital cystic adenomatoid malformation, congenital hyperlucent lung, and pulmonary sequestration).

Cough in childhood, like infants, is most often due to infectious agents. Cystic fibrosis may present with cough at this age, although newborn screening usually allows for this diagnosis earlier. Foreign body aspiration becomes a more common cause of acute cough at this age. Chronic causes of cough include infections (tuberculosis if exposed to infected individuals, *Chlamydia,* and *Mycoplasma),* primary ciliary dyskinesia, chronic sinusitis, aspiration (especially with developmental disabilities), GERD, ETS and other toxic exposures, congenital lung and airway malformations, and the use of angiotensin converting enzyme inhibitor drugs. Functional or habit cough (psychogenic cough) may begin in late childhood but is more common in adolescents. Asthma may present only as cough (cough variant asthma) at almost any age and can be proved with a bronchial challenge, such as methacholine, or by response to a trial of asthma therapy. Acute cough in adolescents is also most often due to infectious agents, but may result from acute toxic exposures, such as primary smoking or exposure to ETS. Postnasal drip and chronic sinusitis are a cause of throat clearing and nighttime–early morning cough. In adolescents with cough, a history of exposure to irritating inhalants should be sought if substance abuse is suspected. Occasionally a congenital malformation, such as a bronchogenic cyst, will not become evident until teen years when recurrent or chronic infection occurs.

Wheezing and Stridor

Wheezing and stridor with respiratory infections (bronchiolitis and croup) are most common during infancy, although CF may also present with chronic wheezing. Infants with disabilities may aspirate silently, and thus a strong index of suspicion should be maintained when recurrent pulmonary symptoms occur in this group of infants. Gastroesophageal reflux disease with retrograde aspiration can occur and may be found with congenital causes of stridor, such as laryngomalacia. When tracheomalacia or bronchomalacia are present, chronic expiratory wheeze is also noted. Rarely, airway lesions, such as laryngeal hemangiomas, laryngeal webs, stenosis, and clefts, are a cause of stridor in infancy. Intermittent stridor beyond early childhood most often occurs in children with atopic dermatitis and is termed *spasmodic croup.* Allergy is a rare cause of wheezing in infancy but is a more common cause of wheezing in childhood. Other causes of wheezing in children include aspirated foreign body, CF, inhalation injury, bronchiectasis from any cause, aspiration syndromes, and mediastinal and airway malformations or neoplasms. Stridor with or without expiratory wheezing is a common finding in vocal cord dysfunction (see Chapter 35), which is transient, non–life-threatening, often associated with exercise, and most common in adolescents. Adolescents can also experience the other etiologies mentioned above for children, although asthma and wheezing as a result of intentional or non-intentional inhalation of irritating aerosols or smoke are the more common in this group.

Chest Pain

Chest pain can originate in chest wall structures or within the lung as a result of inflammation of the lung-covering membranes (pleura). Infants clearly cannot express specific pain, but tenderness on palpation along with skin changes that might be related to trauma can be elicited and noted during a careful examination. Chest wall pain is not uncommonly associated with prolonged and vigorous coughing and is commonly found in children with CF experiencing a pulmonary exacerbation. Other causes of chest pain in children include pleurisy most often associated with coxsackievirus B (pleurodynia) and bacterial pneumonias. Occasionally both GERD and asthma will be causes of chest pain or discomfort in children and adolescents; certainly the acute chest pain associated with sickle cell crisis is well known in pediatrics and should be aggressively treated. Adolescents in athletic activities such as weight lifting can present with acute or chronic chest wall pain localized over the costochondral junctions (costochondritis). Rib fractures due to chest wall trauma or vigorous activities such as competitive rowing can be found in teens. Although spontaneous pneumothorax as a cause of chest pain can occur at other ages, it is most common in adolescents and should be suspected when an otherwise healthy teen complains of sudden onset sharp, unilateral chest pain with shortness of breath (dyspnea). Herpes zoster as a cause of chest wall pain will be readily identifiable by its characteristic rash found along a chest wall dermatome. Rarely, previously undiagnosed coronary artery anomalies and mitral valve prolapse can present in this age group as well as in younger children.

Dyspnea

Increased depth of respiration, often with increased respiratory rate (tachypnea), can occur at any age and is produced by both pulmonary and non-pulmonary causes. Any cause of airway obstruction in infancy can lead to dyspnea, although sudden onset is more likely due to infection or cardiac disease. Acidosis is a cause of non-pulmonary dyspnea and may occur with inborn errors of metabolism or with dehydration. Rarely in infants but more commonly in children and adolescents, dyspnea is associated with ketoacidosis as an initial presentation of diabetes or with inadequate diabetic control. In childhood as well as adolescence, acute asthma becomes a common cause of dyspnea, and acute toxic ingestion (eg, salicylates) can also manifest as dyspnea. Cyanosis and hemoptysis, along with dyspnea, often occur with pulmonary embolism either due to traumatic lower extremity injury, heart disease, or familial or other coagulopathy.

Anxiety (hyperventilation with panic attacks—see Chapter 35) and substance ingestion (eg, suicide attempt with salicylates) are more common in adolescents.

Cyanosis

Central cyanosis (blue mucous membranes) should be distinguished from peripheral cyanosis (blue extremities), as the former is associated with important cardiopulmonary disease. Any pulmonary disease that causes significant mismatching of lung ventilation and perfusion or reduced functional residual capacity (expiratory reserve volume plus residual volume) will lead to oxygen desaturation and, eventually, visible central cyanosis. In newborns this occurs during IRDS (hyaline membrane disease), which reduces functional residual capacity and any significant lung inflammation, such as neonatal pneumonia or meconium aspiration. Space-occupying lesions, such as lung malformations (congenital hyperlucent lung, congenital cystic adenomatoid malformation, pulmonary sequestration, bronchogenic cyst, gastroenteric cyst, etc), may press acutely on the ipsilateral healthy portion of the lung or the contralateral lung leading to decreased ventilation and perfusion. If present prenatally, lung malformations and oligohydramnios can lead to lung hypoplasia, which may cause cyanosis. Any right-to-left shunt due to vascular malformation or intrinsic cardiac disease may lead to cyanosis. In older children and adolescents, cyanosis is most commonly associated with acute pulmonary disease (eg, acute asthma or pneumonia). Cyanosis is a late manifestation of chronic, destructive pulmonary disease such as is found in CF. As a result of increased survival of children with CF, cyanosis is unusual in infancy or childhood. Cyanosis is also a late finding of degenerative neurologic disease such as Duchenne muscular dystrophy. Acute inhalation of smoke or other toxic substances, such as hydrocarbons, can lead to cyanosis stemming from severe acute lung inflammation. A space-occupying thoracic neoplasm may produce enough pressure on surrounding lung or airways to significantly compromise ventilation and perfusion, producing cyanosis.

Key Points

- Careful questioning and listening, with cultural sensitivity, leads to an accurate picture of the patient's condition and how it affects individual and family functioning.
- Genetics and environment play a large role in childhood respiratory disease.
- Information about onset, duration, recurrence, persistence, and triggers helps lead the diagnostician to first determine acuity and chronicity and, second, a likely cause of a pediatric respiratory condition.
- Toxic exposures, particularly ETS or primary smoking, are more important causes of acute and chronic respiratory conditions as children age.
- Asthma is a common cause of chronic cough as well as wheeze.
- Response to previous therapeutic interventions, including medications, can be a valuable clue as to the etiology of an underlying pulmonary condition.

References

1. Homnick D. The respiratory system. In: *The Pediatric Diagnostic Examination*. Greydanus DE, Feinberg AN, Patel DR, Homnick DN, eds. New York, NY: McGraw-Hill; 2007
2. Zitelli BJ, Devis HW. *Atlas of Pediatric Physical Diagnosis*. 4th ed. St Louis, MO: Mosby; 2002
3. Chernick V, Boat TF, Wilmott RW, Bush A, eds. *Kendig's Disorders of the Respiratory Tract in Children*. 7th ed. Philadelphia, PA: Saunders; 2006

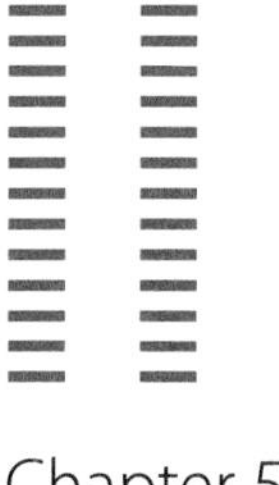

Chapter 5

The Pulmonary Physical Examination

Christopher Harris, MD
Douglas N. Homnick, MD, MPH

Introduction

The clinical encounter begins with a thorough history. Details of the present condition, its time course and past management, other medical and surgical conditions, and family history should be completely reviewed. A social history, environmental history, and complete review of systems along with an immunization history are necessary to completely evaluate a child with a pulmonary complaint.

The pediatric physical examination should vary according to the age and developmental stage of the child. In young children, the passive examination, where possible, is always more productive; for example, a child should be lying down to bring out wheezing by lowering lung volumes and thus reducing airway caliber. Those examinations that are more difficult in a crying child, such as the heart and lungs, should be the first to be accomplished, saving the less-tolerated examinations, such as ears and throat, for last. Young children often are most comfortable when seated in the lap of a parent or caretaker. The time-honored principles of inspection, palpation, auscultation, and percussion apply well to the pulmonary examination of children and youth at any age.[1–3]

Upper Airway

The head, ears, nose, and throat examination is an important part of the respiratory tract examination. Chronic otitis media may be a first sign of immune deficiency and is usually present in children with primary ciliary dyskinesia. Nasal examination is also very important in children presenting with respiratory diseases. Children with allergic conditions, such as allergic rhinitis, often have mucosal pallor or edema along with the presence of clear secretions. Aggressive treatment of upper airway allergies may have a major effect on improving lower airway signs and symptoms.[4] Sinusitis may also be a common problem in children presenting with chronic cough. Because the paranasal sinuses are lined by pseudostratified columnar epithelium (the same cells lining the airway), it stands to reason that conditions affecting the airway may also affect the sinuses.[5] For example, chronic sinusitis is nearly universal in children with cystic fibrosis (CF) and primary ciliary dyskinesia. Patients with allergic rhinitis may also have mucosal edema, preventing the sinus ostia from draining readily. Nasal polyps may also complicate both allergic rhinitis and cystic fibrosis. Polyps, which have a characteristic clear to white bulbous appearance, may be quite large but cause the child relatively few symptoms. This is probably due to the gradual nasal obstruction that occurs with polyp growth.

The diagnosis of sinusitis can be rather difficult to make solely on clinical grounds. Nasal secretions are usually thick and purulent. However, if postnasal drip is present, secretions may not be issuing from the nares. Therefore, the oropharynx should be examined carefully for mucoid material draining from above. Oropharyngeal cobblestoning may be noted with postnasal drip. Sinus tenderness with palpation of the maxillary and frontal sinuses may be helpful in diagnosing a sinus infection in older children. Reports of sinus pressure, especially when the patient bends over, are also commonly noted with sinus infections.

Examination of the mouth and oral cavity is important in respiratory medicine due to congenital anomalies and other conditions that affect sleep. Many dysmorphologies affect oro-facial structures. Common examples include the Pierre-Robin sequence, Stickler syndrome, Treacher-Collins syndrome, and Crouzon syndrome. These infants may present with cleft palate, making early nutritional and feeding intervention of prime importance. Conditions associated with relative or absolute macroglossia, such as Down syndrome, congenital hypothyroidism, and glycogen storage diseases, may place the child at risk of obstruction of the upper airway during sleep. Careful questioning of the caretakers and a low threshold for referral for sleep evaluation and polysomnography are needed in caring for these children. Tonsillar size is also very important to assess in all children, but especially during the preschool years. Frequent infections of the upper respiratory tract during these years cause the lymphoid tissues in the head and neck to proliferate. This hyperplasia, along with the normally sized upper airway, put children at risk for sleep-disordered breathing, including obstructive sleep apnea. In addition, the increasing incidence of obesity among children further contributes to increased risk for obstructive sleep apnea.[6] Therefore, careful inspection of tonsillar size and degree of oropharyngeal filling must be noted in all children, especially for those with sleep-related concerns.

Characterization of the voice is another important part of the pulmonary examination. Lesions in the area of the larynx may impede normal vocal fold function and cause hoarse voice along with inspiratory stridor. For example, respiratory papillomas due to infection with human papillomavirus may cause a hoarse voice. Also, injury to the nerves innervating the larynx may cause vocal disturbance and stridor. Repair of congenital heart defects, especially ligation of the ductus arteriosus, may be associated with at least temporary vocal cord paresis. Of much greater consequence are abnormalities of the central nervous system (CNS) that may compress the brain stem and cranial nerves. Arnold-Chiari malformations are well known to be associated with bilateral vocal cord paralysis. Signs include a soft, breathy voice and stridor. Demonstration of cough by the child should be elicited when there is concern about laryngeal innervation.

Stridor has different causes at different ages and depending on whether it is intermittent or continuous. Inspiratory stridor usually indicates lesions of the glottis or above, and expiratory coarse wheeze or stridor represents lesions below the level of the glottis. Biphasic stridor may occur with severe glottic lesions. Causes of stridor in different age groups are listed in Table 5-1.

Table 5-1. Causes of Stridor in Children and Adolescents

	Intermittent	Persistent
Infant	Aspiration Viral croup Electrolyte abnormality	Laryngeal anomaly Mediastinal mass Vascular ring Lung or gastrointestinal cyst Intubation trauma Neck or surgical trauma to recurrent laryngeal nerve (RLN)
Child	Viral croup Spasmodic croup Aspiration Vocal cord dysfunction (rare)	Vascular ring Laryngeal anomaly Mediastinal mass Inhalation injury Neck or surgical trauma to RLN Foreign body aspiration
Adolescent	Vocal cord dysfunction Spasmodic croup	Mediastinal mass Inhalation injury Neck or surgical trauma to RLN Foreign body aspiration Glottic trauma

Examination of the extremities for clubbing and Schamroth's sign is also important (Figure 5-1). This may be found in chronic lung, heart, and liver disease and is a clue to the chronicity of a respiratory condition in children. Potential causes of digital clubbing are listed in Box 5-1.

Eupnea and Dyspnea

Of primary importance for patients with respiratory complains is the chest and lung examination. **Inspection** of the chest should begin as soon as the examiner enters the room. Findings of respiratory distress depend on age. Increased respiratory rate **(tachypnea)** is often the first indication of respiratory distress at all ages; however, normal rates will vary over a wide range by age (Figure 5-2). Normal respiratory rates are also highly variable in infants and toddlers depending on sleep state. Breathing pattern is also important. **Hyperpnea** (abnormally deep respiration) may accompany acidosis and CNS dysfunction. **Hypopnea** can occur in sleep-disordered breathing and again with CNS disease. **Eupnea** is normal, unlabored breathing and dyspnea is difficulty breathing.

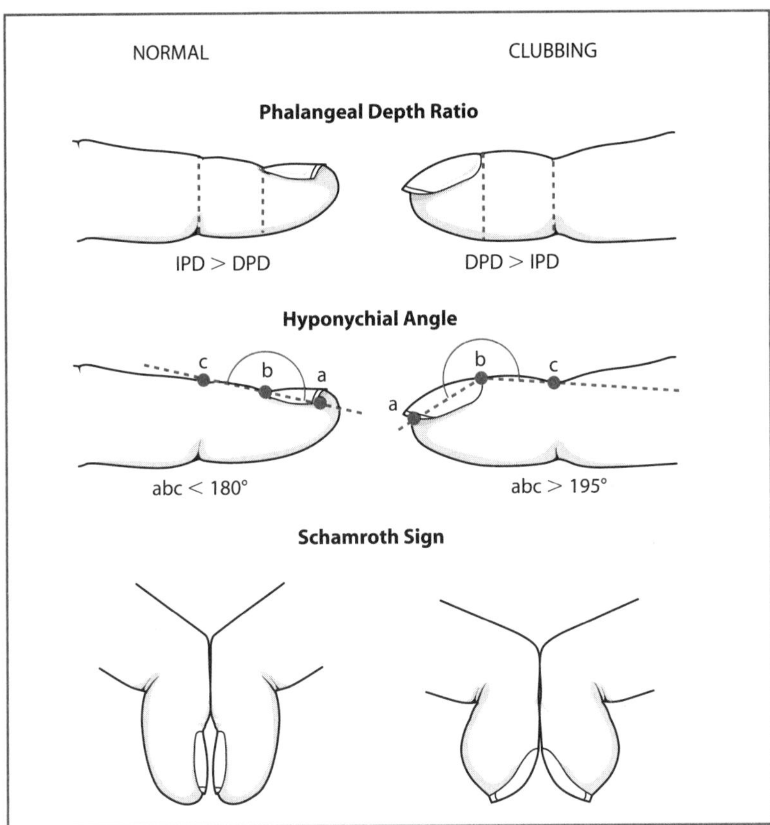

Figure 5-1. Digital clubbing and Schamroth sign. IPD, interphalangeal joint depth; DPD, digital phalangeal joint depth. (From Chernick V, Boat TF, Wilmott RW, Bush A, eds. *Kendig's Disorders of the Respiratory Tract in Children*. 7th ed. Philadelphia, PA: WB Saunders; 2006, with permission from Elsevier.)

Box 5-1. Causes of Clubbing

Pulmonary
- Cystic fibrosis
- Bronchiectasis
- Pulmonary abscess
- Empyema
- Neoplasms
- Interstitial lung disease
- Alveolar proteinosis
- Chronic pneumonia

Cardiac
- Cyanotic congenital heart disease
- Bacterial endocarditis

Gastrointestinal/Hepatic
- Inflammatory bowel disease (ulcerative colitis/Crohn disease)
- Polyposis
- Biliary cirrhosis
- Biliary atresia

Thyrotoxicosis

Familial

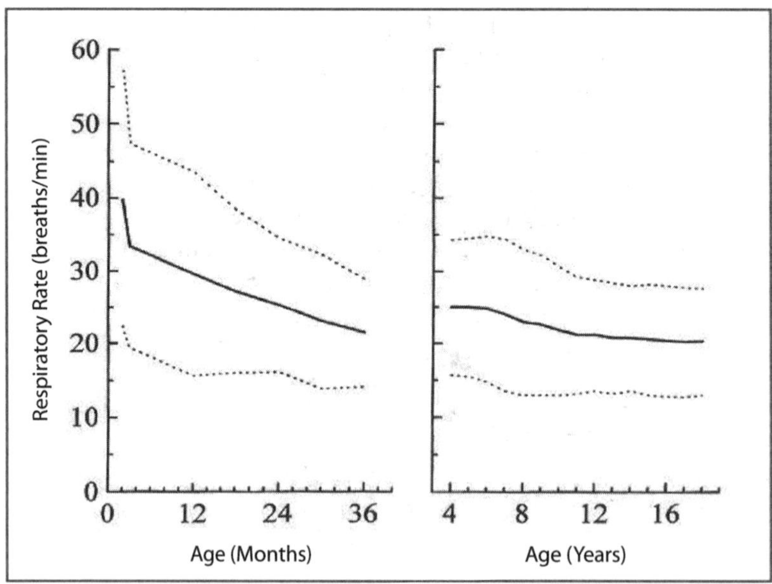

Figure 5-2. Respiratory rates by age. (From Chernick V, Boat TF, Wilmott RW, Bush A, eds. *Kendig's Disorders of the Respiratory Tract in Children.* 7th ed. Philadelphia, PA: WB Saunders; 2006, with permission from Elsevier.)

Dyspnea, which is shortness of breath or difficulty "catching" one's breath, is found with true lung disease, such as acute asthma, but also occurs with hyperventilation secondary to panic attack or panic disorder.

Lungs and Thorax

The highly compliant chest wall of the young infant leads to significant retractions (suprasternal, intercostal, subcostal) with increased respiratory effort. Retractions occur when the skin overlying the neck or chest is drawn in during inspiration. Even with the patient clothed, retractions within the suprasternal notch may be readily apparent in the older child and adolescent. This group may also demonstrate intercostal retractions as well as use of accessory muscles of respiration (sternocleidomastoid and scalene muscles) during periods of respiratory distress. Infants may also demonstrate nasal flaring with respiratory distress.

Inspection and **palpation** of the chest wall may reveal abnormalities. The trachea should normally deviate slightly to the right when a finger is placed in the suprasternal notch. Changes in the position of the trachea may provide important information during the physical examination. In conditions where either air or liquid fill the pleural space, the lung may move away from its normal position with the trachea also shifting in the same direction. Conversely, in complete atelectasis of a lung, the trachea may shift toward the side of collapse. In lung agenesis or hypoplasia the trachea may deviate to the affected side. Absence of a pectoralis muscle is seen in Poland syndrome, and rib or thoracic vertebral anomalies may lead to chest wall asymmetry. Severe scoliosis may lead to respiratory compromise due to restriction of normal lung expansion. This may be accompanied by kyphosis, and both conditions may be seen in children with neuromuscular disease. Pectus carinatum (pigeon breast) or pectus excavatum are both common reasons for referral for evaluation, although they only affect cardiopulmonary functioning when severe (Figure 5-3). In children with significant obstructive sleep apnea, Harrison's groove may develop. This is an indentation along the site of diaphragmatic insertion of the anterior ribs. Further, certain genetic syndromes may be associated with a small thoracic cage. For example, Jeune syndrome, spinal muscular atrophy type I, or other congenital myopathies may show a small bony thorax.

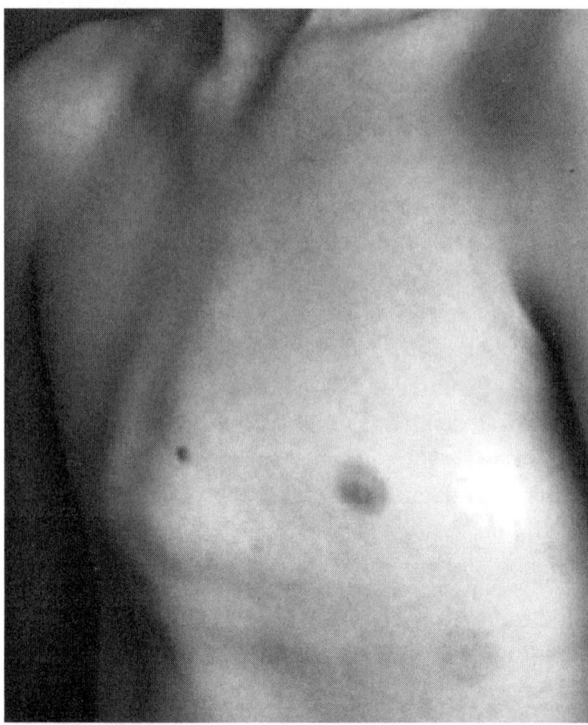

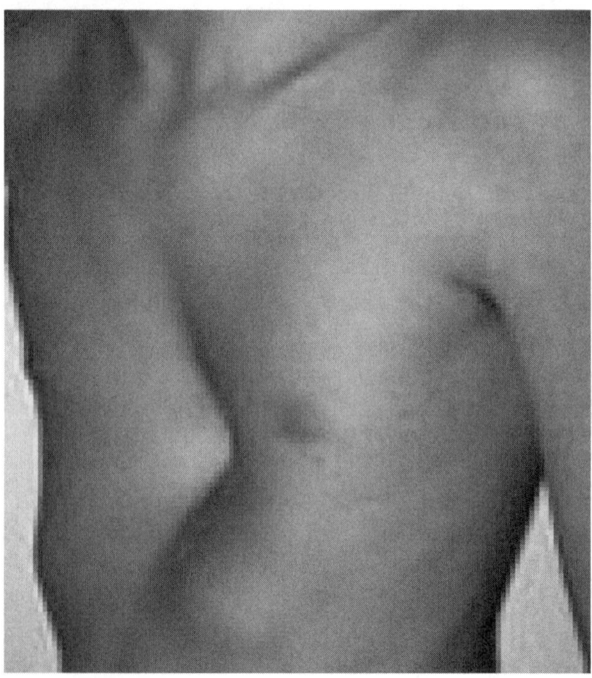

Figure 5-3.
Pectus carinatum (top) and pectus excavatum (bottom).

Percussion of the chest gives the clinician vital information about underlying structures (Figure 5-4). This may be difficult in the small, uncooperative infant, and may precipitate crying. For this reason, percussion and palpation should always follow auscultation in this age group. Usually, normal lungs will provide a resonant note with low pitch and slightly long duration. When pleural effusion, consolidating pneumonia, or an intrathoracic mass is present, the note is flat with high pitch and shorter duration. Conversely, when a pneumothorax has occurred, one will find a high-pitched, loud note. Obstructive lung disease, such as asthma or CF, may also give a hyper-resonant pitch. In particular, when percussing the chest, always remember to compare one side with the other.

Following percussion, **auscultation** of the lungs is performed during physical assessment (except in the infant and small child, when auscultation should precede percussion and palpation). With normal breathing and with larger tidal volumes, normal breath sounds or adventitial sounds may be detected. Normal vesicular breath sounds are low pitched and heard mostly throughout inspiration, continuing approximately one-third of the way into exhalation. During certain clinical conditions, other breath sounds may replace the normal vesicular breath sounds. Bronchial breath sounds are abnormal sounds that are often louder than vesicular breath sounds; they may be shorter on

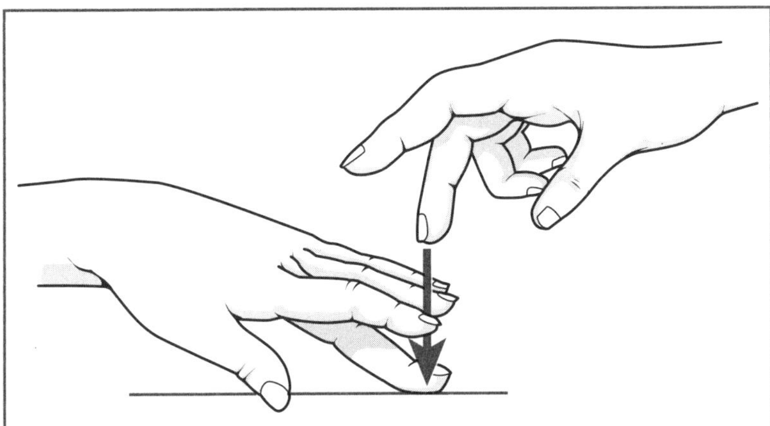

Figure 5-4. Technique of chest percussion in small children. (From Chernick V, Boat TF, Wilmott RW, Bush A, eds. *Kendig's Disorders of the Respiratory Tract in Children.* 7th ed. Philadelphia, PA: WB Saunders; 2006, with permission from Elsevier.)

inspiration and longer on exhalation. Additionally, they may be slightly louder and higher pitched during expiration. These represent sounds of large airways transmitted through lung parenchyma that is consolidated or atelectatic. Three different types are generally acknowledged and agreed on in present medical teaching. First, **crackles** or **rales** are short sounds that are intermittent in character. Two types of crackles are described: Fine crackles are similar to hairs being rubbed together near the ears; coarse crackles, as the name implies, are louder and harsher, more like rubbing together 2 pieces of tissue paper. Fine crackles are more commonly associated with interstitial lung disease. Coarse crackles are often heard in pneumonia or cystic fibrosis. **Wheeze,** the sound most commonly associated with asthma, is a continuous sound and is often musical in nature. **Rhonchi** are also continuous sounds but much lower in pitch and may clear with coughing. These sounds are probably due to secretions in the large airways. A pleural rub may also occasionally be heard on chest examination. More often heard during inspiration, these low-pitched continuous sounds are the result of pleural inflammation. Often described as a creaky noise, they may also sound like leather being stretched.

During auscultation is an opportune time to examine the cardiovascular system. This begins with inspection of mucous membranes and nail beds for signs of central cyanosis. Next, auscultation of the heart tones takes place, and children with congenital heart disease may present with murmurs heard during the entire cardiac cycle. Full characterization of murmurs may require evaluation by a pediatric cardiologist. Dysrhythmias, both bradycardic and tachycardic, may be noted during cardiac auscultation.

Additional Examinations

Additional systems may give important clues to chronic respiratory disease. These include the abdomen, skin, musculoskeletal, and neurologic systems.

The abdominal examination should include accurate assessment of liver and spleen size. Hepatomegaly may be found in patients with CF and may be a potentially life-threatening complication. Cirrhosis may occur due to biliary tract obstruction, leading to hepatocyte damage and subsequent fibrosis. Secondary splenic congestion due to hepatic insufficiency may also occur occasionally and requires expert skill to reliably ascertain fullness in the left upper quadrant of the abdomen. Any mass or fluid in the abdomen may restrict thoracic excursion through elevation of the diaphragm and thus lead to respiratory compromise.

Sequelae of neurologic complications often affect the respiratory system. Severe neurologic dysfunction may interfere with respiratory control, leading to apnea or hypoventilation. Much more commonly, patients are seen with more subtle neurologic involvement, most frequently involving swallowing. Patients with cerebral palsy often are at risk for aspiration pneumonia, and particular care should be paid to the patient's ability to handle oral secretions. Evaluating the strength and duration of an elicited gag reflex may provide clues to aspiration risk because both prolonged and absent gags are abnormal. Silent aspiration can occur often in children with severe neurologic deficits, and a strong index of suspicion should be maintained. Bronchoscopy and radiographic deglutition studies (best with a physical or speech therapist present) can help delineate aspiration risk. Any condition leading to thoracic muscle weakness can lead to progressive respiratory compromise and, eventually, respiratory failure requiring support. At the first sign of sleep disturbance or with recurrent respiratory infection, children with muscle weakness should be referred for pulmonary and sleep evaluation.

Examining the skin may yield important clues to underlying systemic disease with a respiratory component. Eczema in infancy may be associated with food allergy and rarely is associated with respiratory disease. However, as children age, eczema is more often associated with asthma, allergic rhinitis, and inhalation allergy. Severe asthma, with eczema and recurrent *Staphylococcus aureus* infection, occurs with the immunodeficiency of the hyper-IgE syndrome. Cyanosis of nail beds and mucous membranes is always a significant physical finding and should prompt a thorough investigation.

Assessing the musculoskeletal system is the final portion of the physical examination. Many patients with developmental delay or genetic conditions are prone to kyphoscoliosis. Careful examination of the back is of prime importance in children of all ages. Key points to assess include the linearity of the spine, asymmetry of the back and shoulder, and range of motion (flexion, extension, and side-bending). Digital clubbing, if not previously assessed, should be evaluated at this time.

Key Points

- Respiratory rates in children vary over a wide range with activity and age and should be compared with standard tables.
- The heart and lungs are best done first in young children to increase the chance of a good examination.
- Characterization of breath sounds and their location can lead to efficient and accurate diagnosis of acute or chronic pulmonary conditions.
- Children with developmental disabilities can aspirate silently, leading to recurrent pneumonia; therefore, a strong index of suspicion with appropriate testing is in order.
- Other systems affect or are affected by the lungs, including the cardiovascular, neurologic, skin, and musculoskeletal systems, and these must be evaluated along with the pulmonary tract during the pulmonary evaluation. This is especially important in the preparticipation examination for children and teens seeking to undertake athletics. This can be found in detail in the American Academy of Pediatrics publication *Preparticipation Physical Evaluation.*

References

1. Homnick DN. The respiratory system. In: Greydanus DE, Feinberg AN, Patel DR, Homnick DN, eds. *The Pediatric Diagnostic Examination.* New York, NY: McGraw-Hill; 2007
2. Zitelli BJ, Davis HW, eds. *Atlas of Pediatric Physical Diagnosis.* 4th ed. St Louis, MO: Mosby; 2002
3. Chernick V, Boat TF, Wilmott RW, Bush A, eds. *Kendig's Disorders of the Respiratory Tract in Children.* 7th ed. Philadelphia, PA: WB Saunders; 2006
4. Fireman P. Rhinitis and asthma connection: management of coexisting upper airway allergic diseases and asthma. *Allergy Asthma Proc.* 2000;21(4):45–54
5. Slavin RG. The upper and lower airways: the epidemiological and pathophysiological connection. *Allergy Asthma Proc.* 2008;29(6):553–556
6. Tauman R, Gozal D. Obesity and obstructive sleep apnea in children. *Paediatr Respir Rev.* 2006;7(4):247–259

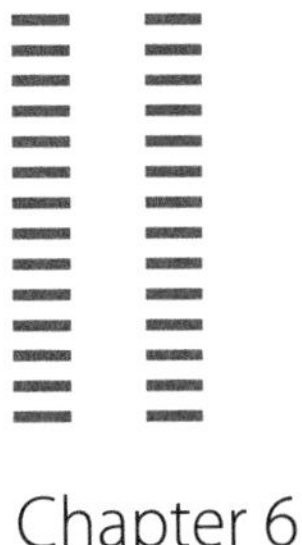

Chapter 6

Pulmonary Function Testing

Carol J. Blaisdell, MD

Pulmonary function testing can be used as an objective measure of lung function in children with known or suspected lung disease. Symptoms of shortness of breath (dyspnea), chest pain, cough, and wheezing have many potential causes. In the clinician's evaluation, the choice of an appropriate objective and reproducible test of lung function may often confirm a working diagnosis. In addition, lung function testing is important for assessing progression of lung disease and response to therapy. Some tests are readily available in the primary care office while others should be conducted in a pulmonary function laboratory. Procedures should follow American Thoracic Society[1] guidelines referenced to healthy populations. Indications for pulmonary function testing are listed in Box 6-1.

Box 6-1. Indications for Pulmonary Function Testing

- To determine the nature of the respiratory dysfunction (obstructive vs restrictive disease)
- To evaluate respiratory function associated with signs and symptoms
- To quantify the extent or progression of known pulmonary disease
- To provide an objective measure to determine the appropriateness of reducing therapy for asthma
- To measure the effect of occupational exposure
- To identify benefits, adverse effects, or consequences of withdrawal of therapy
- To assess the presence of airway hyperreactivity
- To assess preoperative lung function
- As a research objective or measure

Peak Expiratory Flow Rate

The peak expiratory flow rate (PEFR) is a useful measure for monitoring lung function in the primary care management of obstructive lung diseases, particularly asthma; however, it has limitations.[2] It is inexpensive and can be used at the patient's home or workplace, the clinician's office, and in the acute care setting of the emergency department (ED) and hospital. To use a peak flow meter, the child should blow out as quickly as possibly from maximal inhalation with his or her mouth closed tightly on the mouthpiece. The highest of 3 attempts should be recorded. It is important to recognize that PEFR performance is effort dependent and a measure of large-airway dysfunction. Patients who do not keep a tight seal on the mouthpiece will produce a falsely low PEFR, and those who put their tongue in the mouthpiece while exhaling (essentially performing a "blow-dart" maneuver) will have falsely elevated PEFR measurements. Consistency of the values with 3 trials at a time suggests reproducible results that can be interpreted. If there is a greater than 20% variability with 3 efforts performed at one time, the clinician should suspect that there is a problem with the patient's technique.

Normative data for PEFR based on standing height are available to assess flow limitation compared with healthy controls; however, these data vary with PEFR devices used.[2–4] If the values are less than 80% of the expected or the patient's personal best PEFR (see below), airflow obstruction should be suspected. This result could be consistent with subjective complaints of an asthmatic patient or may be unexpected in a patient with poor perception of his or her disease.

In a poorly controlled asthmatic patient who frequently accesses acute care in an ED, the PEFR can be used to set criteria for contacting the clinician for impending asthma exacerbations. The asthma action plan, which defines adjustment in home asthma management in response to early symptoms of asthma (cough, dyspnea, chest pain), may also document the target PEFR for each individual.[5] The convention is to determine the patient's personal best PEFR when asthma is under best control in the clinician's office or with home monitoring and to review these data with the provider.

Using a peak expiratory flow meter to determine whether there is significant airflow obstruction in adolescents who complain of exercise-induced dyspnea can be useful. Peak expiratory flow rate monitoring should be reproducible with a minimum of 3 efforts. However, a change of 20% in the PEFR between before and after exercise that elicits dyspnea is consistent with exercise-induced asthma. Peak expiratory flow rate values of greater than 80% of the personal best or expected for height suggest reasonable control if symptoms are absent. When PEFR decreases to less than 80% of personal best or there is greater than 20% variability from morning to evening PEFR measurements on the same day, then asthma medications should be adjusted. Adjustments that could be made include initiating short-acting β-agonist therapy, such as albuterol; adding a long-acting β-agonist, such as salmeterol or formoterol; or increasing the dose of inhaled corticosteroid. If PEFR measurements decrease to less than 50% of predicted or personal best, and a dose of short-acting β-agonist does not resolve the symptoms and increases the PEFR to 50%, management in an urgent care setting is appropriate, and a short course of systemic corticosteroids is necessary.

Spirometry

Spirometry is the measurement of lung volumes and flows. It is the most useful test for determining if respiratory symptoms are attributable to underlying obstructive versus restrictive lung disease. Abnormal spirometry does not provide a specific diagnosis; rather, it places a patient in a specific physiological category. Normal spirometry results do not exclude lung disease, but they can provide reassurance that the disease is not significantly limiting lung function at rest. The most common obstructive lung disease in children is asthma, affecting about 10% of the US population.[6,7] Cystic fibrosis (CF) is also an obstructive lung disease that often presents to the clinician with recurrent cough, bronchitis, or pneumonia. Restrictive lung diseases include chronic lung diseases that decrease effective lung volumes (eg, bronchopulmonary dysplasia, sickle cell disease), chest wall disorders (eg, pectus deformities, scoliosis), and neuromuscular disorders (eg, Duchenne muscular dystrophy).

Typically a child as young as 6 years can perform spirometry adequately for interpretation. Preschoolers are also able to perform simple maneuvers with good coaching from staff who make the child comfortable and motivated to perform the test.[8] During infancy the raised volume rapid thoracoabdominal compression (RVRTC) technique produces forced expiratory maneuvers in infants that simulate adult-type flow-volume curves. Forced expiratory flows measured by RVRTC in infants with CF are much lower than healthy infants and can be useful for early detection of CF airway dysfunction.[9,10]

Measures of forced vital capacity (FVC), forced expiratory volume in 1 second (FEV_1), and the ratio of these 2 (FEV_1/FVC) are a useful start in distinguishing between obstructive and restrictive lung disorders. Patterns of spirometry results are listed in Table 6-1. The vital capacity is the largest volume of air that a person can inspire or expire from the lungs. The maneuver required to measure FVC involves taking a maximal inhalation and forcefully exhaling with the mouth tightly closed around a mouthpiece with the nose closed with a nose clip until the entire lung volume is exhaled. The volume exhaled in the first second is the FEV_1 (Figure 6-1) and is decreased compared with normal if there is obstruction to exhaled airflow (as with asthma and CF). Flows in the midportion of the forced-exhalation maneuver, forced expiratory flows between 25% and 75% of the FVC (FEF_{25-75}) give an indication of small-airway function and are the first affected in obstructive lung diseases such as asthma and CF.

The results of the expiratory maneuver that generates the measurements of FEV_1 and FVC are displayed most commonly as a flow-volume loop or can be displayed as a volume-versus-time graph (Figure 6-2). In obstructive lung diseases, there may be a reduced rate of airflow at any given lung volume and the FEV_1/FVC is lower than normal. Criteria for assessing for an adequate flow-volume loop include (1) instantaneous start of exhalation and rapid increase in flow

Table 6-1. Patterns of Spirometry Results

Measure	Obstructive	Restrictive
FVC	Normal or increased	Reduced
FRC	Increased	Normal or Reduced
TLC	Increased	Reduced
FEV_1	Decreased	Normal or decreased
FEV_1/FVC	Decreased	Normal or decreased
FEF_{25-75}	Decreased	Normal or decreased

Abbreviations: FEF_{25-75}, forced expiratory flows between 25% and 75% of the FVC; FEV_1, forced expiratory volume in 1 second; FRC, functional reserve capacity; FVC, forced vital capacity; TLC, total lung capacity.

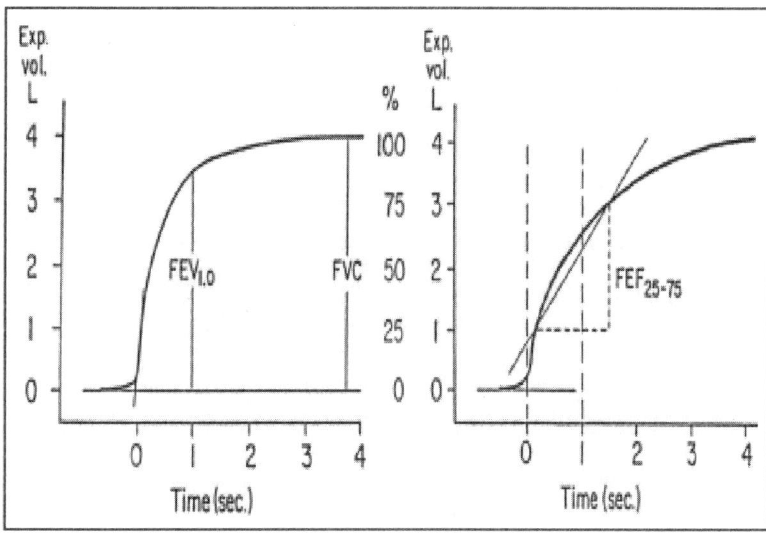

Figure 6-1. What spirometry measures: FVC, FEV_1, FEV_1/FVC%, and FEF_{25-75}, FEV_1. FEF_{25-75}, forced expiratory flows between 25% and 75% of the FVC; FEV_1, forced expiratory volume in 1 second; FVC, forced vital capacity. (From Lemen RJ. Pulmonary function testing in the office, clinic, and home. In: Chernick V, Kendig EL, eds. *Kendig's Disorders of the Respiratory Tract in Children.* 5th ed. Philadelphia, PA: WB Saunders; 1990:150, with permission from Elsevier.)

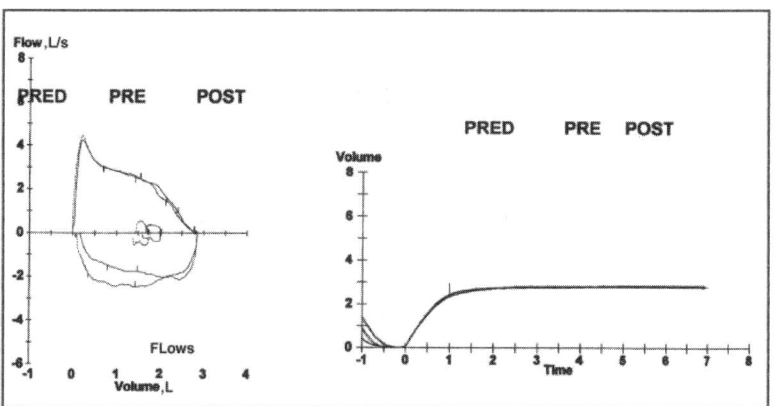

Figure 6-2. Flow-volume loop and volume versus time graph of a spirogram. Pulmonary function testing was performed on a Vmax 6200 (SensorMedics, Yorba Linda, CA) at 4 pm. There was good patient effort on the maneuvers, American Thoracic Society criteria were met, and 2 puffs of albuterol were given via AeroChamber.

to peak; (2) normal sharp peak, indicating maximal effort; (3) smooth, continuous exhalation to zero flow; and (4) reproducible results (Box 6-2, Figure 6-3). An unacceptable flow-volume curve is shown in Figure 6-4, which demonstrates erratic flows on exhalation attributable to coughing. Without a reliable flow-volume loop, the results of the

Box 6-2. Characteristics of Flow-Volume Loops

Acceptable flow-volume loop

- Instantaneous start of exhalation and rapid increase in flow to peak
- Normal sharp peak, indicating maximal effort and no large conducting central airway obstruction
- Smooth, continuous exhalation to residual volume
- Reproducible results

Unacceptable flow-volume loop

- Poor start of exhalation with slow or erratic rise to peak
- Broad or flat peak, which may indicate less-than-optimal effort; if it is smooth and reproducible, it may indicate central conducting airway obstructions
- Erratic exhalation with cough or abrupt flow changes
- Exhalation not complete (ie, flow drops abruptly to zero without a gradual return to zero)
- Curve features are not reproducible

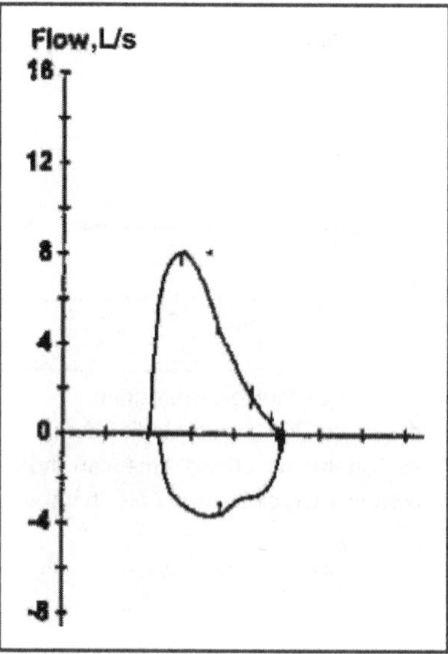

Figure 6-3. Acceptable flow-volume loop: rapid rise on expiration, a normal sharp peak, smooth exhalation, and gradual return to zero flow.

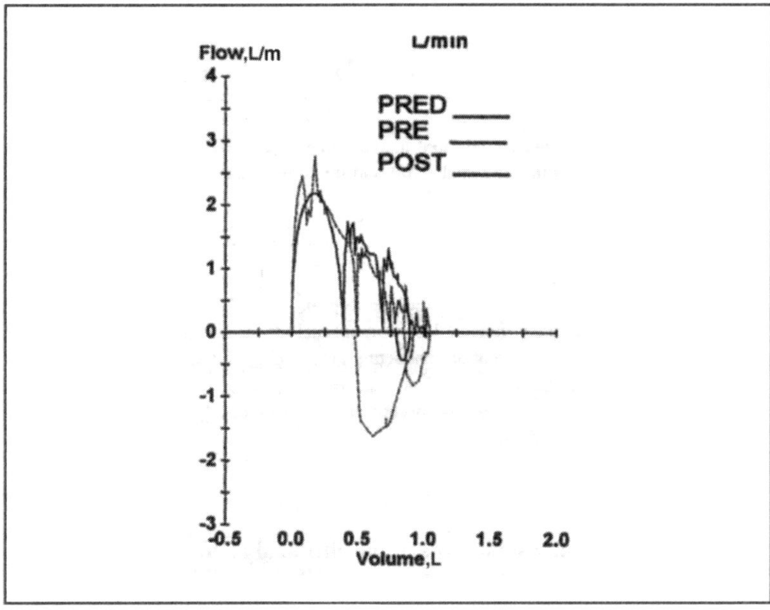

Figure 6-4. Unacceptable flow-volume loop: poor start, erratic exhalation with cough that led to inhalation during expiratory phase, and abrupt return to zero.

spirometric maneuver are in question. The expiratory flow-volume curve provides a more sensitive indication of small-airway obstruction than only evaluating the values measured by spirometry. The early reduction of flow and the flattening of the slope are characteristic of obstruction, which appears as a concave expiratory flow tracing (Figure 6-5). Pulmonary function laboratories should always follow standards set by the American Thoracic Society.

Reference Values

Pulmonary function test results may identify patterns of lung function that are consistent with obstructive or restrictive lung disease. The results should be compared with reference values from healthy populations. "Norms" and standards for interpretation[11,12] should be chosen from a study that used a healthy population similar to the patient. It is important to obtain an accurate standing height (or arm span if the patient cannot stand or has significant scoliosis) because the interpretation of "normal" versus "abnormal" is based on height in addition to age, gender, and race. If the pulmonary function laboratory does not provide a qualitative interpretation of the data, then fixed-

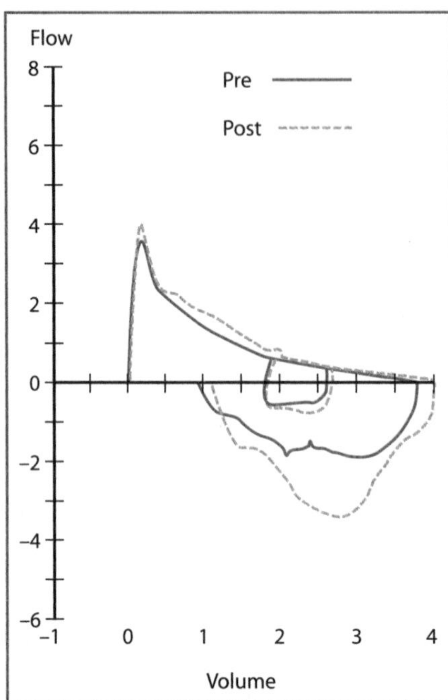

Figure 6-5. Severe airflow obstruction. Shown is a flow- volume loop demonstrating flow limitation at all lung volumes, with concave tracings on the expiratory loop. There was no improvement in flows after use of the bronchodilator. Pre, before bronchodilator; Post, after bronchodilator.

percent predicted cutoffs of less than 80%, 80%, and 60% are reasonable for identifying abnormalities of FVC, FEV_1, and FEF_{25-75}, respectively. Grades of impairment compared with predicted norms are shown in Table 6-2. An FEV_1 or FVC of less than 80% of that predicted is abnormal. If at 70% to 79%, they are considered mildly abnormal; if at 55% to 69%, they are moderately abnormal; and if at 30% to 54%, they are severely abnormal (Table 6-2). An example of how predicted values can vary depending on the reference group used for comparison is represented in Table 6-3. For the spirometry data from the same patient, using National Health and Nutrition Examination Survey III references,[4] FVC and FEV_1 were 64% of that predicted, or moderately abnormal. Using the European Respiratory Society 1993 standards, which do not include black counterparts, the FVC and FEV_1 were 56% and 57% of that predicted, respectively, or moderately severely abnormal.

When comparing results in an individual patient over time it is important to compare absolute volumes and flows and to examine which reference values were used to report the predicted volumes and flows. The use of appropriate references is required not only for spirometry but also for measures of lung volumes and diffusion capacity.

Table 6-2. Grades of Impairment

Grade	FEV_1 or FVC % of Predicted	FEF_{25-75}, % of Predicted	FEV_1/FVC, % of Predicted
Normal	>80	>70	>80
Mild	<80–70	<70–60	<80–60
Moderate	<70–55	<60–40	<60–40
Severe	<55–30	<40–15	<40–25
Extreme	<30	<15	<25

Table 6-3. Differences of Percent-Predicted Values on Spirometry for a Black 15-Year-Old Boy

Subject		Reference[a]	% Predicted[a]	Reference[b]	% Predicted[b]
FVC, L	2.69	4.18	64	4.83	56
FEV_1, L	2.29	3.59	64	3.98	57
FEV_1/FVC	85	86		83	
FEF_{25-75}, L/s	2.48	4.00	62	5.08	49

Abbreviations: FEF_{25-75}, forced expiratory flows between 25% and 75% of the FVC; FEV_1, forced expiratory volume in 1 second; FVC, forced vital capacity.

[a] *National Health and Nutrition Examination Survey III; www.cdc.gov/nchs/nhanes.htm*
[b] *European Community Respiratory Health Survey; www.ecrs.org*

Lung Volumes

When the FVC on a spirometry test is low (<80% of that predicted), a restrictive lung pattern is suggested if the FEV_1/FVC ratio is normal or elevated (>80%). When the FVC is less than 80% and the ratio of FEV_1/FVC is less than 80%, this implies airway obstruction. To confirm a restrictive versus obstructive disease pattern, lung volumes that measure the residual volume (RV), functional reserve capacity (FRC), and total lung capacity can be useful (Figure 6-6). On spirometry, only lung volumes and flow rates within the FVC are measurable: that volume of air that is exhaled or inhaled from maximal inhalation to maximal exhalation, such as the FVC, FEV_1, and FEF_{25-75}. Because RV is the volume of air that cannot be expressed from the lungs after maximal exhalation, it must be measured by an indirect method. The most common methods for measuring lung volumes are helium dilution, nitrogen washout, or body plethysmography (the body box). In practice,

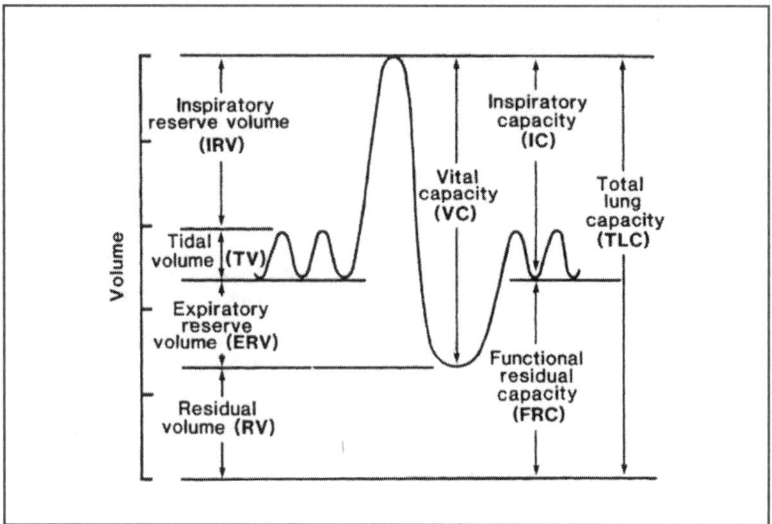

Figure 6-6. Spirogram. Lung volumes: RV, residual volume—amount of air that cannot be exhaled from the lung; ERV (expiratory reserve volume), volume that can be exhaled starting from FRC to RV; FRC, the volume of air in the lungs at the end of the tidal breath, and a combination of ERV and RV; TLC, the total volume of air in the lung on full inspiration. (From Loughlin GM, Eigen H, eds. *Respiratory Disease in Children: Diagnosis and Management.* Baltimore, MD: Williams & Wilkins; 1994:79, with permission from Wolters Kluwer Health.)

the FRC is measured, and RV is calculated from the FRC by measuring the expiratory reserve volume. The helium-dilution and nitrogen-washout methods rely on the mixing of known concentrations of gas with the patient's lung volume at the start of the test, which by convention starts at FRC. If a patient has severe obstructive lung disease, this method is not very accurate, because the gases mix too slowly to reflect accurate volumes or not at all in regions of the lung that have significant air trapping. In this case, use of the body box is more accurate. Pressure changes at the mouth with the patient inside a closed box determine starting volume (FRC). The body box can provide useful information about air trapping (high FRC or RV) in patients with CF but cannot be used successfully if the patient is too obese to fit in the closed box.

When a restrictive lung disease is suspected, such as neuromuscular disorder or sickle cell disease, lung volume testing can provide more detail about the severity of the restrictive changes. These studies take more time than spirometry and must be performed in a pulmonary function laboratory with standardized protocols that follow American Thoracic Society guidelines.

Carbon Monoxide Diffusing Capacity

Carbon monoxide diffusing capacity (DLCO) is the measurement of carbon monoxide (CO) transfer from inspired gas into the pulmonary capillary. The transfer of CO into the blood depends on the alveolar capillary interface (thickness), capillary volume, hemoglobin concentration, and the reaction rates between CO and hemoglobin.[13] For patients with lung disease, the DLCO correlates with disease severity and arterial blood oxygenation, particularly during exercise.[14] Measuring DLCO over time may be useful for patients with the potential for progressive loss of alveolar surface area, such as sickle cell disease (see Figure 6-7), with cancer on chemotherapy or radiation therapy, and after lung resection. Carbon monoxide diffusing capacity is diminished in young adults with a history of prematurity regardless of whether they had a diagnosis of bronchopulmonary dysplasia.[15] This likely reflects inadequate growth of the alveoli after premature birth. Normative data for DLCO are not as comprehensively available for ethnic groups and young ages as for spirometry[13]; however, DLCO of 60% to lower limits of normal for the reference population is considered mildly abnormal, 40% to 60% is considered moderately abnormal, and less than 40% is considered severely abnormal. Trends over time for an individual patient can be evaluated by the clinician to determine if there is progressive loss of alveolar or capillary surface area for gas exchange in certain disease states that need close monitoring, such as patients who are undergoing chemotherapy for cancer, patients with sickle hemoglobinopathy, and patients with interstitial lung disease. Whole-lung irradiation can lead to mild, moderate, and severe changes in DLCO,[16] so monitoring the effects of cancer therapy in children is very important.

Assessing Airway Reactivity

Children who have asthma or a history of early neonatal lung injury (eg, bronchopulmonary dysplasia, bronchiolitis, aspiration syndromes, prolonged mechanical ventilation) may have increased bronchial reactivity. In addition, children with symptoms of dyspnea or chest pain

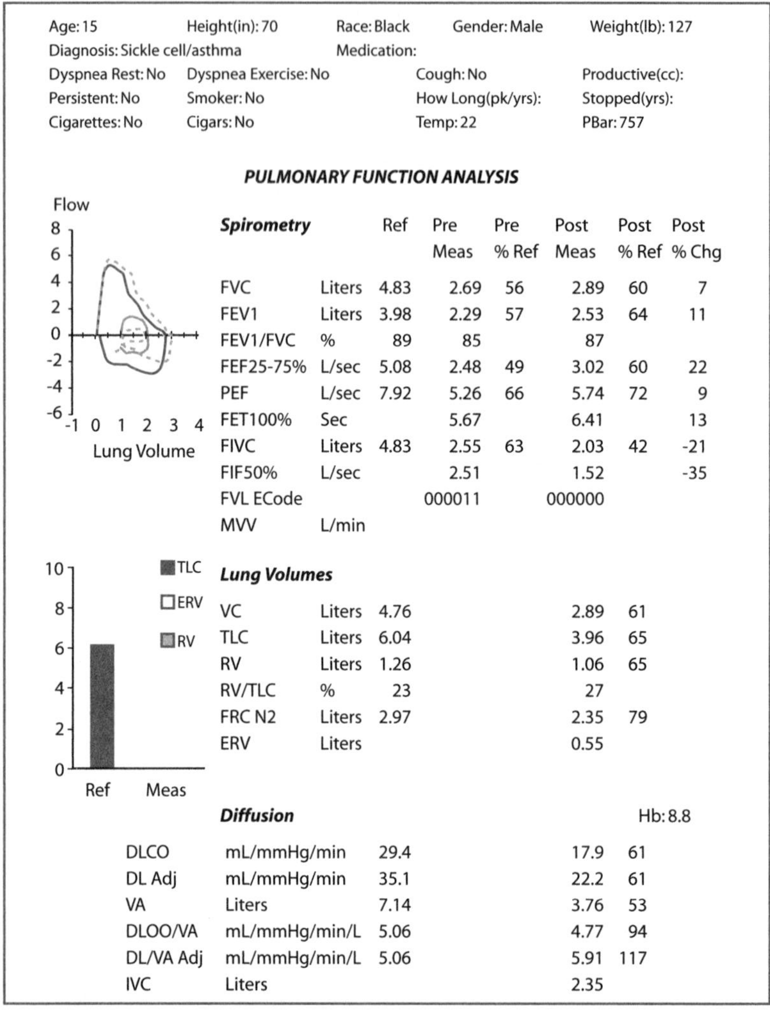

Age: 15	Height(in): 70	Race: Black	Gender: Male	Weight(lb): 127
Diagnosis: Sickle cell/asthma		Medication:		
Dyspnea Rest: No	Dyspnea Exercise: No	Cough: No		Productive(cc):
Persistent: No	Smoker: No	How Long(pk/yrs):		Stopped(yrs):
Cigarettes: No	Cigars: No	Temp: 22		PBar: 757

PULMONARY FUNCTION ANALYSIS

Spirometry		Ref	Pre Meas	Pre % Ref	Post Meas	Post % Ref	Post % Chg
FVC	Liters	4.83	2.69	56	2.89	60	7
FEV1	Liters	3.98	2.29	57	2.53	64	11
FEV1/FVC	%	89	85		87		
FEF25-75%	L/sec	5.08	2.48	49	3.02	60	22
PEF	L/sec	7.92	5.26	66	5.74	72	9
FET100%	Sec		5.67		6.41		13
FIVC	Liters	4.83	2.55	63	2.03	42	-21
FIF50%	L/sec		2.51		1.52		-35
FVL ECode			000011		000000		
MVV	L/min						

Lung Volumes				
VC	Liters	4.76	2.89	61
TLC	Liters	6.04	3.96	65
RV	Liters	1.26	1.06	65
RV/TLC	%	23	27	
FRC N2	Liters	2.97	2.35	79
ERV	Liters		0.55	

Diffusion Hb: 8.8

DLCO	mL/mmHg/min	29.4	17.9	61
DL Adj	mL/mmHg/min	35.1	22.2	61
VA	Liters	7.14	3.76	53
DLOO/VA	mL/mmHg/min/L	5.06	4.77	94
DL/VA Adj	mL/mmHg/min/L	5.06	5.91	117
IVC	Liters		2.35	

Figure 6-7. Example of pulmonary function test: sickle cell disease. Moderate restrictive defect on spirometry is suspected from decreased FVC, normal FEV/FEV$_1$, and confirmed on lung volumes with FVC of 56% predicted and TLC only 65% of predicted. Note also that the DLCO is decreased to 61%, corrected for the patient's anemia (with a hemoglobin [Hb] level of 8.5). This patient has had multiple episodes of acute chest syndrome. Adj, adjusted; DL, lung diffusion; DLCO, carbon monoxide diffusing capacity; ERV, expiratory reserve volume; FEF$_{25-75}$, forced expiratory flows between 25% and 75% of the FVC; FET, forced expired time; FEV$_1$, forced expiratory volume in 1 second; FIF, forced inspiration flow; FIVC, forced inspiratory vital capacity; FRC, functional reserve capacity; FVC, forced vital capacity; FVL, flow-volume loop; IVC, inspiratory reserve volume; MVV, maximum voluntary ventilation; PEF, peak expiratory flow; RV, residual volume; TLC, total lung capacity; VA, alveolar volume; VC, vital capacity.

with normal physical findings and normal spirometry test results at rest may be evaluated by using tests of airway reactivity.[17]

Bronchodilator Testing

Spirometry before and after the use of an aerosolized bronchodilator can evaluate the usefulness of bronchodilator therapy for a patient with known or suspected obstructive lung disease (Figure 6-8).[18] Asthma is the most common reversible obstructive airway disease, and if it is suspected as the cause of a patient's signs and symptoms, bronchodilator testing can help confirm the diagnosis. For patients with neuromuscular disease, the usefulness of bronchodilators can be assessed with spirometry before and after albuterol use. As shown in Figure 6-9, a 13-year-old boy with Duchenne muscular dystrophy had worse expiratory flows after albuterol use (17% worsening of FEV_1 and 67% worsening of FEF_{25-75}), showing that albuterol is not useful in his management. A lack of response to a bronchodilator in a patient with an obstructive pattern on spirometry may represent long-standing airway inflammation and raise the question of other diagnoses, such as CF (see Figure 6-10). Spirometry performed at rest can be repeated 10 to 15 minutes after a standard dose of an inhaled bronchodilator if the patient has not used any bronchodilators for at least 4 hours before testing. Albuterol by metered-dose inhaler (2–4 puffs) with a spacer for adequate dose delivery or 2.5 to 5.0 mg nebulized albuterol should be adequate for assessing bronchodilation. An increase in FVC or FEV_1 of 12% would be considered a significant bronchodilator response and compatible with a diagnosis of asthma regardless of whether the baseline spirometry test demonstrated obstruction or was normal compared with reference values.

Bronchial Challenge Testing

For patients with a history or physical examination suggestive of asthma (eg, cough, dyspnea, chest pain, wheezing), it is not uncommon for a clinician to prescribe a trial of bronchodilator or an anti-inflammatory therapy. However, continued use of a therapy for an unconfirmed diagnosis of asthma can expose the child to unnecessary adverse effects. When an adolescent with unexplained dyspnea, chest pain, or cough has normal spirometry results and an unclear response to bronchodilators, bronchial challenge testing can be used to diag-

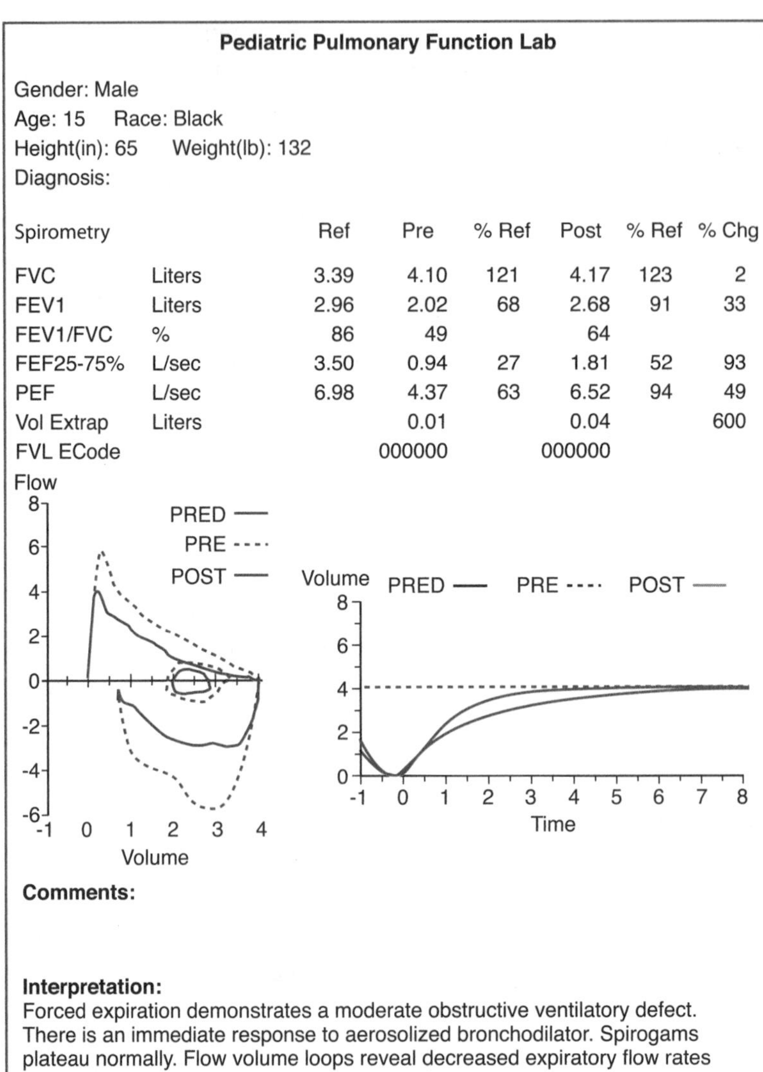

Pediatric Pulmonary Function Lab

Gender: Male
Age: 15 Race: Black
Height(in): 65 Weight(lb): 132
Diagnosis:

Spirometry		Ref	Pre	% Ref	Post	% Ref	% Chg
FVC	Liters	3.39	4.10	121	4.17	123	2
FEV1	Liters	2.96	2.02	68	2.68	91	33
FEV1/FVC	%	86	49		64		
FEF25-75%	L/sec	3.50	0.94	27	1.81	52	93
PEF	L/sec	6.98	4.37	63	6.52	94	49
Vol Extrap	Liters		0.01		0.04		600
FVL ECode			000000		000000		

Comments:

Interpretation:
Forced expiration demonstrates a moderate obstructive ventilatory defect. There is an immediate response to aerosolized bronchodilator. Spirogams plateau normally. Flow volume loops reveal decreased expiratory flow rates at low lung volumes consistent with airway obstruction.

Figure 6-8. Example of pulmonary function test: severe airflow obstruction attributable to asthma due to FEV_1/FVC % of only 49% pre-bronchodilator (pre) with improved but not quite normalized flows after bronchodilator response given FEV_1/FVC % of 64%. FEF_{25-75}, forced expiratory flows between 25% and 75% of the FVC; FEV_1, forced expiratory volume in 1 second; FVC, forced vital capacity; FVL, flow-volume loop; PEF, peak expiratory flow; Pre, before bronchodilator; Pred, predicted; Post, after bronchodilator; Ref, reference; Vol Extrap, extrapolated volume.

DUCHENNE MUSCULAR DYSTROPHY

Age:	13 years	?????TL3097134
Sex/Race:	Male/Caucasian	Room: Out
Height:	63 in 161 cm	1amu/Fre: 39 G/ 749 mmHz
Weight:	142 lbs 65 kg	

				Pre-RX		**Post-RX**		
Spirometry		(BTPS)	PRED	BEST	%PRED	BEST	%PRED	%CHG
FVC	Liters		3.69	0.90	26#	0.95	26	–1
FEV1	Liters		3.17	0.90	38#	0.75	29	–17
FEV1/FVC	%			94		79		–16
FEF25-75%	L/Sec		3.33	2.00	38#	0.66	19	–67
FEF25%	L/Ses			1.34		1.19		–53
FEF50%	L/Sec			2.18		0.72		–67
FEF75%	L/Sec			1.55		0.41		–47
PEF	L/Sec		2.26	2.73	38#	1.48	18	–49
FIVC	Liters		?	0.99	27#	0.98	41	1
PIF	L/Sec			2.24		2.63		0

Figure 6-9. Example of pulmonary function test: Duchenne muscular dystrophy. A severe restrictive pattern is shown, with FVC at only 0.96 L or 26% of that predicted, FEV_1 at 0.90 L or 28% of that predicted, and FEV_1/FVC at 94%, with worsening after bronchodilator (17% decreased FEV_1 [post-Rx]). FEF, forced expiratory flow; FEV_1, forced expiratory volume in 1 second; FIVC, forced inspiratory vital capacity; FVC, forced vital capacity; PEF, peak expiratory flow; PIF, peak inspiratory flow; Pred, predicted; Pre-Rx, before bronchodilator; Post-Rx, after bronchodilator.

CYSTIC FIBROSIS

Age:	21 Years	
Sex/Race:	Female/Caucasian	
Height:	59 in	150 cm
Weight:	86 lbs	39 kg

				Pre-RX		Post-RX		
Spirometry		(BTPS)	PRED	BEST	%PRED	BEST	%PRED	%CHG
FVC	Liters		3.31	1.45 #	44#	1.52 #	46#	5
FEV1	Liters		3.01	0.91 #	30#	0.94 #	31#	3
FEV1/FVC	%		91	63 #	69#	62 #	68#	-2
FEF25-75%	L/Sec		4.02	0.48 #	12#	0.46 #	11#	-4
FEF25%	L/Sec			1.48		1.63		10
FEF50%	L/Sec			0.54		0.56		4
FEF75%	L/Sec			0.20		0.16		-20
PEF	L/Sec			2.60		2.75		6
FIVC	Liters		3.31	1.33 #	40#	1.37 #	41#	3
PIF	L/Sec			2.38		2.64		11

\# = Outside 95% Confidence Interval # = Outside Normal Range
IPS–0L01–05 IPS–0L02–05 N–2103–3

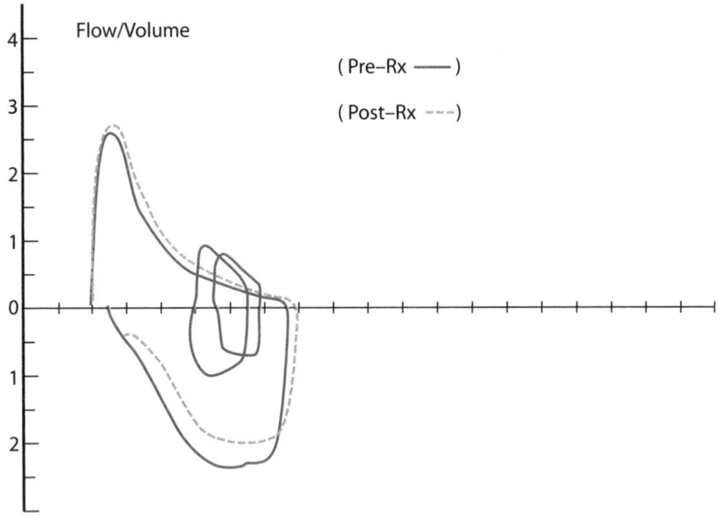

Figure 6-10. Example of pulmonary function test: cystic fibrosis. Shown are severe airflow obstruction (FEV_1 at 30% of that predicted) and a severe restrictive pattern (FVC at 44% of that predicted), with no improvement after bronchodilator administration. Note that flow limitation is worse with forced exhalation compared with tidal breathing at rest. FEF, forced expiratory flow; FEV_1, forced expiratory volume in 1 second; FIVC, forced inspiratory vital capacity; FVC, forced vital capacity; PEF, peak expiratory flow; PIF, peak inspiratory flow; Pred, predicted; Pre-Rx, before bronchodilator; Post-Rx, after bronchodilator.

nose airway hyperreactivity. Airway hyperreactivity is a more sensitive objective marker of asthma in children than PEFR or spirometry at rest or after bronchodilator use.[19]

Inhalation of methacholine is frequently used to determine if airway hyperreactivity is present. Children with asthma will respond to methacholine with a pattern of airway obstruction on spirometry at a lower dose than children who do not have asthma. In addition to asthma, factors that increase bronchial hyperresponsiveness include exposure to environmental antigens, occupational sensitizers, respiratory infections, air pollutants, cigarette smoke, and chemical irritants.[20] After baseline spirometry is measured, the patient inhales increasing doses of methacholine. A change in FEV_1 is the primary outcome measure for methacholine challenge testing. The term PC_{20} (provocative concentration 20) is defined as the exact concentration of methacholine that causes a 20% drop in FEV_1 from the baseline FEV_1. A positive test is one in which the PC_{20} occurs at less than 4.0 mg/mL[16] (Table 6-4). If the patient has a PC_{20} of less than 1.0 mg/mL, he or she has moderate-to-severe bronchial hyperreactivity. If doses of greater than 16 mg/mL methacholine do not cause a 20% drop in FEV_1, then the patient is considered normal, and another cause for the reported symptoms should be sought. Approximately 30% of patients without asthma who have allergic rhinitis will have a PC_{20} in the borderline range (4.0–16 mg/mL). Approximately 90% to 98% of patients with asthma will be hyperreactive to methacholine or histamine (another inhalation challenge agent).[21] Methacholine challenge testing should be performed in a pulmonary function laboratory with experienced personnel, because of the risk of serious airflow obstruction.

Table 6-4. Methacholine Challenge Interpretation of Bronchial Hyperresponsiveness

PC20[a]	Interpretation
>16 mg/mL	Normal
4–16 mg/mL	Borderline
1–4 mg/mL	Mild
<1 mg/mL	Moderate to severe

[a] Provocative concentration of methacholine causing a 20% fall in FEV_1 (forced expiratory volume in 1 second).

Exercise Challenge Testing

Although a little less sensitive than methacholine, bronchial challenge testing can also be accomplished by using exercise on a treadmill or bicycle. The test may be particularly useful for a patient whose respiratory complaints occur primarily with exercise to confirm a suspected diagnosis of exercise-induced asthma bronchoconstriction (EIB). Bronchial challenge can also be used to determine the ability of an adolescent to perform demanding or lifesaving work, and to determine the effectiveness of therapy to prevent symptoms. Exercise-induced asthma bronchoconstriction is present in as many as 95% of children and adolescents with asthma.[22,23] A child or adolescent with suspected EIB whose respiratory symptoms are not prevented by treatment with an inhaled bronchodilator given 15 to 20 minutes before exercise and who has no other manifestations of asthma should be referred for exercise challenge testing to confirm the diagnosis.[17]

Patients are asked to walk or run on a treadmill to reproduce symptoms experienced with exercise. A minimum of 4 minutes at the target heart rate (heart rate is 80%–90% of the predicted maximum, calculated as 220 - age in years, or ventilation at 40% to 60% of the predicted maximum voluntary ventilation, estimated as FEV_1 x 35) is standard.[24] For the bicycle ergometer to produce an adequate test, a target work rate to achieve the target ventilation must be sustained for at least 4 to 6 minutes. Only 50% to 70% of children demonstrate significant bronchoconstriction with cycling so that the treadmill is more likely to provide confirmation of airway hyperreactivity. As with methacholine challenge testing, the change in FEV_1 is the primary outcome variable. Repeated measures of spirometry are performed immediately after exercise and then serially 5, 10, 15, and 20 minutes after completing the exercise. If the FEV_1 is not back to a baseline level by 20 minutes, then another measure at 30 minutes should be taken. Response to a bronchodilator may be assessed if the patient experiences significant dyspnea or the FEV_1 has not returned to within 10% of baseline at 30 minutes. A 10% decrease from the baseline FEV_1 is generally accepted as abnormal,[23,25] although a decrease of 15% is considered by some to be more diagnostic of EIB.[17,26]

Cardiopulmonary Exercise Testing

Cardiopulmonary exercise testing (CPET) involves assessing cardiac and pulmonary function during incremental exercise and includes measuring gas exchange (oxygen consumption, CO production, minute ventilation), electrocardiography, and measuring blood pressure.[27] The clinician requests CPET for patients who complain of shortness of breath, dyspnea on exertion, or exercise intolerance without a clear cause or response to therapeutic trials. It may also be used to assess cardiopulmonary fitness. If the patient has chest pain or symptoms suggestive of cardiovascular disease, a cardiac stress test should be performed by a cardiologist. Exercise challenge testing is more appropriate if the patient complains of chest tightness and wheezing during or after exercise (see Exercise Challenge Testing). Cardiopulmonary exercise testing is useful for a child or adolescent who feels limited by exercise. Limitation can be attributable to impaired lung function; impaired cardiac, pulmonary, or peripheral circulation; or poor conditioning. Patients with asthma, chronic lung disease, or sickle cell disease may have limitations to their oxygenation or ventilatory responses to exercise. See Box 6-3 for indications for CPET.

Box 6-3. Indications for Cardiopulmonary Exercise Testing

- To determine exercise capacity or the cause of any exercise impairment
- To identify abnormal responses to exercise
- To stratify risk and exercise response for training and rehabilitation
- To evaluate results of treatment
- For preoperative assessment
- To evaluate impairment or disability
- To evaluate unexplained dyspnea

Pulse Oximetry

Pulse oximetry is a convenient, in vivo, noninvasive technique for measuring oxygen saturation. Oxygen saturation is determined by the ratio of oxyhemoglobin to the sum of oxyhemoglobin and reduced hemoglobin. Pulse oximeters perform optical measurements across a pulsating arterial bed (the finger, ear) at only 2 wavelengths of light to discriminate oxygenated and deoxygenated hemoglobin. Carboxyhemoglobin and methemoglobin also absorb light at the wavelengths measured by the pulse oximeter and, if abundant, can affect the accuracy of the pulse oximeter. These devices were calibrated by using healthy volunteers with insignificant amounts of dysfunctional hemoglobins.[28]

Pulse oximetry is used widely to assess arterial oxygenation and provides a useful estimate of hypoxia. Oxygen saturations of less than 93% predict a partial pressure of oxygen of less than 70 mm Hg. The pulse oximeter has been validated in various cohorts of patients with presumably normal hemoglobin levels, such as neonates, and in patients with cyanotic heart disease[29]; however, a retrospective review of simultaneous pulse oximetry and arterial blood gas analysis data obtained from patients with sickle cell disease in the ED suggested that the pulse oximeter did not predict hypoxemia well.[30] A prospective study of children and adolescents with sickle cell hemoglobin demonstrated that pulse oximetry overestimated the number of children with hypoxia and could have led to inappropriate treatment with supplemental oxygen.[31]

One cannot rely on the pulse oximeter for assessing oxygenation in an adolescent or young adult with potential smoke inhalation. Carbon monoxide bound to hemoglobin has similar wavelength-absorption characteristics as oxygenated hemoglobin, and patients with smoke inhalation will have a falsely normal pulse oximetry value. In the evaluation of a patient with potential smoke exposure, the measurement of carboxyhemoglobin directly from an arterial blood sample is essential. Methemoglobin causes the pulse oximeter readout to tend toward 85%. If the clinician is aware of the presence of dyshemoglobins in the blood of an individual patient, correlation of an arterial blood sample with pulse oximetry is advisable. It is important to remember that normal oxygen saturation of the blood does not ensure adequate oxygen delivery to the tissues. This is especially true in anemic patients, patients in heart failure, or patients in shock.

Arterial Blood Gas

Arterial blood gas measurements are used to assess oxygenation and ventilation. This subject is covered in Chapter 2.

When to Refer

- If the primary care office does not have access to spirometry, children and adolescents who have asthma or other chronic pulmonary disease should be referred to a pediatric pulmonologist for evaluation at some point in their course.
- If the primary care office performs pulmonary function testing, it is important that there is a mechanism in place to ensure that studies are performed to American Thoracic Society guidelines. This implies that there is a medical director responsible for oversight of the testing.
- Spirometry testing should be used to confirm a suspected diagnosis of asthma (reversible airways obstruction) and periodically used to monitor progression of the disease and its response to therapy.
- Restrictive changes on spirometry should be confirmed with lung volume measurements and if the cause of the low lung volumes is not clear, refer to a pediatric pulmonologist.

Key Points

- Spirometry is useful to distinguish restrictive from obstructive lung disease in order to develop a differential diagnosis in children with chronic respiratory symptoms.
- Pulmonary function testing can provide objective evidence of the severity of pulmonary disease, changes over time, and response to therapies (eg, in disorders such as asthma, CF, sickle cell disease, and muscular dystrophy).
- Although some children can perform spirometry as young as 3 years of age, consistent results are more likely after 6 years of age.
- Measurement of residual volume requires more sophisticated testing than simple spirometry and should be done in a pulmonary function laboratory with experience testing in children.
- Pulmonary function testing may be useful in the primary care office, but oversight and interpretation by the pediatric pulmonologist is helpful, and appropriate normative data for comparison is essential.
- Exercise challenge should be used for evaluating exercise-related symptoms, particularly if lung function measures are normal at rest and there is little or no response to therapy.
- Cardiopulmonary exercise testing can be used to evaluate fitness and/or the etiology of exercise limitations.
- Pulse oximetry is a useful, noninvasive test to measure arterial oxygen saturation, but has limitations (eg, assumes normal adult hemoglobin).

References

1. Miller MR, Crapo R, Hankinson J, et al. General considerations for lung function testing. *Eur Respir J.* 2005;26(1):153–161
2. National Asthma Education and Prevention Program. National Heart, Lung, and Blood Institute of the National Institutes of Health. Expert Panel Report 3: Guidelines for the Diagnosis and Management of Asthma. 2007. http://www.nhlbi.nih.gov/guidelines/asthma/asthgdln.htm
3. Hsu KH, Jenkins DE, Hsi BP, et al. Ventilatory functions of normal children and young adults: Mexican-American, white, and black. I. Spirometry. *J Pediatr.* 1979;95(1):14–23

4. Hankinson JL, Odencrantz JR, Fedan KB. Spirometric reference values from a sample of the general US population. *Am J Respir Crit Care Med.* 1999;159(1):179–187
5. Radeos MS, Camargo CA Jr. Predicted peak expiratory flow: differences across formulae in the literature. *Am J Emerg Med.* 2004;22(7):516–521
6. National Heart, Lung, and Blood Institute. New NHLBI guidelines for the diagnosis and management of asthma. *Lippincott Health Promot Lett.* 1997;2(7):1, 8–9
7. Mannino DM, Homa DM, Akinbami LJ, Moorman JE, Gwynn C, Redd SC. Surveillance for asthma: United States, 1980–1999. *MMWR Surveill Summ.* 2002;51(1):1–13
8. An official American Thoracic Society-European Respiratory Society statement: pulmonary function testing in preschool children. *Am J Respir Crit Care Med.* 2007;175:1304–1345
9. Turner DJ, Lanteri CJ, LeSouef PN, Sly PD. Improved detection of abnormal respiratory function using forced expiration from raised lung volume in infants with cystic fibrosis. *Eur Respir J.* 1994;7:1995–1999
10. Davis S, Jones M, Kisling J, Howard J, Tepper R. Comparison of normal infants and infants with cystic fibrosis using forced expiratory flows breathing air and heliox. *Pediatr Pulmonol.* 2001;31:17–23
11. Pattishall EN. Pulmonary function testing reference values and interpretations in pediatric training programs. *Pediatrics.* 1990;85(5):768–773
12. Pellegrino R, Viegi G, Brusasco V, et al. Interpretative strategies for lung function tests. *Eur Respir J.* 2005;26(5):948–968
13. Macintyre N, Crapo RO, Viegi G, et al. Standardisation of the single-breath determination of carbon monoxide uptake in the lung. *Eur Respir J.* 2005;26(4):720–735
14. Zapletal A, Houstěk J, Samánek M, Copová M, Paul T. Lung function in children and adolescents with idiopathic interstitial pulmonary fibrosis. *Pediatr Pulmonol.* 1985;1(3):154–166
15. Vrijlandt EJ, Gerritsen J, Boezen HM, Grevink RG, Duiverman EJ. Lung function and exercise capacity in young adults born prematurely. *Am J Respir Crit Care Med.* 2006;173(8):890–896
16. Weiner DJ, Maity A, Carlson CA, Ginsberg JP. Pulmonary function abnormalities in children treated with whole lung irradiation. *Pediatr Blood Cancer.* 2006;46(2):222–227
17. Abu-Hasan M, Tannous B, Weinberger M. Exercise-induced dyspnea in children and adolescents: if not asthma then what? *Ann Allergy Asthma Immunol.* 2005;94(3):366–371
18. Miller MR, Hankinson J, Brusasco V, et al. Standardisation of spirometry. *Eur Respir J.* 2005;26(2):319–338
19. Ulrik CS, Postma DS, Backer V. Recognition of asthma in adolescents and young adults: which objective measure is best? *J Asthma.* 2005;42(7):549–554

20. Crapo RO, Casaburi R, Coates AL, et al. Guidelines for methacholine and exercise challenge testing: 1999. This official statement of the American Thoracic Society was adopted by the ATS Board of Directors, July 1999. *Am J Respir Crit Care Med.* 2000;161(1):309–329
21. Chai H, Farr RS, Froehlich LA, et al. Standardization of bronchial inhalation challenge procedures. *J Allergy Clin Immunol.* 1975;56(4):323–327
22. Godfrey S. Exercise-induced asthma: clinical, physiological, and therapeutic implications. *J Allergy Clin Immunol.* 1975;56(1):1–17
23. Backer V, Ulrik CS. Bronchial responsiveness to exercise in a random sample of 494 children and adolescents from Copenhagen. *Clin Exp Allergy.* 1992;22(8):741–747
24. American Thoracic Society. Guidelines for methacholine and exercise challenge testing. *Am J Respir Crit Care Med.* 2000;161:309–329
25. Cropp GJ. Relative sensitivity of different pulmonary function tests in the evaluation of exercise-induced asthma. *Pediatrics.* 1975;56(5 pt 2):860–867
26. Haby MM, Anderson SD, Peat JK, Mellis CM, Toelle BG, Woolcock AJ. An exercise challenge protocol for epidemiological studies of asthma in children: comparison with histamine challenge. *Eur Respir J.* 1994;7(1):43–49
27. American Thoracic Society; American College of Chest Physicians. ATS/ACCP statement on cardiopulmonary exercise testing [published correction appears in *Am J Respir Crit Care Med.* 2003:1451–1452]. *Am J Respir Crit Care Med.* 2003;167(2):211–277
28. Yelderman M, New W Jr. Evaluation of pulse oximetry. *Anesthesiology.* 1983;59(4):349–352
29. Poets CF, Southall DP. Noninvasive monitoring of oxygenation in infants and children: practical considerations and areas of concern. *Pediatrics.* 1994;93(5):737–746
30. Goepp J, Murray C, Walker A, Simone E. Oxygen saturation by pulse oximetry in patients with sickle cell disease: lack of correlation with arterial blood gas measurements [abstract]. *Pediatr Emerg Care.* 1991;7:387
31. Blaisdell CJ, Goodman S, Clark K, Casella JF, Loughlin GM. Pulse oximetry is a poor predictor of hypoxemia in stable children with sickle cell disease. *Arch Pediatr Adolesc Med.* 2000;154(9):900–903

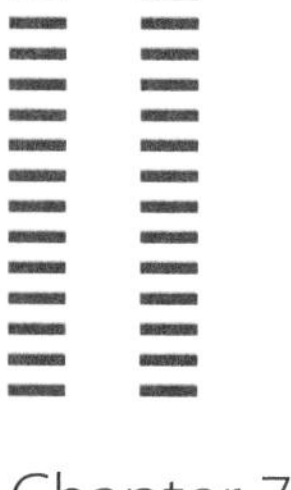

Chapter 7

Pulmonary Imaging

Michael J. Light, MD
Julieta M. Oneto, MD
Ricardo Restrepo, MD

Radiation Exposure in Children

A clinician ordering an imaging test must be familiar with the indications and contraindications of multiple imaging modalities and their alternatives, taking into consideration factors such as radiation exposure, cost, and goal of imaging. A major concern when imaging children is the child's exposure to ionizing radiation. Pediatric radiologists modify imaging parameters to minimize radiation by following standard protocols, particularly for computed tomography (CT) scans. Pediatric radiologists keep in mind the concept of "as low as reasonably achievable" (ALARA) in terms of a child's exposure to radiation during imaging. The Image Gently campaign[1] is an initiative of the Alliance for Radiation Safety in Pediatric Imaging. The campaign goal is to change practice by increasing the awareness of the opportunities to lower radiation dose while imaging children.

Ionizing radiation is used in plain radiographs, fluoroscopy, and CT. Effective dose is a calculated age- and sex-averaged value that is used as a measure to compare detriment from cancer and hereditary effects due to various procedures involving ionizing radiation. Effective dose is expressed in Sieverts (Sv) and is a single dose parameter that reflects the risk of a nonuniform exposure in terms of whole-body exposure. The biological effect of ionizing radiation is represented in the units of Sieverts, which is the product of the absorbed dose and a weighting factor. The weighting factor is a function of the type of radiation and the tissue involved.[2]

Ionizing radiation has the potential to alter DNA directly or by generating free radicals. In the extreme, ionizing radiation causes cell death. In addition, high doses of ionizing radiation are carcinogenic. Medical imaging accounts for an increasing amount of radiation exposure to the general population. In the United States, imaging accounts for about 50% of the total radiation exposure, and of this amount 50% is accounted for by CT scanning. Children are 2 to 10 times more susceptible to radiation of all kinds compared with adults. The risk of cancer from radiation has not been defined, and clinical studies have not been performed to define the risk versus benefit ratio. The theoretical risk of radiation exposure from medical imaging has been suggested from the studies of cancer incidence in survivors of the Hiroshima atomic bomb. Moderate or severe exposure (>100–150 mSv) is clearly a cancer risk, but lower levels are less obvious. The difference in effect on the body between acute and chronic exposure is not fully understood, but it is clear that exposures over a lifetime are cumulative.

The dose of a single chest radiograph is approximately 0.1 mSv, which is equivalent to the natural background radiation that the population is exposed to in 10 days. The effective dose of a standard helical CT ranges from 1.7 mSv in a newborn to 5.4 mSv in an adult. In an effort to decrease radiation, pediatric radiology has developed a low dose protocol that can reduce the radiation dose in, for example, a 5-year-old child from 2.1 to 0.55 mSv.[2,3] More recently, ultra-low dose protocols have been developed for patients with chronic conditions that need continuous follow-up such cystic fibrosis (CF). Such ultra-low dose protocols can have an effective dose as low as 0.14 mSv.[4] With longer life expectancies, children who require repetitive medical imaging are likely to be exposed to more radiation in their lives than they would have received in the past. Children with chronic conditions have a longer life expectancy than in the recent past, and their exposure to medical imaging is higher as well.

Imaging Approach

Several modalities are available to evaluate the chest and its structures in children. In general, chest radiography is the initial imaging approach when a chest anomaly is suspected. General suggestions on choosing imaging technique is found in Table 7-1.

Table 7-1. Imaging Approach by Condition or Suspected Condition

Indication	Imaging Modality
Suspected foreign body	Expiratory radiograph
Suspected pneumothorax	Lateral radiograph with pneumothorax side up
Suspected fluid in pleural space	Lateral decubitus and radiograph
Visualized structural anomalies (chest wall, vascular, tracheobronchial tree, lung parenchyma	Multidetector CT scan
Anomalies of the tracheobronchial tree, evaluate lumen and pulmonary infiltrates that fail to resolve in 10 to 14 days	Virtual bronchoscopy
Chronic unexplained respiratory symptoms with low suspicion for foreign body	Virtual bronchoscopy
Pleural effusion	Ultrasound
Lung abscess	CT scan
Suspected vascular rings	PA and lateral radiograph
Visualized vascular rings	MRI
Characterized vasculature of developmental lung malformations	MRI
Chronic interstitial process	HRCT
Airspace disease	CT scan
Bronchiectasis	HRCT
Asthma complications	CT/HRCT
Measure airway thickness	MDCT
Investigate extent and pattern of bronchiectasis	CT scan
Pneumonia	PA and lateral radiograph
Complicated pneumonia	Ultrasound (pleural effusion), CT scan
Anterior or middle mediastinal mass	CT scan, PET for lymphoma
Posterior mediastinal mass	MRI

Abbreviations: CT, computed tomography; HRCT, high-resolution computed tomography; MDCT, multidetector computed tomography; MRI, magnetic resonance imaging; PA, posteroanterior; PET, positron emission tomography.

Chest Radiograph

The standard order for chest radiograph is the posteroanterior (PA) and lateral views. While a single view saves cost, it has not been shown to be useful because the diaphragm obscures much of the lung field in the PA view, particularly the bases. The radiograph is taken at full inspiration, which may be difficult to time in the young child. Full inspiration typically results in the diaphragm being at the level of the 8th to 10th posterior rib or the 5th to 6th anterior rib. Whenever possible the patient should be imaged in the upright position. On occasion, for example, in evaluating for a foreign body or pneumothorax, an expiratory radiograph may be ordered. The anteroposterior (AP) portable radiograph, taken in bed, may not present as clear an image as that taken in the radiology department, but is of great value in imaging very sick patients. A lateral decubitus radiograph may be ordered to evaluate layering of fluid in the pleural space; however, this has been largely replaced by ultrasound because ultrasound lacks radiation, can be done at the bedside, and evaluates the characteristics of the pleural effusion. The dependent lung in the lateral decubitus radiograph should show increase in density because atelectasis results from the weight of the mediastinum. Failure to show increased density suggests that there is air trapping, which is useful to know if a foreign body is suspected. A lordotic view is taken to view the apices of the lungs.

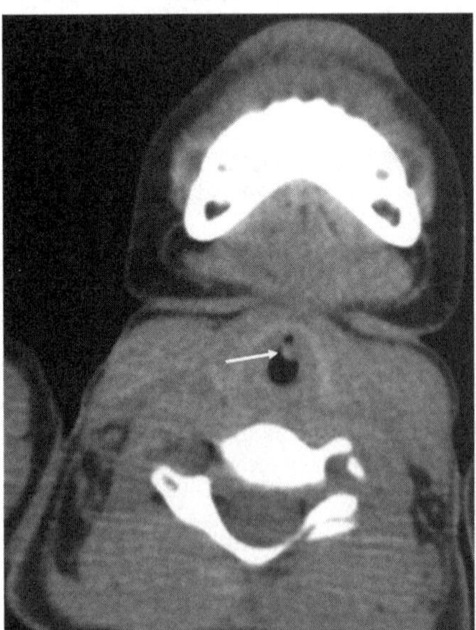

Figure 7-1A. A computed tomography scan of the neck showing laryngeal papillomatosis.

Multidetector CT Scan

Multidetector CT (MDCT) is considered the best modality to characterize in detail the chest wall, vascular structures, tracheobronchial tree, and lung parenchyma. The different post-processing techniques, 2- and 3-dimensional reformations, virtual bronchoscopy, and maximum intensity projections allow detailed characterization of structural anomalies (Figure 7-1A–C).

Computed tomography gives accurate information of the location and extent of involvement, as well as anatomical landmarks and relationship of the abnormality in question.

The main disadvantage of CT is the effect of ionizing radiation. The increased number of detectors on MDCT allows thinner collimation, which shortens the examination and decreases the use of sedation, but increases radiation exposure. When a CT scan is performed in a child, routine adjustments of imaging parameters must be done to minimize radiation with minimal or no compromise of the image quality. These adjustments are routinely performed in pediatric facilities. Manipulations of the scanner parameters to reduce radiation include increasing pitch, decreasing beam energy, and decreasing photon fluence.

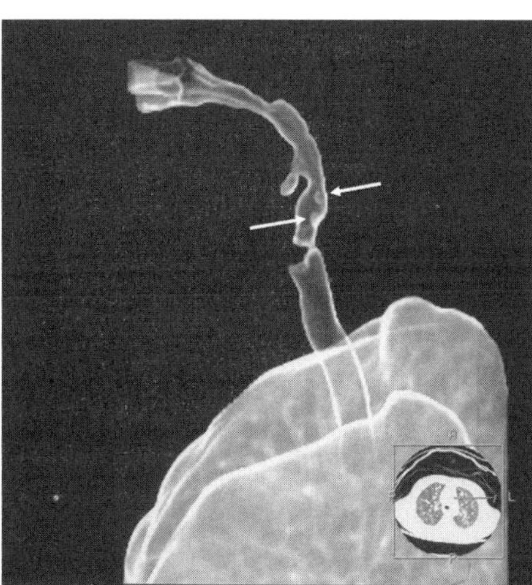

Figure 7-1B. Virtual bronchoscopy of laryngeal papillomatosis.

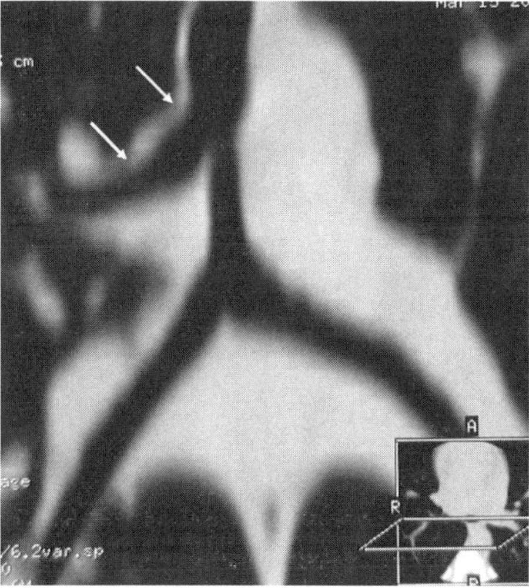

Figure 7-1C. A computed tomography scan showing tracheal bronchus (arrow).

Virtual bronchoscopy (VB) is a relatively new technique that provides an internal rendering of the tracheobronchial walls and lumen.[5] Despite the use of a low-tube-current technique and rapid table speed, the major disadvantage of CT and VB is radiation exposure. Indications for VB include patients with pulmonary infiltrates that fail to resolve in the usual time (10–14 days) and chronic, unexplained respiratory symptoms in a patient who has a low suspicion for foreign body aspiration and normal or nonspecific chest radiograph. The advantages of VB are the ability to evaluate tortuous structures and segmental and subsegmental bronchi, which are hard to evaluate with conventional bronchoscopy given the small size of airways in children. Virtual bronchoscopy also allows evaluation distal to the obstruction and proper visualization of upper lobe bronchi that arise at an acute angle from the major bronchi.[6,7]

Magnetic Resonance Imaging

Magnetic resonance imaging (MRI) is appropriate in certain circumstances; however, the evaluation of the lung parenchyma with this technique is limited. Magnetic resonance imaging may help characterize the vasculature of developmental lung malformations or vascular rings. The use of MR arteriogram provides a very detailed map of the vasculature (Figures 7-2A–C).[3] Magnetic resonance imaging is accurate in evaluating chest wall masses and depicting intraspinal extension of neurogenic lesions in the posterior mediastinum, a feature that helps in the differential diagnosis and treatment. Disadvantages of MRI include its availability and the length of the studies that in some cases require sedation.[8]

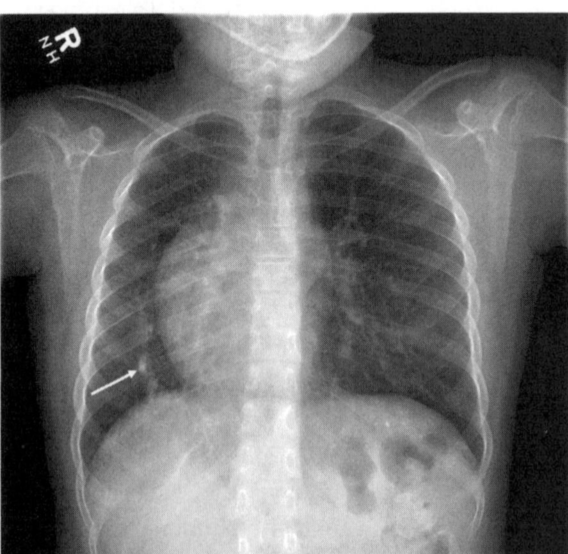

Figure 7-2A. Plain chest radiograph of scimitar syndrome. Arrow shows the vein that drains into the inferior vena cava.

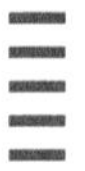

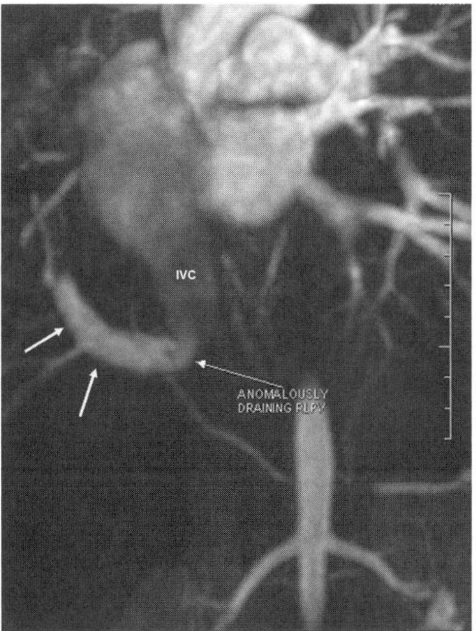

Figure 7-2B. Magnetic resonance imaging of scimitar syndrome. Thick arrows show pulmonary vein draining into inferior vena cava. RLPV, right lower pulmonary vein.

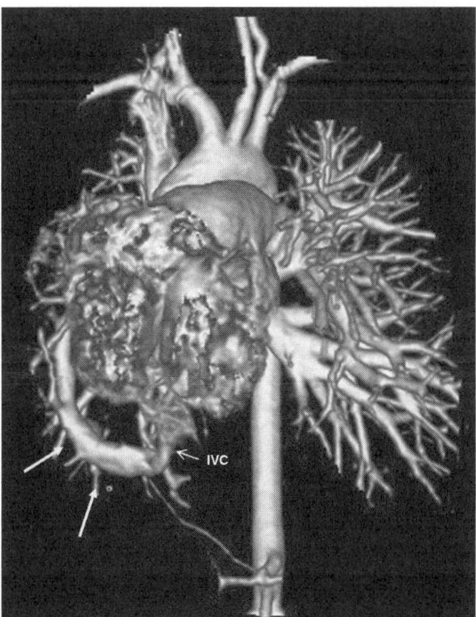

Figure 7-2C. 3-dimensional reconstruction of Figure 7-2B.

Ultrasonography

Ultrasound is preferred in the prenatal and perinatal periods because newborns have cartilaginous bones and larger acoustic windows. For imaging the fetus, ultrasound is of particular value when bronchopulmonary foregut malformations or diaphragmatic hernias are suspected. The role of ultrasound in evaluating chest pathology should not be underestimated in the postnatal period and during childhood. Even though ultrasound's usefulness is limited in evaluating a well-aerated lung due to the poor transmission of the sound waves. However, ultrasound in the presence of consolidations can be useful, allowing the evaluation of the lung parenchyma. Ultrasound is also very helpful in evaluating pleural effusions, providing the best detail of the fluid consistency, demonstrating septations, solid components, or debris that cannot be well characterized on radiographs or CT[9] (Figure 7-3A–B) Assessing mediastinal vascular structures and the thymus is possible with ultrasound using the right acoustic window. For superficial chest wall lesions, ultrasound also can provide information regarding the cystic or solid nature of a mass, the presence of fat or calcification, and the margins and size of the lesion if confined to the superficial tissues. This helps narrowing a differential diagnosis and provides guidance regarding a therapeutic approach. The advan-

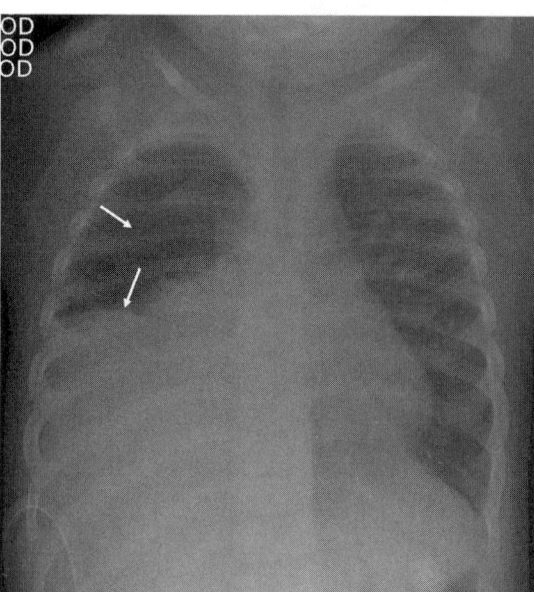

Figure 7-3A. Hydropneumothorax. Note central trachea. Upper arrow shows lung margin and lower arrow shows air-fluid interface.

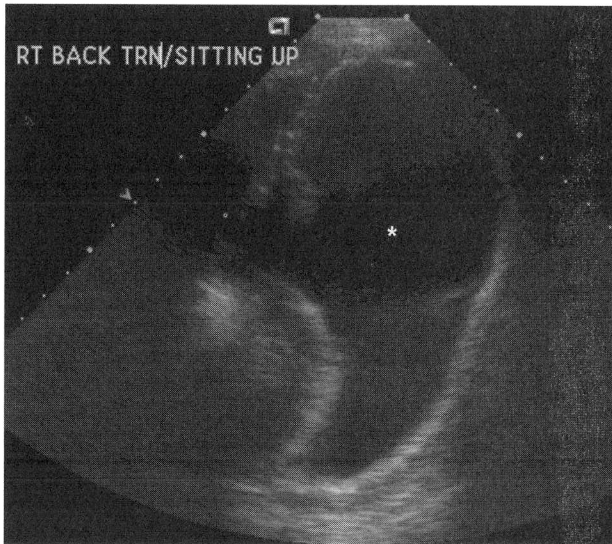

Figure 7-3B. Showing ultrasound of the pleural effusion in Figure 7-3A.

tages of ultrasound include a lack of need for sedation, cost savings when compared with CT, portability, and lack of radiation.[10]

Angiography

Traditionally angiography was the technique of choice for imaging vascular anomalies, particularly when vascular rings, pulmonary sequestration, or hypogenetic lung syndrome is suspected and surgical treatment is considered. Currently, MDCT has replaced the conventional angiogram due to exquisite spatial resolution, lack of invasiveness, and multiplanar reformation capabilities allowing the characterization of other tissues (Figure 7-4A–B).

Ventilation/Perfusion ($\dot{V}/\dot{Q}$) Scan

The $\dot{V}/\dot{Q}$ scan indicates the degree of vascular perfusion of different lobes of the lung and the distribution of ventilation. The ventilation scan is performed as the child inhales xenon through a mask. The perfusion study is performed by injecting nuclear particles that produce microemboli in the parenchyma of the lung, which can indicate the degree of vascular perfusion of the different lobes of the lung. The results are expressed as percentages of ventilation and perfusion.

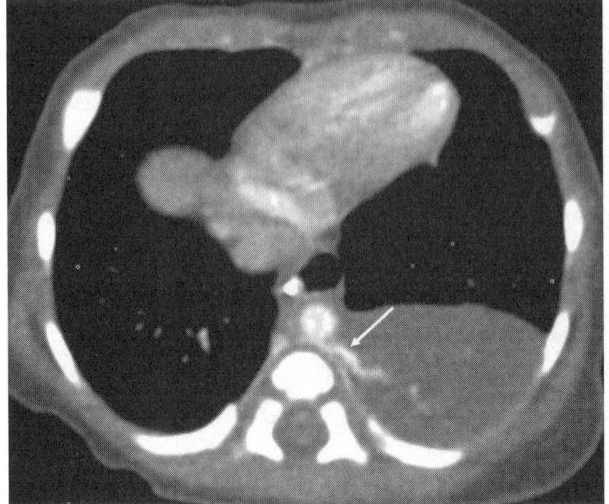

Figure 7-4A. A computed tomography scan shows vessel supplying sequestration (arrow).

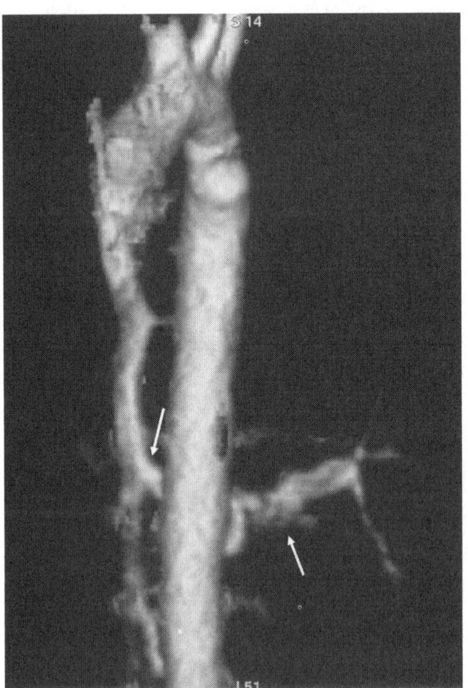

Figure 7-4B. A computed tomography reconstruction of Figure 7-4A showing vessel supplying sequestered lobe.

Chest Radiograph Report

The radiology report is a consultation between the radiologist and the physician who orders the study. It is helpful for the ordering physician to view the images rather than rely on the written or verbal report. It is not only a good exercise, but a good practice because the referring physician has knowledge of the entire clinical history and may aid in the final diagnosis. If necessary the radiologist can be contacted in person or by phone to explain the findings in greater detail. It is important to be aware that the written report is part of the medical record and, as such, may be written in language that requires interpretation. It may be useful to discuss the findings with the radiologist, who may provide additional information that is not in the report. A good example is the statement "these findings are consistent with the diagnosis of pneumonia," which may mean that this is likely a case of pneumonia or alternatively that pneumonia is in the differential diagnosis. Two different radiologists might report the same radiograph as "pneumonia in the right lower lobe" and "there is an infiltrate in the right lower lobe." The radiologist should be able to provide insight to help refine the practitioner's decision for treatment or perhaps recommend additional imaging. It is good practice for radiologists to describe the findings and in the conclusion to mention a brief summary followed by a differential diagnosis in descending order of possibility. The radiologist should be able to provide insight to help refine the practitioner's decision for treatment or perhaps recommend additional imaging.

Access to images has improved markedly in the digital age, so a patient or parent may bring a CD-ROM and ask for an explanation of the findings. The physician may have access to the Picture Archiving and Communications System (PACS), which can archive the radiograph report and images. This helps in the availability of the images and for comparison with previous studies.

Reading the Chest Radiograph

The first step in evaluating the radiograph is to identify the name, the date of birth or medical record number, and note the date of the radiograph, although the widespread use of PACS obviates this step. If prior studies are available, comparison of the findings with previous radiographs helps to identify acute versus chronic abnormalities and change over time.

Radiologists are trained to evaluate the quality and the technique of the study. An appropriate depth of penetration is important for a good radiograph. The thoracic spine should be visible on the PA radiograph above the carina and almost invisible behind the heart. The position of the chest is also important. If there is rotation, the lucency of the 2 lungs will be unequal and will need to be differentiated from alterations in aeration of the lungs. Also in a rotated radiograph, one pulmonary hilum is more exposed and may be misinterpreted as a perihilar opacity. The degree of rotation is assessed by looking for symmetry of the ribs and the position of the ends of the clavicles.

The reading of the chest radiograph needs to be thorough, and radiologists develop their own system to avoid missing any relevant findings. The key to a thorough interpretation is to develop a fixed routine. Clinicians who are not radiologists tend to focus on the obvious abnormality if one is visible and miss other findings that may be important.

Landmarks and Structures

The chest radiograph is a 2-dimensional picture, so objects outside the chest may be superimposed, including monitor leads, jewelry, hair plaits, and other objects that may confuse the picture. An initial broad view should be taken to include the mediastinum, position of the trachea, and the great vessels. The cardiothoracic ratio should be less than 50% in the PA view, but the heart will appear larger than the PA view in a supine or AP view, or using portable radiography. These factors must be considered before making a diagnosis of cardiomegaly, particularly from an AP radiograph. The lung fields should be reviewed from apices to costophrenic angles while comparing right lung to left lung. The right diaphragm is typically higher than the left diaphragm and the outline should be clear and continuous. The costophrenic angles should be sharp; if blunted it may indicate a pleural effusion or sometimes pleural thickening. When a pleural effusion is small, it may be obscured by the overlying lung in an upright radiograph. When a pleural effusion is large enough and free floating, a meniscus sign can be appreciated. On a supine radiograph, a free-floating pleural effusion will layer, causing veiling of the hemithorax. In others words, the involved hemithorax will appear diffusely hazy.

A deviation or shifting of the position of the heart and mediastinum toward one side of the chest may suggest volume loss on that side. If the mediastinum shifts away from the lesion this suggests a space-occupying lesion or pleural effusion. A large tension pneumothorax will shift the mediastinum toward the other side of the chest.

If the hilum is enlarged it may be because of enlarged pulmonary vessels, enlarged lymph nodes, or a mass in the area. Peribronchial thickening (or cuffing) is caused by inflammation or edema of the airways. It is a common finding in children with hyperactive airway disease, especially in preschoolers or in patients with viral lower respiratory infections. Pulmonary edema is also a cause of peribronchial cuffing.

Silhouette Sign

The silhouette sign was first described by Dr Ben Felson and is useful to locate the anatomical position of an abnormality.[11] The silhouette sign is the elimination of the lung and soft tissue interface caused by fluid or a mass in the lung. The most common example of this is the presence of a right middle lobe opacity that obscures the right heart border. If the opacity was in the right lower lobe, the right heart border would be visible (Figure 7-5). In essence, the presence or absence of the silhouette sign is useful to define the anatomical location of the abnormality. Another example of the silhouette

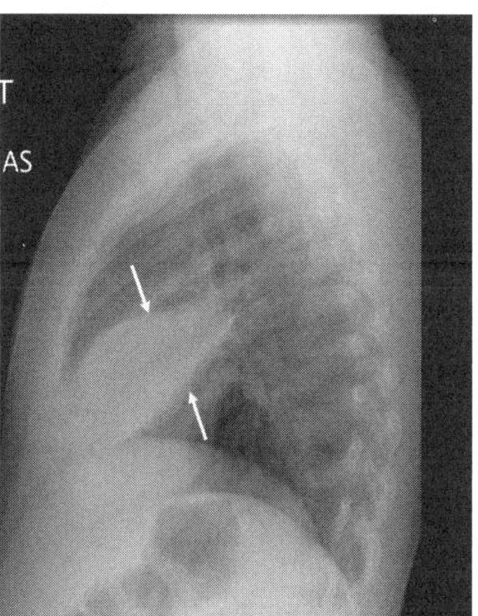

Figure 7-5. Right middle lobe pneumonia obscuring right heart border demonstrating positive silhouette sign. Arrows point to the major and minor fissure.

sign is the lingular opacity overlying and obscuring the left heart border. The silhouette sign is applicable to the heart, aorta, chest wall, and diaphragm.

Other Specific Findings

The following terms are common words used by radiologists to describe findings to reach a differential diagnosis. This thoracic imaging terminology was unified by the Fleischner Society most recently in 2008.[12]

A **bronchogram** refers to the outline of the airway made visible by filling the alveoli with cells or fluid. The air bronchogram is probably best seen in respiratory distress syndrome (RDS) in the neonate but is also seen in the following situations:

- Any condition causing lung consolidation most commonly pneumonia
- Atelectasis
- Acute lung injury (adult RDS)
- Some neoplasms
- Normal expiration

Atelectasis is collapse or incomplete expansion of the lung or part of the lung and is described in Chapter 24. It can be lobar, segmental, or subsegmental depending on the extension, and passive or postprogressive according to the pathophysiology. Atelectasis appears as an increased density on the chest radiograph and is in the differential diagnosis of a parenchymal consolidation.

Infiltrate is a term formerly used to describe an ill-defined opacity in the lung field that almost by definition is not diagnostic of any specific abnormality and should be interpreted with caution. Even though it is still frequently used to refer to a pneumonia by some radiologists, it is not synonymous with this condition. The use of the term infiltrate is currently discouraged and the correct term to be used is an opacity or air space disease.

A **consolidation** is characteristic of lobar pneumonia, and the area may increase in size. If the involved area is airless and decreased in size, it is described as collapse. Areas of consolidation may be seen with pulmonary hemorrhage and vasculitic disorders in addition to the diagnosis of pneumonia. Lobar consolidation is classically seen in pneumococcal pneumonia.

Interstitial as a descriptor has fallen out of favor. By definition, the interstitium is a continuum of connective tissue throughout the lung, including the bronchovascular, the parenchymal/acinar, and the subpleural connective tissue. The correct terms to be used are **reticular pattern** and **reticulo-nodular pattern.** A reticular pattern usually represents interstitial lung disease. Interstitial pneumonia is more typically seen with atypical organisms or viral pneumonia. A nodular pattern is characterized on chest radiographs by the presence of a myriad of tiny round opacities ranging from 2 to 10 mm that are usually widespread. When a reticular pattern is combined with a nodular pattern, it is known as a reticulo-nodular pattern. Recognition of these patterns is critical because each is associated with a subset of diseases that is useful when generating a differential diagnosis.

An **opacity** should be characterized by noting the size and shape, the number and location, the margins, and the homogeneity. Comparison with a previous radiograph is important. **Ground-glass opacities** are partially filled air spaces (with fluid or cells) and interstitial thickening. This is a CT finding seen as hazy lung parenchyma that is not opaque enough to obscure the adjacent interstitial prominence, as opposed to a consolidation. Ground-glass opacities are seen in patients with pulmonary edema, pulmonary hemorrhage, pneumocystis pneumonia, and alveolar proteinosis, among many other entities (Figure 7-6). They are also seen in those with chronic interstitial lung diseases and even as an incidental finding in the dependent portion of the lungs as the result of blood flow redistribution in the horizontal position. In cases of interstitial lung disease, it is considered a marker of active disease suggesting inflammation or alveolitis, which is potentially treatable.[13]

A **micro-nodule** is a discreet opacity in the lung measuring less than 3 mm, whereas nodules are rounded opacities, well- or ill-defined, measuring up to 3 cm in diameter, without regard for contour, border, or intensity. The term mass implies a solid or partially solid lesion that may be caused by infection, by a granuloma such as tuberculosis (TB), or by a tumor (benign or malignant). Vascular anomalies may have the appearance of a nodule and may be caused by arteriovenous malformation and lung infarct, Wegener granulomatosis, or rheumatoid arthritis. The rate of enlargement of a nodule is helpful in diagnosis. If the lesion doubles in size within a month the diagnosis is likely infectious, vascular lesion, or infarction. If the doubling time is 6 to 18 months, it is likely a benign tumor or malignant granuloma; if the doubling time

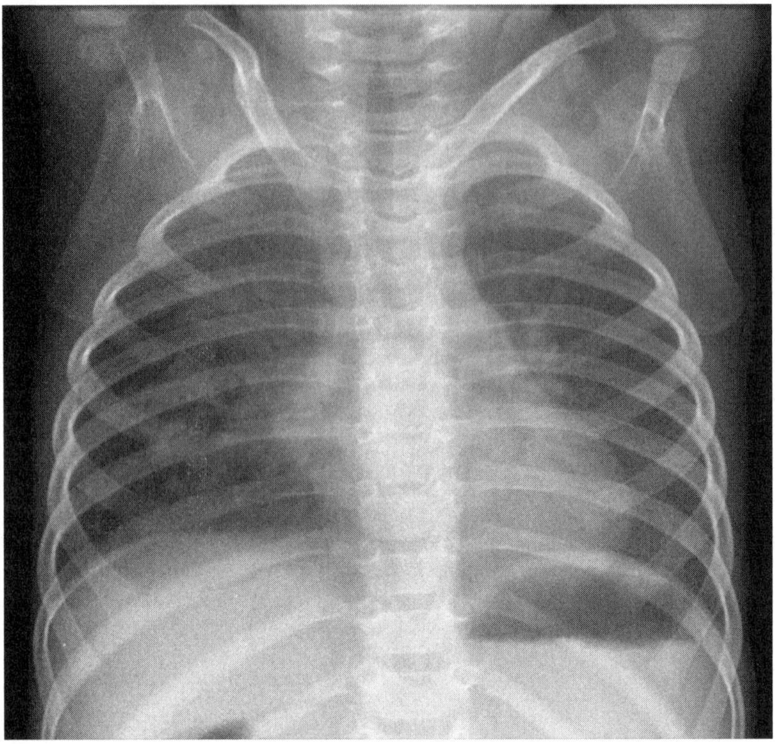

Figure 7-6. Ground-glass appearance of plain chest radiograph.

is more than 24 months, then a benign nodule is likely. The presence of multiple nodules may indicate various etiologies, as shown in Box 7-1.

A **cavity** is essentially a hole in the lung caused by destruction of lung parenchyma. The most common cause in children is infection, and is known as necrotizing pneumonia. The most common cause of necrotizing pneumonia is pneumococcus. Other microorganisms may cause cavitation, including *Staphylococcus aureus, Mycobacterium tuberculosis,* gram-negative bacteria (especially *Klebsiella),* group A streptococcus, anaerobic bacteria, and fungi. It is also seen in non-tuberculous mycobacteria in children with CF. Cavitation can be seen also in those with septic emboli or vasculitis, such as Wegener granulomatosis.

Cystic changes in the lung are seen in the late stages of pulmonary fibrosis, also known as honeycomb lung. Cysts are seen with bronchiectasis, especially saccular bronchiectasis.

Box 7-1. Etiology of Multiple Nodules

- Infection: tuberculosis, fungal infection
- Neoplasm: lymphoma, hamartoma, metastatic lesions
- Rheumatoid: Wegener granulomatosis
- Granuloma: systemic lupus erythematosus

A **pneumatocele** is an air-filled, thin-walled space that is most commonly associated with prior history of pneumonia or trauma. The pathophysiology is unclear but is believed to be either due to focal overinflation or parenchymal necrosis, with a check valve mechanism that may allow it to grow. In most cases, it resolves spontaneously.[14]

A **bleb** is a small gas-containing space within the visceral pleura or subpleural lung smaller than 1 cm, while a **bulla** is 1 cm or larger; however, the distinction is of little clinical significance. They can be associated with other signs of pulmonary emphysema. The cause of blebs and bullae is not known, but they are still meaningful since the possibility of rupture or air leakage may result in a pneumothorax.

A **cyst** is a gas-filled round space surrounded by a thin wall (<2 mm) and without evidence of emphysema, which also may be fluid filled or solid. Cysts are seen in patients with Langerhans cell histiocytosis or in lymphangioleiomatosis. Thicker-walled cysts are seen in the development of end-stage fibrosis (honeycomb lung).

Bronchiectasis is usually considered the irreversible localized or diffuse bronchial dilation secondary to bronchial wall destruction. Three types are described: cystic, cylindrical, and saccular. Cases of reversible or temporary bronchiectasis are related to the reexpansion of a lung that has been collapsed due to infection or atelectasis,[15] also in cases of acute pneumonia, bronchitis, and allergic bronchopulmonary aspergillosis. Its distribution is also important in narrowing the etiology. Upper lobe bronchiectasis is more common in CF and chronic mycotic and mycobacterial infections, the lower lobes are more commonly involved in idiopathic cases, and perihilar or central bronchiectases are frequently seen in those with allergic bronchopulmonary aspergillosis.[16]

Reading the CT Scan

In CT and computed axial tomography, 3 planes can be viewed. The usual chest CT scan is viewed as a cross-section, which implies a horizontal slice from the neck to the abdomen if someone is standing. The sagittal view is from front to back and top to bottom, and the coronal view is side to side and top to bottom. The standard CT of the chest provides continuous images of slices of the lung, whereas a high-resolution CT scan (HRCT) has thin sections with skipped areas between the sections. The parameters used on HRCT are meant to optimize spatial resolution to assess fine parenchymal pattern. The images obtained will be representative of the overall lung parenchyma, but only cover skipped areas and may not image small isolated findings (isolated cavity or nodule, consolidation). It is best used for the evaluation of diffuse parenchymal disease. Examples of diseases well assessed with HRCT are bronchiectasis, CF, immotile cilia syndrome, asthma, Langerhans cell histiocytosis, interstitial pneumonias, allergic bronchopulmonary aspergillosis, recurrent aspiration, and pulmonary infections.[17]

The range of normal findings has considerable overlap with pathology, and care must be taken to avoid overinterpretation. This is particularly true for the ground-glass appearance.[5] Computed tomography scanning has become very sophisticated and provides images that are not overlaid by tissues, as occurs with 2-dimensional radiography, and results in much clearer CT images. Instant reformation in different planes allows the review of the examination on the axial and coronal planes and can help sort out findings that are merely normal structures. The mediastinal structures, especially the vessels, can be evaluated only with intravenous (IV) contrast. The indications for IV contrast administration are many, but in general it is given to evaluate neoplasms in the mediastinum, lung, and chest wall; pulmonary and chest wall abscesses; pleural effusions; congenital developmental lung malformations; and adenopathy. High-resolution CT scan is performed without the administration of IV contrast.

Evaluation of airspace disease by thick section image reconstruction technique in the standard CT scan is usually adequate, whereas chronic interstitial processes are better viewed with HRCT.

Ground-glass attenuation is a hazy attenuation of the lung parenchyma that is from alveolar filling or interstitial thickening, and both may occur[18] (Figure 7-6). The appearance is visible on chest radiograph but is more obvious on CT scan. It is seen with infant RDS, pulmonary edema, interstitial pneumonitis, idiopathic pulmonary fibrosis, and alveolar proteinosis (Figure 7-7).

Tree-in-bud, seen on thin-section CT scans, is the finding of linear branching opacities of similar caliber connecting to small centrolobular nodules of soft tissue representing bronchiolar luminal impaction with mucus, pus, or fluid, which makes the normally invisible peripheral airways visible (Figure 7-8). Tree-in-bud pattern is not visible on the chest radiograph. It is indicative of inflammation and is nonspecific, although certain conditions are associated with the finding. Originally it was used as an indicator of endobronchial spread of TB, but any infectious organism, be it bacterial, viral, fungal, or parasitic, may cause the pattern.[6] It has also been noted in bronchogenic dissemination of atypical mycobacteria and is seen in conditions that result in bronchiectasis, including CF and primary ciliary dyskinesia. The tree-in-bud finding is also seen in allergic bronchopulmonary aspergillosis and connective tissue disorders. Less commonly, certain malignancies can produce this pattern, including gastric breast cancer and renal cancer.[19]

Imaging for Specific Conditions

Allergic Bronchopulmonary Aspergillosis (ABPA)

Allergic bronchopulmonary aspergillosis usually presents in children with long-standing asthma. Aspergillosis infection can be divided into 5 categories according to presentation: (1) saprophytic aspergillosis (aspergilloma in a preexisting cavity), (2) semi-invasive (chronic necrotizing consolidations), (3) hypersensitivity reaction (allergic bronchopulmonary aspergillosis), (4) airway-invasive aspergillosis (tracheobronchitis, bronchopneumonia), and (5) angioinvasive aspergillosis. In ABPA, plugs of inspissated mucus contain aspergillus organisms, which results in bronchial dilatation. Radiologically ABPA may present with a normal chest radiograph or mild hyperinflation. The earlier changes typically are ill-defined opacities, single or multiple, and tubular "finger-in-glove" areas of increased density in a bronchial distribution in the upper lobes. The later stages include bronchiectasis with fibrotic changes.

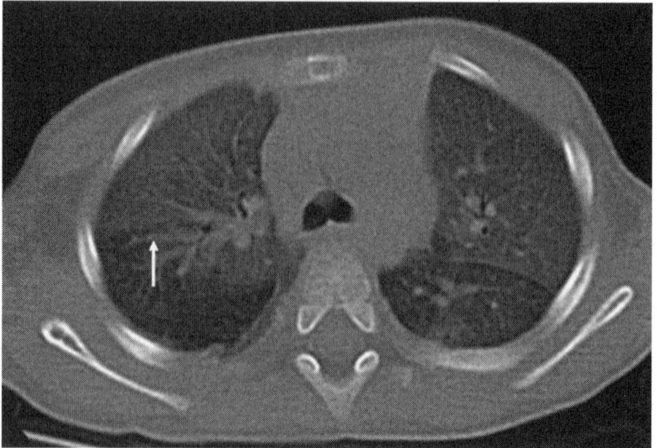

Figure 7-7. Ground-glass appearance of computed tomography scan of alveolar proteinosis.

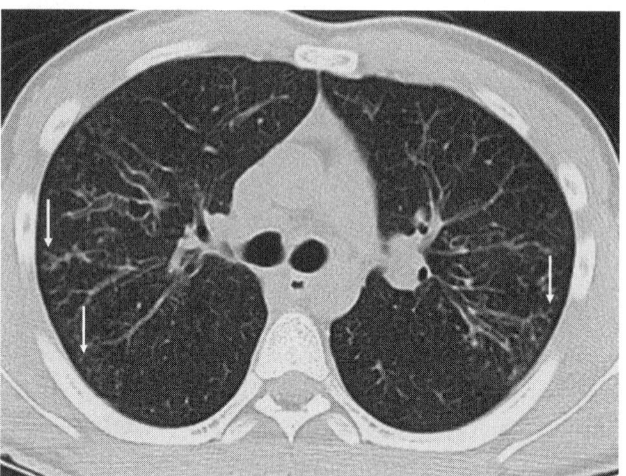

Figure 7-8. A computed tomography scan showing tree-in-bud appearance at the arrows and elsewhere.

In children with debilitating chronic illness, aspergillosis may present as a semi-invasive form with segmental unilateral or bilateral consolidations with or without cavitation; however, the course of the disease takes years and is most commonly seen in adulthood. Airway-invasive and angioinvasive aspergillosis are more common in immunocompromised patients. Airway-invasive disease presents as acute tracheobronchitis with bronchiolitis (tree-in-bud pattern on CT) and bronchopneumonia in a peribronchial distribution. Angioinvasive disease presents as nodules surrounded by a halo of ground-glass attenuation ("halo sign").[20]

Hypersensitivity Pneumonitis

Hypersensitivity pneumonitis, also called extrinsic allergic alveolitis, is the immunologic response to allergens from organic dust of plants or animal origin or chemicals. The presentation is usually divided into acute, subacute, and chronic. Acute hypersensitivity pneumonitis may present in cases as a normal chest radiograph or air space consolidations. The subacute form also may present with a normal chest radiograph, but on HRCT ground-glass opacities and nodules, and sometimes air trapping, can be observed. The chronic presentation manifests as fibrosis that mostly spares the lung bases, as opposed to other causes of fibrosis (idiopathic pulmonary fibrosis, interstitial pneumonias) with other associated findings from the acute or subacute form.[21,22]

Eosinophilic Pneumonia

Acute eosinophilic pneumonia results in diffuse alveolar or alveolar-interstitial opacities with chest radiography. Computed tomography scan shows bilateral patchy areas of ground-glass opacity with septal thickening. There may be additional areas of consolidation or ill-defined nodules.[23,24] The appearance may be similar to hydrostatic pulmonary edema without cardiomegaly. Chronic eosinophilic pneumonia reveals CT findings of airspace opacities predominantly in the upper lobes and peripheral lung fields ranging from ground-glass opacities to consolidations with air bronchograms. The most distinctive radiographic feature is the *photographic negative* of pulmonary edema, which is infrequent and not specific.[25]

Asthma

Most patients with asthma can be diagnosed clinically by medical history and physical examination and tend to respond rapidly to bronchodilator therapy. Therefore, chest radiography is not needed for the initial diagnosis in most children. The value of chest radiography is in diagnosing complications, establishing a precipitating cause for the asthma episode, and excluding alternate diagnoses that resemble asthma (Box 7-2).

Hyperinflation is the most common abnormality and is identified radiographically as hyperexpansion, flattening of the diaphragms, increased retrosternal lucency, anterior bowing of the sternum, and bulging of the intercostal rib spaces. There is poor correlation between the degree of hyperinflation and the severity of the asthma attack or the patient's responsiveness to therapy. Hyperinflation can persist even after symptoms resolve in up to 15% of patients.

The finding of hypoinflation on chest radiography significantly correlates with hospital admission for children aged 6 to 17 years (but not younger children), thus hypoinflation is a poor prognostic sign and may indicate the need for more aggressive therapy.[26] Hypoinflation may result in clinically significant hypoxemia possibly because children with asthma exacerbations may begin to lose their respiratory drive or may exhaust their accessory muscles of respiration. Bronchial wall thickening is usually transient. It is more common in asthmatic patients with superimposed acute viral infections and in those with persistent asthma.

Atelectasis secondary to thickened airway secretions is common and may be lobar, segmental, or subsegmental. The next most common

Box 7-2. Indications for Chest Radiography in Children With Asthma

- Severe respiratory distress
- Unequal breath sounds (to exclude pneumothorax)
- Fever (to exclude pneumonia)
- To detect complications such as atelectasis or pneumomediastinum
- If there is no response to routine treatment
- When other causes of wheezing are suspected, such as a foreign body, endobronchial lesion, vascular ring, or cystic fibrosis

finding in children with complicated asthma is pneumonia. The reported radiographic incidence of pneumonia ranges from 0% to 30%.

Pneumothorax is an uncommon complication in children with asthma, with a reported incidence of 0% to 3%.[27] It is an important complication of mechanical ventilation in children with asthma and should be suspected if there is acute deterioration. The reported incidence of pneumomediastinum in children with asthma ranges from 0% to 15% and may be underreported. There is a bimodal distribution, peaking at ages 4 to 6 and 13 to 18 years. The extent of the pneumomediastinum involved correlates with the severity of the attack. The diagnosis requires a high level of suspicion, since up to 30% of cases may be missed initially by radiography.[28]

Indications for HRCT

High-resolution CT in children with asthma provides additional information of lung pathology, including bronchial wall thickening, narrowing of the bronchial lumen, regions of decreased attenuation and vascularity on inspiratory scans and air trapping on expiratory scans, bronchiectasis, emphysema, atelectasis, pneumonia, and mucus impaction. Combination of inspiratory and expiratory CT reveals the major physiological consequences of small airway diseases. Irreversible findings include bronchiectasis, bronchial wall thickening (because this is caused by inflammation or remodeling rather than only bronchocostriction), fibrotic reactions, and emphysema.[29]

Airway remodeling refers to the thickening of the airway walls due to hypertrophy of smooth muscle, infiltration with inflammatory cells, and mucus gland hyperplasia. Airway wall thickening has been related to the severity of the disease and airflow obstruction. Airway thickness can be measured by HRCT; therefore, the effects of various stimuli and treatments on remodeling can be monitored longitudinally.[30]

Bronchiolitis

Although a chest radiograph is not indicated for children with acute respiratory syncytial virus bronchiolitis, the most typical findings are hyperinflation with flattened diaphragms, increased AP diameter of the chest, and increased lucency in the anterior clear space. There may be prominent peribronchial markings and small opacities, particularly in the lower lobes (Figure 7-9A–B). Pleural effusion does not occur. Changing atelectasis, especially of the right upper lobe, may result from inflammation of the airway.

Bronchiectasis

The finding of parallel lines ("tram track") radiating from the hilum is the hallmark of bronchiectasis on the chest radiograph. The CT scan provides significantly improved images of the degree and extent of bronchiectasis. Ring shadows represent enlarged thickened airways, which may extend well into the lung parenchyma. Cystic bronchiectasis is often accompanied by mucus filled cysts, which may have air-fluid levels. Multiple nodular densities represent mucus plugging of the peripheral airways.

There are 3 patterns of bronchiectasis that can be identified on CT scan. Cylindrical bronchiectasis is the earliest change, with dilation of the airway and mucus plugging. Varicose bronchiectasis demonstrates increased dilation, with ballooning of the airway and reduction of the number of branching airways to the sixth or seventh generation.

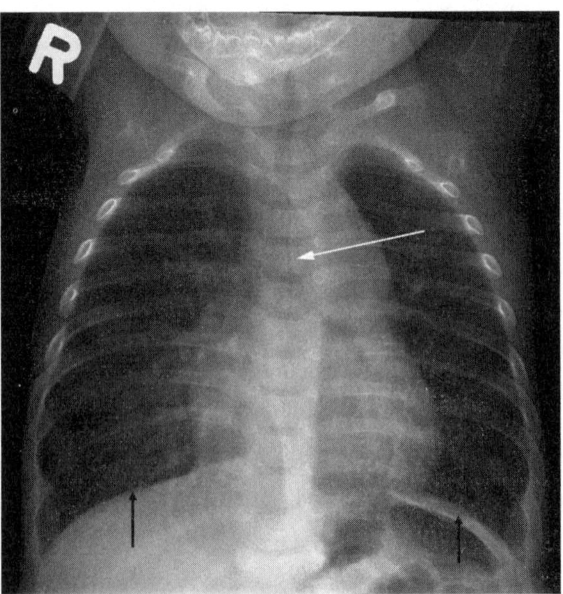

Figure 7-9A. Plain radiograph of bronchiolitis showing flattened diaphragms (black arrows). There is peribronchial thickening. Note herniation of right lung into anterior mediastinum (white arrow).

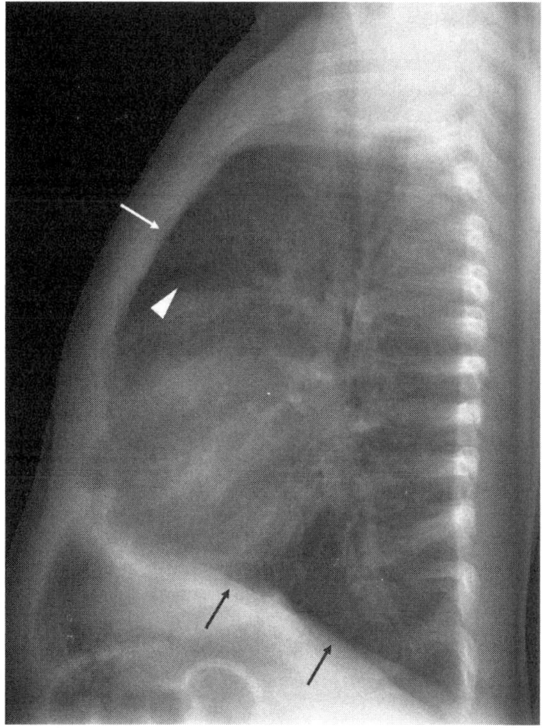

Figure 7-9B. Lateral view of Figure 7-9A showing flat diaphragms (black arrows) and lung in the anterior mediastinum (white arrows).

The most severe form of bronchiectasis is cystic or saccular bronchiectasis. Clusters of cysts may be seen, and on occasion there is a honeycomb appearance.

Congenital Anomalies

Airway Compression Caused by Vascular Anomalies

Vascular rings are congenital anomalies that encircle the esophagus and trachea and typically compress these structures. They are classified as true rings (anatomically complete) or partial rings, though both can have similar clinical presentations. Types of complete vascular rings include double aortic arch and right aortic arch with aberrant left subclavian and left ligamentum arteriosum. Incomplete rings include innominate artery compression and pulmonary artery sling.[31]

Double aortic arch is the most common symptomatic vascular ring. It causes respiratory symptoms earlier in life more frequently than other vascular rings. The second most common vascular ring is the right-sided aortic arch with aberrant left subclavian artery and left-sided ligamentum arteriosus. Other less commonly encountered rings include a right aortic arch with mirror image branching and left-sided ligamentum arteriosus, left aortic arch with aberrant right subclavian artery and right-sided ligamentum arteriosum, and circumflex aorta (the descending aorta crosses behind the esophagus to the opposite side of the arch) with a ligamentum arteriosum on the contralateral side of the arch. The pulmonary artery sling is the anomalous origin of the left pulmonary artery from the right pulmonary artery coursing between the trachea and esophagus to reach the left pulmonary hilum. Pulmonary slings are associated with complete "O-shaped" tracheal rings in 40% to 50% of cases, which narrow the trachea. Other airway abnormalities include bridging bronchus and tracheal bronchus. Multidetector CT (MDCT) angiography as well as MR angiography offer exquisite detail of the vascular anatomy. Association with ipsilateral lung agenesis has been reported.

A diverticulum occurs at the site of aberrant subclavian artery and represents the aortic attachment of a ligamentum arteriosus. The presence of an aortic diverticulum necessitates resection because untreated it may lead to residual obstruction and persistent symptoms.

Posteroanterior and lateral chest radiographs are the typical initial tool for screening for vascular rings. Right-sided or double aortic arch, tracheal narrowing, anterior bowing, and increased retro-tracheal soft tissues are the most common findings. At least one of these findings is reported in greater than 95% of cases. Therefore, the importance of frontal and lateral chest radiographs cannot be underestimated, since a normal chest radiograph significantly decreases the likelihood of finding a vascular ring in a symptomatic patient.

Barium esophagography was considered the most useful study to confirm the diagnosis of a vascular ring. A posterior indentation suggests an aberrant subclavian artery. Bilateral indentation on the AP view suggests a double arch. Anterior pulsatile indentation of the esophagus is virtually pathognomonic of pulmonary artery sling.

Computed tomography and MR angiography are now preferred for confirmation of the vascular ring.[32] Multidetector CT has advantages in that it is widely available and has a short scanning time that can obviate sedation. Computed tomography can evaluate the tracheobronchial tree and lung parenchyma. Magnetic resonance imaging is advantageous in that its multiplanar capabilities depict precisely the vascular anatomy.

Lung Malformations

Congenital developmental lung malformations have been described as a spectrum of disease from lung parenchymal abnormalities with relatively normal vascularity at one end of the spectrum, to vascular abnormalities with relatively preserved parenchyma at the other end.[33,34]

Computed tomography angiogram provides the more comprehensive approach because some of these lesions may have arterial, parenchymal, and tracheobronchial tree abnormalities. Characterizing these structures is important not only to make the diagnosis but for surgical planning and evaluation of complications, such as superimposed infections.

Pulmonary Agenesis/Hypoplasia

Radiographically pulmonary agenesis mimics pneumonectomy. There is hyperinflation of the remaining lung, mediastinal shift, diaphragmatic elevation, and sometimes chest wall deformity.

Bronchial Atresia

Bronchial atresia is considered to be due to intrauterine interruption of bronchial arterial supply. The distal branches can develop normally.

Congenital Lobar Hyperinflation

In children with congenital lobar hyperinflation, previously known as congenital lobar emphysema, the left upper and right middle lobes are the most commonly affected. Radiographically this presents as overinflation with air trapping on expiration (Figure 7-10).

Congenital Pulmonary Airway Malformation

Congenital pulmonary airway malformation, previously known as congenital cystic adenomatoid malformation, represents 25% of all congenital lung anomalies. It consists of adenomatoid proliferation of bronchioles that form cysts instead of normal alveoli. There are 3 most commonly described types: type 1 are cysts measuring 2 to 10 cm (most common); type 2 are cysts of 0.5 to 2 cm; and type 3 are solid-appearing lesions formed by microscopic cysts (Figure 7-11).

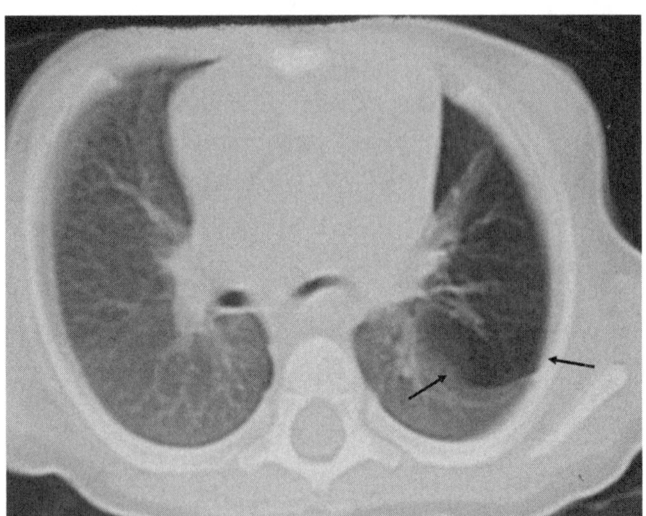

Figure 7-10. A computed tomography scan of lobar emphysema (arrows).

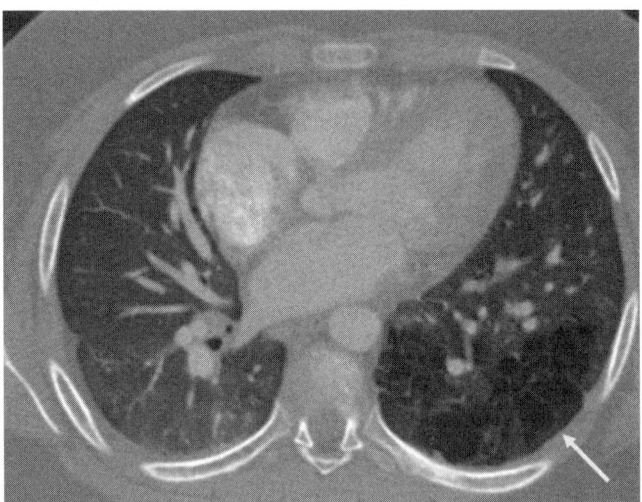

Figure 7-11. A computed tomography scan of congenital pulmonary airway malformation (arrow).

Bronchogenic Cysts

A bronchogenic cyst is usually an incidental finding of a chest radiograph and is in the differential diagnosis of a mediastinal mass. Both CT scan and MRI help to differentiate, but the MRI is more specific. The cyst contains fluid of water density but on occasions the mass is of soft-tissue density, which makes differentiation from lymph nodes or other solid lesions more difficult. The cyst is derived from the foregut and is typically in the aortopulmonary window. More than 65% are mediastinal; when located in the lung parenchyma they are usually in the lower lobes. Bronchogenic cysts can be asymptomatic or present due to superimposed infection simulating a lung abscess.

Pulmonary Sequestration

Pulmonary sequestration is defined as a segment of lung tissue that is separate from the tracheobronchial tree and receives its blood supply from a systemic artery rather than from the pulmonary artery.[35,36] There are 2 types of pulmonary sequestration: intralobar and extralobar (Table 7-2).

Table 7-2. Characteristics of Intralobar and Extralobar Pulmonary Sequestration

Characteristic	Intralobar	Extralobar
Frequency	~75%	~25%
Location	Posterior basal Left>right—2:1	Between lower lobe and diaphragm, also within the diaphragm, lung, hilum, mediastinum, retroperitoneum, upper abdomen, etc Left>right
Arterial supply	Descending thoracic aorta, upper abdominal aorta, splenic or celiac arteries	Aorta, less commonly from splenic, gastric subclavian, intercostals or pulmonary arteries
Venous drainage	>80% to left atrium	Systemic
Chest radiograph	- Normal - Post-obstructive hyperinflation (ventilated by collateral channels) - Mucoid impaction surrounded by hyperinflated lung - Solid mass, if infected	Usually presents as a solid mass since it rarely connects to bronchi
Visceral pleura	Within it	Separated visceral pleura
Bronchial communication	Often present	Sometimes present

Since pulmonary sequestration may present as a consolidation, a history of repeated pneumonias in the same location should raise the suspicion of possible intralobar sequestration.

Computed tomography is a useful method for measuring the volume of pulmonary sequestration.

Dysmorphic Lung Syndrome

Dysmorphic lung syndrome, which includes scimitar syndrome, is characterized by arrested development of either a whole lung (lung-agenesis-hypoplasia complex) or a lobe (lobar agenesis-aplasia complex). Absence of a lobe may be associated with other abnormalities.

Three forms of lobar agenesis have been described: pulmonary agenesis, aplasia, and hypoplasia. Although complete agenesis of a lung has been reported to be twice as common on the left side as it is on the right, in general hypogenetic lung is considered to be almost exclusively on the right (Figure 7-12).

Hypogenetic lung is part of the congenital pulmonary venolobar syndrome, of which major components include hypogenetic lung, partial anomalous pulmonary venous return, absence of a pulmonary artery, pulmonary sequestration, systemic arterialization of the lung, absence of the inferior vena cava, and accessory diaphragm.[37]

Absence of Main Pulmonary Artery

In a child with absence of main pulmonary artery the peripheral pulmonary arteries are usually intact and supplied by systemic collateral circulation, which most often arises from the bronchial arteries. It is more common on the right side. On imaging, the lung and hilum are small; the pulmonary vascularity is decreased rendering a radiolucent lung. Serrated pleural thickening with subpleural bands may represent the systemic collateral vessels.

Pulmonary Arteriovenous Malformation

Pulmonary arteriovenous malformations can be solitary or multiple, as in children with hereditary hemorrhagic telangiectasia or Rendu-Osler-Weber disease. The lesions tend to be recognized with increased age, since time is needed for the flow effects to manifest.

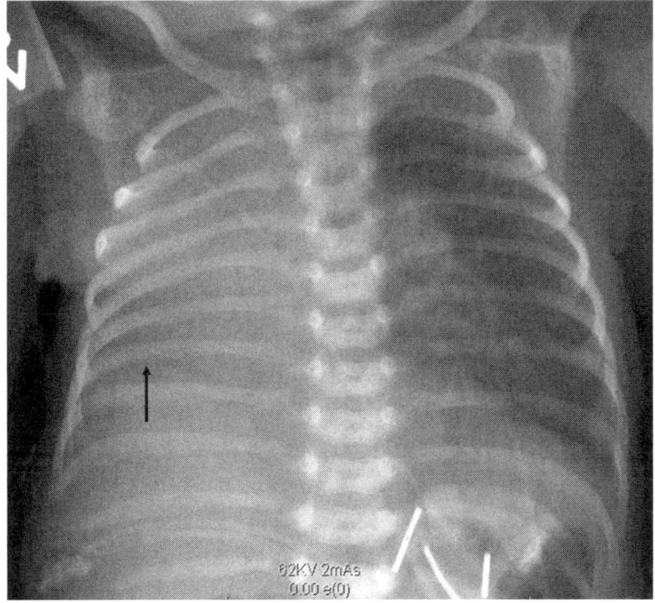

Figure 7-12A. Note the right lung volume loss with mediastinal shift to the right and crowded ribs. Arrow points to the hemidiaphragm, which is still visible due to some aerated lung a the base.

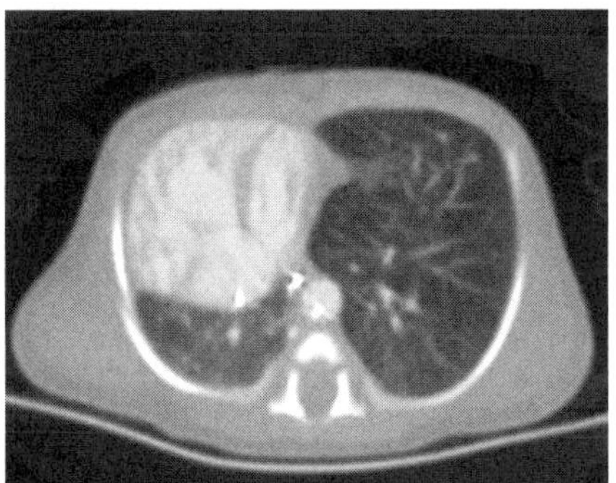

Figure 7-12B. Computed tomography scan showing hypoplastic right lung posterior to the heart.

Pneumonia

Chest radiographs should not be performed routinely in the outpatient management of children suspected of having pneumonia. Radiologic findings are accepted as the reference standard for defining pneumonia, but it is not clear to what extent chest radiographs alter the outcome of childhood pneumonia even though they frequently are used to confirm the presence, site, and extent of pulmonary infiltrates.[38] Besides, Swingler et al[39] also observed that having a chest radiograph significantly increased the likelihood of being prescribed antibiotics. Accepted clinical indications for chest radiography are severe disease, confirmation of nonspecific clinical findings, as well as assessment of complications and exclusion of other thoracic causes of respiratory symptoms.[40]

Computed tomography is not indicated in uncomplicated pneumonia. Computed tomography provides more information than plain radiographs for complicated pneumonias and for assessment prior to procedures. In immunocompromised and hospitalized patients, CT has higher accuracy than plain radiographs detecting early fungal and *Pneumocystis jiroveci* pneumonia.

Ultrasound has an advantage over CT in identification, characterization, and management decisions of complicated effusions. Ultrasound also has an established role in the imaging-guided drainage of pleural fluid. The decision of whether a fluid collection needs to be drained or not is clinical and is indicated if the collections are increasing in size or respiratory function is compromised.[41] If thrombolytic therapy is contemplated, a CT should be considered if there is a suspicion of a bronchopleural fistula. The presence of a fistula is a contraindication to thrombolytic therapy.

Round Pneumonia

Round pneumonia occurs in children younger than 8 years because young children have poorly developed pathways of collateral ventilation (eg, pores of Kohn, channels of Lambert), more closely apposed connective tissue septae, and smaller alveoli than adolescents and adults[42] (Figure 7-13A–B). Round pneumonias clinically present with cough, tachypnea, and malaise followed by an acute febrile illness. Round pneumonias on chest radiographs characteristically are located posteriorly in the lower lobes and touching the pleura or a fissure.

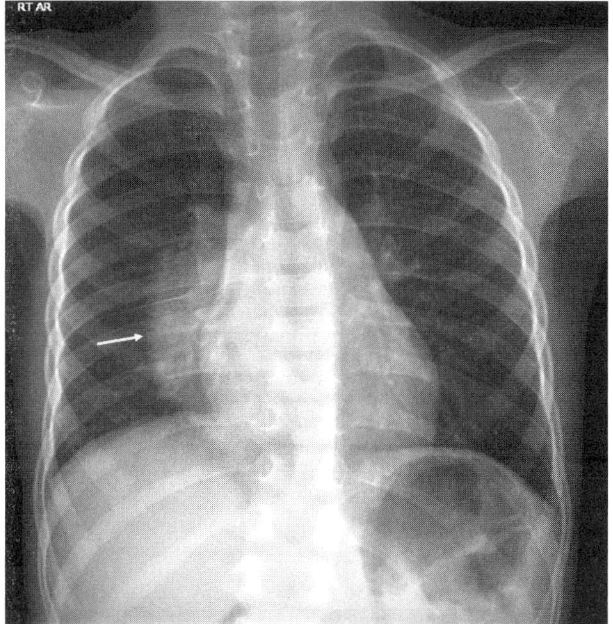

Figure 7-13A. Round pneumonia in right lower lobe, note negative silhouette sign (right heart border visible) and horizontal fissure parallel to the arrow.

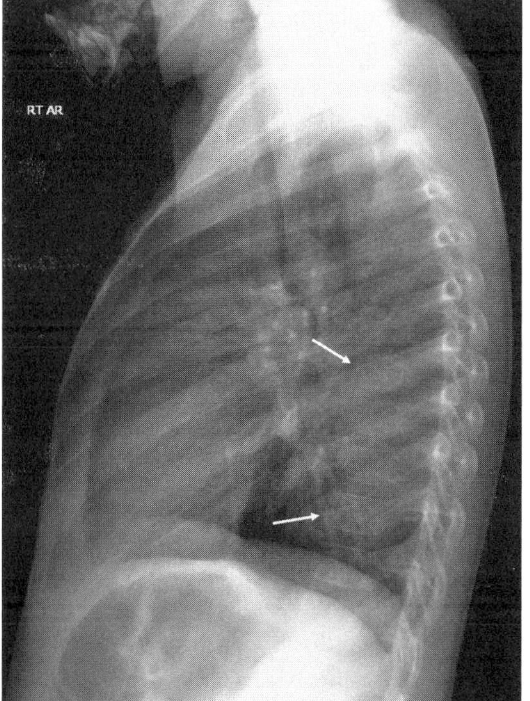

Figure 7-13B. Lateral view of Figure 13A. The arrows delineate the edges of the round pneumonia.

Satellite lesions are not seen in children, while in adults, satellite lesions are found in more than 50% of round pneumonias.[43] In a child younger than 8 years with the typical clinical findings of a pneumonia and a typical radiographic appearance, the diagnosis is almost always a round pneumonia. Round pneumonias are diagnosed on radiographs and, if all the criteria are met, a follow-up chest radiograph to ensure resolution is all that is needed.

Aspiration

Aspiration is of great concern in children because of the frequency with which they place foreign objects in their mouths or noses, and the frequency that young children choke on food items. The most common organic aspirated foreign bodies include peanuts, seeds and nuts, blades of grass, or bone fragments. The most common inorganic bodies are plastic objects (toy fragments, pen caps, dental prostheses) or metallic objects (hairpins, pins, steel filaments). A chest radiograph is the first imaging study performed when aspiration is suspected.[44] Because less than 10% of aspirated foreign bodies are radiopaque, the inhaled object is usually not visible, but indirect findings may assist in supporting the diagnosis. Radiologic findings in the event of an acute aspiration include hyperinflation, air trapping, regional oligemia, atelectasis, or consolidation. The airway is usually either unobstructed or partially obstructed during inspiration but completely obstructed during expiration because the physiological expiratory decrease in bronchial diameter results in air trapping. To improve the accuracy of radiographs, inspiratory and expiratory views in cooperative children may be ordered, and lateral decubitus radiographs may be ordered in younger children (Figure 7-14A–B).[44] However, radiographs are still negative in up to 30% of cases of aspiration.

Multidetector CT is more accurate than chest radiography in detecting radiolucent foreign bodies, and it is suggested in patients with a low clinical suspicion of foreign body aspiration in whom chest radiography is negative.[45] Multidetector CT, as opposed to single slice CT, allows rapid acquisition of volumetric data sets, essential to reduce radiation exposure in children and to avoid sedation. Multidetector CT also has been recommended for children post-bronchoscopy where residual foreign bodies are suspected. Although this is a relatively uncommon complication, retained foreign bodies are described in 1% to 18% of cases. Computed tomography in these children can offer a description

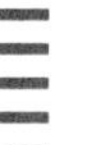

of the pattern of residual obstruction, which would help in future decisions as to whether repeat bronchoscopy is indicated or not.[45]

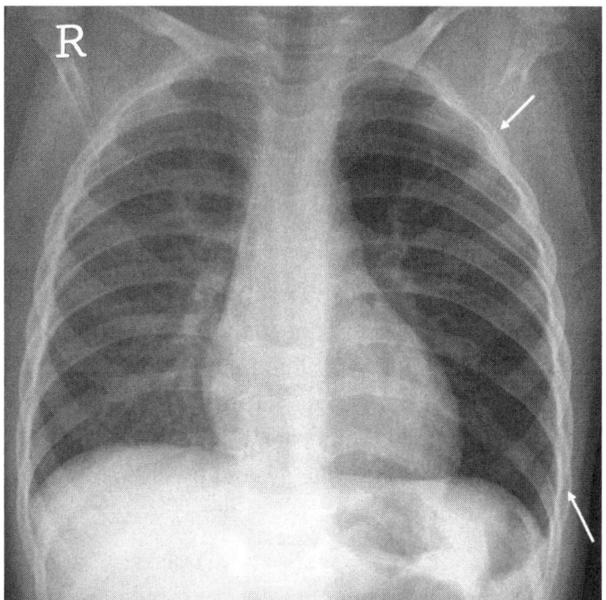

Figure 7-14A. Foreign body aspiration. Left lateral decubitus view with persistent expansion of left lung (white arrows).

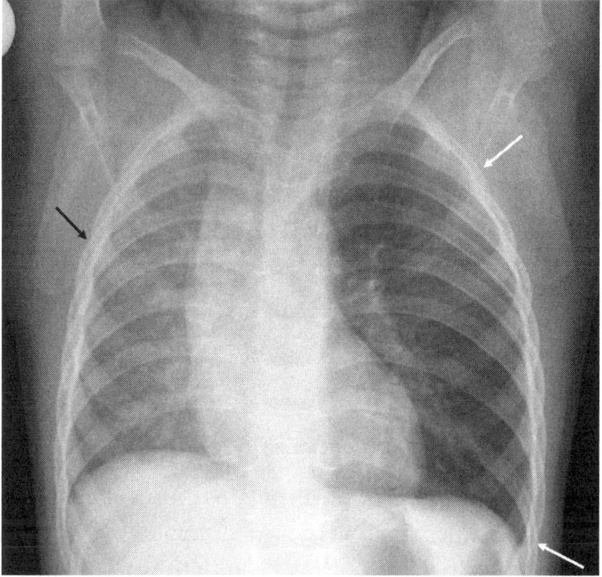

Figure 7-14B. Foreign body aspiration. Right lung normally deflates while on right lateral decubitus (black arrow).

Complications of Pneumonia

Pleural Effusion

The chest radiograph may show pneumonia before the effusion is evident. The earliest sign is blunting of the costophrenic angle. This will be evident on an erect radiograph but not on a supine radiograph. A lateral decubitus radiograph with the affected side down may be helpful in showing small amounts of fluid. If fluid does not shift with a lateral decubitus radiograph it implies loculation of the fluid. If there is an air-fluid level, there is both an effusion and pneumothorax, which is called hydropneumothorax. The presence of a hydropneumothorax in the absence of a recent intervention is suggestive of a bronchopleural fistula. Empyemas on chest radiographs, due to the intra-pleural location, tend to have obtuse angles superiorly and inferiorly on the frontal view. On the lateral view, a distinguishing feature from pulmonary abscess is the decrease in diameter when compared with the frontal view. Lung abscesses tend to have the same AP and transverse diameter on both frontal and lateral views.

Ultrasonography is the best imaging modality to characterize pleural fluid. It can detect fluid before it is evident on the chest radiograph and can easily distinguish between free and loculated fluid. Pleural effusions on ultrasound are classified as simple or complex. Simple effusions are anechoic or black and in most cases represent a transudate. Complex effusions indicate an exudate. Features that make an effusion complex include internal septations, debris, honeycombing, and pleural thickening, all of which are easily depicted on ultrasound.[9] Ultrasound may also be helpful in defining the best site for thoracocentesis and the need for intrapleural fibrinolysis or video-assisted thoracoscopic surgery (Figure 7-15A–B).

Computed tomography scan is not more helpful than ultrasonography in defining the pleural effusion but does have a place in detecting abnormalities in the lung parenchyma.

Lung Abscess

A lung abscess is a thick-walled cavity that contains purulent material as a result of a pulmonary infection that has led to suppurative necrosis of the involved lung parenchyma. Lung abscesses in the early stages present as a consolidation; however, unlike necrotizing pneumonia, abscesses tend to be spherical and well defined, and the diagnosis is

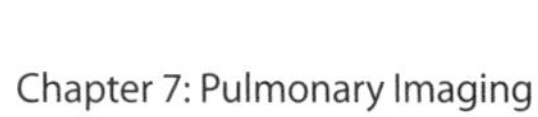

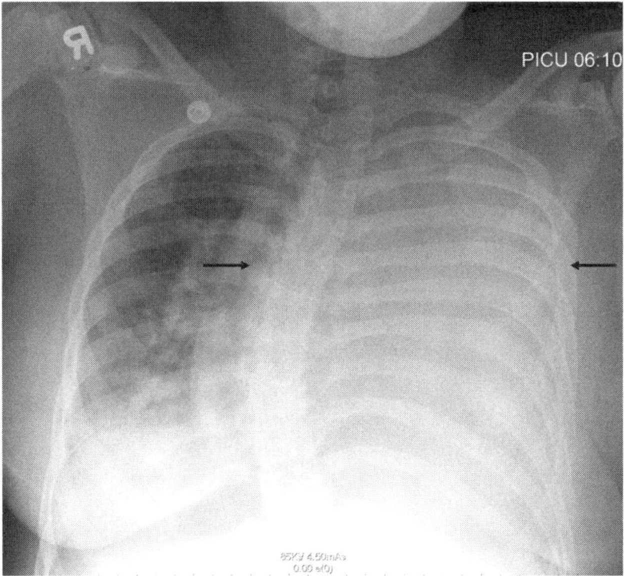

Figure 7-15A. Complicated effusion. Note left arrow shows displaced trachea.

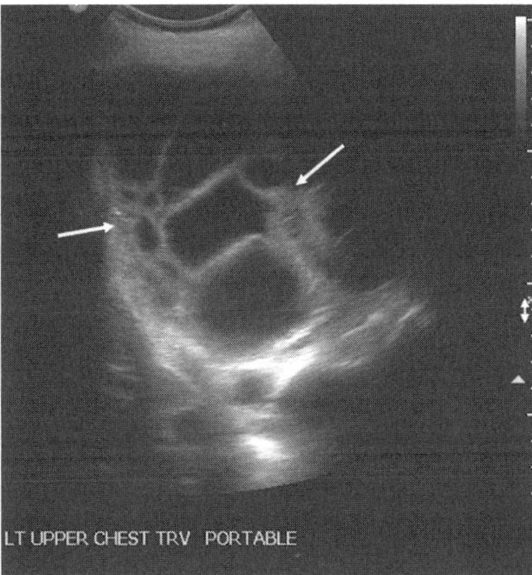

Figure 7-15B. Ultrasound showing septations in effusion.

more obvious when there is a connection between the abscess and draining bronchus, as an air-fluid level will be present. The air-fluid level will only be evident on a lateral decubitus or erect radiograph.[46] The presence of an air-fluid level is not pathognomonic of an abscess, as it can be seen in developmental lung malformations or pneumatoceles with superimposed infection, cavitary pneumonia, cavitating septic emboli, Wegener granulomatosis, and other conditions. To distinguish a lung abscess from other conditions, a contrast CT scan of the chest is the imaging modality of choice[47] (Figure 7-16).

Lung abscess caused by aspiration typically is located in the posterior segments of the upper lobes or superior segments of the lower lobes. When located in the subpleural location, lung abscesses and any consolidation can be identified on ultrasound. In this location, ultrasound can be used as a guiding tool for percutaneous drainage.

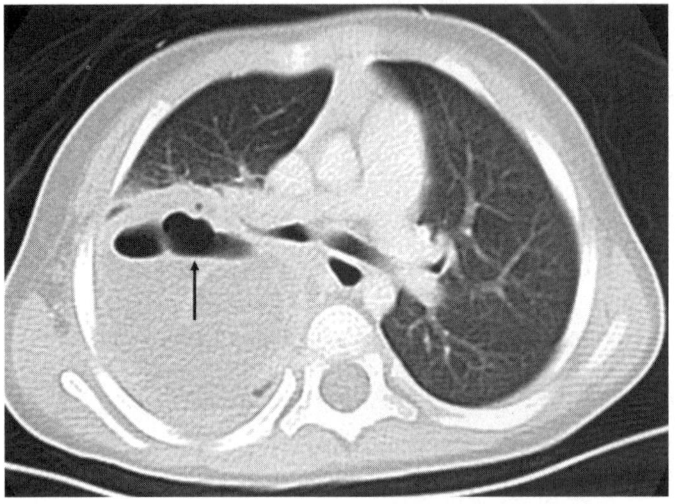

Figure 7-16. A computed tomography scan showing lung abscess with fluid level (arrow).

Necrotizing Pneumonia

Necrotizing pneumonia is a complication of severe pneumonia that demonstrates cavities in the area of pneumonic consolidation due to tissue necrosis. The chest radiograph may show the cavities, but a significant number of children who have CT findings of cavities have no evidence of necrosis on plain radiograph. If the cavity contains air, the chest radiograph may show the cavity, but if it is fluid-filled the plain radiograph may only show consolidation. Different than a pulmonary abscess, the cavities of a necrotizing pneumonia tend to be multiple, tubular or round, and more irregular. In addition, the borders of the consolidation are less distinct. Air bronchogram can be present (Figure 7-17A–C).

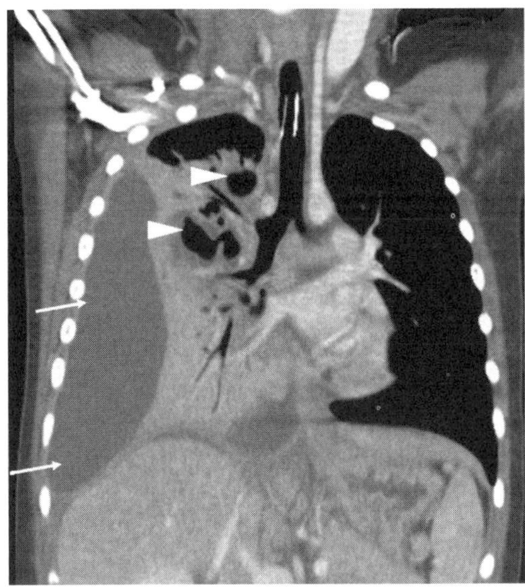

Figure 7-17A. Coronal computed tomography scan showing necrotizing pneumonia. Small arrows show pleural effusion, large arrows point to cavities.

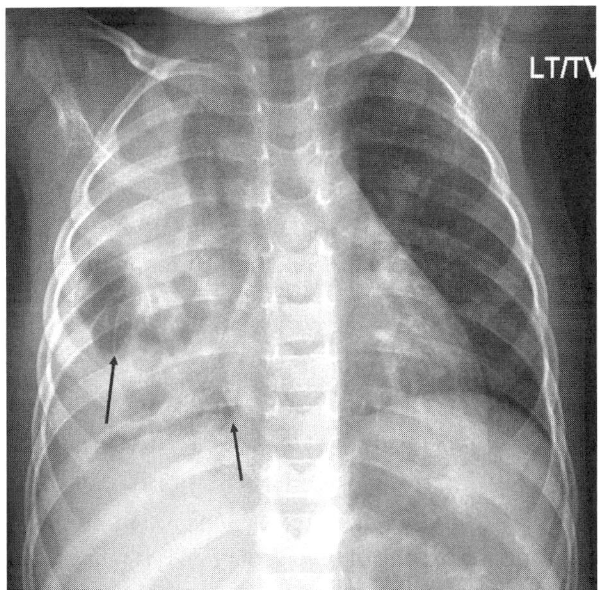

Figure 7-17B. Plain radiograph of necrotizing pneumonia, suggestive of bronchopleural fistula (arrows point to cavitation-necrosis).

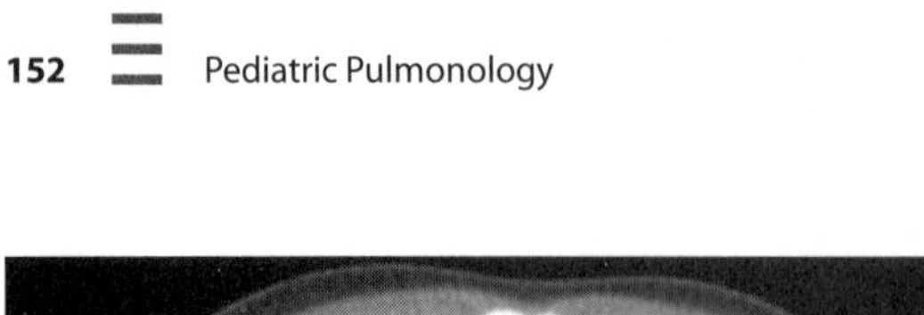

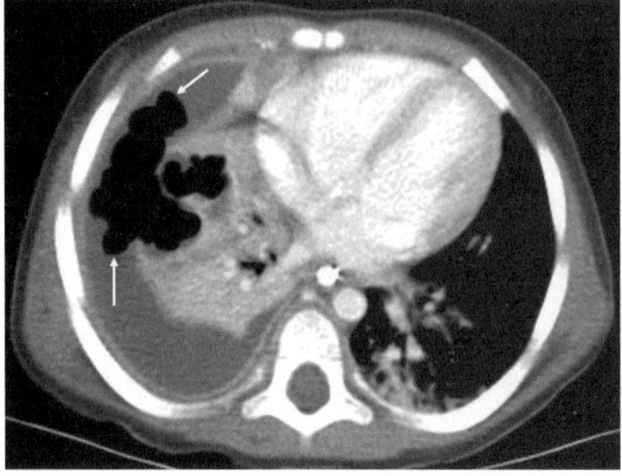

Figure 7-17C. A computed tomography scan of necrotizing pneumonia confirming bronchopleural fistula.

Tuberculosis

Primary Pulmonary TB

The radiographic findings in primary TB are nonspecific. The plain radiograph may be normal, but more commonly there is an area of segmental or lobar consolidation with hilar adenopathy in the adjacent area. Hilar adenopathy is an important finding because it is unusual to see lymphadenopathy in post-primary TB. The lung opacity of primary TB tends to become smaller over time, calcify, and be apparent as a calcified granuloma.

Airway involvement is common in primary TB, and airway compression by the lymphadenopathy may result in atelectasis. This may result in consolidation of the right upper or middle lobe. One of the life-threatening presentations of TB is miliary TB, most common in neonates. It presents as small nodules (usually <2 mm) with uniform distribution in the lungs.

Postprimary Pulmonary TB

Pleural effusion is an important presentation of post-primary TB in adolescents. Miliary TB results from hematogenous spread so that there are diffuse, small (1–2 mm) nodules scattered throughout the lung fields. The characteristic finding of post-primary TB is upper lobe consolidation with cavitation. The findings are usually evident on chest radiography, but CT scan is useful to define the extent of disease, in particular the degree of cavitation.

Pulmonary Non-TB Mycobacterium

The radiologic findings of non-TB mycobacterium (NTM) are nonspecific and similar to TB, fungal infections, and other granulomatous processes. The typical imaging features are

- Multiple small nodules
- Multilobe bronchiectasis
- Tree-in-bud (see above)
- Progressive fibrosis

Most children with pulmonary NTM are those with HIV infection or CF.

Systemic Lupus Erythematosus (SLE)

Pleural effusion is the most common manifestation of SLE, and the effusions are typically small. There may be an associated pericardial effusion. The greatest pulmonary imaging challenge in children with SLE is differentiating pneumonia, pulmonary hemorrhage, and lupus pneumonitis. Computed tomography findings with lung disease, either pneumonia or lupus pneumonitis, include patchy consolidation, especially in the lower lobes, often with a pleural effusion. Lupus pneumonitis has the potential to develop into chronic interstitial pneumonitis with irreversible lung disease and pulmonary fibrosis. Acute alveolitis, recognized by ground-glass appearance, has the potential to be improved by steroids and should be treated promptly to prevent chronic changes.

Interstitial Lung Disease (ILD)

Chest radiography is the usual imaging modality to diagnose children with ILD. It is not specific and therefore usually requires additional imaging studies, especially HRCT scan. The plain chest image may reveal characteristic patterns, including ground-glass opacities, reticular or nodular opacities, and honeycombing. The 3 patterns are consistent with the extent of the disease so that ground-glass opacities are seen with active alveolitis, and honeycombing with advanced disease. The findings are often described as interstitial even though the pathology is primarily alveolar.

High-resolution CT is better than chest radiography at defining the extent of pulmonary disease, and tree-in-bud and patterns of differential aeration may be evident.

Cystic Fibrosis

Chest radiography is not important in diagnosing CF but does allow longitudinal assessment of the progression of pulmonary disease. The findings of CF clearly overlap with other disorders of chronic lung disease. Despite this, the presence of bronchiectasis of unknown etiology is an indication to evaluate the patient for CF. The usefulness of the chest radiograph during an exacerbation of CF is unclear. In this situation the advantage of the chest radiograph is to exclude a pneumothorax, pneumonia, or atelectasis.

More recently the use of CT scan to evaluate inflammation and early lung damage has been confirmed. High-resolution CT scanning allows demonstration of mucus plugging and bronchiectasis to the fifth or sixth generation of bronchi.

Bronchial arteriography is the preferred technique to evaluate major hemoptysis, and the technique is to view all of the bronchial vessels in preparation for embolization. The vessels that are bleeding may not be identified so that all vessels should be embolized, because if only the bleeding vessels are embolized other non-embolized vessels will likely bleed at a later date.

The most widely used scoring system in the United States is the Brasfield system, also called the Birmingham system, that was developed in 1979.[48] Five elements are evaluated as shown in Table 7-3. Scoring of the first 4 elements is 0 to 4, with zero being normal, and the points are subtracted from 25, so that 25 is without abnormality and 3 is the most severe.

There have been several additional scoring systems that have been reviewed and attempts made to provide radiologic and clinical correlation. One of the reasons for deriving scores is to reduce interobserver differences and permit longitudinal following of the clinical course.

Computed tomography findings of CF include air trapping, early evidence of airway inflammation, or bronchiectasis. Mucus plugging, centrilobular nodules, and peribronchial thickening are potentially reversible findings in symptomatic patients. Because children are more sensitive to radiation-induced cancer than adults, special care should be taken, particularly when multiple radiologic examinations in a lifetime will be needed. Computed tomography is used to assess the following conditions:

- Allergic bronchopulmonary aspergillosis
- Atypical mycobacterial infection
- Unexplained clinical deterioration
- Pulmonary embolism
- Severe hemoptysis
- Sinus disease

Table 7-3. Components of Brasfield Score

Category	Definition	Scoring
I. Air trapping	Generalized pulmonary overdistention as sternal bowing, depression of the diaphragm, and/or thoracic kyphosis	0 = absent; 1–4 for increasing severity (4, most severe)
II. Linear markings	Line densities due to prominence of bronchi as parallel line densities, sometimes branching, or as end-on circular densities with thickening of bronchial wall	0 = absent; 1–4 for increasing severity (4, most severe)
III. Nodular cystic lesions	Multiple, discrete, small, rounded densities, ≥0.5, with either radiopaque or radiolucent centers (does not refer to irregular linear markings); confluent nodules not classified as large lesions	0 = absent; 1, 2, 3, or 4 for involvement of 1, 2, 3, or 4 quadrants
IV. Large lesions	Segmental or lobar atelectasis or consolidation; includes acute pneumonia	0 = absent; 3 if segmental or lobar; 5 if large
V. General severity	Impression of overall severity of changes on radiograph	0 = normal; 1–4 for increasing severity of abnormalities; only cardiac enlargement or pneumothorax require 5
Total possible score		25

Mediastinal Masses

The location of medistinal masses in children is shown in Box 7-3.

Anterior Mediastinal Masses

Anterior mediastinal masses represent more than 40% of mediastinal masses, with most of them arising from the thymus or mediastinal lymph nodes.

Thymus

There is extensive variability in the configuration and radiographic appearance of thymic tissue, including the possibility of presenting in an ectopic location. It can usually be recognized in chest radiography: microlobulated borders, ability to see the normal pulmonary architecture through it, and absence of mass effect. If the diagnosis remains uncertain, CT or MRI can aid in its recognition.

The thymus can change in shape and size within hours. An external stimulus, commonly seen in hospitalized patients, can dramatically reduce the size of the thymus. Likewise, thymic rebound represents enlargement/hyperplasia of the thymus in response to withdrawal of myelosuppressive therapy. It typically occurs 6 to 12 months after suspension of therapy, but cases as early as 1 week were described.[49]

Lymphoma

Lymphoma (Hodgkin's and non-Hodgkin's) is the most common true anterior mediastinal mass in children. Mediastinal lymphoma appears

Box 7-3. Location and Types of Mediastinal Masses

Anterior Mediastinum (about 40%)
- Thymus
- Lymphoma
- Germ cell tumor

Middle Mediastinum (about 20%)
- Bronchogenic cyst
- Enteric and neurenteric cyst
- Lymphadenopathy mediastinal
- Pericardial cyst

Posterior Mediastinum (34%)
- Neurogenic mass: neuroblastoma
- Ganglioneuroblastoma, ganglioneuroma
- Schwannoma, neurofibroma

as a hypoattenuating lobulated non-homogeneous mediastinal soft tissue mass. Hilar lymphadenopathy is associated with Hodgkin's lymphoma. In Hodgkin's lymphoma, bulky mediastinal disease has a worse prognosis than in cases where there is a small tumor volume. In non-Hodgkin's lymphoma, tumor bulk does not appear to influence outcome.

Positron emission tomography (PET)/CT is a valuable tool for the initial staging to monitor interim treatment response and assessment of complete response to treatment. Substantial evidence supports that the addition of PET scanning to current staging investigations in lymphoma increases the accuracy of staging and results in change in management.

An International Harmonization Project released consensus recommendations in 2007 to standardize clinical trial parameters for the use of PET. At initial staging, CT should be performed either alone or in combination with PET/CT. Most commonly the latter is preferred to reduce the amount of radiation delivered. If hepatic or splenic disease is also present, then IV contrast should be given to improve the assessment.

Germ Cell Tumors

Germ cell tumors account for up to 20% of anterior mediastinal masses in children. A definite diagnosis of germ cell tumor can be made when the characteristic CT or MRI findings of a complex mass with cystic and solid areas containing fat and irregular calcifications are observed.

Middle Mediastinal Masses

Middle mediastinal masses account for about 20% of mediastinal masses. Foregut duplication cysts include bronchogenic, enteric, and neurenteric cysts, which are developmental malformations of the embryonic foregut. Computed tomography or MRI can be used to confirm diagnosis and characterize the mass. These masses are relatively well marginated, round, or oval with homogeneous water or soft tissue attenuation/signal intensity (due to proteinaceous material) without internal contrast enhancement.[49]

The extension of lymphoma into the middle mediastinum is common. Other causes of lymphadenopathy include metastatic disease, infection/inflammation from granulomatous diseases, or Langerhans cell histiocytosis.

Posterior Mediastinal Masses

Posterior mediastinal masses account for 34% of mediastinal masses. Most (~90%) are neurogenic in origin.[49] Most of the neurogenic masses arise from ganglion cells in the paravertebral sympathetic chain, including neuroblastoma, ganglioneuroblastoma, and ganglioneuroma. The remaining masses are nerve sheath tumors, such as schwannoma and neurofibroma. Chest radiography finds a well circumscribed posterior mediastinal mass with calcifications or adjacent bone erosion (Figure 7-18). Differentiation among the tumor types cannot be done by imaging, and biopsy is needed. Evaluation of the extent of disease, particularly looking for intra-spinal extension, should be performed, and MRI is the modality of choice (Figure 7-19).

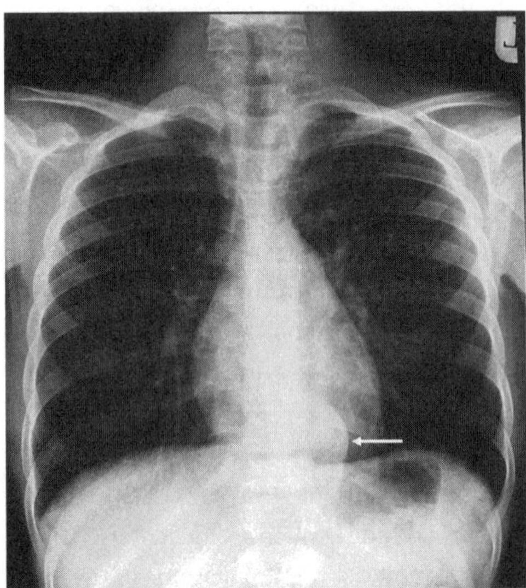

Figure 7-18. Posterior mediastinal mass (arrow) with diaphragm and right heart border visible.

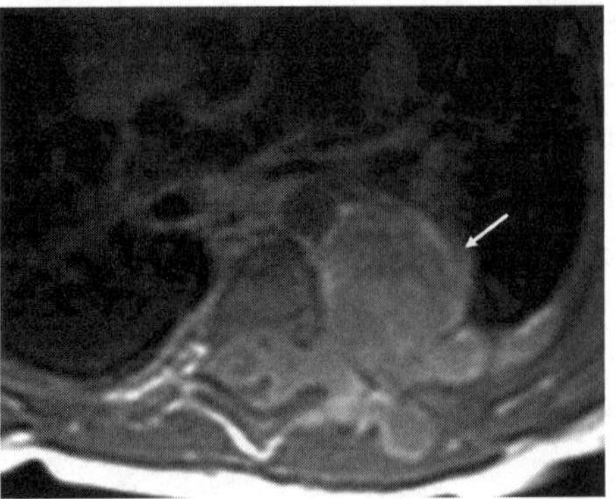

Figure 7-19. Magnetic resonance imaging showing ganglioneuroma.

References

1. Sidhu M, Goske MJ, Connolly B, et al. Image gently, step lightly: promoting radiation safety in pediatric interventional radiology. *Am J Roentgenol.* 2010;195:W299–W301
2. Mettler FA, Huda W, Yoshizumi T, Mahadevappa, M. Effective doses in radiology and diagnostic nuclear medicine: a catalog. *Radiology.* 2008;248:254–263
3. Huda W. Radiation doses and risks in chest computed tomography examinations. *Proc Am Thorac Soc.* 2007;4(4):316–320
4. O'Connor OJ, Vandeleur M, McGarrigle AM, et al. Development of low-dose protocols for thin-section CT assessment of cystic fibrosis in pediatric patients. *Radiology.* 2010;257(3):820–829
5. Heyer CM, Nuesslein TG, Jung D, et al. Tracheobronchial anomalies and stenoses: detection with low-dose multidetector CT with virtual tracheo-bronchoscopy—comparison with flexible tracheobronchoscopy. *Radiology.* 2007;242:542–549
6. Lee EY, Boiselle PM, Cleveland RH. Multidetector CT evaluation of congenital lung anomalies. *Radiology.* 2008;247:632–648
7. Lee EY, Siegel MJ. Pediatric airways disorders: large airways. In: Boiselle PM, Lynch DA, eds. *CT of the Airways.* Totowa, NJ: Humana; 2008:351–380
8. Knisely BL, Broderick LS, Kuhlman JE. MR imaging of the pleura and chest wall. *Magn Reson Imaging Clin N Am.* 2000;8(1):125–141
9. Kim OH, Kim WS, Kim MJ, Jung JY, Suh JH. US in the diagnosis of pediatric chest diseases. *Radiographics.* 2000;20(3):653–671
10. Coley BD. Pediatric chest ultrasound. *Radiol Clin N Am.* 2005;43:405–418
11. Felson B, Felson H. Localization of intrathoracic lesions by means of the postero-anterior roentgenogram; the silhouette sign. *Radiology.* 1950;55(3):363–374
12. Hansell DM, Bankier AA, MacMahon H, McLoud TC, Müller NL, Remy J. Fleischner Society: glossary of terms for thoracic imaging. *Radiology.* 2008;246(3):697–722
13. Remy-Jardin M, Remy J, Giraud F, Wattinne L, Gosselin B. Computed tomography assessment of ground glass opacity: semiology and significance. *J Thorac Imaging.* 1993;8(4):249–264
14. Quigley MJ, Fraser RS. Pulmonary pneumatocele: pathology and pathogenesis. *AJR Am J Roentgenol.* 1988;150(6):1275–1257
15. Field CE. Bronchiectasis in childhood. I. Clinical survey of 160 cases. *Pediatrics.* 1949;4:21–46
16. Habermann TM. *Mayo Clinic Internal Medicine Review, 2006–2007.* 7th ed. Rochester, MN: Mayo Clinic Scientific Press. 2006:851
17. Garcia-Peña P, Lucaya J. HRCT in children: technique and indications. *Eur Radiol.* 2004;14:L13–L30
18. Hansell DM. Thin-section CT of the lungs: the hinterland of normal. *Radiology.* 2010;256:695–711

19. Rossi SE, Franquet T, Volpacchio M, Giménez A, Aguilar G. Tree-in-bud pattern at thin-section CT of the lungs: radiologic-pathologic overview. *Radiographics.* 2005;25(3):789–801
20. Franquet T, Muller N, Gimenez A, Guembe P, de la Torre J, Bague S. Spectrum of pulmonary aspergillosis: histologic, clinical and radiologic findings. *Radiographics.* 2001;21:825–837
21. Flors L, Domingo ML, Leiva-Salinas C, Mazón M, Roselló-Sastre E, Vilar J. Uncommon occupational lung diseases: high-resolution CT findings. *AJR Am J Roentgenol.* 2010;194:W20–W26
22. Silva CI, Müller NL, Lynch DA, et al. Chronic hypersensitivity pneumonitis: differentiation from idiopathic pulmonary fibrosis and nonspecific interstitial pneumonia by using thin-section CT. *Radiology.* 2008;246(1):288–297
23. Daimon T, Johkoh T, Sumikawa H, et al. Acute eosinophilic pneumonia: thin-section CT findings in 29 patients. *Eur J Radiol.* 2008;65:462–467
24. Jung Eun Cheon JE, Lee KS, Jung GS, Chung MH, Cho YD. Acute eosinophilic pneumonia: radiographic and CT findings in six patients. *AJR Am J Roentgenol.* 1996;167:1195–1199
25. Marchand E, Cordier JF. Idiopathic chronic eosinophilic pneumonia. *Orphanet J Rare Dis.* 2006;1:11
26. Spottswood SE, Allison KZ, Lopatina OA, et al. The clinical significance of lung hypoexpansion in acute childhood asthma. *Pediatr Radiol.* 2004;34(4):322–325
27. Woodring JH, Reed JC. Types and mechanisms of pulmonary atelectasis. *J Thorac Imaging.* 1996;11(2):92–108
28. Caceres M, Ali SZ, Braud R, Weiman D, Garrett E. Spontaneous pneumomediastinum: a comparative study and review of the literature. *Ann Thoracic Surg.* 2008;86:962–966
29. de Blic J, Scheinmann P. The use of imaging techniques for assessing severe childhood asthma. *J Allergy Clin Immunol.* 2007;119(4):808–810
30. Aysola RS, Hoffman EZ, Gierada D, et al. Airway remodeling measured by multidetector CT is increased in severe asthma and correlates with pathology. *Chest.* 2008;134;1183–1191
31. Subramanyan R, Venugopalan P, Narayan R. Vascular rings: an important cause of persistent respiratory symptoms in infants and children. *Indian Pediatr.* 2003;40:951–957
32. Browne LP. What is the optimal imaging for vascular rings and slings? *Pediatr Radiol.* 2009;39(2):S191–S195
33. Newman B. Congenital bronchopulmonary foregut malformations: concepts and controversies. *Pediatr Radiol.* 2006;36:773–791
34. Panicek DM, Heitzman ER, Randall PA, et al. The continuum of pulmonary developmental anomalies. *Radiographics.* 1987;7:747–772
35. Yucel O, Gurkok S, Gozubuyuk A, et al. Diagnosis and surgical treatment of pulmonary sequestration. *Thorac Cardiovasc Surg.* 2008;56:154–157

36. Caradonna P, Bellia M, Cannizzaro F, et al. Non-invasive diagnosis in a case of bronchopulmonary sequestration and proposal of diagnostic algorithm. *Monaldi Arch Chest Dis.* 2008;69(3):137–141
37. Woodring JH, Howard TA, Kanga JF. Congenital pulmonary venolobar syndrome revisited. *Radiographics.* 1994;14:349–369
38. Ranganathan SC, Sonnappa S. Pneumonia and other respiratory infections. *Pediatr Clin North Am.* 2009;56:135–156
39. Swingler GH, Hussey GD, Zwarenstein M. Randomised controlled trial of clinical outcome after chest radiograph in ambulatory acute lower-respiratory infection in children. *Lancet.* 1998;351:404–408
40. Westra SJ, Choy G. What imaging should we perform for the diagnosis and management of pulmonary infections? *Pediatr Radiol.* 2009;39(2):S178–S183
41. Calder A, Owens CM. Imaging of parapneumonic pleural effusions and empyema in children. *Pediatr Radiol.* 2009;39:527–537
42. Kim YW, Donnelly LF. Round pneumonia: imaging findings in a large series of children. *Pediatr Radiol.* 2007;37:1235–1240
43. Restrepo R, Palani R, Matapathi UM, Wu YY. Imaging of round pneumonia and mimics in children. *Pediatr Radiol.* 2010;40(12):1931–1940
44. Pinto A, Scaglione M, Pinto F, et al. Tracheobronchial aspiration of foreign bodies: current indications for emergency plan chest radiography. *Radiol Med.* 2006;111:497–506
45. Kosucu P, Ahmetoglu A, Koramaz I, et al. Low-dose MDCT and virtual bronchoscopy in pediatric patients with foreign body aspiration. *AJR Am J Roentgenol.* 2004;183:1771–1777
46. Emanuel B, Shulman ST. Lung abscess in infants and children. *Clin Pediatr.* 1995;34:2–6
47. Patradoon-Ho P, Fitzgerald DA. Lung abscess in children. *Paediatr Respir Rev.* 2007;8(1):77–84
48. Brasfield D, Hicks G, Soong S, Tiller RE. The chest roentgenogram in cystic fibrosis: a new scoring system. *Pediatrics.* 1979;63(1):24–29
49. Lee EY. Evaluation of non-vascular mediastinal masses in infants and children: an evidence-based practical approach. *Pediatr Radiol.* 2009:39 (suppl 2):S184–S190

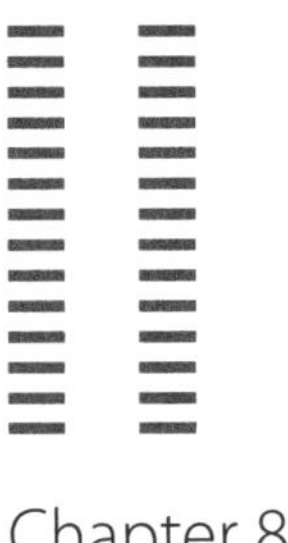

Chapter 8

Bronchoscopy

Samuel Goldfarb, MD
Howard B. Panitch, MD

Case Report 8-1

A 6-month-old infant was noted to have vibratory inspiratory stridor since he was 1 month old. He fed poorly and was observed to have gasping respiration, neck hyperextension, and intermittent upper airway obstruction during sleep. Flexible bronchoscopy under light sedation and with the head in neutral position demonstrated foreshortening of the aryepiglottic folds and prolapse of the arytenoid cartilages during inspiration, causing almost complete obstruction of the glottis. The dynamic airway events correlated with the infant's stridor and clinical airway obstruction. Evaluation of the rest of the airway to the level of the segmental bronchi was normal. A diagnosis of severe laryngomalacia was made. The infant was referred to an otolaryngologist who performed an aryepiglottoplasty, removing some redundant tissue from the arytenoid cartilages. The infant's stridor and obstructive sleep apnea markedly improved, as did his growth. By 12 months of age, his stridor resolved completely and both growth and development were normal.

Introduction

Until relatively recently, direct evaluation of a young child's airway required the skills of a surgeon versed in rigid (open tube) bronchoscopy, with the child under general anesthesia. Flexible bronchoscopy became routinely available in the United States in 1969, but use of the technique was restricted in children because of size limitations of the instruments. By 1980, a commercially available scope that was 3.5 mm in diameter with an integral suction channel and a tip that could be directed was being used to evaluate newborns.[1] With improvements in fiberoptic technology, thinner (eg, 2.8 mm) bronchoscopes could be made without sacrificing functionality or image quality. More recently, digital technology has been applied to bronchoscopic images, and a

3.8-mm pediatric bronchoscope with a video chip in the tip provides high-resolution digital images in an instrument that can be used in most newborns through adolescents. There are also ultrathin scopes ranging from 1.8 to 2.2 mm, but these have neither suction channels nor angulation capabilities, so their use is limited to evaluation of the trachea and proximal main bronchi in children with established artificial airways (endotracheal or tracheostomy tubes).

Choosing Between Flexible and Rigid Bronchoscopy

General Considerations

The flexible bronchoscope complements, but does not replace, the rigid bronchoscope. Each has strengths and weaknesses that must be considered when deciding a particular approach to a patient. Table 8-1 lists some of the relative advantages of each type of procedure. Flexible bronchoscopy is usually performed via a transnasal approach. This allows the head to be kept in a neutral position, and there is no distortion of upper airway structures as the bronchoscope follows the normal contour of the nasopharynx, oropharynx, and hypopharynx. Thus dynamic events that occur in this part of the airway can be

Table 8-1. Relative Advantages of Flexible and Rigid Bronchoscopy

Site/Procedure	Flexible	Rigid
Nasopharynx	++	−/+
Hypopharynx	++	+
Larynx	++	++
Laryngeal function	++	−
Subglottis	+/−	++
Trachea	++	++
Main bronchi	++	++
Lobar bronchi	++	+
Segmental/subsegmental bronchi	++	+/−
Foreign body	−	++
Bronchoalveolar lavage	++	+
Control of bleeding	−	++
Mucosal biopsy	++	++
Transbronchial biopsy	++	+

observed without altering tissue relationships. In contrast, direct laryngoscopy with a rigid bronchoscope or laryngoscope requires hyperextension of the neck and suspension of the base of the tongue for optimal visualization. In this situation, structures that cause noisy breathing could be elevated and the cause of airway obstruction missed.

The transnasal approach, however, causes the flexible bronchoscope to be angulated anteriorly as it approaches the glottis. While anterior structures of the glottis are easily examined, it is more difficult to obtain a thorough evaluation of the intra-arytenoid portion of the glottis, and posterior lesions might be missed. Thus if a lesion like a laryngoesophageal cleft is being considered, rigid bronchoscopy is the preferred technique. Similarly, the subglottic space is better evaluated using a rigid scope than a flexible one.

The flexible bronchoscope can be advanced more distally in the tracheobronchial tree, allowing for better peripheral evaluation of the airway. The diagnostic capabilities of flexible bronchoscopy are broadened when combined with techniques like bronchoalveolar lavage or bronchial brushing, and in select circumstances, transbronchial biopsy. All of these techniques are better accomplished with a flexible scope compared with a rigid one.

Foreign Body

When a retained foreign body in the airway is suspected, the procedure of choice is rigid bronchoscopy under general anesthesia. The rigid bronchoscope has a larger working channel than the flexible scope, allowing for a wide range of instruments specially designed for the safe retrieval of a foreign body. Furthermore, the child's airway and ventilation are carefully controlled, maximizing safety of the procedure. While there are reports of retrieval of a foreign body from the respiratory tract of young children by flexible bronchoscopy,[2] this approach should be the exception rather than the rule. If the presence of a retained foreign body is considered but not highly suspected, however, it is reasonable to perform flexible bronchoscopy as an initial procedure.[3] If a foreign body is in fact present, rigid bronchoscopy can subsequently be used to remove it. This approach can spare most children from general anesthesia and the cost of an operating room.

Hemoptysis and Pulmonary Hemorrhage

Bronchoscopy is occasionally performed in the evaluation and treatment of hemoptysis and pulmonary hemorrhage. When conducted as part of the evaluation of pulmonary bleeding, the procedure should occur after acute bleeding has subsided to maximize the diagnostic yield. If no bleeding site is immediately obvious, or if the diagnosis of pulmonary hemorrhage is uncertain, bronchoalveolar lavage can be performed to look for hemosiderin-laden macrophages. If, on the other hand, bronchoscopy is being entertained to help manage an episode of massive hemoptysis, the procedure of choice is rigid bronchoscopy. In this situation, control of the airway is paramount, and bleeding may be so brisk that visualization will be impaired unless large amounts of blood can be suctioned quickly. The large operating channel of the rigid scope permits such airway clearance, whereas the 1.2-mm channel of the pediatric bronchoscope cannot. If the area of bleeding can be identified, a Fogarty balloon-tipped catheter can be placed under direct visualization in the airway from which blood is emanating to isolate the source and protect other regions of the lung from being soiled.[4]

Indications for Bronchoscopy

Flexible bronchoscopy is used for diagnostic, therapeutic, and research purposes[5] (Box 8-1). It is commonly chosen to evaluate children with chronic stridor or wheezing and chronic or recurrent pulmonary densities, or to determine the cause of pneumonia in children with compromised immune function.[6–7] The procedure is also used in the evaluation of hemoptysis, recurrent aspiration, and chronic cough, and flexible bronchoscopy can be used to examine the airways of children with tracheostomies.

The most common indications for bronchoscopy are stridor or noisy breathing, followed in no particular order by chronic wheezing, atelectasis, and recurrent radiographic densities.[8–12] The frequency and distribution of indications vary by the characteristics of the programs that use bronchoscopy (eg, a program involved in lung transplantation will frequently evaluate patients for airway stenosis at the anastomosis site and perform transbronchial biopsies to assess for signs of rejection, whereas programs associated with large cardiac centers would commonly evaluate patients for airway compression associated with cardiac or pulmonary vascular enlargement).

Box 8-1. Indications for Bronchoscopy

- Noisy breathing
  - Stridor
  - Chronic wheezing (especially homophonous)
  - Voice disturbance (hoarse, decreased amplitude)
- Persistent moist cough
- Persistent radiographic abnormality
- Congenital anomaly
- Recurrent pneumonia
- Atelectasis
- Retained foreign body
- Hemoptysis
- Interstitial lung disease
- Pneumonia in an immunocompromised host
- Tracheostomy evaluation
- Post–lung transplantation evaluation

When the decision to use flexible bronchoscopy as a diagnostic modality is made, the yield is quite good, but varies depending on the indication for the procedure. For instance, Wood[12] found that an abnormality relevant to the primary indication for the procedure was present in 97% of subjects with stridor, but only 46% of those with chronic or recurrent pneumonia. When considering all indications for the procedure, findings related to the primary indication were present in 76% of the 1,000 procedures reviewed. Godfrey et al[10] found the diagnostic yield of bronchoscopy in children younger than 18 years to be 67% of the 200 consecutive procedures reviewed. The groups most likely to have relevant findings included those with noisy breathing (96.2%) and atelectasis (76%). The ability to make a diagnosis related to the indication for bronchoscopy can be enhanced with the addition of bronchoalveolar lavage or biopsy. When cytologic examination and bacterial or fungal culture results were added to findings on inspection, the incidence of clinically meaningful findings rose to 90.5%.[10]

Flexible bronchoscopy can be used therapeutically to remove mucus plugs that cause atelectasis (Figure 8-1), or to instill agents directly into the airway, like DNase in patients with persistent atelectasis[13] or

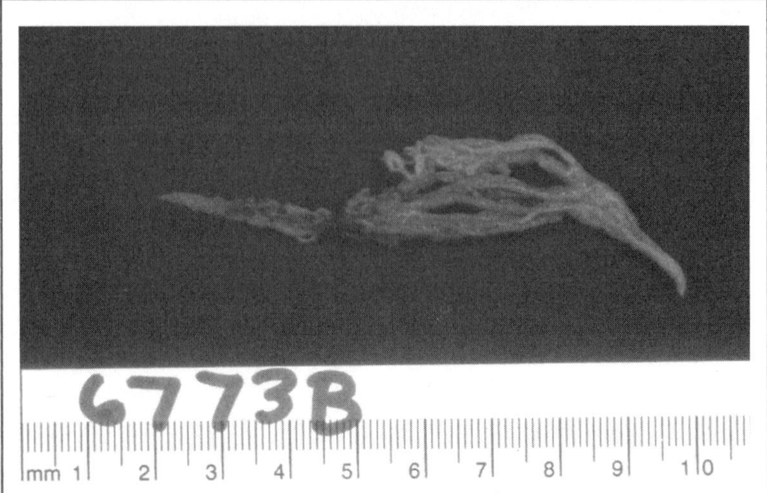

Figure 8-1. Cast of the right lower lobe bronchi removed from a patient with congenital heart disease and respiratory compromise.

surfactant in children with acute respiratory distress syndrome (ARDS).[14] Relief of atelectasis is more likely to occur when no air bronchograms are visible in the atelectatic region, suggesting the presence of a central mucus plug (Figure 8-2). In contrast, if air bronchograms are present (Figure 8-3), it is likely that there are multiple distal mucus plugs that will not be amenable to retrieval via bronchoscopy.

Bronchoscopy with bronchoalveolar lavage has been used as a research tool for evaluating early changes in the lungs of infants with cystic fibrosis.[15–17] Similarly, bronchoalveolar lavage and endobronchial biopsies are shedding new light on the pathophysiology of bronchiolitis and asthma in children.[18–19]

Contraindications for Bronchoscopy

It has been said that the only time bronchoscopy is truly contraindicated is when the information or therapeutic objective can be obtained in a less invasive fashion.[11] There are, however, relative contraindications for which the risk of the procedure must be balanced against the information or therapeutic benefit to be derived. Generally, an uncorrected bleeding diathesis like thrombocytopenia or clotting dysfunction, profound hypoxemia before the procedure, moderate or severe

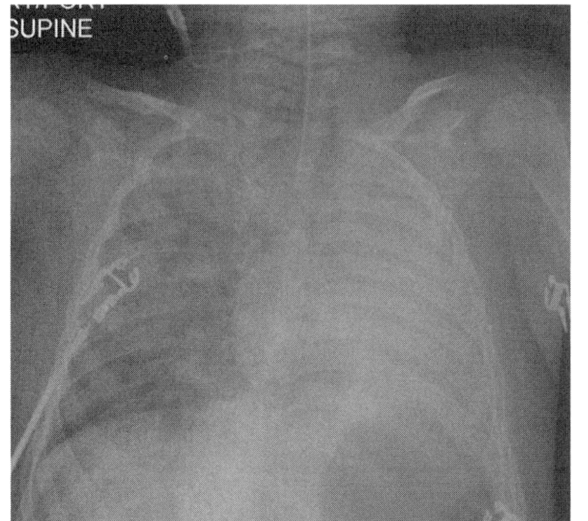

A

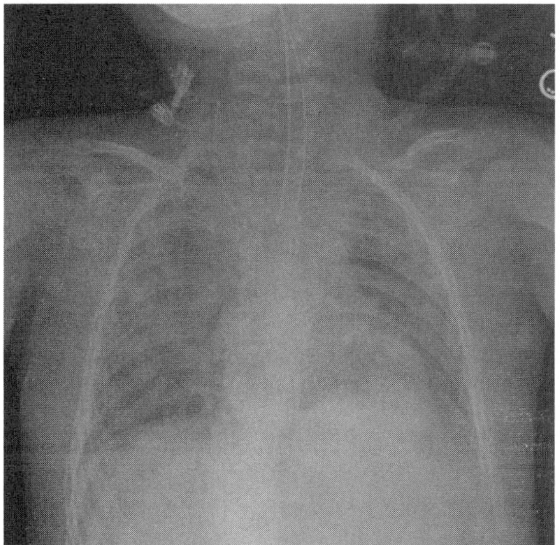

B

Figure 8-2. A. Chest radiograph of a girl with VATER syndrome and acute respiratory failure from adenovirus pneumonia. Note the abrupt ending of an air bronchogram in the distal left main bronchus (arrow), together with left lung atelectasis. **B.** The same patient 24 hours after bronchoscopic removal of a mucus plug from the left main bronchus.

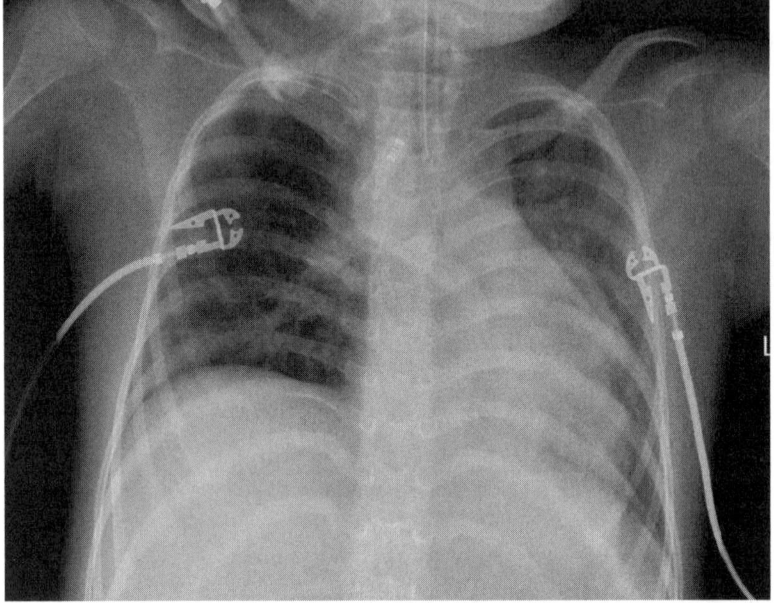

Figure 8-3. Chest radiograph of a 4-year-old boy with myotubular myopathy and left lower lobe atelectasis. Note the air bronchograms within the area of atelectasis, reflecting multiple distal sites of airway obstruction rather than a central mucus plug.

pulmonary hypertension, or severe airway obstruction all should be carefully weighed so that the added risk of the procedure is worth the anticipated outcome to the patient. Occasionally these very conditions are the reason to perform bronchoscopy[11] (eg, if hypoxemia is the result of massive atelectasis or if removing a mucus plug can potentially reverse a condition).

Pathophysiology and Clinical Features in Diagnostic Bronchoscopy

When diagnostic bronchoscopy is performed to evaluate abnormal noises, the diagnostic yield is enhanced if the child creates the noise during the procedure. This may require the examiner to reproduce the situation in which the noise occurs. Thus, if the noise is heard mostly when the child sleeps, as in cases of obstructive sleep apnea, examining the child during sedated quiet sleep is more likely to recreate the airway obstruction and enable the examiner to determine its origin than if the child were minimally sedated. Alternatively, if the noise occurs with increased breathing effort, the child should be only lightly sedated to accentuate breathing effort.

Case Report 8-2

A young athlete was evaluated for possible exercise-related vocal cord dysfunction. To recreate the situation, he was told to hyperventilate with a bronchoscope in place, but this did not reveal any abnormalities. The only time he reported symptoms, however, was during indoor swimming practice and competitions. The examination was repeated while he smelled chlorine bleach and he quickly demonstrated paradoxical vocal fold motion within a few breaths.[20]

In contrast, excessive sedation or breathing effort can lead to erroneous diagnoses. The presence of large airway collapse in an infant making heroic efforts to breathe because of inadequate sedation may be mistaken for tracheomalacia or bronchomalacia. Excessive sedation, or the application of lidocaine to the larynx,[21] can result in dynamic collapse of laryngeal structures and be mistaken for true laryngomalacia. If there is no pre-procedure history of wheezing in the former or stridor in the latter case, such findings are likely artifactual.

Extrathoracic Airway

Intraluminal airway pressure is subatmospheric on inspiration, giving structures in the extrathoracic airway the propensity to collapse. Thus any dynamic lesion will be louder during inspiration. Fixed lesions (ie, those that do not result in a respiratory phase–dependent change in airway caliber, like subglottic stenosis) can cause biphasic noise. The noise created by dynamic lesions depends on the magnitude of the intraluminal pressure drop and the tone or stiffness (compliance) of the airway structures. It may also be positional, as neck hyperextension places longitudinal traction on the extrathoracic airway and can stiffen it to some degree.

Flexible bronchoscopy offers the advantages of examining the extrathoracic airway from the nostril onward, so that any structure in the extrathoracic airway that might cause obstruction or airway vibration should be visible. Furthermore, the patient is examined while the head is in a neutral position. Because the flexible scope follows the contours of the nasopharynx, it does not distort the anatomy of the airway.[22] Sedation can be made lighter or deeper, so that the conditions under which the noise or obstruction is usually present can be replicated.

Extrathoracic lesions that cause noisy breathing or obstruction are identified in most children who undergo bronchoscopy.[10,12,23] When stridor is the indication for evaluation, in the absence of a known history of prolonged airway intubation, the cause is overwhelmingly a congenital lesion.[7,10,23] Of these, laryngomalacia is the most common condition, followed by vocal cord paralysis.[7,12,23] The finding of laryngomalacia during laryngoscopy does not obviate the need to look below the vocal cords: 15% to 21% of patients will have a second airway abnormality noted on more distal evaluation of the airways.[12,23]

A list of common lesions that lead to noisy breathing is shown in Box 8-2. Not all children with noisy breathing, however, require airway evaluation. Bronchoscopy should be reserved for those children whose noisy breathing is progressive, leads to episodes of apnea, and is associated with feeding difficulty and poor growth or sleep disruption and impaired development, or when the history and physical examination raise the possibility of a lesion other than congenital laryngomalacia.[7] Bronchoscopy might also be considered in an infant with laryngomalacia when parental anxiety regarding the noise is so great that confirmation of the diagnosis is necessary to allow for reassurance regarding the natural history of the disorder.

Box 8-2. Lesions Associated With Noisy Breathing

Stridor
- Laryngomalacia
- Subglottic stenosis
- Vocal cord paralysis
- Hemangioma
- Vocal cord dysfunction

Wheezing
- Tracheomalacia or bronchomalacia
- Tracheal stenosis
- Airway compression
  - Vascular
  - Lymph nodes
  - Mediastinal mass
- Bronchitis
- Endobronchial tumor

Intrathoracic Airway

Diagnostic bronchoscopy is undertaken to evaluate chronic wheezing or cough unresponsive to medical therapy, persistent or recurrent radiographic densities in the lung, atelectasis, localized hyperinflation, hemoptysis, suspected recurrent aspiration, or possible retained foreign body. When combined with techniques like bronchoalveolar lavage or transbronchial biopsy, information can also be gleaned about processes in small airways and alveolar spaces. Additionally, biopsies of the airway wall can yield disease-specific information (eg, ciliary ultrastructure and function, or the type of inflammatory cells and degree of remodeling found in chronic asthma).

Evaluating Intrathoracic Airway Collapse

As with evaluation of the extrathoracic airway, the degree of respiratory effort must be considered when evaluating intrathoracic airway collapse. In contrast to extrathoracic obstruction, the forces acting across intrathoracic airway walls favor their narrowing on exhalation. Excessive expiratory effort will cause invagination of the posterior membrane of the trachea and main bronchi; oversedation or paralysis will minimize the collapsing pressures exerted across the airway wall. This makes the diagnosis of primary intrathoracic tracheomalacia or bronchomalacia exceedingly difficult, since all patients can demonstrate some degree of airway collapse with excessive expiratory effort or cough. Furthermore, visual estimates of airway narrowing are highly subjective, and no universally agreed-on definition based on magnitude of airway narrowing exists.[24] When tracheomalacia occurs secondary to another condition, like tracheoesophageal fistula, there is often a larger posterior membrane to anterior cartilage ratio than normal; this is not necessarily true in primary tracheomalacia or tracheomalacia acquired after prolonged mechanical ventilation.

Evaluating Narrowed Intrathoracic Airway

When an intrathoracic airway is narrowed, the endoscopist must determine (1) if the obstruction is dynamic or fixed; (2) if the lesion is intrinsic (web, tumor, mucosal lesion, etc) or extrinsic, and if the narrowing is from extrinsic compression; and (3) whether the compression is pulsatile. Location of the narrowing often is an important clue in the determination of extrinsic compression: the left pulmonary artery crosses over the left main bronchus and proceeds behind the left lower lobe and left upper lobe bronchi, while the right pulmonary artery crosses over the bronchus intermedius (because the right upper lobe bronchus is superior to its attendant pulmonary artery, it is never compressed by it). The aorta will cause a pulsatile compression of the left anterior tracheal wall on its ascent, while the descending aorta can compress the left main bronchus posteriorly.[25] Enlarged lymph nodes encircling the right middle lobe bronchus can narrow the bronchus intermedius, and bronchogenic cysts, which are often subcarinal, can cause compression of main bronchi or widening of the main carina.

Interpreting Other Intrathoracic Bronchoscopy Findings

Often, when bronchoscopy is undertaken for evaluation and treatment of atelectasis, there may be no secretions for removal. Absence of such a finding still may be critical for care decisions (Figure 8-4). Similarly, absence of a suspected retained foreign body is as important as finding one.

It may be difficult to interpret the findings of bronchoalveolar lavage when that modality is used to determine the cause of infection in children with chronic or recurrent radiographic densities, or with a compromised immune system. The bronchoscope is passed through

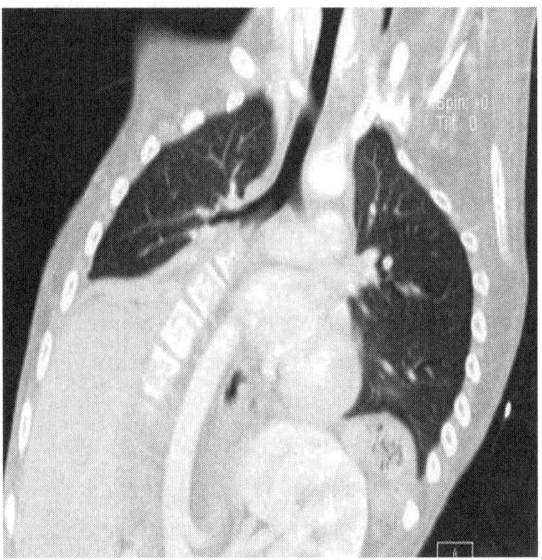

A

B

Figure 8-4. A. Computed tomographic reconstruction of the chest of a 16-year-old boy with Duchenne muscular dystrophy and chronic right lower lobe atelectasis. The air bronchogram ends abruptly (arrow), suggesting a mucus plug. **B.** Bronchoscopic evaluation demonstrated airway narrowing and distortion resulting from the patient's severe scoliosis and chest wall deformity, but no mucus plug.

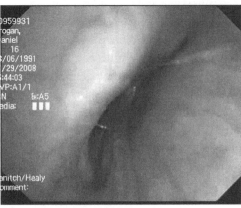

the nose and mouth, compromising sterility of samples. Efforts to avoid suctioning the airway until the scope is below the vocal cords can reduce, but not eliminate, the risk of contamination of specimens. Combining the visual findings on bronchoscopic examination (presence or absence of airway inflammation and secretions) with cell count, cytology, and *quantitative* bacterial culture will strengthen the interpretation of findings (see Diagnostic Procedures). If the proportion of squamous cells is high, or if cultures return showing polymicrobial flora, upper airway contamination of the specimen is likely. If the central airways are inflamed and there are large amounts of secretions in those airways, however, the cells and bacteria may be there because the child chronically aspirates oral secretions.

Diagnostic Procedures

Bronchoalveolar Lavage (BAL) Testing

Bronchoalveolar lavage is used to sample the alveoli for different cell types, including migrated leukocytes and macrophages, invading bacteria, or other infectious pathogens. Analysis can also be performed to evaluate acellular components, including viral particles, cytokines, and proteins. The flexible bronchoscope is advanced into progressively more distal airways until it is "wedged" or unable to be advanced further. The lavage is performed first by instilling normal saline through the working channel of the bronchoscope into the distal airways and airspaces, and then withdrawing it by suction. The amount of saline used for a lavage varies from center to center, from 0.5 to 3.0 mL/kg per aliquot with a maximum of 4 aliquots taken at one procedure. Typically, a protocol is used to limit the total amount of saline that is instilled. In many centers the first sample is discarded as it is believed not to represent alveolar sampling, but rather sampling of bronchial cells. A return of at least 30% to 40% of the aliquot used in the lavage is considered a good sample.[7,26] Bronchoalveolar lavage is performed in the most affected area as determined by radiographic imaging or direct visualization with the bronchoscope. If there is no identified affected area, the right middle lobe or lingula is lavaged in children, while in infants the right lower lobe is lavaged to optimize fluid recovery.[26,27]

Normal Cell Types

Bronchoalveolar lavage is a diagnostic tool that evaluates cellular counts of the lavage fluid (Table 8-2). Absolute number of nucleated cells and red blood cells can be detected. The different types of white blood cells can also be analyzed. In healthy lungs, alveolar macrophages represent roughly 80% to 98% of the cells in the BAL fluid. Other cells that are observed include lymphocytes and neutrophils, representing roughly 2% to 12% and 0% to 5% of the BAL fluid, respectively.[28] There are subtle age-dependent differences in the BAL fluid. A slight increase in neutrophils is observed in patients younger than 12 months when compared with children 12 to 36 months of age. Younger children also can have a greater number of total cells when compared with the adult population.[29] Squamous epithelial cells, when detected in BAL, suggest either contamination by oropharyngeal secretions due to poor technique in performing the BAL or aspiration of upper airway secretions by the subject.

Table 8-2. Cell Types in Bronchoalveolar Lavage Fluid

Cell Types	Normal Percentage in Healthy Patients	Disease Associated With Abnormal Cell Type or Number
Alveolar macrophages	80%–90%	**Lipid-laden macrophages:** aspiration, gastroesophageal reflux
		Hemosiderin-laden macrophages: idiopathic pulmonary hemosiderosis; vascularitis and collagen vascular disease; infections, pulmonary vascular disease, drug-associated
Lymphocytes	2%–12%	**Increased CD4+ cells:** sarcoidosis, Crohn disease
		Increased CD8+ cells: hypersensitivity pneumonia, histiocytosis X, drug-induced pneumonitis, interstitial lung disease (ILD), bronchiolitis obliterans organizing pneumonia
Eosinophils	0%–1%	**Increased eosinophils:** asthma, ILD, drug-associated increase
		Idiopathic increases: Churg-Strauss syndrome, eosinophilic lung disease
Neutrophils	0%–5%	**Increased neutrophils:** ILD, infection, asthma, chronic bronchitis

Abnormal Cell Differentials

The BAL fluid can be examined for pathologic cell types to enhance diagnostic yield. Abnormal cell types and analysis of the ratio of different cell types can be informative. For example, elevated numbers of lipid-laden macrophages, in the proper clinical context, may be associated with aspiration from swallowing dysfunction or from gastroesophageal reflux disease (GERD). Similarly, hemosiderin-laden macrophages reflect a history of pulmonary bleeding.[30] The presence of increased numbers of normal cell types is often nonspecific, but can guide further investigation. Thus increased numbers of eosinophils in the BAL can be associated with multiple disorders, including eosinophilic lung diseases, asthma, Churg-Strauss syndrome, drug reaction, allergic bronchopulmonary aspergillosis, and interstitial lung disease. Increased numbers of neutrophils can be found in infections, asthma, and some interstitial lung diseases. In contrast, an increase in absolute numbers of lymphocytes and variation in T-cell subpopulation ratios (particularly the CD4:CD8 ratio, which is elevated in sarcoidosis and Crohn disease) can help to identify specific diseases. An increase in CD8 lymphocyte populations is associated with hypersensitivity pneumonitis, histiocytosis X, drug-induced pneumonitis, interstitial lung disease associated with collagen vasculitis, and cryptogenic-organizing pneumonia[26,28] (Table 8-2).

In addition to cultures and cell types, BAL fluid can be analyzed for other contents. For example, markers that suggest GERD with microaspiration can be detected in BAL fluid. Several studies have attempted to correlate the presence of pepsin and bile acids in BAL fluid with lung disease from GERD. Detection of either marker has been an important finding in the lung transplant population, as an elevation of either of these indices correlates with onset of bronchiolitis obliterans.[31] Bronchoalveolar lavage fluid can also be analyzed for cytokines. While such measurements currently are largely relegated to research investigations, they can help to assess the impact of different pharmacologic therapies on various lung diseases, particularly inflammatory disease of either infectious or non-infectious etiology. For example, a reduction in measured cytokines in BAL fluid from patients with asthma or cystic fibrosis might be demonstrated after a pharmacologic intervention.[32,33] Some studies have measured immunoglobulin levels in the BAL fluid. When patients with chronic disease were compared with healthy controls, increased levels of immunoglobulin G were observed.[34] While measurements of cytokines or immunoglobulins are not routinely performed in the pediatric patient population, their analysis underscores the importance of the BAL fluid and its usefulness in both research and clinical care.

Microbiology

Testing for bacteria should include direct visualization of the BAL fluid specimen by Gram stain. Such screening not only provides a rapid clue to the type of bacteria that might be present, but it also provides some qualitative assessment of the adequacy of the specimen. Fluid that contains large numbers of squamous cells, for instance, is likely to represent contamination by mouth flora. In contrast, the presence of large numbers of neutrophils supports a diagnosis of acute infection. Bronchoalveolar lavage fluid can be cultured for bacteria, acid-fast bacilli, fungi, and molds based on the clinical history. Quantitative cultures that yield greater than 10^5 colony-forming units offer insight into predominant strains of bacteria present in the lavage, and help to eliminate contaminated samples.

Screening for viruses can also be performed. Polymerase chain reaction (PCR) detection to augment antigen detection and viral cultures has increased the sensitivity of discovering viruses in the lower airways. As an adjunct to these techniques, or if PCR or rapid antigen detection techniques are not available, cytologic examination of the BAL fluid can also identify viral infection of the lung. Inclusion bodies in the cytoplasm or nucleus, balloon cells, syncytial cells, and smudge cells are pathognomonic for agents like herpesvirus, cytomegalovirus, varicella, respiratory syncytial virus, or adenovirus. In addition to using the Gram stain to detect gram-positive or gram-negative organisms, other special stains can be used to find specific pathogens. The Gomori methenamine silver stain is used to detect fungal organisms and *Pneumocystis jiroveci*, while the Ziehl-Neelsen stain is used to detect acid-fast bacilli.

The keys to effective anaerobic bacterial cultures include collecting a contaminant-free specimen and protecting it from oxygen exposure. Bronchoalveolar lavage fluid is aspirated using a sterile syringe that is then tightly capped to prevent entry of air. The specimens should be plated as rapidly as possible onto specially prepared anaerobic culture media. Cultures should be placed in an environment that is free of oxygen at 95°F (35°C) for at least 48 hours before the plates are examined for growth.

Special Studies

Transbronchial Biopsy

Transbronchial biopsies are used in select pediatric populations.[35] By far the largest experience is in the lung transplant population. Transbronchial biopsy is the gold standard for the diagnosis of acute cellular rejection, a common complication in the first 12 months post–lung transplantation. The procedure is performed under fluoroscopic guidance using 1.2-mm or 2.0-mm forceps that are passed though the working channel of the bronchoscope. From 6 to 12 samples are taken for evaluation. These samples can be examined histologically to evaluate for different cell types to establish a diagnosis.[36] Samples can also be cultured if infection is being considered.

Ciliary Biopsy

Ciliary biopsy is an important diagnostic tool for the evaluation of ciliary dyskinesia. To diagnose primary ciliary dyskinesia samples can be taken from the upper and lower airway. Sampling from the upper airway often yields false-positive findings secondary to inflammation from respiratory infections, exposure to tobacco smoke, and allergic rhinitis. Sampling from the lower airway will improve overall yield by eliminating these secondary changes. Bronchoscopic sampling in the lower airway is performed by using either a 1.2-mm or 2.0-mm forceps and sampling the bronchial membrane at the main carina or in close proximity to it. Samples are fixed in glutaraldehyde and sent for evaluation by electron microscopy to assess ciliary ultrastructure. Some centers will also grow or culture cilia samples and/or take samples for direct microscopic evaluation of ciliary motion.

Brushing

Mucosal surface brushing can be used as another method to sample cilia. This method also allows for the sample to be sent for electron microscopy evaluation. The combination of this sampling technique and ciliary biopsy can increase overall yield of diagnostic testing for ciliary dyskinesia. Brushing can be done at the same time as a ciliary biopsy and is used to enhance sampling and reduce sampling error.[37] Mucosal brushing can also be used to sample lesions on the airway wall. The sample can be examined for cytology and also processed for culture. A brush enclosed in a sheath to minimize its contact with contaminating flora as it is passed through the working channel is advanced to the site of interest. Once there, the brush is advanced beyond the protective sheath and rubbed against the mucosa. Once the sample is taken, the brush is returned to its protective sheath. Cytology brush sampling is particularly useful in lung transplant recipients to evaluate the airway and anastomosis site, which in the early postoperative stage is at risk for fungal colonization and subsequent anastomosis site dehiscence.

Therapeutic Bronchoscopy

Medication can be given via a flexible bronchoscope. The administration of exogenous surfactant via bronchoscope has been studied in patient populations with acute lung injury, ARDS, septic shock, and lobar atelectasis. In all of these studies there was some improvement in the treated patients, ranging from reduction of atelectasis or an increase in lung compliance to increased survival compared with groups that did not receive exogenous surfactant.[38]

Epinephrine can be instilled topically to help control bleeding in patients with pulmonary hemorrhage. While the drug is often given blindly through an endotracheal tube, localized deposition to a specific area of concern offers a more directed therapeutic intervention. Another medication that can be given via flexible bronchoscope is dornase alfa. This mucolytic agent has been used in patients with asthma, neuromuscular disease, and more commonly in those with cystic fibrosis to help loosen and remove large mucus plugs that have caused focal or diffuse atelectasis.[13]

Mechanical removal of mucus plugs can also be achieved bronchoscopically. In some instances, particularly in the intensive care unit setting, frequent bronchoscopy can be used for airway clearance. This technique is useful to clear proximal airways, where a chest radiograph shows an abrupt ending of the air bronchogram (Figure 8-2). The technique is not an effective method of airway clearance for processes where air bronchograms can be visualized throughout the area of atelectasis or consolidation (Figure 8-3), as discussed previously. Simple saline washes of the airway through the bronchoscope can also help remove tenacious, thick mucus plugs.

Removal of other foreign bodies is traditionally accomplished with rigid bronchoscopes. While some reports have described foreign body removal with a flexible bronchoscope, it is the general consensus that rigid bronchoscopy is a safer and more efficient mode to remove foreign bodies from the airway, with decreased risk of airway obstruction when removing the foreign body.[2]

Therapeutic Lavage

Pulmonary alveolar proteinosis is a disease in which whole lung lavage is a therapeutic treatment option. This rare disease that occurs in both children and adults is the result of an abnormality in surfactant homeostasis and metabolism, resulting in abnormal accumulation of surfactant in the alveoli. This in turn leads to abnormal gas exchange. Whole lung lavage, whereby each lung is sequentially lavaged in a controlled manner to remove the proteinaceous material filling the airspaces, is a treatment option generally effective at ameliorating symptoms, and is used along with other therapies in this patient population.[39]

Endoscopic Intubation

Endoscopic intubation, in which an endotracheal tube is passed over the flexible bronchoscope to guide its placement under direct visualization, can be used when the standard approach to visualizing the larynx is not feasible or possible. Thus patients with cervical injuries, craniofacial abnormalities, temporomandibular joint limitation, or known previous difficult airway intubations can all benefit from this approach.[40]

Stent Placement

Endobronchial stents can be positioned bronchoscopically in the central airways, as distal as lobar bronchi. There is limited indication for airway stent placement in the pediatric population, typically involving severe cases of airway narrowing that are not amenable to surgical intervention. Patients with severe tracheomalacia, bronchomalacia, or stenosis can benefit from airway stenting when there is significant respiratory compromise. The population in which stenting has been used most commonly is those children with a history of lung transplantation. This cohort can benefit from temporary placement of stents when there is stenosis or malacia at the anastomosis site while it is healing. It is theorized that the temporary placement of a stent can help reshape the area of concern.[41] Limitations of the procedure in the pediatric population include stent sizing and complications from the stent placement. Some stents are easily dislodged with coughing, while others are difficult to remove because of significant growth of granulation tissue.[41,42] Another concern is poor airway clearance of secretions in the area of the stent.

Balloon Dilation of the Airway

Balloon dilation is performed with special balloon catheters. They can be introduced into the affected region through the working channel of the bronchoscope, after which the balloon is inflated under pressure to expand the area. The balloon catheters come in a variety of dimensions and rigidity. Balloon catheters can be used in patients with either congenital or acquired airway stenosis. Often this procedure needs to be repeated at regular intervals to maintain the patency of the airway.[42]

Laser Therapy and Electrosurgery

Laser bronchoscopy uses laser energy delivered via standard bronchoscopes to treat endobronchial disorders. Laser therapy is a widely used tool in adults where the incidence of endobronchial lesions is greater due to a higher prevalence of carcinomas. However, in the pediatric population this technique is helpful in the treatment of bronchial lesions, such as hemangiomas and papillomas, or for the removal of granulation tissue. Another method of treating these causes of obstruction is endobronchial electrosurgery (synonyms: electrocautery or diathermy). This modality employs high-frequency electrical current through a probe to coagulate or vaporize tissue.

Endobronchial Ultrasound (EBUS)

Endobronchial ultrasound is a diagnostic technique for visualizing the tracheobronchial wall and the immediate surrounding structures. Ultrasound waves are transmitted to anatomical structures, and the reflected echoes are transformed into electrical signals, which are converted to a visual image on the monitoring screen. Endobronchial ultrasound is used in the adult population, particularly in the diagnosis of tumors. It can also be used for ultrasound-guided biopsies. It has yet to be used with any frequency in the pediatric population. There is a potential use of EBUS to evaluate airway pathology and also to identify intrapulmonary structures. At this time there are not probes small enough for infants and small children.

Complications of Flexible Bronchoscopy

Flexible bronchoscopy is a safe procedure in practiced hands, but some complications occur with low frequency. Direct trauma to airway mucosa can result in epistaxis or bronchial bleeding; these are typically minor and self-limited problems. Crying, coughing, or phonating while the bronchoscope is positioned between the vocal cords can lead to hoarseness or stridor that is also mild and self-limited, and inadequate topical laryngeal anesthesia can cause laryngospasm. Airway obstruction by the bronchoscope and sedation can impair gas exchange, leading to hypoxemia and hypercapnea. Administration of supplemental oxygen during the procedure usually prevents significant hypoxemia and allows the procedure to be completed safely, and the bronchoscope can be quickly withdrawn from a narrowed airway if its presence causes critical obstruction. Airway instrumentation can elicit vagal responses and cause bradycardia, but this problem is easily avoided by topical application of lidocaine. Passage of the scope through an infected upper airway (ie, if the procedure is performed when the patient has an acute upper respiratory infection) can predispose a child to lower respiratory infection; similarly, meticulous cleaning of equipment is mandatory between procedures to prevent a contaminated scope from infecting other patients. Fever occurs commonly after flexible bronchoscopy, but it is usually transient and resolves after a single dose of antipyretics. Its persistence may indicate significant infection.

Some complications are more likely when procedures like BAL or transbronchial biopsy are also performed. Persistent fever after BAL, especially in the setting of bronchitis, may reflect transient bacteremia or local extension of infection. Sepsis after bronchoscopy, however, is a rare complication. The risk of pneumothorax is increased when transbronchial biopsy is performed, so that any patient undergoing the procedure must be monitored for several hours for the complication.

Key Points

- Fiberoptic bronchoscopy can be used at any age as a diagnostic or therapeutic procedure.
- Foreign body removal usually requires rigid bronchoscopy.
- The most common indication for fiberoptic bronchoscopy is evaluation of noisy breathing.
- Bronchoalveolar lavage is useful to define lower air microbiology and cytology.
- Extensive experience has demonstrated that the procedure is safe in the hands of experienced bronchoscopists.

References

1. Wood RE, Sherman JM. Pediatric flexible bronchoscopy. *Ann Otol Rhinol Laryngol.* 1980;89(5 pt 1):414–4166
2. Ramirez-Figueroa JL, Gochicoa-Rangel LG, Ramírez-San Juan DH, et al. Foreign body removal by flexible fiberoptic bronchoscopy in infants and children. *Pediatr Pulmonol.* 2005;40(5):392–397
3. Righini CA, Morel N, Karkas A, et al. What is the diagnostic value of flexible bronchoscopy in the initial investigation of children with suspected foreign body aspiration? *Int J Pediatr Otorhinolaryngol.* 2007;71(9):1383–1390
4. Karmy-Jones R, Cuschieri J, Vallieres E. Role of bronchoscopy in massive hemoptysis. *Chest Surg Clin N Am.* 2001;11(4):873–906
5. Schellhase DE. Pediatric flexible airway endoscopy. *Curr Opin Pediatr.* 2002;14(3):327–333
6. Midulla F, de Blic J, Barbato A, et al. Flexible endoscopy of paediatric airways. *Eur Respir J.* 2003;22(4):698–708
7. Nicolai T. Pediatric bronchoscopy. *Pediatr Pulmonol.* 2001;31(2):150–164
8. Barbato A, Magarotto M, Crivellaro M, et al. Use of the paediatric bronchoscope, flexible and rigid, in 51 European centres. *Eur Respir J.* 1997;10(8):1761–1766
9. Cerda J, Chacón J, Reichhard C, et al. Flexible fiberoptic bronchoscopy in children with heart diseases: a twelve years experience. *Pediatr Pulmonol.* 2007;42(4):319–324
10. Godfrey S, Avital A, Maayan C, et al. Yield from flexible bronchoscopy in children. *Pediatr Pulmonol.* 1997;23(4):261–269
11. Wood RE. Spelunking in the pediatric airways: explorations with the flexible fiberoptic bronchoscope. *Pediatr Clin North Am.* 1984;31(4):785–799
12. Wood RE. The diagnostic effectiveness of the flexible bronchoscope in children. *Pediatr Pulmonol.* 1985;1(4):188–192

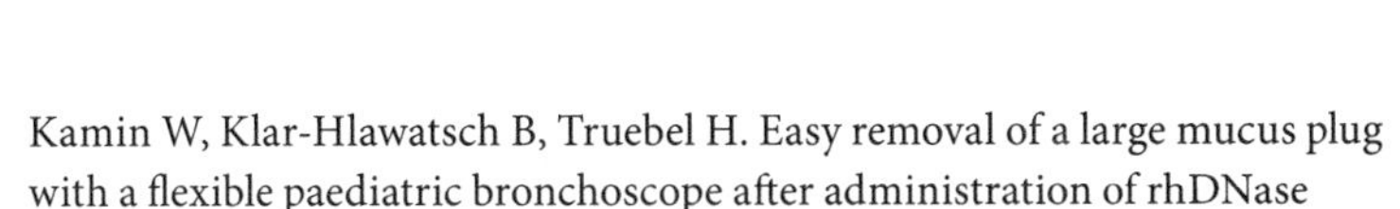

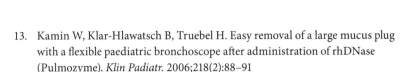

13. Kamin W, Klar-Hlawatsch B, Truebel H. Easy removal of a large mucus plug with a flexible paediatric bronchoscope after administration of rhDNase (Pulmozyme). *Klin Padiatr.* 2006;218(2):88–91
14. Davidson MG, Coutts J, Bell G. Flexible bronchoscopy in pediatric intensive care. *Pediatr Pulmonol.* 2008;43(12):1188–1192
15. Brennan S, Gangell C, Wainwright C, et al. Disease surveillance using bronchoalveolar lavage. *Paediatr Respir Rev.* 2008;9(3):151–159
16. Khan TZ, Wagener JS, Bost T, et al. Early pulmonary inflammation in infants with cystic fibrosis. *Am J Respir Crit Care Med.* 1995;151(4):1075–1082
17. Muhlebach MS, Stewart PW, Leigh MW, et al. Quantitation of inflammatory responses to bacteria in young cystic fibrosis and control patients. *Am J Respir Crit Care Med.* 1999;160(1):186–191
18. Kim ES, Kim SH, Kim KW, et al. Basement membrane thickening and clinical features of children with asthma. *Allergy.* 2007;62(6):635–640
19. Koh YY, Park Y, Lee HJ, et al. Levels of interleukin-2, interferon-gamma, and interleukin-4 in bronchoalveolar lavage fluid from patients with *Mycoplasma pneumonia:* implication of tendency toward increased immunoglobulin E production. *Pediatrics.* 2001;107(3):e39
20. Bhargava S, Panitch HB, Allen JL. Chlorine induced paradoxical vocal cord dysfunction [abstract]. *Chest.* 2000;118:295S
21. Nielson DW, Ku PL, Egger M. Topical lidocaine exaggerates laryngomalacia during flexible bronchoscopy. *Am J Respir Crit Care Med.* 2000;161(1):147–151
22. Wood RE. Evaluation of the upper airway in children. *Curr Opin Pediatr.* 2008;20(3):266–271
23. Zoumalan R, Maddalozzo J, Holinger LD. Etiology of stridor in infants. *Ann Otol Rhinol Laryngol.* 2007;116(5):329–334
24. Boogaard R, Huijsmans SH, Pijnenburg MWH, et al. Tracheomalacia and bronchomalacia in children: incidence and patient characteristics. *Chest.* 2005;128(5):3391–3397
25. Goldman SA, Rimell FL, Meza MP, et al. Diagnosis and management of left main stem bronchus compression. *Ann Otol Rhinol Laryngol.* 1997;106(6):461–465
26. de Blic J, Midulla F, Barbato A, et al. Bronchoalveolar lavage in children. ERS Task Force on bronchoalveolar lavage in children. European Respiratory Society. *Eur Respir J.* 2000;15(1):217–231
27. Baughman RP. Technical aspects of bronchoalveolar lavage: recommendations for a standard procedure. *Semin Respir Crit Care Med.* 2007;28(5):475–485
28. Ratjen F, Bredendiek M, Brendel M, et al. Differential cytology of bronchoalveolar lavage fluid in normal children. *Eur Respir J.* 1994;7(10):1865–1870
29. Midulla F, Villani A, Merolla R, et al. Bronchoalveolar lavage studies in children without parenchymal lung disease: cellular constituents and protein levels. *Pediatr Pulmonol.* 1995;20(2):112–118

30. Ahrens P, Noll C, Kitz R, et al. Lipid-laden alveolar macrophages (LLAM): a useful marker of silent aspiration in children. *Pediatr Pulmonol.* 1999;28(2):83–88
31. Palmer SM, Miralles AP, Howell DN, et al. Gastroesophageal reflux as a reversible cause of allograft dysfunction after lung transplantation. *Chest.* 2000;118(4):1214–1217
32. Cetin I, Özçelik U, Göçmen A, et al. BALF nitrite as an indicator of inflammation in children with cystic fibrosis. *Respiration.* 2004;71(6):625–629
33. Gelfand EW, Cui Z, Takeda K, et al. Fexofenadine modulates T-cell function, preventing allergen-induced airway inflammation and hyperresponsiveness. *J Allergy Clin Immunol.* 2002;110(1):85–95
34. Kitz R, Ahrens P, Zielen S. Immunoglobulin levels in bronchoalveolar lavage fluid of children with chronic chest disease. *Pediatr Pulmonol.* 2000;29(6):443–451
35. Masih AS, Woods GL, Thiele GM, et al. Detection of cytomegalovirus in bronchoalveolar lavage: a comparison of techniques. *Mod Pathol.* 1991;4(1):108–112
36. McWilliams TJ, Williams TJ, Whitford HM, et al. Surveillance bronchoscopy in lung transplant recipients: risk versus benefit. *J Heart Lung Transplant.* 2008;27(11):1203–1209
37. Nuesslein TG, Hufnagel C, Stephan V, et al. Yield of bronchial forceps biopsies in addition to nasal brushing for ciliary function analyses in children. *Klin Padiatr.* 2004;216(4):238–243
38. Willson DF, Thomas NJ, Markovitz BP, et al. Effect of exogenous surfactant (calfactant) in pediatric acute lung injury: a randomized controlled trial. *JAMA.* 2005;293(4):470–476
39. de Blic J. Pulmonary alveolar proteinosis in children. *Paediatr Respir Rev.* 2004;5(4):316–322
40. Elizondo E, Navarro F, Pérez-Romo A, et al. Endotracheal intubation with flexible fiberoptic bronchoscopy in patients with abnormal anatomic conditions of the head and neck. *Ear Nose Throat J.* 2007;86(11):682–684
41. Antón-Pacheco JL, Cabezalí D, Tejedor R, et al. The role of airway stenting in pediatric tracheobronchial obstruction. *Eur J Cardiothorac Surg.* 2008;33(6):1069–1075
42. Törer B, Gülcan H, Oğuzkurt L, et al. Use of balloon-expandable metallic stent in a premature infant with congenital tracheobronchial stenosis. *Pediatr Pulmonol.* 2008;43(4):414–417

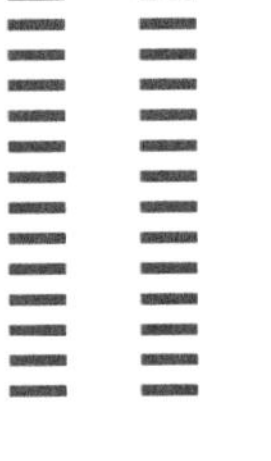

Chapter 9

Allergic Bronchopulmonary Aspergillosis

Richard M. Kravitz, MD

Case Report 9-1

A 13-year-old male with a history of poorly controlled asthma is new to the practice. He averages 2 hospitalizations per year over his lifetime, along with numerous emergency department visits. He has been treated with frequent courses of oral steroids to treat these multiple asthma flares. Previous skin testing was positive for several antigens, but negative for *Aspergillus.*

Medications at the time of his referral included albuterol, low-dose budesonide/formoterol, montelukast, cetirizine, and fluticasone. Pulmonary function testing (PFT) revealed severe obstructive lung disease with a forced expiratory volume in 1 second (FEV_1) of 25% of predicted, which improved to 40% of predicted after bronchodilator treatment. His budesonide/formoterol dose was increased and a steroid burst with taper was prescribed; however, no improvement was noted, with an FEV_1 of only 26% of predicted. An immunoglobulin (Ig) E level was obtained and found to be elevated at 1,960 IU/mL, and a complete blood cell count revealed an absolute eosinophil count of 1,139 IU/μL. These results raised the possibility of allergic bronchopulmonary aspergillosis (ABPA). Further evaluation included repeat skin testing now positive (2+) for *Aspergillus fumigatus;* a repeat IgE level elevated at 2,990 IU/mL; IgE specific to *Aspergillus* positive at 36.5 kU/L; *Aspergillus* precipitins, which were negative; and a chest radiograph that was clear with no evidence of bronchiectasis. Allergy precautions were instituted, theophylline was started, and another steroid burst with taper was prescribed.

One month later, his clinical status and PFTs had improved (FEV_1 was now 50% of predicted) and the IgE level had decreased to 1,340 IU/μL. Another steroid burst was prescribed and itraconazole was added to his regimen. Follow-up 2 weeks later revealed a good clinical interval, with IgE further decreased to 1,030 IU/μL and FEV_1 improved to 64% of predicted.

Case Report 9-2

Patient 2 is a 6-year-old male with cystic fibrosis (CF), poor medication adherence, and infrequent follow-up in the CF clinic. He was clinically doing fair on a respiratory regimen of albuterol and inhaled high-dose tobramycin every other month. He presented to the pulmonary clinic with an increased daily cough and an FEV_1 of 60% of predicted. He was treated with a course of oral cefuroxime. An IgE level was obtained and was elevated at 4,900 IU/mL.

At his next clinic appointment 6 months later, his FEV_1 was unchanged. A repeat IgE was still elevated at 2,500 IU/mL. Skin testing was performed and positive to *A fumigatus*. Oral steroids were started at 2 mg/kg/day for 2 weeks followed by a slow, prolonged tapering period over 2 months. Follow-up 4 months later revealed the patient to be doing better, with his FEV_1 now 72% of predicted.

Over the next few years, the patient had several more exacerbations of coughing and wheezing, for which he received courses of oral antibiotics and/or steroids. IgE levels were monitored and varied between 200 to 4,510 IU/mL. The FEV_1 varied between 40% and 63% of predicted. IgE specific to *Aspergillus* was performed and was positive at 7.54 kU/L. IgG precipitins were performed on 2 occasions, both of which were negative. *Aspergillus* was never recovered from sputum cultures. Chest radiographs consistently showed mild upper lobe bronchiectasis.

The patient is currently doing fair to well; however, he has not remained off oral steroids for long periods.

Introduction

Allergic bronchopulmonary aspergillosis is an IgE-mediated allergic reaction to the mold *A fumigatus*. This ubiquitous mold is usually of little consequence in the immunocompetent host. In patients with an immunodeficiency, however, this mold can infect the lung, leading to an overwhelming infection. In patients with asthma and CF, the host can become colonized with this organism. While no actual infection is present, the body's immune system mounts an IgE-mediated allergic response, which can lead to asthma that is difficult to control, increased pulmonary exacerbations, and worsened bronchiectasis in patients with CF. Failure to recognize this condition can lead to progressive lung disease with significantly decreased pulmonary function and, ultimately, bronchiectasis and pulmonary fibrosis.

Background

The *Aspergillus* species represents a family of molds often found in soil and decaying plant matter.[1–3] There are more than 300 species described, with *A fumigatus* being the most commonly found in human infections.[3] Transmission via inhalation is the most common method of inoculation. No human-to-human spread occurs.[1,2] The conidia (spore) form is infectious, while the hyphae form is what is seen in invasive disease.[4]

Aspergillus infections can take on 1 of 3 forms: allergic, saphrophytic, or invasive.[1,5] Allergic forms include ABPA, hypersensitivity pneumonitis, and IgE-mediated asthma. These represent IgE-mediated reactions to the mold and are seen in immunocompetent hosts. The saprophytic form includes aspergillomas, a situation where the mold grows within preexisting pulmonary cysts or cavities. This represents a nonallergic situation in an immunocompetent host. Finally, the invasive form of the disease is the most severe and life-threatening. These cases are seen in immunocompromised hosts, such as those with prolonged neutropenia (ie, cancer or transplant patients; graft versus host disease) or patients with impaired phagocytosis (eg chronic granulomatous disease).

Etiology

The immunologic cause of ABPA is complicated and not fully elucidated. While several animal models are available to study this allergic-mediated disease, they do not exactly mimic what is seen in humans. Many patients with asthma and CF are sensitized to *A fumigatus*. Approximately 20% to 25% of patients with asthma and up to 60% of patients with CF are skin test positive.[6,7] Up to 80% of patients with CF have IgG antibodies to Aspf14, and 60% to 80% may at one time grow *A fumigatus* in their sputum culture.[4,7,8] Despite this, not all of these patients develop ABPA.

Allergic bronchopulmonary aspergillosis is thought to be a T-helper 2 (Th2)-mediated disease, with interleukin (IL)-4, IL-5, and IgE being important mediators affecting disease progression.[4,6] The working disease model for ABPA is outlined below[1,2,4,6,9–11] and in Figure 9-1.[9]

1. *Aspergillus fumigatus* spores are inhaled. The spores become trapped in the airway surface mucus and eventually germinate.

2. Airway clearance is compromised.
3. *Aspergillus fumigatus* releases virulence factors, allergens (especially Af1), and proteases in genetically susceptible patients, which
   - Disrupt and breakdown airway epithelial barriers.
   - Impair fungicidal proteins and complement.
   - Inhibit phagocytotic killing cells (macrophages and neutrophils).

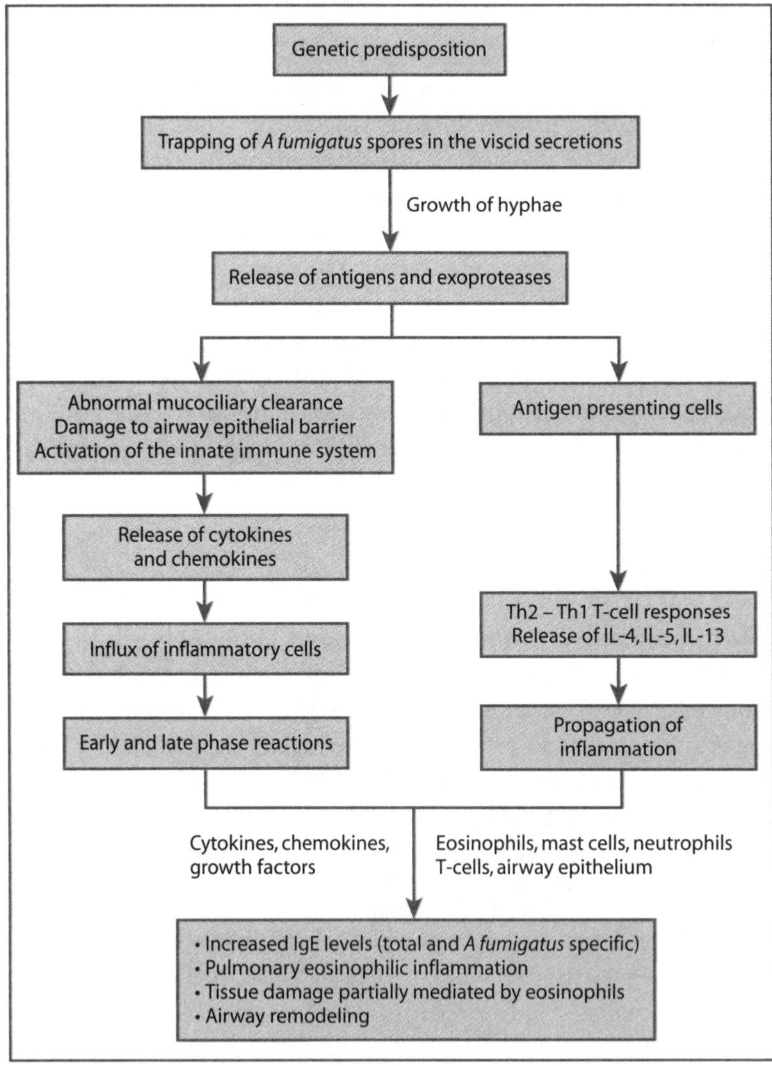

Figure 9-1. Immunology of ABPA. (From Agarwal R. Allergic bronchopulmonary aspergillosis. *Chest.* 2009;135:805–826. Reproduced with permission from the American College of Chest Physicians.)

4. The immune system is activated.
   - Cytokines recruit CD4+ Th2 cells.
   - Interleukin-5 production increases and IL-10 production decreases with subsequent eosinophil infiltration.
   - Interleukin-8 production increases with subsequent neutrophil infiltration.
5. A specific humoral adaptive response occurs with elevation of IgG, IgA, and IgE to *A fumigatus* as well as IL-4 production and nonspecific IgE elevation.

Aspergillus fumigatus spores demonstrate increased binding to inflammatory proteins. In particular, the *Aspergillus* antigens cross-link with the IgE on the mast cells releasing mediators such as histamine, leukotrienes, and platelet-activating factor, which increase vascular permeability and cause smooth muscle constriction. Mast cell cytokines are chemoattractants for eosinophils. Thus a cycle of antigen-mediated stimulation and inflammation is created, ultimately leading to the development of bronchiectasis.

Risk Factors

Certain genetic factors are present that may increase a patient's risk from solely possessing *A fumigatus* sensitivity to developing ABPA. In particular, the presence of HLA-DR2 and DR5 restrictions, IL-4Rα single nucleotide polymorphisms, and IL-10 promoter mutations are associated with the development of ABPA.[5] In a small case series, patients with asthma that were heterozygous for *CFTR* mutations had a higher risk for the development of ABPA, suggesting that this gene has some effect of the organism's immunogenicity.[6,10,12]

There are several other factors that put one at risk for the development of ABPA. In patients with CF, the acquisition of *Pseudomonas aeruginosa* has been associated with a higher incidence of ABPA.[8] *Pseudomonas aeruginosa* is thought to heighten the Th2 response to *A fumigatus* antigens. Colonization of the airway with *P aeruginosa* often precedes the sensitization with *A fumigatus*.[8]

Atopy is also associated with a higher risk for ABPA. Approximately 22% of patients with CF and atopy have ABPA, while 2% of patients with CF who do not also have atopy develop ABPA.[6,10] *Aspergillus fumigatus* colonization is greater in patients with ABPA than those with just atopy.[6] Sensitization to *A fumigatus* is a key factor in the development of ABPA. In patients sensitized to *A fumigatus,* ABPA patients' B cells release more IgE than patients without ABPA. Different *Aspergillus* antigens are associated with different clinical effects. Patients with ABPA develop IgE to antigens Asp2, Asp4, or Asp6, while atopic patients develop IgE to antigens Aspl or Asp3.[6,13]

High levels of *Aspergillus* antibodies are thought to be produced because the *Aspergillus* proteases disrupt the epithelial lining, exposing bronchoalveolar lymph tissue to *Aspergillus* antigens, thus generating a potent immune response.[11] In those with CF, the abnormal mucus traps the spores more effectively, further increasing the antigenic load.

Epidemiology

The prevalence of ABPA is difficult to state, as many studies use different criteria to make the diagnosis. The rate for patients with asthma is about 1% to 2%.[9,10] It is much more common in people with CF, with prevalence varying between 2% to 15%.[4,6,9,10] Several large epidemiological studies in those with CF have further attempted to define the prevalence. The Epidemiologic Study of Cystic Fibrosis published in 1999 looked at 14,210 patients in the United States and Canada and found a rate of 2%,[7] similar to the Cystic Fibrosis Foundation database review in 1995, which found a rate of 2.2%.[14] Reviewing the rate within the United States showed regional variance, with the highest rate in the West (4.0%) and the lowest rate in the Southwest (0.9%).[7] Different criteria used to make the diagnosis of ABPA and the extent to which this diagnosis was sought out are likely explanations for these regional variations and for the lower prevalence rates when compared with other studies. Other confounding features, such as environmental factors, could also not be ruled out. The European Registry of Cystic Fibrosis, published in 2000, covered 9 European countries and 12,447 patients and revealed an ABPA prevalence of 7.8%.[15] This varied country by country, with the highest rate (13.6%) found in Belgium and the lowest rate (2.1%) in Sweden. All 3 of these studies demonstrated higher rates of ABPA in patients older than 5 to 6 years with lower FEV_1 values (<70% of predicted), *Pseudomonas* colonization, and a history of wheezing.

Clinical Presentation

The classic presentation of ABPA is a triad of reversible airway obstruction, recurrent pulmonary infiltrates, and central bronchiectasis. Common symptoms seen in patients with ABPA include wheezing, coughing, and increased mucus production.[5] Other symptoms that may be present include anorexia, malaise, fever, and the expectoration of mucus with brown to black plugs.[5,9] Hemoptysis has also been reported. In patients with asthma, their asthma frequently becomes more difficult to control, while those with CF usually have an increased number of pulmonary exacerbations and a significant deterioration in pulmonary function. Weight loss is often reported. Allergic bronchopulmonary aspergillosis may be easily confused with an exacerbation of the patient's underlying disease process, thus the physician requires a high degree of suspicion to avoid missing the diagnosis of ABPA.

The results of the physical examination are typical for an exacerbation of the patient's underlying illness. Wheezing and a productive cough are often found.[5,10] Clubbing (reports up to 16%) can be seen in patients with ABPA.[5,9] The chest wall can be hyperinflated.[5]

The differential diagnosis of ABPA is broad and includes illnesses that are similar to both asthma and CF.[5,9] Such illnesses include acute processes such as pneumonia (viral or bacterial) or a retained foreign body in the airways. Allergy or inflammatory-mediated illnesses include eosinophilic pneumonia, pulmonary infiltrates with eosinophilia, hypersensitivity pneumonitis, Churg-Strauss syndrome, and sarcoidosis. The differential diagnosis also includes chronic infectious tuberculosis, as well as disorders associated with bronchiectasis, such as ciliary dyskinesia.

Laboratory Studies

There is no single test that can definitively establish the diagnosis of ABPA. There are several tests that may be abnormal in patients with ABPA; however, each of these studies is insufficient to make the diagnosis. To further complicate matters, in select patients many of these tests may actually be normal despite clear evidence that the patient has ABPA. Accordingly, the diagnosis is ultimately made through a combination of history, physical examination, select laboratory studies, and clinical judgment. (Various diagnostic algorithms have been proposed and discussion follows.) Microscopic identification of the mold can be accomplished with 10% potassium hydroxide on a wet mount. For pathologic examination of tissue, silver staining (using Gomori-methenamine or periodic acid-Schiff stains) is recommended, but may be negative in cases of ABPA. Affected tissue may show black staining, dichotomously branching (at a 45-degree angle) hyphae.[1,3] In the airways of patients with ABPA, large mucus plugs (plastic bronchitis[3]) are often found. On examination of these plugs, one can see a variety of inflammatory cells or their breakdown products, including fibrin, Curschmann spirals, Charcot-Leyden crystals, eosinophils, other inflammatory cells, and mold hyphae.[2,9] Examination of the airway tissue itself demonstrates infiltration of the bronchial walls with eosinophils, lymphocytes, and plasma cells.[5] In the more severe or chronic cases, proximal bronchiectasis, especially of the upper lobes, will be evident.[5]

Skin Testing

Because ABPA is an exaggerated IgE-mediated immune response to the presence of *A fumigatus*, a positive immediate skin test (type 1 reaction) is seen as essential for diagnosis in all patients. Various studies consider a positive skin test to be a wheal 4 mm or larger, while others accept a wheal of 3 mm or larger.[6] This disagreement over the appropriate wheal size likely contributes to regional differences in ABPA prevalence. When properly performed in patients with ABPA, an immediate wheal and erythema begins within 1 minute, reaches a maximal size in 10 to 20 minutes, and then resolves within 1 to 2 hours.[5,9] A delayed reaction (type 3) can also be seen 4 to 8 hours later and can occur in 33% of patients.[5,9] As with any type of skin testing, several precautions need to be taken to ensure accurate testing. Anything that can alter a type 1 immunologic response needs to be avoided. Thus the patient should not take antihistamines[13] for an appropriate period before the skin test (72 hours for short-acting antihistamines, such as diphenhydramine, or about 2 weeks for longer-acting agents, such as cetirizine or loratadine), because these could lead to a diminished wheal and flare reaction. Furthermore, it is best that the patient not take steroids at the time of the skin test as they, too, can diminish the type 3 immune response, leading to a false-negative

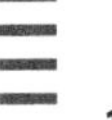

test. As stated earlier, *A fumigatus* is a ubiquitous organism, and many people have been sensitized to it. Approximately 20% to 25% of people with asthma are skin test positive to this mold,[6,7,16] as are 60% of patients with CF.[6–8,16] Because of this, a positive skin test by itself is insufficient to make the diagnosis. On the other hand, a properly performed negative skin test makes the diagnosis highly unlikely.[5]

Blood Work

There are several blood tests that can be abnormal in patients with ABPA. Serum IgE is a key marker of ABPA, both in helping to make the diagnosis as well as assessing for exacerbations. Total serum IgE is markedly elevated in cases of ABPA, with levels often being greater than 1,000 IU/mL in untreated cases. Lower levels (200–500 IU/mL) in patients with CF can be suggestive of ABPA and should be repeated again in 1 to 3 months to assess for persistent elevation. Repeat levels should ideally be performed while the patient is not being treated with steroids.[6] Decreasing IgE levels are a good indication of effective therapy, with levels dropping 35% to 50% within several days of instituting therapy.[9] Doubling of baseline levels are seen in relapses of ABPA. While most patients with ABPA have elevated IgE levels, there is a small subset that may have normal IgE levels despite obvious ABPA. This is thought to be secondary to IgE isotype switching.[8]

IgE and IgG antibodies specific to *Aspergillus* are also useful diagnostic tests. In particular, IgE-specific antibodies are very sensitive markers for ABPA.[13] IgG precipitating antibodies to *Aspergillus* antigens, while a less sensitive test and highly dependent on the antigens used in the assay, is another test that is useful if positive (although a negative study does not eliminate the diagnosis).[9]

Eosinophilia is another nonspecific blood test used in making the diagnosis of ABPA. Patients with ABPA often have an elevated eosinophil count of greater than 1,000 cells/μL.

Culture

Allergic bronchopulmonary aspergillosis represents a hypersensitivity reaction to *A fumigatus,* which colonizes the airways of affected patients. Accordingly, a sputum sample can often yield *A fumigatus* on culture. Because colonization does not always lead to hypersensitivity, a positive sputum culture is not diagnostic of ABPA.[13]

Radiologic Studies

An abnormal chest radiograph is often seen in active cases of ABPA.[5,9] Transient or fixed pulmonary infiltrates are the classic finding. Central bronchiectasis may also be detected. Large bronchial mucus plugs are a pathologic finding of ABPA and manifest themselves on chest film as "finger in glove" opacities or "toothpaste shadows." Tram lines (fine parallel lines radiating from the hila) are another common radiologic finding of ABPA. These infiltrates often improve or resolve with appropriate therapy.[6,17]

Chest computed tomography (CT) scans provide more detail than plain radiographs, but this extra detail is not always needed to make the diagnosis. Computed tomography scans demonstrate the central bronchiectasis of ABPA. This bronchiectasis can be varicose, cylindrical, and cystic in nature, with the varicose and cystic forms typically seen in ABPA.[13] Mucoid impaction can be seen as high attenuation mucus plugs. The sine qua non of ABPA on CT scans is central bronchiectasis and peripheral tapering of the bronchi.[9,17] Other findings include centrilobular nodules and tree-in-bud opacities.

Pulmonary Function Testing

Pulmonary function testing demonstrates obstructive airways disease.[9] This is a non-specific finding, however, because asthma and CF by themselves manifest as obstructive airways disease on PFTs; however, a significant decline in pulmonary function should raise concern of ABPA, particularly if usual interventions are not effective.

Diagnostic Criteria

Because there is no single diagnostic test for ABPA, various authors use different criteria to make the diagnosis. This makes for difficulty in doing epidemiological studies as well as comparing various treatment regimens. In 2003 a consensus statement was created to guide the physician in diagnosing ABPA.[6] Algorithms were created for diagnosis (Figure 9-2) and determining the occurrence of an exacerbation.[9]

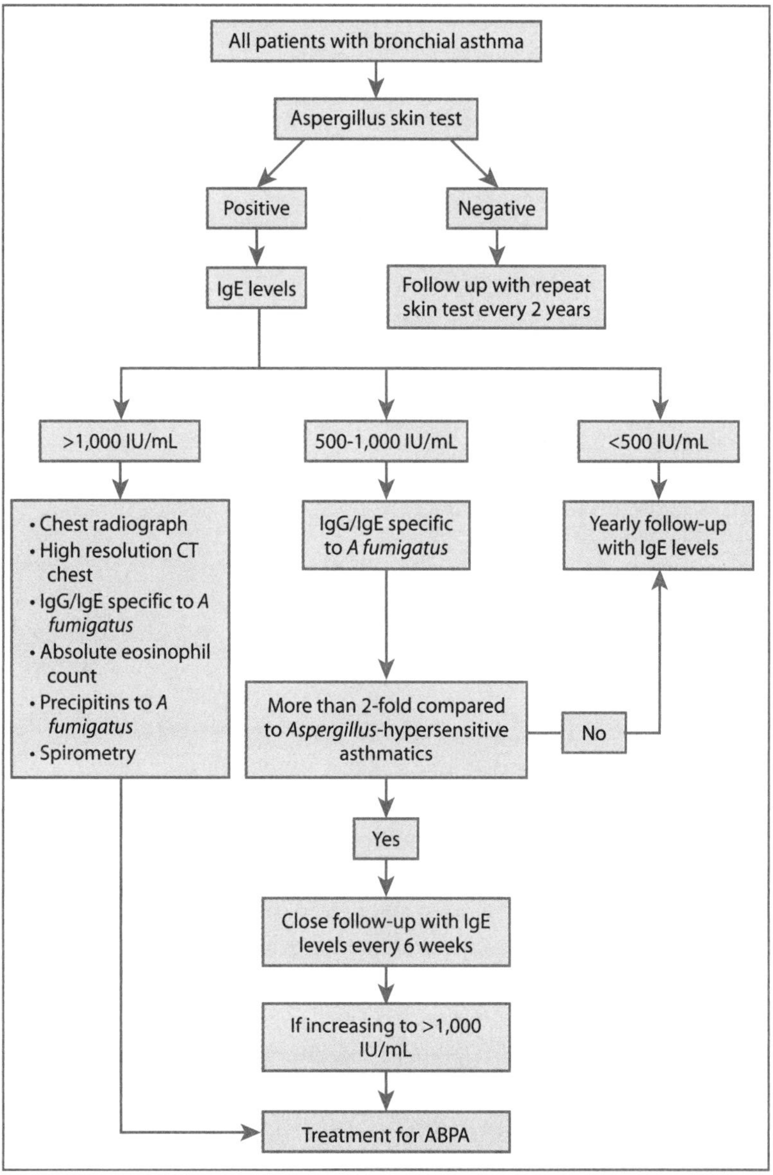

- All patients with bronchial asthma
  - Aspergillus skin test
    - Positive
      - IgE levels
        - >1,000 IU/mL
          - • Chest radiograph
            • High resolution CT chest
            • IgG/IgE specific to *A fumigatus*
            • Absolute eosinophil count
            • Precipitins to *A fumigatus*
            • Spirometry
          - Treatment for ABPA
        - 500-1,000 IU/mL
          - IgG/IgE specific to *A fumigatus*
          - More than 2-fold compared to *Aspergillus*-hypersensitive asthmatics
            - No → Yearly follow-up with IgE levels
            - Yes
              - Close follow-up with IgE levels every 6 weeks
              - If increasing to >1,000 IU/mL
              - Treatment for ABPA
        - <500 IU/mL
          - Yearly follow-up with IgE levels
    - Negative
      - Follow up with repeat skin test every 2 years

Figure 9-2. Algorithm for the diagnosis of allergic bronchopulmonary aspergillosis (ABPA). CT, computed tomography; Ig, immunoglobulin. (From Agarwal R. Allergic bronchopulmonary aspergillosis. *Chest.* 2009;135:805–826. Reproduced with permission from the American College of Chest Physicians.)

The criteria for diagnosing classic ABPA are listed in Box 9-1. The first 5 criteria should be present.[6,10,17]

Box 9-1. Criteria for Diagnosing Classic Allergic Brochopulmonary Aspergillosis in Patients With Asthma[a]

1. Underlying diagnosis of asthma
2. Proximal (central) bronchiectasis
3. Positive skin test to *Aspergillus fumigatus*
4. Elevated total Immunoglobulin (Ig) E (>417 IU/mL or >1,000 ng/mL)[b]
5. Elevated IgE and/or IgG to *A fumigatus*
6. Infiltrates on chest x-ray
7. Positive precipitins to *A fumigatus*
8. Eosinophilia
9. Sputum containing *A fumigatus*

[a] The first 5 criteria should be present.
[b] Recent literature suggests >1,000 IU/mL or 2,400 ng/mL.[9]

In patients with CF, there are 5 criteria which are present in classic cases (Box 9-2).[4,6,10] Because all 5 criteria are not always present, minimum criteria for diagnosing ABPA in patients with CF have been established (Box 9-2).[6] In assessing for these criteria, the physician must make sure that ABPA is the cause of the problem rather than the symptoms representing an exacerbation of the underlying asthma or CF. This can be quite challenging because of the large degree of overlap in these conditions. Confusion can arise both when making the initial diagnosis as well as determining if an exacerbation of ABPA (vs asthma or CF) is occurring. Therefore, referral to a pulmonary or allergy specialist should be considered when the diagnosis of ABPA is suspected.

Box 9-2. Diagnostic Criteria for Allergic Bronchopulmonary Aspergillosis (ABPA) in Patients With Cystic Fibrosis[a]

Classic Diagnostic Criteria

1. Acute or subacute clinical deterioration (cough, wheeze, and other pulmonary symptoms) not explained by another etiology
2. Serum total immunoglobulin (Ig) E levels >1,000 IU/mL
3. Immediate cutaneous reactivity to *Aspergillus* or presence of serum IgE antibody to *Aspergillus fumigatus*
4. Precipitating antibodies to *A fumigatus* or serum IgG antibody to *A fumigatus*
5. New or recent abnormalities on chest radiograph or chest computed tomography (CT) scan that have not cleared with antibiotics and standard physiotherapy

Minimal Diagnostic Criteria

1. Acute or subacute clinical deterioration (cough, wheeze, and other pulmonary symptoms) not explained by another etiology
2. Total serum IgE levels >500 IU/mL (If total IgE level is 200–500 IU/mL, repeat testing in 1–3 months is recommended.)
3. Immediate cutaneous reactivity to *Aspergillus* or presence of serum IgE antibody to *A fumigatus*
4. One of the following: (1) precipitins to *A fumigatus* or demonstration of IgG antibody to *A fumigatus* or (2) new or recent abnormalities on chest radiography (on chest radiography or chest CT scan that have not cleared with antibiotics and standard physiotherapy)

Screening for ABPA in Patients With Cystic Fibrosis (CF)

1. Maintain a high level of suspicion for ABPA in patients with CF.
2. Determine the total serum IgE levels annually. If the total serum IgE level is >500 IU/mL, perform *A fumigatus* skin test or use an IgE antibody to *A fumigatus.* If results are positive, consider diagnosis on the basis of minimal criteria.
3. If the total serum IgE level is 200–500 IU/mL, repeat the measurement if there is increased suspicion for ABPA and perform further diagnostic tests (immediate skin test reactivity to *A fumigatus,* IgE antibody to *A fumigatus, A fumigatus* precipitins, or serum IgG antibody to *A fumigatus,* and chest radiography).

[a] Excerpted with permission from Stevens DA, Moss RB, Kurup VP, et al. Allergic bronchopulmonary aspergillosis in Cystic Fibrosis—State of the Art: Cystic Fibrosis Foundation Consensus Conference. *Clin Infect Dis.* 2003;37(suppl 3):S225–S264.

Staging of ABPA has been developed and can be used in patients with asthma,[9,10,18] though it is not used in patients with CF.[6] Of note, one does not need to pass from Stage 1 through Stage 5 directly; rather, there can be transitioning back and forth between Stages 1 through 3. Staging is summarized in Table 9-1.[17]

To help determine if ABPA is developing or if an exacerbation is occurring, serial monitoring of IgE levels is recommended, especially in patients with CF. Annual measurement of IgE levels should be performed. In patients with no history of ABPA, if the IgE level is greater than 500 IU/mL, then a more formal evaluation for ABPA should be undertaken, including skin testing or IgE specific for *Aspergillus*.[6,10] If positive, a diagnosis of ABPA can be considered using the minimal criteria outlined in Box 9-2. If IgE levels are lower (200–500 IU/mL) and a diagnosis of ABPA or a flare-up is still being entertained, further diagnostic tests (skin testing for *Aspergillus*, IgE and/or IgG specific for *Aspergillus*, precipitins, chest radiographs) should be considered.

Table 9-1. Staging of Allergic Bronchopulmonary Aspergillosis[a]

Stage	Description	Characteristics	Total Serum IgE
I	Acute	Upper lobes or middle lobe, chest radiograph infiltrates, eosinophilia, response to steroid therapy	Sharply elevated
II	Remission	No infiltrate and patient off prednisone for >6 months	Elevated or normal
III	Exacerbation	Upper lobes or middle lobe, similar to Stage 1; chest radiographs clear with steroid treatment	Sharply elevated
IV	Corticosteroid-dependent asthma	Often without infiltrates, but intermittent infiltrates might occur, steroid-dependent asthma, need inhaled corticosteroids	Elevated or normal
V	End stage	Fibrotic, bullous or cavitary lesions, abnormal CT, fixed obstruction seen on PFTs, poor response to steroids	Might be normal

Abbreviations: CT, computed tomography; IgE, immunoglobulin E; PFTs, pulmonary function test.

[a] From Greenberger PA. Allergic bronchopulmonary aspergillosis. *J Allergy Clin Immunol.* 2002;110:685–692, with permission from Elsevier.

Therapy

Treatment of ABPA is directed at modulating the Th2-mediated immune response to *A fumigatus.* While several treatment modalities have been used, steroids appear to be the most effective at downregulating the hyperimmune reaction. Steroids are thought to work by inhibiting phospholipase A2 activity and arachadonic acid metabolism, thus diminishing chemotaxis and tissue infiltration of inflammatory cells. This results in a decrease in IgE levels, lessened eosinophilia, and clearing of pulmonary infiltrates.[6]

While there are a number of different regimens reported, there are several features in common, including aggressive treatment for the first couple of weeks of therapy, slow tapering of the steroid dose over the next several weeks to months, and a universal improvement in the patient's clinical course.[6,13] Immunoglobulin E levels, in general, quickly decrease by 35% to 50% over the first few weeks of therapy.[9,10,17] Chest radiograph infiltrates resolve, or at least improve, over the first 1 to 2 months of therapy. Pulmonary function (particularly FEV_1) improves during this time.

The 2003 consensus statement recommends the following steroid dosing schedule: prednisone at 0.5 to 2.0 mg/kg/day (with a maximum dose of 60 mg/day) for 1 to 2 weeks followed by tapering to every other day dosing for 1 to 2 weeks, and then tapering the dose over the next 2 to 3 months as clinically able.[6] Dose elevation might be needed if symptoms start to worsen. Often, increasing the steroid dose back to the previously effective dosage will bring symptoms under control. Serial IgE levels and follow-up chest radiographs are useful for monitoring the progress of the treatment plan.

Steroids treat the patient's inflammatory burden but do nothing to decrease the antigen load to which the patient's immune system is being exposed. Various antifungal regimens have been used to eradicate, or at least decrease, the disease burden of *A fumigatus.* Unfortunately, this has met with limited success. There have been only a few studies attempted, and most were small in number.[19] The most successful agent used has been itraconazole. This drug has been found effective as a steroid-sparing agent.[20] It acts by inhibiting ergosterol synthesis in the fungal cell membrane, which decreases the organism's growth. In combination, itraconazole and oral steroids are useful at treating exacerbations or relapses of ABPA.[6,19]

As with oral steroids, several dosing regimens have been published, though they share the similar limitations discussed in the steroid studies. The 2003 consensus statement[6] recommends itraconazole at 5 mg/kg (up to 200 mg/dose) once per day. If more than 200 mg/day is indicated, the dose should be split into a twice per day schedule (with a maximum daily dose of 400 mg/day). Treatment with itraconazole is typically continued for 3 to 6 months or longer if symptoms persist or IgE levels remain elevated. A search for and elimination of continued exposure to *Aspergillus* may be helpful in patients with persistently high IgE levels.

Itraconazole has many adverse effects as well as several drug-drug interactions. Hepatic toxicity is problematic, so close monitoring of liver function is warranted. Liver function tests should be obtained before starting therapy and then repeated after 1 month of treatment. Liver function should also be monitored every 3 to 6 months while on therapy or if any liver-related toxicity appears. Levels should also be checked if there is no clinical response to therapy, if there are possible drug-drug interactions, or if there are concerns of poor drug absorption or poor medication adherence.[6]

Common side effects of itraconazole include gastrointestinal upset, fever, rash, headaches, dizziness, and fatigue. Concomitant use of drugs that lower stomach acid (such as histamine-2 blockers or proton pump inhibitors) can decrease absorption. Taking the medication with an acidic drink such as orange juice may aid absorption. Grapefruit juice, however, should be avoided because it interferes with the liver's CYP3A4 enzyme, which can have an effect on itraconazole metabolism.[6] The treatment protocols presented in the consensus statement are summarized in Table 9-2.[6]

Inhaled amphotericin has not been successful. Voriconazole has also been used. Anti-IgE mediated therapy (such as omalizumab) has had limited success, and more study is needed before recommending its routine use.

Table 9-2. Treatment Protocol for Allergic Bronchopulmonary Aspergillosis (ABPA)[a]

Treatment, Factor	Explanation
Corticosteroids	
Indications	All patients except those with steroid toxicity
Initial	0.5–2.0 mg.kg/day po prednisone equivalent, max 60 mg/day, for 1–2 weeks
Begin taper	0.5–2 mg/kg/day every other day for 1–2 weeks
Taper off	Attempt to taper off within 2–3 months
Relapse	Increased corticosteroids, add itraconazole, taper corticosteroids when clinical parameters improve
Itraconazole	
Indications	Slow or poor response to corticosteroids, relapse, corticosteroid-dependent, or corticosteroid toxicity
Dosing	5 mg/kg/day, max dose 400 mg/day po unless itraconazole levels determined; bid dosing required
Duration	3–6 months
Monitor	Liver function tests for all cases; itraconazole serum concentrations if concern of adequate absorption, lack of response, possible drug-drug interaction; serum concentrations of concomitant drugs with potential for drug-drug interaction
Adjunctive therapy	
Inhaled corticosteroids, bronchodilators, other anti-asthma drugs	No evidence for use in ABPA; may be used for the asthma component of ABPA
Environmental manipulation	Attempt to search for and modify mold spore exposure in refractory cases

Abbreviations: bid, twice a day; po, orally.

[a] Reprinted with permission from Stevens DA, Moss RB, Kurup VP, et al. Allergic bronchopulmonary aspergillosis in Cystic Fibrosis—State of the Art: Cystic Fibrosis Foundation Consensus Conference. *Clin Infect Dis.* 2003;37(suppl. 3):S225–S264.

In addition to the use of oral steroids and itraconazole, supportive care of the underlying disease processes (asthma and CF) needs to be used. Chronic anti-inflammatory therapy for asthma is required. While inhaled steroids (such as budesonide or fluticasone) have been attempted to treat the ABPA with questionable success, their use in treating the underlying asthma is not questioned. Supportive care for CF is required and includes nutritional support (pancreatic enzymes and vitamins), aggressive airway clearance (mucolytic agents and chest physiotherapy), and suppressive antibiotics (inhaled tobramycin or aztreonam). Oral or intravenous antibiotics are warranted if a pulmonary exacerbation is occurring. Distinguishing between a classic CF exacerbation versus an ABPA flare can be difficult. If there is not overwhelming evidence that the symptoms are due to an ABPA flare, then aggressive use of antibiotics is indicated. If the patient does not improve, then an ABPA flare needs to be addressed and appropriately treated.

Prognosis

Allergic bronchopulmonary aspergillosis is a chronic and recurrent disease that can often mimic the asthma and/or CF with which it is frequently associated. While therapy is available to successfully treat ABPA, it is not curative and may lead to significant side effects due to the long-term therapy often required. When aggressively treated early in its course, the chance that the disease will progress to end-stage fibrosis is minimized.[5,13] Lifelong monitoring is required to prevent complications and provide for the most beneficial outcome.

Key Points

- The physician should consider the possibility of ABPA in patients with poorly controlled asthma and CF.
- Suspect ABPA
  In children with asthma when
  - Asthma care is under poor control despite being on an appropriate treatment plan.
  - Infiltrates are seen on chest radiography.
  - Atopic dermatitis is present.
  - Elevated IgE levels are present.

  In patients with CF who have
  - Increasing numbers of pulmonary exacerbations
  - Unexplained deterioration in pulmonary function
  - New onset wheezing
  - Increasing IgE levels measured at annual studies
- No single diagnostic test is sufficient to make the diagnosis. Many patients might have positive ABPA-related tests but do not have the illness, while a smaller number of patients might have negative studies and have the illness. **History, physical examination findings, laboratory studies, and clinical judgment are needed to make the diagnosis.**
- Because of the challenges inherent in making the diagnosis of ABPA and its overall low prevalence, all suspected cases are best evaluated and managed by a pediatric pulmonologist.
- Annual screening for ABPA with yearly IgE levels is recommended. IgE levels should also be routinely tested during exacerbations of CF that require intravenous antibiotics to make sure one is not overlooking an ABPA exacerbation.
- Therapy consists of
  - Oral steroids (prednisone)
  - Antifungal therapy (itraconazole)
  - Supportive care
    - In children with asthma: chronic anti-inflammatory therapy
    - In children with CF: nutritional support, airway clearance, appropriate use of antibiotics

References

1. American Academy of Pediatrics. Aspergillosis. In: Pickering LK, Baker CJ, Kimberlin DW, Long SS, eds. *2009 Red Book: Report of the Committee on Infectious Diseases.* 28th ed. Elk Grove Village, IL: American Academy of Pediatrics; 2009:222–224
2. Wark PA, Gibson PG. Allergic bronchopulmonary aspergillosis: new concepts of pathogenesis and treatment. *Respirology.* 2001;6:1–7
3. Kradin RL, Mark EJ. The pathology of pulmonary disorders due to aspergillus ssp. *Arch Pathol Lab Med.* 2008;132:606–614
4. Rapaka RR, Kolls JK. Pathogenesis of allergic bronchopulmonary aspergillosis in cystic fibrosis: current understanding and future directions. *Med Mycol.* 2009;47:S331–S337
5. Knutsen AP, Amin RS, Temprano J, Wilmott RW. Hypersensitivity pneumonitis and eosinophilic pulmonary diseases. In: Chernick V, Boat TF, Wilmott RW, Bush A, eds. *Kendig's Disorders of the Respiratory Tract in Children.* 7th ed. Philadelphia, PA: Saunders Elsevier; 2006:686–704
6. Stevens DA, Moss RB, Kurup VP, et al. Allergic bronchopulmonary aspergillosis in cystic fibrosis-State of the Art: Cystic Fibrosis Foundation Consensus Conference. *Clin Infect Dis.* 2003;37 (suppl 3):S225–S264
7. Geller DE, Kaplowitz H, Light MJ, et al. Allergic bronchopulmonary aspergillosis in cystic fibrosis: reported prevalence, regional distribution, and patient characteristics. *Chest.* 1999;116:639–646
8. Hartl D. Immunologic mechanisms behind the cystic fibrosis-ABPA link. *Med Mycol.* 2009;47:S183–S191
9. Agarwal R. Allergic bronchopulmonary aspergillosis. *Chest.* 2009;135:805–826
10. Moss RB. Pathophysiology and immunology of allergic bronchopulmonary aspergillosis. *Med Mycol.* 2005;43:S203–S206
11. Knutsen AP, Bellone C, Kauffman H. Immunopathogenesis of allergic bronchopulmonary aspergillosis in cystic fibrosis. *J Cyst Fibros.* 2002;1:76–89
12. Miller PW, Hamosh A, Macek M, et al. Cystic fibrosis transmembrane conductance regulator (CFTR) gene mutations in allergic bronchopulmonary aspergillosis. *Am J Hum Genet.* 1996;59:45–51
13. Thia LP, Balfour-Lynn IM. Diagnosing allergic bronchopulmonary aspergillosis in children with cystic fibrosis. *Paediatr Respir Rev.* 2009;10:37–42
14. FitzSimmons SC. Cystic fibrosis foundation patient registry: 1995 annual data report. Bethesda, MD: Cystic Fibrosis Foundation; 1996
15. Mastella G, Rainisio M, Harms HK, et al. Allergic bronchopulmonary aspergillosis in cystic fibrosis. A European epidemiological study. *Eur Respir J.* 2000;16:464–471
16. Schwartz HJ, Greenberger PA. The prevalence of allergic bronchopulmonary aspergillosis in patients with asthma, determined by serologic and radiologic criteria in patients at risk. *J Lab Clin Med.* 1991;117:138–142

17. Greenberger PA. Allergic bronchopulmonary aspergillosis. *J Allergy Clin Immunol.* 2002;110:685–692
18. Patterson ER, Greenberger PA, Radin RC, et al. Allergic bronchopulmonary aspergillosis: staging as an aid to management. *Ann Intern Med.* 1982;96:286–291
19. Wark P, Gibson PG, Wilson A. Azoles for allergic bronchopulmonary aspergillosis associated with asthma (review). *Cochrane Database Syst Rev.* 2004;(3):CD001108
20. Stevens DA, Schwartz HJ, Lee JY, et al. A randomized trial of itraconazole in allergic bronchopulmonary aspergillosis. *N Engl J Med.* 2000;342:756–762

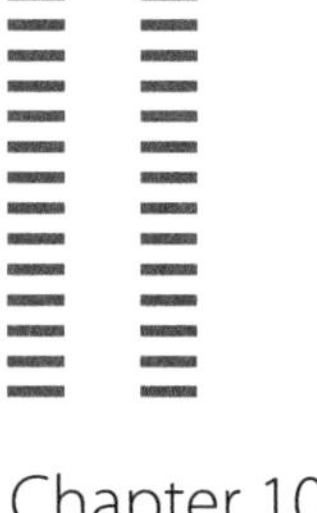

Chapter 10

Hypersensitivity Pneumonitis

Katharine Kevill, MD

Case Report 10-1

A 12-year-old boy presented to the primary care clinic with a 3-month history of cough and shortness of breath when he played soccer. In addition he had lost 7 lbs during this time and had intermittent fevers. The physical examination was remarkable for tachypnea with bibasilar crackles and oxygen saturation of 89%. He was admitted to the hospital and treated with antibiotics. His symptoms improved and he returned home. Within a short time his cough and dyspnea recurred and he was referred to a pulmonologist. Pulmonary function testing revealed a restrictive pattern, and chest radiograph showed increased interstitial markings. An in-depth history revealed that his symptoms started shortly after the family had moved into a house with pigeons nesting in the garden.

Introduction

Hypersensitivity pneumonitis (HP), also called extrinsic allergic alveolitis, results from immunologically mediated inflammation of the lung parenchyma in response to an array of inhaled antigens.[1] Hypersensitivity pneumonitis was first reported in children in 1967 as pigeon breeder's lung.[2] The children had severe interstitial pneumonitis and presented with chronic symptoms of cough, progressive dyspnea, and weight loss, and acute symptoms of fever and chest pain. The children had prolonged exposure to pigeons, either as pets kept in the house or as birds that were bred in a pigeon coop. Before this description, HP was thought to be an adult disease resulting from occupational exposure to environments such as moldy hay (farmer's lung), sugar cane residue (bagassosis), moldy maple bark (maple bark-stripper lung), and pigeon breeding. Since 1967, HP has been described in children as a result of exposure to various other birds (doves, ducks, parakeets) and to specific molds found in areas ranging from a basement shower to hay in a barn.

Clinical Manifestations

The clinical and pathologic manifestations of HP vary with the chronicity of symptoms, with the intensity of the exposure to the offending antigen(s), and with the host response to the antigen. While hypersensitivity pneumonitis has been grouped into acute, subacute, and chronic syndromes,[3–7] a recent study did not support this division into discrete clinical entities.[5] Hypersensitivity pneumonitis is described in the pediatric literature via a series of case reports, many of which describe children who have had symptoms for months or years. Regardless of the duration of symptoms, most adults and children ultimately diagnosed with hypersensitivity pneumonitis present with symptoms of cough, dyspnea, decreased exercise tolerance, and fever. Fatigue and weight loss are common. Crackles are heard on examination in most patients with tachypnea and hypoxemia, and in chronic cases clubbing of the fingers. Wheezing may be heard. Hemoptysis and pneumothorax have also been described at presentation in children. The severity of disease can vary from asymptomatic to severe, with pulmonary fibrosis and even death.

Most children with HP have abnormalities seen on plain chest radiograph,[1] often with reticulonodular shadowing or increased interstitial markings suggestive of interstitial lung disease. High-resolution chest computed tomography (HRCT) is more sensitive than plain radiography for detecting parenchymal lung disease. Pediatric case reports have described ground-glass opacities, centrilobular nodules, and air trapping,[8–12] as well as honeycombing[13] in a case diagnosed late in the disease.

Most pediatric cases that report pulmonary function studies describe restrictive lung disease manifested by decreased lung volumes and often decreased diffusing capacity for carbon monoxide (DLCO). Two large case series of HP in the general population found an incidence of restrictive disease of 53% to 77%, with up to 13% of patients demonstrating a purely obstructive pattern and some patients with mixed restrictive and obstructive findings.[6,7] 26% of patients had air trapping as indicated by an increased residual volume, and 85% had a decreased DLCO.[7] Reversible pulmonary artery hypertension has been described in some children with HP.[11,14] See Table 10-1 for a summary of common and uncommon symptoms.

Table 10-1. Occurrence of Signs and Symptoms in Patients With Hypersensitivity Pneumonitis

	Occurrence			
	Usually	**Often**	**Sometimes**	**Late in Disease**
Symptoms	Cough Dyspnea Fatigue	Weight loss Fever	Hemoptysis	
Signs	Crackles Hypoxemia	Tachypnea Clubbing	Wheezing	
Pulmonary function	Restrictive pattern only Decreased diffusing capacity for carbon monoxide		Obstructive pattern only Mixed obstructive and restrictive pattern	
Plain radiographs	Reticulonodular pattern Increased interstitial markings			
High-resolution chest computed tomography	Nodules in a centrilobular distribution		Ground-glass opacity	Honeycombing Traction bronchiectasis Lobal volume loss
Other complications			Pulmonary artery hypertension Congestive heart failure Pneumothorax	

Epidemiology and Etiology

The incidence of hypersensitivity pneumonitis in children is not known. It is considered a rare, but perhaps underreported, condition. Information comes from case reports in small series of patients, which included approximately 95 cases in total as of the publication of the National Heart, Lung, and Blood Institute and Office of Rare Diseases Workshop statement on HP in 2005.[1] While most pediatric cases of HP have been reported in school-aged children, it has been reported in an infant[15] and in young children.[15,16] The epidemiology of farmer's lung and pigeon breeder's lung has been studied. In England and Finland, the prevalence of farmer's lung has been estimated to range from 10 to 200 per 100,000 inhabitants.[17] The reported prevalence of clinical disease among pigeon breeders ranges 1 per 1,000 to 100 per 1,000.[17]

The list of antigens known to provoke HP is extensive. The antigens are often tied to occupational exposure, with the name of the disease reflecting the profession or hobby of the patient: farmer's lung, bird fancier's lung, maltworker's lung, maple bark-stripper's lung, mushroom worker's lung, hot-tub lung. In a recent review of HP, Lacasse and Cormier[18] divided antigens into 5 categories: bacteria, fungus, mycobacteria, proteins, and chemical products. In pediatric reports, most cases are attributed to proteins in the serum or droppings of birds, including pigeons, doves, parakeets, budgerigars, canaries, and cockatoos. In these cases duration of exposure ranged from weeks to years, with location of exposure often within the house itself or a nearby pigeon coop. The number of birds ranged from one to several hundred.[2,9,11,13,19–27] Exposure to a variety of molds, especially *Aspergillus* species, has been described as a source of HP in children found in locations such as hay in a barn,[28,29] grain dryers kept near the home on a farm,[15] basement shower,[8] standing water under the house,[10] and on a hydroponics plant.[30]

The immunologic pathogenesis of HP is complex and not completely understood. Stiehm et al[2] described features of both immune complex mediated (type III) and T-cell–mediated (type IV) reactions in their cohort. More recent investigations indicate that both types of reactions are necessary. There is no evidence for a role for either immediate type hypersensitivity (type I) or cytotoxic mediated (type II) allergic reactions in the pathogenesis of HP. Atopic individuals are not affected more frequently than non-atopic individuals.[31]

Differential Diagnosis and Evaluation

Diagnosis of HP in children can be difficult, as it is a relatively rare disease with variable manifestations and environmental triggers. Many of the signs and symptoms overlap with a range of infectious and respiratory illnesses (Box 10-1). Diagnosis depends on a high index of suspicion. The diagnosis of HP should be entertained in any child

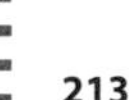

with fulminant respiratory symptoms with hypoxemia and restrictive physiology, rather than more common obstructive physiology, that resolve in the hospital and then recur; prolonged respiratory symptoms of unknown etiology; or restrictive lung disease or interstitial lung disease without a clear cause.

Box 10-1. Differential Diagnosis of Hypersensitivity Pneumonitis in Children

Infectious

- Bacterial pneumonia
- Mycoplasma infection
- Histoplasmosis
- Coccidioidomycosis
- Blastomycosis
- Brucellosis
- Psittacosis
- Legionella infection
- Tuberculosis
- HIV infection

Respiratory

- Asthma
- Cystic fibrosis
- Allergic bronchopulmonary aspergillosis
- Bronchiolitis obliterans, organizing pneumonia
- Recurrent pneumonia
- Interstitial lung disease of childhood of unknown etiology

Other

- Systemic lupus erythematosus
- Sarcoidosis
- Malignancy
- Immune deficiency

There is no definitive test for HP. Multiple diagnostic criteria have been proposed,[1,17,32,33] but currently there is no universally accepted definition. The 4 major criteria detailed by Richerson et al[33] are among the more commonly used: (1) history and physical examination findings and pulmonary function findings indicate interstitial lung disease, (2) radiography is consistent with HP, (3) there is exposure to a recognized cause, and (4) there is antibody to the causative antigen. However, the causative agent is not always known. In a large case series, Hanak et al[6] did not identify the cause in 25% of cases of HP.

Given the prevalence of both respiratory infections and asthma in children, it is not surprising that many children ultimately diagnosed with HP are first treated with antibiotics or with asthma medications. Vigorous bronchodilator therapy may actually increase the hypoxemia characteristic of acute HP disease since the effect of dilating the pulmonary arterial bed in the absence of bronchospasm will increase ventilation/perfusion mismatching by increasing blood flow through poorly ventilated alveoli. Failure to improve with time and treatment or recurrence of symptoms differentiates HP from most acute respiratory illnesses or from asthma. Restrictive lung disease, clubbing, and reduced DLCO are frequent findings in children with HP, but rare in those with asthma. A prolonged course of illness, weight loss, and fevers may prompt an evaluation for tuberculosis, HIV, malignancy, or immune deficiency. A false-positive enzyme-linked immunosorbent assay for HIV has been reported in a boy with symptoms of cough, progressive dyspnea, and weight loss who was eventually diagnosed with HP.[23] Cystic fibrosis (CF) and allergic bronchopulmonary aspergillosis (ABPA) are often considered in these patients. Sweat chloride quantitation and genetic studies permit evaluation for CF. Allergic bronchopulmonary aspergillosis occurs only in those with asthma or CF and is always associated with allergen-specific immunoglobulin (Ig) E to *Aspergillus* detectable by allergy skin test or an in vitro blood test. While a positive test for precipitins to *Aspergillus fumigatus* can be found in both HP and ABPA, eosinophilia is present in ABPA but not HP. Allergic bronchopulmonary aspergillosis typically has a pattern of obstructive lung disease in contrast to HP, which usually manifests as restrictive lung disease. The sequela of ABPA is bronchiectasis of the proximal airways, while long-standing or recurring HP can lead to pulmonary fibrosis.

Evaluation of any patient suspected of HP should include a detailed history, with specific inquiries about exposure to known sources of HP, such as birds and hay. A thorough physical examination is important, with particular evaluation for weight loss, tachypnea, hypoxemia, crackles, and clubbing. Pulmonary function studies, including spirometry, total lung volumes, and diffusing capacity (DLCO) should be performed depending on the child's ability to cooperate. A chest radiograph will usually demonstrate findings consistent with interstitial lung disease. An HRCT is more sensitive, but not specific. Depending on the clinical presentation, one may choose to evaluate the patient for

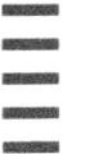

pulmonary artery hypertension, which has been described in HP.[11,14] Laboratory evaluation may reveal neutrophilia or lymphopenia after acute exposure, but eosinophilia is not expected.[33] Elevated levels of IgG, IgM, or IgA subtypes; erythrocyte sedimentation rate; or C-reactive protein may be present occasionally. These findings are not specific and are consistent with acute and chronic inflammation.[33] Elevated IgE or a positive skin prick test does not indicate HP because type I hypersensitivity does not play a role in its pathogenesis.

Positive precipitating antibodies specific to the suspected agent confirm adequate exposure to the agent to generate a humoral immune response and are supportive of a diagnosis (Figure 10-1) but may be present just from exposure.[33] Many exposed but asymptomatic people may have positive precipitins to a given antigen.[14,20] While commercial tests for common serum precipitins are available, negative tests do not rule out the diagnosis of HP, as commercial tests have been found to be inaccurate in some cases[20] or the commercial test may not include the source of exposure.[8,10]

In children where results of evaluation provide a high probability of the diagnosis of HP,[4] proceeding to a bronchoscopy or lung biopsy is not needed. When bronchoscopy is performed, the bronchial alveolar lavage of patients with HP demonstrates a lymphocytosis,[7,10,21,30,34] often with a predominance of CD8 cells in adults, though not always.[34] The

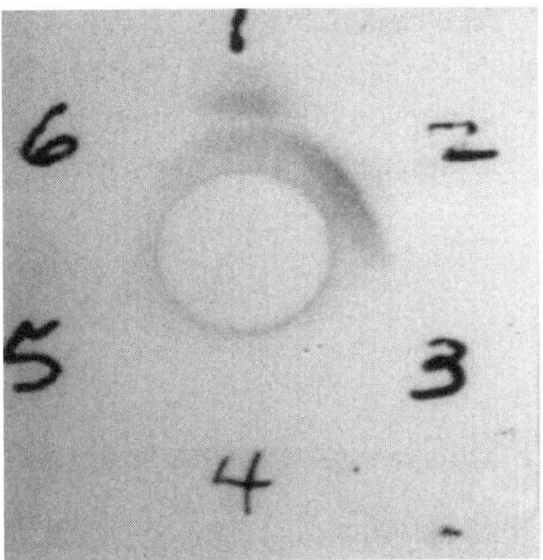

Figure 10-1. Precipitin test. Patient's serum is in center well. Peripheral wells contain (1) pigeon droppings, (2) pigeon serum, (3) chicken serum, (4) canary serum, (5) parakeet serum, and (6) parrot serum. Wells 1 and 2 are positive.

cellular profile may depend on the timing of exposure to the antigen, with CD8 cells predominating after recent exposure.[7]

The lung biopsy histologic findings in children[2,12–14,20,21,29] are consistent with the characteristic findings of bronchiolocentric, interstitial inflammation, composed mostly of lymphocytes.[1] Interstitial non-necrotizing granulomas are found in many cases.[1,20] In individuals with interstitial lung disease of unknown cause, a lung biopsy can prove essential for the diagnosis of HP.[8,20] See Case Report 10-2.

Provocation tests in which the suspected antigen is administered in an aerosolized form have been used to aid the diagnosis of HP and to confirm the environmental trigger. After the exposure, the patient is observed for recurrence of symptoms. Its use is limited by lack of standardized antigens, the possibility of contamination of the aerosol by nonspecific irritants, and the need to administer the test in a specialized center.[1] In some patients, purposeful exposure to the environment in question can be helpful diagnostically, as can a trial period where the patient is not exposed to the suspected trigger.[33]

Treatment and Prognosis

The usual treatment for HP is removing the suspected antigen from the patient's environment. Corticosteroids are indicated for significant symptoms. Outcomes in adults and children depend on cessation of exposure to the trigger. Studies document improvement after the exposure to the antigen in question was halted, but continued or recurrent deterioration in respiratory status when exposure continued.[8,26] Antigens can remain in the home even 18 months after removal of the source, and in some cases, families have moved from their homes to halt exposure.[13,15]

Case Report 10-2

A 10-year-old boy who presented with symptoms of fever, night sweats, chronic cough, and wheezing. No environmental history of exposure to birds, farm animals, or farm materials was obtained. Chest radiograph and pulmonary function testing indicated restrictive lung disease. Commercial serum precipitins were negative. The boy had many features consistent with sarcoidosis, including restrictive lung disease, decreased diffusion capacity, increased angiotensin-converting enzyme levels, a suggestive gallium scan, and a positive response to corticosteroids. A lung biopsy revealed predominant lymphoid interstitial infiltrate with features that distinguished hypersensitivity pneumonitis from sarcoidosis. There was a non-caseating granuloma that was peribronchiolar rather than interstitial in location and composed of poorly organized aggregates of giant cells rather than the large, discrete granulomata characteristic of sarcoidosis. The lung biopsy results prompted further environmental evaluation and ultimately yielded discovery of the inciting antigen.

Adapted from Yee WFH, Castile RG, Cooper A, Roberts M, Patterson R. Diagnosing bird fancier's disease in children. *Pediatrics.* 1990;85(5):848.

Prognosis ranges from complete resolution of symptoms[2] to death,[35] with an increased risk for mortality in those with pulmonary fibrosis documented on lung biopsy at the time of diagnosis.[36] Avoiding the antigenic trigger and administering corticosteroids may or may not improve lung function when fibrosis exists at the time of diagnosis.[13,19]

Few studies address the efficacy of systemic corticosteroid treatment in HP. Available data suggest that corticosteroids hasten the recovery from acute HP but have no beneficial effect on long-term prognosis.[18] There are no clinical trials that address either the necessity of corticosteroids or the optimal dose and duration of treatment in children. Complete resolution of symptoms is described after removal from the antigen alone as well as with removal of antigen and treatment with systemic corticosteroids. Prednisone is the corticosteroid most frequently used, with duration of treatment ranging from weeks to months. Usual starting dose would be 1 to 2 mg/kg for 2 weeks and subsequent dosing depending on response.

Key Points

- Hypersensitivity pneumonitis is a complex disorder with variable presentation.
- Consider a diagnosis of HP in any child with
  - Restrictive lung disease
  - Interstitial lung disease without a clear cause
  - Fulminant respiratory symptoms that resolve in the hospital and then recur
  - Unexplained persistent respiratory symptoms or recurrent pneumonia
  - Bronchiolitis obliterans organizing pneumonia without an underlying risk factor
- Take an environmental history and consider an unknown or not yet described environmental trigger.
- Hypersensitivity pneumonitis is not mediated via IgE. Normal IgE levels or negative skin prick test to a specific antigen are not relevant for the diagnosis.
- If pediatric interstitial lung disease is without a clear etiology, a lung biopsy may prove essential to ascertain the diagnosis.
- Lack of diagnosis and continued exposure to the antigen can lead to end-stage lung disease from pulmonary fibrosis and even death.
- Consider consultation with a pediatric pulmonologist in the evaluation of any child in whom HP is suspected, or in any child treated for asthma whose symptoms don't improve as expected.

References

1. Fink JN, Ortega HG, Reynolds HY, et al. Needs and opportunities for research in hypersensitivity pneumonitis. *Am J Respir Crit Care Med.* 2005;171(7):792–798
2. Stiehm ER, Reed CE, Tooley WH. Pigeon breeder's lung in children. *Pediatrics.* 1967;39(6):904
3. Grech V, Vella C, Lenicker H. Pigeon breeder's lung in childhood: varied clinical picture at presentation. *Pediatr Pulmonol.* 2000;30(2):145–148
4. Lacasse Y, Selman M, Costabel U, et al. Clinical diagnosis of hypersensitivity pneumonitis. *Am J Respir Crit Care Med.* 2003;168(8):952–958
5. Lacasse Y, Selman M, Costabel U, et al. Classification of hypersensitivity pneumonitis: a hypothesis. *Int Arch Allergy Immunol.* 2009;149(2):161–166

6. Hanak V, Golbin JM, Ryu JH. Causes and presenting features in 85 consecutive patients with hypersensitivity pneumonitis. *Mayo Clin Proc.* 2007;82(7):812–816
7. Morell F, Roger A, Reyes L, Cruz MJ, Murio C, Munoz X. Bird fancier's lung: a series of 86 patients. *Medicine (Baltimore).* 2008;87(2):110–130
8. Hogan MB, Patterson R, Pore RS, Corder WT, Wilson NW. Basement shower hypersensitivity pneumonitis secondary to *Epicoccum nigrum. Chest.* 1996;110(3):854–856
9. Yalcin E, Kiper N, Gocmen A, Ozcellk U, Dogru D, Misirligil Z. Pigeon-breeder's disease in a child with selective IgA deficiency. *Pediatr Int.* 2003;45(2):216–218
10. Temprano J, Becker BA, Hutcheson PS, Knutsen AP, Dixit A, Slavin RG. Hypersensitivity pneumonitis secondary to residential exposure to *Aureobasidium pullulans* in 2 siblings. *Ann Allergy Asthma Immunol.* 2007;99(6):562–566
11. Ceviz N, Kaynar H, Olgun H, Onbas O, Misirligil Z. Pigeon breeder's lung in childhood: is family screening necessary? *Pediatr Pulmonol.* 2006;41(3):279–282
12. Lee SK, Kim SS, Nahm DH, et al. Hypersensitivity pneumonitis caused by *Fusarium napiforme* in a home environment. *Allergy.* 2000;55(12):1190–1193
13. Farber HJ, Budson D. A pediatric case of severe chronic interstitial lung disease presenting as spontaneous pneumothorax: blame it on the birds. *Pediatr Asthma Allergy Immunol.* 2000;14(1):75–85
14. Balasubramaniam SK, O'Connell EJ, Yunginger JW, McDougall JC, Sachs MI. Hypersensitivity pneumonitis due to dove antigens in an adolescent. *Clin Pediatr (Phila).* 1987;26(4):174–176
15. Thorshauge H, Fallesen I, Ostergaard PA. Farmer's lung in infants and small children. *Allergy.* 1989;44(2):152–155
16. Wolf SJ, Stillerman A, Weinberger M, Smith W. Chronic interstitial pneumonitis in a 3-year-old child with hypersensitivity to dove antigens. *Pediatrics.* 1987;79(6):1027–1029
17. Demedts M, Wells AU, Anto JM, et al. Interstitial lung diseases: an epidemiological overview. *Eur Respir J Suppl.* 2001;18(32):2S–16S
18. Lacasse Y, Cormier Y. Hypersensitivity pneumonitis. *Orphanet J Rare Dis.* 2006;1:25
19. Purtilo DT, Brem J, Ceccaci L, Cassel C, Fitzpatrick AJ. A family study of pigeon breeders' disease. *J Pediatr.* 1975;86(4):569–571
20. Yee WFH, Castile RG, Cooper A, Roberts M, Patterson R. Diagnosing bird fancier's disease in children. *Pediatrics.* 1990;85(5):848
21. Stauffer Ettlin M, Pache JC, Renevey F, Hanquinet-Ginter S, Guinand S, Barazzone Argiroffo C. Bird breeder's disease: a rare diagnosis in young children. *Eur J Pediatr.* 2006;165(1):55–61
22. Tsai E, Couture D, Hughes DM. A pediatric case of pigeon breeder's disease in Nova Scotia. *Can Respir J.* 1998;5(6):507–510

23. Karakurum M, Doraswamy B, Bennuri SS. Index of suspicion. Case 1. Hypersensitivity pneumonitis. *Pediatr Rev.* 1999;20(2):53–54
24. Reiss JS, Weiss NS, Payette KM, Strimas J. Childhood pigeon breeder's disease. *Ann Allergy.* 1974;32(4):208–212
25. Shannon DC, Andrews JL, Recavarren S, Kazemi H. Pigeon breeder's lung disease and interstitial pulmonary fibrosis. *Am J Dis Child.* 1969;117(5):504–510
26. Dinda P, Chatterjee SS, Riding WD. Pulmonary function studies in bird breeder's lung. *Thorax.* 1969;24(3):374–378
27. Nacar N, Kiper N, Yalcin E, et al. Hypersensitivity pneumonitis in children: pigeon breeder's disease. *Ann Trop Paediatr.* 2004;24(4):349–355
28. Hughes WF, Mattimore JM, Arbesman CE. Farmer's lung in an adolescent boy. *Am J Dis Child.* 1969;118(5):777–780
29. Heersma JR, Emanuel DA, Wenzel FJ, Gray RL. Farmer's lung in a 10-year-old girl. *J Pediatr.* 1969;75(4):704–706
30. Engelhart S, Rietschel E, Exner M, Lange L. Childhood hypersensitivity pneumonitis associated with fungal contamination of indoor hydroponics. *Int J Hygiene Environ Health.* 2009;212(1):18–20
31. Venkatesh P, Wild L. Hypersensitivity pneumonitis in children. *Pediatr Drugs.* 2005;7(4):235–244
32. Schuyler M, Cormier Y. The diagnosis of hypersensitivity pneumonitis. *Chest.* 1997;111(3):534–536
33. Richerson HB, Bernstein IL, Fink JN, et al. Guidelines for the clinical evaluation of hypersensitivity pneumonitis: report of the Subcommittee on Hypersensitivity Pneumonitis. *J Allergy Clin Immunol.* 1989;84(5, part 2):839–844
34. Ratjen F, Costabel U, Griese M, Paul K. Bronchoalveolar lavage fluid findings in children with hypersensitivity pneumonitis. *Eur Respir J.* 2003;21(1):144–148
35. Bang KM, Weissman DN, Pinheiro GA, Antao VC, Wood JM, Syamlal G. Twenty-three years of hypersensitivity pneumonitis mortality surveillance in the United States. *Am J Ind Med.* 2006;49(12):997–1004
36. Vourlekis JS, Schwarz MI, Cherniack RM, et al. The effect of pulmonary fibrosis on survival in patients with hypersensitivity pneumonitis. *Am J Med.* 2004;116(10):662–668

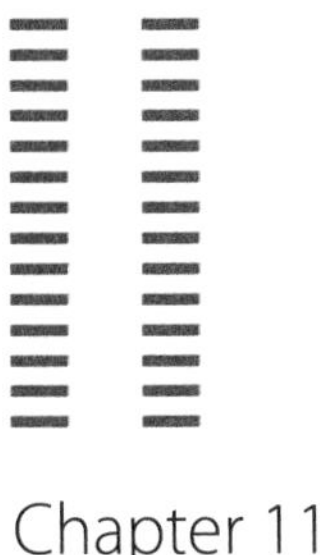

Chapter 11

Eosinophilic Pneumonia

Peter H. Michelson, MD

Introduction

A wide variety of respiratory illnesses cause elevations in peripheral blood eosinophil leukocyte numbers, but eosinophilic pneumonia is a specific condition characterized by infiltration of eosinophils into the lung parenchyma.[1,2] Eosinophilic pneumonia is either an acute or chronic condition.

Acute Eosinophilic Pneumonia

Although no specific causative agent has been determined, acute eosinophilic pneumonia (AEP) has been reported following exposures to multiple agents, including a number of medications, industrial agents, and tobacco smoke.[3] Recently environmental triggers have been reported with an unidentified toxin-induced AEP in US military personnel in Iraq,[4] as well as in rescue workers exposed following the terrorist attack of the World Trade Center.[5]

The clinical features of AEP include acute onset fever, severe hypoxemia, dyspnea, and cough. Diffuse pulmonary infiltrates are seen on chest radiograph.[2,6] In children, the onset of symptoms is rapid, resulting most commonly in respiratory failure requiring mechanical ventilation.[7] Because this condition closely simulates acute respiratory distress syndrome, aggressive supportive interventions are recommended while the initial diagnostic steps are undertaken.[3] Fluid stabilization, ventilatory support, and the initiation of broad-spectrum antibiotics are usually recommended. For diagnosis, bronchoscopy with bronchoalveolar lavage (BAL) is indicated to obtain a lower airway sample and to document the eosinophilia.[8,9]

Chronic Eosinophilic Pneumonia

Chronic eosinophilic pneumonia (CEP) is less commonly seen in children and differs from AEP in that it has an older age of onset; CEP is associated with an increase in the incidence of both asthma and atopy.[10,11] Symptoms of CEP are similar to AEP but absent the severe hypoxemia and acute respiratory failure. Patients with CEP progress more slowly, often extending months from the initial presentation. Although patients progress with subacute illness for weeks, when symptoms progress, BAL examination is also indicated to evaluate for CEP and has replaced open lung biopsy as the predominant diagnostic procedure. If there is concern about associated extrapulmonary manifestations or organ involvement, then systemic eosinophilic syndromes need to be considered with the appropriate blood work, and tissue sampling pursued.[12]

Presentation

Acute

Patients with AEP typically present with acute onset fever, dyspnea, and cough.[3] The age at presentation ranges from adolescence to young adult. The average onset of symptoms prior to diagnosis is approximately 4 days.[13] In addition to the acuity of presentation, the severity of the hypoxemia and the lack of a confirmed diagnosis of the respiratory distress are features of AEP. Pope-Harman et al[9] have proposed diagnostic criteria, which are listed in Box 11-1. To assess for lung eosinophilia,

Box 11-1. Diagnostic Criteria for Acute Eosinophilic Pneumonia[a]

- Acute onset (presentation within 7 days of onset of symptoms)
- Fever
- Bilateral infiltrates on chest radiograph
- Severe hypoxemia (arterial oxygen partial pressure on room air ≤60 mm Hg)
- Lung eosinophilia (bronchoalveolar lavage differential eosinophil cell count of ≥25%)
- No laboratory evidence of infection
- No history of hypersensitivity to drugs or other known causes of acute eosinophilic lung disease

[a] Adapted from Pope-Harman AL, Davis WB, Allen ED, Christoforidis AJ, Allen JN. Acute eosinophilic pneumonia. A summary of 15 cases and review of the literature. *Medicine (Baltimore).* 1996;75:334–342, with permission from Wolters Kluwer Health.

bronchoscopy with BAL is needed to document a differential cell count of 25% or greater, which has been proposed to be one of the diagnostic criteria for AEP, as well as to confirm no other infectious etiology.[9,14,15] The approach to evaluation of AEP is shown in Box 11-2.

Box 11-2. Evaluation of Acute Eosinophilic Pneumonia

History

Previously healthy individual
Acute onset dyspnea
Recent outdoor activity with extensive dust exposure
Possible recent tobacco use

Presentation

Cough
Fever
Chest pain
Tachypnea
Tachycardia
Crackles on physical examination

Laboratory Evaluation

Bilateral infiltrates on chest x-ray
Computed tomography with ground-glass opacities
Room air arterial oxygen partial pressure <60 mm Hg
Bronchoalveolar lavage (BAL) eosinophilia ≥25%
Negative infectious workup

Diagnostic Criteria

Acute onset of symptoms within 7 days of presentation
Fever
Bilateral infiltrates on chest radiograph
Severe hypoxemia
BAL or pulmonary eosinophilia
No other known cause of acute eosinophilia

Treatment

Systemic steroids

Although reports of AEP have included children aged 15 to 20 years,[3] the predominance of cases of AEP occur in adults, with a reported mean of 30 years and a maximum reported age at diagnosis of 86 years. Presentations are typical across all age ranges with no consistent association of asthma and only an inconsistent history of atopy. Tobacco use has been commonly linked, with some studies reporting up to two-thirds of patients with a history of tobacco use, many with recent initiation of smoking. In considering the very high rate of tobacco use contrasted with the rarity of AEP, a direct causative relationship is unlikely, but further investigation of this link is needed.[16] More likely, lung injury, perhaps enhanced by or associated with tobacco use, likely contributes to the development of AEP in a predisposed patient population.[17]

Exposures that have been reported to result in AEP include dust during outdoor activities, tear gas, workplace renovations, medications, and fungal exposure.[18] More recently there have been reports of AEP in firefighters exposed to World Trade Center dust[5] and in military personnel exposed to sand and possibly other toxins in Iraq.[4] One case of AEP was reported in a patient with HIV disease, although no specific infectious or medication trigger was identified.[19] As many have reported exposure to dusty outdoor activities, a hypersensitivity response to inhaled antigens has been suggested.[20]

Chronic

Chronic eosinophilic pneumonitis presents in a more progressive fashion than AEP, with the duration of symptoms reported for months.[1] Symptoms at presentation include chest pain, dyspnea, and cough, with a history of atopy and asthma reported in as many as two-thirds of patients.[17] The mean age at presentation is in the fifth decade; there is a female predominance and most patients report no history of tobacco use.[21]

Diagnostic Testing

Chest radiography typically shows bilateral infiltrates with alveolar, interstitial, or mixed alveolar and interstitial infiltrates.[18] Pleural effusions are not uncommon and persist during the recovery period. Although computed tomography findings of nodular infiltrates with ground-glass opacities have been reported,[8,17] these findings are not required to make the diagnosis. Conditions that merit consideration and mimic those radiologic findings include viral or atypical bacterial pneumonia, pulmonary hemorrhage, and diffuse alveolar damage.

Neither elevation of the peripheral white blood cell count or isolated eosinophilia have been consistently reported.[3] Obtaining BAL is critical to confirm lower airway eosinophilia. Cell differential examination of the BAL is required to make the diagnosis, with eosinophil differentials ranging up to greater than 50%. Diagnostic criteria require a differential greater than or equal to 25% eosinophils, which precludes the need for open lung biopsy.[9] This eosinophilia may also exist in the pleural fluid and sputum.[2]

In addition to cell differential determination, characterization of the hypoxemia is needed for the diagnosis. Either pulse oximetry or arterial oxygen determination is needed in addition to the radiograph, BAL cell count, and differential and examination findings to meet the established diagnostic requirements. Until bronchoscopy cultures are completed and negative, AEP can only be suggested but not confirmed.[18]

The workup of CEP is made difficult by its slow onset of symptoms and exclusion of other diagnoses. In this condition, pulmonary function testing may be indicated and a more complete assessment of extrapulmonary manifestations is recommended. Bronchoalveolar lavage or sputum examination for eosinophil markers of eosinophil degranulation will help to confirm the diagnosis.[12,22] Additional laboratory characteristics reported in CEP include elevated erythrocyte sedimentation rate and C-reactive protein, as well as a marked increase in immunoglobulin E in approximately half of the patients.[17]

Pathophysiology

The respiratory distress or respiratory failure associated with AEP seems to be most directly related to the influx of eosinophils.[23] Although peripheral eosinophilia is not universally present, eosinophilic infiltration into the lung parenchyma is what is responsible for the radiologic findings of infiltrates and hypoxemia characteristic of AEP. The immunologic response appears to involve both lymphocyte and eosinophilic recruitment.[24] Activated T lymphocytes secrete chemokines and interleukin-5, which recruit eosinophils and inhibit their apoptosis.[25] Once localized to the pulmonary interstitium, these cells degranulate further, releasing inflammatory mediators such as major basic protein, eosinophilic cationic protein, and leukotrienes.[26] These products have been implicated in causing the pathologic findings of interstitial infiltration, airway inflammation, and exudate deposition seen when biopsies are performed.[27]

Treatment

Treating acute eosinophilic pneumonia caused by exposure to medication or related to illness should primarily address treatment of the underlying cause. This should result in effective treatment of the lung disease. If this fails to resolve the symptoms, corticosteroids provide rapid successful resolution of the pulmonary pathology.[9] Either oral prednisolone or intravenous (IV) methylprednisolone is most commonly prescribed and is continued for 1 month after symptoms resolve or when the chest radiograph normalizes.[3] In most patients, this usually results in 4 to 6 weeks of steroids total. Additional treatment options have included inhaled corticosteroids and bronchodilators, especially if the symptoms involve airflow obstruction.[28]

Initial therapy for AEP includes supportive therapy of supplemental oxygen, IV antibiotics, and fluid management.[3,28] While the diagnosis is evolving, therapy should be broad and conservative. If respiratory failure ensues, ventilator support, initially with bi-level positive airway pressure and progressing to intubation and ventilation, is indicated. With rapid responses to corticosteroids reported, there is rarely a need for long periods of mechanical ventilator support.[18]

Most treatment regimens for both AEP and CEP begin with IV corticosteroids with doses up to 1 g/day in divided doses. Steroid dosing is usually tapered once symptoms resolve but, depending on the severity of presentation, the duration of treatment may extend past 6 weeks and last up to 3 months.[3] Relapse has not been reported in AEP responsive to corticosteroids. Chronic eosinophilic pneumonia is similarly responsive to the initial course of treatment, but in this condition, relapse is more common[17] and may require reinitiation of steroid therapy, with some chronic dosing often being maintained.

Key Points

- Acute eosinophilic pneumonia is marked by acute onset of respiratory distress, the severity of the hypoxemia, the presence of eosinophils on BAL, and lack of other causes of the respiratory failure.
- Acute eosinophilic pneumonia is significant for the short duration of symptoms prior to presentation and the rapid deterioration to respiratory failure, which may require mechanical ventilation.
- Treatment for AEP is high-dose steroids; recovery is rapid with no clinical sequelae.
- Acute eosinophilic pneumonia is distinguished from CEP by its rapid progression; the severity of the hypoxemia; and the lack of history of hypersensitivity to medications, asthma, or atopy.
- Chronic eosinophilic pneumonia differs in its infrequent need for mechanical ventilation and the high frequency of relapse on the withdrawal of corticosteroids.

References

1. Wechsler ME. Pulmonary eosinophilic syndromes. *Immunol Allergy Clin North Am.* 2007;27(3):477–492
2. Cottin V, Cordier JF. Eosinophilic pneumonias. *Allergy.* 2005;60(7):841–857
3. Janz DR, O'Neal HRJ, Ely EW. Acute eosinophilic pneumonia: a case report and review of the literature. *Crit Care Med.* 2009;37(4):1470–1474
4. Shorr AF, Scoville SL, Cersovsky SB, et al. Acute eosinophilic pneumonia among US military personnel deployed in or near Iraq. *JAMA.* 2004;292(24):2997–3005
5. Rom WN, Weiden M, Garcia R, et al. Acute eosinophilic pneumonia in a New York City firefighter exposed to World Trade Center dust. *Am J Respir Crit Care Med.* 2002;166(6):797–800
6. Allen J, Pacht ER, Gadek JE, Davis WB. Acute eosinophilic pneumonia as a reversible cause of noninfectious respiratory failure. *N Engl J Med.* 1989;321(9):569–574
7. Alp H, Daum RS, Abrahams C, Wylam ME. Acute eosinophilic pneumonia: a cause of reversible, severe, noninfectious respiratory failure. *J Pediatr.* 1998;132(3):540–543

8. Jeong YJ, Kim K-I, Seo IJ, et al. Eosinophilic lung diseases: a clinical, radiologic, and pathologic overview. *Radiographics.* 2007;27(3):617–637
9. Pope-Harman AL, Davis WB, Allen ED, Christoforidis AJ, Allen JN. Acute eosinophilic pneumonia. A summary of 15 cases and review of the literature. *Medicine (Baltimore).* 1996;75(6):334–342
10. Wubbel C, Fulmer D, Sherman J. Chronic eosinophilic pneumonia: a case report and national survey. *Chest.* 2003;123(5):1763–1766
11. O'Sullivan BP, Nimkin K, Gang DL. A fifteen-year-old boy with eosinophilia and pulmonary infiltrates. *J Pediatr.* 1993;123(4):660–666
12. Durieu J, Wallaert B, Tonnel AB. Long-term follow-up of pulmonary function in chronic eosinophilic pneumonia. Groupe d'Etude en Pathologie Interstitielle de la Societe de Pathologie Thoracique du Nord. *Eur Respir J.* 1997;10(2):286–291
13. Oermann CM, Panesar KS, Langston C, et al. Pulmonary infiltrates with eosinophilia syndromes in children. *J Pediatr.* 2000;136(3):351–358
14. Ogawa H, Fujimura M, Matsuda T, Nakamura H, Kumabashiri I, Kitagawa S. Transient wheeze. Eosinophilic bronchobronchiolitis in acute eosinophilic pneumonia. *Chest.* 1993;104(2):493–496
15. Hayakawa H, Sato A, Toyoshima M, Imokawa S, Taniguchi M. A clinical study of idiopathic eosinophilic pneumonia. *Chest.* 1994;105(5):1462–1466
16. Uchiyama H, Suda T, Nakamura Y, et al. Alterations in smoking habits are associated with acute eosinophilic pneumonia. *Chest.* 2008;133(5):1174–1180
17. Mason RJ, Broaddus VC, Martin T, et al, eds. *Murray and Nadel's Textbook of Respiratory Medicine.* 4th ed. Philadelphia, PA: WB Saunders; 2005
18. Philit F, Etienne-Mastroianni B, Parrot A, Guerin C, Robert D, Cordier JF. Idiopathic acute eosinophilic pneumonia: a study of 22 patients. *Am J Respir Crit Care Med.* 2002;166(9):1235–1239
19. Glazer CS, Cohen LB, Schwarz MI. Acute eosinophilic pneumonia in AIDS. *Chest.* 2001;120(5):1732–1735
20. Iwami T, Umemoto S, Ikeda K, Yamada H, Matsuzaki M. A case of acute eosinophilic pneumonia. *Chest.* 1996;110(6):1618–1621
21. Marchand E, Reynaud-Gaubert M, Lauque D, Durieu J, Tonnel AB, Cordier JF. Idiopathic chronic eosinophilic pneumonia. A clinical and follow-up study of 62 cases. The Groupe d'Etudes et de Recherche sur les Maladies "Orphelines" Pulmonaires (GERM"O"P). *Medicine (Baltimore).* 1998;77(5):299–312
22. Jederlinic P, Sicilian L, Gaensler EA. Chronic eosinophilic pneumonia: a report of 19 cases and a review of the literature. *Medicine (Baltimore).* 1988;67(3):154–162
23. Sarnaik A. Acute eosinophilic pneumonia: a treatable cause of severe acute respiratory failure. *Crit Care Med.* 1999;27(9):2069–2070

24. Katoh S, Matsumoto N, Fukushima K, et al. Elevated chemokine levels in bronchoalveolar lavage fluid of patients with eosinophilic pneumonia. *J Allergy Clin Immunol.* 2000;106(4):730–736
25. Taniguchi H, Kadota J, Fujii T, et al. Activation of lymphocytes and increased interleukin-5 levels in bronchoalveolar lavage fluid in acute eosinophilic pneumonia. *Eur Respir J.* 1999;13(1):217–220
26. Godding V, Bodart E, Delos M, et al. Mechanisms of acute eosinophilic inflammation in a case of acute eosinophilic pneumonia in a 14-year-old girl. *Clin Exp Allergy.* 1998;28(4):504–509
27. Katz U, Shoenfeld Y. Pulmonary eosinophilia. *Clin Rev Allergy Immunol.* 2008;34(3):367–371

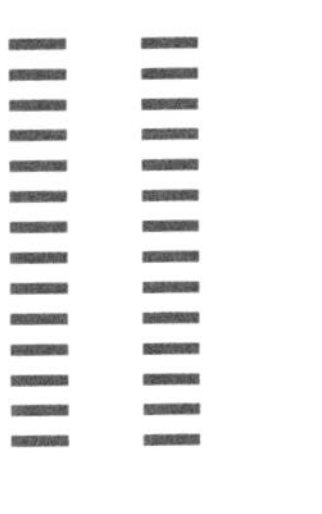

Chapter 12

Asthma

Miles Weinberger, MD

Introduction

Asthma is the most common medical diagnosis among hospitalized children. In the United States, asthma accounts for about 15% of non-surgical admissions to the hospital in children and adolescents. Asthma is also one of the leading causes for emergency care requirements; one of the leading causes for missed school; and a cause for considerable morbidity, disability, and occasional mortality at all ages.[1]

Despite these statistics, convincing data indicate that this failure of asthma management is not the result of inadequate therapeutic potential, but instead represents ineffective delivery of medical care.[2,3] Guidelines proposed by the National Asthma Education and Prevention Program have been published as expert panel reports beginning in 1991, with updates in 1997, 2002, and 2007.[4–6] Several specialist-guided and team-directed model programs involving primary care physicians have been shown to positively affect the outcomes of children with asthma.[7–9] However, the greatest degree of effectiveness for asthma management has been documented for care programs directed by subspecialists that use continuity of care, an organized plan for effective therapeutic decisions, and patient education to carry out the plan.[2,10–13] Even among particularly difficult groups of patients where socioeconomic factors complicate care, controlled clinical trials have demonstrated that specialized programs substantially improve outcome.[2,12]

Case Reports 12-1

J.L. is a 3-year-old boy who has had repeated episodes of prolonged coughing and occasional labored breathing since infancy. Between episodes he is completely well. Symptoms have been most frequent in the autumn and much less frequent during the summer months. He appears healthy and has been growing and developing normally. His episodic respiratory symptoms are often preceded by rhinorrhea. Respiratory symptoms have at times lasted several weeks. He has had multiple visits to his physician and local emergency department (ED), and has required several hospitalizations.

P.K. is an 8-year-old boy who had atopic dermatitis in infancy but has not been troubled by that since 3 years of age. Last fall he had episodes of wheezing and cough that abated during the winter but recurred the past year with greater severity and chronicity. Cough and wheezing were also associated with troublesome nasal stuffiness resulting in snoring and restless sleep.

L.M. is a 13-year-old girl who for the past year has had progressively severe wheezing and dyspnea, even with casual activity. While this is relieved by albuterol, the symptoms limit activity and at times interfere with sleep. She has seen an allergist who found no evidence for allergy.

C.P. is a 14-year-old girl who has been an accomplished athlete involved in competitive basketball, cross-country, track, and soccer since age 12. For the past year, she has been experiencing dyspnea during competitive activity, requiring her to frequently rest and briefly sit out during the competitive activity. She has no other history of respiratory problems. She has been diagnosed with exercise-induced asthma and was given an albuterol inhaler to use before exercise. The albuterol has not relieved her symptoms.

Diagnosis of Asthma

When presented with a child who has persistent, recurrent, newly experienced asthma symptoms, the most pertinent issues are how to confirm the diagnosis of suspected asthma and when to consider alternate diagnoses.

The diagnosis of asthma has no lower age limit. However, the diagnosis of asthma in the young child has been particularly associated with controversy.[14] Misdiagnosis, by calling acute exacerbations bronchitis or pneumonia, and alternative diagnostic terminology, such as reactive airways disease,[15] is a frequent consequence of this. Symptoms resulting from airway inflammation associated with asthma are frequently misdiagnosed as pneumonia and bronchitis.[16] This results in ineffective and unnecessary use of antibiotics.[17,18] On the other hand, asthma is also overdiagnosed, which also results in unnecessary and ineffective medication.[19–22]

Asthma is characterized by hyperresponsiveness of the airways to various stimuli resulting in airway obstruction that is reversible to a substantial degree either spontaneously or as a result of treatment. The airway obstruction is a result of varying degrees of bronchospasm and inflammation. Inflammation results in mucosal edema and mucus secretion (Figure 12-1).

Asthma should be considered when children have the following symptoms:

- Recurrent or chronic wheezing most prominent on expiration
- Recurrent or chronic coughing
- Repeated diagnoses of bronchitis
- Repeated diagnoses of pneumonia not clinically consistent with pyogenic infection

The diagnosis of asthma is most efficiently confirmed by demonstrating improvement of symptoms or spirometric measurement of airway obstruction to an inhaled $ß_2$-agonist or a 5- to 10-day course of high-dose oral corticosteroids. Children who do not become either asymptomatic or who do not have substantial reversal of airway obstruction with these measures may be referred to an appropriate subspecialist for further investigation of other medical or functional disorders that

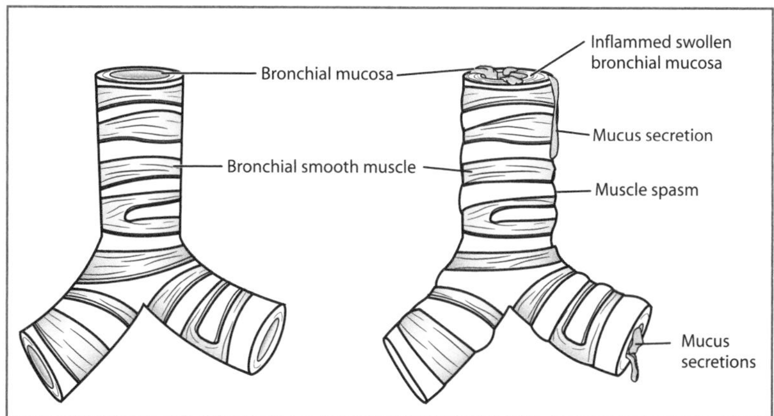

Figure 12-1. The 2 components of airway obstruction in asthma: bronchospasm and inflammation with mucosal edema and mucus secretions illustrated on the right. The normal airway is illustrated on the left.

can cause similar symptoms.[22] These include disorders such as cystic fibrosis, primary ciliary dyskinesia, tracheal or bronchial malacia, foreign body aspiration, vocal cord dysfunction, hyperventilation, or habit cough syndrome. Avoid making the diagnosis of asthma until there have been 3 distinct episodes of wheezing or prolonged cough with at least one response to anti-asthmatic medications.

Clinical Characterization of Asthma

Phenotypic Patterns

Because of the heterogeneous nature of asthma, simply making the diagnosis of asthma is not sufficient for the development of the most appropriate treatment plan. Planning effective and efficient strategies for managing asthma requires identifying the clinical pattern of disease. These clinical patterns or phenotypes can generally be determined by a brief history that addresses the following questions:

- What is the age of onset of lower respiratory symptoms?
- Are symptoms of asthma *only* associated with the clinical symptoms of a viral respiratory infection?
- Are there extended periods between episodes of respiratory symptoms where there is no cough or wheeze?
- Is there a seasonal variation in symptoms, and does the season match those of inhalant allergens for which the patient has allergen-specific immunoglobulin E (IgE)?
- Are respiratory symptoms related to specific environmental exposures?
- Are lower respiratory symptoms occurring daily for extended periods?

From the responses to those questions, a clinical pattern of asthma can be determined.

Intermittent Asthma

Intermittent asthma is characterized by episodic symptoms. Commonly, the asthma is triggered solely by viral respiratory infections with completely asymptomatic periods between the viral respiratory infections. Typically parents will say, "every time he/she gets a cold, it goes into his/her chest." Generally, this pattern of asthma begins in the first 1 or 2 years of life. The typical course is the onset of coryza from a common cold virus followed by cough, wheezing, and respiratory distress of varying severity that progresses over the next 1 to 2 days.

The duration of symptoms without effective intervention can be days, weeks, or months. During asymptomatic periods between colds, these patients have no evidence of airway inflammation when examined by bronchoalveolar lavage.[23]

The frequency of colds in preschoolers is increased for those in child care or where there is an older sibling in school. The seasonal pattern for this asthma phenotype parallels the seasonal pattern of cold viruses that begin with the onset of the school year and continue throughout the fall, winter, and spring (Figure 12-2).[24] An average of 7 colds per year with 15% of children experiencing 12 or more colds per year[25] can result in the appearance of almost continuous symptoms, but summer is generally associated with an abatement of symptoms in children. Asthma is limited to exacerbations from viral respiratory infection. Distinguishing this pattern of asthma from a chronic or seasonal allergic pattern is important because, unlike the latter, the most effective of maintenance therapies will not prevent the viral respiratory infection–induced asthma that characterizes this common intermittent pattern.[26–28]

The absence of allergen-specific IgE in an infant or toddler with a pattern of intermittent viral respiratory infection–induced asthma is generally predictive of a future associated with a greatly reduced frequency of symptoms or remission over time. While most infants and toddlers with asthma have this intermittent viral respiratory infection–induced pattern, allergy testing is effective in identifying those who have an allergic component currently contributing to their disease or those who are at risk for more persistent symptoms in the future.[29] Contrary to the belief of some, there is no age limitation for allergy testing, and some children can have evidence for inhalant allergy contributing to asthma even in infancy (Figure 12-3).

Persistent Asthma

Children with persistent (chronic) asthma experience virtually daily year-round symptoms and, in the absence of effective maintenance therapy, do not have extended symptom-free periods. These children may have begun with the viral respiratory infection–induced intermittent pattern of symptoms with subsequent evolution to persistent daily symptoms. Most, but not all, have an allergic component to their asthma.[30]

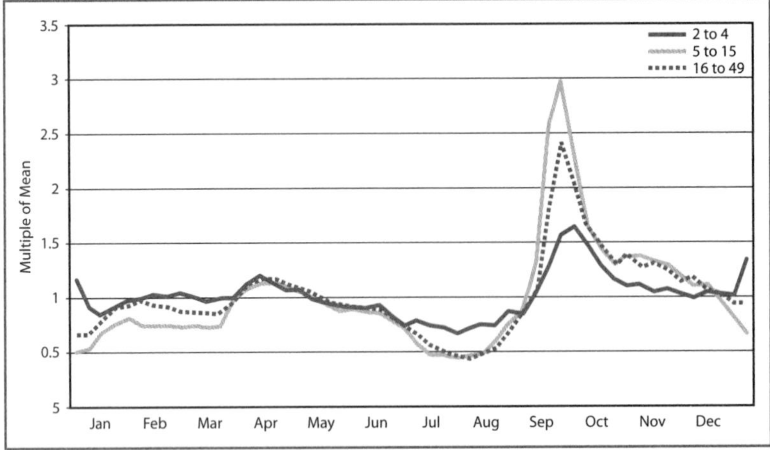

Figure 12-2. Typical autumnal increase in asthma at the beginning of the school year with the younger school-aged children beginning first followed by their older and younger siblings. (From Johnston NW, Johnston SL, Norman GR, Dai J, Sears MR. The September epidemic of asthma hospitalization: school children as disease vectors. *J Allergy Clin Immunol.* 2006;117:557–562, with permission from Elsevier.)

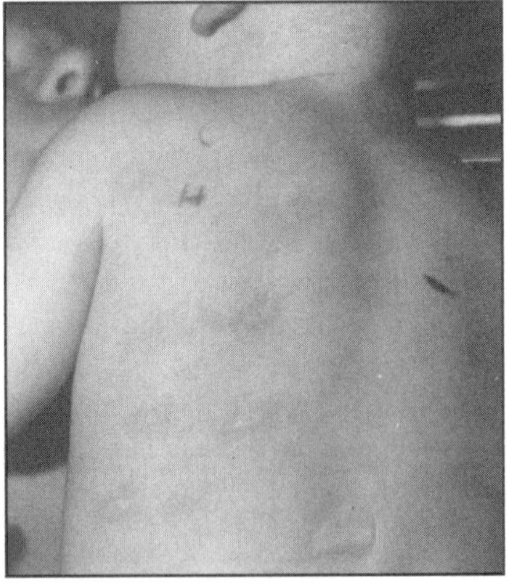

Figure 12-3. This 11-month-old infant was hospitalized at 9 months of age with severe acute asthma preceded by rhinoconjunctivitis during the peak of the grass pollen season in a Northern California valley area, where grass pollen is a major inhalant allergen. The typical wheal and flare of the multiple related species of grass pollen native to that area are seen on the left side of the infant's back. They are much larger than the histamine control (H) with no reactivity to the diluent control (C). Skin tests on the right side of the back to other common inhalant allergens were all negative. While immunotherapy using injections of allergenic extracts is rarely indicated at this age, this infant illustrates a striking exception where benefit could reasonably be expected.

Seasonal Allergic Asthma

Children with seasonal allergic asthma experience virtually daily symptoms during an inhalant allergy season. For example, in the North Central United States, this is most commonly from outdoor molds that grow on decaying vegetation from early spring through late fall, with peaks particularly in the spring and fall. In the valley areas of the Pacific Northwest and Northern California, grass pollens are the major allergens causing seasonal allergic asthma, generally accompanied by rhinoconjunctivitis. Allergens and seasonal patterns will vary with the geographic region. In other parts of the world, seasonal symptoms may be from molds, pollens, flying insects, or a combination of those airborne allergens.

There is potential overlap among these clinical patterns. For example, patients with chronic disease often have intermittent exacerbations from viral respiratory illness and may have seasonal allergic exacerbations. Nonetheless, identification of the clinical pattern contributes to the determination of a therapeutic strategy.

Consider these phenotypes in addressing the case reports described previously.

J.S., the 3-year-old boy with episodic respiratory symptoms that parallel the seasonal increase in common cold viruses, illustrates the most common pattern of intermittent asthma in the preschool-aged child. Most have fewer symptoms by school age, with perhaps about half remitting completely. However, many continue to have episodic asthma associated with viral respiratory infections into adult life. The decrease in the frequency of viral illnesses may explain the decrease in episodic asthma. About 20% of children with episodic respiratory symptoms demonstrate evidence of atopy and progress to more persistent symptoms. The presence or absence of atopy in J.S. could be used to provide prognostic information regarding the likelihood that he will have fewer symptoms with age or develop persistent symptoms. J.S. is unlikely to benefit from maintenance medication with an inhaled corticosteroid. Early intervention with inhaled bronchodilators and a short course of prednisolone is likely to minimize the risk of further ED visits and hospitalization.

P.K., who has atopic eczema and later developed seasonal asthma and rhinitis, exhibits a classical atopic triad. Atopic dermatitis is an eczematous rash commonly associated with the propensity to make allergen-specific IgE to ingestants and inhalants. While P.K. followed the pattern typical of two-thirds of children with atopic dermatitis by remitting after age 3, he progressed later to a seasonal pattern of asthma and rhinitis triggered by inhalant allergens during the growing season. Use of an inhaled corticosteroid during the growing season is likely to provide substantial benefit to P.K. Regular seasonal use of an intranasal steroid is also indicated for this child because of the nasal stuffiness, which is contributing to snoring and restless sleep.

L.M., the girl who developed a later onset of progressive wheezing and dyspnea, is illustrative of one type of nonallergic persistent asthma, which is more common in girls than boys. While different in clinical pattern from the first 2 vignettes in that there is neither a history of lower respiratory illness with viral respiratory infections in the past nor is there evidence of atopy, she nonetheless has asthma that is likely to be responsive to maintenance therapy with an inhaled corticosteroid.

C.P. is the active young athlete with exercise-induced dyspnea during her athletic activities. With no other respiratory symptoms, past or present, and no response to pre-activity use of albuterol, it is not likely she has asthma, and further use of medications for asthma is unlikely to be beneficial. She would benefit from a treadmill exercise challenge study that reproduces her symptoms and determines what is occurring physiologically at the time of symptoms.[20,31]

Severity

Asthma can vary in severity from trivial to life-threatening. Questions to assess severity include

- Do respiratory symptoms interfere with sleep?
- Do respiratory symptoms interfere with activity?
- What is the frequency of use of rescue medication with bronchodilator and systemic corticosteroids?
- With what frequency is urgent care required—a physician's office or ED? What is the frequency of hospitalization?
- How often was there a requirement for intensive care?
- What is the requirement for ventilatory assistance?
- Have there been any acute life-threatening events?

Treatment of Asthma

Treatment of asthma can be divided into 2 therapeutic strategies: intervention measures for acute symptoms (Table 12-1) and maintenance measures for prevention of future symptoms (Table 12-2).

Intervention Medication

An inhaled ß$_2$-agonist is typically the initial intervention for acute symptoms (Table 12-1). While older children can generally use a metered-dose inhaler (MDI) successfully, commonly nebulizers are used for young children and in EDs in the United States. However, the MDI with a valved holding chamber can provide equal or better efficacy for young children, even in the emergency care setting.[32,33] The simplicity, more rapid administration, lower cost, and greater portability of the MDI with a valved holding chamber has made this the method of choice for aerosol administration in children with asthma who are younger than 6 years, with the caveat that parents be properly trained and demonstrate the appropriate use of these devices prior to going home. Whether nebulizer or MDI with a valved holding chamber is used, proper instruction and a tight-fitting mask for those too young to seal their mouth on a mouthpiece are essential. A crying child gets little medication by either method. While providing rapid bronchodilatation, the ß$_2$-agonists do not alter the inflammatory component of asthma that contributes to airway obstruction by causing mucosal edema and mucus secretions.

Albuterol is the most common ß$_2$-agonist. A closely related pharmacologic agent that is essentially a therapeutic equivalent to albuterol, pirbuterol, is present in the Maxair Autohaler (Graceway Pharmaceuticals). That device activates with an inspiratory effort, eliminating the need to coordinate manual activation with inspiration. Marketing of the active optical isomer of albuterol, levalbuterol, has focused on the potential for the traditional racemic preparation of albuterol to have adverse effects that are not present with levalbuterol. However, clinical studies have not supported this claim,[34,35] and levalbuterol should be considered as therapeutically equivalent to the racemic preparation when given in dosage equivalent to the levalbuterol component of racemic albuterol (ie, half of the milligram quantity of racemic albuterol is levalbuterol).[36] One study suggesting therapeutic advantage

Table 12-1. Intervention Medication: Dosage and Decisions for Usual Treatment of Acute Symptoms of Asthma

Medication	Dosage	When to Use
Albuterol, levalbuterol, or pirbuterol by metered-dose inhaler	2–4 inhalations is usual, but up to 6 inhalations can be used (one at a time) and is equivalent to the most common dosage by nebulizer	As needed for cough, wheezing, labored breathing. Scheduled use has no advantage over as-needed use and may be deleterious for some patients. Repeated requirements for bronchodilator use during exacerbations generally warrants a short course of an oral corticosteroid.
Prednisone, prednisolone, methylprednisolone, dexamethasone as tablets. Liquid formulations and oral disintegrating tablets of prednisolone for young children. *(Parenteral forms indicated only when concerned about oral retention.)*	Dosage as prednisone or prednisolone. 1–2 mg/kg/twice daily, maximum 40 mg, twice daily. Higher doses for status asthmaticus.	When bronchodilator sub-responsiveness is identified by incomplete resolution of symptoms and signs from even repeat use of the bronchodilator. Continue until asymptomatic; reevaluate if not improving within 5 days or asymptomatic within 10 days. Don't taper.[a–c]
Ipratropium aerosol	0.5 mg with 2.5–5 mg albuterol by nebulizer	Indicated for severe acute asthma in the emergency department or hospital when response to a β_2-agonist is inadequate for relief of respiratory distress.

[a] Weinberger M. Commentary—corticosteroids for exacerbations of asthma: current status of the controversy. *Pediatrics.* 1988;81:726–729.

[b] Weinberger M. Corticosteroids for exacerbations of asthma: problems and solutions. *J Pediatr.* 2000;136:276–278.

[c] Ducharme FM, Chabot G, Polychronakos C, et al. Safety profile of frequent short courses of oral glucocorticoids in acute pediatric asthma: impact on bone metabolism, bone density, and adrenal function. *Pediatrics.* 2003;111:376–383.

Table 12-2. Maintenance Medication: Initial Dosage and Decisions for Treatment of Persistent Symptoms of Chronic or Seasonal Allergic Asthma[a]

Medication	Dosage	When to Use
Inhaled corticosteroid	Flovent 44 HFA MDI, 2 inhalations bid or Flovent 100 Diskus, 1 inhalation bid QVAR 40 (beclomethasone microaerosol HFA MDI), 2 inhalations bid Pulmicort Flexhaler (budesonide dry powder inhaler), 1 inhalation bid Asmanex 110 Twisthaler, 1 inhalation bid	First-line medication for persistent symptoms; use the Flovent or QVAR MDI with a valved holding chamber and mask for infants and toddlers—most can use a chamber without a mask by age 4; the dry powder inhaler formulations[b] can be used effectively in most by age 6.
Montelukast	4-mg sprinkle, 4- & 5-mg chewable, or 10-mg tablets (similar blood levels for each), once daily	An alternative to an inhaled corticosteroid for mild persistent symptoms; modest additional benefit as add-on to inhaled corticosteroids.
Long-acting β_2-agonist	Advair 100/50 Diskus (fluticasone/salmeterol dry powder inhaler), 1 inhalation bid or Advair 45/21 HFA MDI, 2 inhalations bid, or Symbicort 80/4.5 (budesonide/formoterol) HFA MDI, 2 inhalations bid	When a conventional dose of inhaled corticosteroid does not maintain control; monitoring for the occasional patient made worse from the addition of long-acting β_2-agonist is essential.
Slow-release theophylline	Begin with 10 mg/kg/day divided bid to a maximum of 150 mg bid; increase in increments to 16 mg/kg/day to a maximum of 300 mg bid; monitor serum theophylline concentrations to attain peak serum concentrations of 10–15 µg/mL[c]	As an additive agent to an inhaled corticosteroid for the occasional patient where a long-acting β_2-agonist worsens rather than improves asthma control. Awareness of drug interactions and effect of fever on theophylline levels is essential for safety.[d]

Abbreviations: bid, twice a day; MDI, metered-dose inhaler.

[a] Acute exacerbations, especially when induced by viral respiratory infection, require the intervention measures in Table 12-1.

[b] Asmanex Twisthaler, Flovent Diskus, Pulmicort Flexhaler.

[d] Walker S, Monteil M, Phelan K, et al. Anti-IgE for chronic asthma in adults and children. *Cochrane Database Syst Rev.* 2006;Apr 19:CD003559.

[c] Weinberger M, Hendeles L. Theophylline in asthma. *N Engl J Med.* 1996;334:1380–1388.

over racemic albuterol for children with acute asthma seen in an ED[37] was not supported in 2 subsequent studies.[38,39]

Because the $ß_2$-agonists do not alter the inflammatory component of airway obstruction, anti-inflammatory therapy is essential to relieve airway obstruction that is subresponsive to bronchodilators. Inhaled corticosteroids, even in high doses, have been shown to be relatively ineffective for acute exacerbations of asthma,[40] most of which are caused by viral respiratory infections.[41] In contrast to the little or no effect of inhaled corticosteroids on acute exacerbations of asthma, several studies have demonstrated that early aggressive use of systemic steroids provides impressive clinical benefit for children having an acute exacerbation of asthma.[42–46]

Early administration of systemic corticosteroids for acute asthma permits earlier discharge from the hospital,[42] decreases the likelihood of admission of patients seen for emergency care of asthma,[43,44] and prevents progression of exacerbations of asthma in ambulatory patients at risk for requiring urgent care.[45,46] These courses of oral corticosteroids average 5 to 7 days and should not exceed 10 days and tapering is not indicated.[47–49] Additionally, administration of oral corticosteroids during the early symptoms of a viral respiratory infection may prevent progression to severe acute asthma in children who have previously required hospitalization.[46] Despite controversies regarding the use of oral corticosteroids,[50] data now support early administration of systemic corticosteroids for acute exacerbations of asthma.[51] Repeated short courses of oral corticosteroids for viral respiratory infection–induced exacerbations in young children do not appear to cause sustained adverse effects.[52]

The most appropriate place to treat acute symptoms of asthma is where they occur: at home, at school, or at play. Treatment in the doctor's office, ED, or hospital should generally be considered damage control for treatment failure. The most effective measures for treating acute asthma are inhaled and oral medications. These measures are more effective when used before the need for urgent medical care rather than waiting until evaluation and treatment are performed in the ED, clinic, or physician's office.

When care is required in the emergency care setting, ipratropium, an anticholinergic aerosol, has been of value added to inhaled albuterol for severe acute asthma not fully responsive to albuterol alone.[53] However, it has no documented clinical role in ambulatory patients. Intravenous magnesium also may have some value for severe acute asthma, although routine use is not indicated.[54,55] Oxygen is indicated to correct hypoxemia. Measuring pH and partial pressure of carbon dioxide (Pco_2) is indicated when hypoxemia is present. Early in the course of acute asthma, ventilation/perfusion ($\dot{V}/\dot{Q}$) mismatching causes hypoxemia. As airway obstruction progresses, Pco_2 may gradually increase. This constitutes respiratory failure. While $\dot{V}/\dot{Q}$ mismatching requires only continued oxygen and pharmacologic intervention measures, respiratory failure requires admission to an intensive care setting where assisted ventilation is available if sufficiently rapid reversal of the airway obstruction does not occur.

Maintenance Medication

Maintenance medication (Table 12-2) is indicated for those with persistent asthma and for those with prolonged seasonal allergic asthma. The goal is to use acceptably safe daily medication that effectively suppresses asthmatic symptoms and maintains normal lung function. Inhaled corticosteroids are the most effective medications for children with persistent asthma. These agents can be effectively delivered, even to preschool-aged children, by both MDI via a valved holding chamber and by nebulizer.[56–58] Although an aerosol corticosteroid is available as a nebulizer solution (Pulmicort Respules), there is no evidence that this offers any therapeutic advantage over the simpler and more rapid administration from a pressurized MDI with a valved holding chamber. Whichever inhaled corticosteroid preparation is used, individualized instruction is essential for efficacy. For infants and toddlers, a tight-fitting mask[59] and quiet breathing are required for effective delivery—a crying child gets little delivery of aerosolized medication to the lungs.[60]

Although there is evidence for dose-related systemic effects,[61] conventional low doses of inhaled corticosteroids have an established safety record.[62,63] A minimal degree of hypothalamic-pituitary axis suppression and a small degree of transient growth suppression is detectable at modest doses, but neither clinically detectable adverse effects nor sustained effect on growth are apparent except at higher doses.[64] Montelukast has potential benefit for some with milder manifestations of asthma[65] and also has some additive effect with inhaled corticosteroids.[66] However, the additive effect of montelukast does not appear to be as great as is seen with a long-acting inhaled $ß_2$-agonist (LABA).[66] Adding a LABA to an inhaled corticosteroid is generally more effective than a higher dose of the inhaled steroid.[67,68] However, concerns have been raised regarding tolerance to the subsequent bronchoprotective effect of inhaled $ß_2$-agonists with continued stimulation of the $ß_2$-adrenergic receptors.[69,70]

A small subset of patients appears to be at particular risk for adverse effects from LABAs. Increased fatalities associated with LABAs have been reported and resulted in a US Food and Drug Administration black box warning regarding this class of medications.[71,72] A report of 2 patients who had life-threatening symptoms poorly responsive to $ß_2$-agonist bronchodilators while receiving salmeterol had dramatic improvement after stopping the salmeterol.[73] This was consistent with studies showing that certain genetic polymorphisms of the $ß_2$-receptor were associated with down-regulation of that receptor during regular administration of $ß_2$-adrenergic agents.[74–78] Theophylline is an alternative additive agent with similar efficacy to the addition of a LABA, though less convenient to use.[79] Rational medication selection and careful monitoring of the patient with regularly scheduled return visits permits optimal control.

Immunotherapy (allergy shots) can reduce asthma symptoms in highly selected cases where the symptoms can be convincingly related to a limited number of well-defined inhalant allergens to which immunotherapy has been shown to be of benefit.[80,81] The monoclonal anti-IgE preparation omalizumab (Xolair) may treat the allergic component of asthma. Although quite costly, severely symptomatic children with asthma that has a major allergic component may benefit substantially from this medication.[82]

Environmental Considerations

The primary care physician should assess the child's environment and its role in contributing to asthma symptoms. See Box 12-1 for questions to clarify environmental issues.

Rural homes, especially those on farms, can result in more intense exposure to outdoor molds during procedures that stir up decaying vegetation, such as harvesting. Very old homes may be plagued by indoor mold, especially if there is a basement with dampness or water leakage. Forced air heating can distribute aeroallergens throughout

Box 12-1. Questions to Clarify Environmental Issues

- Urban or rural home?
- Age of home?
- Presence of a basement and dampness or water leakage problems?
- Forced air heating system; central air conditioning?
- Pets in home?
- Smokers in home?
- Nearby industrial or agricultural source of air pollution?

the home but also provides an opportunity to use a high-efficiency air filter to minimize aeroallergens in the indoor environment. Pets are a common contributing factor to asthma, but they should not be blamed for symptoms without demonstrating allergen-specific IgE and obtaining a convincing history that exposure contributes to morbidity.

Indoor fireplaces and outdoor bonfires or leaf burning are important non-allergenic major irritants that contribute to asthmatic symptoms. Exposure to tobacco smoke is a major irritant that increases the frequency and severity of acute and chronic asthma symptoms (Figure 12-4).

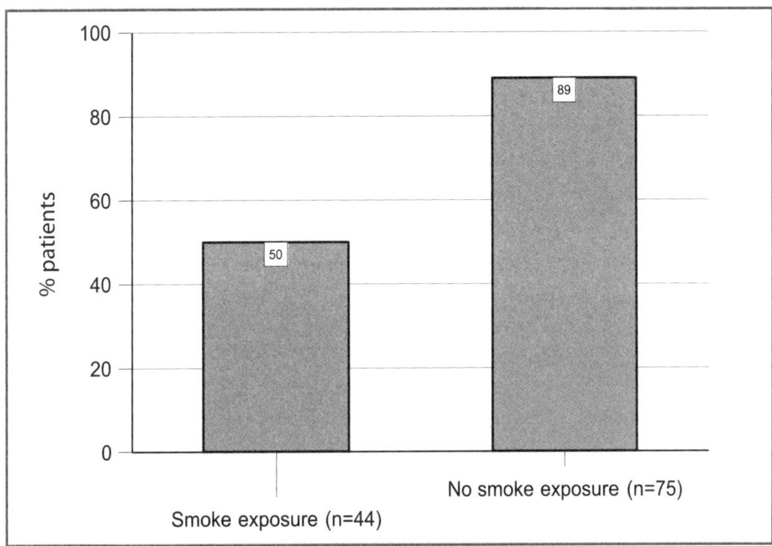

Figure 12-4. Patients meeting criteria for control of asthma during a 1-year period of observation (defined in Box 12-1) during care in a specialty care program among those exposed or not exposed to cigarette smoke. Cigarette smoke exposure was associated with a significantly lower likelihood of meeting criteria for control despite receiving care at the same specialty clinic ($P<0.001$). (Based on data from Najada et al.[3])

Clinically important aeroallergens vary with the region and include pollens, outdoor and indoor molds, animal dander, cockroaches, and dust mites. Knowledge of allergen-specific IgE in the patient and the aerobiology of the patient's environment are essential to assess the importance of environmental factors.

Treating Exercise-Induced Asthma

Bronchospasm induced by exercise is a common component of active asthma. If baseline pulmonary function is normal or near normal, either naturally or with maintenance medication, exercise-induced bronchospasm can be readily prevented for most patients by pretreating with an inhaled bronchodilator, such as albuterol or pirbuterol. If a bronchodilator does not block exercise-induced bronchospasm, then alternate diagnoses need to be pursued.[20,31] An uncommon but serious reason for the loss of bronchoprotective effect from bronchodilators is as a result of the regular use of long-acting bronchodilators, such as salmeterol or formoterol.[73]

Treating Difficult Asthma

Asthma symptoms may be difficult to control because (1) the asthma responds poorly to therapeutic measures, (2) there is non-adherence to the prescribed treatment, or (3) the child does not have asthma.[22] When asthma responds poorly to treatment, consider that the first of these reasons is the least common. The most common cause is that the medication is not being taken or is not being taken properly. Check the technique of inhaler administration. Check pharmacy refills to determine if a maintenance corticosteroid inhaler is being refilled at intervals consistent with regular use, but also consider that the problem is appropriateness of diagnosis.[22]

Hospitalization

While hospitalization for asthma leads all other medical causes at many hospitals, treatment is essentially the same as that which would have prevented most hospitalizations had the treatment been performed earlier (ie, aerosol bronchodilators and systemic corticosteroids). The additional essential care provided by hospitalization is the ability to ensure that medications are effectively given and the ability to monitor and provide assisted ventilation if needed. Hospitalization occurs when dyspnea or hypoxemia is not responsive to home or emergency care. The decision to hospitalize may be influenced by social factors in addition to the severity of the physiological abnormality.

High doses of systemic corticosteroids (Table 12-1) should be given for any child with asthma that requires an ED visit or hospitalization for asthma. Inhaled albuterol can be given repeatedly whenever there is an increase in the work of breathing, and continuous nebulization of albuterol has been associated with a decreasing need for assisted ventilation. The addition of ipratropium provides clinical benefit for those with severe airway obstruction that does not respond adequately to albuterol alone. Discharge from the hospital should occur once the level of care is such that it can be continued at home. There is no indication to continue hospitalization until all wheezing is gone. Once improvement is well established, deterioration is highly unlikely.

Treating Comorbidities

Treating comorbidities may benefit the control of chronic asthma. There is a great deal of controversy regarding the role of sinusitis and gastroesophageal reflux (GER) as comorbidities that contribute to asthma. While both sinusitis and GER are associated with asthma, the evidence that treating them benefits asthma is anecdotal only and not evidence-based.[83–85] While chronic rhinitis should be treated with topical nasal steroids in patients experiencing discomfort from nasal congestion, and GER should be treated in those experiencing the associated substernal discomfort, there is little reason to expect clinically important benefit for the asthma itself. Symptoms attributed to sinusitis are predominantly those of rhinitis, and there is little correlation between radiologic evidence of sinusitis and clinical symptoms.[83,86–88]

Monitoring the Clinical Course

Successful management of asthma does not stop with writing the prescriptions. There should rarely be a need to see the patient during acute symptoms, since the patient or family should have been taught with verbal and written instructions successful management by use of the inhaled bronchodilator for symptom relief and early intervention with a short course of systemic corticosteroid for an exacerbation identified by subresponsiveness to the inhaled $ß_2$-agonist. However, scheduled return visits are essential to review adherence to the treatment plan, to check inhaler technique, to assess if the patient meets criteria for control (Box 12-2), and to make adjustments in treatment when appropriate to meet those criteria with the least amount of medication.

Box 12-2. Criteria for Control of Asthma

- Absence of hospitalization
- Absence of urgent care requirements
- Absence of interference with sleep
- Absence of interference with activity
- Infrequent use of inhaled $ß_2$-agonists for acute symptoms
- Infrequent use of oral corticosteroids
- Normal or near normal pulmonary function by spirometry

While some believe the peak flow meter is a useful means to monitor a patient, the weight of evidence indicates that symptom monitoring (and consequent need for intervention with an inhaled $ß_2$-agonist) has been demonstrated to be generally equal to[89,90] or better[91,92] than peak flow monitoring in providing early warning of an exacerbation that requires intervention. The only situations where a home peak flow meter might be useful are for the occasional under-perceiver, who usually has very severe chronic asthma and who doesn't recognize worsening airway obstruction, or the over-perceiver, who confuses anxiety or hyperventilation with asthma.

There is current interest in the use of exhaled nitric oxide as a marker of asthmatic inflammation.[93,94] Although the commercial device available to measure exhaled nitric oxide may have some clinical usefulness, particularly in children who present with atypical asthma, such as with chronic cough, troublesome asthmatic inflammation is generally adequately detectable by the presence of active symptoms and the measurement of the extent to which pulmonary function does not fully reverse with a bronchodilator.

General medical care for asthma should include routine immunizations. The varicella vaccine is particularly important because of the small but serious risk of disseminated varicella that has been reported when an infection occurs during a course of high-dose systemic corticosteroids as may be necessary for exacerbations of asthma.[95] A yearly influenza vaccine is now a general recommendation for children and is especially appropriate for children with asthma.[96] A small risk from influenza vaccine is present for those with allergy to egg. However, the presence of clinically important adverse affects appears unlikely.[97]

The best decision-making by the physician will fail unless the family or patient is adequately educated about the benefits and risks, if any, of each medication and in the implementation of the treatment plan.[98] Particularly important is having a simple written action plan that deals with periods of increased symptoms and exacerbations (Box 12-3). There is no advantage to complex plans with traffic light cartoon illustrations, although some parents may find these useful to organize their approach to treating asthma exacerbations at home.[99] Seasonal allergic

Box 12-3. Intervention Action Plan Handout for an Acute Exacerbation of Asthma

Acute symptoms of asthma including cough, wheeze, or shortness of breath should be dealt with promptly. They are particularly likely with a viral respiratory infection (common cold). Increasing cough following a day of runny nose is often the first sign of asthma triggered by a viral respiratory infection. While regularly taken medication will not prevent the acute flare of asthma from a viral respiratory infection, prompt intervention can shorten the course and generally prevent the need for urgent medical care or hospitalization.

First: Use your inhaled bronchodilator.

If symptoms stop completely: Repeat inhaled bronchodilator when necessary; consider a short course of oral corticosteroid after third dose for acute symptoms within 8 hours or if more than 4 in 24 hours *(other than for preventive use before exercise).*

If symptoms are not completely relieved: Repeat inhaled bronchodilator.

If symptoms still not completely relieved: A short course of oral corticosteroids may be needed. If uncertain what to do, call us for advice at (telephone number). Otherwise, take first dose of oral corticosteroid and contact us at the same number. *(Dosage and instructions should already be on hand.) The response to oral corticosteroids is slow.* ***For patients who have required emergency care or hospitalization, oral corticosteroid should be started at least 12 to 24 hours before symptoms become severe.***

Once corticosteroids are begun, inhaled bronchodilator can be repeated when needed. Maintenance medications should be continued.

Continued increase in the frequency of inhaled bronchodilator use or continued difficulty breathing may require hospitalization. Call us at the number above if there is continued difficulty breathing. Frequent intervention treatment for episodes of asthma requires reassessment of the management plan.

increases in symptoms may warrant an increase in or additional maintenance medication. Viral respiratory infection–induced symptoms are likely to require a short course of oral corticosteroids.

Evaluating and Managing Difficult Asthma

Difficult asthma is that which does not meet criteria for control despite appropriate therapy. The reason for such poor control is variable. In some cases, the asthma is truly poorly responsive to usual measures. However, more often, the poor control is because of poor adherence to the medical regimen. When poorly controlled symptoms of asthma are present despite appropriately prescribed medication, adherence to the prescribed medication can be verified by asking for a record of medication refills from their pharmacy. For example, a month's supply of the maintenance medication that lasted 6 months can readily explain inadequate control. The technique of using inhaled medication can also be an issue. Observing technique during a routine office visit can be revealing and provides an opportunity for appropriate education. In some cases, poor control is because the patient doesn't have asthma at all—the symptoms are from some other problem with symptoms that mimic those of asthma[22] (see comments in the section Diagnosis of Asthma). Placing the difficult-to-treat patient in a hospital for a period for around-the-clock observation may be necessary in some cases to sort out these various confounding problems.

Natural History of Asthma

Parents frequently ask if their child will outgrow asthma. In the preschool-aged child with episodic wheezing, the presence of atopy identified by the presence of allergen-specific IgE is highly associated with continued symptoms throughout childhood, while those with no presence of a potential allergic component are likely to have marked reduction or cessation of asthmatic symptoms by school age (Figure 12-5).[100]

The long-term clinical course of asthma in young children has been impressively examined in a prospective study with repeated evaluations for 35 years.[101] In 1963 all children aged 6 to 7 years in Melbourne, Australia, had a medical examination on entering school that included a short questionnaire and interview. As part of that questionnaire, parents were asked if their child had experienced episodes

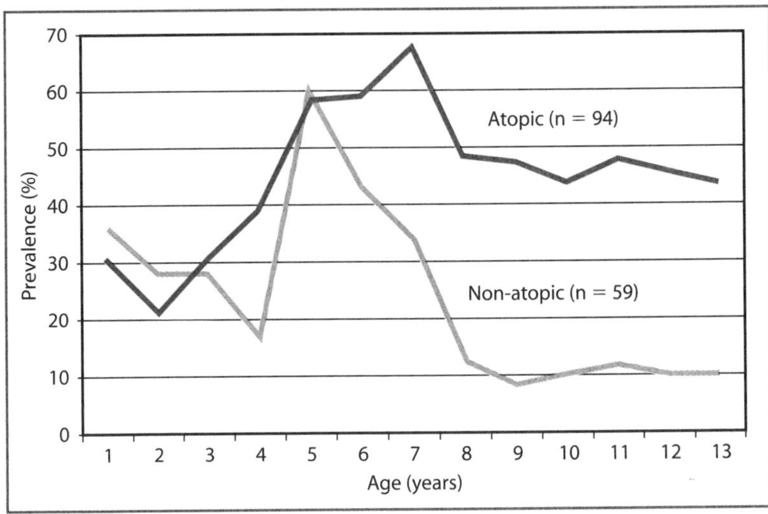

Figure 12-5. Prevalence of symptoms by age in atopic and non-atopic asthma. (From Illi S, von Mutius E, Lau S, Niggemann B, Gruber C, Wahn U. Perennial allergen sensitization early in life and chronic asthma in children: a birth cohort study. *Lancet.* 2006;368:763–770, with permission from Elsevier.)

of wheezing or asthma and whether that had been associated with symptoms of a viral respiratory infection. Based on that survey, overall community prevalence for asthma symptoms in childhood was estimated to be about 20%, a rate similar to that described more recently in the United States.[102,103] A stratified sample was then randomly selected the following year from the approximately 30,000 seven-year-old children in the survey. This included 105 second graders who had never wheezed to serve as controls, 75 with less than 5 episodes of previous wheezing with viral respiratory infections, 104 with 5 or more episodes of previous wheezing with viral respiratory infections, and 113 with recurrent wheezing not limited to association with viral respiratory infections. The investigators also entered 83 children from the same population who had severe chronic asthma since before age 3 years with persistent symptoms, barrel chest deformity, and/or forced expiratory volume in 1 second that was 50% or less than the forced vital capacity. The children were reevaluated at ages 14, 21, 28, 35, and 42 years (Figure 12-6).[101]

Seventy-five percent of the sample followed longitudinally had infrequent episodes while 25% had frequent episodes. Forty percent of the initial children with asthma were free of respiratory symptoms by age

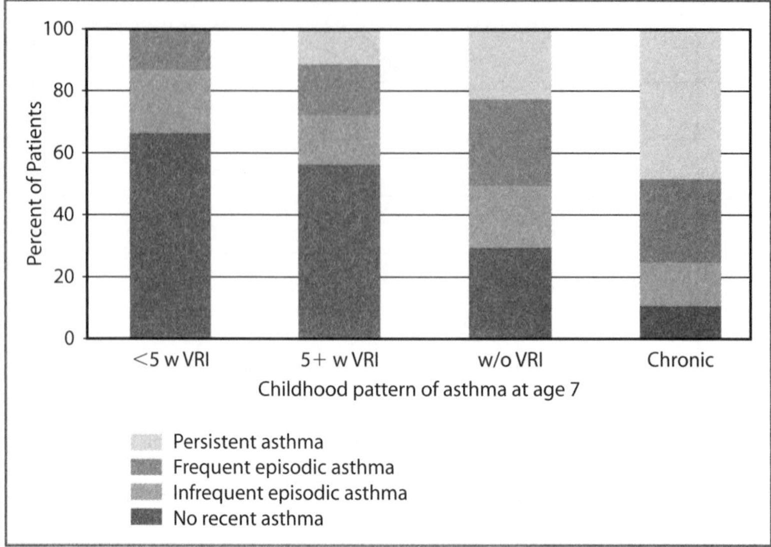

Figure 12-6. Clinical expression of childhood asthma at age 42 years. VRI, viral respiratory infection. (From Phelan PD, Robertson CF, Olinsky A. The Melbourne Asthma Study: 1964–1999. *J Allergy Clin Immunol.* 2002;109:189–194, with permission from Elsevier.)

10, and 50% were asymptomatic by age 14. The remainder continued into adult life, but symptoms were frequently not troublesome, present only with viral respiratory infections or exercise for many. However, 10% who had ceased wheezing in childhood had recurrences as young adults, and some of those had troublesome symptoms. The group with severe persistent asthma had growth failure and delayed puberty but eventually attained normal adult height. While 50% of that group with severe persistent asthma improved considerably at puberty, only 5% became totally asymptomatic.

When the subjects were examined at 42 years of age, a correlation between the nature of the symptoms in childhood and the subsequent outcome was apparent. More than half of those with symptoms of asthma limited to an association with viral respiratory infection prior to age 7 were asymptomatic at age 42. Others were still having episodic asthma, and a few had developed persistent asthma. The frequency of all patterns of active asthma at age 42 years was greater among those in whom wheezing without viral respiratory infections had been reported in childhood. About half of those with severe persistent asthma as children continued to have persistent symptoms at age 42, with only 11% of that group reporting no recent asthma.

There has been speculation that early treatment with inhaled corticosteroids could modify the course of subsequent asthma. The hypothesis that inhaled steroids given for episodic wheeze might alter the subsequent course of asthma was examined in a randomized, double-blind study of infants without demonstrable benefit either for acute symptoms or the frequency of recurrent episodes.[104] This hypothesis also has been tested in a group of 2- and 3-year-old children at high risk for persistent asthma randomly assigned to receive fluticasone aerosol or placebo over a 1-year period. While symptoms were significantly less in the inhaled corticosteroid–treated group, the frequency of asthmatic symptoms became identical to the placebo-treated group once the inhaled corticosteroids were stopped, indicating the absence of any sustained effect on the disease.[105]

Key Points

Introduction

- Asthma is the most common chronic disease of children.
- Asthma causes more hospitalizations than any other medical problem in children.
- Asthma is associated with rhinitis and atopic dermatitis as important comorbidities.

Clinical characteristics of asthma

- Asthma is both underdiagnosed and overdiagnosed.
- Intermittent asthma is most commonly a viral respiratory infection–induced phenotype in preschool-aged children but is seen at all ages.
- Persistent asthma phenotype is characterized by the absence of extended symptom-free periods.
- Seasonal allergic phenotype is characterized by being limited to seasons that correspond to allergen-specific IgE to seasonal inhalant allergens.

Severity of asthma

- Interference with activity from exercise limitation
- Interference with sleep from repeated nocturnal awakening
- Frequency of requirements for intervention measures, inhaled bronchodilators, and oral corticosteroids

Key Points (continued)

Management of asthma

- Intervention measures for relief of acute symptoms are albuterol and oral corticosteroids.
- Maintenance medications for those with chronic or extended seasonal symptoms include inhaled corticosteroids, long-acting bronchodilators, leukotriene modifiers, immunotherapy, and anti-IgE.

Monitoring the clinical course of asthma

- The patient's awareness of symptoms is essential to early intervention to prevent progression of exacerbations.
- Scheduled follow-up appointments for assessment and education are required to evaluate adequacy of treatment and assess adherence to the treatment plan.

Evaluating and managing difficult asthma

- Distinguishing between poor adherence and incorrect diagnosis may require observation of the patient's inhaler use technique, family education, or even temporary hospitalization.

Natural history of asthma

- Many children will outgrow symptoms of asthma by adolescence. A significant number of children will continue to have asthma symptoms well into adulthood, even if they appear to have ceased wheezing during adolescence.
- Children who wheeze without an associated viral respiratory infection have a greater likelihood of asthma symptoms that persist into adulthood.

References

1. Mannino DM, Homa DM, Akinbami LJ, et al. Surveillance for asthma—United States, 1980–1999. *MMWR Surveill Summ.* 2002;(5)1:1–13
2. Kelly CS, Morrow AL, Shults J, et al. Outcomes evaluation of a comprehensive intervention program for asthmatic children enrolled in Medicaid. *Pediatrics.* 2000;105:1029–1035
3. Najada A, Abu-Hasan M, Weinberger M. Outcome of asthma in children and adolescents at a specialty based care program. *Ann Allergy Asthma Immunol.* 2001;87:335–343

4. National Heart, Lung, and Blood Institute. *National Asthma Education and Prevention Program Expert Panel Report 2: Guidelines for the Diagnosis and Management of Asthma*. Bethesda, MD: National Institutes of Health; 1997. NIH Publication No. 97-4051
5. National Heart, Lung, and Blood Institute. *National Asthma Education Program Updates on Selected Topics from Expert Panel Report 2:. Guidelines for the Diagnosis and Management of Asthma*. Bethesda, MD: National Institutes of Health; 2002. NIH Publication No. 02-5074
6. National Heart, Lung, and blood Institute. *National Asthma Education Program Expert Panel Report 3 (EPR-3). Guidelines for the Diagnosis and Management of Asthma*. Bethesda, MD: National Institutes of Health; 2007. NIH Publication No. 08-5846
7. Cloutier MM, Wakefield DB, Sangeloty-Higgins PS, et al. Asthma guideline use by pediatricians in private practices and asthma morbidity. *Pediatrics*. 2006;118:1880–1887
8. Guarnaccia S, Lombardi A, Gaffurini A, et al. Application and implementation of the GINA asthma guidelines by specialist and primary care physicians: a longitudinal follow-up study on 264 children. *Prim Care Respir J*. 2007;16:357–362
9. Fox P, Porter PG, Lob SH, et al. Improving asthma-related health outcomes among low-income, multiethnic school-aged children: results of a demonstration project that combined continuous quality improvement and community health worker strategies. *Pediatrics*. 2007;120:e902–e911
10. Fireman P, Friday GA, Gira GC, et al. Teaching self-management skills to asthmatic children and their parents in an ambulatory care setting. *Pediatrics*. 1981;68:341–348
11. Bucknall CE, Robertson C, Moran F, et al. Differences in hospital asthma management. *Lancet*. 1988;1:748–750
12. Mayo PH, Richman J, Harris HW. Results of a program to reduce admissions for adult asthma. *Ann Intern Med*. 1990;112:864–871
13. Kelso TM, Abou-Shala N, Heilker BM, et al. Comprehensive long-term management program for asthma: effect on outcomes in adult African-Americans. *Am J Med Sci*. 1996;311:272–280
14. Weinberger M, Abu-Hasan M. Asthma in preschool children. In: Chernick V, Boat TF, Wilmott RW, Bush A, eds. *Kendig's Disorders of the Respiratory Tract in Children*. 7th ed. Philadelphia, PA: Saunders Elsevier; 2006:795–807
15. Fahy JV, O'Byrne PM. Reactive airways disease: a lazy term of uncertain meaning that should be abandoned. *Am J Respir Crit Care Med*. 2000;163:822–823
16. Joseph CL, Foxman B, Leickly FE, et al. Prevalence of possible undiagnosed asthma and associated morbidity among urban schoolchildren. *J Pediatr*. 1996;129:735–742
17. Shapiro GG, Eggleston PA, Pierson WE, et al. Double-blind study of the effectiveness of a broad spectrum antibiotic in status asthmaticus. *Pediatrics*. 1974;53:867–872

18. Glauber JH, Fuhlbrigge AL, Finkelstein JA, et al. Relationship between asthma medication and antibiotic use. *Chest.* 2001;120:1485–1492
19. Hammo AH, Weinberger M. Exercise induced hyperventilation: a pseudo-asthma syndrome. *Ann Allergy Asthma Immunol.* 1999;82:574–578
20. Abu-Hasan M, Tannous B, Weinberger M. Exercise-induced dyspnea in children and adolescents: if not asthma then what? *Ann Allergy Asthma Immunol.* 2005;94:366–371
21. Seear M, Wensley D, West N. How accurate is the diagnosis of exercise induced asthma among Vancouver school children. *Arch Dis Child.* 2005;90:898–902
22. Weinberger M, Abu-Hasan M. Pseudo-asthma: when cough, wheezing, and dyspnea are not asthma. *Pediatrics.* 2007;120:855–864
23. Maclennan C, Hutchinson P, Holdsworth S, et al. Airway inflammation in asymptomatic children with episodic wheeze. *Pediatr Pulmonol.* 2006;41:577–583
24. Johnston NW, Johnston SL, Norman GR, et al. The September epidemic of asthma hospitalization: school children as disease vectors. *J Allergy Clin Immunol.* 2006;117:557–562
25. Rosenstein N, Phillips WR, Gerber MA, et al. The common cold—principles of judicious use of antimicrobial agents. *Pediatrics.* 1998;101:181–184
26. Wilson N, Sloper K, Silverman M. Effect of continuous treatment with topical corticosteroid on episodic viral wheeze in preschool children. *Arch Dis Child.* 1995;72:317–320
27. Doull IJ. Limitations of maintenance therapy for viral respiratory infection-induced asthma. *J Pediatr.* 2003;142:S21–S25
28. McKean M, Ducharme F. Inhaled steroids for episodic viral wheeze of childhood. *Cochrane Database Syst Rev.* 2000;(2):CD001107
29. Sherrill D, Stein R, Kurzius-Spencer M, et al. On early sensitization to allergens and development of respiratory symptoms. *Clin Exp Allergy.* 1999;29:905–911
30. Wright AL. Epidemiology of asthma and recurrent wheeze in childhood. *Clin Rev Allergy Immunol.* 2002;22(1):33–44
31. Weinberger M, Abu-Hasan M. Perceptions and pathophysiology of dyspnea and exercise-tolerance. *Pediatr Clin North Am.* 2009;56:33–48
32. Delgado A, Chou KJ, Silver EJ, et al. Nebulizers vs metered-dose inhalers with spacers for bronchodilator therapy to treat wheezing in children aged 2 to 24 months in a pediatric emergency department. *Arch Pediatr Adolesc Med.* 2003;157:76–80
33. Castro-Rodriguez JA, Rodrigo GJ. Beta-agonists through metered-dose inhaler with valved holding chamber versus nebulizer for acute exacerbation of wheezing or asthma in children under 5 years of age: a systematic review with meta-analysis. *J Pediatr.* 2004;145:172–177
34. Ahrens RC, Weinberger M. Levalbuterol and racemic albuterol: are there therapeutic differences [editorial]? *J Allergy Clin Immunol.* 2001;106:681–684

35. Weinberger M. Is there any advantage to using levalbuterol in the treatment of asthma? *Clin Pulm Med.* 2004;11:129–134
36. A levalbuterol metered-dose inhaler (Xopenex HFA) for asthma. *Med Lett Drugs Ther.* 2006;48(1230):21–22
37. Carl JC, Myers TR, Kirchner HL, et al. Comparison of racemic albuterol and levalbuterol for treatment of acute asthma. *J Pediatr.* 2003;143:731–736
38. Qureshi F, Zaritsky A, Welch C, et al. Clinical efficacy of racemic albuterol versus levalbuterol for the treatment of acute pediatric asthma. *Ann Emerg Med.* 2005;46:29–36
39. Hardasmalani MD, DeBari V, Bithoney WG, et al. Levalbuterol versus racemic albuterol in the treatment of acute exacerbation of asthma in children. *Pediatr Emerg Care.* 2005;21:415–419
40 Hendeles L, Sherman J. Are inhaled corticosteroids effective for acute exacerbations of asthma in children? *J Pediatr.* 2003;142:S26–S33
41. Lemanske RF. Viruses and asthma: inception, exacerbation, and possible prevention. *J Pediatr.* 2003;142:S3–S8
42. Storr J, Barrell E, Barry W, et al. Effect of a single oral dose of prednisolone in acute childhood asthma. *Lancet.* 1987;1:879–882
43. Tal A, Levy N, Bearman JE. Methylprednisolone therapy for acute asthma in infants and toddlers: a controlled clinical trial. *Pediatrics.* 1990;86:350–356
44. Scarfone RJ, Fuchs SM, Nager AL, et al. Controlled trial of oral prednisone in the emergency department treatment of children with acute asthma. *Pediatrics.* 1993;92:513–518
45. Harris JB, Weinberger M, Nassif E, et al. Early intervention with short courses of prednisone to prevent progression of asthma in ambulatory patients incompletely responsive to bronchodilators. *J Pediatr.* 1987;110:627–644
46. Brunette MG, Lands L, Thibodeau LP. Childhood asthma: prevention of attacks with short-term corticosteroid treatment of upper respiratory tract infection. *Pediatrics.* 1988;81:624–629
47. Lederle FA, Pluhar RE, Joseph AM, et al. Tapering of corticosteroid therapy following exacerbation of asthma. A randomized, double-blind, placebo-controlled trial. *Arch Intern Med.* 1987;147:2201–2203
48. O'Driscoll BR, Kalra S, Wilson M, et al. Double-blind trial of steroid tapering in acute asthma. *Lancet.* 1993;341:324–327
49. Karan RS, Pandhi P, Behera D, et al. A comparison of non-tapering vs. tapering prednisolone in acute exacerbation of asthma involving use of the low-dose ACTH test. *Int J Glin Pharmacol Ther.* 2002;40:256–262
50. Weinberger M. Commentary—corticosteroids for exacerbations of asthma: current status of the controversy. *Pediatrics.* 1988;81:726–729
51. Weinberger M. Corticosteroids for exacerbations of asthma: problems and solutions. *J Pediatr.* 2000;136:276–278

52. Ducharme FM, Chabot G, Polychronakos C, et al. Safety profile of frequent short courses of oral glucocorticoids in acute pediatric asthma: impact on bone metabolism, bone density, and adrenal function. *Pediatrics.* 2003;111:376–383
53. Streetman DD, Bhatt-Mehta V, Johnson CE. Management of acute, severe asthma in children. *Ann Pharmacother.* 2002;36:1249–1260
54. Scarfone RJ, Loiselle JM, Joffe MD, et al. A randomized trial of magnesium in the emergency department treatment of children with asthma. *Ann Emerg Med.* 2000;36:572–578
55. Ciarallo L, Brousseau D, Reinert S. Higher-dose intravenous magnesium therapy for children with moderate to severe acute asthma. *Arch Pediatr Adolesc Med.* 2000:154:979–983
56. Baker JW, Mellon M, Wald J, et al. A multiple-dosing placebo-controlled study of budesonide inhalation suspension given once or twice daily for treatment of persistent asthma in young children and infants. *Pediatrics.* 1999;103:414–421
57. Nielsen KG, Bisgaard H. The effect of inhaled budesonide on symptoms, lung function, and cold air and methacholine responsiveness in 2- to 5-year-old asthmatic children. *Am J Respir Crit Care Med.* 2000;162:1500–1506
58. Chavasse RJ, Bastian-Lee Y, Richter H, et al. Persistent wheezing in infants with an atopic tendency responds to inhaled fluticasone. *Arch Dis Child.* 2001;85:143–148
59. Smaldone GC, Berg E, Nikander K. Variation in pediatric aerosol delivery: importance of facemask. *J Aerosol Med.* 2005;18:354–363
60. Iles R, Lister P, Edmunds AT. Crying significantly reduces absorption of aerosolized drug in infants. *Arch Dis Child.* 1999;81:163–165
61. Eid N, Morton R, Olds B, et al. Decreased morning serum cortisol levels in children with asthma treated with inhaled fluticasone propionate. *Pediatrics.* 2002;109:217–221
62. Allen DB. Inhaled corticosteroid therapy for asthma in preschool children: growth issues. *Pediatrics.* 2002;109:373–380
63. Kelly HW, Nelson HS. Potential adverse effects of the inhaled corticosteroids. *J Allergy Clin Immunol.* 2003;112:469–478
64. Doull IJ. The effect of asthma and its treatment on growth. *Arch Dis Child.* 2004;89:60–63
65. Muijsers RB, Noble S. Spotlight on montelukast in asthma in children 2 to 14 years of age. *Am J Respir Med.* 2002;1:225–228
66. Ram FS, Cates CJ, Ducharme FM. Long-acting beta2-agonists versus anti-leukotrienes as add-on therapy to inhaled corticosteroids for chronic asthma. *Cochrane Database Syst Rev.* 2005;Jan 25(1):CD003137
67. Greening AP, Ind P, Northfield M, et al. Added salmeterol versus higher-dose corticosteroid in asthma patients with symptoms on existing inhaled corticosteroid (Allen & Hanburys Limited UK Study Group). *Lancet.* 1994;344:219–324

68. Woolcock A, Lundback B, Ringdal N, et al. Comparison of addition of salmeterol to inhaled steroids with doubling of the dose of inhaled steroid. *Am J Respir Crit Care Med.* 1996;153:1481–1488
69. Anderson SD, Caillaud C, Brannan JD. β2 agonists and exercise-induced asthma. *Clin Rev Allergy Immunol.* 2006;31:163–180
70. Haney S, Hancox RJ. Recovery from bronchoconstriction and bronchodilator tolerance. *Clin Rev Allergy Immunol.* 2006;31:81–196
71. Castle W, Fuller R, Hall J, et al. Serevent nationwide surveillance study: comparison of salmeterol with salbutamol in asthmatic patients who require regular bronchodilator treatment. *BMJ.* 1993;306:1034–1037
72. Nelson HS, Weiss ST, Bleecker ER, et al. The salmeterol multicenter asthma research trial: a comparison of usual pharmacotherapy for asthma or usual pharmacotherapy plus salmeterol. *Chest.* 2006;129:5–26
73. Weinberger M, Abu-Hasan M. Life threatening asthma during treatment with salmeterol. *N Engl J Med.* 2006;335:852–853
74. Israel E, Drazen JM, Liggett SB, et al. The effect of polymorphism of the beta2-adrenergic receptor on the response to regular use of albuterol in asthma. *Am J Respir Crit Care Med.* 2000;162:75–80
75. Lee DK, Currie GP, Hall IP, et al. The arginine-16 beta2-adrenoceptor polymorphism predisposes to bronchoprotective subsensitivity in patients treated with formoterol and salmeterol. *Br J Glin Pharmacol.* 2004;57:68–75
76. Israel E, Chinchilli VM, Ford JG, et al. Use of regularly scheduled albuterol treatment in asthma: genotype-stratified, randomized, placebo-controlled cross-over trial. *Lancet.* 2004;364:1505–1512
77. Wechsler ME, Lehman E, Lazarus SC, et al. β-adrenergic receptor polymorphisms and response to salmeterol. *Am J Respir Crit Care Med.* 2006;173:519–526
78. Palmer CNA, Lipworth BJ, Ismail T, et al. Arginine-16 3 2 adrenoceptor genotye predisposes to exacerbations in young asthmatics taking regular salmeterol. *Thorax.* 2006;61:940–944
79. Weinberger M, Hendeles L. Theophylline in asthma. *N Engl J Med.* 1996;334:1380–1388
80. Reid MJ, Moss RB, Hsu YP, et al. Seasonal asthma in northern California: allergic causes and efficacy of immunotherapy. *J Allergy Glin Immunol.* 1986;78:590–600
81. Roberts G, Hurley C, Turcanu V, et al. Grass pollen immunotherapy as an effective therapy for childhood seasonal allergic asthma. *J Allergy Clin Immunol.* 2006;117:263–268
82. Walker S, Monteil M, Phelan K, et al. Anti-IgE for chronic asthma in adults and children. *Cochrane Database Syst Rev.* 2006;Apr 19:CD003559
83. Zimmerman B, Stringer D, Feanny S, et al. Prevalence of abnormalities found by sinus x-rays in childhood asthma: lack of relation to severity of asthma. *J Allergy Glin Immunol.* 1987;80:(3 pt 1):268–273

84. Weinberger M. Gastroesophageal reflux is not a significant cause of lung disease in children. *Pediatr Pulmonol.* 2004;S26:194–196
85. Gibson PG, Henry RL, Coughlan JL. Gastro-oesophageal reflux treatment for asthma in adults and children. *Cochrane Database Syst Rev.* 1999;(2):CD001496
86. Shopfner CE, Rossi JO. Roentgen evaluation of the paranasal sinuses in children. *Am J Roentgenol Radium Ther Nucl Med.* 1973;118:176–186
87. Glasier CM, Ascher DP, Williams KD. Incidental paranasal sinus abnormalities on CT of children: clinical correlation. *AJNR.* 1986;7:861–864
88. Diament MJ, Senac MO, Gilsanz V, et al. Prevalence of incidental paranasal sinuses opacification in pediatric patients: a CT study. *J Comput Assist Tomogr.* 1987;11:426–431
89. Malo JL, L'Archeveque J, Trudeau C, et al. Should we monitor peak expiratory flow rates or record symptoms with a simple diary in the management of asthma? *J Allergy Clin Immunol.* 1993;91:702–709
90. Legge JS. Peak-expiratory-flow meters and asthma self-management. *Lancet.* 1996;347:1709–1710
91. Clough JB, Sly PD. Association between lower respiratory tract symptoms and falls in peak expiratory flow in children. *Eur Respir J.* 1995;8:718–722
92. Chan-Yeung M, Chang JH, Manfreda J, et al. Changes in peak flow, symptom score, and the use of medications during acute exacerbations of asthma. *Am J Respir Crit Care Med.* 1996;154:889–893
93. Ratnawati R, Thomas PS. Exhaled nitric oxide in paediatric asthma. *Chronic Respir Dis.* 2005;2:163–174
94. Taylor DR, Pijnenburg MW, Smith AD, et al. Exhaled nitric oxide measurements: clinical application and interpretation. *Thorax.* 2006;61(9):817–827
95. Silk HJ, Guay-Woodford L, Perez-Atayde AR, et al. Fatal varicella in steroid-dependent asthma. *J Allergy Clin Immunol.* 1988;81:47–51
96. Brownstein JS, Kleinman KP, Mandl KD. Identifying pediatric age groups for influenza vaccination using a real-time regional surveillance system. *Am J Epidemiol.* 2005;162:686–693
97. James JM, Zeiger RS, Lester MR, et al. Safe administration of influenza vaccine to patients with egg allergy. *J Pediatr.* 1998;133(5):624–628
98. Weinberger M. Managing asthma for patients and families. 2006. http://www.uihealthcare.com/topics/medicaldepartments/pediatrics/asthma/index.html. Accessed November 10, 2010
99. Gibson P, Powell H. Written action plans for asthma: an evidence-based review of the key components. *Thorax.* 2004;59:94–99
100. Illi S, von Mutius E, Lau S, et al. Perennial allergen sensitization early in life and chronic asthma in children: a birth cohort study. *Lancet.* 2006;368:763–770
101. Phelan PD, Roberson CF, Olinsky A. The Melbourne asthma study: 1964–1999. *J Allergy Clin Immunol.* 2002;109:189–194

102. Grant EN, Daugherty SR, Moy JN, et al. Prevalence and burden of illness for asthma and related symptoms among kindergartners in Chicago public schools. *Ann Allergy Asthma Immunol.* 1999;83:113–120
103. Yawn BP, Wollan P, Kurland M, et al. A longitudinal study of the prevalence of asthma in a community population of school-age children. *J Pediatr.* 2002;140:576–581
104. Bisgaard H, Hermansen MN, Loland L, et al. Intermittent inhaled corticosteroids in infants with episodic wheezing. *N Engl J Med.* 2006;354:1998–2005
105. Guilbert TW, Morgan WJ, Zeiger RS, et al. Long-term inhaled corticosteroids in preschool children at high risk for asthma. *N Engl J Med.* 2006:354:1985–1997

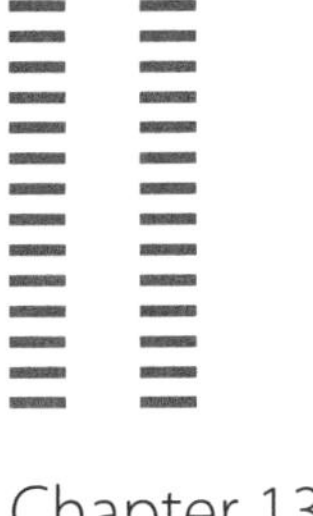

Chapter 13

Congenital Abnormalities of the Upper Airway

James W. Schroeder Jr, MD
Susanna McColley, MD

Introduction

Obstructive congenital lesions of the upper airway produce turbulent airflow according to the laws of fluid dynamics. This rapid, turbulent airflow across a narrowed segment of the respiratory tract produces distinctive sounds that are diagnostically useful to the clinician. The location of the obstruction dictates the phase, tone, and nature of the sound, and these direct the differential diagnosis. *Stertor* describes the low-pitched inspiratory snoring sound typically produced by nasal or nasopharyngeal obstruction. *Stridor* typically originates from the larynx, upper trachea, or hypopharynx. *Wheezing* is the expiratory sound produced by the turbulent flow of air through constricted small airways (bronchioles). This sound is similar to, and frequently mistaken for, other intrathoracic conditions such as bronchomalacia, tracheomalacia, or foreign bodies in the tracheobronchial tree.[1]

The timing of the noisy breathing can be particularly useful in determining the location of a congenital abnormality of the upper airway. As outlined in Holinger's "laws" of airway obstruction,[2] the severity of the noisy breathing in relation to the sleep-wake cycle is important. In general, when the noise is worse during sleep, the obstruction is nasal or pharyngeal. This is especially true with tonsil and adenoid obstruction. If the symptoms are worse when the child is awake or exacerbated by exertion, the obstruction is typically laryngeal, tracheal, or bronchial. These rules are helpful in locating the lesion during the initial assessment. However, they are generalizations and like most rules they have exceptions. For example, the initial presentation of a child with recurrent respiratory papillomatosis of the larynx is progressive upper airway obstruction during sleep rather than on exertion.

The phase of breathing in which the noises occur can also be diagnostic. Stertor is typically an inspiratory sound that occurs due to turbulent airflow over a fixed or positional obstruction in the nasal cavity or pharynx. In infants, who are obligate nasal breathers, this turbulence will be greatest during inhalation. During exhalation the infant will be able to use the oral cavity or will be able to displace non-fixed lesions and decrease or bypass the obstruction. Stridor is most often an inspiratory sound. Based on Bernoulli's principle, a narrowing at the level of the larynx will cause the air flowing through the narrowing to increase in speed and therefore decrease the pressure in this area. This in turn causes the narrowed area to narrow even further, increasing the obstruction and the stridor. During exhalation the opposite occurs. The non-fixed laryngeal lesion is forced laterally, opening the obstruction, and decreasing the noise. However, if the laryngeal lesion is fixed, such as in the subglottis where the cricoid cartilage forms a complete ring, the lesion will not move during exhalation and there will be a biphasic (inspiratory and expiratory) stridor. Intrathoracic lesions (tracheomalacia and bronchomalacia) create an expiratory sound (wheezing) due to the exaggerated collapse of the airways during exhalation when the pleural pressure increases and compresses the bronchioles. During inhalation, when the pleural pressure decreases, the bronchioles enlarge and no sound is produced.

Assessment

When assessing a child with a suspected congenital anomaly of the upper airway it is important to determine the severity and location of the obstruction. The severity of mild to moderate chronic persistent obstruction must be assessed in the presence of acute symptoms of respiratory distress (increased work of breathing, retractions, nasal flaring, and cyanosis). The mnemonic SPECS-R[3] is a useful tool to organize history taking and to determine the need for endoscopy in the operating room. This technique incorporates the parents' subjective interpretation of the child's obstruction along with a more objective measurement of the child's eating and sleeping behavior (Box 13-1). Radiography is also a helpful tool in assessing these children.

Box 13-1. Subjective Interpretation of Airway Obstruction

S: Severity—parents' subjective impression
P: Progression of the obstruction over time
E: Eating or feeding difficulties; aspiration; failure to thrive
C: Cyanotic episodes; apparent life-threatening events
S: Sleep obstruction so severe that retractions occur during sleep
R: Radiology-specific abnormalities detected by radiographs

Congenital Nasal Anomalies

Newborns are obligate nasal breathers. Therefore, an obstructive lesion of the nasal cavity can cause significant respiratory distress in an infant. The symptoms do not vary based on the location of the lesion in the nasal cavity. In general, the respiratory distress caused by nasal obstruction is worse at rest and can be relieved with crying because the oral cavity is open. Some common congenital nasal anomalies are listed in Box 13-2.

Box 13-2. Congenital Anomalies of the Upper Airway

Congenital nasal anomalies
- Piriform aperture stenosis
- Choanal atresia
- Nasolacrimal duct cyst
- Nasal dermoids, gliomas, encephaloceles

Craniofacial Abnormalities
- Crouzon syndrome
- Apert syndrome
- Pierre Robin sequence
- Down syndrome

Congenital Lesions of the Tongue
- Vascular malformations
- Tumors (rhabdomyosarcoma)
- Tongue base
  - Ectopic thyroid
  - Lingual thyroid
  - Thyroglossal duct cyst

Congenital Laryngeal Anomalies
- Laryngomalacia
- Laryngocele
- Saccular cysts
- Vocal cord paralysis
- Subglottic stenosis

Piriform Aperture Stenosis

Piriform aperture stenosis is caused by overgrowth of the medial maxilla. This condition is often not readily noticed on physical examination and can be diagnosed by a craniofacial computed tomography (CT) scan demonstrating a narrowed piriform aperture in relation to the posterior choana.[4] This can also be seen in conjunction with a mega-incisor, which may be associated with holoprosencephaly.[5] These children should be evaluated with neuroimaging as well as for other endocrine abnormalities associated with an abnormal pituitary adrenal axis. Piriform aperture stenosis causing significant respiratory distress can be corrected surgically through a sublabial incision.

Choanal Atresia

Choanal atresia is an uncommon disorder that is the most common cause of complete nasal obstruction in the neonate. It occurs when the posterior choanae fail to develop properly. The published incidence varies from 1 in 5,000 to 1 in 8,000 live births.[6] Both sexes are affected, but reports suggest a female predominance of 2 to 1. Unilateral cases are more common than bilateral cases, and bony atresia (90%) is more common than membranous atresia (10%). However, some publications suggest that mixed bony-membranous anomalies may have the highest incidence.[7] The condition can be diagnosed by the failure to pass a 6 French catheter more than 32 mm past the anterior nares. Axial CT and nasal endoscopy confirm the diagnosis. Orotracheal intubation or an oral airway device must be used to relieve the obstruction until the patient is a candidate for surgery. Unilateral atresia may not be noticed until later in life. Choanal atresia is associated with other congenital anomalies 43% to 72% of the time.[8] It is most commonly seen as part of CHARGE association, which includes coloboma of the eye, heart defects, atresia (choanal), retarded growth and development, genitourinary hypoplasia, and ear anomalies. Non-syndromic choanal atresia is usually sporadic and most likely multifactorial. Surgical correction can be performed via a transoral transpalatal approach or, more commonly, through a transnasal endoscopic approach that often requires postoperative stenting followed by repeat dilations.

Nasolacrimal Duct Cyst

The nasolacrimal duct is patent in 30% of newborns. It becomes patent for most newborns during the first month of life.[9] If the nasolacrimal apparatus fails to canalize, a mucocele (nasolacrimal duct cyst) can develop and expand into the nose from under the inferior turbinate and enter the inferior meatus anteriorly, causing nasal airway obstruction. The cyst can occasionally be seen via anterior rhinoscopy, but the diagnosis is confirmed by nasal endoscopy after nasal decongestion and/or CT scan. The cyst can become infected and cause swelling and erythema of the medial canthus and purulent orbital discharge. Treatment consists of endoscopic marsupialization and nasolacrimal duct probing.

Nasal Dermoids, Gliomas, and Encephaloceles

Nasal dermoids, gliomas, and encephaloceles are congenital midline nasal lesions that are believed to result from abnormal closure of the anterior neuropore. All encephaloceles and many dermoids and gliomas communicate with the central nervous system. Therefore, no congenital nasal mass or polyp in a child should be manipulated until intracranial communication is ruled out. Computed tomography and magnetic resonance imaging (MRI) are required for diagnosis and surgical planning. Dermoid sinuses and cysts generally occur in the nasal midline and can present as a fistulous tract or a mass anywhere from the nasal tip to the glabella.[10] Hair or sebaceous material may protrude from the pit, and patients may present with drainage. Gliomas and encephaloceles are similar in clinical appearance and histology. Gliomas are unencapsulated collections of glial cells that may retain attachments to the dura. Encephaloceles are herniations of the meninges with or without brain tissue through the skull base and communicate with the subarachnoid space.[11] They usually present early in life but can be unrecognized until adulthood. Unlike dermoids, they do not routinely occur in the midline, nor do they connect to a sinus tract to the skin. These lesions are surgically removed jointly by an otolaryngologist and neurosurgeon using a combination of external and endoscopic approaches.

Craniofacial Abnormalities

Craniofacial abnormalities can be associated with airway compromise by obstructing the nose, nasopharynx, oropharynx, or hypopharynx (Box 13-2). Crouzon syndrome (craniofacial dysostosis) is defined by craniosynostosis and maxillary hypoplasia. The resulting midface hypoplasia and high-arched palate can lead to nasal obstruction. Severe cases can warrant intubation or tracheotomy. Apert syndrome (acrocephalosyndactyly) is also marked by severe maxillary hypoplasia resulting in proptosis and relative prognathism. The underdeveloped nose and high-arched palate result in significant nasal obstruction. Apert syndrome is also associated with syndactyly of the hands. Pierre Robin sequence (cleft palate, micrognathia, and glossoptosis) can cause severe pharyngeal airway obstruction at birth. In mild cases prone positioning can help. In more severe cases an oral airway or intubation may be needed to bypass the obstruction caused by the base of the tongue. Mandibular distraction can eliminate the obstruction by pulling the tongue base forward and relieving the glossoptosis. A tracheostomy is occasionally needed until the distraction is completed or the mandible has grown sufficiently. This sequence can be associated with Stickler syndrome, and genetic workup is required.

Down syndrome occurs in approximately 1 in 700 live births and is the most common congenital chromosomal anomaly.[12] There are multiple head and neck morphological abnormalities in these children that predispose them to disease. This includes midface hypoplasia, which is characterized by malformation of the eustachian tube, a shortened palate, macroglossia, and a narrowing of the oropharynx and nasopharynx.[13] In combination with systemic hypotonia, these abnormalities underlie the high incidence of recurrent otitis media and obstructive sleep apnea in children with Down syndrome. Obstructive sleep apnea is the most common cause of upper airway obstruction in children older than 1 year. Nearly 50% of parents of these children do not report a sleep disturbance despite abnormal findings on a sleep study. The true incidence of obstructive sleep apnea is unknown, and a high level of suspicion should be maintained.

Congenital Lesions of the Tongue

Macroglossia

Macroglossia can also be caused by vascular malformations, muscular enlargement, and tumors. Lymphangiomas or hemangiomas of the tongue may cause significant airway obstruction present at birth. Lymphangiomas are the most common cause of macroglossia in children and are apparent at birth in 60% of cases.[14] Symptoms include dysphagia; drooling; disarticulation; and a dried, fissured tongue. In cases of severe obstruction intubation or tracheostomy may be required followed by a surgical reduction of the tongue. In children, tumors of the tongue are rare but rhabdomyosarcoma can occur, and 20% of these tumors that occur in the head and neck present in the tongue[14] (Box 13-2).

Congenital Lesions of the Base of the Tongue

Congenital lesions of the base of the tongue are rare and include ectopic thyroid tissue, most commonly a lingual thyroid, and thyroglossal duct cysts. A lingual thyroid can present with upper airway obstruction in a newborn or as part of the workup for congenital hypothyroidism. Seventy percent to 100% of children with ectopic thyroid tissue in the tongue have no other thyroid tissue present.[15] Diagnosis can be confirmed with CT, ultrasonography, or MRI. Radionuclide scans will help localize functioning thyroid tissue. The ectopic thyroid tissue is subject to the same pathologic changes as normal thyroid tissue but it is usually associated with hypothyroidism. Treatment includes suppression therapy to prevent enlargement, hypothyroidism, and malignancy.[16] Radioactive iodine-131 ablation has also been described.[16] However, when the obstruction is not corrected by suppression therapy or if malignancy is suspected, surgical excision is the treatment of choice. This can be accomplished through transoral and transcervical approaches.

Thyroglossal Duct Cysts

Thyroglossal duct cysts are the most common malformations found in the neck and account for 70% of congenital cervical abnormalities. Although they can present at any age, most are detected in the first 2 decades of life, making them primarily a pediatric disease.[17] Thyroglossal duct cysts usually present as a midline cervical mass that lies either directly above the hyoid bone or just below it. The mass typically moves with protrusion of the tongue. Besides the cosmetic deformity associated with these lesions, they can become recurrently infected and, therefore, surgical excision is the treatment of choice. The cyst is removed through a midline cervical incision along with the central portion of the hyoid bone as well as the associated tract in the base of tongue. This is called the Sistrunk procedure.

Congenital Laryngeal Anomalies

Laryngomalacia

Laryngomalacia is the most common cause of inspiratory stridor in infants. Symptoms typically begin 1 to 3 weeks after birth and usually progress over several months. It is caused, in part, by decreased laryngeal tone leading to supraglottic collapse during inspiration.[18] Gastroesophogeal reflux disease and neurologic disease influence the severity of the disease and, thereby, the clinical course.[18] A greater disease severity is associated with low Apgar scores. The diagnosis is made primarily based on symptoms that include stridor, dysphagia, apnea, cyanosis, and failure to thrive. Awake flexible fiberoptic laryngoscopy is used to confirm the diagnosis. In otherwise healthy children, laryngomalacia typically resolves by 1 year of age without surgical intervention. However, in 15% to 20% of patients symptoms are severe enough to cause progressive respiratory distress, cyanosis, or failure to thrive.[19] In these patients, supraglottoplasty is considered. This procedure has replaced tracheostomy as the initial surgical intervention in infants with severe laryngomalacia. It may be performed using cold knife instrumentation, laser, or microdebrider techniques. All techniques focus on directed removal of the redundant cuneiform cartilages, the lysis of tight aryepiglottic folds, and the occasional removal of obstructing portions of the epiglottis. Potential complications include persistent airway obstruction requiring further surgery, supraglottic stenosis, dysphasia, aspiration, and death.[20] Supraglottoplasty is more than 90% successful in relieving upper airway obstruction caused by severe laryngomalacia.[20]

Laryngocele and Saccular Cysts

A laryngocele is an abnormal dilation or herniation of the laryngeal saccule, which rises vertically between the false vocal cord, the base of the epiglottis, and the inner surface of the thyroid cartilage. It communicates with the lumen of the larynx and is filled with air. An internal laryngocele is confined to the interior of the larynx and extends posterosuperiorly into the area of the false vocal cord and aryepiglottic fold, causing a mass that can be seen by direct or indirect laryngoscopy. An external laryngocele extends cephalad to protrude laterally into the neck through the thyrohyoid membrane presenting as a neck mass.[21] A laryngocele may be solely congenital; it may represent a congenital defect made apparent or exacerbated by habitual, increased intralaryngeal pressure; or it may be acquired solely on the basis of prolonged increased intralaryngeal pressure. A saccular cyst is distinguished from the laryngocele in that the lumen is isolated from the interior of the larynx and it does not contain air. These cysts result from a developmental failure of the saccular orifice to maintain patency.[21] Inflammation, trauma, and tumors may occlude the orifice as well. Therefore, saccular cysts can be congenital or acquired.

In infants and children, laryngoceles cause hoarseness and dyspnea that may increase with crying. Saccular cysts cause respiratory distress and stridor. The diagnosis of laryngocele is made by a soft tissue posteroanterior radiograph of the neck. If the laryngocele is not distended at the time of the film, the image of the larynx will be normal. Saccular cysts are diagnosed by direct laryngoscopy. Cysts can be treated endoscopically by repeat needle aspiration or by excision through marsupialization or unroofing. External excision through a lateral horizontal cervical incision can be used in recurrent cases.[21]

Paralysis of the Vocal Cords

Paralysis of the vocal cords in infants is the third most common cause of stridor in infants, after laryngomalacia and subglottic stenosis.[1] In approximately 40% of cases, bilateral vocal cord paralysis in infants is the result of central congenital anomalies.[22] It is found most commonly in association with myelomeningocele, Arnold-Chiari malformation, and hydrocephalus. Unilateral vocal cord paralysis is most often iatrogenic as a result of surgical treatment for gastrointestinal (tracheoesophageal fistula) and cardiovascular (patent ductus arteriosis repair) anomalies. Unilateral vocal cord paralysis is seen most often on the left because of the longer course of the recurrent laryngeal nerve on this side. Internal trauma, such as with an endotracheal tube or nasogastric tube, and external trauma, as in strangulation injury or motor vehicle accidents, may lead to vocal cord paralysis.

Bilateral vocal cord paralysis presents with a high-pitched, inspiratory stridor and respiratory distress. The vocal cords are drawn together during inspiration causing stridor, but are pushed apart during exhalation relieving the obstruction. Children with unilateral vocal cord paralysis experience aspiration leading to cough and a weak, breathy cry. Airway obstruction and stridor are less common in these patients because the paralyzed vocal cord tends to stay fixed in a lateral position. The diagnosis is confirmed using flexible fiberoptic laryngoscopy without anesthesia. Once the diagnosis is made, determining the cause should include pediatric neurology and cardiology consultations. It may include chest and neurologic imaging depending on the patient's history.

Vocal cord paralysis in infants usually resolves spontaneously within 6 to 12 months.[22] If it does not resolve within 2 to 3 years it is unlikely to do so. Treatment is based on the severity of the symptoms in the patient. In patients with bilateral vocal cord paralysis and respiratory distress, a trial of intubation may be warranted to allow a chance for spontaneous recovery. If this does not occur, a tracheostomy may be considered. Procedures that widen the posterior glottis to relieve the obstruction include laryngotracheal reconstruction using an endoscopically placed posterior glottic cartilage graft, arytenoidectomy, or arytenoid lateralization. These procedures are successful in reducing the obstruction. However, they may worsen the patient's voice quality and they may result in aspiration that can become severe. In cases of unilateral vocal cord paralysis where aspiration and a hoarse cry are the main symptoms, vocal cord medialization is often used. This is most commonly performed endoscopically through an injection technique. A temporary injectable material, such as Gelfoam or endogenous fat, may be injected into the larynx to medialize the vocal cord and decrease aspiration. The material will absorb in 3 to 6 months and, if it was successful, another injection with a more permanent substance can be used. The main complication is over-injection, leading to postoperative respiratory distress. This is most often temporary.

Congenital Subglottic Stenosis

Congenital subglottic stenosis is the second most common cause of stridor in neonates.[1] The subglottis is the narrowest part of the upper airway in a child. Subglottic stenosis is a narrowing of the subglottic larynx, which is the space extending from the undersurface of the true vocal cords to the inferior margin of the cricoid cartilage. It typically causes respiratory distress and biphasic stridor. In mild cases, the child may present with recurrent croup before the age of 1 year. The edema and thickened secretions of the common cold further narrow an already marginal airway that leads to croup-like symptoms. The stenosis can be caused by an abnormally shaped cricoid cartilage; by a tracheal ring that becomes trapped underneath the cricoid cartilage; or by soft tissue thickening caused by ductal cysts, submucosal gland hyperplasia, or fibrosis.[23] The diagnosis can be made by posteroanterior and lateral airway radiographs and it is confirmed by endoscopy. During diagnostic laryngoscopy and bronchoscopy the subglottic larynx is visualized directly and sized objectively using an endotracheal tube. The percentage of stenosis is determined by comparing the size of the patient's larynx to a standard of laryngeal dimensions based on age.[24] The degree of stenosis will help dictate treatment. Children with stenosis greater than 50% tend to be more symptomatic and more often require treatment. Surgical options include laryngotracheal reconstruction and cricotracheal resection. Laryngotracheal reconstruction involves augmenting the subglottis with an anterior or posterior cartilage graft placed in the cricoid cartilage. This can be performed via an open technique through a cervical neck incision or endoscopically through the oral cavity depending on the type and degree of stenosis. A cricotracheal resection involves removing most of the stenosed cricoid cartilage and re-anastomosing the trachea to the larynx. The postoperative care is critical and often requires multiple bronchoscopies to ensure patency and to prevent repeat stenosis.

Key Points

- Rapid, turbulent airflow across a narrowed segment of the respiratory tract leads to the production of various distinctive sounds that are diagnostically very useful to the clinician.
- Stridor is the low-pitched inspiratory, snoring sound typically produced by nasal or nasopharyngeal obstruction.
- Stridor typically originates from the larynx, upper trachea, or hypopharynx.
- Wheezing is the expiratory sound produced by turbulent flow of air through constricted bronchioles.
- The mnemonic SPECS-R is a useful tool to organize history taking and to determine the need for endoscopy.
- Piriform aperture stenosis seen in conjunction with a mega-incisor may be associated with the holoprosencephaly.
- Choanal atresia can be diagnosed by the failure to pass a 6 French catheter more than 32 mm past the anterior nares.
- No congenital nasal mass or polyp in a child should be manipulated until intracranial communication is ruled out.
- Crouzon and Apert syndromes are defined by craniosynostosis and maxillary hypoplasia, which can result in severe upper airway obstruction.
- Pierre Robin sequence (cleft palate, micrognathia, and glossoptosis) can cause severe pharyngeal airway obstruction that presents at birth.
- Lymphangiomas are the most common cause of macroglossia in children. They are apparent at birth in 60% of cases.

Key Points (continued)

- Congenital lesions of the base of the tongue are rare and include ectopic thyroid tissue, lingual thyroid (most common), and thyroglossal duct cysts.
- Thyroglossal duct cysts are the most common malformations found in the neck and account for 70% of congenital cervical abnormalities.
- Laryngomalacia is the most common cause of inspiratory stridor in infants and typically begins 1 to 3 weeks after birth and resolves by about 1 year.
  - Subglottic stenosis is the second most common cause of stridor in neonates.
  - It typically presents with respiratory distress and biphasic stridor.
  - In mild cases, the child may present with recurrent croup before the age of 1 year.
- Paralysis of the vocal cords is the third most common cause of stridor in infants. Bilateral paralysis in infants is the result of central congenital anomalies in approximately 40% of cases.
- Unilateral vocal cord paralysis is often iatrogenic as a result of surgical treatment for gastrointestinal and cardiovascular anomalies.
- Vocal cord paralysis in infants usually resolves within 6 to 12 months. If it does not resolve within 2 to 3 years it is unlikely to do so.

References

1. Holinger LD. Etiology of stridor. *Ann Otol Rhinol Laryngol.* 1980;89:397
2. Holinger LD. Evaluation of stridor and wheezing. In: Holinger LD, ed. *Pediatric Laryngology & Bronchoesphogology.* New York, NY: Lippincott–Raven; 1997:41–28
3. Holinger LD. Diagnostic endoscopy of the pediatric airway. *Laryngoscope.* 1989;99:346
4. Bignault A, Castillo M. Congenital nasal piriform aperture stenosis. *Am J Neuroradiol.* 1994;15:877
5. Cohen M Jr. Perspectives on holoprosencephaly: part 1. Epidemiology, genetics and syndromology. *Teratology.* 1989;40:211
6. Gujrathi CS, Daniel SJ, James AL, et al. Management of bilateral choanal atresia in the neonate: an instructional review. *Int J Pediar Otorhinolaryngol.* 2004;68:399–407
7. Sadek SA. Congenital bilateral choanal atresia. *Int J Pediatr Otorhinolaryngol.* 1998;42:247–256
8. Stahl R, Jurkiewicz M. Congenital posterior choanal atresia. *Pediatrics.* 1985:429–436
9. Lusk RP, Muntz HR. Nasal obstruction in the neonate secondary to nasolacrimal duct cysts. *Int J Pediatr Otorhinolaryngol.* 1987;13:315
10. Frodel J, Larrabee W, Raisis J. The nasal dermoid. *Otlaryngol Head Neck Surg.* 1989;101:392
11. Hengerer A. *Congenital Anomalies of the Nose: Their Embryology, Diagnosis and Management* [monograph]. Philadelphia, PA: American Academy of Otolaryngology Head and Neck Surgery; 1987
12. Down syndrome prevalence at birth—United States, 1983–1990. *MMWR Morb Mortal Wkly Rep.* 1994;43:617–622
13. Mitchel R, Call E, Kelly J. Ear, nose and throat disorders in children with Down syndrome. *Laryngoscope.* 2003;113:259–163
14. Weiss LS, White JA. Macroglossia: a review. *J La State Med Soc.* 1990;142:13
15. Maddern BR. Lingual thyroid in a young infant presenting as airway obstruction: report of a case. *Int J Pediatr Otorhinolaryngol.* 1990;19:79
16. Kansal P, Sakati N, Rifai A, et al. Lingual thyroid. Diagnosis and treatment. *Arch Intern Med.* 1987;147:2046
17. Maddalozzo J, Venkatesan T, Gupta P. Complications associated with the Sistrunk procedure. 2001 *Laryngoscope.* 111:119–123
18. Thompson D. Abnormal sensorymotor integrative function of the larynx in congenital laryngomalacia: a new theory of etiology. *Laryngoscope.* 2007;117:1–33
19. Olney D, Greinwald J, Smith R, et al. Laryngomalacia and its treatment. *Laryngoscope.* 1999;109(11):1770–1775
20. Schroeder J, Thakkar K, Poznanovic S, et al. Aspiration following CO2 laser assisted supraglottoplasty. *Int J Ped Otorhinolaryngol.* 2008;77:985–990

21. Holinger LD, Barnes DR, Smid LJ. Laryngocele and saccular cysts. *Ann Otol Rhinol Laryngol.* 1978;87:675
22. Holinger LD, Holinger PC, Holinger PH. Etiology of bilateral abductor vocal cord paralysis. A review of 389 cases. *Ann Otol Rhinol Laryngol.* 1976;85:428
23. Holinger P, Johnson K, Schiller F. Congenital anomalies of the larynx. *Ann Otol Rhinol Laryngol.* 1954;63:581
24. Myer C, O'Connor D, Cotton R. Proposed grading system for subglottic stenosis based on endotracheal tube sizes. *Ann Otol Rhinol Laryngol.* 1994;108:319

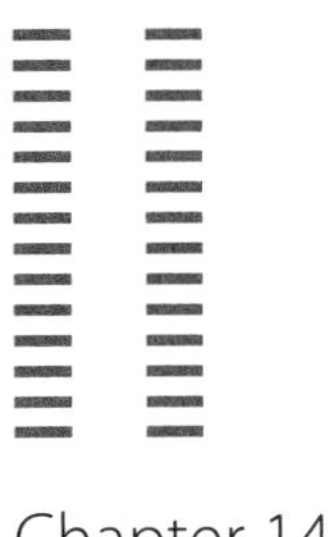

Chapter 14

Congenital Lung Anomalies

Brian O'Sullivan, MD
T. Bernard Kinane, MD

Although major congenital lung malformations are often presented as separate entities, there is great overlap between these abnormalities. Congenital lung malformations represent a spectrum of disorders arising from errors in formation of the airways or vascular supply of the lung. A single congenital abnormality may not fit neatly into one category.

The "wheel" theory of airway and vessel malinosculations (Figure 14-1) helps to understand the malformations.[1] In this approach, the developmental interactions of bronchial, acinar, and vascular components are interpreted along a continuum. A congenital abnormality may be isolated to large airways (eg, bronchomalacia), involve abnormalities in both bronchial and vascular development (pulmonary sequestration), or involve the vasculature only, without any airway involvement (vascular rings). Although a unified nomenclature based on this model makes the most sense taxonomically, in practice, clinicians still refer to the malformations by specific names.

Lung Growth and Development

Lung development occurs in 5 stages: embryonic (0–5 weeks postconception), pseudoglandular (6–16 weeks), canalicular (17–24 weeks), saccular (24–38 weeks), and alveolar (38 weeks to years) (Figure 14-2).[2,3] Differentiation of the bronchial tree is complete by the end of the pseudoglandular period (16 weeks of gestation). Thus events that disrupt development before 16 weeks of gestation will affect airway development, whereas events occurring after 16 weeks will affect development of terminal respiratory bronchioles and alveoli (the acinus). See also Chapter 1, Pulmonary Anatomy.

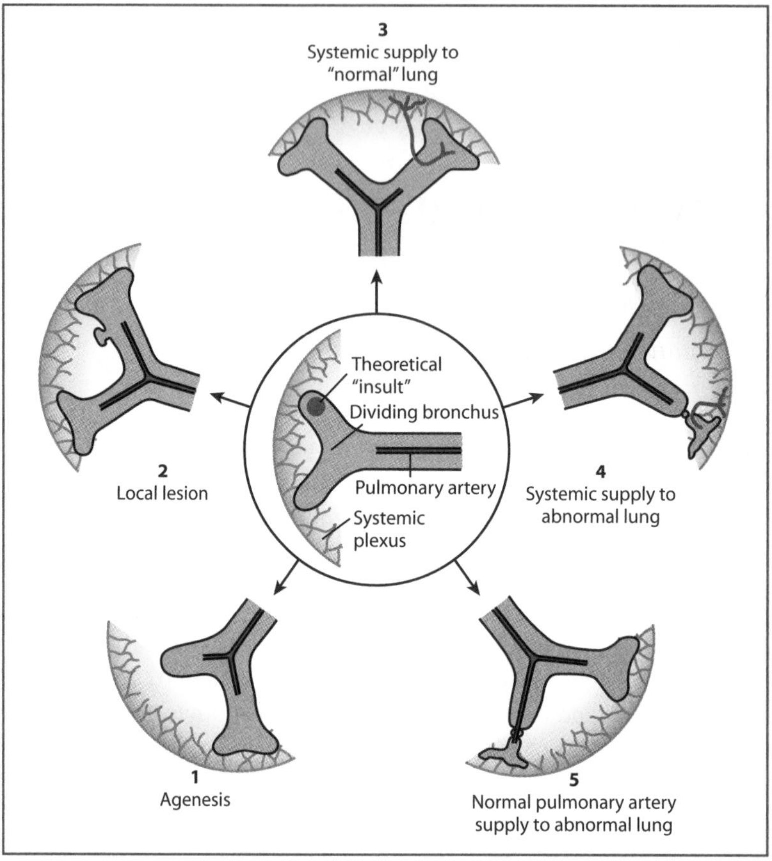

Figure 14-1. Wheel theory of abnormal lung development. **1.** agenesis of lung segment, **2.** budding lesion of airway (eg, bronchogenic cyst), **3.** systemic blood supply to normal lung segment, **4.** systemic blood supply to abnormal lung (eg, sequestration), **5.** normal blood supply to abnormal lung segment. (Reprinted from Clements BS, Warner JO. Pulmonary sequestration and related congenital bronchopulmonary-vascular malformations: nomenclature and classification based on anatomical and embryological considerations. *Thorax.* 1987;42:401–408, with permission from BMJ Publishing Group Ltd.)

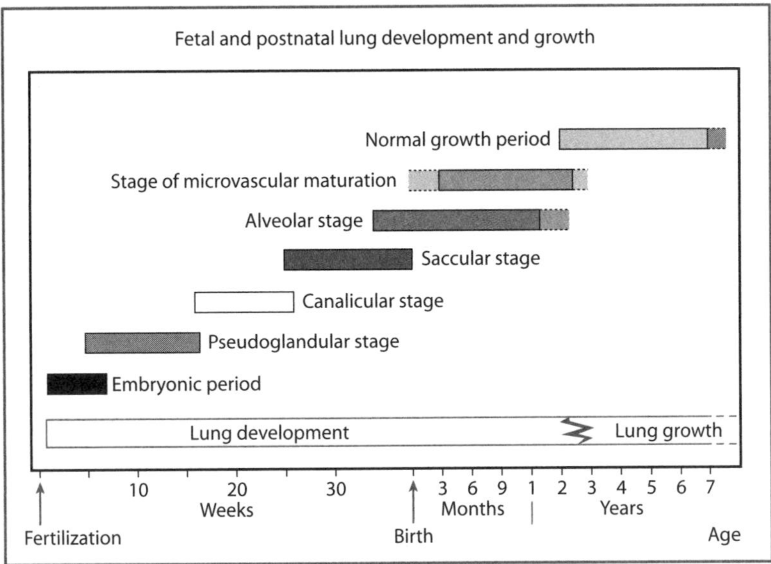

Figure 14-2. Intrauterine stages of lung development. Airway branching is complete by the end of the pseudoglandular phase (16 weeks, postconception). (Reprinted from Zeltner TB, Burri PH. The postnatal development and growth of the human lung. II. Morphology. *Respir Physiol.* 1987;67:269–282, with permission from Elsevier.)

Laryngomalacia

Laryngomalacia is the most commonly seen developmental abnormality of the respiratory tree. Laryngomalacia is a result of inadequate support of supraglottic tissue and should not be confused with tracheomalacia, which results in collapse of the subglottic trachea. Tissue supporting the epiglottis and arytenoid processes in infants is less firm than in older children and adults, and collapse of these structures into the glottic chink during inspiration is common (Figure 14-3). The resultant narrowing of the airway and vibration of the surrounding tissue leads to a characteristic inspiratory crowing sound. Mild laryngomalacia is extremely common and may be seen in up to 10% to 20% of newborns. Stridor due to laryngomalacia is generally noted within the first days to weeks of life, may worsen as the infant grows and is able to generate greater negative inspiratory pressures, and resolves by 12 to 18 months of age. Classically, the stridor is worse when the child is active or in the supine position and diminishes with rest and sleep. Gastroesophageal reflux can be associated with laryngomalacia either

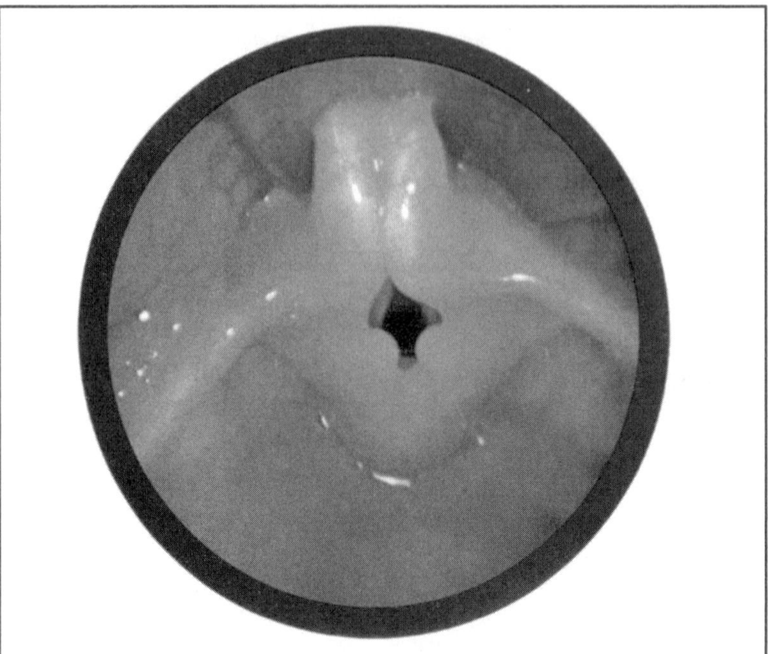

Figure 14-3. Laryngomalacia. Note curled epiglottis and prolapse of arytenoid processes into the glottic chink. (Reprinted with permission from Benjamin B. *Atlas of Paediatric Endoscopy: Upper Respiratory Tract and Oesophagus.* Oxford: Oxford University Press; 1981.)

as a causative factor producing swelling of the supraglottic tissue or as a result of the wide swings seen in thoracoabdominal pressures due to upper airway obstruction. Treating the associated reflux may decrease the degree of stridor. The diagnosis of laryngomalacia can often be made on clinical grounds alone or with the aid of laryngoscopy. Direct bronchoscopy of the lower airway is rarely indicated in uncomplicated laryngomalacia.[4]

Therapy is generally supportive with reassurance to the parents that the problem will resolve over time. In a minority of cases, laryngomalacia may cause severe respiratory embarrassment, increased work of breathing, and failure to thrive due to an inability to feed and breathe at the same time. Children with laryngomalacia should be seen frequently to assess growth. Failure to thrive is an indication for surgical intervention to release the short aryepiglottic folds and remove redundant mucosa (supraglottoplasty). Rarely, a tracheotomy tube will need to be placed until the upper airway structures mature.

Tracheobronchial Abnormalities

Disorders of the large airways include tracheobronchomalacia, tracheomegaly, and tracheal bronchus. Of these, tracheal bronchus, an aberrant lobar bronchus arising above the carina, which supplies 1 or all 3 of the right upper lobe segments, is most common, occurring in up to about 2% of people (Figure 14-4).[5] In most instances, tracheal bronchus is a benign variant of no clinical significance. However, if the orifice of the tracheal bronchus is small and easily plugged, it can lead to recurrent right upper lobe pneumonia. Similarly, obstruction of the tracheal bronchus by an endotracheal tube can lead to problems with mechanical ventilation.

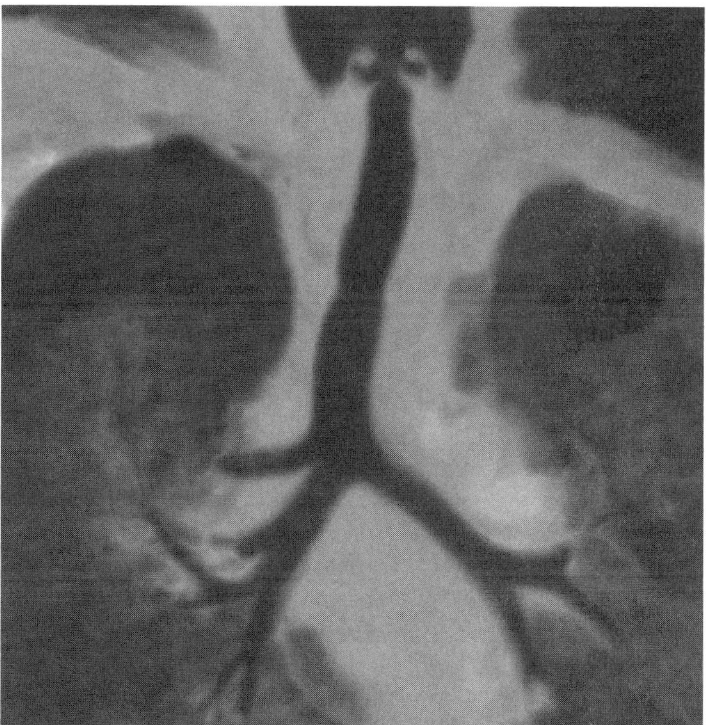

Figure 14-4. Coronal computed tomogram demonstrating takeoff of tracheal bronchus to right upper lobe above the main carina.

Tracheomalacia and bronchomalacia may be primary or secondary to other congenital anomalies. Mass lesions, such as vascular rings and bronchogenic cysts, can cause indentation and malacia of the developing tracheobronchial tree with resultant airway collapse with shifts in intraluminal pressure during the respiratory cycle. Primary tracheobronchomalacia occurs in about 1 in 2,000 infants and may be misdiagnosed initially as asthma.[6,7] A wheeze caused by narrowing of a single large intrathoracic airway during expiration differs from the wheezing of an asthmatic subject. The child with asthma has many small airways involved, all to a differing degree, such that the wheeze will be orchestral (polyphonic) and vary in pitch and intensity when auscultating different chest regions. The child with tracheobronchomalacia has narrowing of a single large airway during expiration (when pleural pressure exceeds intraluminal pressure), leading to a monophonic (homophonous) wheeze that has the same characteristics throughout the chest. A fixed lesion causing constant large airway narrowing will cause noisy breathing during inspiration and expiration.

Children with tracheomalacia or bronchomalacia can present with intractable cough caused by contact between the membranous and cartilaginous portions of the airway. Such children are at risk for respiratory illness and protracted symptoms, and may have exercise limitation even with growth. Many children with tracheobronchomalacia need no intervention. As the child grows the airway cartilage stiffens and the lumen diameter increases, thus decreasing the absolute degree and significance of narrowing. In severely symptomatic children, continuous positive airway pressure may stent the airway open sufficiently. Some have advocated use of medications that increase smooth muscle tone.[8] If medical management fails and intervention is required, tracheotomy with use of an elongated tracheotomy tube or placement of a bronchial stent may be necessary.[9]

A much less common tracheal abnormality is tracheobronchomegaly (Mounier-Kuhn syndrome), which results from absence or atrophy of elastic fibers and smooth muscle in the wall of the airways. The loss of tracheal wall support leads to dilatation and development of diverticula. Mounier-Kuhn syndrome has been seen in association with other disorders of connective tissue, including Ehlers-Danlos syndrome and cutis laxa.[10] Mounier-Kuhn syndrome usually presents in the third or fourth decade of life, which has led to some debate as to whether it is a congenital or acquired anomaly. The weakened and dilated walls of the large airways collapse during forced exhalation (cough), decreasing mucociliary clearance and increasing the probability of repeated infections.[10] Involvement of smaller, more peripheral airways will lead to bronchiectasis. Acquired forms of tracheomegaly result from intubation and high-pressure ventilation of neonates. Plain chest radiographs may lead to suspicion of the diagnosis, but computed tomography (CT) with comparison to normal tracheal diameter for age is necessary to make the diagnosis. A CT scan is diagnostic if the trachea is more than 3 standard deviations above mean reference values.[11]

Tracheoesophageal Fistula

Tracheoesophageal fistula (TEF) represents an early embryological defect in foregut differentiation. The incidence of these malformations is approximately 1 in 3,000 births.[12] The rate is increased in multiple birth pregnancies and Caucasians. A genetic basis is plausible, and the reoccurrence rate is about 2% in children of an affected parent. Most cases of TEF, however, are sporadic. Tracheoesophageal fistula can occur in association with chromosomal abnormalities such as trisomies (18 and 21) and deletions of 22q11, and an increased incidence occurs in DiGeorge syndrome, Pierre Robin syndrome, Holt Oram syndrome, and Feingold syndrome.

There are several types of TEF (Figure 14-5). Esophageal atresia with distal TEF accounts for 86% of cases. In this form, the proximal esophagus is dilated and usually ends high in the mediastinum. The distal esophagus is usually much smaller in diameter and usually communicates with the distal trachea via a fistula to a point about 2 cm proximal to the carina (Figure 14-5A). The distance between the proximal pouch and distal esophagus can vary. Isolated esophageal atresia without fistula accounts for 10% of cases. In this formation, the proximal esophagus ends high in the posterior mediastinum. The distal esophagus usually ends low in the mediastinum just above the diaphragm. The distance between the 2 ends is significant and usually does not allow for a primary repair (Figure 14-5E).

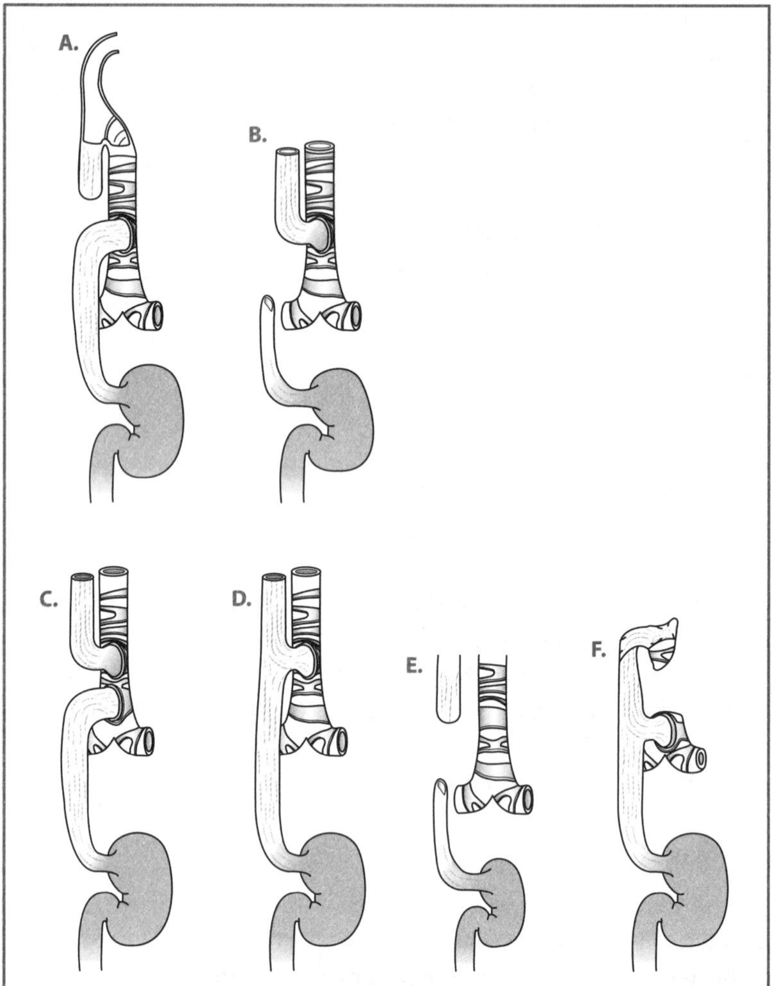

Figure 14-5. Types of tracheoesophageal fistulae. **A.** Proximal esophageal pouch with distal fistula; **B.** proximal fistula with distal isolated esophagus; **C.** disrupted esophagus with proximal and distal fistula; **D.** H-type fistula; **E.** esophageal atresia without fistula; **F.** upper and lower fistula without esophageal atresia.

H-type TEF accounts for approximately 4% of cases. In this case both the esophagus and trachea are continuous from cephalad to caudad, but there is a fistulous connection between the 2 tubular structures. The fistula is very narrow and usually is found in the lower cervical region. Usually there is a single fistula, but multiple fistulae have been described (Figure 14-5D).

The mechanism that underlies tracheoesophageal malformation is the subject of intensive investigation. Formation of the trachea is a multistage process. Initially, a groove forms in the posterior foregut, the sulcus laryngotrachealis, then a septum separates the groove, thus forming the primitive trachea and esophagus.[3] Both genetic and environmental factors are likely to contribute to developmental abnormalities affecting this separation and subsequent formation of a normal trachea and esophagus. Fifty percent or more of infants with tracheoesophageal malformation have at least one other congenital abnormality.[13] Esophageal atresia without a fistula has the highest incidence of associated abnormalities, and H-type fistula has the lowest. Tracheoesophageal fistula has been associated with a number of syndromes including the VATER association (vertebral, anorectal, tracheoesophageal, and renal or radial abnormalities), VACTERL association (C cardiac, L limb), and the CHARGE association (coloboma, heart defects, atresia choanal, retarded growth and development, genital hypoplasia, and ear deformities).

The classical presentation of a child with esophageal atresia is coughing, choking, and aspiration during the first feed. These infants also have excessive salivation because they cannot swallow their saliva. A plain radiograph of the chest is usually diagnostic and should show the tip of a nasogastric catheter curled up in the upper pouch at the level of thoracic vertebra 3. Associated findings on the radiograph provide insight into which type of malformation is present. If air is present in the stomach, the presence of a distal TEF is probable (Figure 14-5C). Alternatively, the lack of gastrointestinal air suggests isolated atresia. H-type fistulas may not present until a child is several months of age and is noted to have chronic coughing or choking with feeding and recurrent pneumonia. A persistently distended abdomen caused by air in the intestinal tract may be seen as well. The diagnosis is made by performing a barium study with contrast material infused through a nasogastric tube under gentle pressure to distend the esophagus in the distal to proximal direction (Figure 14-6).

Surgical correction of the esophageal abnormality is mandatory. Preoperative management is critical. A suction tube (Replogle catheter) should be placed in the upper pouch to prevent aspiration. Likewise, the child should be positioned upright to prevent reflux into the trachea through the distal fistula. Surgery can normally be performed

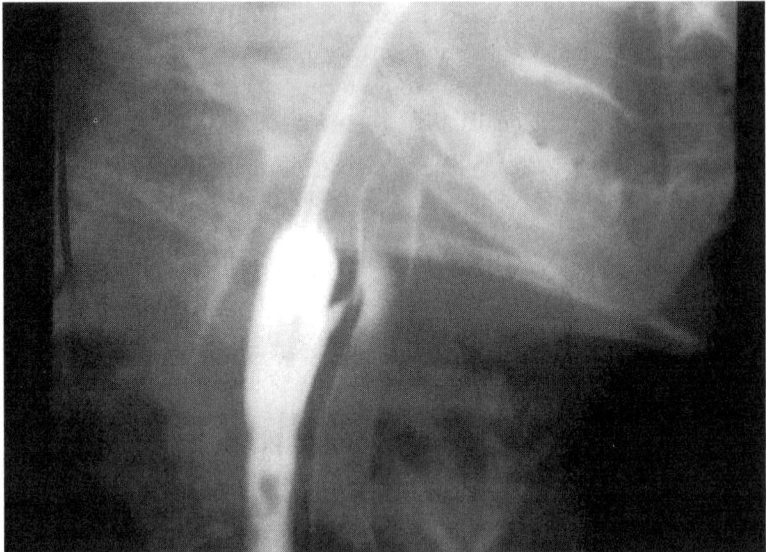

Figure 14-6. Barium swallow demonstrating H-type tracheoesophageal fistula. Note contrast in distended esophagus with movement of the agent across the fistula outlining the trachea.

electively. The exception is when an infant with a distal fistula is in severe respiratory distress requiring ventilatory support. High-pressure gas delivered to the trachea can cross the fistula and may lead to dangerous inflation of the stomach with possible gastric rupture. In such cases surgery should be performed emergently.

Most defects can be corrected in one procedure. A number of strategies have been developed to facilitate a primary anastomosis and ligation of the fistula. In children with pure esophageal atresia there may be a long gap between the 2 esophageal remnants, so the surgical procedure is modified. Many procedures have been developed to apply tension on the esophageal ends over a period of 6 to 10 days to approximate the pouches and allow a primary anastomosis. Rarely, patients require the placement of a large bowel graft.

Complications of these surgeries are expected. Early complications include anastomosis leakage, anastomotic stricture, and recurrent fistulae. Leaks occur in about 20% of cases, and one-third of these events leads to a major disruption and may require emergency surgery. Anastomotic strictures occur in about a third of patients and respond to 1 or 2 dilatations. Recurrent TEF occurs in about 10% of cases and is frequently overlooked. It should be considered if the infant has respiratory symptoms around feeds or has recurring pneumonia after initial corrective surgery.

Late complications include gastroesophageal reflux, tracheomalacia, and esophageal dysmotility. Gastroesophageal reflux occurs in 40% of cases, and a significant proportion of these cases will need surgical management. Reflux can occur after any type of repair but is most frequent when there is tension across the anastomosis site. Aggressive antireflux medical therapy is required. Long-term respiratory complications are common, with 40% of patients having wheezing and brassy cough at 15 years of age.[14,15] Most studies suggest that tracheomalacia occurs in about 15% of cases, but a higher number is probable. The extent of malacia can be quite variable, probably reflecting a defect in formation of tracheal cartilage and smooth muscle. Most cases can be managed medically with inhaled ipratropium bromide. Generally, the tracheomalacia improves with time.

Pulmonary Agenesis or Hypoplasia

The most severe form of lung malformation is agenesis of both lungs. This malformation is believed to be a result of loss of development of the trachea or the main pulmonary arteries. Obviously, complete pulmonary agenesis is incompatible with life. However, lesser degrees of agenesis, such as absence of one lung or one lobe, are seen. Complete agenesis of the right lung carries a worse prognosis than agenesis of the left lung due to greater displacement of the mediastinum and heart, with increased torsion on the great vessels and remaining bronchus. Pulmonary agenesis of single lobes is uncommon, but when present is predominantly a right-sided event, with the right upper lobe and right middle affected together.[16] Pulmonary agenesis is often associated with other congenital abnormalities, particularly cardiac defects, and a diagnosis of agenesis should trigger a careful assessment for other somatic malformations.

Hypoplasia of the right lung or agenesis of a lobe therein with anomalous pulmonary venous blood flow to the inferior vena cava is known as scimitar syndrome, the name deriving from the curved, scimitar sword-like appearance of the vein descending through the diaphragm to the vena cava (Figure 14-7). This syndrome may present with a

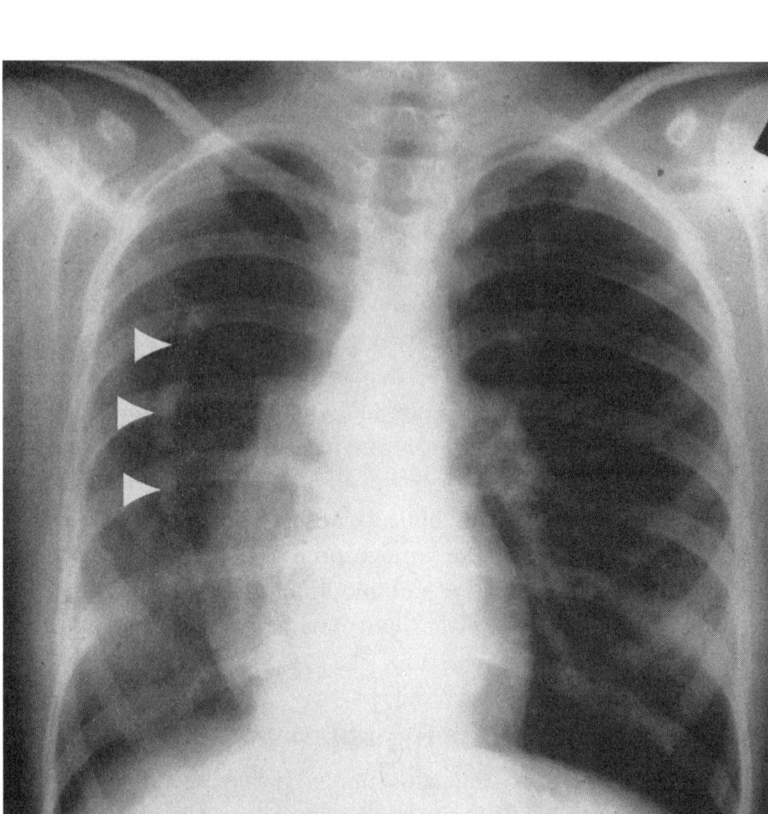

Figure 14-7. Scimitar syndrome. The right lung is smaller than the left and a large, anomalous vein is draining the right lung to the subdiaphragmatic inferior vena cava (arrowheads).

variety of vascular abnormalities, including systemic arterial supply to the right lower lobe, agenesis of the right pulmonary artery, and congenital heart defects. Two forms, the infantile and adult form, have been reported, the distinction based on age of presentation. The infantile form is diagnosed in the first months of life and is associated with more severe cardiac defects or congestive heart failure due to high output failure through the systemic vessels feeding the right lung, whereas the adult form with pulmonary hypoplasia and aberrant venous drainage may be asymptomatic and only discovered serendipitously.[17,18] Immediate attention to the underlying cardiac problems is essential with presentation in the newborn period. Older children or adults in whom the scimitar syndrome is diagnosed as an incidental finding may not require any intervention at all.

Generalized pulmonary hypoplasia is more common than agenesis of a single lung or lobe. It is associated with a variety of intrauterine insults, including (1) hydrops fetalis; (2) renal anomalies; (3) hernia, including diaphragmatic and omphalocele; (4) skeletal anomalies; and (5) amniotic fluid abnormalities, particularly oligohydramnios.[19] Mild pulmonary hypoplasia may cause tachypnea without serious associated lung disease, which may improve over time as the lungs achieve "catch-up" growth. More severe pulmonary hypoplasia may necessitate aggressive ventilatory support in the newborn period.

Of particular interest is the association between amniotic fluid abnormalities and pulmonary hypoplasia. Abnormalities that result in reduced or absent urine formation (renal agenesis) or oligohydramnios (eg, premature rupture of membranes) lead to physical restriction of fetal breathing movements and limited chest wall development. The earlier in gestation these problems occur, the more severe the pulmonary hypoplasia. The premature rupture of membranes late in pregnancy may have little or no effect on pulmonary function, whereas extremely early rupture of membranes will result in severe pulmonary compromise. The degree of pulmonary hypoplasia depends on the degree of oligohydramnios, its duration, and the gestational age (stage of lung development) at which it occurs. The most severe form of oligohydramnios and pulmonary hypoplasia is Potter syndrome, named for Edith Potter who in 1946 described the association of renal agenesis, unusual flattened facies, club feet, intrauterine growth retardation, and pulmonary hypoplasia.[20] The absence of urine production due to renal agenesis leads to severe oligohydramnios throughout pregnancy and associated compression defects in the fetus.

Bronchogenic Cysts

Bronchogenic cysts are the most common cysts of infancy, accounting for about 5% of mediastinal masses in infants and children. Many remain asymptomatic and are detected only incidentally later in life, so the true incidence of these cysts is unknown. Bronchogenic cysts are formed when a piece of bronchial tissue separates from the developing airway. In most cases there is no connection between the bronchogenic cyst and the normal airway, but such a connection can be seen and may lead to chronic, recurrent infection of the cyst.[21] There is overlap between bronchogenic and esophageal cysts, since both represent abnormalities in foregut differentiation. A cleft develops between the developing trachea and esophagus at approximately day 28 postconception. Abnormalities in budding around this time can result in cysts with both bronchial and esophageal characteristics. Generally, bronchogenic cysts are thin-walled and lined with ciliated respiratory epithelium. The cysts may contain mucoid material and frequently have cartilage in their walls (Figure 14-8).

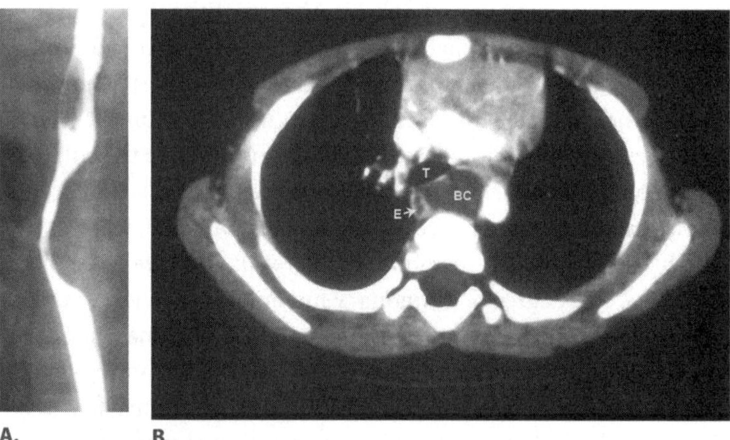

A. B.

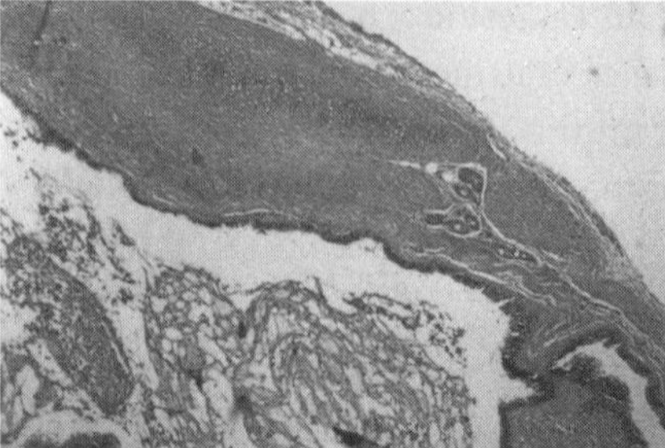

C.

Figure 14-8. A. Barium swallow demonstrates compression of the esophagus by a bronchogenic cyst. **B.** Computed tomography scan shows bronchogenic cyst (BC) compressing trachea (T) and esophagus (E). **C.** Photomicrograph of a bronchogenic cyst demonstrating cartilage in the cyst wall with lung remnants within the cyst.

Bronchogenic cysts are usually found in the peritracheal region, with a predisposition to the right side.[21,22] Less commonly, bronchogenic cysts can be found within the lung parenchyma. This likely represents a difference between early splitting off of the cyst from the tracheobronchial bud (central lesions) versus later differentiation (peripheral lesions). If the abnormal buds are pinched off and migrate before the closure of the diaphragm at 6 weeks of gestation, the cysts may be found outside of the chest cavity.[23]

Bronchogenic cysts may be asymptomatic, minimally symptomatic, or cause extreme respiratory embarrassment. The degree of symptoms depends on the location of the cyst. Infants have compressible tracheobronchial cartilage, and a mass-occupying lesion in the peritracheal area will cause airway narrowing and noisy breathing. Compression of the esophagus can lead to concomitant feeding problems. More peripheral bronchogenic cysts will be less symptomatic, but may cause recurrent infections, especially if there is communication with the bronchial tree. Rare cases of compression of vascular structures, including coronary arteries, have been reported.[24] Bronchogenic cysts do not have a known association with other congenital malformations, but may be seen in conjunction with other malformations of lung development. Diagnosis is generally made by barium esophagram and CT scan.

Therapy for a bronchogenic cyst consists of surgical removal of the cyst if it is causing symptoms. Therapy for asymptomatic cysts, often detected incidentally, is less clear. Many experts believe that surgical resection of asymptomatic cysts is indicated for pathologic examination, because there is a chance the cyst may cause future symptoms, including infection and hemorrhage later in life, and that there is an inherent oncogenic risk to the lesion. In fact, there have been several case reports of different types of cancer being detected within bronchogenic cysts, including large-cell carcinoma, bronchoalveolar carcinoma, and carcinoid tumor.[25–28] Other experts believe that all mediastinal cysts should not be treated surgically, citing concerns regarding the reliability of some of the reports of malignant transformation and putting into perspective the low incidence of malignancies in simple cysts.[29] A definitive answer to the question of what to do with a bronchogenic cyst is not available due to the rarity of the lesion and the reports of only small series of patients. At present, surgical excision remains the most common way to deal with these lesions.

Congenital Cystic Adenomatoid Malformation

Congenital cystic adenomatoid malformation (CCAM) of the lung, characterized by a multicystic mass of pulmonary tissue, is an uncommon malformation. Congenital cystic adenomatoid malformations are thought to reflect an overgrowth of bronchi at various stages in lung development. The size of the cyst offers insight into the pathogenesis. These malformations were classified by Stocker et al[30] into 3 histological types.

- Type I, the most common form (70%) is composed of variable-sized cysts, with at least one dominant cyst greater than 2 cm in diameter.
- Type II contains multiple cysts less than 2 cm in diameter and represents 20% of cases.
- Type III is the solid, adenomatoid form and represents 10% of cases.

Recently, CCAM classification has been redefined and renamed to congenital pulmonary airway malformations (CPAM), types 0 through IV.[31] This is similar to Stocker and colleagues' original description except for a type 0 defect, which is acinar dysplasia, and type IV, which is an unlined cystic lesion. Type I is thought to arise from bronchial overgrowth, as type II is bronchiolar in origin, type III is bronchiolar or alveolar in origin, and type IV is distal acinar in origin.

Congenital cystic adenomatoid malformations are quite rare. These lesions are almost always unilateral, although bilateral lesions occur in approximately 10% of cases. They affect the left and right side equally. Associations with other congenital malformations have been described, in particular with congenital heart disease and congenital diaphragmatic hernia.

Cystic adenomatoid malformations are frequently diagnosed as a result of a prenatal ultrasound. Additionally, they may present as an incidental finding, as an unresolving pneumonia, or as a pneumothorax. These lesions have to be differentiated from other cystic lesions, including diaphragmatic hernia, cystic hygroma, bronchogenic and enteric cysts, and bronchopulmonary sequestration.

Overall, prognosis of prenatal CCAMs is based on size and growth characteristics. Seventy percent of those resolve or decrease in size prior to birth, 10% remain unchanged, and 20% increase in size.

About 10% of infants with a prenatal diagnosis of CCAM develop hydrops fetalis and have a poor outcome. In those lesions that persist postnatally, there is a risk of superinfection. There may be an increased risk of tumor formation in the type I and IV CCAMs. Pleuropulmonary blastoma (PPB) is a malignancy that may be indistinguishable from CCAM on radiographic studies; however, a genetic predisposition and a family history of malignancy is often present in patients with PPB and helps identify the at-risk population.[32] Twenty-one cases of bronchoalveolar carcinoma have been reported in patients with CPAM but, in most of these cases, the bronchoalveolar carcinoma was an incidental finding in a cyst resected for other reasons.

Surgery is indicated if CCAM leads to hydrops, if there is recurring infection, or if there is an increased familial cancer risk. Surgery should also be considered if the diagnosis of PPB is entertained, since surgical resection of an early stage blastoma is curative and histologic examination will be necessary to differentiate PPB from CCAM.

Congenital cystic adenomatoid malformation is one of the rare indications for fetal surgery. The approach depends on the type of lesion. In those in which there is a dominant cyst, hydrops may respond to cyst aspiration and, if it recurs, to thoracoamniotic shunting. In a solid type of CCAM, open fetal surgery for resection of the CCAM may be indicated. The survival rate of such surgeries is 61%.[33]

Congenital Lobar Emphysema

Strictly speaking, the term congenital lobar emphysema (CLE) is a misnomer, and this condition is better referred to as an infantile large, hyperlucent lobe. The exact cause of this lesion remains obscure. The lung parenchyma is not truly emphysematous since there is not destruction of alveolar walls, nor is the condition uniformly present antenatally, although it likely has its origins in a prenatal condition. Abnormalities of the bronchi leading to partial obstruction or collapse on expiration, with resultant ball-valve effect and air or amniotic fluid trapping in the peripheral lung, are often invoked as a causative feature but, in fact, such bronchial defects are identified in no more than a third of children with CLE.[34,35] Microscopic evaluation of excised lobar emphysema tissue shows 1 of 2 patterns. In classical CLE there is a hyperexpanded lobe with a normal number of enlarged alveoli. In about 30% of cases CLE presents with a polyalveolar lobe, which consists of an enlarged lobe containing many more than the normal number of alveoli.[35,36] Congenital lobar emphysema most frequently affects the left upper lobe, followed by the right middle lobe and right upper lobe.[34,35] The lower lobes are rarely involved. Multiple lobes may be enlarged, but it is extremely unusual to have bilateral lesions.

Clinically, CLE presents in the immediate newborn period in most cases, with symptoms typical of a space-occupying mass: tachypnea, dyspnea, decreased breath sounds on the affected side, and wheezing. More than half of all cases present in the first week of life due to respiratory distress, and more than 80 will present by 6 months of age. Occasionally a child will remain asymptomatic and CLE will be diagnosed incidentally when a chest radiograph is obtained for an unrelated reason. In the newborn period, CLE may resemble neonatal pneumothorax or CCAM. The lesion may present as a fluid-filled mass that then becomes hyperlucent as retained fetal lung liquid is cleared. Delayed clearance of lung fluid is most common in the polyalveolar form of CLE.[35,36] In older children, the differential diagnosis should include foreign body aspiration with post-obstructive hyperinflation.

Radiographic studies show hyperinflation of a lobe with compression of the ipsalateral lung and herniation of the emphysematous lung across the anterior mediastinum. The contralateral lung may be compressed and atelectatic due to the mass effect of the hyperinflated lung. The diagnosis depends on being able to recognize which lung is abnormal. The small lung may be hypoplastic or atelectatic with compensatory hyperinflation of the other normal lung. Alternately, the large lung may be emphysematous with corresponding compression of the smaller lung. While this distinction is not always easy, CT or ventilation/perfusion scans can be helpful in distinguishing the healthy from the affected lung (Figure 14-9).

With the increased use of prenatal ultrasonography and fetal magnetic resonance imaging (MRI), there has been an increase in detection of CLE during fetal life. Follow-up shows spontaneous resolution in some cases, although postpartum symptoms may occur even in children whose lesions seem to have disappeared before birth.[37] Knowledge of the ability of CLE to regress spontaneously has led to a more conservative management approach. Previously, it was felt that once detected an emphysematous lobe must be removed to relieve respiratory distress and to allow the healthy lobes to grow normally. Surgery remains

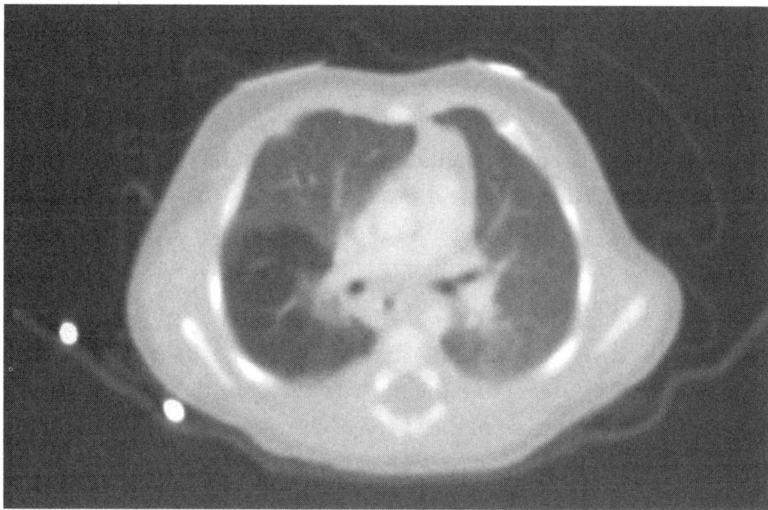

Figure 14-9. Computed tomography scan of a child with congenital lobar emphysema. There is hyperlucency and decreased lung markings in the right-sided lesion.

the treatment of choice for the child with severe respiratory distress; however, it is increasingly apparent that infants with mild to moderate symptoms can be managed medically. Some infants symptomatic at birth do not require surgery.[38]

Congenital Diaphragmatic Hernia

Congenital diaphragmatic hernia (CDH) is a major congenital defect and the classical hernia, Bochdalek hernia, is through a posterolateral defect in the diaphragm. A recent population-based study from Atlanta places the incidence at approximately 2.4 per 10,000 live births,[39] with increased frequency in premature and male infants. Eighty percent of diaphragmatic hernias are left-sided and 20% are right-sided. The expected recurrence risk in a first-degree relative is slightly greater than 2%. Deletions in various chromosomes have been described in patients with congenital diaphragmatic hernia. The incidence of associated abnormalities is about 30%, with skeletal and cardiac abnormalities being the most common.[40,41] Cardiac malformations tend to affect the outflow tracts and include tetralogy of Fallot and transposition of the great vessels. Congenital diaphragmatic hernia occurs in the context of a number of syndromes, including trisomies 21, 18, and 13; Fryns syndrome; Beckwith-Wiedemann syndrome; and Goldenhar syndrome.

The pathophysiology of congenital diaphragmatic hernia is complex. The diaphragm is formed in 2 stages. The septum transversum forms from the area of the inferior portion of the pericardial cavity. This septum separates the peritoneal and thoracic cavities. This septum ultimately forms the central tendon. However, lateral foramina persist and are called pleuroperitoneal canals. Normally, these canals are closed by pleuroperitoneal membranes. It is through these canals that the usual Bochdalek hernia protrudes. The left-sided hernia may contain stomach, small bowel, spleen, and even kidney.

The hernia is covered by a membrane in 10% of cases. The extension of the abdominal viscera into the thoracic cavity results in significant lung hypoplasia by virtue of the space-occupying effect. If the hernia occurs before 16 weeks of gestation there will be a reduction in the number of bronchial branches. Whether early or late, the hernia decreases acinar development of both the ipsilateral and contralateral lung, and thus gas-exchange surface area is reduced. Vascular abnormalities are striking, with reduced numbers of pulmonary arterial branches and muscular thickening of the arteries. These vascular abnormalities increase the risk of the affected infant having pulmonary hypertension and developing persistent fetal circulation.

The diagnosis of CDH is considered when respiratory distress occurs at birth. The degree of distress depends on the degree of pulmonary hypertension and hypoplasia. In infants where a great deal of abdominal viscera are displaced into the thorax, the abdomen is flat (scaphoid) and there is asymmetrical distension of the chest. Respiratory distress may increase as the gastrointestinal tract fills with swallowed air. The presence of bowel sounds over the thorax and the absence of breath sounds on the affected side are frequently described.

The diagnosis is often made during a routine prenatal ultrasound. Ultrasound can detect diaphragmatic hernias as early as 12 weeks of gestation, but they are usually found at 24 weeks of gestation. Polyhydramnios is reported in 75% of cases. After birth the diagnosis is confirmed by plain chest radiograph. Common findings are bowel in the chest cavity and deviation of the mediastinum. The diagnosis is usually obvious, but other diagnoses should be considered, including congenital cystic disease of the lung and agenesis of the lung. Once the diagnosis is confirmed, it is important to screen for associated anomalies using echocardiography and ultrasound of the head and kidneys.

Early therapy is directed at improving respiratory status. Although defects in surfactant have been described, a role for prenatal steroid therapy or surfactant administration at birth has not been established.[42,43] Fetal surgery to enhance lung development is no longer used because recent studies demonstrated no benefit.[44] Initial resuscitation should involve endotracheal intubation and placement of a nasogastric tube to abrogate expansion of the stomach and small bowel by swallowed air. Once intubated, mechanical ventilation is used as a bridge to surgical repair. A number of ventilatory strategies can keep the preductal arterial Po_2 (partial pressure of oxygen) greater than 60 mm Hg, including varying from high rates with low positive end-expiratory pressure (PEEP) to lower rates with higher PEEP. Central to most strategies is the use of the pressure-cycled ventilators with strict monitoring of tidal volume and preductal oxygen saturations. If extensive support is needed, this suggests that lung hypoplasia or pulmonary hypertension is significant. Indeed, a number of indices have been established to quantify this support and thus help predict ultimate outcome. These indices include a ventilatory index and an oxygenation index. Nitric oxide (NO) is a successful therapy for pulmonary artery hypertension, but in children with congenital diaphragmatic hernia the results are mixed; however, a therapeutic trial is appropriate when pulmonary artery hypertension is significant.[45] Extracorporeal membrane oxygenation (ECMO) is indicated if conventional or high-frequency ventilation and NO therapies are not beneficial.

Surgery for CDH is no longer considered an emergency intervention. With advances in intensive care medicine, surgery can be elective, allowing for appropriate time to look for other congenital abnormalities that may alter the surgical approach. If the diaphragmatic defect is large, it may be closed with a prosthetic patch or a local flap from the chest wall or abdominal wall. The abdominal cavity may be hypoplastic due to relocation of the bowel into the thorax during development. With return of the viscera it may not be possible to close the abdomen. In these cases the skin is approximated, and after a few months the abdominal wall defect can be closed.

Outcomes of CDH have improved dramatically in recent years, and survival rates of 80% to 90% are frequently described.[46] Pulmonary function tests are frequently abnormal but improve over time; long-term follow-up found that 50% of patients had normal lung function by 10 years of age.[47] Increased bronchial reactivity, as demonstrated by wheezing with respiratory tract infections, can be a persistent problem. Neurodevelopmental abnormalities are common, particularly when ECMO has been used. Additionally, gastroesophageal reflux is frequently seen and needs to be addressed medically.

A less common form of CDH is the Morgagni hernia. This hernia occurs at either side of the midline just behind the sternum, where the septum transversum joins the chest wall. Occasionally these hernias are bilateral and give rise to a large central defect. Morgagni hernias are rarely symptomatic and can present at any age. These hernias may be associated with other abnormalities, particularly malrotation of the gut. Operative repair is relatively straightforward via a transverse upper abdominal incision, where the diaphragm is attached to the posterior rectal sheath. These hernias may also be amenable to laparoscopic and thoracoscopic approaches.

Another frequently seen diaphragmatic defect is eventration of the diaphragm. In congenital eventration there is a thin, membranous diaphragm with some protrusion into the thoracic cavity. Although usually benign, a large eventration may present with similar symptoms as CDH. In the acquired form there is paralysis of the phrenic nerve either due to birth trauma or surgical trauma. The distribution of the muscle fibers in the diaphragm is normal in the acquired form; however, in the congenital form the muscle is distributed around the rim of the diaphragm. Generally, eventrations are identified as an incidental finding or because of mild respiratory symptoms during respiratory tract infections. Occasionally there is intolerance of rigorous exercise. The diagnosis is confirmed by fluoroscopy of the chest. On fluoroscopy there is paradoxical movement, with the diaphragm on the affected side rising on inspiration. Most eventrations are small, and surgical repair is not necessary. When the defect is large or symptomatic, plication of the thinned-out diaphragm can optimize lung growth and development.

Pulmonary Sequestration

Of all the lesions discussed here, perhaps pulmonary sequestration is the most complex, least clear, and most controversial in terminology, origin, and description. Classical extra-lobar pulmonary sequestration consists of an isolated segment of lung tissue with no connection to the tracheobronchial tree, invested in its own pleura, fed by a systemic artery, and drained via a systemic vein.[48] However, pulmonary sequestration is often associated with multiple variants of this schema and may be seen in combination with other pulmonary anomalies, such as CCAM, bronchogenic cyst, and scimitar syndrome.[49] Intralobar sequestration was initially thought to be an acquired lesion consisting of neovascularization via a systemic artery to an area of chronically inflamed lung parenchyma (generally due to recurrent infection). More recently it has become apparent that intralobar sequestration can be a congenital problem unrelated to recurrent infection.

Using the malinosculation classification of Clements and Warner,[1] pulmonary sequestration can be seen as a spectrum of diseases, which can involve any or all 4 of the major components of lung tissue: airways, arterial blood supply, venous drainage, and lung parenchyma. Thus, in classical extra-lobar sequestration, all 4 components are abnormal, whereas in intralobar sequestration the arterial blood supply may be the only abnormality. Given the myriad variations of sequestration, and given the frequent association with other intrapulmonary lesions, some experts believe a more proper name for pulmonary sequestration is congenital bronchopulmonary foregut malformation. Most pediatrics experts prefer using a more specific term, which allows for the differentiation of problems that pediatricians and surgeons need in order to make clinical decisions. The more specific term is used with the understanding that each lesion has its own variations and associated anomalies.

Extra-lobar sequestrations of the lung are predominantly left-sided (65%) and are usually found between the lower lobe and the diaphragm, but can be located anywhere in the thorax and occasionally even subdiaphragmatically.[48] Blood supply is directly from the thoracic or abdominal aorta in 80% of cases and arises from branches of smaller systemic vessels in the remainder. Venous drainage is generally to the right atrium, creating a left-to-right shunt. On cut section the sequestrum contains irregularly formed bronchi, alveolar ducts, and alveoli and may even have cystic elements, confirming the maldevelopment of lung parenchyma in addition to the airway and blood vessel abnormalities.

Extra-lobar sequestrations appear as triangular-shaped opacities and can be seen on chest radiographs in the retrocardiac area. Computed tomography and MRI allow for much better characterization of the lesions and frequently demonstrate the abnormal systemic blood supply to the area.[50,51] It should be remembered that feeder vessels may not be visible if their diameter is below the limit of resolution of the scanning technique. Resolution is improved by using helical CT scanning and post-processing workstations, which allows visualization of even small aortic branches.

Extra-lobar sequestrations may be incidental findings consisting of a retrocardiac mass on a chest radiograph obtained for other reasons, may present with respiratory distress in the newborn period, or may become infected at some time after the newborn period. Infection is generally due to hematogenous spread of bacteria unless there is a connection to a bronchus or to the esophagus. Repeat infection or abscess formation may occur and is an indication for surgical resection. Tachypnea in the newborn period may be due to mass effect, high output cardiac failure, or associated cardiac or pulmonary congenital defects. Treatment for an extra-lobar sequestration is usually surgical removal, given the need to confirm the lesion histologically, prevent future infection or bleeding, and allow for normal lung growth. Treatment with arterial embolization and recognition of spontaneous involution of some lesions have led to questioning the need for surgery in all cases.[52,53]

Vascular Rings

Vascular rings represent a wide spectrum of abnormalities that frequently include the aortic arch, the pulmonary arteries, and brachiocephalic vessels. Most infants with vascular rings are asymptomatic, but if symptoms arise they relate to the degree of compression of the respiratory and gastrointestinal tract. If vascular rings cause symptoms, presentation is in the first few months of life in most infants. Symptoms can be variable, including stridor, arching of the neck, unusual postures during sleep, a brassy or seal-like cough, and apnea. These symptoms are not unique to vascular rings and, accordingly, infants with rings are frequently initially diagnosed as having esophageal reflux, laryngotracheomalacia, or reactive airways disease. Dysphagia occurs when the child transitions to solid foods if constriction of the esophagus is severe. Indeed, an infant may refuse solid foods. Interestingly, dysphagia can present later in life when the arteries calcify.

The overall incidence of vascular rings is unknown, since many may remain asymptomatic and go undiagnosed, but are thought to comprise 1% to 2% of congenital heart defects. Vascular rings are classified into complete rings, incomplete rings, and pulmonary slings. These vascular abnormalities usually occur in isolation, but 10% to 15% are associated with congenital heart disease.[54]

There are a number of types of complete rings, including double aortic arch and right arch with the ring formed by ligamentum/ductus or aberrant left subclavian branching. A double aortic arch occurs when the right dorsal aortic arch does not regress. Thus the 2 arches encircle the trachea and the esophagus (Figure 14-10). The right arch is predominant in about 75% of cases. This form usually presents in infancy and is confirmed by echocardiography and CT. Although the MRI is superior for vascular imaging, long scan time and required sedation make CT a more appropriate choice for infants. Surgery is indicated when the child is symptomatic. Surgery involves ligation of the nondominant arch while preserving brachiocephalic blood flow. There is often associated tracheomalacia from in utero compression of the trachea, and many infants have persistent respiratory symptoms after surgery.

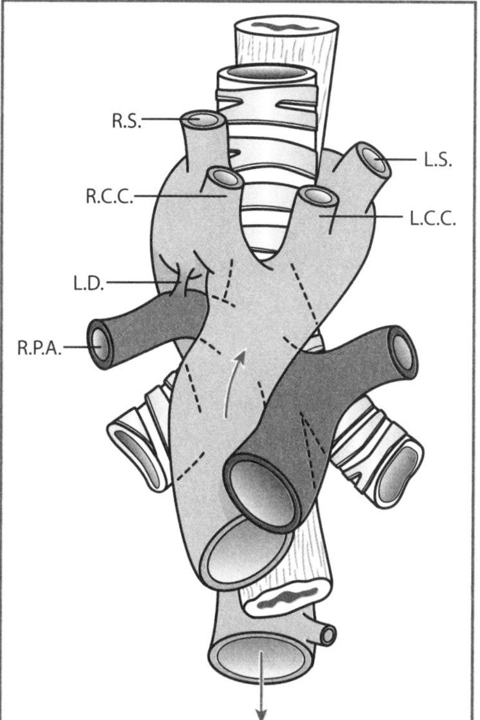

Figure 14-10. Double aortic arch encircling the trachea and esophagus. LCC, left common carotid artery; LD, ligamentum arteriosa; LS, left subclavian; RCC, right common carotid artery; RPA, right pulmonary artery. RS, right subclavian.

A right-sided aortic arch may occur in isolation or may form part of a ring. In one ring formation (Figure 14-11), the right arch traces around the back of the esophagus and there is an aberrant left subclavian artery from the descending aorta. The ring is closed by the ligamentum arteriosum, which bridges the pulmonary artery and the left subclavian artery. In another form of right-sided arch rings, called mirror imaging, an aberrant left innominate artery reaches across the front of the trachea. The arch still traces behind the aorta, and the ring is completed by the ligamentum arteriosum arising from the descending aorta rather than the aberrant subclavian artery to the pulmonary artery. Another form of vascular ring maintains a less complete ring where the ligamentum arteriosum arises from the mirror image left subclavian/innominate artery to the pulmonary artery. These arches

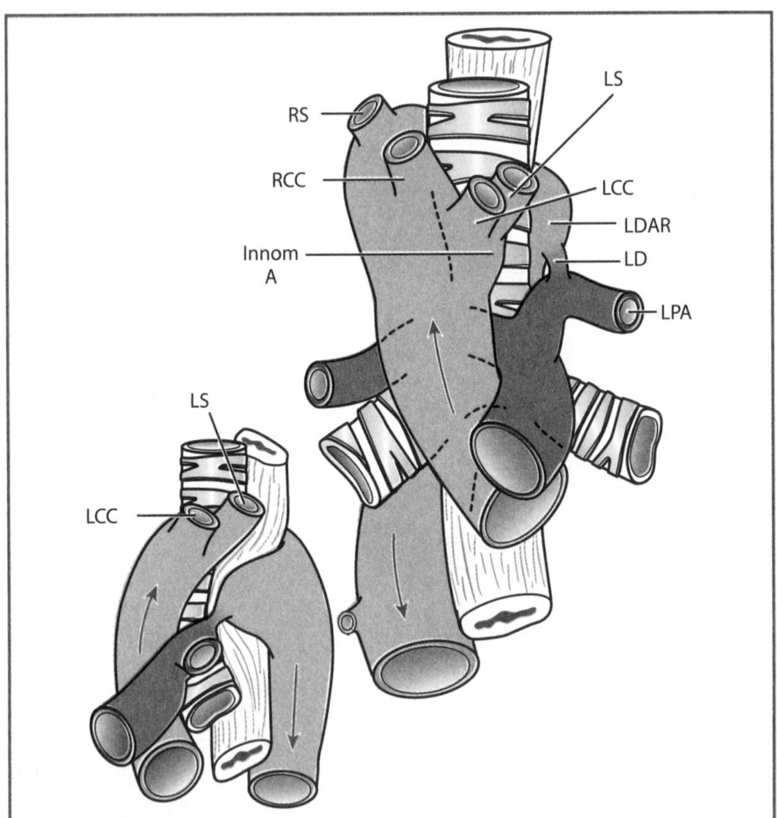

Figure 14-11. Isolated right aortic arch with ductus arteriosa arising from diverticulum of Kommerell. Innom A, innominate artery; LD, ligamentum arteriosa; LDAR, left dorsal aortic root (diverticulum of Kommerell); LPA, left pulmonary artery; PT, pulmonary trunk.

may be complicated by a Kommerell diverticulum at the site where the ligamentum arteriosum joins the aorta. Surgery is recommended in symptomatic vascular rings. It involves ligation of the ligamentum arteriosum. If a Kommerell diverticulum is present, then a resection or aortopexy surgery may be required.

Incomplete vascular rings do not form closed, constricting lesions, but may still impinge on the airway or esophagus. Anomalous innominate artery compression is considered to exist if the artery arises from the aortic arch to the left of midline and causes tracheal compression. Usually this causes no or mild symptoms and no surgery is indicated. Only when symptoms are severe should surgery be considered since in most untreated cases symptoms ameliorate over time. Another simple ring involves an aberrant right subclavian artery. It arises from the descending aorta and traces behind the esophagus. It rarely causes symptoms, but can be associated with feeding problems.

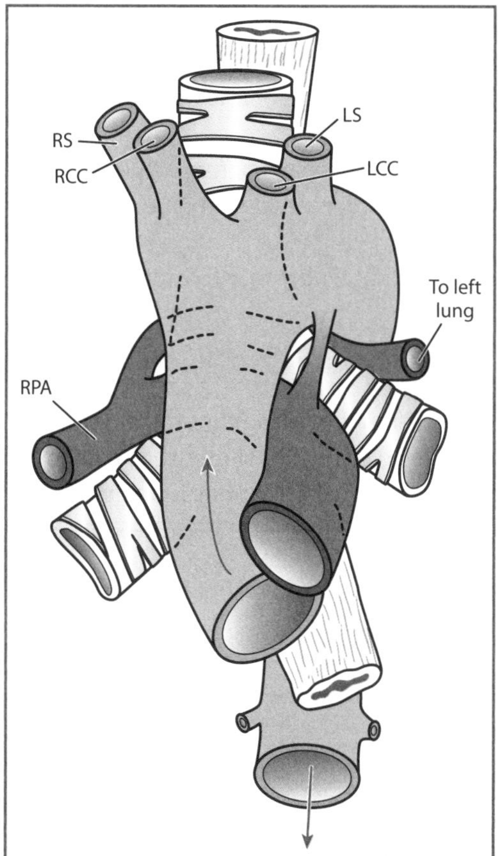

Figure 14-12. Pulmonary sling. The left pulmonary artery arises from the right pulmonary artery and courses behind the trachea and in front of the esophagus. LCC, left common carotid artery; LS, left subclavian; PT, pulmonary trunk; RCC, right common carotid aartery; RPA, right pulmonary artery; RS, right subclavian.

Pulmonary slings are an unusual form of vascular compression. In this condition, the left pulmonary artery arises from the right pulmonary artery and travels between the trachea and esophagus (Figure 14-12). Pulmonary slings are associated with complete tracheal rings and tracheal stenosis in about one-third of cases.[55] Surgery is usually indicated and may involve tracheal reconstruction. Generally, the long-term prognosis after surgical correction is favorable. However, after surgery there is usually some tracheomalacia that results in a lingering cough and noisy breathing, which should improve in time.

Key Points

- Pulmonary congenital malformations arise from errors in fetal lung development.
- Pulmonary malformations can involve the airways, pulmonary parenchyma, blood vessels, or any combination of the 3.
- Lung abnormalities that arise from errors before 16 weeks of gestation affect airway development; those after 16 weeks affect acinar development.
- Some lesions detected by prenatal ultrasound resolve spontaneously.
- Symptomatic congenital abnormalities require surgical intervention.
- Although there have been reports of malignant transformation within some of these lesions, the absolute risk of cancer associated with congenital lung malformations is unknown.

References

1. Clements BS, Warner JO. Pulmonary sequestration and related congenital bronchopulmonary-vascular malformations: nomenclature and classification based on anatomical and embryological considerations. *Thorax.* 1987;42:401–408
2. Cardoso WV, Lu J. Regulation of early lung morphogenesis: questions, facts and controversies. *Development.* 2006;133:1611–1624
3. Kinane TB. Lung development and implications for hypoplasia found in congenital diaphragmatic hernia. *Am J Med Genet C Semin Med Genet.* 2007;145C(2):117–124
4. O'Sullivan BP, Finger L, Zwerdling RG. Use of nasopharyngoscopy in the evaluation of children with noisy breathing. *Chest.* 2004;125:1265–1269
5. O'Sullivan BP, Frassica JJ, Rayder SM. Tracheal bronchus. *Chest.* 1998;113:537–540

6. Finder JD. Primary bronchomalacia in infants and children. *J Pediatr.* 1997;130:59–66
7. Boogaard R, Huijsmans SH, Pijnenburg MW, Tiddens HA, de Jongste JC, Merkus PJ. Tracheomalacia and bronchomalacia in children: incidence and patient characteristics. *Chest.* 2005;128:3391–3397
8. Panitch HB, Keklikian EN, Motley RA, Wolfson MR, Schidlow DV. Effect of altering smooth muscle tone on maximal expiratory flows in patients with tracheomalacia. *Pediatr Pulmonol.* 1990;9:170–176
9. Carden KA, Boiselle PM, Waltz DA, Ernst A. Tracheomalacia and tracheobronchomalacia in children and adults. *Chest.* 2005;127:984–1005
10. Benesch M, Eber E, Pfleger A, Zach MS. Recurrent lower respiratory tract infections in a 14-year-old boy with tracheobronchomegaly (Mounier-Kuhn syndrome). *Pediatr Pulmonol.* 2000;29:476–479
11. Griscom NT, Wohl MEB. Dimensions of the growing trachea related to age and gender. *AJR Am J Roentgenol.* 1985;146:233–237
12. Torfs CP, Curry CJ, Bateson TF. Population-based study of tracheoesophageal fistula and esophageal atresia. *Teratology.* 1995;52:220–232
13. Spitz L. Oesophageal atresia. *Orphanet J Rare Dis.* 2007;2:24
14. Kovesi T, Rubin S. Long-term complications of congenital esophageal atresia and/or tracheoesophageal fistula. *Chest.* 2004;126:915–925
15. Malmström K, Lohi J, Lindahl H, et al. Longitudinal follow-up of bronchial inflammation, respiratory symptoms, and pulmonary function in adolescents after repair of esophageal atresia with tracheoesophageal fistula. *J Pediatr.* 2008;153:396–401.e1
16. Felson B. Pulmonary agenesis and related anomalies. *Semin Roentgenol.* 1972;7:17–30
17. Dupuis C, Charaf LAC, Brevière G-M, Abou P, Rémy-Jardin M, Helmius G. The "adult" form of the scimitar syndrome. *Am J Cardiol.* 1992;70:502–507
18. Dupuis C, Charaf LAC, Breviere G-M, Abou P. "Infantile" form of the scimitar syndrome with pulmonary hypertension. *Am J Cardiol.* 1993;71:1326–1330
19. Nakamura Y, Harada K, Yamamoto I, et al. Human pulmonary hypoplasia. *Arch Pathol Lab Med.* 1992;116:635–642
20. Potter EL. Bilateral renal agenesis. *J Pediatr.* 1946;29:68–76
21. Abel RM, Bush A, Chitty LS, Harcourt J, Nicholson AG. Congenital lung disease. In: Chernick V, Boat TF, Wilmott RW, Bush A, eds. *Kendig's Disorders of the Respiratory Tract in Children.* Philadelphia, PA: Saunders Elsevier, 2006:280–316
22. Ribet ME, Copin MC, Gosselin B. Bronchogenic cysts of the mediastinum. *J Thorac Cardiovasc Surg.* 1995;109:1003–1010
23. Itoh H, Shitamura T, Kataoka H, et al. Retroperitoneal bronchogenic cyst: report of a case and literature review. *Pathol International.* 1999;49:152–155

24. Azeem F, Rathwell C, Awad WI. A near fatal presentation of a bronchogenic cyst compressing the left main coronary artery. *J Thorac Cardiovasc Surg.* 2008;135:1395–1396
25. Jakopovic M, Slobodnjak Z, Krizanac S, Samarzija M. Large cell carcinoma arising in bronchogenic cyst. *J Thorac Cardiovasc Surg.* 2005;130:610–612
26. Servais E, Paul S, Port JL, Altorki NK, Lee PC. Carcinoid tumor nested within a bronchogenic cyst. *J Thorac Cardiovasc Surg.* 2008;136:227–228
27. Endo C, Imai T, Nakagawa H, Ebina A, Kaimori M. Bronchioloalveolar carcinoma arising in a bronchogenic cyst. *Ann Thorac Surg.* 2000;69:933–935
28. Okada Y, Mori H, Maeda T, Obashi A, Itoh Y, Doi K. Congenital mediastinal bronchogenic cyst with malignant transformation: an autopsy report. *Pathol Int.* 1996;46:594–600
29. Ponn RB. Simple mediastinal cysts: resect them all? *Chest.* 2003;124:4–6
30. Stocker JT, Madewell JE, Drake RM. Congenital cystic adenomatoid malformation of the lung. *Hum Pathol.* 1977;3:155–171
31. Stocker JT. Congenital pulmonary airway malformation—a new name for and an expanded classification of congenital cystic adenomatoid malformation of the lung. *Histopathology.* 2002;41:424–431
32. Priest JR, Williams GM, Hill DA, Dehner LP, Jaffe A. Pulmonary cysts in early childhood and the risk of malignancy. *Pediatr Pulmonol.* 2009;44(1):14–30
33. Crombleholme TM, Coleman B, Hedrick H, et al. Cystic adenomatoid malformation volume ratio predicts outcome in prenatally diagnosed cystic adenomatoid malformation of the lung. *J Pediatr Surg.* 2002;37(3):331–338
34. Özçelik U, Göçmen A, Kiper N, Dogru D, Dilber E, Günes Yalcin E. Congenital lobar emphysema: evaluation and long-term follow-up of thirty cases at a single center. *Pediatr Pulmonol.* 2003;35:384–391
35. Mani H, Suarez E, Stocker JT. The morphologic spectrum of infantile lobar emphysema: a study of 33 cases. *Paediatr Respir Rev.* 2004;5:S313–S320
36. Cleveland RH, Weber B. Retained fetal lung liquid in congenital lobar emphysema: a possible predictor of polyalveolar lobe. *Pediatr Radiol.* 1993;23:291–295
37. Olutoye OO, Coleman BG, Hubbard AM, Adzick NS. Prenatal diagnosis and management of congenital lobar emphysema. *J Pediatr Surg.* 2000;35:792–795
38. Mei-Zahav M, Konen O, Manson D, Langer JC. Is congenital lobar emphysema a surgical disease? *J Pediatr Surg.* 2006;41:1058–1061
39. Dott MM, Wong LY, Rasmussen SA. Population-based study of congenital diaphragmatic hernia: risk factors and survival in Metropolitan Atlanta, 1968–1999. *Birth Defects Res A Clin Mol Teratol.* 2003;67:261–267
40. Migliazza L, Xia H, Diez-Pardo JA, Tovar JA. Skeletal malformations associated with congenital diaphragmatic hernia: experimental and human studies. *J Pediatr Surg.* 1999;34:1624–1629

41. Migliazza L, Otten C, Xia H, Rodriguez JI, Diez-Pardo JA, Tovar JA. Cardiovascular malformations in congenital diaphragmatic hernia: human and experimental studies. *J Pediatr Surg.* 1999;34(9):1352–1358
42. Ford WD, Kirby CP, Wilkinson CS, Furness ME, Slater AJ. Antenatal betamethasone and favourable outcomes in fetuses with 'poor prognosis' diaphragmatic hernia. *Pediatr Surg Int.* 2002;18:244–246
43. Kay S, Laberge JM, Flageole H, Richardson S, Belanger S, Piedboeuf B. Use of antenatal steroids to counteract the negative effects of tracheal occlusion in the fetal lamb model. *Pediatr Res.* 2001;50:495–501
44. Harrison MR, Keller RL, Hawgood SB, et al. A randomized trial of fetal endoscopic tracheal occlusion for severe fetal congenital diaphragmatic hernia. *N Engl J Med.* 2003;349(20):1916–1924
45. Kinsella JP, Ivy DD, Abman SH. Pulmonary vasodilator therapy in congenital diaphragmatic hernia: acute, late, and chronic pulmonary hypertension. *Semin Perinatol.* 2005;29:123–128
46. Weber TR, Kountzman B, Dillon PA, Silen ML. Improved survival in congenital diaphragmatic hernia with evolving therapeutic strategies. *Arch Surg.* 1998;133(5):498–502; discussion 502–503
47. Muratore CS, Kharasch V, Lund DP, et al. Pulmonary morbidity in 100 survivors of congenital diaphragmatic hernia monitored in a multidisciplinary clinic. *J Pediatr Surg.* 2001;36:133–140
48. Stocker JT. Sequestration of the lung. *Semin Diagn Pathol.* 1986;3:106–121
49. Bratu I, Flageole H, Chen M-F, Di Lorenzo M, Yazbeck S, Laberge J-M. The multiple facets of pulmonary sequestration. *J Pediatr Surg.* 2001;36:784–790
50. Au V, Chan J, Chan F. Pulmonary sequestration diagnosed by contrast enhanced three-dimensional MR angiography. *Br J Radiol.* 1999;72:709–711
51. Ko S-F, Ng S-H, Lee T-Y, et al. Noninvasive imaging of bronchopulmonary sequestration. *Am J Roentgenol.* 2000;175:1005–1012
52. Garcia-Pena P, Lucaya J, Hendry GMA, Duran C. Spontaneous involution of pulmonary sequestration in children: a report of two cases and review of the literature. *Pediatr Radiol.* 1998;28:266–270
53. Nayar P, Thakral C, Sajwani M. Congenital lobar emphysema and sequestration—treatment by embolization. *Pediatr Surg Int.* 2005;21:727–729
54. van Son JA, Julsrud PR, Hagler DJ, et al. Surgical treatment of vascular rings: the Mayo Clinic experience. *Mayo Clin Proc.* 1993;68:1056–1063
55. Berdon WE, Baker DH, Wung JT, et al. Complete cartilage-ring tracheal stenosis associated with anomalous left pulmonary artery: the ring-sling complex. *Radiology.* 1984;152:57–64

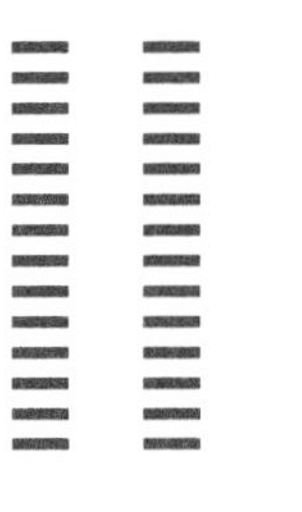

Chapter 15

Chest Wall and Spinal Deformities

Oscar Henry Mayer, MD
Julian L. Allen, MD

Introduction

Mechanics of Breathing: Inspiration Versus Expiration

The act of breathing is sometimes compared with the movement of a piston because of the cyclical cephalad and caudal motion of the diaphragm, and the chest wall is seen as a passive participant; however, this view is too simplistic. The chest wall is very dynamic during breathing and is critical in maintaining resting lung volume, optimizing lung mechanics, allowing normal respiratory growth, and protecting the thoracic organs.

In healthy children, inspiration begins from functional residual capacity (FRC), which is the point in the respiratory cycle when the outward recoil of the rib cage and the inward recoil of the lungs are equal and opposite. The diaphragm contracts and moves caudally, increasing intra-abdominal pressure, and displacing the abdominal contents and the lower edges of the rib cage outward. This caudal motion of the diaphragm, along with outward and cephalad rotation of the ribs, produces increasingly negative intrathoracic pressure and a gradient favoring airflow down the respiratory tract from the mouth to the alveoli (Figure 15-1A).

While inspiration is an active process, exhalation is largely passive. After the muscles of inspiration relax, the inward recoil of the lungs produces positive pressure in the alveoli that favors expiratory flow down the pressure gradient to the mouth, as the lung volume decreases to FRC (Figure 15-1B).

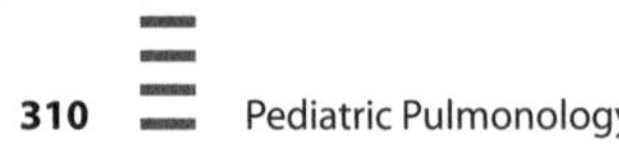

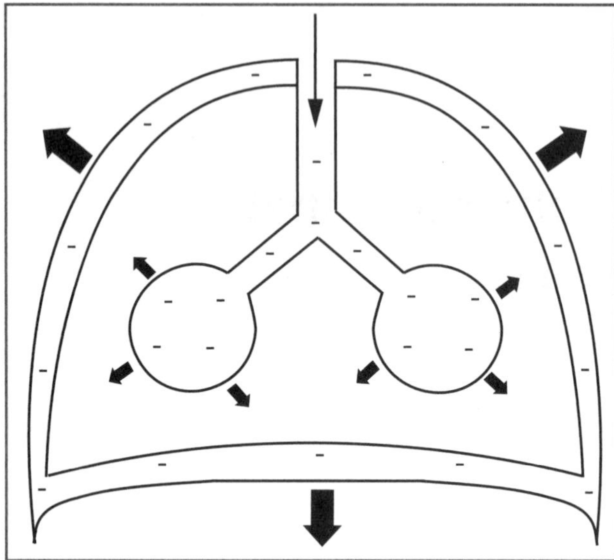

A

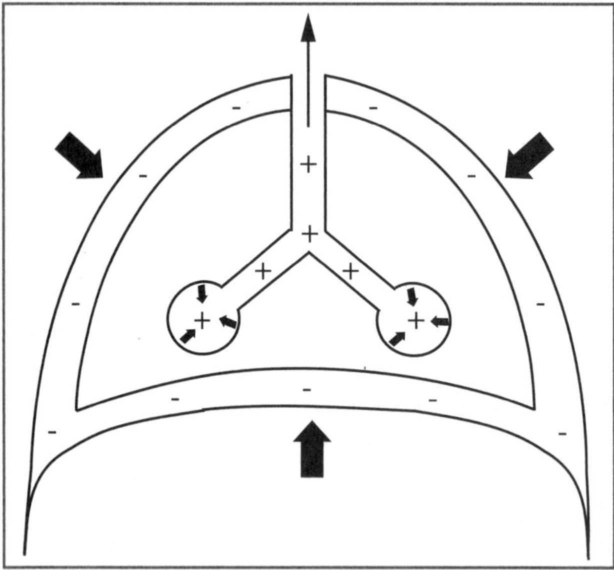

B

Figure 15-1. Representation of the motion of the alveoli, diaphragm, and chest wall during **(A)** inspiration and **(B)** exhalation.

Mechanics of Breathing: Area of Apposition

The extent of downward excursion of the diaphragm depends on the area of apposition of the diaphragm to the rib cage, or the portion of the diaphragm aligned vertically along the inner surface of the chest wall (Figure 15-2A). As the portion of the diaphragm in the area of apposition contracts, the diaphragm moves caudally. The area of apposition comprises one-quarter to three-quarters of the total surface area of the rib cage in adults.[1] It is somewhat less in children and substantially less in infants. In a child with significant lung disease with hyperinflation, the diaphragm will be positioned in a lower and flatter position and the area of apposition can be much smaller. Furthermore, with a smaller area of apposition and a flatter diaphragm the radius of curvature of the diaphragm will be larger (Figure 15-2B) and, by the Law of Laplace, the force-generating capacity of the diaphragm will be lower.

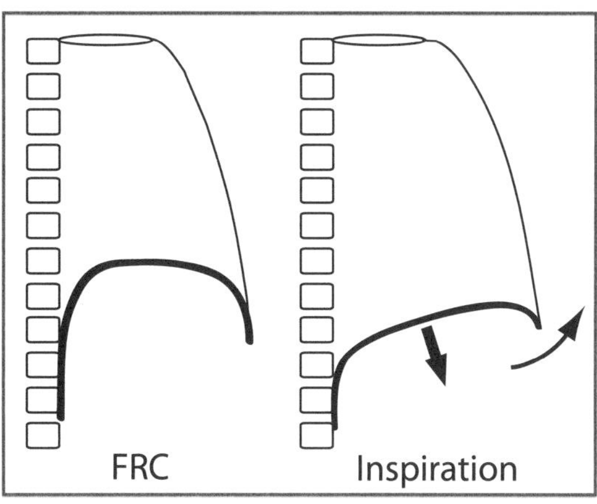

A

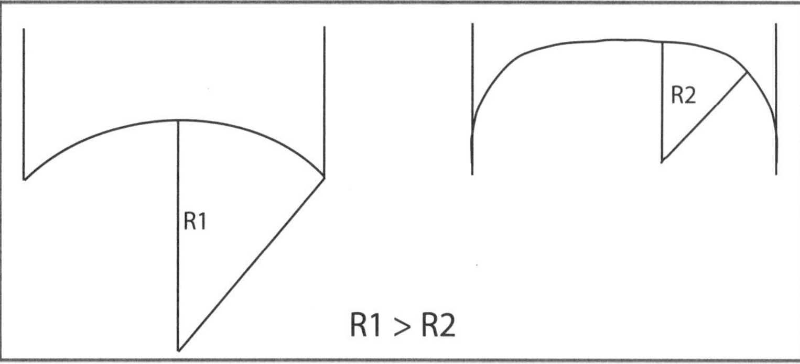

B

Figure 15-2. **(A)** Area of apposition at functional residual capacity (FRC) and during inspiration and **(B)** radius of curvature of the diaphragm in 2 different orientations with R1 > R2.

Mechanics of Breathing: Thoracoabdominal Mechanics

During restful breathing in a healthy child the abdominal and rib cage excursion are nearly coincident (Figure 15-3A). With respiratory disease, such as increased airway resistance or chest wall compliance, the abdominal excursion will lead the chest wall excursion (thoracoabdominal asynchrony). This is easily visible during a respiratory examination and can increase to the far end of the spectrum to completely asynchronous or paradoxical respiration, with the abdomen moving outward as the chest wall is moving inward (Figure 15-3B).

When airway resistance increases, the pressure gradient needed to overcome the resistance and generate flow is higher, and it takes longer to generate outward chest wall motion. A highly compliant rib cage will move inward while the abdomen moves outward at the onset of inspiration because of the progressively negative intrathoracic pressure (Figure 15-3B). This condition can be seen in some neonates and young infants; children with neuromuscular disease, especially spinal muscular atrophy type 1; and children with chest wall disorders.

To increase inspiration, the diaphragm will contract more caudally and the scalene and sternocleidomastoid muscles will contract to further elevate the superior rib cage. With forceful exhalation from total lung capacity (TLC), such as coughing, the abdominal muscles contract pushing the abdominal contents inward and upward elevating the diaphragm, while the internal intercostal muscles contract to augment the inward recoil of the chest wall and lungs.

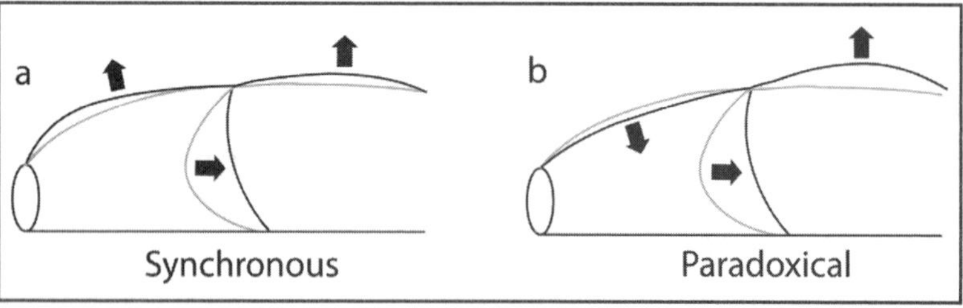

Figure 15-3. Thoracoabdominal motion during inspiration from functional residual capacity with **(A)** synchronous and **(B)** asynchronous conditions.

Pathophysiology

Structural Changes Resulting From Growth and Development

In neonates, lung compliance is low and chest wall compliance is high compared with older children and adults.[2–6] In addition the ribs are more horizontal in infants compared with children and adults in whom the ribs slope more caudally.[7]

Through early childhood lung compliance increases as the alveoli develop and lung volume increases; however, lung compliance and lung volume increase at roughly the same rate such that when lung compliance is normalized for lung growth it remains constant.[8] However, chest wall compliance normalized to lung volume decreases through childhood as the chest stiffens due to a combination of rib ossification and increasing chest wall muscle mass.[9,10] In adulthood, chest wall compliance decreases further as the costal cartilage also progressively calcifies.[10]

Functional Consequences of Developmental and Structural Changes

A highly compliant chest wall has clear advantages in the birthing process by allowing distortion during the movement through the birth canal. In neonates and infants, this high degree of chest wall compliance creates mechanical disadvantages. First, the negative intrathoracic pressure produced during inspiration can move the highly compliant chest wall inward (Figure 15-3B). Second, infants have low *lung* compliance relative to their *chest wall* compliance, which produces a lower FRC relative to that in older children and adults. The lower FRC may be at or below the point when airways close and atelectasis occurs (the closing volume). If closing volume occurs during tidal breathing, before any inspiratory flow can occur, pressure needs to be applied to the respiratory system to raise lung volume above the closing volume to open the closed airways. This increases work of breathing without benefit because the energy used to inflate the lung above closing volume does not produce inspiratory flow.

To compensate for this mechanical inefficiency, infants will often slow expiration, using glottic narrowing, ending at an end-expiratory lung volume (EELV) higher than FRC and above the closing volume.[11,12] Actively maintaining EELV above FRC and closing volume minimizes the work of breathing.

Finally, a highly compliant chest wall may move outward during cough due to the highly positive intrathoracic pressure during a forced exhalation thereby decreasing cough efficiency.

Under normal circumstances the outward excursion of the rib cage provides about 35% of the volume of inspiration in a newborn,[13] with the remainder coming from abdominal excursion. The relative rib cage excursion increases to the adult value of 65% of inspiratory volume early in the second year of life.[13]

While a chest wall with high compliance may move inward during inspiration (Figure 15-3B), a chest wall with low compliance moves very little. To maintain an acceptable tidal volume the diaphragm will contract further and the lungs will expand more caudally and less outward. This can cause a number of problems.

First, inspiratory reserve volume (IRV), the volume that can be recruited during a maximal inspiration, will be lower (Figure 15-4)

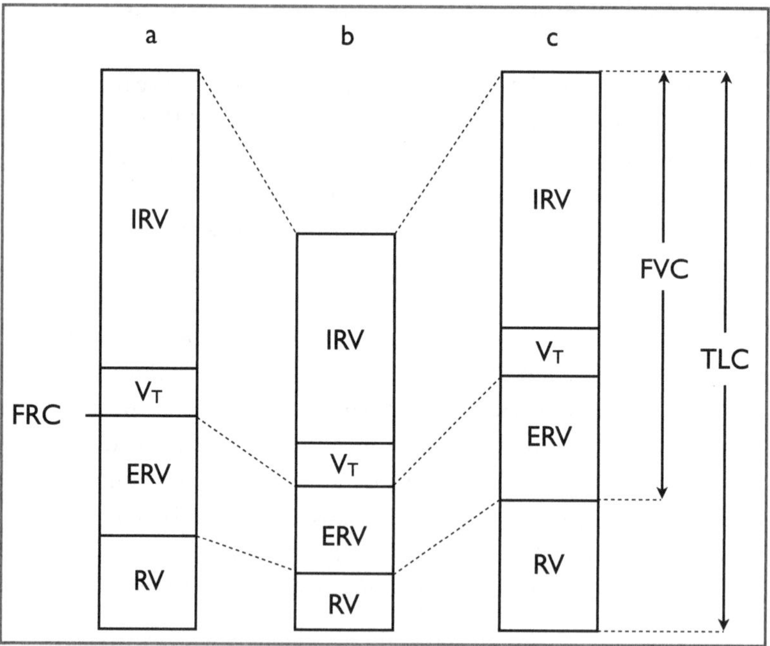

Figure 15-4.
Lung volumes in **(A)** normal condition, **(B)** restrictive lung disease, and **(C)** obstructive lung disease. ERV, expiratory reserve volume; FRC, functional residual capacity; IRV, inspiratory reserve volume; RV, residual volume; TLC, total lung capacity; Vt, tidal volume.

as will forced vital capacity (FVC), the volume of air that can move through the lungs during maximal inspiration and expiration.

Second, since the diaphragm is contracting more during inspiration, it is working harder and is at risk for fatigue.

Third, cough and airway clearance can be compromised since FVC and IRV will be lower, which limits how deeply air is inhaled into the lungs and beyond airway secretions.

Methods for Assessing Chest Wall Function

Physical Examination

It is very important to qualitatively assess chest wall function by observation. Scoliosis is often thought of as a uniplanar defect with a curve that is in the coronal plane based on the radiographic appearance; however, there can also be more complicated multi-planar kyphoscoliosis and rotational scoliosis.

It is important to first assess the back statically and look for gross asymmetry. Scoliosis can often be seen by visually examining the spine and tracing it with a finger while a patient is standing upright. Shoulder asymmetry and unilateral scapular or rib bulging can be a sign of scoliosis with significant spinal rotation. Examining the spine with the patient bending at the waist and reaching for his or her toes can show more subtle scoliosis and right-to-left asymmetry.

It is then important to evaluate the extent and symmetry of thoracoabdominal excursion. This can be qualitatively assessed using the thumb excursion test[14] by placing the fingers of each hand on the left and right scapula with the thumbs placed on either side of the spine. In a healthy patient the thumbs should move laterally the same amount. Auscultation of the right and left lungs can discriminate asymmetrical aeration due to airway compression or atelectasis.

The relative excursion of the convex and concave chest is variable and is based on the mobility of the chest wall and the position and extent of compression of the lungs in the concave and convex chest.[15,16] In unilateral diaphragm dysfunction due to paralysis or eventration, the contralateral chest should move normally while the ipsilateral chest may move very little if at all, due to the asymmetrical diaphragm motion. With a flail chest there will be a marked asymmetry in chest wall excursion; the unaffected side will move outward during inspiration and the affected side will move inward.

Thoracoabdominal asynchrony, the difference in timing between chest wall and abdominal excursion, is also important to assess and is a measure of overall respiratory mechanics,[17–18] not specific for obstructive or restrictive lung disease.

With a poorly compliant or stiff chest wall, the abdomen moves outward and there is a delay before outward chest wall movement. It takes more intra-abdominal pressure to move the lower chest wall and more accessory inspiratory muscle contraction to expand the chest wall.

A highly compliant abdomen will have a greater outward abdominal excursion during inspiration, but still should lead the thorax on inspiration. On forced expiration the abdominal contraction can be irregular based on the characteristics of the initial defect, as with gastroschisis and omphalocele; the subsequent repair; and the amount of residual muscle mass.

Diaphragm fatigue, dysfunction, or unilateral paralysis can limit the caudal movement of the diaphragm during inspiration. To compensate, the chest wall excursion is greater, can occur before any abdominal motion, and will be more important in inspiration than typical. Depending on severity, a patient may have asynchronous respiration with outward chest wall motion coincident with inward abdominal motion. This can occur due to negative intrathoracic pressure pulling the diaphragm cephalad during inspiration.

Quantitative Assessment of Chest Wall Motion

The qualitative assessment of thoracoabdominal motion that is done during the observation portion of the physical examination can be quantitated using respiratory inductive plethysmography (RIP). During RIP thoracoabdominal motion is measured by timing the maximal thoracic and abdominal excursion during respiration using inductance bands that measure the cross-sectional area of the chest wall and abdomen.[17–19] The exact delay between abdominal and thoracic excursion and the relative excursion of each compartment can be measured.[17–19]

Lung Function Testing

Conventional lung function testing can be stratified into 2 different types: (1) forced flow measurements by spirometry to evaluate for obstructive lung disease and (2) static lung volume measurement by plethysmography or gas dilution to evaluate for restrictive lung disease (see Chapter 6). In children with obstructive lung disease, the forced expiratory flow in 1 second (FEV_1), the forced expiratory flow between 25% and 75% of FVC, and/or the FEV_1/FVC can be low. In those with restrictive lung disease, however, the FEV_1/FVC is usually normal, and there is always a low TLC. Though FVC should be low in those children with restrictive lung disease, it can be low in those with obstructive lung disease due to air trapping and increased residual volume (RV), so a low TLC is needed to definitively diagnose restrictive lung disease. Forced vital capacity can be monitored as an index of severity thereafter.

In patients with scoliosis, TLC decreases as the spinal curvature increases; however, TLC can be within the normal range.[20] Patients with more complicated rotational kyphoscoliosis or constrictive scoliosis, such as in thoracic insufficiency syndrome (TIS), can have a marked restrictive defect.[21] When evaluating the lung function of a patient with scoliosis, it is important to normalize the results using arm span as a surrogate for height to avoid underrepresenting the restrictive defect (Figure 15-5A). There are well-documented tables with normal values for upper/lower body ratio.[22,23] This ratio is abnormal in patients with chest wall or spinal disease, with the upper body being shorter relative to the lower body. Since the height of a patient with scoliosis may be shorter than the idealized height due to the curve and a shorter spine, using height, to normalize lung volume will give an inappropriate (low) normal value, and lung volume as a percent of predicted will then be falsely high (Figure 15-5B). Since arm span is not affected by spinal growth it will more accurately represent the potential, idealized height, and metabolic demand. However, lung volume normalized to height can still be useful. This correction will normalize for chest size and, if low is consistent with an intrinsic restrictive lung disease, separate from any external compression.

Respiratory Muscle Strength

Respiratory muscle strength is measured by recording the maximal inspiratory pressure (MIP) and maximal expiratory pressure (MEP) using manometry. The MIP is the maximal sustained pressure that can be maintained for 1 second when inhaling maximally against a closed shutter from RV or from FRC. It is critical to measure at the same volume or the comparisons will not be accurate. The MEP is the maximal sustained pressure that can be maintained for 1 second when exhaling maximally against a closed shutter from TLC. In adolescents with scoliosis, inefficient coupling between the muscle and chest wall reduces respiratory muscle strength. The degree of weakness partly depends on the severity of the curve.[24] Children with severe scoliosis have a similar activation of respiratory muscles as children with respiratory failure caused by obstructive lung disease.[25]

Age: 9
Gender: Female
Race: African American   Height: 158 cm   BMI: 11.9   Weight: 29.6 Kg

Note: Height and/or Weight and/or BMI is <3 %tile or >97 %tile for age.

Spirometry (BTPS) ATS ✓

		Ref	Pre	% Ref	Z-score
FVC	L	2.66	1.37	52	-3.16
FEV_1	L	2.31	1.29	56	-2.92
FEV_1 / FVC	%	90	94	104	0.67
FEF_{25-75}	L/s	2.70	2.25	83	-0.57
PEFR	L/s	5.27	3.22	61	-1.78
FET	sec		3.07		
FIF50	L/s		1.92		
FEF_{50} / FIF_{50}			1.36		
FEV.5	L	1.57	1.10	70	
Back Volume			0.05		

Lung Volumes (Box) ATS ✓

		Ref	Pre	% Ref	Z-score
TLC	L	3.51	1.99	57	-3.61
VC	L	2.59	1.37	53	-0.87
FRC	L	1.83	1.00	55	-2.67
ERV	L	0.91	0.38	42	
RV	L	0.92	0.62	67	-1.16
RV/TLC	%	26	31	119	0.36

A

Figure 15-5A. Spirometry and static lung volume measurements in a child with scoliosis with normalization using **(A)** arm span or **(B)** height. ERV, expiratory reserve volume; FEF_{25-75}, forced expiratory flows between 25% and 75% of the FVC; FEF_{50}, forced expiratory flow at 50%; FET, forced expiratory time; $FEV_{.5}$, forced expiratory volume in 0.5 seconds; FEV_1, forced expiratory volume in 1 second; FIF_{50}, forced inspiratory flow at 50%; FRC, functional reserve capacity; FVC, forced vital capacity; PEFR, peak expiratory flow rate; RV, residual volume; TLC, total lung capacity; VC, vital capacity.

Age: 9
Gender: Female **DOB:** 10/11/1999 **BMI:** 20.6
Race: African American **Height:** 120 cm **Weight:** 29.6 Kg

Note: Height and/or Weight and/or BMI is <3 %tile or >97 %tile for age.

Spirometry (BTPS) ATS ✓

		Ref	Pre	% Ref	Z-score
FVC	L	1.23	**1.37**	111	0.59
FEV!	L	1.16	**1.29**	111	0.65
FEV! / FVC	%	90	**94**	104	0.67
FEF@%_&%	L/s	1.79	**2.25**	126	1.01
PEFR	L/s	3.19	**3.22**	101	0.05
FET	sec		**3.07**		
FIF50	L/s		**1.92**		
FEF%) / FIF%)			**1.36**		
FEV.5	L	0.96	**1.10**	115	
Back Volume			**0.05**		

Lung Volumes (Box) ATS ✓

		Ref	Pre	% Ref	Z-score
TLC	L	1.79	**1.99**	111	0.93
VC	L	1.21	**1.37**	113	0.24
FRC	L	0.99	**1.00**	101	0.06
ERV	L	0.41	**0.38**	93	
RV	L	0.58	**0.62**	107	0.25
RV/TLC	%	32	**31**	97	-0.06

B

Structural Abnormalities

A list of structural abnormalities of the chest wall is found in Box 15-1.

Pectus Excavatum and Carinatum

Clinical Features

Pectus excavatum accounts for about 90% of chest wall defects,[26] with an incidence of between 1 in 400 to 1,000.[27] While abnormal lung function is rare in most patients with pectus excavatum, subjective complaints of pulmonary difficulty are much more common.[28]

Box 15-1. Structural Abnormalities of the Chest Wall

Pectus Deformity
- Pectus excavatum
- Pectus carinatum

Scoliosis
- Spinal deformity
- Rib cage deformity
    - Flail chest
    - Rib fusion
    - Neuromuscular disease (eg, spinal muscular atrophy)
- Idiopathic

Thoracic Insufficiency Syndrome
- Congenital constricted chest wall syndrome
    - Progressive congenital scoliosis and spinal disorders
        - Hemivertebra
        - Wedge vertebra
        - Bar vertebra
        - Segmental fusion
        - Fused ribs
    - Hypoplastic chest wall
        - Jeune syndrome
        - Jarcho-Levin syndrome
        - Ellis-van Creveld syndrome
        - Achondroplasia
        - Campomelic dysplasia
        - Osteogenesis imperfecta
        - Hypophosphatemia
- Neuromuscular scoliosis
- Flail chest
    - Absent ribs
    - Iatrogenic/trauma
        - Rib resection

Patients with pectus excavatum commonly have cardiac deviation to the left, and occasionally will have conduction abnormalities as a result of the distortion.[27] Exercise testing is more effective in diagnosing cardiopulmonary limitation,[27,29] which is still a rare complaint. However, when there is exertional limitation, it is typically due to cardiac limitation as opposed to pulmonary limitation.[30–32] Pectus excavatum is usually sporadic[27] but is associated with connective tissue defects, such as Marfan syndrome, Ehlers-Danlos syndrome, and osteogenesis imperfecta,[33] and progressive neuromuscular defects, such as spinal muscular atrophy. While pectus excavatum can present early in life, it commonly gets worse through adolescence.[34]

Computed tomography (CT) scans of the chest can be very helpful in clearly defining the defect and the severity. Haller et al[35] developed criteria for evaluating the severity of pectus excavatum via chest CT scan using the ratio of the lateral chest diameter to the sternum-spine distance, or the pectus severity (Haller) index (PSI) (Figure 15-6). In pectus excavatum, a PSI of 2.5 or less is considered normal, and the higher the PSI, the worse the defect. Patients with an index ratio of 3.25 or higher are likely to undergo corrective surgery.[36] Computed tomography scanning has also been used to define the amount of cardiac distortion from the pectus defect.[37] If there is cardiac distortion, then it is important for the patient to get an echocardiogram and a thorough cardiac evaluation.

Pectus carinatum is less common, with a North American incidence of 1 in 1,500.[38] Pulmonary, cardiac, or exercise limitation is extremely rare, and physical appearance is by far the most common concern.[39] As with pectus excavatum, there are also a number of associated disorders such as Marfan syndrome, Noonan syndrome, and osteogenesis imperfecta that can be present with pectus carinatum.[40] Chest CT scanning is also useful in defining the defect and, opposite of pectus excavatum, the lower the pectus severity index (<2.0), the more severe the disease,[41] since the defect is one of protrusion instead of invagination.

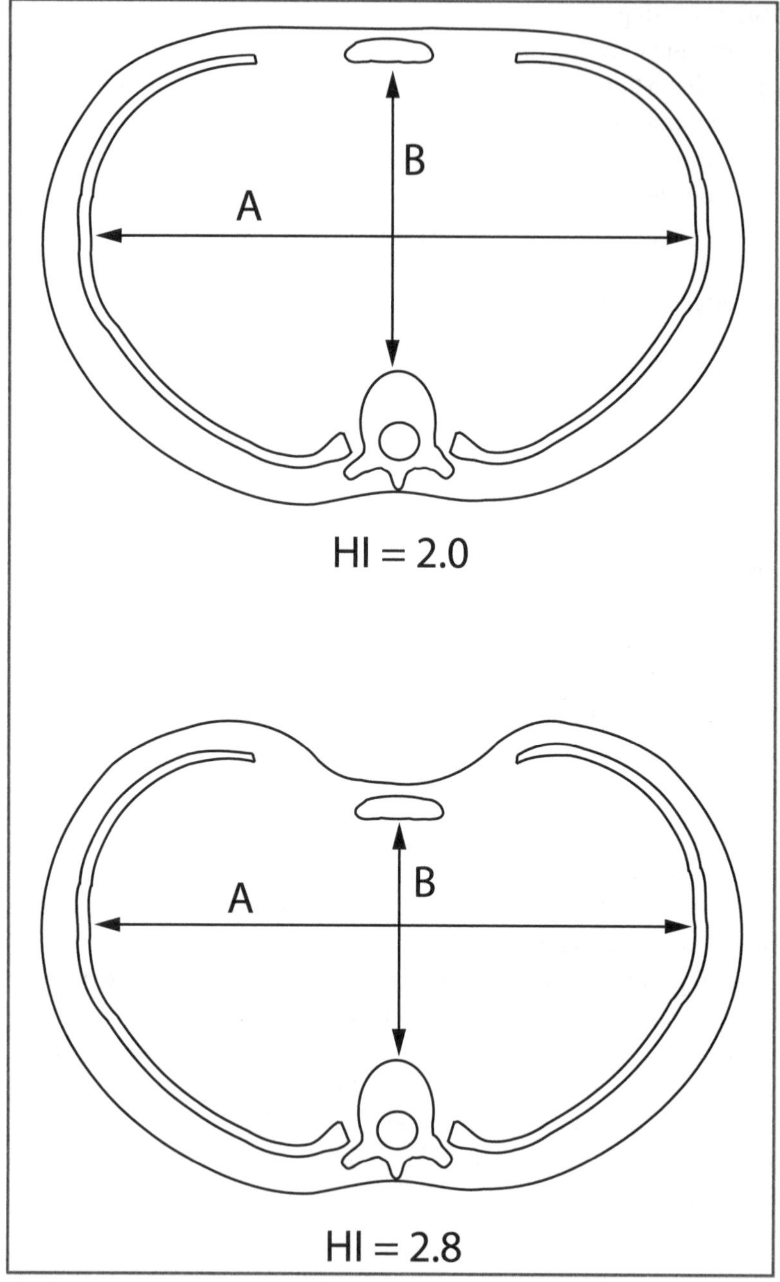

Figure 15-6. Haller index (HI) for grading pectus excavatum. The index is the ratio of the transverse rib-to-rib diameter **(A)** to the distance between the spine and sternum **(B)**.

Medical Management

Chest bracing is not used for patients with pectus excavatum, but physical therapy has been used in conjunction with surgery for patients with significant postural abnormalities.[42,43] Part of the challenge in using nonsurgical repair is that the defect is an invagination as opposed to a protuberance, as with pectus carinatum. Alternately, pectus carinatum can respond well to bracing, and may prevent the need for surgery.[44,45]

Surgical Management

The impact of pectus excavatum on lung function is variable, as is the improvement in lung function after surgical correction. There are 2 main surgical procedures that are used for correcting pectus excavatum: the modified Ravitch procedure and the Nuss procedure.

In the modified Ravitch procedure a number of cartilage segments are resected, leaving the perichondrium in place.[27] A sternal support, usually a metallic strut, is placed between the anterior edges of the rib cage and through the sternum, with the sternum repositioned normally. After 2 to 3 years the strut is removed. In the past, aggressive and extensive cartilage resection and sternal remodeling were performed. This practice has since been severely modified due to cases of severe asphyxiating thoracic dystrophy, believed to be due to the disruption of sternal and cartilage growth, thereby limiting future chest wall growth.[45] However, recent modifications to the technique to perform a limited cartilage resection and recommendations to perform the procedure in children no younger than 8 years have largely eliminated this concern.

The Nuss procedure, or minimally invasive pectus excavatum repair, uses a titanium rod that is bent to the corrected contour of the chest wall. It is inserted into the pleural space through a small axillary thoracotomy, passed through the retrosternal space anterior to the heart, and through the contralateral chest at the same level of the entry point. It is then rotated anteriorly to press the sternum outward at the level of the maximal invagination and sutured in place on the outside of the chest wall[46] (Figure 15-7A–D). The rod is kept in place as a brace until the sternum has remolded and usually is removed after 2 years, usually with a permanent repair.

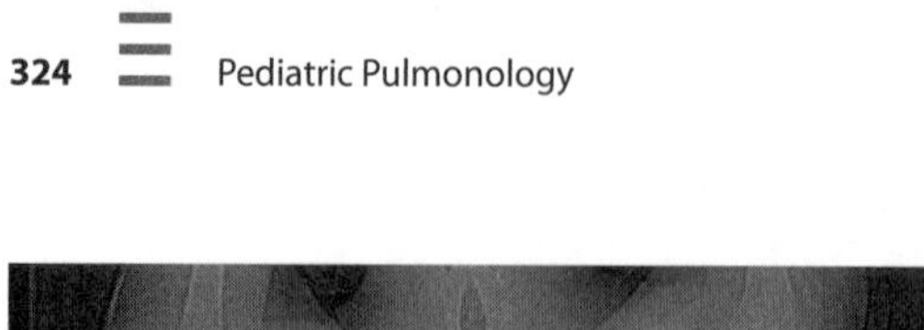

A

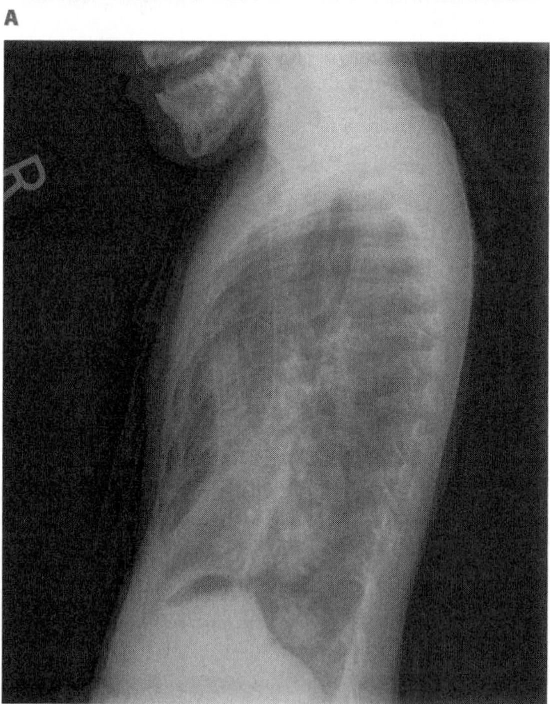

B

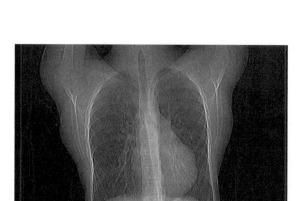

Figure 15-7. Pectus excavatum repair by the Nuss procedure with **(A)** anteroposterior (AP) and **(B)** lateral chest radiographs pre-insertion, and post-insertion **(C)** AP and **(D)** lateral radiographs.

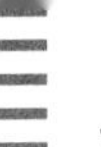

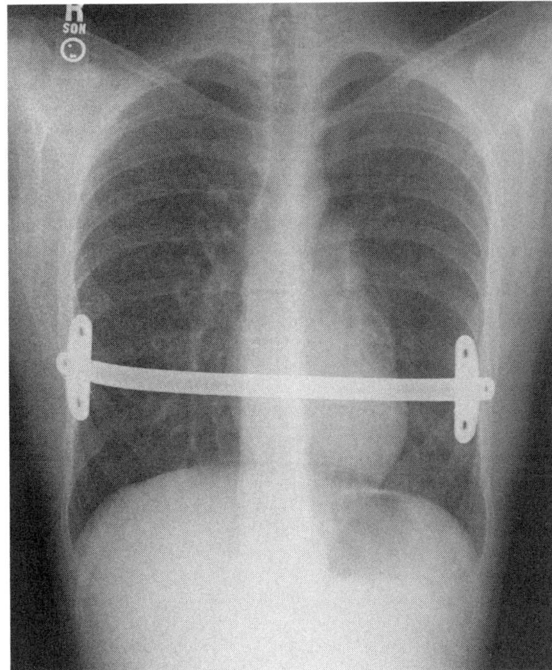

C

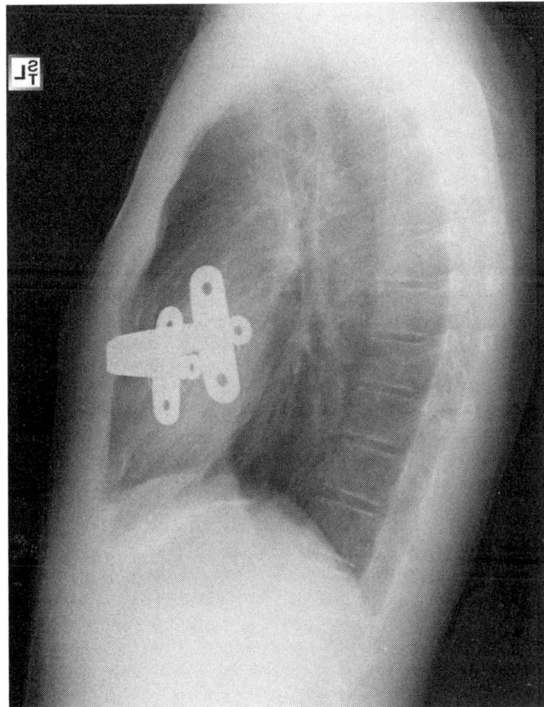

D

While there are some centers with data demonstrating a modest increase in lung function after pectus repair, the results are quite variable.[29–32,41,46]

Scoliosis

Clinical Features

Scoliosis can decrease chest wall compliance and lung compliance in the concave chest, thereby worsening respiratory mechanics. As scoliosis progresses, the convex chest can become hyperexpanded due to the lateral rotation of the chest and stretching of the intercostal muscles (Figure 15-8), further limiting chest wall excursion and worsening chest wall compliance.

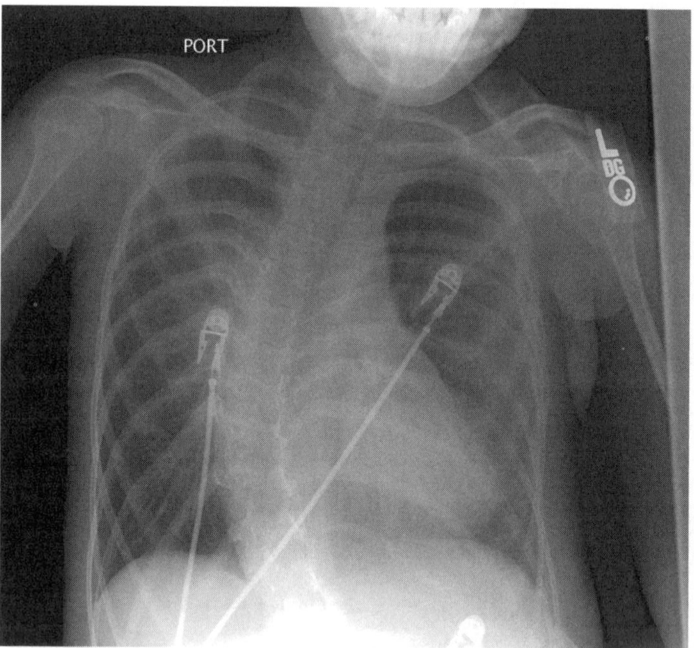

Figure 15-8. Scoliosis: The compression of the lung and chest wall on the concave side of the chest and the hyper-expansion of the chest on the convex side in a teenager with spinal muscular atrophy type 2.

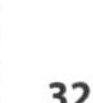

More complex scoliosis with significant transverse chest wall rotation (Figure 15-9A–D) can significantly distort the chest wall in the transverse plane. In doing so the diaphragm can rotate radially and flatten and increase the radius of curvature; however, the clinical significance of this has not been demonstrated. Bronchial compression can also occur due to compression by the rotated anterior edge of the vertebral body.[47]

The cause of scoliosis can be described in 1 of 3 ways based on the cause and outcome: (1) spinal instability or abnormality with asymmetrical growth; (2) rib cage deformity with either absence of ribs, rib fusion, or general lateral instability from muscle weakness; or (3) idiopathic, in which there is no clear cause.

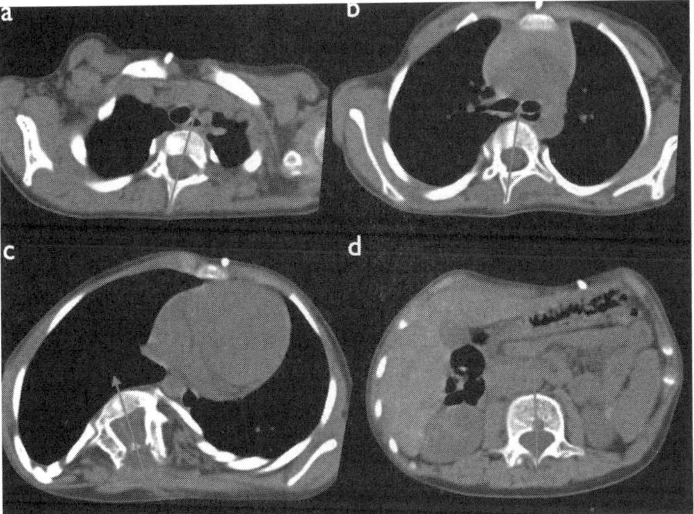

Figure 15-9. Rotation of the spine and diaphragm in complicated scoliosis with transverse images from the **(A)** apex of the lung, **(B)** the carina, **(C)** the lower thorax, and **(D)** at the lower edge of the liver.

In children with hemivertebrae or asymmetrical vertebra, such as wedge or bar vertebra, scoliosis will serve as a nidus for the curve because spinal integrity is disrupted at that point (Figure 15-10). A bar vertebra or unilateral fusion provides a tethering point around which vertical spinal growth is asymmetrical and produces scoliosis (Figure 15-10). In children with absent ribs, lateral chest wall support will be deficient and the lateral chest wall will collapse, creating an ipsilateral scoliosis (Figure 15-11A). Rib fusion that causes a tethering point around which the spine will grow asymmetrically can cause scoliosis (Figure 15-11B). In children with neuromuscular disease, the

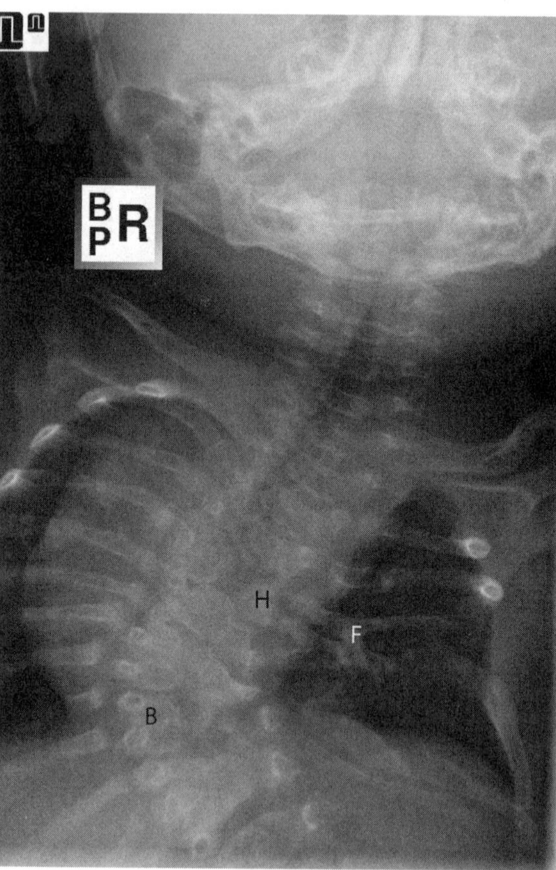

Figure 15-10. Chest radiograph demonstrating scoliosis due to an underlying spinal disorder with hemivertebrae **(H)**, bar vertebra **(B)**, and rib fusion **(F)**.

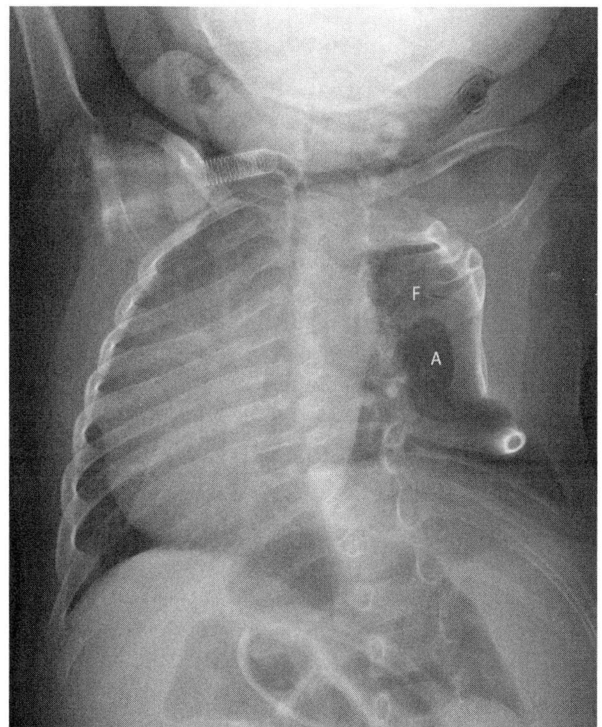

A

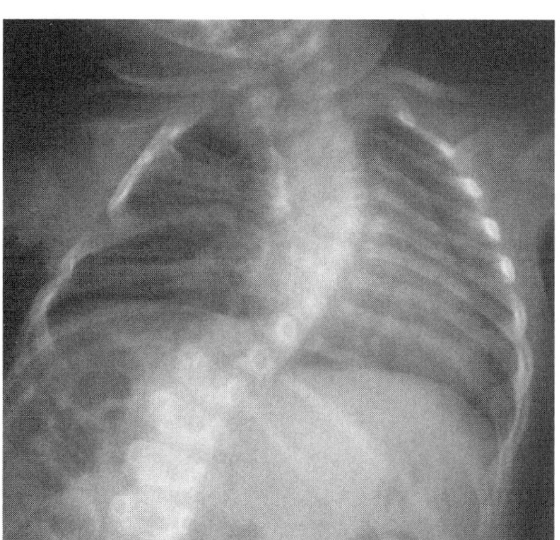
B

Figure 15-11. Scoliosis due to eg, **(A)** rib fusion (F in radiograph) and rib absence (A in radiograph) **(B)** rib fusion. (Courtesy of Dr Robert Campbell.)

biomechanics of the thorax are abnormal, often with weak rib-to-rib support and eventual unilateral or bilateral collapse, with severe caudal rotation of the ribs in the convex chest, as is often seen in spinal muscular atrophy type 1 (Figure 15-12). Finally, idiopathic scoliosis can occur in children with no clear underlying musculoskeletal abnormality. Often the scoliosis is asymptomatic and noticed incidentally as part of a well visit or on a chest radiograph.

Medical Management

Before recommending surgery, bracing can be used to align the spine in a more favorable midline position, or as close to it as possible. While in many situations, bracing is seen as a temporizing procedure and not a cure,[48] it can be successful in preventing scoliosis curve progression in skeletally immature patients with curves of less than 40 degrees,[48,49] and in occasional situations may obviate the need for surgery.[48]

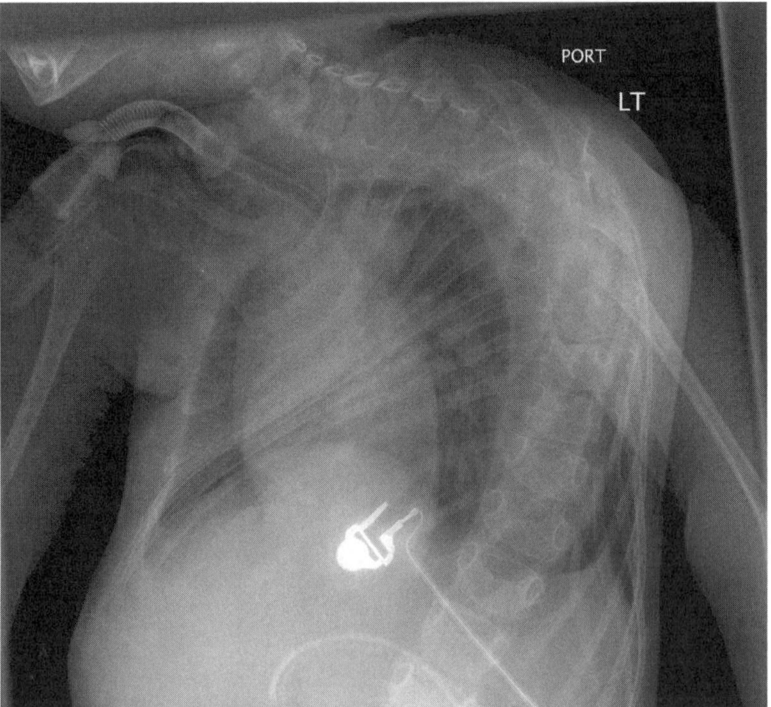

Figure 15-12. Neuromuscular scoliosis due to spinal muscular atrophy type 1 with caudal rotation of the ribs in the right chest.

Surgical Management

The decision to treat scoliosis is made on the basis of clinical symptoms, severity of scoliosis, and the rapidity of progression, with 50 degrees of curve being the point at which surgical intervention is often considered.[48] The definitive surgical treatment is spinal fusion rods along each edge of the spine using metal suture material to connect to the spinal lamina (Figure 15-13A–B), pedicle screws placed into the vertebral bodies, or laminar hooks over the spinal lamina. Though this provides mechanical stability, it prevents further spine growth within the fused region, and limits FVC commensurate with both length of fusion and height of the superior fusion point.[50] This clearly limits the utility of the procedure in younger children. In these children growth can be maintained with nonsurgical interventions, such as bracing the abdomen and part of the thorax intermittently to keep the spine aligned properly.

The longitudinal pulmonary outcome of scoliosis surgery is chiefly determined by the preoperative FVC and, to a lesser extent, by the surgical approach, with the posterior approach without thoracotomy being more favorable than the anterior approach via thoracotomy.[20] There are a number of potential complicating factors. There is the potential for a secondary lordosis, "crank-shaft abnormality," with posterior-only spinal fusion due to continued anterior spinal growth and arrested posterior spine growth. The alternative of a thoracotomy and anterior fusion has been associated with a decrease in lung function.[37]

It is hard to make a definitive statement on the utility of spinal fusion in correcting lung function, since lung function is not the only outcome measure. With that, however, there is little expectation of significant improvement in vital capacity as a percent of predicted after scoliosis surgery, since the act of fusion limits further spine growth and worsening of scoliosis at the expense of lung growth, and in some situations loss of lung function.[37,51] Therefore, the decision to perform spinal fusion is a balance between supporting growth and minimizing the further loss of lung function.

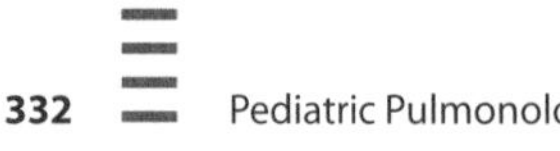

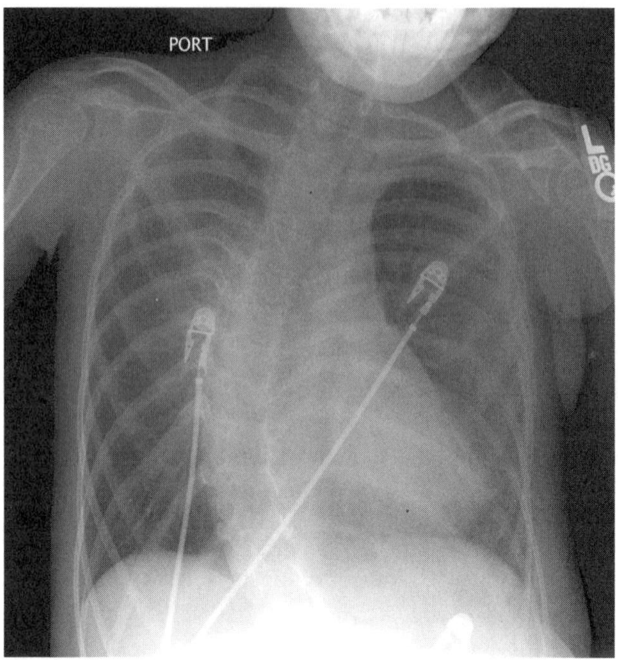

A

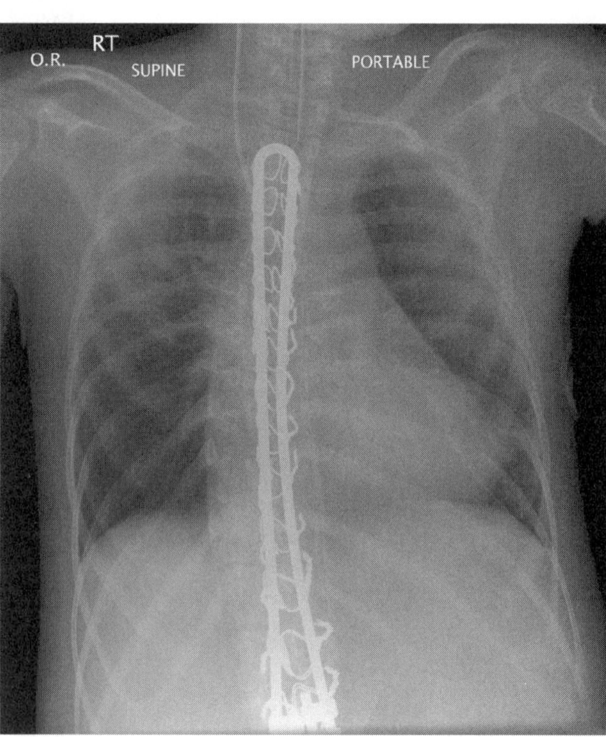

B

Figure 15-13. A child with spinal muscular atrophy type 2 **(A)** before and **(B)** after spinal fusion.

A separate approach is to use growing rods (Figure 15-14A–B) along the spine to support the spine, as is done with spinal fusion, but with serial lengthening of the rods commensurate with expected spine growth.[52] While spine growth can be kept in the normal range,[52] the impact on future lung function is not yet known. These rods must be transitioned to a static rod to fuse the spine after growth is complete. The definitive spinal fusion may be more challenging in this approach due to residual perispinal scarring from the growing rods.

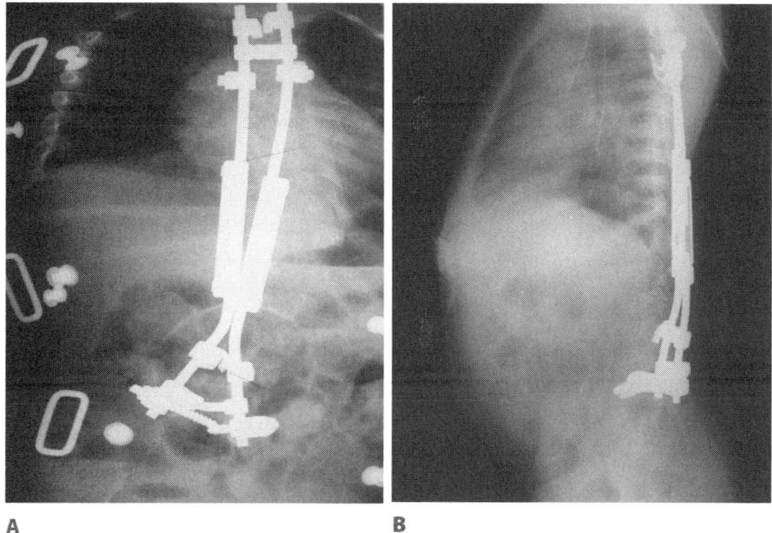

Figure 15-14. Growing rods in a child with scoliosis in the **(A)** anteroposterior and **(B)** lateral projections. (Courtesy of Dr Robert Campbell.)

Thoracic Insufficiency Syndrome

Clinical Features

Thoracic insufficiency syndrome encompasses a wide range of complex thoracospinal disorders in which the chest wall and spine cannot support normal respiration and lung growth.[14] Thoracic insufficiency syndrome is different from idiopathic scoliosis in that patents with TIS typically have a more rapid loss of lung function that can cause severe pulmonary morbidity or respiratory failure if untreated. While TIS represents a number of disparate conditions, there are 3 phenotypic categories of TIS: congenital constricted chest wall syndrome, progressive spinal deformity, and flail chest.[53]

Congenital constricted chest wall syndrome has 2 subtypes: progressive congenital thoracic scoliosis and hypoplastic thorax syndromes.[14,53] Progressive congenital thoracic scoliosis can result from abnormal rib segmentation, or rib fusion (Figure 15-11B), with or without a skeletal abnormality.[14,53] In congenital cases clinical symptoms can occur quite early and may be severe. Primary rib defects, such as rib fusion, can also occur.

Hypoplastic thorax disorders can occur due to defects in cartilage (achondroplasia, campomelic dysplasia), costal growth abnormalities (Ellis-van Creveld, Jeune [Figure 15-15]), or spinal growth abnormalities (Jarcho-Levin [Figure 15-16]).[14,53] Similarly, the thorax can be hypoplastic with osteogenesis imperfecta type 2 and with hypophosphatemia due to undermineralized bone causing easy fracture, disrupted healing, and poor thoracic growth. Over time the chest does not grow with the rest of the body and the increasing metabolic need.

Progressive spinal deformity is progressive scoliosis due to neuromuscular disease (Figure 15-12) or a primary vertebral abnormality, such as bar vertebra, segmental fusion, hemivertebrae, or wedge vertebra[14,53] (Figure 15-10), without rib abnormalities. In congenital cases clinical symptoms can occur quite early and may be severe.

Flail chest can occur due to a congenital defect with absent ribs (Figure 15-11A) and may also be associated with a variety of different spinal defects. It can also occur as a result of chest wall surgery to remove a portion of the chest wall or as a result of trauma.

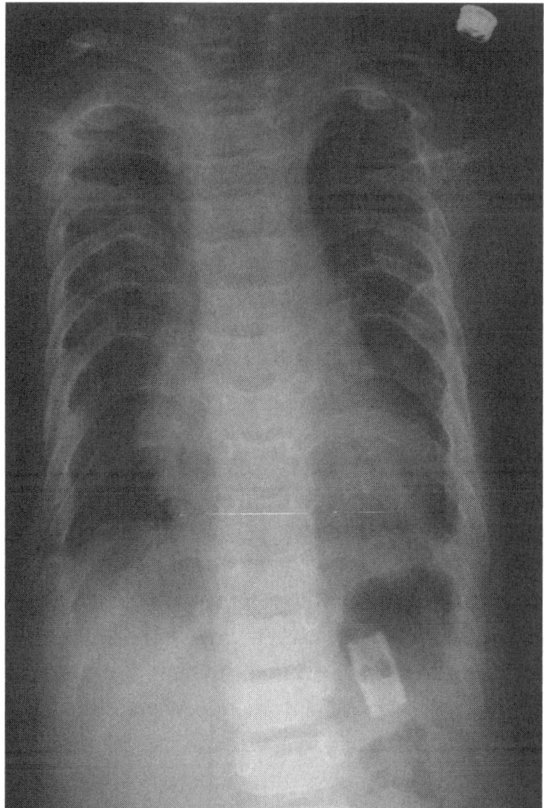

Figure 15-15. Hypoplastic thorax in Jeune syndrome. (Courtesy of Dr Robert Campbell.)

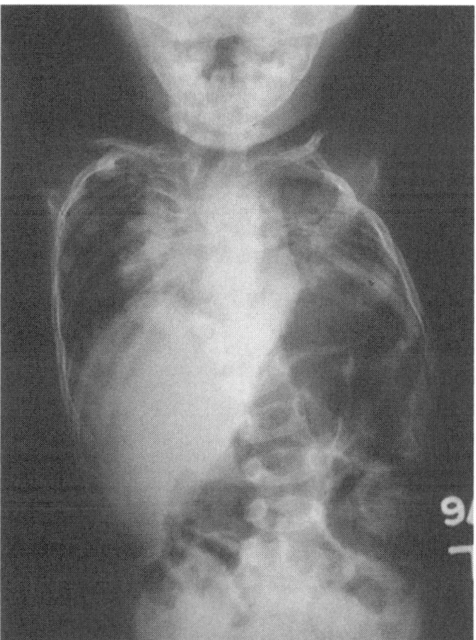

Figure 15-16. Jarcho-Levin syndrome. (Courtesy of Dr Robert Campbell.)

Medical Management

While there is no medical therapy that can effectively treat TIS, nutritional support and noninvasive or invasive ventilation can be critical in helping a patient grow to the point in which surgery would be most feasible. With the chest wall expansion and spinal straightening, as described below, proper soft tissue mass is needed to close the newly expanded chest wall and to cover the vertical expandable prosthetic titanium rib (VEPTR).[53] If this is not done, there can be a higher risk for complications, such as skin and soft tissue breakdown at the site of the repair.

Surgical Management

Thoracic insufficiency syndrome poses surgical challenges that go well beyond stabilizing the spine, and with the early age that many patients with TIS present, fusion is not a viable option. The combination of early onset of thoracospinal disease with TIS spurred the development of the VEPTR. This model provides spinal support and is expandable to allow normal longitudinal growth, as with the growing rod model. However, the VEPTR has the additional advantage of lateral support in a variety of different ways based on the placement of the devices[14] (Figure 15-17A–B). It can also be used to correct rotational scoliosis and a variety of types of complicated thoracospinal disorders,[53] such as flail chest; scoliosis with fused ribs or with absent ribs; and scoliosis with major vertebral abnormalities that destabilize the spine, such as bar vertebra, hemivertebrae, or wedge vertebra. The expansions are typically done every 6 to 8 months during a day-surgery procedure to maintain a normal spinal growth velocity while providing spinal and thoracic stability.[52]

Because TIS is a constellation of heterogeneous conditions, which have similar morbidity, optimal timing for correction is based on a combination of the severity of the underlying thoracospinal defect and the associated respiratory morbidity. Thus the ideal insertion time of the VEPTR is variable and individualized to the patient. While there is clearly a benefit in surgically treating TIS early to minimize progression, there are no data that give a clear link between age of surgery and long-term prognosis.

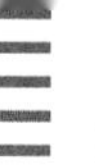

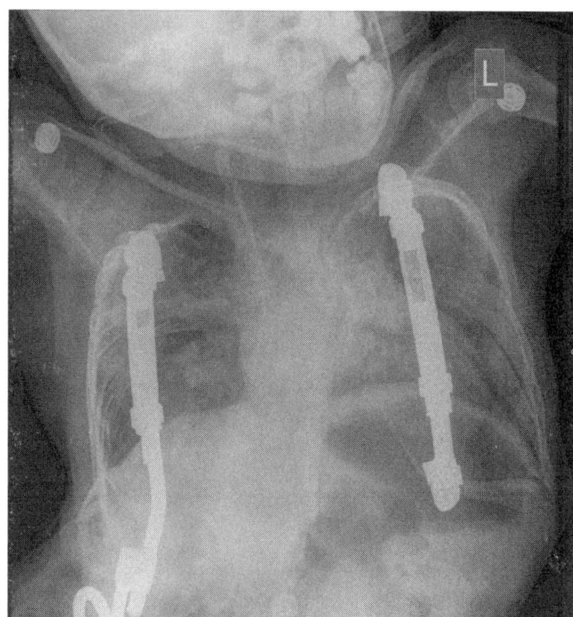

A

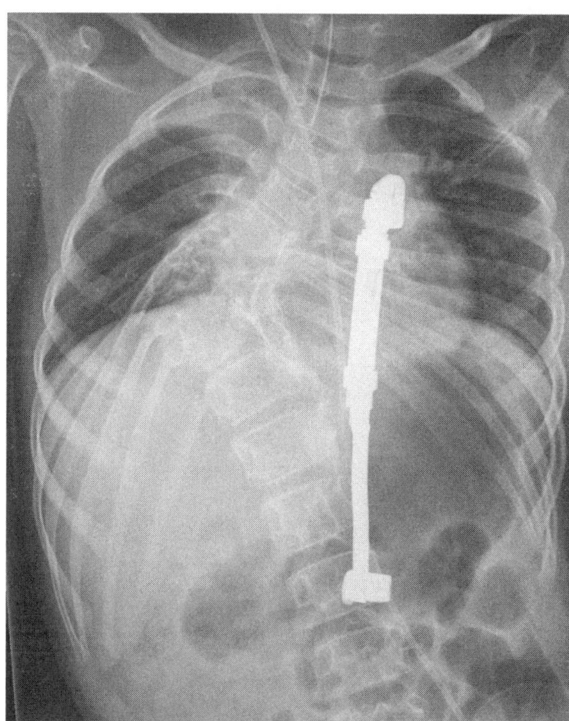

B

Figure 15-17. Vertical expandable prosthetic titanium rib placement in the **(A)** rib to rib (right) and rib to iliac crest (left) and **(B)** rib to spine orientations. (Courtesy of Dr Robert Campbell.)

The VEPTR can be used in patients with a hypoplastic chest, such as with Jarcho-Levin syndrome and Jeune syndrome. With Jarcho-Levin syndrome, the VEPTR supports the spine and places a longitudinal traction force to encourage growth (Figure 15-18A–B). In Jeune syndrome, the VEPTR provides a lateral tethering point for the rib cage to expand after a series of rib osteotomies and outward traction leaving the periosteum in place (Figure 15-19A–B). There is also an alternative approach, lateral thoracic expansion technique, in which there are a series of staggered rib osteotomies with fusion of the alternating longer lengths of rib to expand the chest wall circumference[54] (Figure 15-20). Unlike the VEPTR, in which the device is lengthened about every 6 months, the lateral thoracic expansion technique is a single procedure that is not repeated.

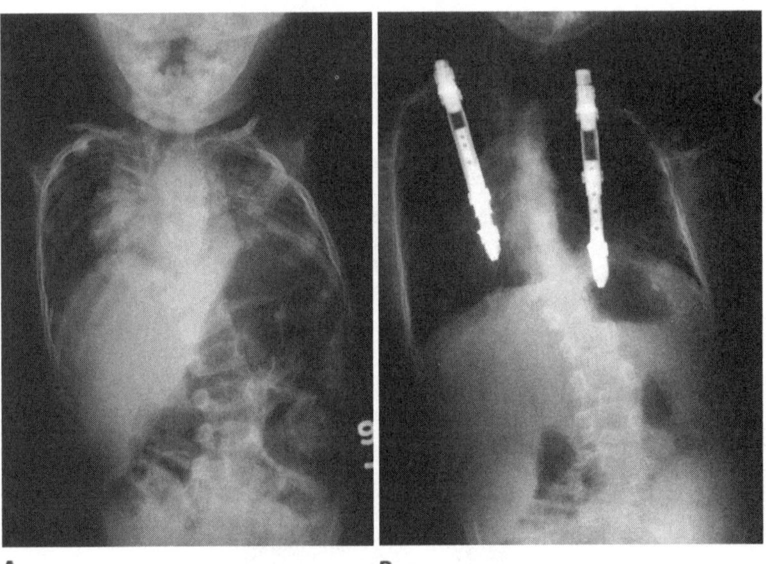

Figure 15-18. Jarcho-Levin syndrome **(A)** before and **(B)** after repair with the vertical expandable prosthetic titanium rib.

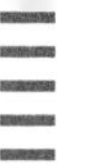

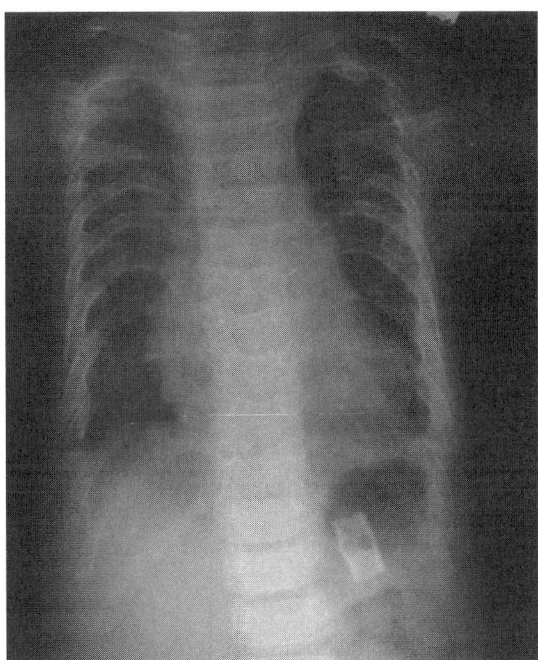

A

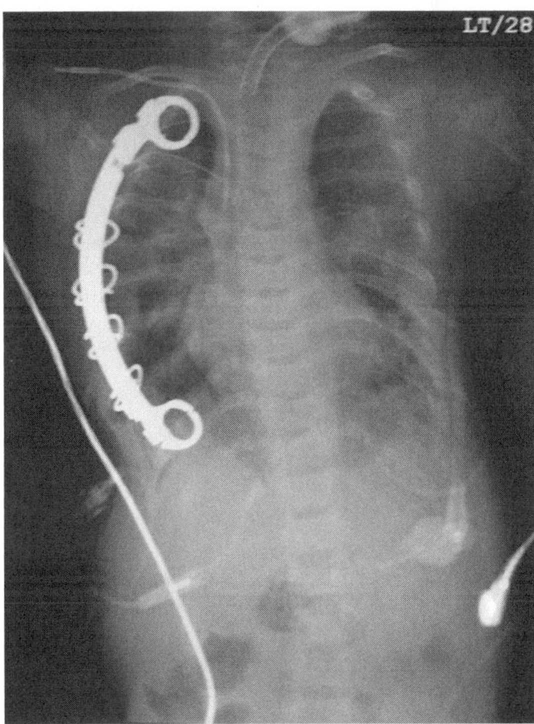

B

Figure 15-19. Jeune syndrome **(A)** before and **(B)** after vertical expandable prosthetic titanium rib insertion. (Courtesy of Dr Robert Campbell.)

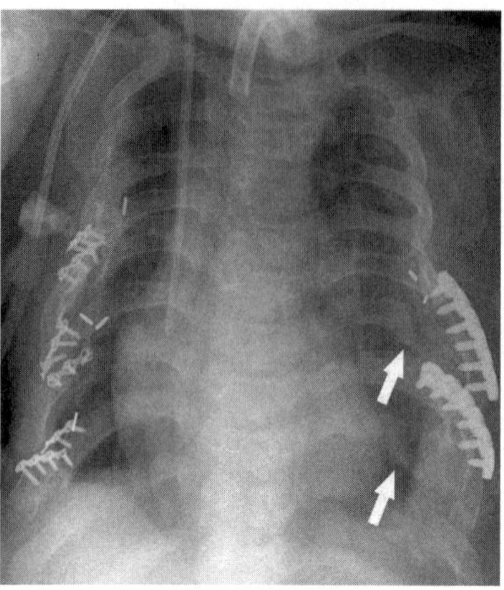

Figure 15-20. Jeune syndrome repair by the lateral thoracic expansion technique, with white arrows pointing to the free rib segments with growth of new bone.

Muscular Abnormalities

A list of muscular abnormalities is found in Box 15-2. Diaphragm weakness is common in Duchenne muscular dystrophy, and chest wall weakness and abnormal mechanics are prominent in both spinal muscular atrophy and Duchenne muscular dystrophy, and can be seen in the congenital muscular dystrophies, and can lead to significant thoracospinal disease. These conditions will be discussed in Chapter 45.

Gastroschisis and Omphalocele

Gastroschisis and omphalocele cause lateral and midline defects, respectively, in the abdominal musculature, and after successful closure the abdomen is devoid of muscle and highly compliant. Prune

Box 15-2. Muscular Defects

- Congenital diaphragmatic hernia
- Abdominal wall defects
- Gastroschisis
- Omphalocele
- Prune-belly syndrome (Eagle-Barrett syndrome)

belly syndrome or Eagle-Barrett syndrome has a similar outcome, but is associated with urinary tract obstruction and massive dilation of the urinary tract and abdomen, affecting mesenchymal development and abdominal muscle structure. These defects can affect respiration in 2 ways. First, the high abdominal compliance means that caudal diaphragm movement during inspiration will displace the abdominal contents outward more, with less resistance from the abdominal wall. As a result there will be a smaller increase in intra-abdominal pressure and less outward excursion of the lower rib cage. Second, the paucity of abdominal muscle limits forceful exhalation and reduces cough effectiveness.

Congenital Diaphragmatic Hernia

Congenital diaphragmatic hernia (CDH) occurs when the pleuroperitoneal canal fails to close during early fetal development. The primary morbidity from CDH is related to pulmonary hypoplasia or other organ system defects.[55–57] Diaphragm function and muscle strength, based on maximal inspiratory pressures,[58] is directly related to the size of the diaphragm defect and synthetic patch needed for the repair. However, in a cohort of 25 patients with CDH, diaphragm function was adequate for unsupported respiration, even considering the associated pulmonary hypoplasia and airway disease.[58]

Abdominal wall defects and CDHs are repaired surgically; however, the chronic respiratory failure and pulmonary hypertension that are often seen coincidently can require substantial medical therapy, both before and after definitive surgical repair.

Key Points

- Normal respiration involves coordination between diaphragm contraction and abdominal and chest wall motion. Chest wall abnormalities can significantly compromise respiratory system function by interfering with these functions.
- The central tenet of treating thoracospinal defects is to prevent the progression, stabilize the chest and spine, and support normal growth. While the likelihood for a significant improvement in lung function remains low, it is possible to prevent or minimize further decline in lung function.

References

1. de Troyer A, Loring S. Action of the respiratory muscles. Section 3: the respiratory system. In: Maklem PT, Mead J, eds. *Mechanics of Breathing.* Bethesda, MD: American Physiological Society; 1986:443–461. *Handbook of Physiology;* vol 3
2. Davis GM, Coates AL, Papageorgiou A, Bureau MA. Direct measurement of static chest wall compliance in animal and human neonates. *J Appl Physiol.* 1988;65(3):1093–1098
3. Gerhardt T, Bancalari E. Chest wall compliance in full-term and premature infants. *Acta Paediatr Scand.* 1980;69(3):359–364
4. Reynolds RN, Etsten BE. Mechanics of respiration in apneic anesthetized infants. *Anesthesiology.* 1966;27(1):13–19
5. Richard CC, Bachman L. Lung and chest wall compliance in apneic paralyzed infants. *J Clin Ivest.* 1961;40:273–278
6. Papastamelos C, Panitch HB, England SE, Allen JL. Developmental changes in chest wall compliance in infancy and early childhood. *J Appl Physiol.* 1995;78(1):179–184
7. Openshaw P, Edwards S, Helms P. Changes in rib cage geometry during childhood. *Thorax.* 1984;39(8):624–627
8. Gerhardt T, Hehre D, Feller R, Reifenberg L, Bancalari E. Pulmonary mechanics in normal infants and young children during first 5 years of life. *Pediatr Pulmonol.* 1987;3(5):309–316
9. Davidson MB. The relationship between diaphragm and body weight in the rat. *Growth.* 1968;32(3):221–223
10. Mittman C, Edelman N, Norris A, Shock N. Relationship between chest wall and pulmonary compliance and age. *J Appl Physiol.* 1965;20(6):1211–1216

11. England S. Laryngeal function. In: Chernick V, Mellins RB, ed. *Basic Mechanisms of Pediatric Respiratory Disease: Cellular and Integrative.* Philadelphia, PA: BC Decker; 1991
12. Kosch P, Hutchison A, Wozniak J, Carlo W, Stark A. Posterior cricoarytenoid and diaphragm activities during tidal breathing in neonates. *J Appl Physiol.* 1988;64(5):1968–1978
13. Hershenson M, Colin A, Wohl M, Stark A. Changes in the contribution of the ribcage to tidal breathing during infancy. *Am Rev Respir Dis.* 1990;141:922–925
14. Campbell RM Jr, Smith MD, Mayes TC, et al. The characteristics of thoracic insufficiency syndrome associated with fused ribs and congenital scoliosis. *J Bone Joint Surg Am.* 2003;85-A(3):399–408
15. Delelis D, Basse-Cathalinat B, Arnaud D, Lavignolle B. Xenon 133 pulmonary scintigraphy. Its significance in the preoperative evaluation of pulmonary function in adolescents with kyphoscoliosis prior to vertebral arthrodesis [in French]. *Anesth Analg (Paris).* 1977;34(5):929–942
16. Grau M, Leisner B, Rohloff R, Fink U, Moser E, Matzen KA, Hausinger K. Functional scintigraphy of pulmonary ventilation with 133Xe in juvenile scoliosis (author's transl) [in German]. *Nuklearmedizin.* 1981;20(4):178–182
17. Allen JL, Greenspan JS, Deoras KS, Keklikian E, Wolfson MR, Shaffer T. Interactions between chest wall motion and lung mechanics in normal infants and infants with bronchopulmonary dysplasia. *Pediatr Pulmonol.* 1991;11:37–43
18. Allen JL, Wolfson MR, McDowell K, Shaffer T. Thoracoabdominal asynchrony in infants with airflow obstruction. *Am Rev Respir Dis.* 1990;141:337–342
19. Mayer O, Clayton R, McDonough J, Allen J. Respiratory inductance plethysmography (RIP) to assess respiratory function in healthy three to five year old children. *Am J Respir Crit Care Med.* 2001;163:A372
20. Newton PO, Perry A, Bastrom TP, et al. Predictors of change in postoperative pulmonary function in adolescent idiopathic scoliosis: a prospective study of 254 patients. *Spine.* 2007;32(17):1875–1882
21. Mayer OH, Redding G. Early changes in pulmonary function after vertical expandable prosthetic titanium rib insertion in children with thoracic insufficiency syndrome. *J Pediatr Orthop.* 2009;29(1):35–38
22. Pearson VV. *Genetics.* Gunn VL, Nechyba C, eds. Philadelphia, PA: Mosby; 2002
23. Turan S, Bereket A, Omar A, Berber M, Ozen A, Bekiroglu N. Upper segment/lower segment ratio and armspan-height difference in healthy Turkish children. *Acta Paediatr.* 2005;94(4):407–413
24. Laghi F, Tobin MJ. Disorders of the respiratory muscles. *Am J Respir Crit Care Med.* 2003;168(1):10–48

25. Estenne M, Derom E, de Troyer A. Neck and abdominal muscle activity in patients with severe thoracic scoliosis. *Am J Respir Crit Care Med.* 1998;158(2):452–457
26. Fokin AA, Steuerwald NM, Ahrens WA, Allen KE. Anatomical, histologic, and genetic characteristics of congenital chest wall deformities. *Semin Thorac Cardiovasc Surg.* 2009;21:44–57
27. Fonkalsrud EW. 912 open pectus excavatum repairs: changing trends, lessons learned: one surgeon's experience. *World J Surg.* 2009;33:180–190
28. Bay V, Farthmann E, Naegele U. Unoperated funnel chest in middle and advanced age: evaluation of indications for operation. *J Pediatr Surg.* 1970;5:606–609
29. Malek MH, Berger DE, Marelich WD, Coburn JW, Beck TW, Housh TJ. Pulmonary function following surgical repair of pectus excavatum: a meta-analysis. *Eur J Cardiothorac Surg.* 2006;30:637–643
30. Malek MH, Fonkalsrud EW, Cooper CB. Ventilatory and cardiovascular responses to exercise in patients with pectus excavatum. *Chest.* 2003;124:870–882
31. Quigley PM, Haller JA Jr, Jelus KL, Loughlin GM, Marcus CL. Cardiorespiratory function before and after corrective surgery in pectus excavatum. *J Pediatr.* 1996;128(5 pt 1):638–643
32. Borowitz D, Cerny F, Zallen G, et al. Pulmonary function and exercise response in patients with pectus excavatum after Nuss repair. *J Pediatr Surg.* 2003;38(4):544–547
33. Williams AW, Crabbe DC. Pectus deformities of the anterior chest wall. *Paediatr Respir Rev.* 2003;4:237–242
34. Nuss D, Kelly RE. Minimally invasive surgical correction of chest wall deformities in children (Nuss procedure). *Adv Pediatr.* 2008;55:395–410
35. Haller JA Jr, Kramer SS, Lietman SA. Use of CT scans in selection of patients for pectus excavatum surgery: a preliminary report. *J Pediatr Surg.* 1987;22(10):904–906
36. Nakagawa Y, Uemura S, Nakaoka T, Yano T, Tanaka N. Evaluation of the Nuss procedure using pre- and postoperative computed tomographic index. *J Pediatr Surg.* 2008;43(3):518–521
37. Kim HC, Park HJ, Ham SY, et al. Development of automatized new indices for radiological assessment of chest-wall deformity and its quantitative evaluation. *Med Biol Eng Comput.* 2008;46:815–823
38. Shamberger RC. Congenital chest wall deformities. In: O'Neill J, Rowe MI, Grosfeld JL, et al, eds. *Pediatric Surgery.* 5th ed. Mosby; 1998:787
39. Robicsek F. Surgical treatment of pectus carinatum. *Chest Surg Clin N Am.* 2000;10:357
40. Kotzot D, Schwabegger AH. Etiology of chest wall deformities—a genetic review for the treating physician. *J Pediatr Surg.* 2009;44:2004–2011
41. Fonkalsrud EW. Surgical correction of pectus carinatum: lessons learned from 260 patients. *J Pediatr Surg.* 2008;43:1235–1243

42. Schoenmakers MA, Gulmans VA, Bax NM, Helders PJ. Physiotherapy as an adjuvant to the surgical treatment of anterior chest wall deformities: a necessity? A prospective descriptive study in 21 patients. *J Pediatr Surg.* 2000;35:1440–1443
43. Egan JC, DuBois JJ, Morphy M, Samples TL, Lindell B. Compressive orthotics in the treatment of asymmetric pectus carinatum: a preliminary report with an objective radiographic marker. *J Pediatr Surg.* 2000;35:1183–1186
44. Frey AS, Garcia VF, Brown RL, et al. Nonoperative management of pectus carinatum. *J Pediatr Surg.* 2006;41:40–45; discussion 40–45
45. Haller JA, Colombani PM, Humphries CT, Azizkhan RG, Loughlin GM. Chest wall constriction after too extensive and too early operations for pectus excavatum. *Ann Thorac Surg.* 1996;61:1618–1624; discussion 1625
46. Nuss D, Kelly RE Jr, Croitoru DP, Katz ME. A 10-year review of a minimally invasive technique for the correction of pectus excavatum. *J Pediatr Surg.* 1998;33(4):545–552
47. Colin AA, Allen JL, Berde CB, Griscom NT, Hall JE, Young LW. Radiological case of the month. Bronchial compression and ventilatory dysfunction in scoliosis. *Am J Dis Child.* 1988;142(5):545–546
48. Shaughnessy WJ. Advances in scoliosis brace treatment for adolescent idiopathic scoliosis. *Orthop Clin North Am.* 2007;38(4):469–475, v
49. Jarvis J, Garbedian S, Swamy G. Juvenile idiopathic scoliosis: the effectiveness of part-time bracing. *Spine.* 2008;33(10):1074–1078
50. Karol LA, Johnston C, Mladenov K, Schochet P, Walters P, Browne RH. Pulmonary function following early thoracic fusion in non-neuromuscular scoliosis. *J Bone Joint Surg Am.* 2008;90:1272–1281
51. Wong CA, Cole AA, Watson L, Webb JK, Johnston ID, Kinnear WJ. Pulmonary function before and after anterior spinal surgery in adult idiopathic scoliosis. *Thorax.* 1996;51:534–536
52. Thompson GH, Akbarnia BA, Campbell RM Jr. Growing rod techniques in early-onset scoliosis. *J Pediatr Orthop.* 2007;27(3):354–361
53. Campbell RM Jr, Smith MD. Thoracic insufficiency syndrome and exotic scoliosis. *J Bone Joint Surg Am.* 2007;89 (suppl 1):108–122
54. Davis JT, Long FR, Adler BH, Castile RG, Weinstein S. Lateral thoracic expansion for Jeune syndrome: evidence of rib healing and new bone formation. *Ann Thorac Surg.* 2004;77(2):445–448
55. Chatrath RR, el-Shafie M, Jones RS. Fate of hypoplastic lungs after repair of congenital diaphragmatic hernia. *Arch Dis Child.* 1971;46:633–635
56. Lally KP. Congenital diaphragmatic hernia. *Curr Opin Pediatr.* 2002;14(4):486–490
57. Rottier R, Tibboel D. Fetal lung and diaphragm development in congenital diaphragmatic hernia. *Semin Perinatol.* 2005;29(2):86–93
58. Panitch H, Hedrick H, Rintoul N, Weiner D. Pulmonary function in infants with congenital diaphragmatic hernia. *Proc Am Thoracic Soc.* 2005;2:A187

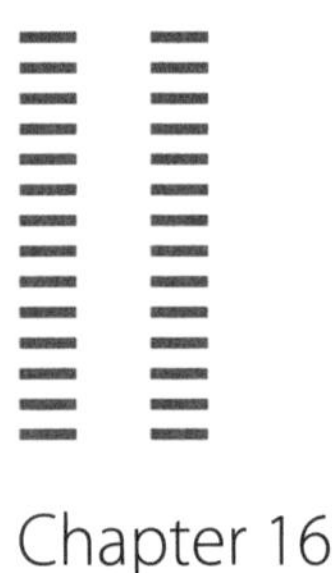

Chapter 16

Croup, Epiglottitis, and Bacterial Tracheitis

Girish D. Sharma, MD
Carol Conrad, MD

Croup

Case Report 16-1

A 2-year-old boy with history of mild upper respiratory symptoms for 2 days develops sudden onset of barky, croupy cough at 2:00 am. His voice is hoarse. When taken to the emergency department (ED), he develops intermittent inspiratory stridor when agitated. He is afebrile and tachycardic. His oxyhemoglobin saturation in room air is normal, and he has minimal retractions and no cyanosis. Lung auscultation reveals good and equal air exchange bilaterally, with coarse sounds but no wheeze or crackles. There is a history of similar complaints 2 months ago when he had similar symptoms and, as his parents prepared to take to him to the ED, there was sudden resolution of symptoms during the car trip. That time, he was observed for a short time in the ED before being discharged. A diagnosis of croup is suspected.

Introduction

Croup, or acute laryngotracheobronchitis, is an early childhood viral syndrome characterized by acute laryngeal and subglottic swelling resulting in the sudden onset of barky cough, inspiratory stridor, hoarse voice, and respiratory distress. Onset of these symptoms in a young child with acute worsening usually in the early hours of the morning and associated disruption of family routine may lead to significant anxiety in both child and caretaker.

Etiology

The cause of croup is primarily parainfluenza type 1.[1] Other viruses implicated in the etiology are parainfluenza types 2 and 3, influenza A and B, adenovirus, respiratory syncytial virus, rhinovirus, measles, human metapneumovirus, and coronavirus. Most patients presenting with mild symptoms and mild fever have acute laryngotracheitis. Presence of a high-grade fever, significant respiratory distress, and toxemia point to a bacterial cause, such as bacterial tracheitis or laryngotracheobronchitis.[2]

Pathophysiology

In mild cases there is noninflammatory edema in the subglottic region. In more severe cases (acute laryngotracheitis), there is inflammation and edema of the subglottic area and lateral wall of the trachea characterized by cellular infiltration with lymphocytes, neutrophils, histiocytes, and plasma cells. The inflammation and edema of the subglottic region results in narrowing and clinical presentation of barky, brassy cough; hoarse voice; stridor; and respiratory distress with retractions. Subglottic and upper tracheal narrowing is responsible for the typical "steeple sign" on radiograph (Figure 16-1). The fluctuation in the severity of symptoms, nocturnal worsening, and tendency of some children to develop severe and recurrent episodes of croup may be related to whether the child is agitated or calm,[3] low levels of endogenous cortisol,[4] and tendency of some children for having intrinsically narrower subglottic space,[5] respectively. Host factors, such as allergies, may play a role in recurrent croup.[6]

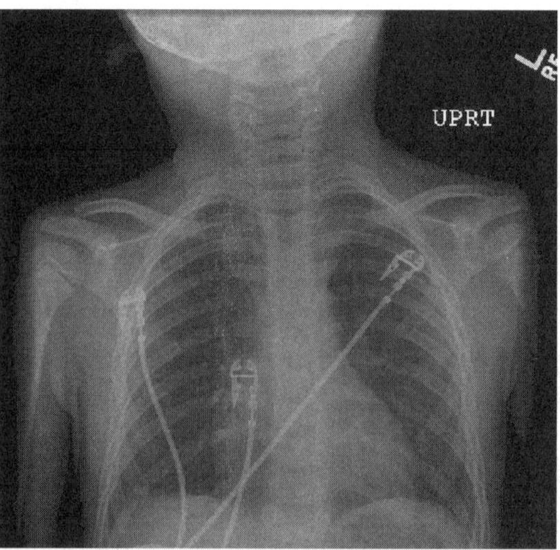

Figure 16-1. Radiograph of an airway of a patient presenting with croup. Note the typical steeple sign due to upper tracheal and subglottic narrowing.

Epidemiology

Most patients with viral croup are younger than 6 years and more typically are between 3 months and 3 years of age. The incidence in males is 1.5 times higher, and the disease tends to occur most commonly September to December in the northern hemisphere. The incidence has been reported to correlate with parainfluenza virus prevalence.[7]

Clinical Features

Typically the child with croup has mild upper respiratory symptoms for 12 to 48 hours before the abrupt onset of characteristic barky cough, respiratory distress, stridor, and hoarse voice. Usually the onset of these symptoms is during the early hours of the morning. The symptoms are generally short-lived, and most children have resolution of the barky cough within 48 hours. The symptoms are worse if the child is agitated. There may be diminished breath sounds, rhonchi, and scattered crackles.

Differential Diagnosis

The differential diagnosis of croup includes retropharyngeal or peritonsillar abscess, which is identified by a typical swelling of the local area. Other diagnoses to rule out include angioneurotic edema, allergic reaction, and foreign body, which are identified by a corroborative history and sudden onset.

Unlike viral croup, the diagnosis of spasmodic croup (laryngismus stridulus) usually describes the croup-like cough that occurs in an older age group, tends to be recurrent, and is thought to be allergic in origin. It is treated with steroids and tends to be benign even though it can be persistent.

Modern vaccination practices have resulted in a drastic reduction in the prevalence of laryngeal diphtheria, a highly contagious infection that should be considered in unimmunized patients with possible exposure. It can affect all ages. There is usually a prodromal phase of pharyngitis, and the illness is characterized by hoarseness, barking cough, usually dysphagia, minimal to severe inspiratory stridor, fever, and membranous pharyngitis. *Clostridium diphtheriae* is identified on smear and culture of the membrane.

Assessment of Severity

Table 16-1 summarizes the classification of clinical features in mild, moderate, and severe croup.

Table 16-1. Classification of Severity of Croup

	Severity		
Clinical Feature	**Mild**	**Moderate**	**Severe**
Cough	Occasional barking	Frequent barking	Frequent barking
Stridor	None at rest	Audible at rest	Prominent inspiratory
Retractions	None or mild	Suprasternal	Marked sternal
Agitation	None	None or little	Significant with distress

Investigations

Radiographs

Usually a radiograph is not indicated because the clinical picture is straightforward and there is appropriate response to treatment. Moreover the child may be more agitated during a visit to the radiology department, resulting in further worsening of clinical condition. In the event that there is an atypical clinical picture and the diagnosis is uncertain, an anteroposterior and lateral soft tissue neck radiograph shows a typical "steeple sign" consistent with the diagnosis of croup (Figure 16-1) or differentiates it from an alternative diagnosis, such as epiglottitis.[8]

Management

General

Effort should be made to make the child comfortable and to reduce agitation because agitation can significantly worsen the condition. Sitting the child comfortably in the lap of a parent or caregiver is usually the best way to examine the child.

Figure 16-2 shows an algorithm to treat croup in pediatric practice. It is important to be aware that children who have a compromised airway, such as subglottic stenosis, may experience worse symptoms and may require endotracheal intubation or tracheostomy.

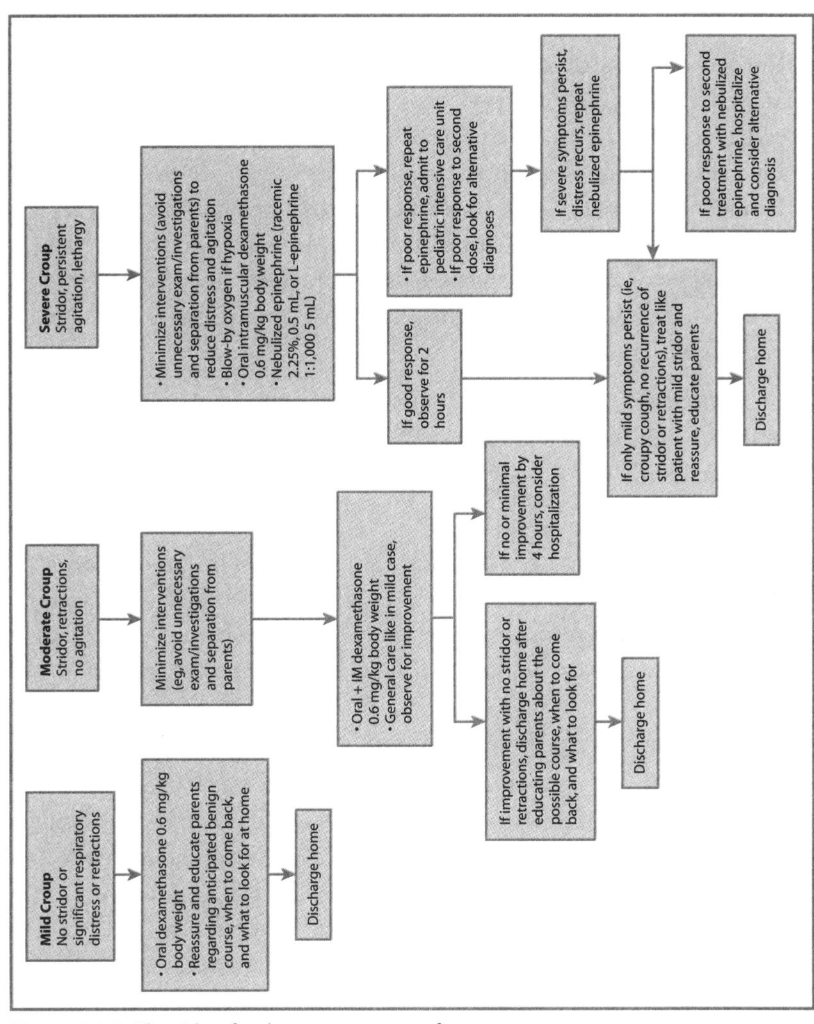

Figure 16-2. Algorithm for the management of croup.

Corticosteroids

Corticosteroids are routinely used in the treatment of croup. A meta-analysis of 24 studies using corticosteroids for the treatment of croup concluded that dexamethasone and budesonide are effective in relieving the symptoms of croup as early as 6 hours after treatment, fewer co-interventions were used, and the length of hospital stay was reduced in patients treated with corticosteroids.[9] Similar results were reported by a Cochrane database systemic review, which also showed fewer return visits and/or readmissions and reduced lengths of stay in patients with mild croup.[10]

In children with mild croup, oral dexamethasone in a dose of 0.6 mg/kg of body weight results in consistent, small but clinically significant improvement.[11] If the child is vomiting, intramuscular dexamethasone is indicated.

In moderately severe cases of croup a single dose of intramuscular dexamethasone in doses of 0.6 mg/kg body weight or nebulized budesonide 4 mg resulted in significant reduction in hospitalization. Dexamethasone was associated with greater clinical improvement at 5 hours.[12]

Epinephrine

Though nebulized racemic epinephrine has been traditionally used to treat croup, nebulized epinephrine 1/1,000 was found to be as effective and safe.[13] The usual dose is 0.5 mL of 2.25% racemic epinephrine or 5 mL of 1/1,000 epinephrine via nebulizer. The effect in the form of improved croup score tends to last for 1 hour and essentially disappears in 2 hours. Therefore, children with croup who have received epinephrine should continue to be monitored for recurrence of symptoms, and can be discharged home if the symptoms do not recur within 2 to 4 hours of treatment.[14,15] Symptoms that occur once the epinephrine wears off are not likely a rebound phenomenon, but a recurrence of the original symptoms. If more than 2 doses of epinephrine are needed, it is likely that the child should be hospitalized.

Oxygen Supplementation

Oxygen supplementation may be used in the unlikely situation of hypoxia. The clinical practice guidelines developed by Alberta Clinical Practice Guidelines Working Group recommend blow-by oxygen in children with respiratory distress.[8]

Humidified Air

Though humidified air has been used for a long time, there is no published evidence to suggest that administration of humidified air results in substantial improvement.[16] A recent Cochrane Collaboration review of data with systemic review and meta-analysis of 3 studies[17] concluded that there is no significant improvement in croup score of children managed in an emergency setting with mild to moderate croup, and there is insufficient evidence to exclude either a small beneficial or a harmful effect with its use.

Heliox

Heliox is a combination of inert gas helium with oxygen. Since low-density helium (vs nitrogen present in air) converts turbulent flow into laminar flow through a narrow airway, some have advocated its use. Heliox provides no benefit compared with standard treatment[18] and, because of the limitation of use in children requiring higher oxygen concentration, its use is not recommended for children with severe croup.[5]

Other Medications

Other medications, such as decongestants, short-acting β_2-agonists, antitussives, and analgesics, have no physiological basis for their use. Sedatives should not be prescribed.

When to Refer

- Cases of croup that are associated with excessive tachycardia may be associated with impending respiratory failure.
- In addition, persistence of symptoms for several days may merit referral for ear, nose, and throat (ENT)/pediatric pulmonologist evaluation.

When to Admit

- Severe respiratory distress, particularly if there is hypoxia (hypoxia is unusual in benign croup)
- Inability to eat or drink
- Acute care requiring 2 or more nebulizations of epinephrine

Epiglottitis

Case Report 16-2

A 4-year-old boy who was previously healthy and received all immunizations expected for his age is brought into the ED for evaluation of fever and sore throat. He refuses to eat or talk. He has a temperature of 39.5°C and oxygen saturation is 94% while breathing room air. He appears ill, is drooling, and prefers to sit alone and prop himself up and forward onto his hands, in a tripod position. The examination reveals inspiratory stridor and suprasternal retractions.

The differential diagnosis is short, and clinical suspicion for impending respiratory failure due to acute epiglottitis should be quite high. In this case, consultation with the otolaryngology and anesthesiology teams should be initiated, and the child taken to the operating room for endotracheal intubation. Ideally a protocol for team mobilization for this situation should be determined in advance and standardized as an interdisciplinary policy.

Introduction

Acute epiglottitis, also known as supraglottitis, is a potentially life-threatening infection of the supraglottic structures, which can lead to sudden, fatal airway obstruction if treatment is delayed. Classically, the disease does not involve the subglottic or tracheal mucosa. If treatment is delayed, it may rapidly progress to complete airway obstruction with cardiorespiratory arrest.

Epidemiology

Historically, acute epiglottitis was initially described as a disease of adults, but in the 1960s it was recognized primarily as a pediatric disease, with an incidence of 1 per 100,000 children by 1993.[19] Invasive disease due to *Haemophilus influenzae* occurred at a rate of 116 per 100,000 children in 1986, and this is the organism most often cultured in children with epiglottitis. After the introduction of the conjugate vaccine against *H influenzae* type b (Hib) in 1985, the incidence of invasive disease due to *H influenzae* decreased dramatically,[20] and there was a concomitant and dramatic decline in the incidence of acute epiglottitis in children.[21–23]

Causative Organisms

As the frequency of Hib disease has decreased, the cause of epiglottitis has shifted toward other causative organisms. Today, most cases are thought to be caused by other bacteria, such as *Streptococcus pneumoniae* and other *Streptococcus* species, *Staphylococcus aureus, Moraxella catarrhalis, Pseudomonas* species, *Candida albicans, Klebsiella pneumoniae, Pasturella multocida,* and *Neisseria* species.[22,24] Bacterial superinfection of viral infections also occurs, particularly with herpes simplex, parainfluenza, varicella-zoster, and Epstein-Barr.[23,24]

Epiglottitis tends to occur throughout the year, but mainly during the 6-month period from December to May in the northern hemisphere. It previously occurred equally in males and females, with a slight male predominance between the ages of 2 and 6 years of age,[25] though more recently the epidemiology has shifted toward significantly older patients[26] and should be a consideration at any age.

Clinical Presentation

The onset of epiglottitis is usually abrupt, preceded by a minor upper respiratory infection in some cases. The onset is characterized by high fever, toxic appearance, and sore throat that progresses over a few hours to dysphagia, drooling, and respiratory distress. The patient appears anxious and irritable. Stridor is a late finding. Breathing becomes noisy, and the voice and cry are muffled as swelling of the aryepiglottic folds and supralaryngeal mucosa obstructs the glottic inlet. The patient tends to sit forward in the "sniffing" position with the neck hyperextended in order to increase airway patency. Complete airway obstruction may occur at any time without any preceding deterioration in clinical signs.

Diagnosis

A very high index of suspicion must be maintained, and epiglottitis should be considered in every child with apparent acute upper airway obstruction who has a high fever and sore throat, and especially when those signs have developed over a few hours. A lateral neck radiograph can be helpful, though it only should be attempted if the patient is stable and the diagnosis is in doubt, because the disease can progress rapidly. Therapeutic trials of inhaled medicines, such as corticosteroids or racemic epinephrine, should not be initiated, as time is wasted and it may irritate the child, leading to complete obstruction of the airway. Additionally, direct visualization of the epiglottis should not be undertaken until the child is undergoing tracheal intubation.

Epiglottitis must be differentiated from other causes of acute upper airway obstruction, including viral croup (laryngotracheobronchitis), spasmodic croup, and bacterial tracheitis. Trauma and accidental causes are easily ruled out by the history. Foreign body aspiration should be considered as well, and this diagnosis may be suggested by a history of choking while eating or of playing with small objects in the mouth, the absence of fever, or visualization of an object in the airway on inspection.

Management

Most fatalities occur within the first few hours after the patient has arrived at the hospital. All deaths result from complete airway obstruction. Once the diagnosis is made, there should be no delay in establishing an artificial airway. If there is time, the child should be intubated in the operating room under general anesthesia by personnel who can perform emergency tracheostomy in case intubation fails. Corticosteroids and epinephrine have been used in the past; however, there is no solid evidence that these medications are helpful in cases of epiglottitis.

Approximately 10% to 25% of cases may be managed by observation, though these are older patients, with larger airways, and mortality is a risk. Box 16-1 describes an appropriate treatment protocol.

Box 16-1. Management of Suspected Epiglottitis

1. Avoid disturbance until an airway is secured. Allow the child to sit up and stay in his parent's arms to avoid agitation.
2. Provide 100% oxygen via blow-by administration.
3. Perform a radiologic study of the lateral neck, only if the child appears stable and the diagnosis of epiglottitis is in doubt.
4. Notify and assemble the epiglottitis team.
5. Intubate in the operating room; tracheotomy if unable to intubate.
6. Provide sedation (after intubation), critical care if tracheostomy is required.
7. Intravenous antibiotics may effectively control inflammation and infection. Antibiotics are usually prescribed to treat the most common types of bacteria. Blood cultures are usually obtained with the premise that any organism found growing in the blood can be attributed as the cause of the epiglottitis, even though *Haemophilus influenzae* (which has a recovery rate of 80%–100% from the blood) is now a very uncommon cause of epiglottitis.

When to Refer

As soon as epiglottitis is suspected, the child should be referred to the nearest pediatric ED, with surgical and anesthesia expertise available.

When to Admit

All children who are suspected of having epiglottitis should be admitted to the hospital for intravenous antibiotic treatment and intensive care monitoring. The surgical specialist (pediatric ENT, pediatric surgeon, etc) and anesthesiologist should be contacted immediately. In some institutions rapid responders may include a skilled flexible bronchoscopist. The medical and surgical team should be ready to emergently place an endotracheal tube, and also be ready for emergent tracheotomy. It is best for the surgeons to visualize the airway when in the operating room.

Bacterial Tracheitis

Case Report 16-3
A 4-year-old-boy arrived in the ED with cyanosis and a very productive cough. The history reveals a mild case of croup 1 week prior. The previous day he developed a high fever with rapidly progressive symptoms of cough and respiratory distress. Respiratory failure was diagnosed and he was intubated, and purulent secretions were aspirated from the airway. A diagnosis of bacterial tracheitis was made.

Introduction

Bacterial tracheitis is a serious and potentially life-threatening cause of acute upper airway obstruction. Bacterial tracheitis has also been referred to as membranous croup, bacterial croup, and pseudomembranous croup.

Epidemiology

Until recently, viral croup and epiglottitis have been considered the main causes of infectious upper airway obstruction.[27] Immunization against *H influenzae*[28] and treatment of viral croup with nebulized or systemic corticosteroids[9–12] have changed the incidence, morbidity, and mortality of upper airway obstruction. Bacterial tracheitis has assumed predominance over that of epiglottitis as the most common cause of acute upper airway obstruction in children older than 2 years. Bacterial tracheitis generally affects children between 4 weeks to 13 years of age, with a mean age of 4 years. The number of cases increases during the fall and winter when viral croup is more prevalent.

Causative Organisms

The pathogenesis of bacterial tracheitis remains controversial. Bacterial tracheitis often occurs as a secondary bacterial infection complicating a preexisting viral infection, including parainfluenza, adenovirus, and influenza A or B. Bacteria can gain access to the tracheal epithelium after a viral infection compromises epithelial integrity. Tracheal epithelial inflammation causes mucosal damage and predisposes to bacterial adherence to the compromised epithelial cells of the trachea. The usual protective and defensive response of the epithelial cells is weakened and results in mucus hypersecretion as well as inflammatory cell chemotaxis, and allows for thick mucopurulent secretions to accumulate. Prior to 1985, when the Hib conjugate vaccine was introduced, *H influenzae* was one of the primary causative organisms, but as of 1997 the predominant organisms identified include *S aureus, M catarrhalis, Streptococcus* species, and oral anaerobes.[29]

Presentation

Bacterial tracheitis can be distinguished from croup by patient age and symptom severity[30] (Table 16-2). Children with bacterial tracheitis tend to be older (preschoolers) compared with those with viral croup (toddlers). A sign more characteristic of bacterial tracheitis is toxic appearance and high fever. Patients with both bacterial tracheitis and viral croup can present with a prodrome of fever, barky cough, and stridor. In contrast to croup, in bacterial tracheitis, symptoms worsen over time. The presenting symptoms are shown in Box 16-2.

Diagnosis

Lateral and anteroposterior radiographs of neck and chest may be helpful in diagnosis. Findings on plain-film radiographs include subglottic narrowing, a ragged edge to the usually smooth tracheal air column, and a hazy density within the tracheal lumen. The epiglottis and supraglottic structures appear normal on neck films. The steeple sign characteristically seen in croup may also be evident.

Table 16-2. Comparison of Epiglottitis, Viral Croup, and Bacterial Tracheitis

Factor	Epiglottitis	Viral Croup	Bacterial Tracheitis
Age	2–6 yrs	3 mos–3 yrs	4 weeks–13 yrs
Organism	Various	Parainfluenza 1, 3	*Staphylococcus aureus,* *Streptococcus* species *Moraxella catarrhalis*
Season	All year	Late spring, late fall	All year
Clinical presentation	Child sitting Toxic Drooling Dysphagia Muffled voice	Child lying down Nontoxic Barking cough Hoarseness	Toxic Barking cough
Onset prodrome	Rapid; over a few hours	Variable; few hours to 4 days	Variable; few hours to 5 days
Stridor	Less common	Common	Common
Fever	High	Low-grade	High
Chest retractions	Less common	Common	Common
Lateral neck film	Swollen epiglottis	Subglottic narrowing	Pseudomembrane
Progression	Rapid	Usually slow	Usually slow
Recurrence	Rare	Common	Rare

Box 16-2. Presentation of Bacterial Tracheitis

- Fever, which may be high
- Stridor, inspiratory that may also be expiratory
- Seal-like brassy cough
- Hoarseness
- Dyspnea with retractions, nasal flaring
- Cyanosis
- May progress rapidly to respiratory failure

The most definitive procedure is to visualize the trachea endoscopically. The supraglottic structures will appear normal, but subglottic edema is the prominent feature, and ulcerations and copious purulent secretions will be present. These secretions should be cultured so that the causative agent may be effectively treated with antibiotics.

Management

Children with bacterial tracheitis must be monitored very closely and, often, tracheal intubation with mechanical ventilation is necessary in the event of respiratory collapse or an inability to mobilize secretions effectively. Using an endotracheal tube one size smaller than usual is recommended to reduce trauma to the subglottic area. Careful attention to the suctioning and mobilization of secretions is essential. Occlusion of the endotracheal tube has been reported as the most frequent cause of death in intubated and mechanically ventilated children with bacterial tracheitis. Some otolaryngologists have advocated for expectant placement of tracheotomy tubes in children with bacterial tracheitis for this reason. Humidification of the inspired air helps prevent mucus plugging of the endotracheal tube. Antibiotics and supportive care are essential for full recovery. Antibiotics should be initiated with nafcillin or oxacillin (200 mg/kg/day divided every 6 hours for either agent) in conjunction with a third-generation cephalosporin, such as ceftriaxone (50 mg/kg daily). The addition of vancomycin should be considered if resistant organisms are present in the local community or if there is multisystem involvement.

Complications

Complications associated with bacterial tracheitis include toxic shock syndrome, septic shock, postintubation pulmonary edema, acute respiratory distress syndrome, and subglottic stenosis.[31] Most children recover, and there is no reason to suspect an underlying immunodeficiency. It is rare for a child to have a second episode of bacterial tracheitis.

Key Points

- The differential diagnosis for children who have stridulous breathing should include croup, epiglottitis, and bacterial tracheitis.
- Most patients with croup can be managed as outpatients.
- When symptoms are severe, croup should be differentiated from alternative causes, such as epiglottitis or bacterial tracheitis.
- Corticosteroids are the established treatment of choice for croup.
- If epiglottitis is suspected, the child should be admitted to the hospital. A pediatric otolaryngologist or anesthesiologist should be contacted immediately and should be the only physicians to attempt to visualize the airway.
- Children who have croup tend to have a sudden onset of hoarseness and barking cough, but do not appear toxic, as do those who have epiglottitis or bacterial tracheitis.
- Children with bacterial tracheitis have high fever and typically require endotracheal intubation and mechanical ventilation.

References

1. Henrickson KJ, Hoover S, Kehl KS, et al. National disease burden of respiratory viruses detected in children by polymerase chain reaction. *Pediatr Infect Dis J.* 2004;23:S11–S18
2. Cherry JD. Croup. *N Engl J Med.* 2008;358:384–391
3. Johnson D, Williamson J. Croup; duration of symptoms and impact on family functioning. *Pediatr Res.* 2001;49:83A
4. Geelhoed G. Croup. *Pediatr Pulmonol.* 1997;23(5)370–374
5. Bjornson CL, Johnson DW. Croup. *Lancet.* 2008;371:329–339
6. Arslan Z, Cipe FE, Ozmen S, Kondolot M, Piskin IE, Yuney A. Evaluation of allergic sensitization and gastroesophageal reflux disease in children with recurrent croup. *Pediatr Int.* 2009;51(5):666–665
7. Marx A, Torok T, Holdman R, et al. Pediatric hospitalizations for croup (laryngotracheobronchitis): biennial increase associated with human parainfluenza virus 1 epidemics. *J Infect Dis.* 1997;176:1423–1427
8. Worrall G. Croup. *Can Fam Physician.* 2008;54(4):573–574. http://www.ncbi.nlm.nih.gov/pmc/articles/PMC2294095
9. Ausejo M, Saenz A, Pham BA, et al. The effectiveness of glucocorticoids in treating croup: meta-analysis. *BMJ.* 1999;319;595–600

10. Russell K, Wiebe N, Saenz A, et al. Glucocorticoids for croup. *Cochrane Database Syst Rev.* 2003;(4):CD001955
11. Bjornson CL, Klassen TP, Williamson J, et al. A randomized trial of a single dose of oral dexamethasone for mild croup. *N Engl J Med.* 2004;351:1306–1311s
12. Johnson DW, Jacobson S, Edney PC, et al. A comparison of nebulized budesonide, intramuscular dexamethasone, and placebo for moderately severe croup. *N Engl J Med.* 1998;339:498–503
13. Waisman Y, Klein B, Boenning D, et al. Prospective randomized double-blind study comparing L-epinephrine and racemic epinephrine aerosols in the treatment of laryngotracheitis (croup). *Pediatrics.* 1992;89:302–306
14. Kelley P, Simon J. Racemic epinephrine use in croup and disposition. *Am J Emerg Med.* 1992;10:181–183
15. Corneli H, Bolte R. Outpatient use of racemic epinephrine in croup. *Am Fam Physician.* 1992;46:683–684
16. Johnson D. Croup. In: Moyer V, ed. *Clinical Evidence.* London: BMJ Publishing Group Ltd; 2004:401–226
17. Moore M, Little P. Humidified air inhalation for treating croup: a systemic review and meta-analysis. *Fam Pract.* 2007;24:295–301
18. Weber J, Chudnofsky C, Younger J, et al. A randomized comparison of helium-oxygen mixture (heliox) and racemic epinephrine for the treatment of moderate to severe croup. *Pediatrics.* 2001;197:e96
19. Carey MJ. Epiglottitis in adults. *Am J Emerg Med.* 1996;14:421–424
20. Broadhurst LE, Erickson RL, Kelley PW. Decreases in invasive *Haemophilus influenzae* diseases in US army children, 1984 through 1991. *JAMA.* 1993:269(2):227–231
21. Kessler A, Wetmore RF, Marsh RR. Childhood epiglottitis in recent years. *Int J Pediatr Otorhinolaryngol.* 1993;25:155–162
22. Wenger JD. Epidemiology of *Haemophilus influenzae* type B disease and impact of *Haemophilus influenzae* type B conjugate vaccines in the United States and Canada. *Pediatr Infect Dis J.* 1998;17:S132–S136
23. Senior BA, Radkowski D, McArthur C, et al. Changing patterns in pediatric supraglottitis: a multi-institutional review, 1980 to 1992. *Laryngoscope.* 1994;104(11 pt 1):1314–1322
24. Ward MA. Emergency department management of acute respiratory infections. *Sem Respir Infect.* 2002;17:65–71
25. Baxter JD. Acute epiglottitis in children. *Laryngoscope.* 1967:77:1358–1367
26. Shah RK, Roberson DW, Jones DT. Epiglottitis in the *Hemophilus influenzae* type B vaccine era: changing times. *Laryngoscope.* 2004;114:557–560
27. Hopkins A, Hahiri, T, Salerno R, et al. Changing epidemiology of life-threatening upper airway infections: the reemergence of bacterial tracheitis. *Pediatrics.* 2006;118:1418–1421

28. Centers for Disease Control and Prevention. Progress toward elimination of *Haemophilus influenzae* type b invasive disease among infants and children: United States, 1998–2000. *MMWR Morb Mortal Wkly Rep.* 2002;51(11):234–237
29. Brook I. Aerobic and anaerobic microbiology of bacterial tracheitis in children. *Pediatr Emerg Care.* 1997;113:16–18
30. Bernstein T, Brilli R, Jacobs B. Is bacterial tracheitis changing? A 14-month experience in a pediatric intensive care unit. *Clin Infect Dis.* 1998;27(3):458–462
31. Burns JA, Brown J, Ogle JW. Group A streptococcal tracheitis associated with toxic shock syndrome. *Pediatr Infect Dis J.* 1998;17(10):933–935

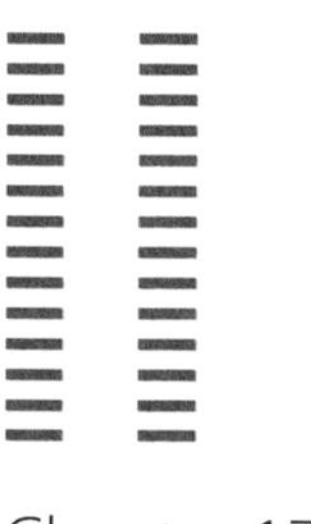

Chapter 17

Bronchiectasis

Paul C. Stillwell, MD

Case Report 17-1

A 30-month-old girl has had a hacking cough since early infancy and recurrent pneumonia. The cough was often associated with wheezing. She has experienced at least 5 episodes of pneumonia, documented radiographically. She was born with a tracheoesophageal fistula that was repaired at day 1 of life. She had normal growth parameters and vital signs with a room air oxygen saturation of 97%. There were no crackles or wheezes, and there was no prolongation of the expiratory phase. She had no digital clubbing.

A high-resolution computed tomography (CT) scan shows patches of bronchiectasis primarily in the left lower lobe region with loss of volume. A flexible bronchoscopy shows a well-healed fistula repair and copious amounts of purulent endobronchial secretions. The airway culture is positive for *Haemophilus influenzae* and negative for fungus and acid-fast bacteria. The pH probe is positive for acid reflux.

The recommended treatment is antibiotics directed against the *H influenzae,* a proton-pump inhibitor for the gastroesophageal reflux, and high-frequency external chest oscillation to facilitate airway clearance. With these therapies the recurrent pneumonias resolve and her cough is nearly extinct.

Introduction

Bronchiectasis is the dilatation of bronchi and bronchioles associated with airway wall thickening.[1,2] The most common cause in children is cystic fibrosis (CF), but the other potential underlying causes are numerous (Table 17-1). The most commonly identified causes have considerable geographic variability based on the risk of serious infections and the particular diagnostic expertise of the regional medical centers.[3] Even after extensive evaluation for an underlying cause, bronchiectasis is idiopathic in a high percentage of patients.[1-3] Bronchiectasis is the final common pathway of airway injury followed by

Table 17-1. Disease Processes Associated With Bronchiectasis and Potential Evaluations

Disease Process	Possible Diagnosis	Evaluation
Impaired mucociliary clearance	Cystic fibrosis	Sweat test; DNA analysis
	Primary ciliary dyskinesia	Ciliary biopsy (electron microscopy); DNA analysis
Infections	*Mycobacterium tuberculosis*	Skin test; acid fast stain and culture; interferon-γ release assay
	Atypical mycobacteria	Acid fast stain and culture
	Measles	Serology
	Pertussis	Direct fluorescent-antibody serology
	Mycoplasma	Serology
	HIV	Serology
	Varicella	Serology
	Adenovirus	Serology
	Severe pneumonia	Cultures
	Necrotizing pneumonia	Cultures
Immunodeficiency	Humoral or cellular immunodeficiency	Immunoglobulins; complement levels; cell-mediated immunity tests
	Neutrophil dysfunction	Nitroblue tetrazolium
Airway injury or toxin	Dysphagia with aspiration	Modified barium swallow
	Esophageal reflux	Esophagram; pH/impedance probe; milk scan
	Inhalational injury	History
Immunologic	Allergic bronchopulmonary aspergillosis	Specific immunoglobulin IgE and IgG;
	Connective tissue disease	Various
	Inflammatory bowel disease	Endoscopy; bronchoscopy
Congenital/ connective tissue abnormality	Tracheobronchomegaly	Computed tomography (CT) scan; bronchoscopy
	Airway cartilage deficiency	CT scan; bronchoscopy
	Marfan syndrome	Clinical criteria
	Yellow nail syndrome	Clinical criteria
	Young syndrome	Sperm count
	Alpha-1 antitrypsin deficiency	Alpha-1 antitrypsin levels; Pi type
Obstructed airways	Retained foreign body	Bronchoscopy
	Endobronchial tumor	Bronchoscopy
	Extrinsic compression	CT scan; bronchoscopy

acute and chronic inflammation. It can occur in one or a few lung segments, or it can be generalized throughout all segments. If the airway injury is severe or recurrent, the airway damage becomes irreversible and self-sustaining.

Clinical Manifestations

The child with bronchiectasis presents with a chronic "wet" or productive cough and recurrent "chest infections." Some children may have recurrent wheezing. A small percentage may have hemoptysis.[2,3] Recurrent or persistent pneumonia can also be a presenting feature of bronchiectasis. The chest examination of the child with bronchiectasis may be normal until significant airway abnormalities are present. As the disease advances the intensity of breath sounds may be decreased and inspiratory crackles may be present. Expiratory wheezing may be present when severe airway damage has occurred. The examination may be more prominently abnormal during acute exacerbations of the bronchiectasis, and less so after resolution. The abnormal findings may be localized if the bronchiectasis is segmental. Other examination findings may be present depending on the underlying cause of the bronchiectasis (eg, failure to thrive in patients with CF). Digital clubbing can occur with moderate and severe bronchiectasis.

Pulmonary function testing (PFT) performed in children old enough to cooperate may show an obstructive pattern, a restrictive pattern, or a combination of both.[4] The spirometric abnormalities in children with bronchiectasis due to CF are generally correlated with disease severity and progression,[5] but the utility of spirometry in monitoring non-CF bronchiectasis is less certain.[6] Because of ready availability and absence of risk, PFT is commonly used to monitor the airway function in children with bronchiectasis. However, the abnormalities that may be present with bronchiectasis are not specific to this diagnosis. An evaluation for bronchiectasis should be considered for children with persistent or progressive PFT abnormalities. Figure 17-1 shows an example of flow-volume loops of a child with severe non-CF bronchiectasis.

The chest radiograph (Figure 17-2) may show increased interstitial markings, but may also appear normal until the bronchiectasis is extensive. A definitive diagnosis of bronchiectasis is made by high-resolution chest CT (HRCT) (Figure 17-3A and 17-3B), which has largely supplanted bronchograms as a diagnostic tool.[1] The radiographic findings on chest radiography and CT scan are outlined in Box 17-1.[7]

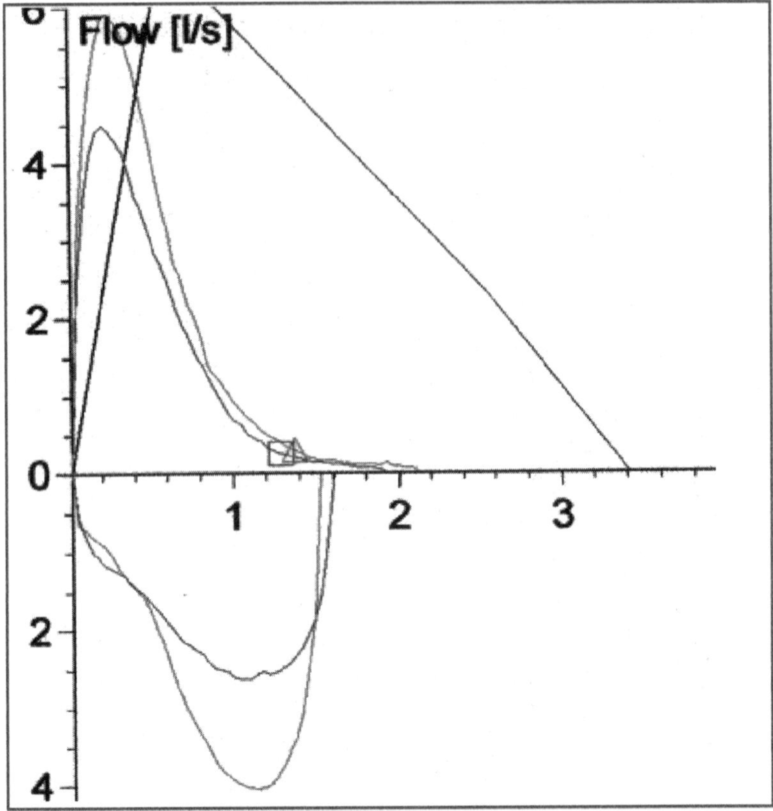

Figure 17-1. Example of a flow-volume loop in bronchiectasis. Flow-volume loop with volume on the horizontal axis and flow on the vertical axis. Expiratory flow is above the volume axis and inspiratory flow is below the volume axis. The biggest expiratory loop is the predicted, the smallest is the pre-bronchodilator loop, and the middle-sized loop is after bronchodilator. The expiratory loop is concave with regard to the volume axis, indicating abnormal airflow obstruction. This demonstrates a mixed restrictive and obstructive abnormality with modest bronchodilator improvement, which in a child with chronic cough should expand the differential diagnosis beyond asthma. A bronchodilator response of ≥15% would be more typical of asthma. FVC, forced vital capacity; FEV_1, forced expiratory volume in 1 second; PEFR, peak expiratory flow rate; FEF_{25-75}, forced expiratory flow between 25% and 75% of the vital capacity.

FVC = 1.91 L (56% predicted); improved 9.4% post-bronchodilator
FEV_1 = 1.26 L (41% predicted); improved 7% post-bronchodilator
FEV_1/FVC ratio = 0.66
PEFR = 4.47 L/s (% predicted); improved % post-bronchodilator
FEF_{25-75} = 0.50 L/s (13% predicted); decreased 10% post-bronchodilator

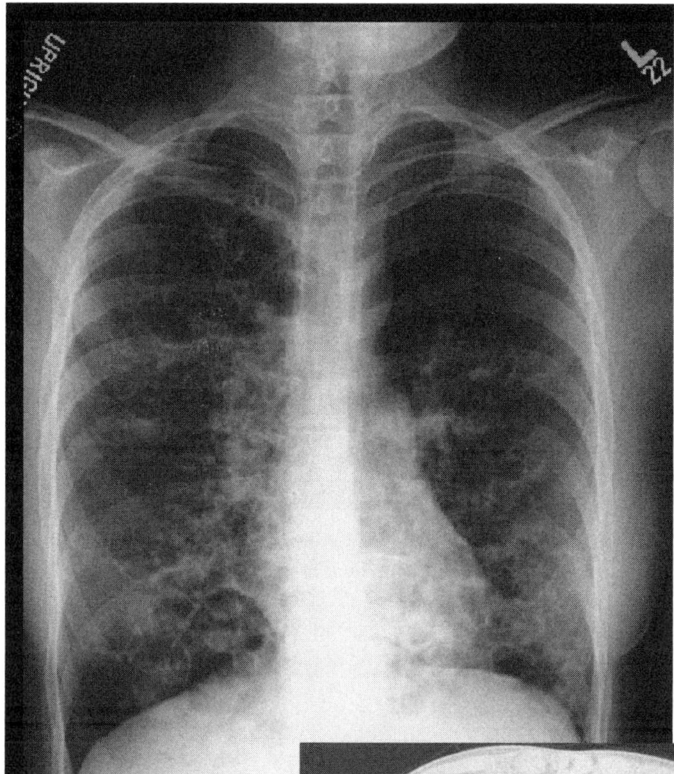

Figure 17-2. Example of bronchiectasis on chest radiograph (frontal and lateral). Frontal and lateral chest radiograph in a 16-year-old girl with severe bronchiectasis following adenovirus pneumonia in early childhood. There are diffuse increased interstitial markings, multiple thin-walled cavitary lesions, and overinflation.

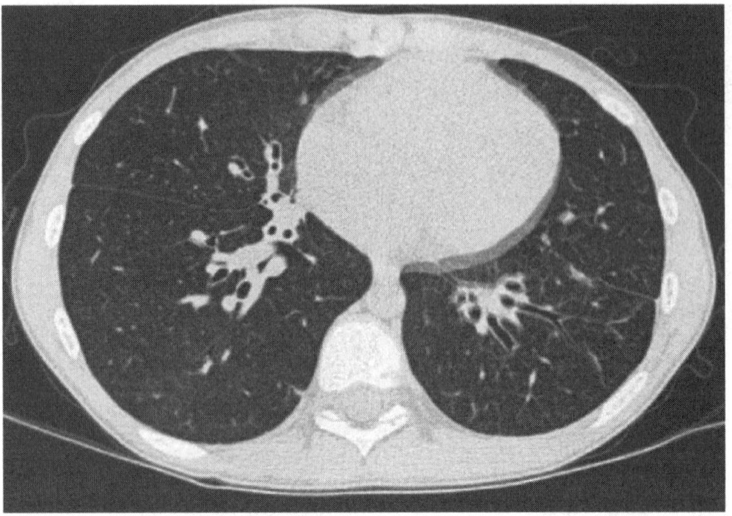

Figure 17-3A. Examples of bronchiectasis on high-resolution computed tomography (HRCT): generalized. HRCT scan demonstrating diffuse bronchiectasis with thickened airway walls, dilated airway lumens, extension of the airway markings too far into the periphery, and centrilobular opacities. The patient is a 12-year-old boy with immunoglobulin A deficiency as the underlying cause of the bronchiectasis.

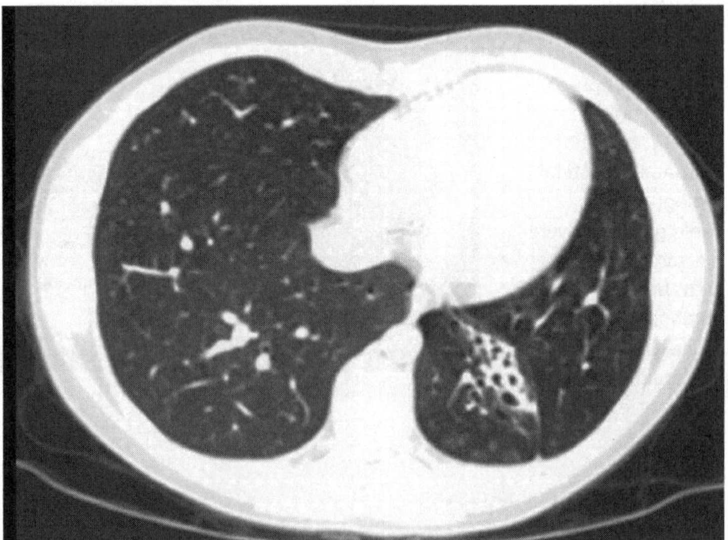

Figure 17-3B. Example of bronchiectasis on HRCT: segmental. HRCT scan demonstrating segmental bronchiectasis of the left lower lobe. There are thickened airway walls, dilated airway lumens, and loss of volume. The patient was an 11-year-old girl with idiopathic segmental bronchiectasis.

Box 17-1. Radiographic Findings in Bronchiectasis

Chest Radiograph Findings
- Increased interstitial markings
- Thickened airway walls
- Dilated airway lumen
- Hyperinflation may be seen

High-resolution Chest Computed Tomography Findings
- Airway lumen greater than adjacent blood vessel ("signet ring")
- Tram-track markings
- Extension of airway markings to periphery
- Lack of tapering of airways toward periphery
- Mucus plugging and centrilobular opacities ("tree in bud")
- Mosaic pattern of perfusion
- Focal air-trapping (best seen on expiratory views)
- Mucus plugging

A chest CT scan should be considered to evaluate bronchiectasis for children with persistent productive cough, chronically abnormal chest radiographs, chronically abnormal chest auscultation, or persistent PFT abnormality.

Pathophysiology

The initial airway injury leading to bronchiectasis can be from a variety of insults, but the most common is an infection.[1] A mucosal injury or an underlying immunodeficiency allows an initial infection, and perpetuation of the host response eventually leads to airway damage. The cellular response is predominantly neutrophilic, and ongoing inflammation produces increased mucus secretion, thickened mucus, and airway edema. It is unclear in most cases why the enhanced host response persists (unlike acute bronchitis, which resolves), unless there is repeated injury such as may occur with repeated chronic aspiration or repeated airway infections. The combination of dilated airway walls, mucosal inflammation, and thickened secretions impairs mucociliary clearance, which impairs clearance of the infection and increases the risk of subsequent infection. Eventually the airway damage becomes irreversible and self-perpetuating.[1,2,8]

Microscopic examination of the bronchiectatic airway reveals thickened airway walls, mucosal gland enlargement, cellular (usually neutrophilic) infiltration, dilated cross-sectional airway lumen, and excessive secretions.[1] If not previously treated with antibiotics, bacteria may be evident on special stains. Excessive pro-inflammatory mediators are present in the bronchoalveolar lavage fluids.[1]

Evaluation

Once bronchiectasis has been documented, an underlying cause should be sought (Table 17-1). If the history or examination suggests a specific cause, the initial evaluation can be targeted to that cause (eg, sweat test if steatorrhea is present). More commonly several tests are necessary and are usually performed progressing from least invasive to more invasive. All children with bronchiectasis should have a sweat chloride test to assess for CF (even if newborn screening was negative). Screening for immunodeficiency should include quantitative immunoglobulins, white blood cell counts with differential, and total complement levels. More advanced immune studies would include assessment of response to immunizations, evaluation of cell-mediated immunity, and neutrophil function tests. Allergic bronchopulmonary aspergillosis and connective tissue diseases can be assessed by specific immunologic studies. *Mycobacterium tuberculosis* infection can be assessed by skin test, interferon-γ release assay in those older than 5 years, and culture at the time of bronchoscopy. Risks for aspiration can be assessed by modified barium swallow to assess swallowing coordination and an upper gastrointestinal barium study to assess for gastroesophageal reflux. Other tests to assess the risks for aspiration include the esophageal pH/impedance probe and radionuclide milk scans. Primary ciliary dyskinesia can be assessed by electron microscopy of ciliary ultrastructure, ciliary wave form analysis, nasal exhaled nitric oxide, and DNA analysis; these are usually accomplished at a referral center. Flexible bronchoscopy allows assessment of airway obstruction, visual inspection of the airway mucosa, and collection of airway secretions and bronchoalveolar lavage (BAL) fluid. The BAL fluid can be analyzed by stains and cultures for a variety of infections, as well as cell counts with differential and other specialized stains.

Management

Once the clinical suspicion of bronchiectasis is confirmed by HRCT scan, an evaluation for the specific underlying disease should be undertaken (Table 17-1). If a specific disease can be identified, therapy directed at that process should be initiated or intensified. Therapeutic options for CF have undergone sophisticated evaluation to help direct appropriate management choices,[9] but randomized clinical prospective studies for non-CF bronchiectasis in children are lacking. Much of the treatment offered for non-CF bronchiectasis is extrapolated from data acquired in patients with CF.[10]

Antibiotics targeting bacteria isolated from sputum or bronchoscopy samples may be beneficial in treating bronchiectasis, similar to treatment for CF airway infections. The most frequent bacteria isolated with non-CF bronchiectasis include *Streptococcus pneumoniae, Haemophilus influenzae, Moraxella catarrhalis,* and *Staphylococcus aureus.* Patients with CF have greater risk of *Pseudomonas aeruginosa* airway infection than patients with non-CF bronchiectasis. Antibiotics for acute exacerbations of bronchiectasis are documented to help reverse the acute illness.[1,10] The role for chronic antibiotic therapy for non-CF bronchiectasis is not well established.[1,10] Inhaled antibiotics have documented benefit for patients with CF, and may have benefit in non-CF bronchiectasis as well, depending on the organisms in the airway.[1,9,10] Airway clearance therapy using a variety of techniques is commonly prescribed with perceived anecdotal benefit. Some individuals may respond to inhaled bronchodilators, and even if there is no documented increase in airflow after bronchodilator on PFTs, the bronchodilator may have a positive effect on mucociliary clearance.[1,10] Inhaled corticosteroids have shown some benefit in some adult subjects with bronchiectasis,[1,10] but their role in CF has recently been challenged with conflicting evidence.[9] Other anti-inflammatory treatments show promising benefit in CF, but there is limited evidence of benefit in non-CF bronchiectasis, particularly in children.[10] Oral macrolide therapy, used as an anti-inflammatory rather than as an antibiotic, has shown some benefit in small trials for adults with non-CF bronchiectasis.[1,10]

Mucolytic treatments with rhDNase has documented benefit for patients with CF,[9] but may have a detrimental effect for patients with non-CF bronchiectasis (based on adult studies).[1] Nebulized hypertonic saline, recently shown to benefit patients with CF,[9] has received limited study in patients with non-CF bronchiectasis to date.

Hospitalization to intensify antibiotic therapy and airway clearance might be indicated for an exacerbation in patients with non-CF bronchiectasis, an approach that has documented benefit for patients with

CF. Anecdotal experience suggests the same benefit can be achieved for children with non-CF bronchiectasis. Patients with large volumes of hemoptysis, hypoxia, or rapidly declining pulmonary function require hospitalization.

Surgical resection of limited or segmental bronchiectasis may be necessary if massive hemoptysis occurs, but recent evidence suggests in the absence of hemoptysis that aggressive medical management can provide similar improvement to surgical intervention in non-CF bronchiectasis.[11] Double lung transplantation may be an option for patients with severe progressive bronchiectasis that does not respond well to medical management.[10] Lung transplantation has commonly been offered as an option for end-stage bronchiectatic lung disease due to CF, although the benefits have recently been questioned.[12]

Prognosis

Improved understanding of CF lung disease and vigorous evaluation of new and old treatment options have steadily increased the median age of survival.[9] The rate of progression of non-CF bronchiectasis and prognosis for survival is likely related to the underlying cause and treatment of that process.[1,10] Survival of patients with non-CF bronchiectasis is generally expected to be considerably longer than for patients with CF bronchiectasis.[10] The presence of chronic *P aeruginosa* airway infection negatively affects survival of patients with both CF and non-CF bronchiectasis.[1,10]

Key Points

- Bronchiectasis in children can be caused by a wide variety of underlying causes.
- Often no cause for the bronchiectasis is found, and these cases are considered idiopathic.
- Bronchiectasis should be suspected if a child has chronic cough and recurrent chest infections.
- An HRCT scan should be performed to definitively establish the diagnosis of bronchiectasis.
- Once bronchiectasis is confirmed, an underlying cause should be sought.
- The management of patients with non-CF bronchiectasis has largely been determined by expert opinion and data extrapolated from CF studies.

References

1. O'Donnell AE. Bronchiectasis. *Chest.* 2008;134:815–823
2. Dagli E. Non cystic fibrosis bronchiectasis. *Paediatr Respir Rev.* 2000;1:64–70
3. Li AM, Sonnappa S, Lex C, et al. Non-CF bronchiectasis: does knowing the aetiology lead to changes in management? *Eur Respir J.* 2005;26:8–14
4. Pifferi M, Caramella D, Bulleri A, et al. Pediatric bronchiectasis: correlation of HRCT, ventilation and perfusion scintigraphy, and pulmonary function testing. *Pediatr Pulmonol.* 2004;38:298–393
5. VanDevanter DR, Rasoulivan L, Murphy TM, et al. Trends in the clinical characteristics of the US cystic fibrosis patient population from 1995 to 2005. *Pediatr Pulmonol.* 2008;43:739–744
6. Twiss J, Stewart AW, Byrnes CA. Longitudinal pulmonary function of childhood bronchiectasis and comparison with cystic fibrosis. 2006;61:414–418
7. Rossi UG, Owens CM. The radiology of chronic lung disease in children. *Arch Dis Child.* 2005;90:601–607
8. Boren EJ, Teuber SS, Gershwin ME. A review of non-cystic fibrosis pediatric bronchiectasis. *Clin Rev Allergy Immunol.* 2008;34(2):260–273
9. Flume PA, O'Sullivan BP, Robinson KA, et al. Cystic fibrosis pulmonary guidelines: chronic medication for maintenance of lung health. *Am J Respir Crit Care Med.* 2007;176:957–969
10. Rosen MJ. Chronic cough due to bronchiectasis (ACCP Evidence-based Clinical Practice Guidelines). *Chest.* 2006;129:122S–131S
11. Karadag B, Karakoc F, Ersu R, et al. Non-cystic fibrosis bronchiectasis in children: a persisting problem in developing countries. *Respiration.* 2005;72:233–238
12. Allen J, Visner G. Lung transplantation in cystic fibrosis—primum non nocere? *N Engl J Med.* 2007;357:2186–2188

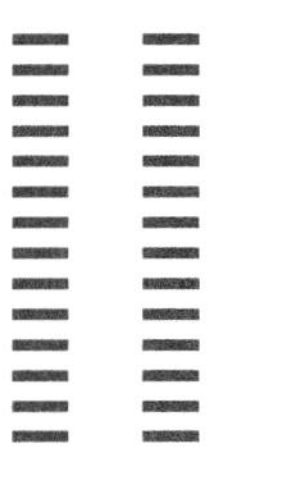

Chapter 18

Bronchiolitis

Miles M. Weinberger, MD

Introduction

Bronchiolitis is an isolated episode in an infant of a symptomatic airway obstruction associated with lower respiratory tract infection. An infant with bronchiolitis typically presents with increased work of breathing manifested by retractions and associated with polyphonic wheezing heard audibly with or without a stethoscope. The term bronchiolitis should not be applied to repeated episodes of wheezing that are seen in infants and toddlers with upper respiratory infections.

Epidemiology

As many as 3% of all US infants are hospitalized annually for bronchiolitis, making this clinical problem the leading cause of hospitalization during the first year of life.[1] While respiratory syncytial virus (RSV) predominates as a cause of bronchiolitis, many respiratory viruses are associated with bronchiolitis.[2] Regardless of the viral cause, a predictable seasonal pattern occurs for bronchiolitis, although there is some variability from year to year[3,4] and with region.[5]

Clinical Presentation

The prodrome of bronchiolitis is a typical-appearing upper respiratory tract infection, with mild rhinorrhea and occasionally a low-grade fever. Progression then occurs over 1 to 2 days to cough, retractions (see Figure 18-1), tachypnea, and prolonged expiratory phase with wheezing and inspiratory crackles. The tachypnea and increased work of breathing can result in poor feeding. Otitis media, usually nonbacterial, is often present. A varying degree of hypoxemia can occur, and hypercapnia can be found in severe cases.

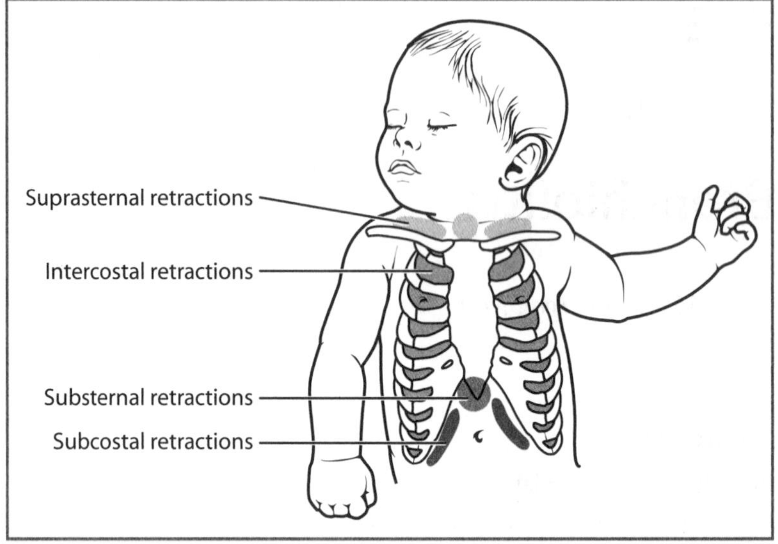

Figure 18-1. Retractions in infants and young children. The location of retractions is an important clue to the cause and severity of respiratory distress. Suprasternal retractions predominate when infants have extra- thoracic obstruction. Subcostal and substernal retractions usually result from lower respiratory tract disorders. Suprasternal retractions occur in upper respiratory tract disorders. Alone, mild intercostal retractions may be normal. However, intercostal retractions accompanied by subcostal and substernal retractions may indicate moderate respiratory distress. Deep suprasternal retractions typically indicate severe distress.

Depending on the duration of symptoms and oral intake, dehydration may be present manifested by poor tearing, dry mucous membranes, and poor skin turgor. Crackles and wheezing may be present on auscultation. Wheezing may be audible without a stethoscope.

Antigen tests of nasal washings provide rapid (usually within 30 min) and accurate (sensitivity 87%–91%, specificity 96%–100%) detection of RSV during the peak season. Respiratory viral panels, cultures for RSV or other viruses, or detection by direct fluorescent antibody or polymerase chain reaction may be useful for epidemiologic and educational purposes. However, they add to the cost and provide no useful information for patient care.

Pulse oximetry can identify the presence of sufficient hypoxemia to warrant supplemental oxygen. Blood gas measurement can provide partial pressure of carbon dioxide (Pco_2) measurement, which is essential to distinguish hypoxia caused by ventilation/perfusion ($\dot{V}/\dot{Q}$) mismatching from that caused by hypoventilation and hypercarbic respiratory failure.

A complete blood cell count is seldom useful since the white blood cell count is usually within normal limits. Urine specific gravity may provide useful information regarding fluid balance and possible dehydration. Serum chemistries are not affected directly by the infection but may aid in assessing and managing dehydration.

Radiologic findings are nonspecific and typically demonstrate hyperinflation with flattened diaphragms and increased anteroposterior diameter with precordial air from air trapping. Patchy infiltrates and focal atelectasis may also be present. None of those findings alter therapy. Consequently, chest radiographs are not routinely necessary when the clinical presentation is typical of bronchiolitis.[6]

Pathophysiology

The virus initially replicates in the epithelium of the upper respiratory tract, but in the susceptible young infant it spreads rapidly to the lower tract airways. The pathologic findings in bronchiolitis are primarily in the respiratory epithelium with generalized involvement. Inflammatory changes of variable severity are observed in most small bronchi and bronchioles. Peribronchiolar infiltration, mostly with mononuclear cells, and edema of the submucosa and adventitia occur. Necrosis and sloughing of the bronchiolar epithelium occur with gradual recovery. Plugs of necrotic material and fibrin may completely or partially obstruct the small airways. Smooth muscle constriction does not appear to be important in the obstruction.

Infants are particularly vulnerable to obstruction because mucosal inflammation causes relatively greater compromise of their small-lumen airways, and changes in resistance are proportional to the cube of changes in the radius of the airway. In areas peripheral to sites of partial obstruction, air becomes trapped by a process similar to a ball-valve mechanism. The negative intrapleural pressure exerted during inspiration allows air to flow beyond the point of partial obstruction. However, on expiration, the size of the lumen decreases with the positive intrathoracic pressure, thereby resulting in increased obstruction and hyperinflation. Thus, although airflow is impeded during both inspiration and expiration, the latter is more affected and prolonged.

In areas peripheral to complete obstruction, the trapped air eventually becomes absorbed, which results in multiple areas of atelectasis. This absorptive atelectasis is greatly accelerated when the child is breathing a high concentration of oxygen. A presumed reason why infants have increased susceptibility to the development of atelectasis or hyperinflation is that collateral channels that maintain alveolar expansion in the presence of airway obstruction are not well developed early in life.

Natural History

Virtually all infants contract RSV during the first 2 years of life, most during the first year. An estimated 20% develop bronchiolitis from an RSV infection, while others develop upper respiratory symptoms, coryza, or the symptoms of a common cold. Of those with bronchiolitis, most do not require hospitalization. Nonetheless, bronchiolitis is the leading cause of hospitalization during the first year of life beyond the neonatal period.

Of those who do get bronchiolitis, an estimated 25% to 50% have similar recurrent symptoms, consistent with a phenotype of asthma characterized by being induced by recurrent viral respiratory infection.[7,8] Those who develop bronchiolitis appear to differ from those who do not in genetic factors that involve innate immunity.[9–11] Thus, while all children get viral respiratory infections, it is primarily genetic susceptibility that contributes to both bronchiolitis and recurrent symptoms of asthma exacerbations from viral respiratory infections. Exposure to tobacco smoke during pregnancy and after birth appears to be an environmental contributing factor that increases the risk of bronchiolitis.[12–14]

Management

Bronchodilators

The role of bronchodilators in treating bronchiolitis has long been controversial. Their widespread use undoubtedly relates to the similarity between the symptoms of bronchiolitis and asthma. Recent studies have not shown a clear clinical benefit from the use of either epinephrine or albuterol. A meta-analysis of randomized controlled trials evaluating the efficacy of bronchodilators for the treatment of acute viral bronchiolitis concluded the short-term benefit of epinephrine among outpatients might be greater than for albuterol, but there was insufficient evidence to support routine use of either among inpatients.[15]

A reasonable conclusion from studies over the last 30 years on the use of bronchodilators in treating bronchiolitis is that some patients may have some degree of transient benefit from bronchodilators but the effects are generally insufficient to provide clinically relevant benefit. The beneficial effects of epinephrine appear to stem from the α-adrenergic effect of vasoconstriction, perhaps resulting in decreasing mucosal edema. Nevertheless, the rapid metabolism of epinephrine makes it an unlikely agent to substantially alter the clinical course of bronchiolitis, even when transient clinical benefit is apparent. A trial administration of an aerosol bronchodilator, albuterol or epinephrine, may be useful in decision-making regarding subsequent use for symptom relief. However, since neither epinephrine nor albuterol has been associated with improving the clinical course of hospitalized patients with bronchiolitis, there is no support for the common practice of scheduled use of either of these bronchodilators.

Corticosteroids

The use of corticosteroids, as with bronchodilators, is driven by the similar clinical presentations of bronchiolitis and asthma. Multiple studies in hospitalized children demonstrated no effect of systemic corticosteroids on the outcome of bronchiolitis.[16–21] However, a meta-analysis that included many of these studies concluded that there was a modest but statistically significant improvement in clinical symptoms, length of stay, and duration of symptoms.[22] The mean difference in length of stay or duration of symptoms from the pooled analysis was 0.43 days less among those who received corticosteroids.

Studies in outpatients who did not require hospitalization when initially seen in the emergency department (ED) have suggested that treatment with corticosteroids in that population may provide clinical benefit. Significantly lower symptom scores on day 2 were seen following 2 mg/kg/day of prednisolone given for 5 days to infants who could be discharged from the ED.[23] A randomized, double-blind placebo-controlled trial among 230 children who received 2 mg/kg/day of prednisolone or placebo for 3 days found the mean duration of respiratory distress to be 2 days in the placebo-treated group and only 1 day in the corticosteroid-treated group for the 123 children who had to be initially admitted to the hospital and the others who remained as outpatients.[24] While that study included patients who had previous wheezing episodes in addition to those for whom wheezing was a first-time event, the authors specified that there were similar results for those who wheezed for the first time as for those who had previous wheezing events.

Studies conflict on the benefits of the use of the dexamethasone in treating children seen in the ED for bronchiolitis. An initial dose of 1 mg/kg of dexamethasone or placebo in a double-blind, randomized, placebo-controlled trial involving 70 children resulted in 44% of the 34 children who received dexamethasone requiring hospitalization 4 or more hours after receiving the placebo while only 19% of the 36 patients who received the active medication were hospitalized ($P = 0.039$).[25] A much larger multicenter investigation using a nearly identical treatment plan showed no significant benefit from dexamethasone.[26]

The conflicting studies of corticosteroids may be a function of the timing of treatment in the course of bronchiolitis. Early treatment might have clinical benefit that cannot occur once the airways are plugged with cellular debris.[27] This theory is supported by the considerably shorter duration of symptoms reported in the initial report showing decreased hospitalization following 1 mg/kg dexamethasone in the ED[25] compared with the subsequent larger multicenter study based on the same protocol (Table 18-1).[26] The mean duration of symptoms before treatment in the ED were 1.7 and 3.7 days, respectively. Thus, early in the course of bronchiolitis, inflammation may be susceptible to treatment by corticosteroids, whereas once there is extensive mechanical plugging of multiple airways from cellular debris, corticosteroids have little or no effect. However, other differences in participants in the 2 studies included a somewhat older mean age, 6.5 versus 5.1 months, in the initial study and a greater percentage with a family history of atopy in the initial study. It is conceivable that those variables might also contribute to a greater likelihood of response to systemic corticosteroids.

Antibiotics

While bronchiolitis is a potentially serious and occasionally life-threatening respiratory illness, the cause of bronchiolitis in an infant with a typical clinical presentation is a respiratory virus (Figure 18-2). As such, antibiotics are not of routine value for bronchiolitis.

Table 18-1. Differences Between 2 Studies of 1 mg/kg Dexamethasone on Presentation to an ED[a]

Characteristics	Schuh et al[b]	Multicenter[c]
No. of children	70	600
Mean age (months)	6.5	5.1
Hospitalized after 4 hours	Dex 19% Plac 44% (P = 0.03)	Dex 41% Plac 40% (P = 0.74)
Family history of atopy	Dex 83% Plac 53%	Dex 56% Plac 60%
Prior duration of symptoms (days)	Dex 1.7 Plac 1.8	Dex 3.7 Plac 3.8

Abbreviations: Dex, dexamethasone; ED, emergency department; Plac, placebo.
[a]The different outcomes were also associated with differences in the frequency of atopy in the family and in the duration of symptoms.
[b]Refers to the initial study by that author.[25]
[c]Refers to the subsequent large study attempting to reproduce the results of the Schuh study.[26]

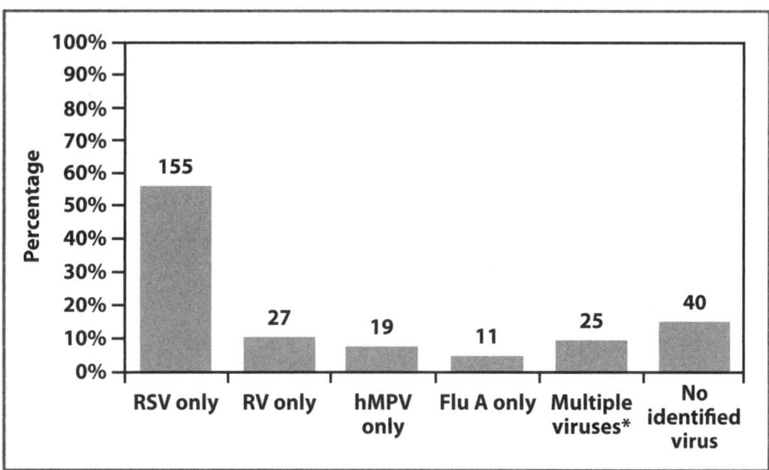

Figure 18-2. Viral causes of bronchiolitis in young children. Children younger than 2 years with the identified viruses present to an emergency department with bronchiolitis. The X axis represents the percentage of children with the identified virus. The number of children with the virus is indicated above the bar. RSV, respiratory syncytial virus; RV, rhinovirus; hMPV, human metapneumovirus; Flu A, influenza A.

*Multiple virus combinations included all possible combinations of 2 viruses and one patient with RSV, RV, and Flu A.

(From Mansbach JM, McAdam AJ, Clark S, et al. Prospective multicenter study of the viral etiology of bronchiolitis in the emergency department. *Soc Acad Emerg Med.* 2008;15:111–118, with permission from John Wiley & Sons, Inc.)

Consistent with the absence of a rationale for routine antibiotic use in infants with bronchiolitis, a Cochrane review concluded there was no evidence to support their use.[28] The most common indication for antibiotics was for urinary tract infections found in febrile RSV-positive infants during the first 2 months of life.[29]

Leukotriene Modifiers

An early report suggesting that montelukast provided benefit for post-RSV wheezing[30] was not supported by 2 subsequent trials that showed no benefit.[31,32] Based on the published data, there is no indication for treating bronchiolitis with leukotriene modifiers.

Antiviral Agents

While an antiviral agent, ribavirin (Virazole), has been marketed for RSV, its very modest effect[33] and the need for prolonged aerosol administration has resulted in limited use primarily to immunocompromised patients. Development of effective and safe orally administered antivirals would be of considerable benefit in the treatment and prevention of RSV for initial infections in infants at risk and perhaps also for repetitive episodes of asthma induced by RSV in young children with that predisposition. Multiple agents with high and selective viral inhibitory activity in cell culture with low cytotoxicity are in the discovery and preclinical stages, but none are yet approved by the US Food and Drug Administration.[34]

Hypertonic Saline

The Cochrane review of 4 studies concluded that 3% hypertonic saline aerosol improved the clinical course of bronchiolitis.[35] Using 0.9% saline as a control, clinical improvement was apparent during the first 3 days of treatment, and a mean difference in hospital stay of 0.94 days ($P = 0.00006$) was found for those who received 3% hypertonic saline 3 times daily. A subsequent study, also in hospitalized infants, supported the same degree of benefit.[36] While 1 of the 4 studies in the Cochrane review documented efficacy also in ambulatory patients, no decrease in the already low frequency of hospitalization was demonstrated, suggesting that the use of hypertonic saline was of questionable cost-effectiveness in patients not requiring hospitalization.[37]

Prophylaxis

Passive immunity is used for at least partial prophylaxis of bronchiolitis in high-risk infants. Double-blind studies of palivizumab have shown reduction in hospitalizations by about 50% for high-risk infants with prematurity, chronic lung disease, or congenital heart disease. Other products for passively administered anti-RSV antibody are at various stages of development.[34]

Hospitalization

Since bronchiolitis is generally a self-limited illness for which specific treatments are of unclear effectiveness, the primary reasons for admission are poor oral intake, dehydration, and concern that the degree of respiratory distress may result in respiratory failure and the need for assisted ventilation. If the caretakers are unable to assess the severity of illness or there is concern of their reliability to monitor the infant, then hospitalization may be indicated. The frequent use of pulse oximetry in office or ED assessment has been associated with an increase in the frequency of hospitalization for bronchiolitis because of the perceived need for supplemental oxygen.

If there is a concern regarding the potential for respiratory failure, hospitalization at a facility with a pediatric intensive care unit is the preferred site. The potential for respiratory failure can be assessed by the presence of hypoxemia detected by pulse oximetry and a blood gas (capillary or venous) indicating an increased $P\text{CO}_2$. Assessing $P\text{CO}_2$ is essential to distinguish $\dot{V}/\dot{Q}$ mismatching from respiratory failure that may require assisted ventilation.

In-Hospital Management

Since there is little documented evidence that pharmacologic measures have any clinically important effect on symptoms, length of stay, or duration of symptoms, treatment is predominantly supportive.[38,39] This includes oxygenation, hydration, and ventilation if needed. Not routinely indicated are chest radiography, which doesn't influence treatment, and testing for RSV antigen, since the clinical course and treatment are independent of which respiratory virus is causing the bronchiolitis. The recent data supporting the clinical effect of 3%

hypertonic saline indicate this treatment has the potential to somewhat decrease the duration of hospitalization.[35,36]

Evaluation for bacterial infection is rarely indicated but may be considered in select situations, such as temperature greater than 38°C, particularly in infants younger than 2 months. Chest physiotherapy and cool mist are not indicated. The scheduled use of bronchodilators, routine use of antibiotics, routine use of corticosteroids by any route, antihistamines, and decongestants are not indicated. Cardiorespiratory monitoring should be considered for all patients during the acute stage. Monitoring, including continuous oximetry, may be discontinued as status improves since excessive monitoring does not improve outcome and can prolong hospitalization.[40] Respiratory and contact isolation should be routine to prevent nosocomial spread of infection.

Discharge

Infants may be discharged when they are sufficiently comfortable to take full oral feeds for at least 12 hours, oxygenation when checked by pulse oximetry is at least 90%, and the social situation provides no concerns about care. Discharge instructions should include advice regarding tobacco smoke exposure and the risk of recurrent similar respiratory symptoms, especially if there is a family history of asthma or recurrent episodes of prolonged lower respiratory symptoms, cough, or labored breathing in the parents or siblings during preschool-aged years.

Key Points

- Respiratory Distress
  - Retraction
  - Tachypnea
  - Grunting
  - Cyanosis
- Decision to Hospitalize
  - Severe respiratory distress
  - Hypoxemia
  - Poor oral intake
  - Social situation
- Treatment and Monitoring
  - Measure pulse oximetry until clinically stable and then only spot checks with vital signs.
  - Bronchodilator, if given, may be albuterol or racemic epinephrine as a trial, but only with physician assessment of respiratory distress level before and after. If there is improvement, the bronchodilator can be repeated as needed.
  - Routine scheduled bronchodilators are not indicated.
  - Hydration and nutrition as needed.
- Criteria for Discharge
  - Oxygen saturation stable on room air ≥90% with normal to low $P{CO_2}$
  - Good oral intake
  - No social contraindications (distance from medical care and parental capability may delay discharge)
- Discharge Planning
  - Counseling regarding smoking cessation if needed
  - Counseling regarding risk for recurrent episodes (influenced by family history)

References

1. Shay DK, Holman RC, Newman RD, Liu LL, Stout JW, Anderson LJ. Bronchiolitis-associated hospitalizations. *JAMA.* 1999;282:1440–1446
2. Mansbach JM, McAdam AJ, Clark S, et al. Prospective multicenter study of the viral etiology of bronchiolitis in the emergency department. *Acad Emerg Med.* 2008;15:111–117
3. Holman RC, Curns AT, Cheek JE, et al. Respiratory syncytial virus hospitalizations among American Indian and Alaska native infants and the general United States infant population. *Pediatrics.* 2004;114:e437–e444
4. Canducci F, Debiaggi M, Samaolo M, et al. Two-year prospective study of single infections and co-infections by respiratory syncytial virus and viruses identified recently in infants with acute respiratory disease. *J Med Virol.* 2008;80:716–723
5. Fowlkes AL, Fry AM, Anderson LJ. Respiratory syncytial virus activity—United States, 2005–2006. *MMWR Morb Mortal Wkly Rep.* 2006;55:1277–1279
6. Schuh S, Lalani A, Allen U, Manson D, Babyn P, Stephens D. Evaluation of the utility of radiography in acute bronchiolitis. *J Pediatr.* 2007;150(4):429–433
7. Weinberger M. Clinical patterns and natural history of asthma. *J Pediatr.* 2003;142:S15–S20
8. Weinberger M, Solé D. The natural history of childhood asthma. In: Pawankar R, Holgate S, Rosenwaser L, eds. *Allergy Frontiers: Epigenetics to Future Perspectives.* Vol 5. New York, NY: Springer; 2010:511–530
9. Janssen R, Bont L, Siezen CLE, et al. Genetic susceptibility to respiratory syncytial virus bronchiolitis is predominantly associated with innate immune genes. *J Infect Dis.* 2007;196:826–834
10. Smyth RL. Innate immunity in respiratory syncytial virus bronchiolitis. *Exp Lung Res.* 2008;33:543–547
11. Hayley S, Wark P. Innate immune response to viral infection of the lungs. *Paediatr Respir Rev.* 2008;9:243–250
12. Gürkan F, Kiral A, Dağli E, Karakoç F. The effect of passive smoking on the development of respiratory syncytial virus bronchiolitis. *Eur J Epidemiol.* 2000;16:465–468
13. Bradley JP, Bacharier LB, Bonfiglio J, et al. Severity of respiratory syncytial virus bronchiolitis is affected by cigarette smoke exposure and atopy. *Pediatrics.* 2005;115:e7–e14
14. Carroll KN, Gebretsadik T, Griffin MR, et al. Maternal asthma and maternal smoking are associated with increased risk of bronchiolitis during infancy. *Pediatrics.* 2007;119:1104–1112
15. Harling L, Wiebe N, Russel K, Patel H, Klassen TP. A meta-analysis of randomized controlled trials evaluating the efficacy of epinephrine for the treatment of acute viral bronchiolitis. *Arch Pediatr Adolesc Med.* 2003;157:956–964

16. Van Woensel JBM, Wolfs RFW, van Aalderen WMC, Brand PLP, Kimpen JLL. Randomized double blind placebo controlled trial of prednisolone in children admitted to hospital with respiratory syncytial virus bronchiolitis. *Thorax.* 1997;52:634–637
17. Dabbous IA, Tkachyk JS, Stamm SJ. A double blind study on the effects of corticosteroids in the treatment of bronchiolitis. *Pediatrics.* 1966;37:477–484
18. Springer C, Bar-Yishay E, Uwayyed K, Avital A, Vilozni D, Godfrey S. Corticosteroids do not affect the clinical or physiological status of infants with bronchiolitis. *Pediatr Pulmonol.* 1990;9:181–185
19. Roosevelt G, Sheeehan K, Grupp-Phelan J, Tanz RR, Listernick R. Dexamethasone in bronchiolitis: a randomized controlled trial. *Lancet.* 1996;348:292–295
20. Klassen TP, Sutcliffe T, Watters LK, Wells GA, Allen UD, Li MM. Dexamethasone in salbutamol-treated inpatients with acute bronchiolitis: a randomized, controlled trial. *J Pediatr.* 1997;130:191–196
21. De Boeck K, Van der Aa N, Van Lierde S, Corbeel L, Eeckels R. Respiratory syncytial virus bronchiolitis: a double-blind dexamethasone efficacy study. *J Pediatr.* 1997;131:919–921
22. Garrison MM, Christakis DA, Harvey E, Cummings P, Davis RL. Systemic corticosteroids in infant bronchiolitis: a meta-analysis. *Pediatrics.* 2000;105:e44
23. Goebel J, Estrada B, Quinonez J, Nagji N, Sanford D, Boerth RC. Prednisolone plus albuterol versus albuterol alone in mild to moderate bronchiolitis. *Clin Pediatr.* 2000;39:213–220
24. Csonka P, Kaila M, Laippala P, Iso-Mustajärvi M, Vesikari T, Ashorn P. Oral prednisolone in the acute management of children age 6 to 35 months with viral respiratory infection-induced lower airway disease: a randomized, placebo-controlled trial. *J Pediatr.* 2003;143:725–730
25. Schuh S, Coates AL, Binnie R, et al. Efficacy of oral dexamethasone in outpatients with acute bronchiolitis. *J Pediatr.* 2002;140;27–32
26. Corneli HM, Zorc JJ, Majahan P, et al. A multicenter, randomized controlled trial of dexamethasone for bronchiolitis. *N Engl J Med.* 2007;357:331–339
27. Weinberger M. Should corticosteroids be used for first-time young wheezers? *J Allergy Clin Immunol.* 2007;119:567–569
28. Spurling GK, Fonseka K, Doust J, Del Mar C. Antibiotics for bronchiolitis in children. *Cochrane Database Syst Rev.* 2007;(1):CD005189
29. Levine DA, Platt SL, Dayan PS, et al. Risk of serious bacterial infection in young febrile infants with respiratory syncytial virus infections. *Pediatrics.* 2004;113:1728–1734
30. Bisgaard H. A randomized trial of montelukast in respiratory syncytial virus postbronchiolitis. *Am J Respir Crit Care Med.* 2004;169:542–543
31. Bisgaard H, Flores-Nunez A, Goh A, et al. Study of montelukast for the treatment of respiratory symptoms of post-respiratory syncytial virus bronchiolitis in children. *Am J Respir Crit Care Med.* 2008;178:854–860

32. Amirav I, Luder AS, Kruger N. A double-blind, placebo-controlled, randomized trial of montelukast for acute bronchiolitis. *Pediatrics.* 2008;122:e1249–e1255
33. Ventre K, Randolph AG. Ribavirin for respiratory syncytial virus infection of the lower respiratory tract in infants and young children. *Cochrane Database Syst Rev.* 2007;(1):CD000181
34. Maggon K, Barik S. New drugs and treatment for respiratory syncytial virus. *Rev Med Virol.* 2004;14:149–168
35. Zhang L, Mendoza-Sassi RA, Wainwright C, Klassen TP. Nebulized hypertonic solution for acute bronchiolitis in infants (review). *Cochrane Database Syst Rev.* 2008;(4):CD006458
36. Luo Z, Liu E, Luo J, et al. Nebulized hypertonic saline/salbutamol solution treatment in hospitalized children with mild to moderate bronchiolitis. *Pediatr Int.* 2010;52:199–202
37. Sarrell EM, Tal G, Witzling M, et al. Nebulized 3% hypertonic saline solution treatment in ambulatory children with viral bronchiolitis decreases symptoms. *Chest.* 2002;122;2015–2020
38. American Academy of Pediatrics Subcommittee on Diagnosis and Management of Bronchiolitis. Diagnosis and management of bronchiolitis. *Pediatrics.* 2006;118:1774–1793
39. Yanney MP, Vyas HG. The treatment of bronchiolitis. *Arch Dis Child.* 2008;93:793–798
40. Schroeder AR, Marmor AK, Pantell RH, Newman TB. Impact of pulse oximetry and oxygen therapy on length of stay in bronchiolitis hospitalization. *Arch Pediatr Adolesc Med.* 2004;158:527–530

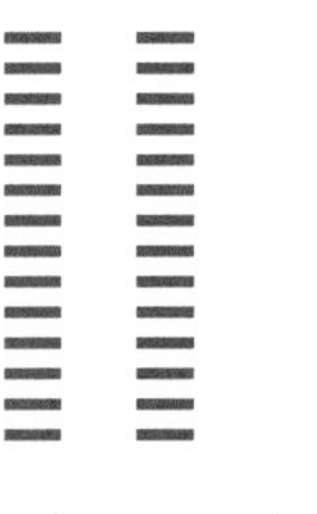

Chapter 19

Pneumonia

Michael J. Light, MD

Introduction

Community-acquired pneumonia (CAP) is a common problem worldwide and causes considerable mortality. In North America, the annual incidence is reported to be 34 to 40 cases per 1,000 in children younger than 5 years. The incidence among adolescents is about 7 per 1,000 between 12 and 15 years of age. In developing countries pneumonia is even more common. The mortality rates are high, with 4 million deaths per year, which means pneumonia is the number one cause of death in adolescents in developing countries.

Community-acquired pneumonia is defined as pneumonia that is acquired outside the hospital environment, whereas nosocomial pneumonia is that which is acquired in the hospital environment. The diagnosis of pneumonia is usually made on the basis of signs and symptoms and supported by a radiologic diagnosis. The World Health Organization (WHO) has defined pneumonia on the basis of the clinical findings because chest radiology is not readily accessible in many parts of the world.[1]

The agents that cause pneumonia are varied and include bacteria, viruses, fungi, and protozoal organisms. It can also be caused by aspiration and exposure to toxic substances, for example chlorine.

Pathology

The pathology of pneumonia is described as either

- Lobar
- Bronchopneumonia
- Interstitial
- Miliary

Lobar pneumonia has 4 stages. The initial stage is congestion, where the alveoli are filled with fibrinous fluid, neutrophils, and bacteria. This stage occurs within 24 hours of infection. The second stage usually occurs on days 2 to 3 and is called red hepatization. The lung reddens and is of the consistency of liver. The alveoli are filled with fibrinous inflammatory exudates with increased numbers of neutrophils, and red cells that contribute to the color. The consolidated lobe is airless and evident on chest radiography. The pleura is usually thickened and a pleural rub may be heard. The next stage is called grey hepatization, where the alveoli are filled with fibrin threads and neutrophils and the red cells are much fewer in number. The lung is still stiff and the alveolar walls are thickened and fibrosed. The fourth stage is that of resolution as the inflammatory exudates are resorbed.

Bronchopneumonia is more patchy and, as the name suggests, there is suppurative inflammation of the bronchi and surrounding alveoli. The exudates fill bronchi and bronchioles and affect the adjacent alveoli while the distant alveoli may be free of exudates. The patchy consolidation may affect one or several lobes and is usually bilateral. The lobes more involved include the dependent lung zones and the bases.

Interstitial pneumonia results from inflammation that is within the alveolar wall rather than the alveolar air space. The infiltrate tends to be lymphocytes and macrophages, and hyaline membranes may line the alveolar spaces.

An additional category is miliary, which occurs with hematogenous spread to the lung, which leads to multiple discrete lesions often throughout both lungs.

Bacterial pneumonia often follows a viral upper respiratory infection. Lobar pneumonia is most commonly bacterial, including atypical bacteria. Bronchopneumonia may be bacterial, atypical, or viral. Interstitial pneumonia may result from measles and pertussis, as well as noninfectious causes including aspiration. Miliary pulmonary infection is most commonly seen in tuberculosis, histoplasmosis, and coccidioidomycosis. Immunocompromised patients are at risk for miliary herpesvirus, cytomegalovirus, or varicella-zoster virus.

Etiology

It is difficult to study the causes of pneumonia because there is so much diversity in the causes, and what is found in one community may not apply to another community. A study of 154 hospitalized children with CAP looking carefully for etiology showed that it was caused by identifiable bacteria in approximately 60% of cases, of which 73% were caused by *Streptococcus pneumoniae*. A viral etiology was found in 45% of cases, and of these 23% had concurrent bacterial and viral disease. They also found *Mycoplasma* sp. in 14% and *Chlamydophila (Chlamydia) pneumoniae* in 9%.[2]

Clinical Features

The symptoms and signs of pneumonia vary from subtle to highly suspicious. Table 19-1 shows age-related symptoms and signs that suggest the diagnosis of pneumonia. In a pediatric emergency department study in the United States, the finding of respiratory rate alone and clinical impression of tachypnea did not discriminate between those who had radiographic evidence of pneumonia and those who did not, whereas the children who exceeded the WHO respiratory rate thresholds were more likely to have pneumonia.[3] The most common presentation is cough and fever, which is very nonspecific. The appearance of the child is important with signs of respiratory distress, including

Table 19-1. Symptoms and Signs of Pneumonia

	≤2 months	2–12 months	1–5 years	>5 years
Respiratory rate WHO threshold	≥60/min	≥50/min	≥40/min	≥30/min
Symptoms and signs	Cough Poor feeding Apnea Tachypnea Grunting Nasal flaring Retractions	Cough Fever Poor feeding Tachypnea Grunting Rhinorrhea Nasal flaring Retractions	Cough Fever Rhinorrhea Chest pain Tachypnea Retractions	Cough Fever Headache Pleuritic pain Abdominal pain Tachypnea Retractions
Auscultation	Crackles Wheeze	Wheeze Crackles	Crackles Wheeze Pleural rub	Crackles Wheeze Pleural rub

Abbreviation: WHO, World Health Organization.

retractions and nasal flaring, and abnormal auscultation will aid the clinician in arriving at the diagnosis of pneumonia.

Diagnosis

The microbiological diagnosis of pneumonia is difficult to prove in many cases without extensive investigation. The age of the child will suggest the most likely etiology, and it is also helpful to be aware of which organisms are in the community at the time. Pneumonia in the pediatric population is most common in infants and toddlers and least common in adolescents.

Box 19-1 lists the more likely cause of pneumonia based on age.

Infants to School Age (1–4 Years of Age)

After 1 month of age cough is the most common presentation of pneumonia. A viral upper respiratory illness commonly precedes the pneumonia. If the pneumonia is bacterial a significant fever is usually present, whereas in viral or atypical infections the fever may be low-grade. Generally, though, the height of the fever is a poor indicator of etiology. Most cases of pneumonia are viral, and respiratory syncytial virus (RSV) is the most common pathogen. Although RSV principally causes bronchiolitis, it is also a common cause of pneumonia. After 2 years of age RSV does not cause lower respiratory tract infection except in immunocompromised (especially transplant) patients. Parainfluenza type 3 occurs year-round, with peaks in the spring, and types 1 and 2 are typically seen in the fall.

Box 19-1. Age-Related Etiology of Pneumonia in the Immunocompetent Child

≤2 Months	2–12 Months	1–4 Years	5–12 Years	≥12 Years
Group B streptococcus	Pneumococcus	Pneumococcus	Mycoplasma	Mycoplasma
Pneumococcus	RSV	Parainfluenza	Pneumococcus	*Chlamydophila pneumoniae*
Staphylococcus aureus	Parainfluenza	Influenza	Group A streptococcus	Pneumococcus
Listeria monocytogenes	Influenza	Adenovirus	Viruses	Group A streptococcus
	Adenovirus	RSV		Viruses
	hMPV	hMPV		
	Chlamydia trachomatis	Mycoplasma		
	Pertussis			

Abbreviations: hMPV, human metapneumovirus; RSV, respiratory syncytial virus.

From 5 Years of Age to Adolescence

The most common cause of bacterial pneumonia is *S pneumoniae,* but mycoplasma is increasingly being diagnosed as the cause of CAP. Group A streptococcus is also increasingly being diagnosed. Various viruses cause pneumonia, including adenovirus, influenza, parainfluenza, and RSV (in the immunocompromised and transplant patient).

Laboratory Findings

As previously noted, the diagnosis of pneumonia is clinical and is supported by the radiographic changes if an x-ray is performed. Laboratory investigation is usually of limited value in the outpatient evaluation of a child with pneumonia.

Complete blood cell count may reveal an elevated white count greater than 20,000 with pneumococcal pneumonia. Atypical lymphocytes may be found with viral infections, but the finding is nonspecific. It is not considered essential to attempt to find the etiologic agent routinely in children who have been previously well. Pneumonia in children does not usually have bacteremia, and blood culture is not routinely required in immunocompetent children unless they are hospitalized.[4] If the child is critically ill or immunocompromised, blood culture is more likely to be positive. Sputum culture, including Gram stain, and sensitivity may be considered in the older child. If the child does not respond to initial therapy within 72 hours or if there is a rapid progression of symptoms, further testing may be indicated.

Elevation of C-reactive protein may predict more severe disease, but it does not differentiate bacterial from viral pneumonia.

If the child has a pleural effusion and has not received antibiotics, a pleural tap should be considered. If antibiotics have been given, the yield from pleural tap is low. Polymerase chain reaction (PCR), if available, may be helpful with further etiologic diagnosis.

Imaging

The standard imaging for diagnosis of pneumonia is 2-view plain chest radiograph. It is not possible to differentiate between viral or bacterial disease.[5] Lobar pneumonia, with disease restricted to the involved lobe, may be suspicious for bacterial pneumonia. Perihilar scattered infiltrates, hyperinflation, and hilar adenopathy are more likely in viral pneumonia than bacterial pneumonia. Round pneumonia, seen in younger children, is likely of bacterial etiology, including *S pneumoniae*, *Staphylococcus aureus* and *Klebsiella* sp. A computed tomography (CT) scan or ultrasound is indicated if there are complications, as discussed in Chapter 7, Chapter 20, and Chapter 28.

Bacterial Causes of Pneumonia

Bacterial pneumonia is an important cause of death if untreated, especially in developing countries. Although most children with bacterial pneumonia improve without sequelae, children with a preexisting condition may be at increased risk for morbidity, including subsequent infections because of scarring in the lungs. The immune status of the child also impacts the risk of mortality and morbidity.

Gram-positive

Pneumococcus

Streptococcus pneumoniae was the most common bacterial cause of lower respiratory infection before the institution of the pneumococcal vaccine in 2000. Since 2000 there has been a reduction of invasive pneumococcal disease by 80% for children younger than 2 years, and this finding may increase since 13-valent pneumococcal conjugate vaccine (PCV) replaced PCV-7 in the routine childhood immunization schedule and became available in 2010.[6] Surveillance is also indicated for non-vaccine serotypes. Although invasive pneumococcal disease has decreased, complicated pneumonia has increased significantly across the United States,[7] and these cases tend to be due to non-vaccine serotypes.

Pneumococci are gram-positive diplococci, and many people are colonized in the upper respiratory tract. Transmission is by droplet, and the incubation period is short (sometimes 1–3 days). Populations at more risk for invasive pneumococcal disease (pneumonia, meningitis, and sepsis) are shown in Box 19-2.

Pneumococcal pneumonia may be preceded by a mild upper respiratory infection. Infants may present with a sudden rise in fever, possibly a seizure, and diarrhea and vomiting. Cough may be absent, but evidence of respiratory distress includes tachypnea, nasal flaring, and perioral cyanosis. The older child usually presents with fever, chills, dyspnea, and pleuritic chest pain. Older children may have sputum production, and streaks of blood may be apparent in the sputum.

Box 19-2. Children at Increased Risk for Invasive Pneumococcal Disease

- Children younger than 36 months
- Children with sickle cell disease
- Children with asplenia
- Children with HIV
- Children with cochlear implants
- Children with chronic disease including asthma, immune deficiency (including transplants), cardiac disease, pulmonary disease, renal insufficiency, and diabetes mellitus are at presumed high risk but the data are insufficient to calculate rates.

Examination of the chest may not be abnormal in the infant and small child. The older child will usually demonstrate crackles and dullness to percussion with bronchial breathing over the involved lobe. Friction rub is not often elicited. Abdominal pain in the older child is a common symptom.

Laboratory findings also are not consistent. Although not recommended in the outpatient setting, a white blood cell count over 20,000/μL with the clinical picture of pneumonia is certainly suspicious of pneumococcal disease. The yield from blood culture is low but the sputum findings of many polymorphonuclear leukocytes with gram-positive diplococci is almost diagnostic. Young age is a barrier to sputum collection. Antigen detection is not considered useful for diagnosis except for pleural fluid.

The chest radiograph in children with pneumococcal pneumonia may initially demonstrate a lobar pattern and then extend beyond the lobar boundaries. It is the most common cause of "round pneumonia" pattern. On occasion, the markings may be patchy or interstitial. As discussed in Chapter 7, the chest radiograph is not consistently able to confirm the diagnosis of a bacterial or viral pneumonia because of the overlap between findings.

The clinical course of pneumococcal pneumonia is usually rapid, with response to antibiotics causing reduction of fever within a few hours. In children with CAP proven or suspected to be of bacterial origin who are treated as outpatients, amoxicillin or amoxicillin-clavulanate is recommended. In school-aged children (>5 years), the addition of a macrolide for coverage of atypical organisms is advised. In children ill enough to warrant hospitalization, the use of penicillin, or ceftriaxone and the addition of a macrolide is usually appropriate, and decisions for therapy should take into account local resistance patterns and immunization history. Complications may be systemic, with meningitis, carditis, peritonitis, and septic arthritis resulting from bacteremia. Pulmonary complications include pleural effusion and empyema. Inappropriate secretion of antidiuretic hormone is common and may cause significant reduction of serum sodium.

Group A Streptococcus

Also known as *Streptococcus pyogenes*, group A ß-hemolytic streptococcus is an uncommon etiology for pneumonia. It is important because the clinical course is aggressive and may result in necrotizing pneumonia. The clinical appearance of the child is that of fever, chills, lethargy, cough, and dyspnea. The most common radiographic pattern is a patchy bronchopneumonia, but in a minority of cases there is lobar consolidation. Cavitation may occur, as well as pleural effusion with progression to fibrinopurulent empyema.

The response to antibiotics tends to be slow, even with sensitive organisms. Complications are common and include pneumothorax, pneumatoceles, bronchiectasis, and bronchopleural fistula. Penicillin is the treatment of choice, although ampicillin is an alternative.

Staphylococcal Pneumonia

Staphylococcus aureus is an uncommon cause of pneumonia in immunocompetent children, but it does occur in infancy. It also occurs more commonly after influenza infection and other upper respiratory viral infections. Staphylococci are gram-positive organisms that occur in clusters. Pneumonia results from inhalation of organisms or from bacteremic spread. The clinical picture varies from a mild respiratory infection with fever, cough, and tachypnea to a rapidly progressive illness with dyspnea, cyanosis, and septic shock. The initial radiographic appearance is multiple nodular infiltrates, usually unilateral, which in a few days become cavitary and, subsequently, pneumatoceles form. Pneumothorax is common, especially in ventilated infants, and empyema is present in most cases.

The scenario described in the previous paragraph would be likely diagnosed as *S aureus* in an infant, but if the same findings were present in an older child other organisms would be more likely, including

Escherichia coli, Pseudomonas, or *Klebsiella.* It is likely that the relative prevalence from pneumococcus to *S aureus* is increasing in older children and that there are increasing numbers of children with pneumonia caused by methicillin-resistant *S aureus* (MRSA).[8,9] Schultz et al also compared complications between MRSA and methicillin-sensitive *S aureus* and found similar complication rates.[8]

If staphylococcal pneumonia is suspected, the increased prevalence of MRSA may require vancomycin or clindamycin for initial treatment until the sensitivities are known.

Gram-negative

Pseudomonas aeruginosa

Pseudomonas is a gram-negative bacterium that has a predilection to moist environments. It is common to acquire *Pseudomonas* with colonization in more than 50% of humans, and *Pseudomonas* often causes nosocomial infection. It is an unusual cause of pneumonia in healthy children. Pneumonia caused by *Pseudomonas* is a common complication of patients with endotracheal tubes or tracheostomy. It is the dominant organism in cystic fibrosis (CF). It occurs more frequently in children with HIV infection, neutropenia, and complement deficiency[10] and those who are immunosuppressed. It is the most common cause of pneumonia in the intensive care environment. It has been reported following exposure in hot tub spas.

Although the typical color of sputum produced in pseudomonal pneumonia is green, this color may be seen with pneumococcal and *Haemophilus* infections. The progression of *Pseudomonas* pneumonia to necrotizing bronchopneumonia may be rapid if untreated. Pleural effusion is common and the pneumonia may have a lobar or diffuse bilateral bronchopneumonia radiographic pattern.

Treatment of *Pseudomonas* pneumonia should be with 2 antibiotics, usually an aminoglycoside and a ß-lactam antibiotic. For children with chronic *Pseudomonas* infection there is a major problem of resistance to antibiotics, especially those with CF.

Burkholderia cepacia

Pseudomonas cepacia was described initially by Walter Burkholder in 1949 and is now named *Burkholderia cepacia.* It is an important pathogen in CF causing pneumonia and has been reported to cause pneumonia in immunocompromised patients. *Burkholderia cepacia* does not cause pneumonia in healthy children.

Klebsiella Pneumonia

Klebsiella pneumoniae is a gram-negative rod-shaped bacillus, and clinically the most important member of the *Klebsiella* genus of Enterobacteriaceae.

Clinical Features

Pneumonia as a result of *K pneumoniae* is typically a nosocomial infection. It may also be community-acquired, although rare in otherwise healthy children. Pneumonia tends to occur in immunocompromised or debilitated children. It is associated with an acute onset with fever and chills. The cough is productive and yields abundant thick sputum that is typically blood-tinged and is known as red currant jelly sputum. Pneumonia is usually complicated, and abscess formation, cavitation, and empyema are common. Infection is more commonly unilateral, occurring typically in the upper lobes.

Management

Hospitalization is indicated, including for CAP, because even with treatment there is significant mortality. Many *Klebsiella* organisms are resistant to multiple bacteria so, rather than monotherapy, multiple antibiotics are indicated until antibiotic sensitivities are available. The potential choice is wide, including third generation cephalosporins (eg, cefotaxime or ceftriaxone), carbapenems (eg, meropenem), aminoglycosides, and quinolones. Infectious disease consultation is recommended.

Legionella Pneumonia

Legionnaires' disease was first recognized in 1976 at an American Legion convention in Philadelphia. The organism that caused an outbreak of pneumonia was identified as a gram-negative bacillus, *Legionella pneumophila*. While an unusual cause of pneumonia in children, it is important to recognize. It is more common in children who are immunosuppressed, and more than one-third of children in pediatric cases have been younger than 1 year. Transmission occurs by aerosolization and inhalation or aspiration of water containing the organism. It has been linked to contaminated water in hospitals and respiratory therapy equipment, as well as cooling towers; central air conditioning systems; evaporative coolers; hot water systems, including showers and hot tub spas; and ice-making machines. The disease is particularly prevalent in hotels, cruise ships, and hospitals that have outdated cooling systems. The incubation period is 2 to 10 days, and for milder disease, Pontiac fever, the incubation period is 1 to 2 days.

Clinical Features

Legionnaires' disease presents with fever, chills, and cough, which is initially nonproductive. Constitutional symptoms include headache, muscle ache, and sometimes ataxia (loss of coordination) and diarrhea or vomiting. The lung examination typically reveals crackles.

Blood test may reveal abnormal hepatic or renal function, and hyponatremia is common. Chest radiograph typically shows unilateral or bilateral bronchopneumonia.

Management

Clues to the diagnosis are the constitutional symptoms and the laboratory abnormalities including hyponatremia. Detection of *L pneumophila* serogroup 1 is aided by detecting *Legionella* antigen in the urine.

Azithromycin is the drug of choice for children with suspected or confirmed *Legionella* pneumonia. It is initially recommended to give azithromycin intravenously, converting to orally when the child responds. If disease is severe or unresponsive to treatment, addition of rifampin is recommended. Fluoroquinolones are bactericidal and can be used in adolescents and adults.

Anaerobic Organisms

The most common anaerobic gram-negative bacilli (AGNB) to cause pneumonia are the pigmented *Prevotella* spp. The *Prevotella* spp. are important components of the bacterial florae of the mouth, nose, and nasopharynx. They are not often cultured because of the difficulty in specimen collection and growing in the microbiology laboratory. Anaerobic organisms are common causes of chronic sinusitis, chronic mastoiditis, chronic otitis media, and retropharyngeal abscess.

Pneumonia caused by anerobic organisms results from aspiration of upper airway or gastric secretions. Severe gingival disease is a risk factor. Following aspiration there may be progression from pneumonia to necrotizing pneumonia, and AGNB is an important cause of lung abscess.[11] Frequently, AGNB may be recovered in culture along with Enterobacteriacae, *Pseudomonas,* and *S aureus.*

The *Prevotella* are resistant to penicillin and typically susceptible to metronidazole and carbapenems.

Atypical Pneumonia

The term atypical pneumonia is applied because the organism that causes the pneumonia does not fit the category of bacteria or viruses. The agents that cause atypical pneumonia include *Mycoplasma pneumoniae, Chlamydia trachomatis, Chlamydophila pneumoniae,* and *Chlamydophila psittaci.*

Mycoplasma

Mycoplasma pneumoniae is the commonest cause of community-acquired pneumonia in children older than 5 years, often called "walking pneumonia." It is not rare in children younger than 5 years.[12] The true incidence is unknown because many cases are treated empirically without confirmation of the diagnosis. There are no geographic limitations, and infection occurs year-round. There may be epidemics every 3 to 7 years, and outbreaks occur in schools and universities.

Mycoplasma pneumoniae is called mycoplasma because of the plasticity of the bacterial forms, which resemble fungal elements. Instead of a cell wall there is a cell membrane containing sterols, which are not present in bacteria or viruses. Unlike viruses they do not require a cell to replicate and can grow in cell-free media, and they contain both RNA and DNA.

Clinical Features

Mycoplasma pneumoniae infections usually start with an upper respiratory infection (URI) with pharyngitis, cough, headache, and myalgias. There may be fever, which is usually less than 102°F. The cough is initially nonproductive and can be severe and debilitating. Blood streaking of the sputum is not uncommon, and the coughing may cause chest pain that is non-pleuritic. In 5% to 10% of children the URI progresses to bronchitis or pneumonia. Pleural effusion occurs in 5% to 20% of patients. Cutaneous manifestations are common and include macular-papular rash and erythema nodosum. Extrapulmonary symptoms are not uncommon and include bullous myringitis, which supports the diagnosis of mycoplasma.

In sickle cell anemia the mycoplasma infection may be severe and is considered an important cause of acute chest syndrome.[13] It also can be severe in Down syndrome, especially in those with congenital cardiac disease. Both mycoplasma and chlamydophila cause exacerbations of asthma in children and adolescents.

The physical examination usually reveals oropharyngeal inflammation. The chest examination may be relatively benign, with few crackles and rhonchi, at the same time that a chest radiograph shows significant findings of pneumonia. Wheezing may occur, particularly if the child has asthma.

Laboratory

Cold agglutinins are not recommended to confirm the diagnosis as they are nonspecific (about 75%). Mycoplasma immunoglobulin (Ig) M and IgG may be useful to confirm the diagnosis, with sensitivity approximately 98% if both are done. Immunoglobulin M may be negative in the first week of illness, and may be indicative of past infection.[12] It is likely that in the future, diagnosis using PCR will be available clinically, which will expedite the results.

Imaging

Infiltrates are more likely to be bilateral than unilateral. There may be lobar, multifocal, or diffuse disease with reticular infiltrates.[11] Pleural effusions are present in about 20%, and hilar adenopathy is seen in 7% to 22%.

Management

Recommended treatment for mycoplasma pneumonia is macrolide antibiotics, although there are now reports of macrolide resistance. Tetracycline is active, in particular doxycycline, and can be used for adolescents, but not for children younger than 8 years. The newer fluoroquinolones are effective, but not as effective as macrolides.

The lack of cell wall predicts that ß-lactams are not effective, nor is trimethoprim. Most cases of CAP improve in a matter of days with no residual findings.

Chlamydia trachomatis

Chlamydia trachomatis is an important cause of sexually transmitted infection and trachoma. Although uncommon in the United States, trachoma is the most common cause of blindness in the world. *C trachomatis* causes pneumonia, especially in infants. Approximately 5% to 22% of pregnant women have *C trachomatis* of the cervix, and 30% to 50% of these will show culture evidence of infection. The infection in the newborn is conjunctivitis with or without nasopharyngitis, which in some cases results in neonatal pneumonia.

Clinical Features

Most infants with *C trachomatis* pneumonia have a history of conjunctivitis, nasal stuffiness, and cough with tachypnea. This pneumonia is characteristically afebrile. The chest examination reveals scattered crackles; wheezing is absent.

Imaging

The chest radiograph is either a lobar or interstitial pattern.

Management

The recommendation to treat infants with *C trachomatis* pneumonia is erythromycin 50 mg/kg/day divided by 4 for 14 days.

Chlamydophila psittaci

Chlamydophila psittaci causes psittacosis or ornithosis following exposure to infected birds. Ornithosis is the preferred name because it can be caused by any bird, including parrots, chickens, ducks, turkeys, pigeons, and sparrows. It is transmitted from birds to humans by either direct contact or aerosolization. It is much less common since the imposition of quarantine for a period of 30 days for imported birds and the introduction of bird feed laced with antibiotics.

It is quite difficult to diagnose and it is possible that it is more common than appreciated. The most common disease is a mild pneumonia, but it can produce a more fulminant illness. There is fever without elevation of the pulse, which is usually associated with fever. The clues to the diagnosis include splenomegaly, a blanching erythematous maculopapular rash, and signs of hepatitis, disseminated intravascular coagulation, or meningoencephalitis, any of which may be present.

Chlamydophila pneumoniae

Chlamydophila pneumoniae causes a mild pneumonia or bronchitis in older children, adolescents, and adults. Approximately 50% of young adults have serologic evidence of prior infection. *Chlamydophila pneumoniae* is estimated to cause 10% to 20% of CAP. It is transmitted from person to person by respiratory secretion transfer. The incubation period is approximately 3 to 4 weeks.

Initially there is an upper respiratory infection, and many have no further symptoms. The symptoms can be prolonged, and helpful in the diagnosis is the presence of hoarseness and headache; fever is uncommon. The physical examination reveals crackles and rhonchi. Even with treatment, *C pneumoniae* tends to respond more slowly than mycoplasma, which may also be a clue to the diagnosis. It also tends to recur if therapy is stopped too early. Mortality of 9.8% has been reported in patients with sickle cell disease.[13]

Other Causes of Bacterial Pneumonia

Tularemia, anthrax, and plague are uncommon bacterial syndromes in which pneumonia may be a prominent feature; they should raise the suspicion of bioterrorism.

Viral Causes of Pneumonia

Viral infections are the most common cause of symptomatic disease in children. The number of respiratory infections per year may be 5 to 10 or even more, with most being upper respiratory infections. Most cases of pneumonia are diagnosed clinically, but there is an increasing ability to find an etiologic agent as new biotechnology facilitates the diagnosis of viral infections. As noted previously, secondary bacterial infection occurs in about one-third of cases of viral pneumonia. Although immunocompromised children are at higher risk for the opportunistic infections, such as cytomegalovirus, varicella-zoster virus, herpes, and measles, they are also at risk of seasonal pneumonias, including RSV, influenza, and parainfluenza. The symptoms of viral pneumonia are similar to bacterial pneumonia, although there is less chest pain or rigors with viral pneumonia.

Respiratory Syncytial Virus

Respiratory syncytial virus is the most important cause of lower respiratory infection in the first 2 years of life. By 2 years of age, more than 94% of children will have serologic evidence of RSV infection. During the RSV season, RSV will be the cause of more than 90% of infants hospitalized with bronchiolitis. The differentiation between bronchiolitis and pneumonia can be difficult, so the designation of lower respiratory tract infection due to RSV may be easier than trying to define whether there is one or both diagnoses. Infants with RSV pneumonia tend to have less wheezing, less hyperinflation, and more crackles.

The clinical scenario is similar to bronchiolitis (see Chapter 18), with an upper respiratory prodrome followed by worsening cough and increasing respiratory distress. As noted, wheezing tends to be less prominent and there may be crackles on examination. The radiographic appearance of lobar consolidation (especially right upper lobe) or a bronchopneumonia pattern supports the diagnosis of pneumonia.

Most infants with RSV pneumonia recover in a few days, but a small percentage progress to respiratory failure. Infants younger than 2 months and those with significant respiratory distress or apnea should be hospitalized.

Influenza Virus

The influenza virus is a single-stranded RNA virus that is a common cause of pneumonia, especially in the very young and very old. It occurs in epidemic form in the winter months, and chronically ill children are at more risk for serious illness. Pandemics in the last 100 years include the 1918–1919 Spanish pandemic (influenza virus subtype H1), the 1957 pandemic (subtype H2N2), the 1968–1969 pandemic (Hong Kong subtype H3N2), the Russian pandemic in 1977 (subtype H1N1), and the novel influenza A (H1N1) pandemic of 2009–2010 . The incubation period is 1 to 5 days following exposure to the virus.

The presentation of influenza is characteristic with high fever, chills, muscle aches, and headache, although young children may have more nonspecific symptoms. The illness starts as an upper respiratory infection with rhinitis, pharyngitis, and initially nonproductive cough. Young children may also have conjunctivitis and gastrointestinal symptoms. Pneumonia is associated with increasing respiratory symptoms and hypoxemia. Secondary bacterial infection is common following influenza pneumonia.

Positive A or B influenza virus can be determined by immunofluorescence or hemagglutination techniques, although during the recent H1N1 pandemic these tests were not very helpful in diagnosis.

Symptoms last for several days and are treated with over-the-counter medications. Aspirin is not recommended because of the association with Reye syndrome.

Oseltamivir (Tamiflu) is approved for oral administration in persons older than 1 year with influenza A or B who have been symptomatic for no more than 2 days. Most recently Tamiflu can be given to infants younger than 1 year with reduced dosage. Neither zanamivir nor oseltamivir is approved for prophylaxis of influenza infection. Oseltamivir resistance emerged in the United States during the 2008–2009 influenza season. However, by 2009, most influenza A viruses and all influenza B viruses were noted to be resistant to these agents.

H1N1 Influenza

Following an outbreak of influenza in Mexico in 2009, the WHO raised the pandemic alert to phase 6, implying a global pandemic. The virus that evolved was a combination of swine, avian, and human influenza genes. The epidemiology was different than in previous pandemics because the population at risk for severe disease and mortality was highest in pregnant women. In addition, the population aged 5 to 59 years was associated with more severe disease than the very young or very old. On August 10, 2010, the WHO declared an end to the 2009 H1N1 pandemic globally, although they and the Centers for Disease Control and Prevention (CDC) warn that the virus is likely to circulate during subsequent influenza seasons. The 2010 influenza vaccine provides coverage for both seasonal and H1N1 influenza, and it is recommended that everyone 6 months and older get vaccinated.

Human Parainfluenza Virus

Human parainfluenza virus (HPIV)-1, HPIV-2, and HPIV-3 cause croup; HPIV-1 and HPIV-3 cause lower respiratory tract infection, including bronchiolitis, bronchitis, and pneumonia. Outbreaks of

HPIV-3 occur during spring and summer. Almost all children have been infected and, as immunity is short-lived, repeated infections occur. Human parainfluenza virus is spread via droplet and fomite exposure.

Morbidity and mortality from HPIV lower respiratory tract infection is uncommon in the United States. It is a significant cause of mortality in developing countries, especially following secondary bacterial infection in malnourished children.

Adenovirus

Adenovirus is an enveloped DNA virus that causes both upper and lower respiratory infection. Most cases are mild, self-limited upper respiratory infections. The population at risk for severe disease is the immunocompromised, including the post-transplant patient, especially patients who have received hematopoietic stem cell as well as solid organ transplants. Treatment is symptomatic. Cidofovir has been used.

Human Metapneumovirus

Human metapneumovirus was first described in the Netherlands in 2001.[14] It is in the same family as RSV and HPIV (the Paramyxoviridae family). In the pediatric population the infections are similar to RSV, although the illness tends to milder and the children tend to be older. The symptoms include rhinorrhea, cough, tachypnea, and wheeze. The signs include retractions, crackles, and wheeze. The clinical manifestations are similar to RSV bronchiolitis, but pneumonia and respiratory failure may occur.

Coronavirus

Coronavirus made headlines in 2003 when the severe acute respiratory distress syndrome was the cause of life-threatening pneumonia.[15] The virus quickly spread from China to the rest of the world, affecting 8,000 patients in 29 countries, and caused 774 deaths. As a result of intensive infection control measures, the global transmission was halted in 2003. It is speculated that subsequent variant strains of coronavirus will cause increased cases of pneumonia in the future.

Varicella-zoster Virus

Varicella-zoster virus is a herpesvirus that causes chickenpox and has the potential to reactivate as shingles. Risk factors for varicella pneumonia include high-dose steroids (1–2 mg/kg/day for >2 weeks), malignancy (including leukemia), and other immunocompromised states (including HIV). Varicella pneumonia causes significant mortality and is associated with severe invasive group A streptococcal disease. The viremia is treated with acyclovir, and children with varicella pneumonia should be hospitalized.

Measles Virus

Measles virus is another member of the Paramyxoviridae family. It causes a febrile illness with morbilliform rash; pneumonia can occur. Children who are unvaccinated, malnourished, or immunocompromised are at risk for severe lower respiratory tract infection.

Cytomegalovirus

Cytomegalovirus is a virus in the herpes group. Cytomegalovirus pneumonia is a major cause of pneumonia in immunocompromised children, including those with transplant, HIV, and malignancy. The typical scenario is 2 to 3 months post-transplant there is cough and fever, and severe dyspnea and hypoxia result. The symptoms are nonspecific, and the lung involvement is an interstitial pneumonia. The chest radiograph shows bilateral interstitial infiltrates. Pulmonary symptoms may be accompanied by gastrointestinal disease, especially diarrhea, and chorioretinitis.

Ganciclovir is used as prophylaxis in transplant patients at risk (eg, a seropositive donor and seronegative recipient). It is also beneficial for symptomatic patients with pneumonia.

Herpes Simplex Virus

Herpes simplex virus infection is also seen in immunocompromised and transplant patients. The highest risk group is those patients that are severely neutropenic or lymphopenic. Pneumonia may result from transmission from the upper to the lower airway or as a result of viremia from oral or genital lesions. Treatment is with acyclovir 5 mg/kg every 8 hours intravenously or 400 mg orally 5 times per day.

Fungal Causes of Pneumonia

Aspergillus

Aspergillus spp. are common on decaying material everywhere. There are more than 900 species, but *Aspergillus fumigatus* is responsible for about 90% of infections in humans. They are dichotomously branching septate hyphae. The spores or conidia are small, 2 to 3 microns, and easily inhaled into the lower respiratory tract. Three forms of disease are associated with aspergillus: invasive aspergillosis, allergic bronchopulmonary aspergillosis (see Chapter 9), and aspergilloma within a cavity. This section will discuss pneumonia due to aspergillus. Opportunistic infections result when children are neutropenic or immunocompromised. Both profound (polymorphs <100 μL) and prolonged (>12–15 days) neutropenia are high risk for developing invasive aspergillosis. It is common post-transplant, in children with cancer, and with chronic granulomatous disease (CGD).

Clinical Features

Eighty percent to 90% of patients with acute invasive aspergillosis will have pulmonary disease. Nonproductive cough with fever, shortness of breath, blood in the sputum, and pleuritic chest pain are the main symptoms. Twenty-five percent of children may have minimal physical signs, others may present with hypoxemia. Chronic invasive pulmonary aspergillosis is associated with diabetes mellitus, CGD, and HIV.

Diagnosis

Hyphae may be evident microscopically but this does not prove the diagnosis, as other fungi may have a similar appearance. Culture of sputum or bronchoalveolar lavage fluid will not provide a definitive diagnosis, as it is important to be aware that these specimens may be positive in those who are colonized with aspergillus. Evidence of invasive aspergillosis is supported by the finding of galactomannan (GM) in these fluids, and this test has been approved by the US Food and Drug Administration. The negative predictive value of GM is highly specific; however, GM is not positive in 100% of patients with pulmonary aspergillosis.

Imaging

Plain chest x-ray of invasive aspergillosis reveals wedge-shaped infiltrates and cavities, and CT may be helpful for the early diagnosis of invasive aspergillosis. The halo sign, which is ground-glass attenuation surrounding a soft tissue nodule, is characteristic and cavitation may follow.

Management

Voriconazole has become the treatment of choice for invasive aspergillosis. Rapid institution of treatment is necessary because invasive aspergillosis can be rapidly progressive. Posaconazole or amphotericin B may be considered if there is a possibility of mucor. In addition, caspofungin has also been approved for treatment of invasive aspergillosis if there is resistance or intolerance to other therapies. Consultation with infectious diseases is indicated.

Candida

Candida spp., especially *Candida albicans,* are the most common fungal infections to cause disease in humans. Disease caused by *Candida* spp. includes cutaneous, gastrointestinal, oropharyngeal (thrush), and vulvovaginal candidiasis. The respiratory tract is frequently colonized with *Candida* spp. and may result in tracheobronchitis or pneumonia. Invasive candidiasis results from host defects and other risk factors, including CGD, diabetes, and immune deficiency states.

Candida pneumonia is associated with disseminated candidiasis, and the lungs are rarely the only organ involved. The most common form is multiple lung abscesses as a result of hematologic spread of *Candida.* The physical signs include fever, dyspnea, and evidence of sepsis. The lung examination is variable, from non-contributory to rhonchi, crackles, and wheeze.

Fluconazole is the treatment of choice, initially intravenous (IV), and with improvement can be switched to oral. If it is unclear whether there are other molds involved, voriconazole may be a better alternative. With more severe infections and in high-risk patients, echinocandins, such as caspofungin, may be a better selection, especially if the infection is non-albicans, such as *Candida glabrata.*

Blastomycosis

Blastomyces dermatitidis is a thermal dimorphic fungus, and the conidia (spores) that convert to yeast are infectious to humans. In the United States, the states most likely to be the site of infection are adjacent to the Mississippi and Ohio rivers and the Great Lakes. The conidia are inhaled and deposited in the lungs. Incubation time is variable but averages 4 to 6 weeks.

Clinical Features

Children are most likely to be infected if they have HIV infection or are immunocompromised, including transplant patients. About 50% of infected children will be asymptomatic. Those who are symptomatic have flu-like symptoms with fever, chills, night sweats, weight loss, and myalgia. The pulmonary symptoms include productive cough, wheezing, and chest pain. There is an acute form as well as a chronic form, which may last 2 to 6 months and is associated with weight loss and cough. Either acute or chronic pulmonary blastomycosis has the potential for a more severe course with life-threatening infection, which may disseminate to the skin, central nervous system, and bone.

Diagnosis

The sputum is full of polymorphonuclear cells and has a high yield for fungal stain, and the fungus grows from culture of sputum, tracheal aspirate, bronchoalveolar lavage, cerebrospinal fluid, and urine. Direct identification of the fungus is possible by experienced personnel. Children who do not expectorate sputum may need bronchoscopy or lung biopsy to confirm the diagnosis.

Imaging

The chest radiograph shows infiltrates, reticulonodular pattern, and pleural effusion, and in some cases cavitation is evident.

Coccidioidomycosis

Coccidioides spp. are dimorphic fungi endemic in the soil of southwestern United States, Mexico, and Central and South America. Inhalation of spores, even one spore, results in an acute pulmonary infection. It is not spread from person to person. There is increased risk when the soil is disrupted, for example by earthquake or farming, particularly when the soil is dry. The incubation period is 10 to 16 days, although the range is 7 to 30 days.

Clinical Features

The most important part of the history is the story of travel or residence in an endemic area, and the exposure can be as simple as driving

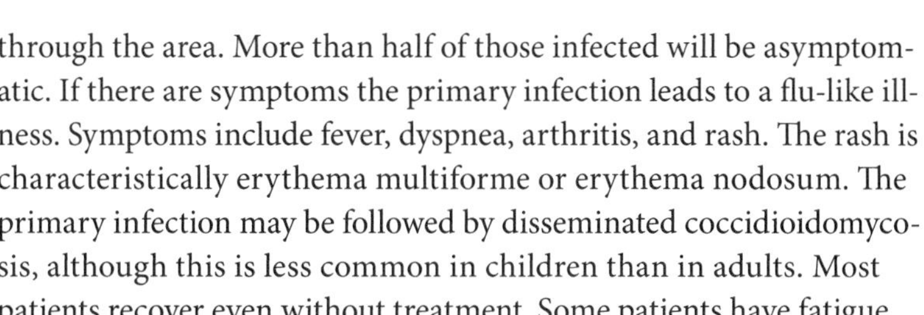

through the area. More than half of those infected will be asymptomatic. If there are symptoms the primary infection leads to a flu-like illness. Symptoms include fever, dyspnea, arthritis, and rash. The rash is characteristically erythema multiforme or erythema nodosum. The primary infection may be followed by disseminated coccidioidomycosis, although this is less common in children than in adults. Most patients recover even without treatment. Some patients have fatigue that lasts for months.

Diagnosis

Coccidioidal IgM appears within 1 to 3 weeks of onset of symptoms and lasts for 3 to 4 months.

Imaging

Chest radiograph findings tend to be nonspecific with infiltrates, hilar adenopathy, and small pleural effusions. A small percentage of patients have nodules or cavities early on, and 5% to 10% have persistent pulmonary nodules or cavities. The cavities tend to be thin-walled and resolve spontaneously. On occasion the cavities expand. If they are larger than 6 cm, they are at risk for rupture, and surgery is indicated.

Treatment

Most patients do not require treatment, but the following are considerations for treatment:

- Continuous fever for longer than 1 month
- Night sweats for longer than 3 weeks
- Weight loss greater than 10%
- Large (>50% of one lung) or bilateral pulmonary infiltrates
- Primary infection during infancy
- Primary infection during pregnancy, especially in the third trimester, or immediately postpartum
- Immunosuppression
- Diabetes mellitus or preexisting cardiopulmonary disease

Treatment of acute pulmonary coccidioidomycosis includes oral azoles, such as fluconazole. During pregnancy amphotericin B is preferred because the azoles may be teratogenic. Although uncommon in children, disseminated disease or those with progressive fibrocavitary disease may require prolonged treatment up to 1 year.

Histoplasmosis

Histoplasma capsulatum is a dimorphic fungus that is endemic in the central United States and other parts of the world that have warm, humid soil and large populations of migratory birds or chickens. It is the most common pulmonary mycosis of humans. It can occur at any age. The geographic distribution is the central United States, specifically the Ohio and Mississippi river valleys, and it is endemic in Central and South America, the Caribbean, Africa, and Asia.

Clinical Features

The clinical features of histoplasmosis depend on the size of the inoculum, the immune status of the host, and the presence of lung disease. The exposure increases if there is major disturbance of soil, as with construction projects and proximity to chicken coops, especially those with rotten wood. The incubation period is 9 to 17 days, and the acute illness is characterized by flu-like symptoms of fever, chills, muscle aches, nonproductive cough, and chest pain. The acute symptoms may be mild (lasting less than a week) to severe (lasting 2–3 weeks). There are varied clinical manifestations, again varying with the immune status.

Severe acute pulmonary syndrome results from exposure to a large inoculum and starts with an acute flu-like syndrome, with fever chills and myalgias. Pulmonary symptoms develop with cough, dyspnea, and hypoxemia. The chest examination includes diffuse fine crackles with possibly a pleural rub. There may be rapid progression to acute respiratory distress syndrome. Some patients develop a single pulmonary nodule in the lung parenchyma, which has the appearance of a coin lesion on chest radiograph. It is usually asymptomatic.

Mediastinal obstructive syndrome results from hilar lymphadenopathy, which may be large enough to compress surrounding structures, including the airway, the great vessels, and the esophagus.

Management

Acute pulmonary histoplasmosis that is asymptomatic or mild requires no treatment. If the symptoms are prolonged for more than 4 weeks, oral itraconazole for 6 to 12 weeks is indicated. If there is severe infection, treatment should be initiated with amphotericin B for 1 to 2 weeks followed by a year of itraconazole.

Pneumocystis Pneumonia

Pneumocystis carinii pneumonia led to the abbreviation PCP. *Pneumocystis carinii* was originally classified as a trypanosome and later as a protozoan, and now as a unicellular fungus. It has recently been renamed *Pneumocystis jiroveci* because *P carinii* is not found in humans. The accepted abbreviation is still PCP. Pneumocystis pneumonia is the most common opportunistic infection in patients with HIV and is common in transplant patients. The routine use of prophylaxis has reduced the prevalence of PCP.

Clinical Features

The symptoms and signs of PCP are nonspecific, so a high index of suspicion is necessary in patients who are HIV-infected or immunocompromised, especially if they are not taking prophylactic measures (see below). The symptoms are typically shortness of breath, fever, and nonproductive cough, with chills and weight loss. The signs are tachypnea and tachycardia. Auscultation may reveal some crackles, but often there are no adventitious signs. The main finding supportive of the diagnosis is hypoxemia. The typical radiographic appearance is diffuse bilateral infiltrates extending out from the hilum. In the early stages the chest radiograph may be normal and later there may be pneumatoceles. Pleural effusion is uncommon. High-resolution CT may be helpful, as patchy areas of ground-glass appearance are suggestive, particularly in the patient with HIV.

Expectorated sputum usually does not yield a satisfactory specimen; induced sputum production with hypertonic saline is the quickest way to make the diagnosis. Bronchoalveolar lavage is the most common procedure performed. The diagnosis is confirmed by various stains, including silver stains, that show the cysts.

The choice of treatment depends on the degree of hypoxemia. The treatment of choice is trimethoprim-sulfamethoxazole (TS), and oral therapy is used for mild cases, although most patients will require IV treatment at least at first. Intravenous pentamidine is an alternative choice for treatment, especially if there is a reaction to TS. Duration of treatment should be 21 days for patients with HIV and 14 days for patients without HIV, and similar durations should be given based on severity of disease (mild vs severe).

Chemoprophylaxis against PCP is indicated for patients with HIV and those who are immunocompromised, especially transplant patients and those with both primary and acquired immunodeficiency. The standard regimen is 3 consecutive days per week of oral TS. If this is not tolerated, nebulized pentamidine is an alternative. Infectious disease and pulmonary consultation are recommended.

Management of CAP

A sample algorithm for the management of CAP is shown in Figure 19-1. If the clinical impression of pneumonia is high, it is thought that a bacterial etiology is likely, and antibiotics are indicated, the choice of antibiotic will vary depending on age and organisms that are in the community.[16] The "Evidence-Based Care Guideline for Children with Community Acquired Pneumonia (CAP)" from Cincinnati Children's Hospital Medical Center can be reviewed.[17] Additionally, the Infectious Diseases Society of America in conjunction with the Pediatric Infectious Diseases Society have drafted guidelines for the management of CAP in infants and children older than 3 months. These guidelines should be published in 2011.[18]

From 2 months to 5 years it is recommended to prescribe high-dose amoxicillin 80 to 90 mg/kg/day for 7 days. As previously noted, 17% to 35% of *S pneumoniae* isolates from CAP in the United States are resistant to penicillin G[19] and 15% are resistant to macrolides,[20] which may indicate an alternative when bacterial pneumonia is suspected. For hospitalized patients with uncomplicated pneumonia, ampicillin, penicillin or, alternatively, a third generation cephalosporin is preferred. Consultation with infectious disease specialists will assist in this decision.

Although mycoplasma infection does occur in children younger than 5 years, a macrolide may not be the best antibiotic choice for empiric treatment at this age, in part because many *S pneumoniae* are now resistant to macrolides or azides. If the child is vomiting or otherwise may be unable to take oral medications, the recommendation is a single initial dose of ceftriaxone prior to attempting oral antibiotics. For children age 5 years and older it is recommended that a macrolide be used to treat CAP in the outpatient setting with either 7 to 14 days of erythromycin or 5 days of azithromycin. Doxycycline for children older than 7 years and levofloxacin for older adolescents are alternatives. It is recommended that practitioners follow up children diagnosed with pneumonia within 1 to 3 days.

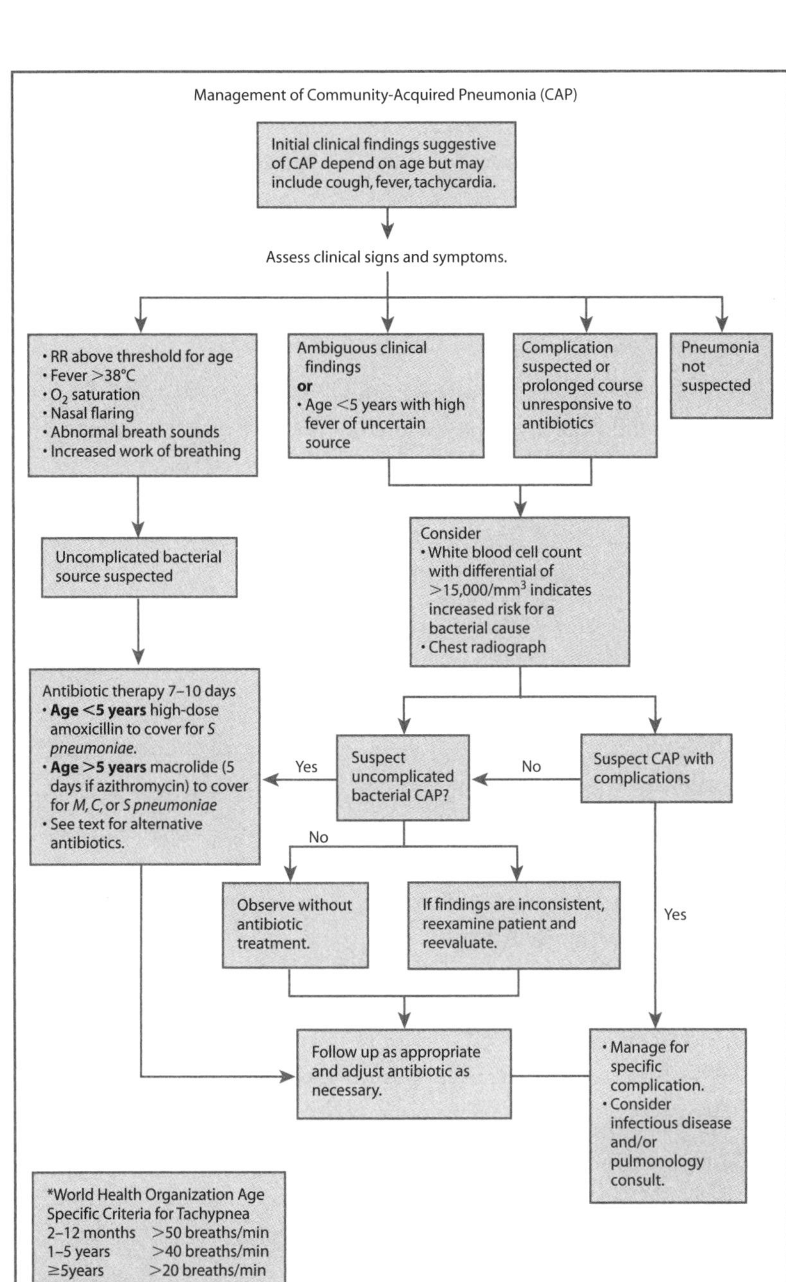

Figure 19-1. Management of community-acquired pneumonia (CAP). M, *Mycoplasma;* C, *Chlamydophila;* S, *Streptococcus.*

Prevention of Pneumonia

Heptavalent pneumococcal vaccine was recommended in 2000 for children in the United States to reduce the incidence of pneumococcal pneumonia. The original vaccine, which contained 7 serotypes, was highly effective, but two-thirds of the invasive pneumococcal disease was caused by 6 serotypes not included in this vaccine. Subsequently 13-valent PCV was approved in February 2010 and is recommended for all children from 2 months through 5 years of age.

The CDC recommends that all individuals aged 6 months and older get a seasonal flu vaccine. The seasonal flu vaccine protects against 3 influenza viruses that research indicates will be most common during the upcoming season. The 2010–2011 flu vaccine will protect against 2009 novel influenza A (H1N1) and 2 other influenza viruses (an influenza A [H3N2] virus and an influenza B virus).

The CDC also recommends that people in contact with certain groups of children get a seasonal flu vaccine in order to better protect the child (or children) in their lives from the flu.

The CDC recommends that the following contacts of children receive seasonal influenza vaccination:

- Close contacts of children younger than 5 years (people who live with them), especially those younger than 6 months
- Out-of-home caregivers (nannies, child care providers, etc) of children younger than 5 years
- People who live with or have other close contact with a child or children of any age with a chronic health problem (asthma, diabetes, etc)
- All health care workers, to keep from spreading the flu to their patients

Additional considerations are *Haemophilus influenzae* type B vaccine and varicella vaccine.

When to Refer

Most children with CAP will not require consultation. If there are complications, such as pleural effusion or prolonged hypoxia, consultation with a pulmonologist may be indicated. If the child has a chronic illness, consultation with the specialist who is involved in their long-term care may be helpful. Consultation with infectious

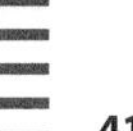

diseases or allergy is indicated when allergies, comorbid conditions, or unresponsiveness to antibiotics are present.

When to Admit

Children with pneumonia and a chronic illness, for example if they are immunocompromised, may require hospitalization. If the degree of respiratory distress is significant, if there is hypoxia, and if they appear septic, they may require hospitalization. Currently, validated screening systems do not exist to help predict which children with pneumonia should be hospitalized. Hospitalization is indicated with the following:

- Oxygen saturation consistently less than 90% (definite)
- Suspected sepsis (definite)
- Severe dehydration (definite)
- Inability to drink fluids (possible)
- Moderate or severe respiratory distress (possible)
- Failed outpatient antibiotic treatment (clinical judgment)
- Home circumstance or social situation raises concerns (likely)
- Infants younger than 6 months (unless ideal caretaker)

Key Points

- The WHO guidelines for tachypnea in children suggest which children may be more likely to be diagnosed with pneumonia.
- The etiology of pneumonia is closely related to the age of the child.
- Imaging studies do not differentiate viral from bacterial lower respiratory tract infections.
- Chest x-ray is not necessary to make the diagnosis of pneumonia.
- A CT scan is indicated for evaluation of complications of pneumonia.
- Ultrasound is useful to characterize pleural effusion or empyema.
- Management depends on the age of the child and the likely diagnosis.

References

1. Puumalainen T, Quiambao B, Abucejo-Ladesma E, et al. Clinical case review: a method to improve identification of true clinical and radiographic pneumonia in children meeting the World Health Organization definition for pneumonia. *BMC Infect Dis.* 2008;8:95
2. Michelow IC, Olsen K, Lozano J, et al. Epidemiology and clinical characteristics of community-acquired pneumonia in hospitalized children. *Pediatrics.* 2004;113(4):701–707
3. Shah S, Bachur R, Kim D, Neuman MI. Lack of predictive value of tachypnea in the diagnosis of pneumonia in children. *Pediatr Infect Dis J.* 2010;29(5):406–409
4. Wubbel L, Muniz L, Ahmed A, et al. Etiology and treatment of community-acquired pneumonia in ambulatory children. *Pediatr Infect Dis J.* 1999;18(2):98–104
5. Courtoy I, Lande AE, Turner RB. Accuracy of radiographic differentiation of bacterial from nonbacterial pneumonia. *Clin Pediatr (Phila).* 1989;28(6):261–264
6. FDA News Release. FDA Approves Pneumococcal Disease Vaccine with Broader Protection. February 24, 2010. http://www.fda.gov/NewsEvents/Newsroom/PressAnnouncements/ucm201758.htm. Accessed November 18, 2010
7. Li ST, Tancredi DJ. Empyema hospitalizations increased in US children despite pneumococcal conjugate vaccine. *Pediatrics.* 2010;125(1):26–33
8. Schultz KD, Fan LL, Pinsky J, et al. The changing face of pleural empyemas in children: epidemiology and management. *Pediatrics.* 2004;113(6):1735–1740
9. Alfaro C, Fergie J, Purcell K. Emergence of community-acquired methicillin-resistant *Staphylococcus aureus* in complicated parapneumonic effusions *Pediatr Infect Dis J.* 2005;24(3):274–276
10. Younger JG, Shankar-Sinha S, Mickiewicz M, et al. Murine complement interactions with *Pseudomonas aeruginosa* and their consequences during pneumonia. *Am J Respir Cell Mol Biol.* 2003;29(4):432–438
11. Marik PE. Aspiration pneumonitis and aspiration pneumonia. *N Engl J Med.* 2001;344(9):665–671
12. Waris ME, Toikka P, Saarinen T, et al. Diagnosis of *Mycoplasma pneumoniae* pneumonia in children. *J Clin Microbiol.* 1998;36(11):3155–3159
13. Neumayr L, Lennette E, Kelly D, et al. Mycoplasma disease and acute chest syndrome in sickle cell disease. *Pediatrics.* 2003;112(1 pt 1):87–95
14. van den Hoogen BG, de Jong JC, Groen J, et al. A newly discovered human pneumovirus isolated from young children with respiratory tract disease. *Nat Med.* 2001;7(6):719–724
15. Poon LL, Guan Y, Nicholls JM, et al. The etiology, origins, and diagnosis of severe acute respiratory syndrome. *Lancet Infect Dis.* 2004;4(11):663–671

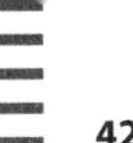

16. Fine MJ, Smith MA, Carson CA, et al. Prognosis and outcomes of patients with community-acquired pneumonia. A meta-analysis. *JAMA.* 1996;275(2):134–141
17. Community Acquired Pneumonia Guideline Team, Cincinnati Children's Hospital Medical Center. Evidence-based guideline for medical management of community-acquired pneumonia in children 60 days to 17 years of age. Guideline 14. Cincinnati, OH: Cincinnati Children's Hospital Medical Center; 2005:1–16. http://www.cincinnatichildrens.org/assets/0/78/1067/2709/2777/2793/9199/1633ae60-cbd1-4fbd-bba4-cb687fbb1d42.pdf
18. Bradley JS, Byington CL, Shah SS, et al. The management of community-acquired pneumonia (CAP) in infants and children older than 3 months of age: clinical practice guidelines by the Pediatric Infectious Diseases Society (PIDS) and the Infectious Diseases Society of America (IDSA). *Clin Infect Dis.* In press
19. Gordon KA, Biedenbach DJ, Jones RN. Comparison of *Streptococcus pneumoniae* and *Haemophilus influenzae* susceptibilities from community-acquired respiratory tract infections and hospitalized patients with pneumonia: five-year results for the SENTRY Antimicrobial Surveillance Program. *Diagn Microbiol Infect Dis.* 2003;46(4):285–289
20. Hsieh SC, Kuo YT, Chern MS, et al. Mycoplasma pneumonia: clinical and radiographic features in 39 children. *Pediatr Int.* 2007;49(3):363–367

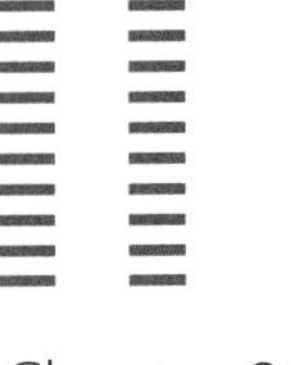

Chapter 20

The Complications of Pneumonia

Jonathan Steinfeld, MD

Case Report 20-1

A 3-year-old girl with an unremarkable medical history presents to her pediatrician with a fever, tachypnea, and cough for 2 days. She has been drinking well and does not appear to be in pain. Crackles are heard at the left base of the lungs. A chest radiograph confirms a left lower lobe consolidation with a small effusion. Outpatient therapy is started with high-dose amoxicillin and supportive therapy. After 2 days the tachypnea has improved but the cough and the fever persist. She now complains of pain and points to her chest. Her parents call her pediatrician, who recommends that she go to the emergency department (ED) for further evaluation. At the ED her temperature is 39.1°C, her respiratory rate is 35 breaths per minute, and her pulse oximetry is 92% in room air. A second chest radiograph shows increased consolidation of the left lower lobe infiltrate and the left-sided pleural effusion has not changed.

She is admitted to the hospital on intravenous (IV) ampicillin and supplemental oxygen. Surgery is consulted, but the decision is made not to insert a chest tube due to the small size of the effusion. After 2 days of treatment in the hospital with IV ampicillin, her pain persists and she remains febrile. A computed tomography (CT) scan is done, which demonstrates a large left lower lobe consolidation with a moderate-sized pleural effusion. There are several small lucent areas within the consolidation. Video-assisted thoracoscopic surgery is performed to place a chest tube. Necrotic lung tissue is removed from the left lower lobe. Purulent pleural fluid is sent for bacterial culture, but no organisms grow. Antibiotic therapy is broadened after surgery to treat resistant *Streptococcus pneumoniae* with vancomycin. On the third postoperative day she is finally afebrile; in addition, the chest tube has stopped draining and is removed. Her supplemental oxygen requirement resolves the next day. Intravenous antibiotics are continued until her cough improves. She is sent home after 12 days in the hospital on 2 more weeks of high-dose amoxicillin and is seen by her pediatrician 1 week after discharge. Two months after discharge she is seen by her pediatrician again. Her cough has resolved, she has been afebrile since discharge, and her activity level is back to normal. A repeat chest radiograph is completely normal with no residual infiltrate.

Case Report 20-2

A 12-year-old boy with an unremarkable medical history has had a cough for 2 days. His fever started yesterday. He has a good appetite and continues to take fluids well. His parents take him to the local ED. His temperature is 38.5°C, his respiratory rate is 30 breaths per minute with retractions, and his oxygen saturation is 91% in room air. He has diminished breath sounds at his right apex. A chest radiograph shows a right upper lobe consolidation without an effusion. A blood culture, complete blood cell count, and electrolytes are done. His white blood cell count is elevated and his serum sodium is 131 mmol/L. Additional labs are sent, which show a decreased serum osmolality and increased urinary sodium levels. He is admitted to the hospital on supplemental oxygen and IV ampicillin, and his fluid intake is limited to 500 mL per 24 hours. Electrolytes are checked every 12 hours. Two days later he is afebrile and his electrolytes are normal. He is discharged home on high-dose amoxicillin with follow-up arranged with his pediatrician.

Introduction

Despite prompt, appropriate treatment, many children will experience complications from pneumonia.

The most clinically significant complication of pneumonia is a parapneumonic effusion (PPE) with empyema. An empyema is the last stage of a PPE, but these terms are sometimes used interchangeably. Other less common complications are lung abscesses, necrotizing pneumonia, pneumatoceles, and bronchopleural fistulas. While these complications are a direct extension of infection, in other complications, such as hyponatremia, the mechanism of action is not clear.

The relative incidence of complicated pneumonia in children appears to be increasing.[1–3] One multicenter study showed that in patients admitted for pneumonia secondary to *S pneumoniae* there was an increase in the percentage of complicated pneumonia from 22.6% to 53%.[2] In a review of 10 years at Texas Children's Hospital in Houston, the incidence of admissions for empyema increased from 5.8 (per 10,000 admissions) to a peak of 23 before dropping to 12.6 in the last period of the study.[4] Of note, Texas Children's was included in the aforementioned multicenter trial, which ended in the same year that they saw their peak incidence of empyema (1999).

Complications of pneumonia may arise due to either an aggressive infectious organism or increased susceptibility in the patient. Unfortunately, since many children are unable to produce sputum samples from the lower airways it can be difficult to determine exactly what the infectious organism is. In addition, many children are diagnosed clinically as outpatients without the aid of radiographic testing. Typically, the cause of pneumonia is only discovered in hospitalized patients. In a recent prospective study of 154 hospitalized patients, despite aggressive testing, the cause was only identified in 79% of the patients.[5] See Chapter 19 for a more extensive discussion on the organisms responsible for community-acquired pneumonia (CAP).

Despite the advent of the 7-valent conjugated pneumococcal vaccine (PCV7), *S pneumoniae* remains the most common cause of bacterial CAP as well as complicated pneumonia.[5] Children with complicated *S pneumoniae* pneumonia are older (median age 45 months vs 27 months), more likely to be Caucasian, and more likely to have been given antibiotics before diagnosis; possibly antibiotics were able to partially suppress the infection but could not prevent progression to a complicated pneumonia.[2] Surprisingly, patients with underlying diseases, such as genetic disorders, hemoglobinopathies, central nervous system disorders, leukemia, HIV, gastrointestinal disorders, and heart disease, have not been found to have an increased risk for complicated pneumonia.[2]

While both *Mycoplasma pneumoniae* and *Chlamydophila pneumoniae* are important causes of CAP in the developed world,[3] they are not commonly found to be the responsible organisms in patients with complications of pneumonia.

While viruses are the leading cause of pneumonia in children, most viral infections are self-limiting. However, patients may develop a bacterial coinfection, and pneumonias caused by mixed viral and bacterial coinfection are often responsible for prolonged hospitalizations.[5] In children who die from bacterial coinfection of influenza, *Staphylococcus aureus* is the most common coinfecting bacterial organism. Increasingly, pneumonia is caused by methicillin-resistant *S aureus* as well as less common causative agents, including mycobacterial and fungal organisms. See Chapter 19.

Parapneumonic Effusion

The incidence of PPE and empyema is 3.3 per 100,000 pediatric patients.[1] The prevalence is seasonal, with 50% occurring in the winter months. The bacteria that cause PPE also commonly cause CAP. In the late 1980s and early 1990s, *S pneumoniae* was isolated in 40% of cases—far more than any other bacteria.[1] In more recent studies, *S pneumoniae* is still the most common cause of PPE,[6,7] especially serotypes 1 and 14,[2] but other bacteria such as *S aureus* have increased in incidence.[8] After *S pneumoniae* and *S aureus,* group A streptococcus is the third most common pathogen for effusions or empyemas from CAP.[4]

Aspiration from the oropharynx is typically the entry site for bacteria into the lungs. From there, infection develops as pneumonia in the periphery and the dependent lobes with extension toward the hilum. After several days, a PPE may develop. The presence of foreign organisms in the lung leads to activated neutrophils, which attempt to destroy the bacteria. Subsequent damage to the endothelium leads to increased capillary permeability. Extravascular fluid increases the interstitial-pleural pressure gradient and shifts fluid to the pleural space. Pleural fluid is constantly created and removed by the pleural lymphatics; however, if this increase in fluid cannot be cleared, then a pleural effusion forms.[9] This is the exudative stage, and it can typically be treated with antibiotics alone.

The fibrinopurulent stage develops 5 to 10 days later. Intravascular clotting proteins enter the pleural space and prevent fibrinolysis. Fibrinous adhesions form in the pleural space, and neutrophils and bacteria are typically present. Pus may be present, but the lung is still expandable.[9]

A true organized empyema is the last stage of a PPE. This stage may be 10 to 21 days after the fibrinopurulent stage. Pus and fibrinous adhesions lead to visceral pleural fibrosis, which traps the lung parenchyma and prevents full lung expansion.[9]

Clinical Presentation

Symptoms in a patient with a PPE may be similar to patients with pneumonia and include fever, cough, shortness of breath, decreased exercise tolerance, decreased appetite, abdominal pain, halitosis, lethargy, and malaise. Additional signs are pleuritic chest pain and splinting of the affected side.[10] Patients with PPEs typically have more febrile days before diagnosis and take longer to defervesce after treatment.[2]

A second pattern of presentation may be a patient who has already been diagnosed with pneumonia but appears to have failed treatment.

Patients who are febrile or still appear ill 48 hours after admission for pneumonia should be evaluated for PPE.[11]

On physical examination, patients with PPE often appear quite unwell. They may be in significant pain and discomfort, especially when asked to move or take deep breaths. Since PPEs are more frequently unilateral, asymmetry is a common finding. Patients may have unilateral decreased chest wall expansion, dullness to percussion, splinting, cyanosis, and decreased breath sounds.[10] Careful attention must be paid to the oxygen saturation, because levels below 92% indicate severe disease.[11]

Diagnosis

Chest radiographs are the simplest method of diagnosing a PPE (Figure 20-1). The costophrenic angle is often obscured, and an ascending rim of fluid may be seen along the lateral chest wall. Supine films may not have this meniscus sign and instead often show a homogeneous opacity over the entire lung field, also known as a white out. It can be difficult to differentiate these films from severe atelectasis, and further investigation may be necessary.[10] A lateral decubitus view is helpful in showing the fluid layer, unless the fluid is thick and organized.

Ultrasonography of the chest is an excellent, non-traumatic, ionizing radiation-free method of evaluating children for a PPE. An ultrasound can approximate the size of the effusion, discover if the pleural fluid is freely flowing, and determine the fluid's echogenicity.[11] In addition, chest ultrasonography can be used to help guide any invasive diagnostic or therapeutic procedures.[10] The major limitations in the use of ultrasonography are that it cannot be used to determine the stage of the effusion,[10] and it may not be consistently available in some hospitals.

While chest CT scans may be useful in the evaluation of patients with suspected complicated pneumonia,[12] they do not add to a well-performed and interpreted ultrasound.[10] Chest CT scans do not reliably distinguish empyema and are not helpful in guiding medical management in patients with known effusions.[13]

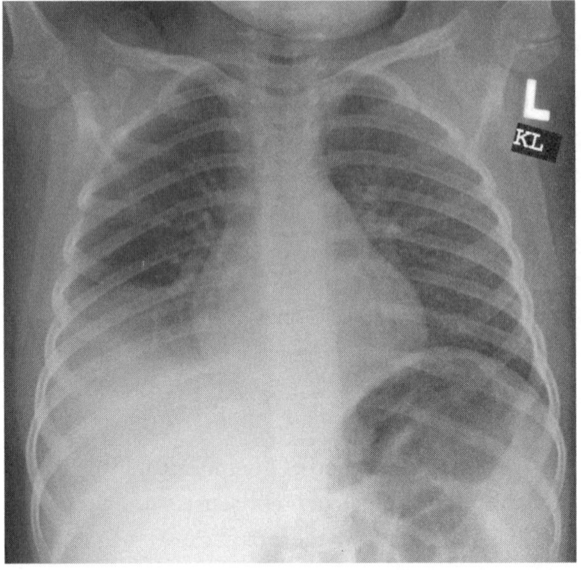

A

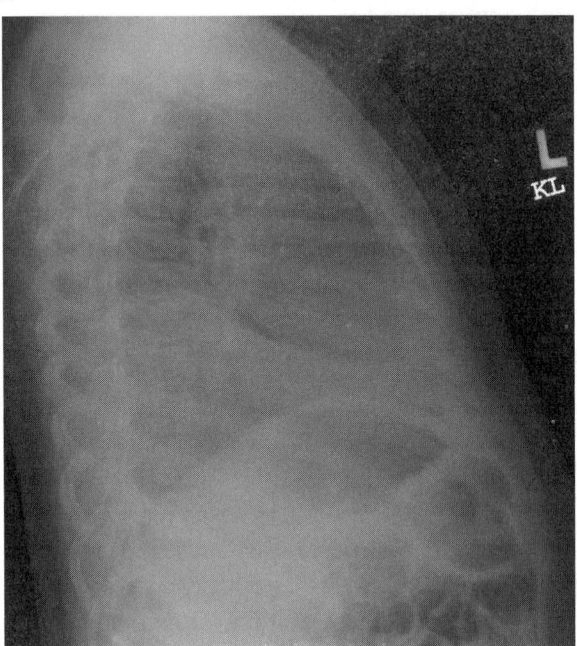

B

Figure 20-1. This 6-year-old patient presented to the emergency department with fever, cough, upper abdominal pain, and lower rib pain on the right side. **A.** A chest radiograph shows right lower lobe airspace disease with a pleural effusion. **B.** The lateral film shows increased opacity due to fluid. **C.** A computed tomography (CT) scan clarifies the pleural effusion and demonstrates right middle and lower lobe pneumonia with significant compressive atelectasis. **D.** The coronal view of the CT scan shows the patient's scoliosis due to right-sided pain.

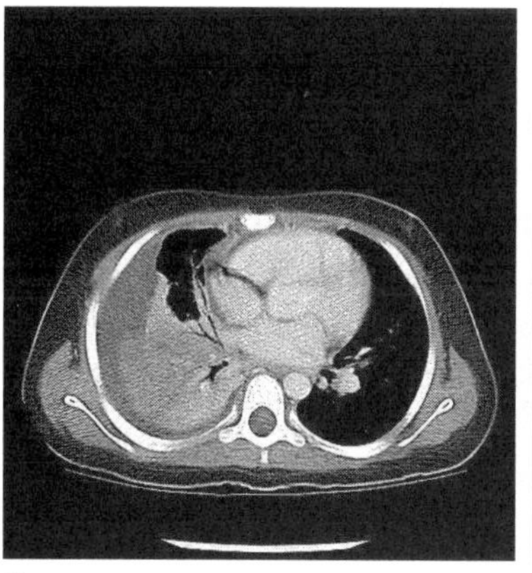
C

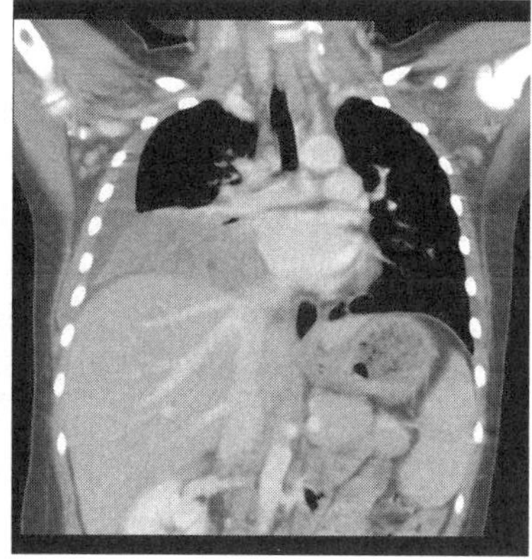
D

Management

Significant debate exists regarding the appropriate management of PPE in children. While there have been many clinical trials in adults, there have been very few in children, and extrapolating data from adults to children is inappropriate. Adults are more likely to have underlying lung disease and have a much higher mortality rate. On the other hand, children typically do not have other medical problems and have excellent outcomes.[10]

Since multiple pediatric specialists, including pulmonologists, surgeons, and infectious disease specialists, may contribute to the optimal management of children with complicated PPE, the ideal setting for the care of these children is a pediatric tertiary care center.

There are currently 2 main approaches to PPE. Conservative therapy consists of IV antibiotics and observation. Antibiotics should be tailored to treat the most common causes of pneumonia and should take into consideration local community sensitivities. (See Chapter 19 for a complete discussion of antimicrobial therapy.) If the effusion increases or if there is respiratory compromise, then a chest tube should be inserted with or without fibrinolytics. Patients who worsen or do not improve should be treated with video-assisted thoracoscopic surgery (VATS) to break up loculations, remove the fibrinous "peel," and allow infectious material to drain.

A second, more aggressive approach is to perform VATS along with IV antibiotics within the first 48 hours of an effusion. One benefit of an early pleural tap or VATS is that it is more likely to identify an infectious organism, which can be used to tailor antibiotic therapy.[3] Patients who have early VATS have a shorter hospital stay compared with patients who have had their VATS more than 48 hours after diagnosis.[4] Early VATS compared with chest tube insertion in a small randomized controlled trial showed a significant decrease in length of stay and chest tube duration in the VATS group.[14] However, in a larger prospectively randomized trial, when early VATS is compared with early chest tube insertion with urokinase (and salvage VATS if needed) there is no difference in length of stay or other outcomes despite a significantly higher cost of care for the VATS group.[15]

To help physicians manage these patients, the British Thoracic Society (BTS) has provided guidelines based on published evidence and the clinical experience of expert specialists.[10] Their extensive recommendations include an algorithm for the management of pleural infections in children (Figure 20-2). Until more research is done, the BTS guidelines are the most complete reference for management. One caveat regarding fibrinolytics is that while urokinase has been frequently studied and used in the United Kingdom, it is not currently available in the United States. Streptokinase and tissue plasminogen activator have been used as substitutes.[16]

See Chapter 19 for details on treating pneumonia.

Prognosis

Most patients return to their usual state of health in 4 weeks. Follow-up chest radiographs at 3 to 6 months should reveal normal results.[17] Typically, well-grown children with no previous bacterial infections will not require a full immune workup.[10] Children who do not quickly recover or who have atypical medical histories may require further specialist evaluation.

Lung Abscess

A lung abscess is a thick-walled area of necrotic lung tissue 2 cm or greater in diameter caused by an infection. Primary lung abscesses develop from either direct aspiration or a progression of infected lung tissue. Secondary lung abscesses develop in children who have an underlying medical condition that predisposes them to pulmonary infections.[17] Children who are at higher risk of pulmonary aspiration,

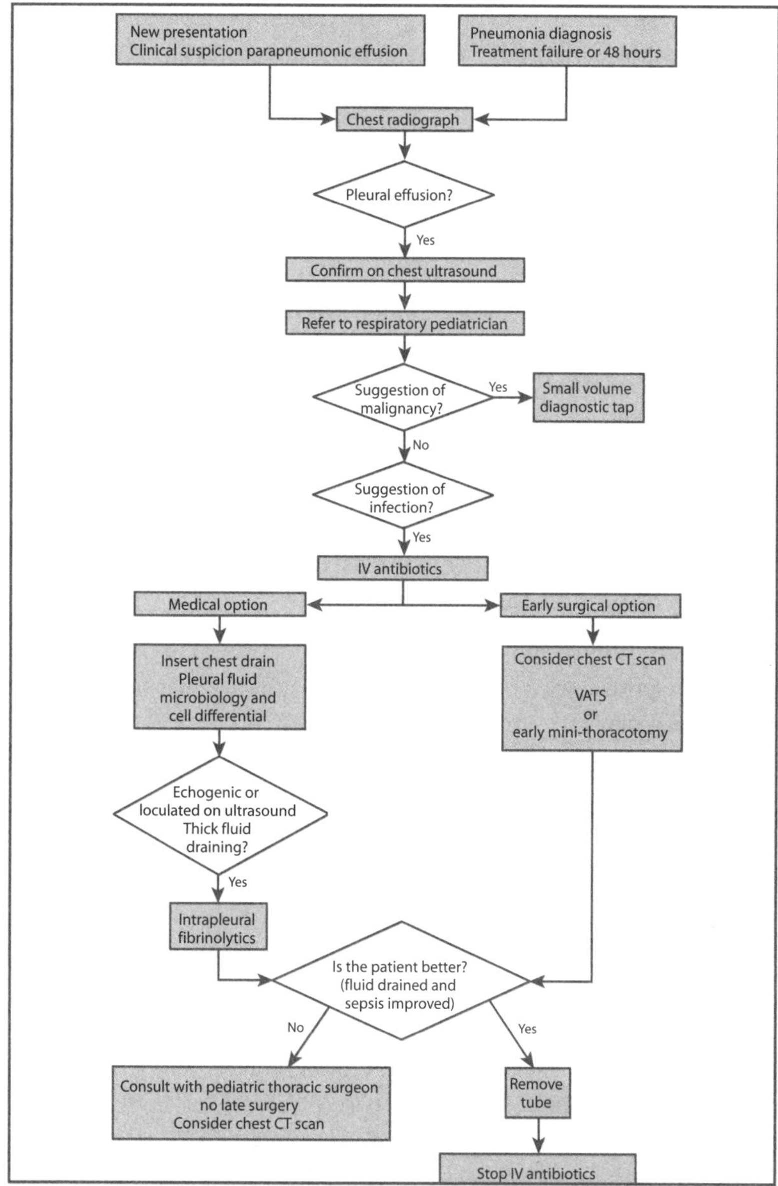

Figure 20-2. Algorithm for the management of pleural infection in children from the British Thoracic Society guidelines. CT, computed tomography; IV, intravenous; VATS, video-assisted thoracoscopic surgery. (From Balfour-Lynn IM, Abrahamson E, Cohen G, et al. BTS guidelines for the management of pleural infection in children. *Thorax*. 2005;60(suppl 1):i1–i21, with permission from BMJ Publishing Group, Ltd.)

such as those with a developmental delay, swallowing dysfunction, or muscle weakness, may develop secondary lung abscesses.[18] Secondary lung abscesses have also been described in patients with immunodeficiencies, either congenital or acquired.[19] Children with cystic fibrosis typically have more generalized lung infections, but they have been known to develop localized pulmonary abscesses as well.

Clinical Presentation

Fever and cough are the most common symptoms, followed by dyspnea, chest pain, anorexia, purulent sputum production, rhinorrhea, and malaise/lethargy.[18–20] The physical examination is similar to uncomplicated pneumonia with fever, tachypnea, decreased breath sounds, and isolated crackles. Chest radiographs may show what appears to be a consolidation. The presence of an air-fluid level indicates free-flowing fluid and an abscess. Since a supine film may not show an air-fluid level, radiographs must be taken with the patient either in a decubitus or upright position.

Doppler ultrasonography can be a useful complement to chest radiography. The procedure is painless and radiation-free, and can be done without sedation.

Some institutions prefer a chest CT to look for other complications of pneumonia as well.[18] Either study can be used for interventional radiology to perform a needle aspiration or place a chest tube for diagnosis and drainage if this is desired. Magnetic resonance imaging does not provide any advantage to either of these studies.

Management

All patients with lung abscesses should be hospitalized to administer IV antibiotics. The choice of which antibiotic and for how long may vary from institution to institution based on local susceptibilities, availability, and if a specimen is obtained by interventional radiology. Antibiotic therapy for primary abscesses should target *S pneumoniae, S aureus,* other staphylococci, and gram-negative bacilli. Therapy for secondary abscesses should be broadened to include oral anaerobes.[19,20] Patients at high risk for aspiration should start with antibiotics targeting both CAP as well as oral anaerobes. Immunocompromised patients will require broad-spectrum antibiotic therapy, possibly including antifungal drugs, until there is clinical improvement or an organism is isolated.[19]

The standard of care for primary lung abscesses is conservative therapy with IV antibiotics.[21] A 2- to 3-week IV course followed by oral therapy for 4 to 8 weeks has been widely adopted.[20] Patients should remain hospitalized until their fever has resolved and their radiographic appearance has improved. Fortunately, in many cases, chest radiographs alone can be used to monitor the infectious fluid inside the abscess. As mentioned previously, secondary lung infections may require longer courses of IV antibiotics, and each case must be considered individually.

Recently, there has been an increasing role for interventional radiology. At this time there is insufficient research to provide stronger recommendations, but at least one institution has reported a decreased length of stay with routine CT-guided pigtail catheter insertion on presentation.[18]

Surgery has been used in isolated cases for patients who have failed medical therapy. It carries significant risks and is not currently recommended as a standard therapy.[18]

Prognosis

There are very few data regarding children with lung abscesses. Prognosis is likely very good for primary lung abscesses, while the outcome for secondary lung abscesses is affected by their predisposing conditions.[18,19] One long-term study of children who were treated with antibiotics alone showed that, aside from patients with asthma, there were no pulmonary function abnormalities approximately 9 years after treatment. Many of these children did show resolution of the abscess on chest radiographs; however, this took anywhere from 6 weeks to 5 years.[21]

Necrotizing Pneumonia and Bronchopleural Fistulas

Necrotizing pneumonia and bronchopleural fistulas are considered rare events in children; however, there has been some concern that the incidence is higher than previously thought.[7] While a solitary cavitary lesion is defined as an abscess, multiple cavitary lesions are characteristic of necrotizing pneumonia. These cavitary lesions are necrotic foci, and they represent lung parenchyma that is nonviable. The progressive infection often occurs simultaneously with progression of empyema, and almost all cases have an associated PPE.[22–24] Bronchopleural fistulas may develop as either a cause or sequelae of these lesions, as there is local spread of infection. The epidemiology and pathophysiology of necrotizing pneumonia in children is not completely understood at this time; however, it may develop due to either a particularly invasive organism or due to an exaggerated host-defense response.[23] Most patients with necrotic disease have already been treated with antibiotics. This may explain why an infectious organism is rarely recovered from pleural fluid or the blood. When bacteria are isolated, it is typically *S pneumoniae* and sometimes *S aureus*.[7,22,24]

Clinical Presentation

Children with necrotizing pneumonia have similar presenting signs and symptoms as uncomplicated pneumonia.[22] Patients will present with a pulmonary consolidation and a pleural effusion. Their symptoms may rapidly progress despite appropriate antibiotic treatment. While a chest radiograph will show an infiltrate and effusion, a chest CT may demonstrate multiple cavitary lesions within the consolidation[22] (Figure 20-3 and Figure 20-4).

A bronchopleural fistula should be suspected in any patient who produces sputum only when lying in one position.[25] An upright chest radiograph may show an air-fluid level in the pleural space, and a chest CT can help confirm the diagnosis.

Management

Appropriate parenteral antibiotic therapy must be initiated in the hospital. To ensure a rapid response to treatment, antibiotics should start with coverage for CAP, including resistant *S pneumoniae*. If an organism is isolated, then antibiotics may be tailored accordingly. The standard of care has been to give IV antibiotics for a prolonged course; many patients require weeks of therapy and some experts advocate for an additional course of oral antibiotics following IV therapy. Of note, shorter courses of treatment have been used with good outcomes in some case reports.[22] Supportive therapy is a key element of therapy because many children are critically ill and require mechanical ventilation. Many patients need to be admitted to the intensive care unit until they show clinical improvement, including resolution of fever, decreased work of breathing, and decreased supplemental oxygen requirement. Patients have been reported to have prolonged fevers despite antibiotic therapy for as long as 20 days.[26]

Most patients will require a thoracotomy tube for drainage; the use of VATS to debride the necrotic tissue is common but controversial.[7,22,24]

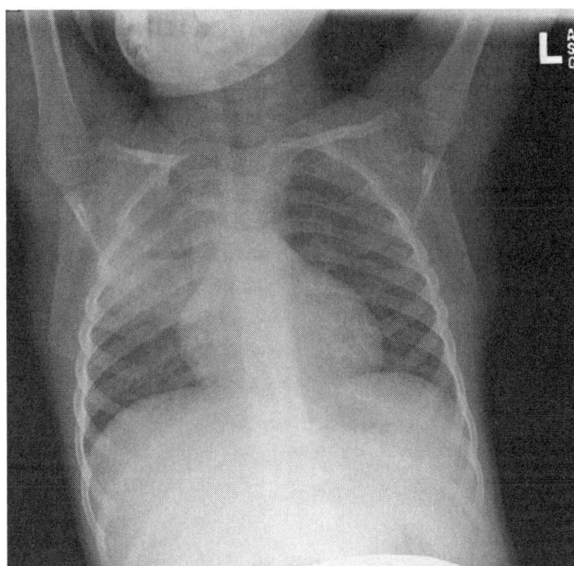

A

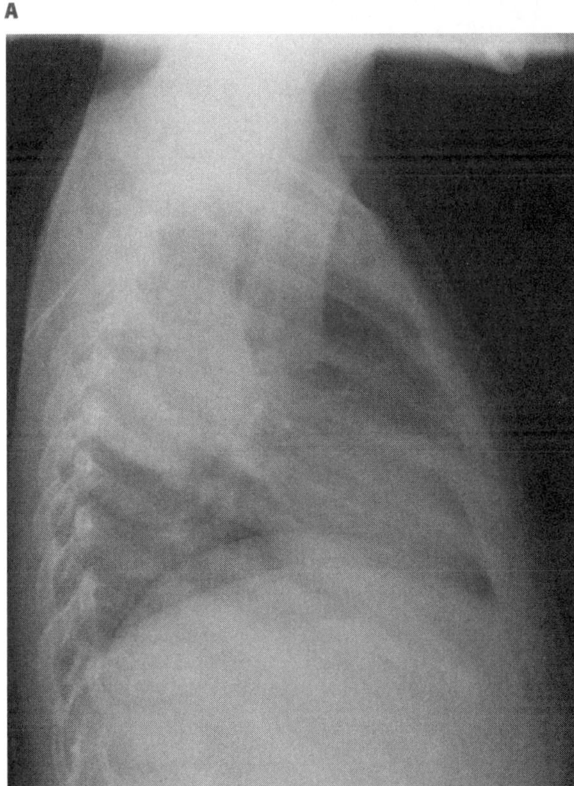

B

Figure 20-3.
This is a 4-year-old male who presented with a history of methicillin- resistant *Staphylococcus aureus* and increasing cough and intermittent fevers. **A, B.** Chest radiographs showed a cavitary lesion with an air-fluid level in the right upper lobe.

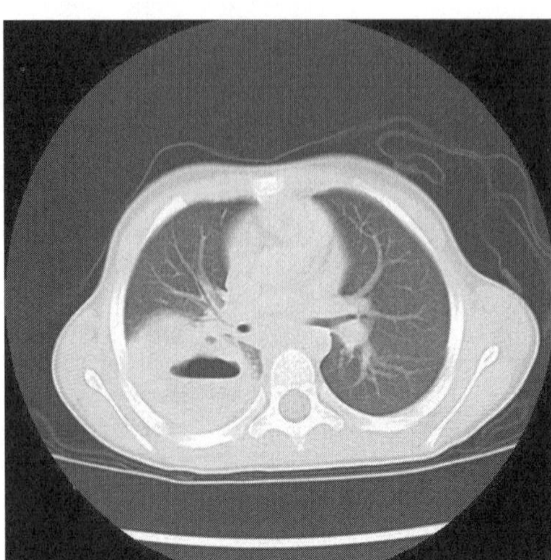

C

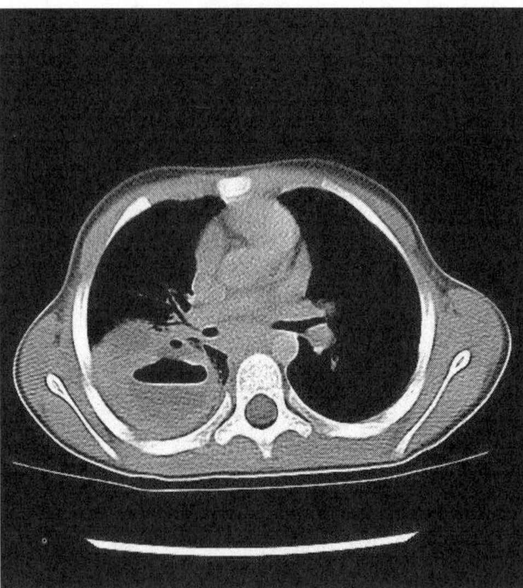

D

Figure 20-3.
C, D. A computed tomography scan demonstrated a multilocular cavitary lesion in the right upper lobe consistent with necrotizing pneumonia. He was treated with intravenous antibiotics followed by a prolonged oral course of antibiotics.

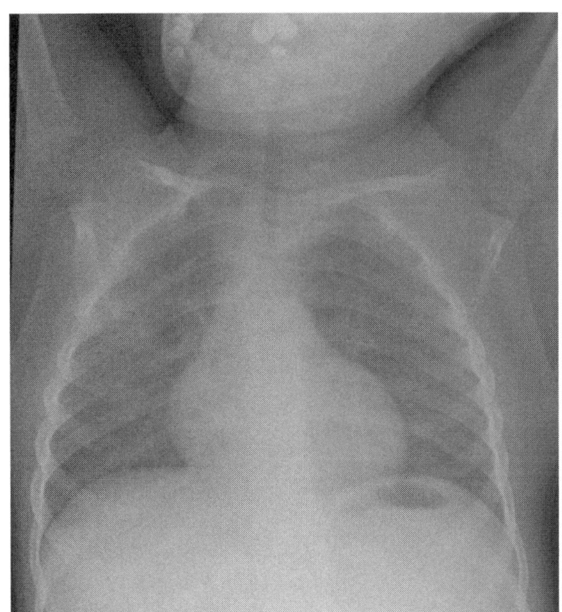

E

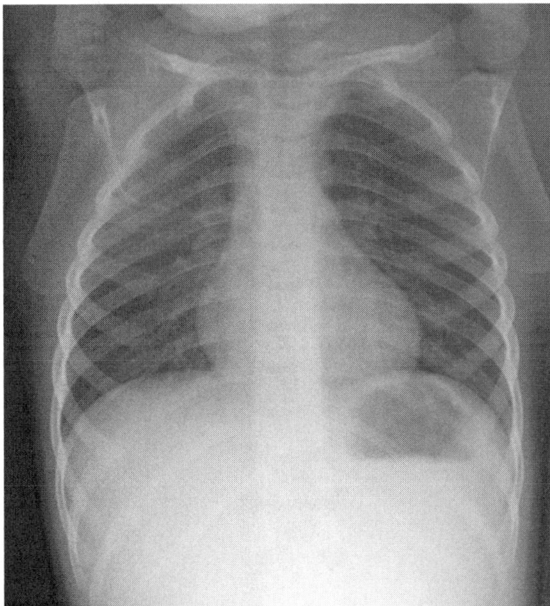

F

Figure 20-3.
E, F. After 1 month he demonstrated good radiologic improvement, with almost complete resolution after 3 months.

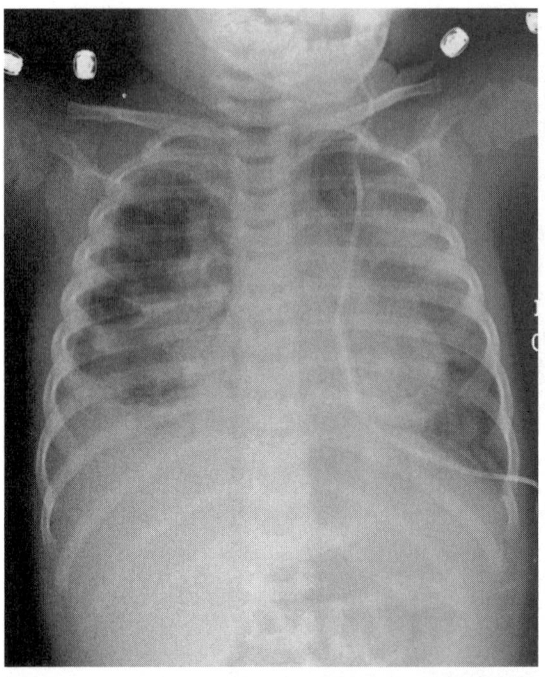

A

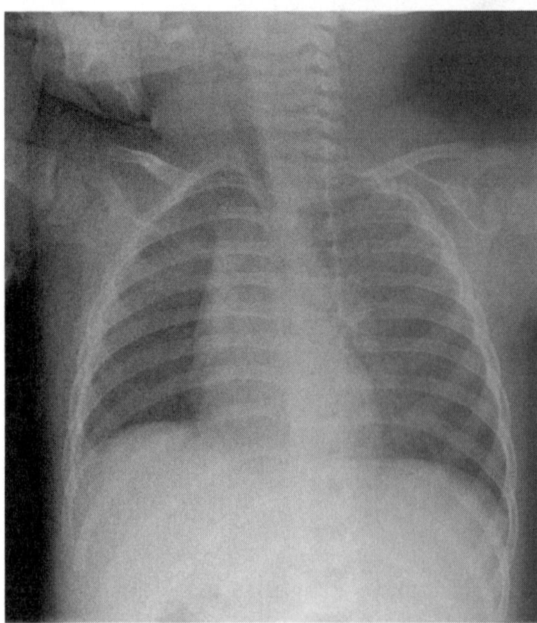

B

Figure 20-4.
This 3-year-old girl presented with fever, cough, and tachypnea. She was treated for community-acquired pneumonia. **A.** After she failed to defervesce she was found to have a parapneumonic effusion and necrotizing pneumonia. She was treated with intravenous antibiotics and video-assisted thoracoscopic surgery. After a prolonged hospitalization, including several days on the high-frequency oscillating ventilator, she was discharged home on oral antibiotics. **B.** A follow-up chest radiograph 2 months later shows almost complete resolution.

Patients who have developed a bronchopleural fistula will require prolonged drainage and subsequently a longer hospital stay.[7]

Prognosis

The mortality rate for necrotizing pneumonia is as high as 5.5% to 7%, although survivors typically are discharged in good health.[23,24] Most patients will have complete radiologic resolution at 1 to 3 months.[24,27]

Pneumatocele

Pneumatoceles develop after bacterial pneumonia has led to bronchiolar and alveolar necrosis. A communication is then made between the areas of the lung used for gas exchange and the interstitial space. The result is a thin-walled, air-filled, intraparenchymal air cyst. Pneumatoceles can be further divided into uncomplicated and complicated cases based on their clinical manifestations.[28] It is possible that pneumatoceles, which are rare in adults and occur more frequently in younger children, are more common in underdeveloped lungs. One theory is that the pores of Kohn, which allow collateral ventilation, are not fully developed and therefore air cannot escape from an obstructed region.[29]

Pneumatoceles are more common in children younger than 3 years.[29] Although bacteria are not always recovered, *S aureus* is frequently determined to be the responsible organism.[28]

Clinical Presentation

Patients with pneumatoceles secondary to pneumonia may not have any additional findings. Complicated pneumatoceles may have persistent fevers, coughing, or tachypnea despite adequate medical therapy.[28]

Pneumatoceles can typically be diagnosed by plain radiographs (Figure 20-5). At times a CT scan may be required to determine the thickness of the walls of the cyst or to look for bronchopleural fistulas. A new air-fluid level in the cyst may indicate an infected pneumatocele, which may require drainage.

Management

Most pneumatoceles caused by infection will self-resolve in fewer than 6 months with treatment of the underlying pneumonia.[28,29] Children with uncomplicated cases who have few clinical complaints, minimal

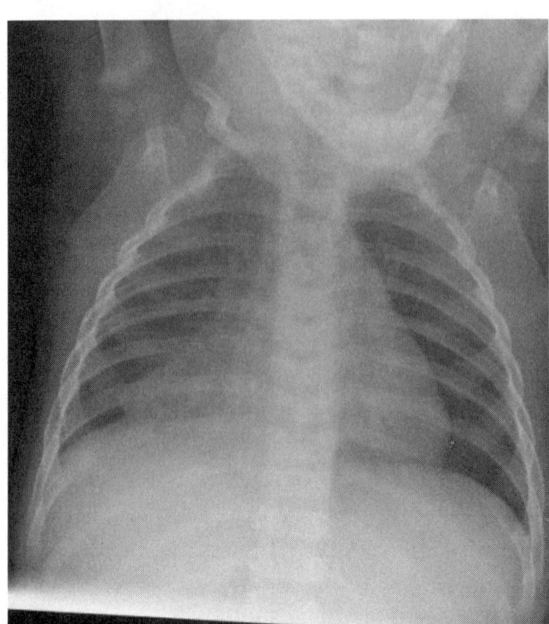

A

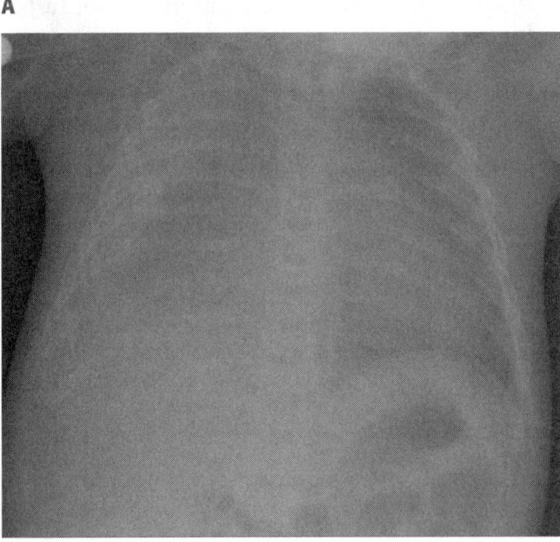

B

Figure 20-5. This 6-month-old patient initially presented with fever and tachypnea. **A.** His initial chest radiograph shows right-sided pneumonia. **B.** Subsequent film shows an effusion.

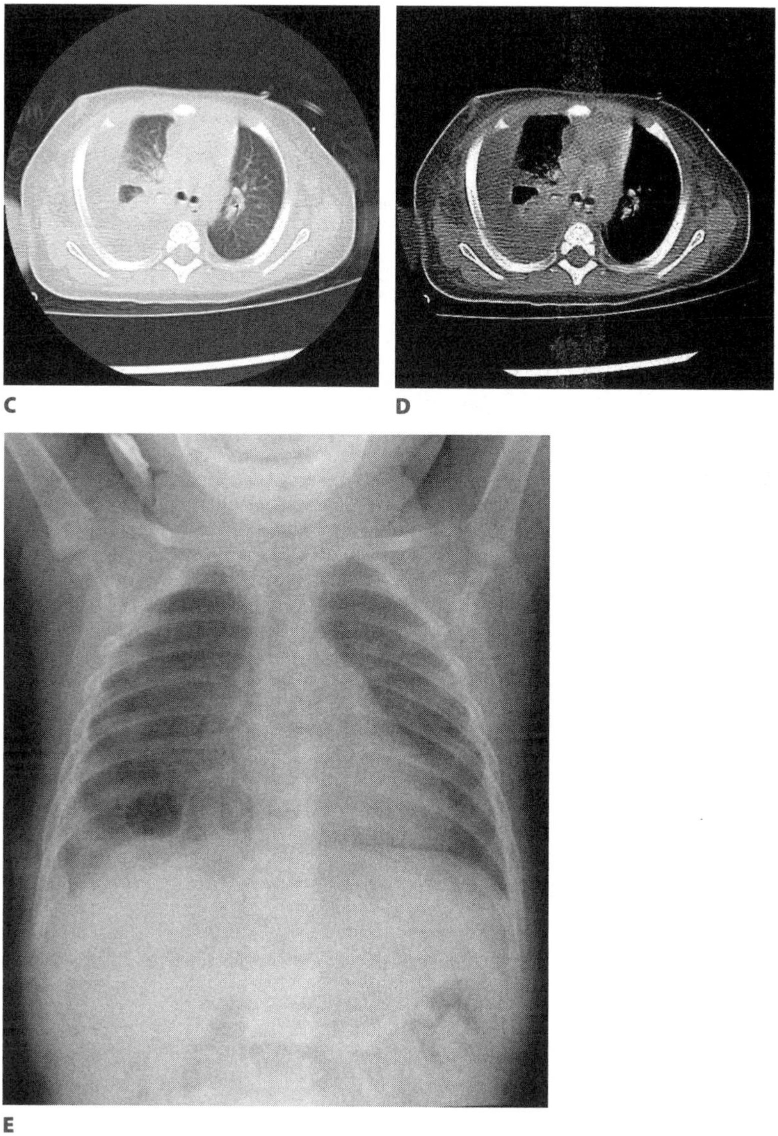

C

D

E

Figure 20-5. C, D. A computed tomography scan shows a freely flowing effusion. This patient underwent video-assisted thoracoscopic surgery, and methicillin-resistant *Staphylococcus aureus* was recovered from cultures of pleural fluid. **E.** Follow-up radiographs demonstrated pneumatoceles on the right side. The patient was in good health and was discharged home. Several days later he presented with increased work of breathing.

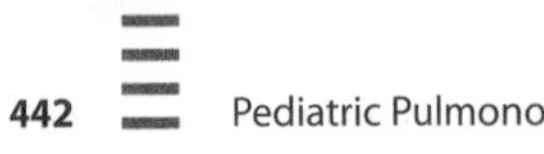

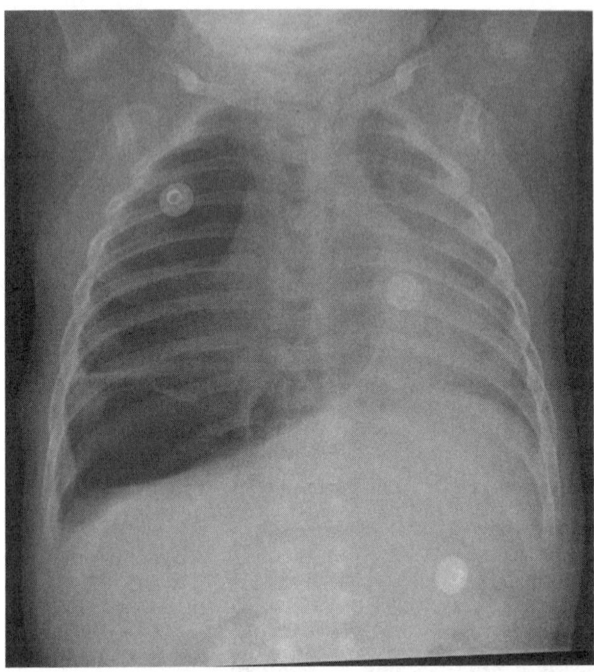

F

Figure 20-5.
F. A radiograph showed a right-sided tension pneumothorax, which was treated with needle decompression and a chest tube.
G. A radiograph 7 weeks later showed good radiologic recovery.

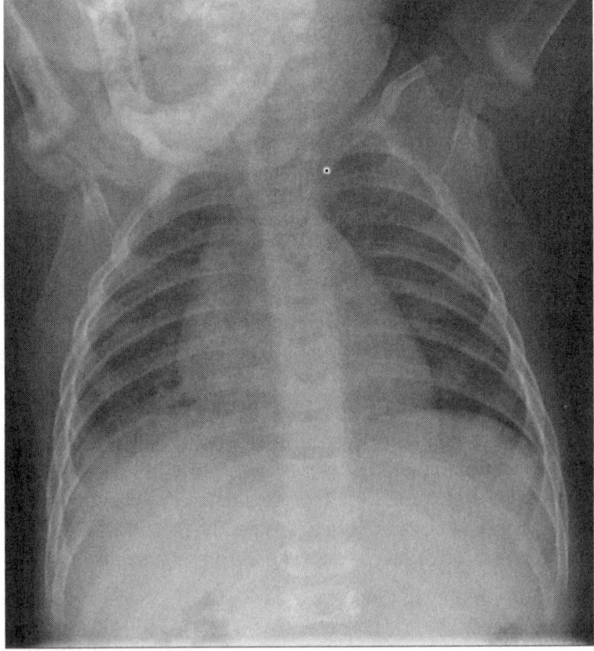

G

atelectasis, and involvement of less than 50% of the hemithorax can be observed with the expectation of spontaneous clinical improvement.[28]

Complicated pneumatoceles are more rare. These patients may have fevers, cough, tachypnea, localized infection, significant atelectasis, bronchopleural fistulae, and thicker walls. The pneumatocele also may involve more than 50% of the hemithorax. These patients may have some improvement after 6 months, but often require additional intervention. There is a risk of bronchopleural fistula formation and pneumothorax leading to rapid respiratory compromise, so close follow-up is advocated. Imamoğlu and colleagues[28] have advocated for early image guided catheter drainage in complicated cases. They have found that a delay in intervention may allow the thin wall of the pneumatocele to thicken and then require surgical excision. Figure 20-6 is a clinical guideline for pneumatocele management.[28]

Prognosis

Simple pneumatoceles have an excellent prognosis and typically resolve without treatment. Typically there are no visible sequelae on radiographs in 2 months, though some patients may require as long as 6 months to fully recover.[28,29] Complicated pneumatoceles, as noted previously, may require more intervention and have a less predictable prognosis. Patients who did require image-guided catheter drainage or surgery had a good prognosis afterward and did not experience recurrence of pneumatoceles.[28]

Hyponatremia

In the 1920s it was recognized that many children with pneumonia retained water,[30] and later an association with hyponatremia was discovered.[31] The incidence of hyponatremia (serum sodium <135 mmol/L) in children with pneumonia has been found to be approximately 42% to 45% of patients.[31,32]

Hyponatremia seen in children with pneumonia is often caused by the syndrome of inappropriate secretion of antidiuretic hormone (SIADH). Patients continue to drink despite elevated levels of antidiuretic hormone.[33] With excessive water retention the serum becomes increasingly hypo-osmolar, and a relative hyponatremia develops. The reason for this increase in antidiuretic hormone has not been extensively studied and is not known at this time.

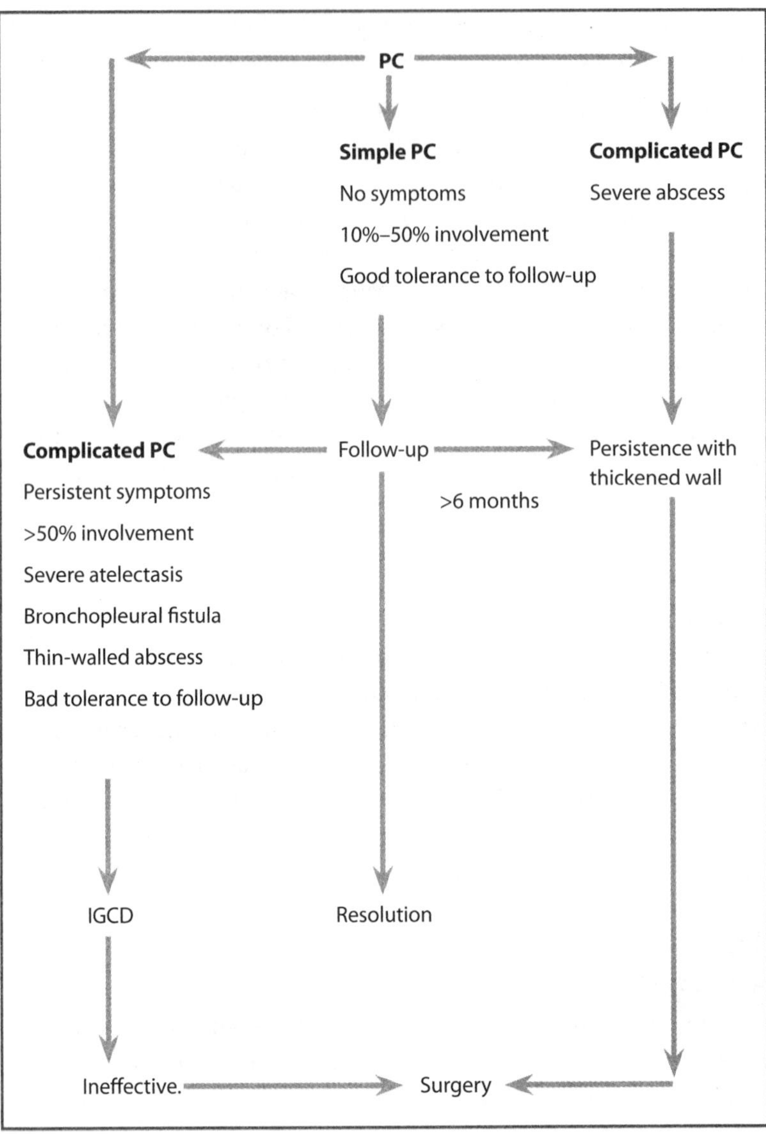

Figure 20-6. Algorithm for the management of pneumatoceles. IGCD, image-guided catheter drainage; PC, pneumatocele. (From Imamoğlu M, Cay A, Koşucu P, et al. Pneumatoceles in postpneumonic empyema: an algorithmic approach. *J Pediatr Surg.* 2005;40(7):1111–1117, with permission from Elsevier.)

Clinical Presentation

Patients with SIADH due to pneumonia develop a normovolemic hyponatremia. These patients do not gain excessive weight, do not develop edema, and are typically asymptomatic unless their sodium levels drop below 120 to 125 mmol/L for several days.[33]

No association has been found between the presence of hyponatremia and the pattern of pneumonia on chest radiograph or the cause of the infection.[32] The diagnosis can be made by evaluating serum electrolytes. Hyponatremia accompanied by decreased plasma osmolality may be enough for the diagnosis. Increased urine sodium excretion and urine osmolality greater than plasma osmolality may aid the diagnosis.[32]

Management

Treatment for hyponatremia in pneumonia consists of confirmation of SIADH and fluid restriction. Once it is clear that the patient has normovolemic hyponatremia they should receive less than full volume maintenance fluids, and any oral intake must be carefully measured. If IV fluids are used, then they should be limited to one-half of maintenance requirements, and older patients may have their oral intake limited to 500 to 1,000 mL/24 hours. Patients will continue to attempt to drink, since the regulatory mechanisms for osmoregulation are not strong enough to control their thirst.[33] If patients are too uncomfortable with fluid restriction, then drug therapy may be used. Hypertonic saline, or even normal saline, infusions should be reserved only for patients with significant symptoms or symptomatic hyponatremia for less than 3 days.[34]

Patients whose hyponatremia is lower than 130 mmol/L and who have chronic hyponatremia or patients in whom the diagnosis is in question require a nephrology consultation. Most patients with SIADH due to pneumonia will be asymptomatic since their hyponatremia is mild. Signs of severe hyponatremia (<120 mmol/L) are lethargy, anorexia, nausea, irritability, headache, muscle weakness, or cramps. Patients with these symptoms should have serum electrolytes and a nephrology evaluation immediately.

Prognosis

Hyponatremia in children with pneumonia in some developed countries has been reported to be mild and resolves with the treatment of the underlying pneumonia. In other countries, hyponatremia in children with pneumonia has been associated with prolonged hospital stays, increased complications, and a higher mortality rate. While similar findings have been found in adults with CAP in the United States, there has not been sufficient research in children to draw any definitive conclusions.

When to Refer

Due to the complicated nature of the infection and the need for a multidisciplinary approach, children with PPE and empyemas should be referred and admitted to a children's hospital. Pediatric specialists, specifically surgeons, pulmonologists, and infectious disease specialists, should be involved in their care. After discharge these patients should follow up with pediatric pulmonology specialists for pulmonary function testing and chest radiographs to ensure that they improve without further complications.

Lung abscesses are frequently treated with IV antibiotics alone and therefore may be treated at local children's inpatient centers, unless there is significant respiratory compromise. More complicated cases may require a transfer to a children's hospital for pediatric pulmonology, pediatric surgery, and possibly interventional radiology. Complicated cases require a referral to pediatric pulmonology after discharge.

Necrotizing pneumonia and bronchopleural fistulas should be referred and transferred to a children's hospital. Like PPE, these patients often require a multidisciplinary approach and long-term follow-up with pediatric pulmonology specialists after discharge.

Complicated pneumatoceles should be referred to a children's hospital for management by pediatric pulmonology and surgery specialists. Uncomplicated cases have a very good prognosis and may be followed as an outpatient by pediatric pulmonology specialists.

Hyponatremia with pneumonia is a very common complication that does not typically require a referral to a children's hospital. Pediatricians should manage the care of these patients but, unless there are significant symptoms or their sodium is below 125 mmol/L, specialists may not need to be involved. If the hyponatremia is due to SIADH, then it should resolve without treatment and the patient does not need to follow up with a pediatric nephrologist or pulmonologist.

When to Admit

Many of the complications of pneumonia are diagnosed in patients who have failed outpatient therapy or patients who are already hospitalized. All of these patients should be treated with IV antibiotics, and many will require further medical and/or surgical treatment. Experienced pediatric interventional radiologists or surgeons should be involved in the care of any patient who may need chest tube placement or surgical intervention, such as VATS. It is important to note that surgical consultation does not obligate the surgeon to perform a procedure. Pediatric surgeons, interventional radiologists, pediatric pulmonologists, and pediatric infectious disease specialists should, as a team, help determine the best approach for the patient.

Key Points

Complications of Pneumonia

- Typically require hospitalization
- Are usually caused by the most common causes of CAP
- Frequently require multidisciplinary care at a children's hospital
- Even in very ill children the long-term prognosis is generally very good

Recommended Resources

Balfour-Lynn IM, Abrahamson E, Cohen G, et al. BTS guidelines for the management of pleural infection in children. *Thorax.* 2005;60(suppl 1):i1–i21

Taussig LM, Landau LI, eds. *Pediatric Respiratory Medicine.* 2nd ed. Philadelphia, PA: Mosby; 2008

Acknowledgment

Special thanks to Dr Polly Koch from the radiology department at St Christopher's Hospital for Children, for providing many of the images for this chapter.

References

1. Hardier W, Bucolic R, Garcia VG, et al. Pneumococcal pleural empyemas in children. *Clin Infect Dis.* 1996;22(6):1057–1063
2. Tan TQ, Mason EO Jr, Wald ER, et al. Clinical characteristics of children with complicated pneumonia caused by *Streptococcus pneumoniae. Pediatrics.* 2002;110(1 pt 1):1–6
3. Colin AA. Pneumonia in the developed world. *Paediatr Respir Rev.* 2006;7(suppl 1):S138–S140
4. Schultz KD, Fan LL, Ponsky J, et al. The changing face of pleural empyemas in children: epidemiology and management. *Pediatrics.* 2004;113(6):1735–1740
5. Michelow IC, Olsen K, Lozano J, et al. Epidemiology and clinical characteristics of community-acquired pneumonia in hospitalized children. *Pediatrics.* 2002;113(4):701–707
6. Eastham KM, Freeman R, Kearns AM, et al. Clinical features, etiology and outcome of empyema in children in the north east of England. *Thorax.* 2004;59(6):522–525
7. Ampul N, Eastham KM, Freeman R, et al. Activatory lung disease complicating empyema in children. *Pediatr Pulmonol.* 2006;41(8):750–753
8. Buckingham SC, King MD, Miller ML, et al. Incidence and etiologies of complicated parapneumonic effusions in children, 1996 to 2001. *Pediatr Infect Dis J.* 2003;22(6):499–504
9. Sahn SA. Diagnosis and management of parapneumonic effusions and empyema. *Clin Infect Dis.* 2007;45(11):1480–1486
10. Balfour-Lynn IM, Abrahamson E, Cohen G, et al. BTS guidelines for the management of pleural infection in children. *Thorax.* 2005;60(suppl 1):i1–i21
11. Gould IM. BTS guidelines on CAP. Community acquired pneumonia. *Thorax.* 2002;57(7):657
12. Donnelley FL, Lobsterman LA. The yield of CT of children who have complicated pneumonia and noncontributory chest radiography. *AJR Am J Roentgenol.* 1998;170(6):1627–1631
13. Donnelley LF, Lobsterman LA. CT appearance of parapneumonic effusions in children: findings are not specific for empyema. *AJR Am J Roentgenol.* 1997;169(1):179–182
14. Kurt BA, Winterhalter KM, Connors RH, Betz BW, Winters JW. Therapy of parapneumonic effusions in children: video-assisted thoracoscopic surgery versus conventional thoracostomy drainage. *Pediatrics.* 2006;118(3):e547–e553
15. Snapper S, Cohen G, Owens CM, et al. Comparison of urokinase and video-assisted thoracoscopic surgery for treatment of childhood empyema. *Am J Respir Crit Care Med.* 2006;174(2):221–227
16. Breonesin D, Thomson AH. How should we manage empyema: antibiotics alone, fibrinolytics, or primary video-assisted thoracoscopic surgery (VATS)? *Semin Respir Crit Care Med.* 2007;28(3):322–332

17. Cham PC, Huang LM, Wu PS, et al. Clinical management and outcome of childhood lung abscess: a 16-year experience. *J Microbiol Immunol Infect.* 2005;38(3):183–188
18. Parazoon-Ho P, Fitzgerald DA. Lung abscess in children. *Paediatr Respir Rev.* 2007;8(1):77–84
19. Yen CC, Tang RB, Chen SJ, et al. Pediatric lung abscess: a retrospective review of 23 cases. *J Microbiol Immunol Infect.* 2004;37(1):45–49
20. Tan TQ, Sellheim DK, Kaplan SL, et al. Pediatric lung abscess: clinical management and outcome. *Pediatr Infect Dis J.* 1995;14(1):51–55
21. Asher MI, Spier S, Bland M, et al. Primary lung abscess in childhood: the long-term outcome of conservative management. *Am J Dis Child.* 1982;136(6):491–494
22. McCarthy VP, Patamasucon P, Gaines T, et al. Necrotizing pneumococcal pneumonia in childhood. *Pediatr Pulmonol.* 1999;28(3):217–221
23. Hacimustafaoglu M, Celebi S, Sarimehmet HJ, et al. Necrotizing pneumonia in children. *Acta Paediatr.* 2004;93(9):1172–1177
24. Hsieh YC, Hsiao CH, Tsao PN, et al. Necrotizing pneumococcal pneumonia in children: the role of pulmonary gangrene. *Pediatr Pulmonol.* 2006;41(7):623–629
25. Crawford SE, Daum RS. Bacterial pneumonia, lung abscess, and empyema. In: Taussig LM, Landau LI, eds. *Pediatric Respiratory Medicine.* 2nd ed. Philadelphia, PA: Mosby; 2008:501–553
26. Kerem E, Bar Ziv Y, Rudenski B, et al. Bacteremic necrotizing pneumococcal pneumonia in children. *Am J Respir Crit Care Med.* 1994;149(1):242–244
27. Sawicki GS, Lu FL, Valim C, Cleveland RH, Colin AA. Necrotising pneumonia is an increasingly detected complication of pneumonia in children. *Eur Respir J.* 2008;31(6):1285–1291
28. Imamoğlu M, Cay A, Koşucu P, et al. Pneumatoceles in postpneumonic empyema: an algorithmic approach. *J Pediatr Surg.* 2005;40(7):1111–1117
29. Kunyoshi V, Cataneo DC, Cataneo AJ. Complicated pneumonias with empyema and/or pneumatocele in children. *Pediatr Surg Int.* 2006;22(2):186–190
30. Lussky H, Friedstein H. Water retention in pneumonia. *Am J Dis Child.* 1920;19:337–343
31. Shann F, Germer S. Hyponatraemia associated with pneumonia or bacterial meningitis. *Arch Dis Child.* 1985;60(10):963–966
32. Don M, Valerio G, Korppi M, et al. Hyponatremia in pediatric community-acquired pneumonia. *Pediatr Nephrol.* 2008;23(12):2247–2253
33. Baylis PH. The syndrome of inappropriate antidiuretic hormone secretion. *Int J Biochem Cell Biol.* 2003;35(11):1495–1499
34. Singhi S, Dhawan A. Frequency and significance of electrolyte abnormalities in pneumonia. *Indian Pediatr.* 1992;29(6):735–740

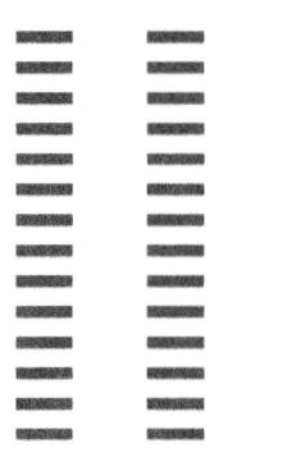

Chapter 21

Recurrent Pneumonia

Paul C. Stillwell, MD

Introduction

Recurrent pneumonia is arbitrarily defined as 3 or more episodes of pneumonia in a lifetime or 2 episodes within a 6-month period.[1–3] In pediatric practice chest radiographs are not consistently used to diagnose pneumonia. The diagnosis of pneumonia is commonly made based on clinical history and physical examination findings alone, despite recommendations for radiographic confirmation in community-acquired pneumonia.[4] It is also common practice to not obtain a follow-up radiograph to document resolution of the pneumonia if the patient returns to their usual state of health. This makes it difficult to determine if there has actually been recurrent pneumonia or whether the problem is really persistent rather than recurrent.[3]

The differential diagnosis of a persistent radiographic abnormality is somewhat different than that for recurrent pneumonia. The lack of consistent radiographic confirmation for each episode also makes it difficult to ascertain whether the abnormality recurs in the same lung segments or in a variety of different segments.[3] From a global perspective, where pneumonia in underdeveloped countries is a major childhood killer, the clinical findings of fever and rapid respiratory rate are sufficient to diagnose pneumonia and institute appropriate intervention.[5] Even the British Thoracic Society guidelines for the management of community-acquired pneumonia in childhood do not recommend chest radiography for mild, uncomplicated acute lower respiratory tract infection.[6] Because early identification of and treatment directed at a potential underlying cause of recurring pneumonia may be beneficial for long-term lung health, the practitioner should consider radiographic confirmation for patients who seem to have frequent lower respiratory tract symptoms.[1–3] Recurrent pneumonia can certainly lead to persistent lung injury and radiographic abnormalities if not prevented.

Pathophysiology

Box 21-1 categorizes conditions causing recurrent pneumonia in children. A careful history, physical examination, and review of the radiographs will help tailor the investigation to identify the underlying cause.[1–3]

A number of immune-mediated diseases can cause recurrent pneumonia in children. Fortunately most are uncommon. Associated symptoms and signs may provide a clue to the underlying diagnosis. Congenital anomalies and airway obstructions most commonly present as persistent radiographic abnormalities, but they may present as recurrent pneumonia if there is an overlying recurrent infection in or adjacent to the abnormality, or if follow-up radiographs are not taken.[7]

If the recurrent pneumonia is due to immune deficiency, and the patient does not have significant infections outside the respiratory tract, then the immunodeficiency is likely to be a B-cell problem. The infectious agent is often a common respiratory tract pathogen. Immunoglobulin (Ig) G deficiency, IgG subclass deficiency, and IgA deficiency are all associated with recurrent sinopulmonary infections. If the child has poor growth and serious infections in other organ systems, the immunodeficiency is more likely to be in the T-cell–mediated system or in the phagocytic portion of the immune system. These infections can be due to common respiratory pathogens or opportunistic pathogens.[3]

The mechanism of recurrent pneumonia in the child with asthma is likely mucus plugging during acute asthma exacerbations. The usual trigger is a viral upper respiratory tract infection, which may cause a fever as well. The constellation of fever, respiratory difficulty, abnormal auscultation, and an abnormal chest radiograph leads to the diagnosis of pneumonia. Many children with asthma as the cause of their recurrent pneumonia will have cough and wheeze acutely, and may have asthma symptoms apart from viral infections (eg, allergen, irritant, or exercise triggers). Improved asthma control often eliminates or reduces the episodes of pneumonia.[3]

Box 21-1. Conditions Leading to Recurrent Pneumonia in Children

Immune Deficiency (congenital or acquired)

- Abnormal cell mediated immunity (T cell)
- Hypogammaglobulinemia (B cell)
- Neutrophil/macrophage dysfunction
- Mucosal surface immunodeficiency (immunoglobulin [Ig] A deficiency, IgG subclass deficiency)
- Syndromes associated with immunodeficiency

Impaired Mucociliary Clearance

- Asthma
- Cystic fibrosis
- Primary ciliary dyskinesia
- Tracheomalacia/bronchomalacia
- Restricted chest wall (weakness, immobility, uncoordinated cough)

Mechanical Abnormalities

- Aspiration
- Intrinsic obstruction (tumor, retained foreign body)
- Extrinsic compression (tumor, adenopathy, enlarged cardiac structure)

Systemic and Immune-Mediated Diseases

- Hypersensitivity pneumonitis
- Collagen vascular disease
- Idiopathic hemosiderosis
- Renal-pulmonary syndromes
- Granulomatous diseases
- Allergic bronchopulmonary aspergillosis
- Pulmonary alveolar proteinosis
- Acute chest syndrome (in sickle cell disease)

Congenital Anomaly

- Bronchogenic cyst
- Sequestration
- Esophageal duplication
- Cystic adenomatoid malformation
- Congenital lobar overdistention
- Tracheal bronchus (or other abnormal tracheobronchial branching)

Non-Pulmonary Causes

- Pulmonary edema
- Lymphangiectasis
- Diaphragmatic hernia
- Mediastinal mass
- Anomalous pulmonary venous return

The child with cystic fibrosis (CF) may present with a history of recurrent pneumonia.[8] Cystic fibrosis as the cause of recurrent pneumonia should be considered if there is associated steatorrhea and/or failure to thrive. However, approximately 10% to 15% of patients with CF are pancreatic sufficient, so the patient may not have growth failure.[9] Most states now have newborn screening for CF, which should identify 95% or more of the patients with CF. Even if the child has had a negative newborn screen, the diagnosis of CF should be considered for children with recurrent pneumonia.[9]

Patients with primary ciliary dyskinesia (PCD) may have recurrent pneumonia starting in the neonatal period. Approximately 50% will have associated dextrocardia and abdominal situs inversus. Chronic and recurrent otitis media and sinus infections are almost universal for patients with PCD. The diagnosis is usually made by documenting ciliary abnormalities on electron micrographs. More recently available DNA analysis and exhaled nitric oxide studies may help establish the diagnosis of PCD.[10]

Children with reduced cough efficiency may have recurrent pneumonias because they have poor control of normal secretions. This occurs commonly in children with neurologic deficits (eg, cerebral palsy) and weakness (eg, muscular dystrophy) but can also occur in children with other types of chest wall restriction, such as kyphoscoliosis.[3] Excessive dynamic collapse of the trachea or main stem bronchi (tracheomalacia/bronchomalacia) may also impair mucus clearance. In addition to recurrent pneumonia these children may have stridor or wheezing. The etiology of tracheomalacia and bronchomalacia is usually unknown, and the collapse usually improves with age, although patients with prior surgery for a tracheoesophageal fistula commonly have dynamic airway collapse that persists.[11,12]

Aspiration is a common cause of recurrent pneumonia in children.[1-3] It can occur while swallowing directly or after esophageal reflux. Children with neurologic abnormalities are at particular risk, although neurologically normal children can aspirate as well. Any child with gastroesophageal reflux (GER) is at risk for aspiration during periods of decreased consciousness (such as sleep) and while recumbent.[13] It is controversial whether or not aspiration of normal oral secretions causes recurrent pneumonia. Laryngeal clefts and H-type tracheoesophageal fistulas are rare causes of aspiration.

Evaluation of the Child With Recurrent Pneumonia

A careful history and physical examination should lead to a concise differential diagnosis, and the subsequent laboratory evaluation can then be tailored for the most likely underlying condition. Box 21-2 lists common diagnostic tools often of help in evaluating the child with recurrent pneumonia.[1–3]

The first step is to gather all the chest radiographs for review. It is often helpful to have all the radiographs interpreted by a pediatric radiologist who has access to all the images at the same time and has a clinical summary. Certain patterns may suggest other tests or simply a different therapeutic approach. For example, the child whose chest radiographs repeatedly show overinflation, diffuse increased peribronchial markings, and subsegmental atelectasis with normal findings in between may not need additional studies but more aggressive asthma management.

If a defect in the immune system is suspected, initial screening studies should be considered, such as a complete blood cell count, white cell differential, quantitative immunoglobulins (IgG, IgM, and IgA), and perhaps IgG subclasses. More extensive evaluations might include T- and B-cell numbers, antibody response to immunizations, total complement, and measurement of neutrophil function.[1–3]

Box 21-2. Diagnostic Evaluation of the Child With Recurrent Pneumonia

- Screening for immunodeficiency
- Testing for cystic fibrosis (sweat chloride test, DNA analysis)
- Testing for primary ciliary dyskinesia (electron microscopy studies, DNA analysis, fractional exhaled nitric oxide)
- Modified barium swallow (with speech therapist present)
- Esophogram and upper gastrointestinal series
- Other tests for reflux and aspiration
    - Gastric emptying study
    - Radioactive lung scintiscan
    - pH/impedance probe
- Pulmonary function testing
    - Flow-volume loops before and after bronchodilator
    - Lung volume studies
    - Diffusion capacity
    - Challenge tests (exercise, methacholine, cold air)
- Chest computed tomography
- Flexible bronchoscopy with bronchoalveolar lavage

The standard test for CF is the sweat chloride determination. Even if the newborn screen was negative for CF, a sweat test should be performed for any child with recurrent pneumonia unless there is a clear alternative explanation. DNA analysis is another available diagnostic test for CF. Specialized tests, such as the mucosal electrical potential difference, are not commonly available.[9]

The traditional test for PCD is electron microscopic evaluation of the ciliary ultrastructure. Cilia from respiratory mucosa can be obtained by mucosal biopsy, brushing the mucosa with a cytology brush, or curette scraping of the nasal mucosa. Patients with PCD usually have a decreased exhaled nitric oxide. DNA analysis for mutations causing PCD has recently become available, but the recognized mutations are present in less than 50% of the subjects with PCD. Assessment of the ciliary wave form and beat frequency by microscopic examination on live cilia can also document ciliary dyskinesia, but this test is not definitive nor commonly available.[10]

Aspiration can be identified with certainty only if contrast material is identified in the airway during a modified barium swallow or upper gastrointestinal series. If GER is identified without evidence for aspiration, additional testing may be pursued to determine if there is a link between GER and recurrent pneumonia. Milk scintiscan is one test that can document aspiration after reflux, but it is insensitive.[14] The use of the lipid index, which is a semiquantification of lipid-laden macrophages obtained during bronchoalveolar lavage, to document aspiration is controversial.[15]

Computed tomography (CT) of the chest is helpful in identifying congenital lung anomalies; chronic airway damage, such as bronchiectasis; bronchial obstruction; and tracheobronchial branching pattern abnormality.[16] Because of the high radiation exposure with CT scanning, this test should be ordered after prudent consideration and performed with pediatric-specific algorithms to reduce the total radiation dose.[16] Flexible bronchoscopy is useful for identifying airway abnormalities and for sampling lower airway and alveolar samples. Mucosal biopsy for ciliary electron microscopy to assess primary ciliary dyskinesia can be obtained during bronchoscopy. Bronchoalveolar lavage is useful to assess acute and chronic infection, evaluate opportunistic infection in the immunocompromised patient, and assess for lipid-laden macrophages.

Treatment

If a specific underlying etiology for the recurrent pneumonia can be identified, therapy should be directed at that etiology. If the underlying etiology is asthma, comprehensive and aggressive management of the asthma usually stops the recurrence of the pneumonia. Similarly, stopping aspiration from occurring usually prevents the recurrence of the pneumonia. Some children will be at risk for recurring pneumonias despite appropriate therapy. An example might be the neurologically challenged child with impaired secretion control. Assisting these patients with airway clearance techniques may minimize the frequency of their pneumonia. There are several options for assisting airway clearance, such as nebulized bronchodilators, nebulized corticosteroids, chest physical therapy with postural drainage, high-frequency chest wall oscillation, and cough assist devices. There are some pharmacologic treatments targeted for patients with CF that have not been extensively studied in other lung diseases, such as nebulized antibiotics, dornase alpha, and hypertonic saline. Other lung-protective strategies should be recommended, such as complete childhood immunization; annual influenza immunization; and avoidance of toxicities, such as environmental tobacco poisoning.

Key Points

- A careful history and physical examination, coupled with radiographic documentation of suspected lower respiratory tract infections, allow a stepwise evaluation plan to discover an underlying cause for the recurrent pneumonia if one exists.
- Treatment is directed at a specific cause once identified. Every effort should be made to protect and preserve lung function.

References

1. Kaplan KA, Beierle EA, Faro A, et al. Recurrent pneumonia in children: a case report and approach to diagnosis. *Clin Pediatr (Phila).* 2006;45(1):15–22
2. Panitch HB. Evaluation of recurrent pneumonia. *Pediatr Infect Dis J.* 2005;24(3):265–266
3. Vaughn D, Katkin JP. Chronic and recurrent pneumonias in children. *Semin Respir Infect.* 2002;17(1):72–84
4. McIntosh K. Community-acquired pneumonia in children. *N Engl J Med.* 2002;346:429–437
5. Durbin WJ, Stille C. Pneumonia. *Pediatr Rev.* 2008;29(5):147–158
6. British Thoracic Society. BTS guidelines for the management of community acquired pneumonia in childhood. *Thorax.* 2002;57:1–24
7. Mendeloff EN. Sequestrations, congenital cystic adenomatoid malformations, and congenital lobar emphysema. *Semin Thorac Cardiovasc Surg.* 2004;16(3):2009–2014
8. Gibson RL, Burns JL, Ramsey BW. Pathophysiology and management of pulmonary infections in cystic fibrosis. *Am J Respir Crit Care Med.* 2003;168:918–951
9. Farrell PM, Rosenstsein BJ, White TB, et al. Guidelines for diagnosis of cystic fibrosis in newborns through older adults: Cystic Fibrosis Foundation Consensus report. *J Pediatr.* 2008;153:S4–S14
10. Noone PG, Leigh MW, Sannuti A, et al. Primary ciliary dyskinesia: diagnostic and phenotypic features. *Am J Respir Crit Care Med.* 2004;169:459–467
11. Yalcin E, Dogru D, Ozcelik U, et al. Tracheomalacia and bronchomalacia in 34 children: clinical and radiologic profiles and associations with other diseases. *Clin Pediatr (Phila).* 2005;44(9):777–781
12. Kovesi T, Rubin S. Long-term complications of congenital esophageal atresia and/or tracheoesophageal fistula. *Chest.* 2004;126(3):914–925
13. Sheikh S, Allen E, Shell R, et al. Chronic aspiration without gastroesophageal reflux as a cause of chronic respiratory symptoms in neurologically normal infants. *Chest.* 2001;120(4):1190–1195
14. Ravelli AM, Panarotto MB, Verdoni L, et al. Pulmonary aspiration shown by scintigraphy in gastroesophageal reflux-related respiratory disease. *Chest.* 2006;130(5):1520–1526
15. Colombo JL, Hallberg TK. Pulmonary aspiration and lipid-laden macrophages: in search of gold (standards). *Pediatr Pulmonol.* 1999;28(2):79–82
16. Copley SJ. Application of computed tomography in childhood respiratory infections. *Br Med Bull.* 2002;61:263–279

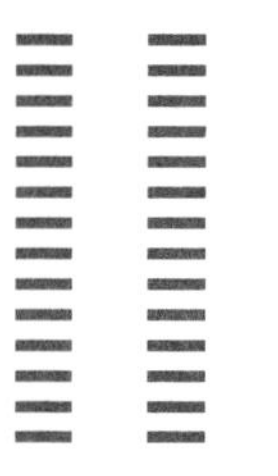

Chapter 22

Tuberculosis

Carol Conrad, MD

Introduction

Tuberculosis (TB) is an infectious disease that has coevolved with humans and has been described at least since the Neolithic times, 10,000 BC, when the development of human technology and farming began. Tuberculosis is typically caused by *Mycobacterium tuberculosis* and occasionally by *Mycobacterium bovis* and *Mycobacterium africanum*. The lungs are the major site of *M tuberculosis* infection (TB), though other modes of infection with *M tuberculosis* can occur on contamination of an open wound, such as could occur with infection of an insect bite or an abrasion of the skin. Congenital infection occurs either transplacentally or by inhalation of infected amniotic fluid at the time of delivery. *Mycobacterium bovis* infection results primarily from ingestion of unpasteurized milk or dairy products that contain *M bovis* and more likely will cause cervical lymphadenitis, gastrointestinal disease, and meningitis, although latent infection can progress to pulmonary disease. Infection by *M bovis*, representing about 1% to 2% of TB cases, is more likely to occur in developing countries where control of TB in cattle and pasteurization of milk are not available and may occur in children of families entering the United States from endemic countries.

Worldwide, TB remains one of the leading causes of death from infectious disease. An estimated 2 billion persons (ie, one-third of the world's population) are infected with *M tuberculosis*. After approximately 30 years of decline, the number of TB cases reported in the United States increased 20% during 1985–1992. In 2005 approximately 8.8 million persons became ill from TB, and 1.6 million died from the disease. Although the 2009 TB rate (3.8 cases per 100,000 population) was the lowest recorded in the United States since national reporting began in

1953, the average annual decline has slowed since 2000 (Figure 22-1). Today there is much concern about the multidrug-resistant (MDR) TB (resistant to both isoniazid and rifampin), and extensively drug-resistant (XDR) (resistant to isoniazid; rifampin; fluoroquinolones; and at least one second-line injectable agent, such as amikacin, kanamycin, and/or capreomycin). The emergence of these species poses a serious threat to disease control, and is particularly concerning in southern Africa, China, India, and the former Soviet Union. Because of regional problems such as drought, famine, and war, mass migration from these countries has contributed to the increasing incidence of MDR strains in Western Europe[1] and the United States.[2] In 2010 the World Health Organization (WHO) published a global surveillance and report of MDR-TB and XDR-TB. They report that in 2008 an estimated 390,000 to 510,000 cases of MDR-TB emerged globally (best estimate: 440,000 cases). Among all incident TB cases globally, 3.6% are estimated to have MDR-TB. Almost 50% of MDR-TB cases worldwide are estimated to occur in China and India. In 2008 MDR-TB caused an estimated 150,000 deaths. Combining data from these countries, 5.4% of MDR-TB cases were found to have XDR-TB globally. To date,

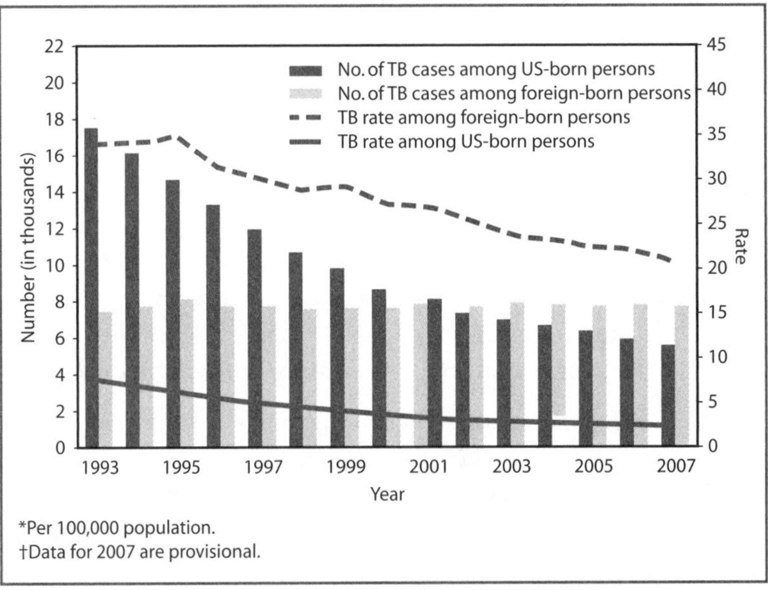

Figure 22-1. Number and rate* of tuberculosis (TB) cases among US- and foreign-born persons, by year reported—United States, 1993–2007.† (From Centers for Disease Control and Prevention. Trends in tuberculosis—United States, 2007. *MMWR Recomm Rep.* 2008;57[11]:281–285.)

a cumulative total of 58 countries have confirmed at least one case of XDR-TB.[3]

Almost all cases of TB are acquired through person-to-person contact via droplet nuclei formed by sneezing, coughing, or phonating. The tubercle bacilli establish infection in the lung after droplets containing 2 or 3 bacilli (small enough [5–10 μm] to reach the alveolar space) are inhaled. If the bacterial clusters contain more bacilli, the droplets are larger and will not cause infection, because the droplet will be cleared quickly by mucociliary transport defense mechanisms of the larger airways. Whether a particle that reaches the alveoli will cause infection or disease depends on the virulence of the bacilli and the killing activity of the host macrophages.

Primary Infection

The initial host defense in the alveoli involves phagocytosis by the macrophages. However, a tubercle bacillus can multiply slowly within the macrophage without being killed. Once bacterial numbers are large enough (10^3–10^4 organisms), a cellular response is elicited by macrophage activation. At the slow rate of replication by *M tuberculosis,* this process takes about 4 to 8 weeks. A *tubercle,* or *granuloma,* is a formation of an epithelioid cluster of macrophages with phagocytosed bacilli, and is the primary focus that represents infection. The infection spreads through the lymphatics to the hilar lymph nodes. A Ghon complex consists of the primary focus, lymphangitis, and regional hilar lymph node inflammation associated with it. These are generally located in the middle or lower lobes of the lungs. The spread of infection is contained by stimulation of cell-mediated immunity (CMI) processes. The granuloma will proceed to fibrosis and calcification and produce an isolated, calcified spot on the chest radiograph.

Dissemination

Bacilli can escape before a sufficient immune response has been elicited if the innate defense system of the host fails to mount an effective cell-mediated response for eliminating the infection. The bacilli proliferate inside alveolar macrophages and kill the cells. Dying cells release TB bacilli into the surrounding lung parenchyma and cause progressive destruction of the lung. Bacilli can spread mechanically by erosion of the caseating lesions into the lung airways or cavities can form. Once bacilli are present within the airspaces, the host becomes infectious to others, and infection is spread via droplet nuclei created when coughing, etc. In an infected population, bacilli may also be spread hematogenously and seed other portions of the lungs or other organs. This can result in the formation of numerous small granulomata. These have the appearance of small nodules on the chest radiograph and indicate the presence of miliary TB. Symptomatic hematogenous spread is rare, except in immunocompromised patients.

As CMI develops, so does the ability to test for TB infection. For example, the reaction to the skin test occurs as a result of delayed-type hypersensitivity (DTH), in which sensitized T-helper (CD4+) cells move to the site of antigen deposition and release lymphokines and result in the indurated area characteristic of the purified protein derivative (PPD) skin test. The skin test reaction and other tests for TB infection are discussed in detail later.

The nature of pathologic findings in infected persons is relative to the antigen load and the degree of hypersensitivity elicited. If few antigens are present and hypersensitivity is active, the classic tubercle develops, characterized by the presence of organized lymphocytes, macrophages, giant cells (Langerhans), and fibroblasts that result in the formation of the classic tuberculous granuloma. A large bacterial load can overwhelm the immune system. The resulting hypersensitivity reaction can be destructive to cells and surrounding tissues. In some of the granulomata, incomplete necrosis occurs. Caseation is a process that occurs through the release of hydrolytic, destructive enzymes; reactive oxygen species; and cytotoxic lymphokines, producing the classic caseating granuloma described by pathologists. The TB bacillus can replicate at a very high rate in a liquefaction process such as this, which further increases antigen load and the destructive response by the host immune system. Healing can occur only when growth of the tubercle bacilli is inhibited. With caseous, liquefied cavities, the body isolates lesions with a primarily fibrotic process.

Clinical Presentation

Primary Pulmonary Disease

Tuberculous infection is different from tuberculous disease. Most initial infections are asymptomatic and controlled by cell-mediated immunity. When infection is present, the child manifests a positive tuberculin skin test (TST) but there is no clinical, radiographic, or laboratory evidence that indicates the occurrence of organ involvement. Approximately 10% of children who become infected with *M tuberculosis* develop manifestations of disease, with infants and postpubertal adolescents at highest risk.

Pulmonary disease is the most common presentation of TB in children. Fever is the most frequent symptom of disease, but cough is less commonly present. Symptoms are highly variable in children and also include weight loss or poor weight gain, night sweats, and chills. Pulmonary disease due to TB should be considered if a fever of 38°C has persisted for at least 2 weeks and other causes have been treated or excluded, or if a child develops a chronic unremitting cough that does not improve with treatment and has lasted for more than 3 weeks. Additionally, if weight loss or failure to thrive are notable on examination of the child's growth chart, TB should be considered as growth delay may be a manifestation of disease. These signs and symptoms are nonspecific, thus a history obtained of an exposure to an infected person and a positive skin test will direct the differential diagnosis toward TB. However, a negative test for TB infection (skin test or blood-based test) does not rule out TB. If other features are suggestive of TB, the diagnosis should be considered, even if the test for TB infection is negative. These findings, along with the characteristic abnormalities of a pulmonary infiltrate associated with hilar lymph node enlargement seen on chest radiograph, nearly confirms the diagnosis. However, children less frequently demonstrate infiltrates on radiographic evaluation than adults, but more frequently demonstrate regional lymphadenopathy, lymphohematogenous spread, and calcified lesions than do adults. Approximately one-third of patients develop a pleural effusion that is visible on the chest radiograph in addition to the Ghon complex previously described. Lymphadenopathy may be robust and can cause bronchial compression with resultant atelectasis of the associated bronchial segment. In short, any patient, adult or child, with pneumonia, pleural effusion, cavitary lesion, or mass lesion in the lung that does not improve with standard antibacterial therapy should be evaluated for TB.

Once infected, infants younger than 1 year are at highest risk to develop disseminated TB (10%–20%) as well as pulmonary TB (30%–40%). The risk for dissemination decreases as the age increases, with the 5- to 10-year-old age group demonstrating the least risk for developing disease[4–7] (Table 22-1). Infants and children who develop disseminated disease will develop symptoms related to the organ affected. The most common sites of extrapulmonary disease in children are the superficial lymph nodes and the central nervous system. Neonates have the highest risk of progression of TB disease with meningeal involvement and are likely to present with seizures or stroke associated with high fevers.

Approximately 5% of infected individuals develop disease within the first 5 years of infection if it is not treated. The likelihood of developing disease decreases as time passes, but another 5% of infected individuals will manifest disease after the 5 years, particularly if immunocompetence is lost. Thorough evaluation of infants and young children is important due to their higher rate of progression to symptomatic TB. Disease in other organs appears to follow a specific timetable of presentation characteristic to the organ: Meningitis usually occurs within 3 to 6 months of infection, pleuritis develops within 3 to 9 months, bone and joint disease will develop within 1 to 3 years, and renal disease within 5 to 25 years after the initial infection.

After infection, several factors influence the balance of risk between latent TB infection or progression to active disease, including age,[8] and nutritional,[9] vaccination,[10] and immune status.[11] Studies in animal and human hosts have shown reduced microbial killing and diminished monocyte recruitment to the site of infection in infants compared with adults. Thus impairment of innate pulmonary defenses in the neonate and infant might allow mycobacteria to overwhelm the effects of the

Table 22-1. Risk of Pulmonary and Extrapulmonary Disease in Children Following Infection With *Mycobacterium tuberculosis*[a]

	Risk of Disease Following Primary Infection		
	Disseminated TB/ TB meningitis	**Pulmonary TB**	**No Disease**
<1 year	10%–20%	30%–40%	50%
1–2 years	2%–5%	10%–20%	75%–80%
2–5 years	0.5%	5%	95%
5–10 years	<0.5%	2%	98%
>10 years	<0.5%	10%–20%	80%–90%

Abbreviation: TB, tuberculosis.

[a] Adapted with permission from Marais BJ, Gie RP, Schaaf HS, et al. The natural history of childhood intrathoracic tuberculosis: a critical review of literature from the pre-chemotherapy era. *Int J Tuberc Lung Dis.* 2004;8:392–402.

innate immune system before the initiation of an antigen-specific immune response. Active surveillance data from areas where antibiotic treatment is scarce but infection rates are high suggest that most children develop radiologic abnormalities following infection, including 60% to 80% of children younger than 2 years. Overall, in this study, the risk of progression to disease was highest in infants and individuals in their late teens, with the lowest risk in children aged between 5 and 10 years.[3]

Reactivation Disease

Reactivation of latent disease is primarily a phenomenon that occurs in adolescents and adults. Reactivation TB results when the persistent bacteria in a host suddenly proliferate. While immunosuppression is clearly associated with reactivation TB, it is not clear what host and pathogen factors specifically maintain the infection in a latent state for many years and what triggers the latent infection to become overt (Box 22-1). Primary TB generally resolves spontaneously, but reactivation disease may occur in 50% to 60% of patients who do not receive appropriate antibiotic therapy. Reactivation TB begins insidiously over a period of weeks to months. Cough is common with a slow increase in sputum production. Constitutional symptoms of fever, weight loss, anorexia, and night sweats are frequent, and episodes of streaky hemoptysis are not unusual in this stage. Reactivation tends to be a phenomenon related to reinitiation of bacillus replication, rupture of dormant lesions, and release of caseating material into the bronchi and parenchyma, causing cavity formation. This form of TB is the classic upper lobe, cavitating disease.

In contrast to primary disease, the disease process in reactivation TB tends to be localized; there is little regional lymph node involvement and less caseation. The lesion typically occurs at the lung apices. Disseminated disease is unusual, unless the host is severely immune suppressed.

Box 22-1. Immunosuppressive Conditions Associated With Reactivation Tuberculosis

- HIV infection and AIDS
- Solid organ transplant recipient
- Diabetes mellitus
- Lymphoma
- Corticosteroid use
- Diminution in cell-mediated immunity

Chronic Disease/Latent Infection

Of the 10% of children acutely infected with TB who develop TB disease, a certain proportion will develop chronic disease but most recover spontaneously. It is unknown what the proportion of children is who will develop chronic disease since treatment for TB infection is generally aggressively approached. The chronic disease is characterized by repeated episodes of spontaneous healing by fibrotic changes around the lesions and tissue breakdown. Healing by complete spontaneous eradication of the bacilli is rare. If bacterial growth continues to remain unchecked, the bacilli may spread hematogenously to produce disseminated TB.

Extrapulmonary Disease

Approximately 15% of patients with active TB also present with TB disease in an extrapulmonary site, and the risk is increased in immunocompromised patients as well as children younger than 2 years. The most commonly involved sites include, in order of frequency, lymph nodes, pleural space, heart, skin, genitourinary tract, bone and joint sites, meninges, and in the peritoneum-gastrointestinal tract.

Diagnosis

Skin Testing

The American Academy of Pediatrics (AAP) suggests that a TST be placed to determine latent TB infection if any of the following are true[12]:

- Contacts of people with confirmed or suspected contagious TB (contact investigation).
- Children with radiographic or clinical findings suggesting TB disease.
- The child has drunk unpasteurized milk, or eaten unpasteurized cheese.
- Children emigrating from countries with endemic infection (eg, Asia, Middle East, Africa, Latin America, countries of the former Soviet Union), including international adoptees.
- Children with travel histories to countries with endemic infection and substantial contact with indigenous people from such countries.

- Annual skin testing is indicated in children with HIV infection and in incarcerated adolescents.
- An initial skin test should be performed before initiation of immunosuppressive therapy, including prolonged steroid administration, use of tumor necrosis factor-α antagonists, or other immunosuppressive therapy in any child requiring these treatments.

The TST is the only practical tool for diagnosing latent TB infection (LTBI) in asymptomatic children; however, for those older than 5 years, interferon-γ release assays (IGRAs) are now available for diagnosis (see section on improving immunologic diagnosis). The preferred skin test is the Mantoux test, which contains 5 tuberculin units of PPD administered intradermally. The estimated sensitivity of TST tests ranges from 80% to 96%. Mantoux tests should be read within 48 to 72 hours of placement by measuring the largest diameter of induration (not redness) and is best done by experienced health care professionals.

Causes of false-negative TST reactions include

1. Infections (eg, early TB infection [<12 weeks], active TB, HIV, measles, varicella, typhoid fever, brucellosis, typhus, leprosy, blastomycosis).
2. Live virus vaccines can suppress tuberculin reactivity for 4 to 6 weeks. Live virus vaccines can be administered at the same visit as TST; if they are not administered on the same day, they should be separated by at least 6 weeks.
3. Medical conditions (eg, chronic renal failure, malignancies, sarcoidosis, poor nutrition) and glucocorticoid therapy (if initiated before the TST was placed).
4. Technical factors (eg, inadequate dose, improper storage, failure to administer intradermally, improperly timed reading).

Causes of false-positive TST reactions may occur in children who have been exposed to nontuberculous mycobacteria, have received whole-blood transfusions from donors with positive TST, or if the individual reading the test is inexperienced or biased. False-positive reactions also may occur in children who have received bacille Calmette-Guérin (BCG) vaccine; nonetheless, receipt of BCG vaccine is not a contraindication to TST testing, and interpretation of TST is not affected by receipt of BCG. Interpretation of the TST depends on the child's risk factors.

Interpreting Skin Test Results

A wide spectrum of results occurs in the general population from PPD skin testing. Reactions depend in part on the type of exposure to TB among tested populations. People with a history of contact and subsequent infection with TB frequently exhibit a prominent reaction to the skin test. In this population, the median diameter of induration is 16 to 17 mm, and there are few reactions smaller than 10 mm. In comparison, the general population without a significant history of TB contact demonstrates a different distribution of reactivity, with reactions varying from none (no infection) to reactions with induration less than 10 mm. Cross reaction to other *Mycobacteria* is commonly associated with this type of reaction (Figure 22-2).

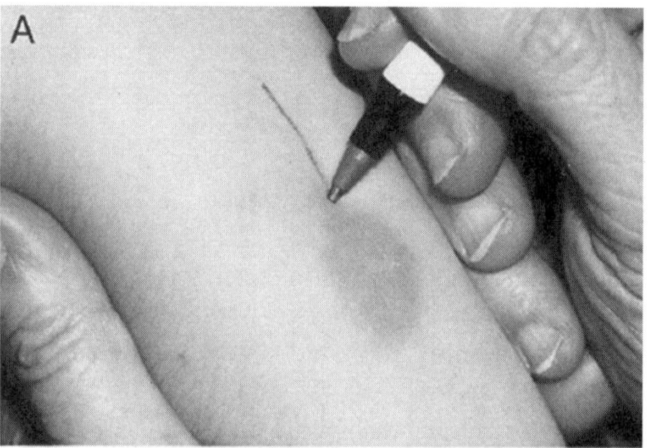

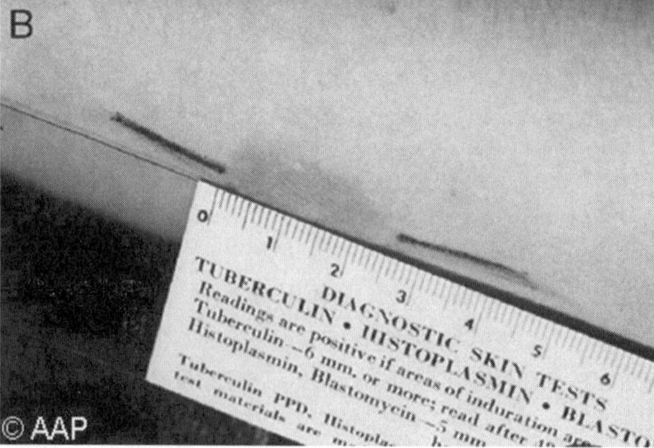

Figure 22-2. Positive skin test for tuberculosis.

Because of these results, the American Thoracic Society and the Centers for Disease Control and Prevention have recommended different criteria or demarcation points for the determination of a positive reaction based on the prior probability or likelihood of true infection with *M tuberculosis* (Box 22-2). Figure 22-3 is a flow chart regarding the evaluation of a child exposed to a person with contagious TB.

Box 22-2 Definition of Positive TST Results in Infants, Children, and Adolescents[a,b]

Induration 5 mm or Greater

Children in close contact with known or suspected contagious people with tuberculosis (TB) disease

Children suspected to have TB diseases

- Findings on chest radiograph consistent with active or previous tuberculosis disease
- Clinical evidence of TB disease[c]

Children receiving immunosuppressive therapy[d] or with immunosuppressive conditions, including HIV infection

Induration 10 mm or Greater

Children at increased risk of disseminated TB disease

- Children younger than 4 years
- Children with other medical conditions, including Hodgkin's disease, lymphoma, diabetes mellitus, chronic renal failure, or malnutrition
- Children with likelihood of increased exposure to TB disease
- Children born in high-prevalence regions of the world
- Children frequently exposed to adults who are HIV infected, homeless, users of illicit drugs, residents of nursing homes, incarcerated or institutionalized, or migrant farm workers
- Children who travel to high-prevalence regions of the world

Induration 15 mm or Greater

Children 4 years of age or older without any risk factors

[a] From: American Academy of Pediatrics. Pickering LK, Baker CJ, Kimberlin DW, Long SS, eds. *Red Book: 2009 Report of the Committee on Infectious Diseases.* 28th ed. Elk Grove Village, IL: American Academy of Pediatrics; 2009:281.

[b] These definitions apply regardless of previous bacille Calmette-Guérin immunization; erythema alone at tuberculin skin test site does not indicate a positive test result. Tests should be read 48 to 72 hours after placement.

[c] Evidence by physical examination or laboratory assessment that would include TB in the working differential diagnosis (eg, meningitis).

[d] Including immunosuppressive doses of corticosteroids

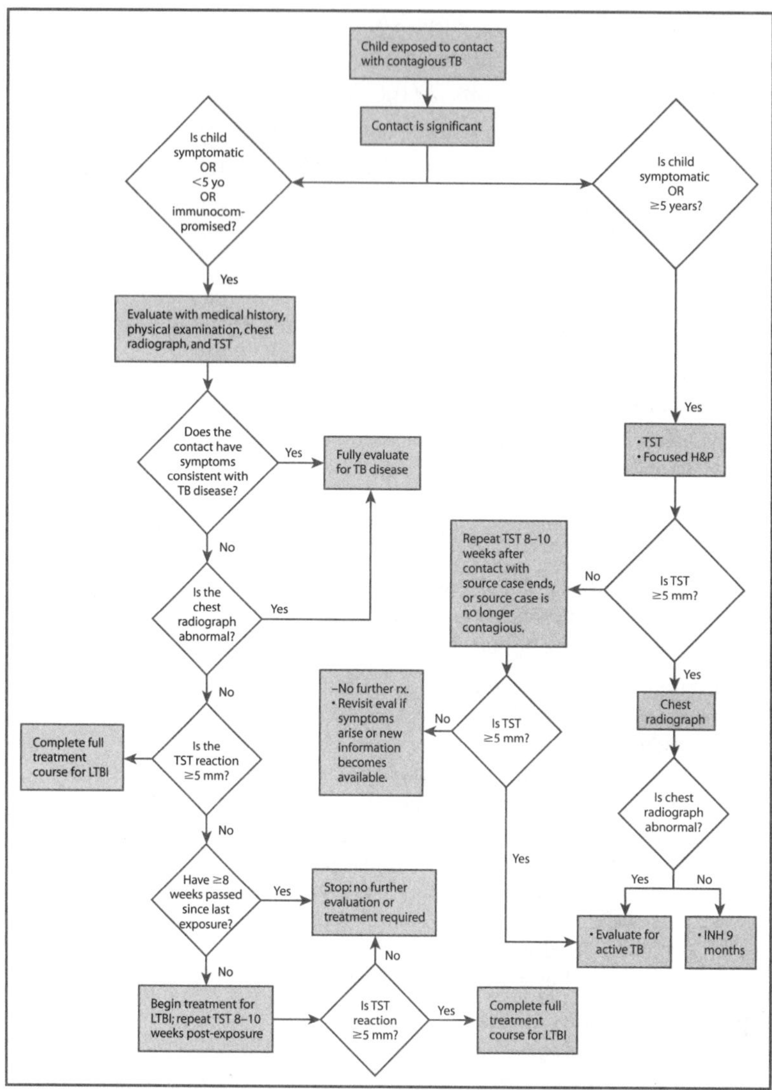

Figure 22-3. Evaluation of a child exposed to a person with contagious tuberculosis (TB). INH, isoniazid; LTBI, latent tuberculosis infection; TST, tuberculin skin test.

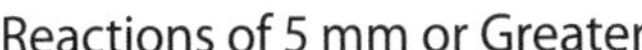

Reactions of 5 mm or Greater

A tuberculin test with induration of 5 mm or greater should be considered positive in individuals who are at highest risk for developing active TB if they become infected with *M tuberculosis.* Such populations include persons who are HIV positive, recent contacts of TB case patients, patients with fibrotic changes on chest radiographs consistent with prior TB, patients with organ transplants, other immunosuppressed patients receiving the equivalent of more than 15 mg/day of prednisone for 1 month or more, and patients planning to take tumor necrosis factor-α inhibitors.

Reactions of 10 mm or Greater

A reaction with induration of 10 mm or greater should be considered positive for individuals who have an increased probability of infection or who have conditions (other than HIV or pharmacologic immunosuppression) that increase the risk for TB, including recent (within the last 5 years) immigrants from high-prevalence countries, such as areas of Eastern Europe, Latin America, Asia, and Africa; injection drug users who are HIV-negative or with an unknown HIV status; persons with clinical conditions that place them at high risk for active disease such as silicosis, chronic kidney disease, hematologic disorders such as leukemia and lymphoma, other specific malignancies (eg, carcinoma of the head or neck and lung), weight loss of 10% or greater of ideal body weight, gastrectomy, and jejunoileal bypass; children younger than 4 years; and infants, children, and adolescents exposed to adults at high risk for active TB.

Reactions of 15 mm or Greater

Routine tuberculin testing is not recommended for populations at low risk for TB exposure or reactivation. However, if these persons are tested because of entry into a work site where a high risk for exposure to TB is anticipated and a longitudinal tuberculin testing program is in place, a criterion of induration of 15 mm or greater is considered a positive response.

Effect of BCG Vaccine

Bacille Calmette-Guérin vaccination often results in tuberculin conversion; most vaccine recipients develop tuberculin reactions 10 mm or greater within 8 to 12 weeks following vaccination. For individuals who receive BCG vaccination in the neonatal period, tuberculin reactions diminish relatively rapidly; among more than 1,000 individuals who received vaccination in the first year of life, no effect on tuberculin reactions 10 mm or greater could be detected after 10 to 25 years.

For individuals who first receive BCG after the first year of life or receive a second dose of BCG, however, tuberculin reactions wane more slowly. In a study that included more than 1,000 individuals with history of BCG vaccination, those vaccinated between the ages of 6 and 10 years had a higher rate of persistent tuberculin reaction than those vaccinated at the ages of 2 and 5 years (20%–25% versus 10%–15%, respectively).[13] Even though distinguishing between tuberculin reactions caused by vaccination with BCG from those caused by natural mycobacterial infections is a difficult challenge, a history of prior BCG vaccination is not a valid basis for dismissing positive reactions. Positive results should prompt evaluation for latent or active infection according to the interpretation guidelines outlined above. Repeated PPD testing or 2-step testing can boost BCG-induced sensitivity. If the TST is positive to cause a concern for infection, an IGRA may assist to distinguish reactivity caused by BCG sensitization versus that from latent TB infection, see Improving Immunological Diagnosis on page 480. However, the usefulness of this test has not been verified in children younger than 5 years, and a search for the organism in sputum, gastric aspirates, or bronchoalveolar lavage may be necessary.

Purified Protein Derivative

Purified protein derivative is prepared by precipitation of protein components from culture filtrate of *M tuberculosis*. The precipitation removes some of the large carbohydrate antigens. Purified protein derivative is more specific for the detection of TB infection than is old tuberculin. The 2 commercially available preparations in the United States, Aplisol and Tubersol, provoke equivalent Mantoux test responses among HIV-negative patients with recent, culture-proven TB. A person infected with *M tuberculosis* will react to intradermal injection of tuberculin with a DTH response. Cellular infiltration by T cells in combination with other recruited inflammatory cells results in maximal induration at 48 to 72 hours after inoculation with intradermal antigen. A period of 2 to 12 weeks after primary infection is generally required for skin test conversion to occur. The ability to mount such a response is usually maintained for many years, although reactivity may wane over time.

Sputum Analysis

It is somewhat difficult to make a diagnosis of TB in children, in view of the fact that they tend to be unable to expectorate and the bacterial load within the sputum is low, since there is a generally low incidence of cavitary disease in the pediatric population. However, if endobronchial caseating lesions are present and caseating lymph nodes have eroded into a bronchus, the bacterial load and likelihood of smear positivity increases. Nonetheless, children tend to swallow sputum rather than expectorate it, so in general, the bacteriologic specimens must be collected by obtaining early morning gastric aspirate washings. This requires overnight fasting with collection on 3 consecutive days and is often best done during a hospitalization. Even so, the rate of positive confirmation with acid-fast bacilli staining using this method is only 10% to 15% and, unfortunately, cultures are negative approximately 70% of the time. All specimens obtained should be sent for bacteriologic evaluation, and nontuberculous mycobacteria should also be considered with a positive smear.

Without definitive diagnosis, treatment is based on exposure history, clinical features, the TST, and radiography.

Improving Analysis of Specimens Obtained

The method of obtaining sputum by induction with nebulization of hypertonic saline has been reported to induce a higher yield of *M tuberculosis,* but may be somewhat impractical outside of hospital settings, and infection control procedures must be strictly adhered to.[14]

More recently, there have been some advances in bacteriologic and molecular methods for the detection of *M tuberculosis* in patient samples that aim to identify drug resistance in parallel with detection of the bacterium. These methods include the microscopic observation drug susceptibility assay (MODS),[15] more sensitive polymerase chain reaction techniques,[16] or phage-based tests such as FASTPlaque (Biotec Laboratories).[17] In adults, MODS seems to be at least as sensitive as gold-standard liquid culture methods. Data comparing its performance in children are more limited, but MODS has been assessed in a pediatric hospital setting and found to be more sensitive than solid media.[18]

Improving Immunologic Diagnosis

In addition to the traditional TST, which is known to lack both sensitivity and specificity, blood-based assays have recently become available. These T cell assays rely on stimulation of host blood cells with *M tuberculosis*–specific antigens and measure production of interferon-γ. These are termed T cell–based IGRAs. Several studies have compared the 2 available commercial assays, the T-Spot.TB (Oxford Immunotec) and Quantiferon-TB Gold (Cellestis), with the TST for both detection of active disease and latent TB infection.[19,20] T cell assays have proven to be more specific than the TST, but like the TST are unable to distinguish between active disease and latent TB infection. Interpretation therefore depends on the clinical context. A few studies have presented pediatric data of T cell assays; however, none have provided an assessment of age-related performance, and reservations remain regarding their performance in very young children and in immunocompromised populations, such as those with HIV.[21]

The AAP recommendations for the use of IGRAs in children include the following:

At this time, neither an IGRA nor the TST can be considered a gold standard for diagnosis of LTBI. Current recommendations for use of IGRAs in children are as follows:

- For immune-competent children 5 years of age and older, IGRAs can be used in place of a TST to confirm cases of TB or cases of LTBI and likely will yield fewer false-positive test results.
- Children with a positive result from an IGRA should be considered infected with *M tuberculosis* complex. A negative IGRA result cannot universally be interpreted as absence of infection.
- Because of their higher specificity and lack of cross-reaction with BCG, IGRAs may be useful in children who have received BCG vaccine. Interferon-γ release assays may be useful to determine whether a BCG-immunized child with a reactive TST more likely has LTBI or has a false-positive TST reaction caused by the BCG.
- Interferon-γ release assays cannot be recommended routinely for use in children younger than 5 years or for immune-compromised children of any age because of a lack of published data about their utility with these groups.
- Indeterminate IGRA results do not exclude TB infection and should not be used to make clinical decisions.

The PPD has been found to be a very poor indicator of TB infection in young children with HIV. Although studies from South Africa[22] indicated increased sensitivity of the T-Spot assay compared with TST, the data were not stratified by CD4 count. The costs and technical demands of IGRAs will probably limit their wider use in resource-poor settings, where better tests are most needed.

Treatment of Positive TST and Negative Chest Radiograph (Latent TB)

Infection, with no evidence of active disease, caused by *M tuberculosis* in a low-risk patient can be treated with single drug therapy. Isoniazid is the drug of choice and is prescribed for a minimum of 9 months. For patients unable to take isoniazid or who are known to have been exposed to isoniazid-resistant *M tuberculosis,* rifampin daily for 6 months is an alternative therapy (Table 22-2).

Treatment of TB Disease

Because TB in infants and children younger than 4 years is more likely to disseminate, treatment should be started as soon as the diagnosis is suspected. Asymptomatic children with a positive PPD skin test and an abnormal chest radiograph should receive combination chemotherapy, usually with isoniazid, rifampin, and pyrazinamide as initial therapy. But some consideration must be given to the risk group

Table 22-2. Treatment of Latent Tuberculosis With No Disease

Drug	Duration Criteria for Completion	Dose (Maximum)	
Isoniazid	Daily for 9 months 270 doses within 12 months	**Weight**	**Dose (daily)**
		<2.5 kg	25 mg
		2.5–3.0 kg	30 mg
		>3.0–≤5.0 kg	50 mg
		>5.0–≤7.5 kg	75 mg
		>7.5–≤10 kg	100 mg
		>10.0–≤15 kg	150 mg
		>15–≤20 kg	200 mg
		>20 kg	300 mg

Table 22-3. Treatment of Tuberculosis Disease (Suspects/Cases)

Consult CDC Guidelines for the Treatment of Active TB Disease for Alternative Anti-TB Regimens					
Drug	**Dosage**	**Interval**	**Side Effects**	**Monitoring**	**Comments**
Isoniazid	Adults: 300 mg Children: 10–15 mg/kg up to 300 mg	qd	Hepatitis, peripheral neuropathy, mild CNS effects, skin rash, increased Dilantin levels, increased tacrolimus levels.	LFTs (transaminases) once; more if history of chronic liver disease or other hepatotoxic drugs. This is not normally needed for children unless signs of hepatitis occur during therapy.	Give pyridoxine 25–50 mg/day to prevent neuropathy in elderly, IDDM, nutritional deficiency, pregnancy, HIV, and renal disease; exclusively breastfed infants; and children on meat and milk-deficient diets.
Rifampin	Adults: 10 mg/kg up to 600 mg Children: 10–20 mg/kg up to 600 mg. For <45 kg, use 450 mg.	qd	Orange discoloration of secretions, cholestatic hepatitis, febrile (flu-like reaction), thrombocytopenia, drug interactions, skin rash.	Baseline CBC count. LFTs once; more if history of chronic liver disease or other hepatotoxic drugs.	Warn patient about orange discoloration of urine and other body secretions, such as tears. Can discolor contact lenses. Induces hepatic microsomal enzymes.
Ethambutol	Adults: 15–25 mg/kg Children: 20–25 mg/kg (2.5-g max for all ages)	qd	Optic neuritis very rare at 15 mg/kg if renal function is normal. Reversible if discontinued. Skin rash.	Red-green color discrimination and visual acuity should be done at baseline and monthly.	Dose adjustment needed for renal disease.
Pyrazinamide	Adults: 20–25 mg/kg Children: 30–40 mg/kg (2-g max for all ages)	qd	Hepatitis, GI upset, hyperuricemia, arthralgia, photosensitive dermatitis.	LFTs at start and monthly. Uric acid if renal disease.	Dose adjustment needed for renal disease. Safety not established in pregnancy.

Abbreviations: CBC, complete blood cell; CDC, Centers for Disease Control and Prevention; CNS, central nervous system; GI, gastrointestinal; HIV, human immunodeficiency virus; IDDM, insulin-dependent diabetes mellitus; LFT, liver function test; TB, tuberculosis; qd, every day.

to which the individual belongs before deciding on a treatment regimen. Although TB originating in the United States has a very low incidence of infection with MDR and XDR strains of *M tuberculosis,* the risk of MDR is much higher in most foreign countries. Therefore, all children from a foreign country where there is not a known contact with an *M tuberculosis* isolate available for drug testing should be started on 4-drug therapy, usually with the addition of ethambutol as the fourth drug. When the risk of infection with MDR or XDR organisms exists, all effort must be given to obtaining culture and antibiotic sensitivities of the organism.

For patients who exhibit drug intolerance or who are infected with minimally resistant organisms, alternative regimens can be substituted. *Mycobacteria* can develop drug resistance rapidly, particularly when single-drug regimens are used. To avoid the development of drug resistance, a 2-drug combination is the minimum recommended for treatment of disease and is only recommended for those patients who absolutely cannot tolerate a more rigorous regimen. (See Table 22-3 and Table 22-4 for typical dosing regimens, alternate regimens, and medication toxicities).

Therapies for TB tend to be associated with multiple toxicities. Isoniazid and rifampin are often associated with liver toxicity, and thus laboratory evaluation for evidence of hepatitis should be undertaken at least once in the first month of treatment, and more frequently for patients who have a history of hepatitis or renal insufficiency (those who are treated with streptomycin or other aminoglycosides). However, routine monitoring of transaminase levels in children taking isoniazid alone is not recommended by the AAP, except in the case of severe and disseminated disease. Additionally, rifampin may accelerate elimination of drugs metabolized by the CYP450 complex in the liver, resulting in the need to alter dosing regimens of those medications. Rifampin will discolor urine and tears an orange color and should be cautioned. Soft contact lenses will be permanently stained. Ethambutol is associated with optic neuritis in addition to the above other typical toxicities, thus follow-up to assess changes in visual acuity may be necessary. Finally, these medications are not generally available in liquid or suspension form, thus increasing the likelihood that therapies may not be consistently ingested.

Table 22-4. Tuberculosis Treatment Regimens

Standard Regimen	Duration	Comments
Initial Phase INH+RIF+EMB+PZA	First 2 months	For all children in whom an INH-susceptible infection is not proven
Continuation Phase INH+RIF	Months 3 through 6[a]	If sensitive to all first-line drugs
INH+RIF+EMB+PZA INH+RIF+EMB	2 months Months 3–6	If culture is negative and chest radiograph improved
Alternative Regimens[b]		
RIF+EMB+PZA	6–9 months	Use if INH-resistant
INH+EMB+PZA	9–12 months	Use if RIF-resistant

Abbreviations: EMB, ethambutol; INH, isoniazid; RIF, rifampin; PZA, pyrazinamide.

[a] Patient with cavitary disease, extensive disease, or positive cultures after 2 months should continue treatment for a total of 9 months, or 6 months beyond the date of culture conversion if culture positivity is prolonged. Expert consultation is recommended.

[b] With advice from a tuberculosis specialist.

Directly Observed Therapy

Since TB is highly contagious and the mortality rate due to TB is high, and poor adherence to the multidrug regimen can lead to multidrug resistance, directly observed therapy (DOT) medication administration systems have been developed. With DOT, a health care worker is assigned to watch the patient swallow every dose. Directly observed therapy should be used for all children with TB. Directly observed therapy may be performed in any setting including medical (eg, public health, facilities, the home, and school, etc) by trained personnel. The lack of pediatric dosage forms of most anti-TB medications necessitates using crushed pills and suspensions. Even when drugs are given under DOT, tolerance of the medications must be monitored closely. Parents should not be relied on to supervise DOT. If a patient experiences toxicity from the medications, this can be detected early. Directly observed therapy also provides for ongoing patient education. In some patients, the multidrug regimen for TB can be given 3 times weekly, rather than daily. Directly observed therapy services increase the likelihood of successful treatment of TB, decreasing mortality due to TB, and preventing the spread of MDR-TB in the United States. This system has also proved successful in other countries where access to medical care is limited.

Prognosis and When to Refer/Admit

In general, the prognosis for patients infected with TB is good, but mortality rates rise when patients have comorbidities such as malnutrition, disseminated disease, or immunodeficiency (especially HIV) and increases dramatically if patients are infected with MDR-TB. Globally, the mortality rate for MDR-positive TB cases in 2008 (HIV-negative) was estimated at 26% (range: 16%–58%).[3] The high mortality rate due to MDR-TB can eventually be addressed if resources to provide adequate prevention, diagnosis, treatment, and care are present. In the United States, while a significant portion of the population is medically and economically indigent, most cases are likely detected at some point in the disease course. In Africa and China, most cases are undetected and these patients do not receive adequate care. A global decline in MDR-TB mortality can be affected as the coverage and quality of DOT and treatment programs improve globally. Systematic infection control measures have the potential to greatly reduce transmission in hospitals and other clinical settings, and therefore the mortality of MDR-TB.

Control of TB

Control of TB requires a concerted and consistent public health effort involving state and local health departments, individual health care providers, and other institutions, including hospitals and incarceration units. The local health department often plays a significant role in the following areas once a TB case is identified:

- Thorough investigation of contacts of an index case and ensuring that contacts receive appropriate testing for evidence of infection
- Ensuring that the index case receives appropriate standard therapy or therapy for MDR-TB based on laboratory evaluation and that all infected contacts receive appropriate evaluation, monitoring, and therapy
- Providing a mechanism so that all patients receive DOT for TB
- Ensuring that all patients receive regular monitoring to secondary effects of anti-TB therapy
- Ensuring that high-risk groups such as those incarcerated, HIV-positive individuals, and health care workers, receive regular screening for TB
- Ensuring that children and adults return to school and the workplace as soon as able after treatment for TB is initiated

Most children, particularly those younger than 10 years, are not contagious. Exceptions are children with (1) cavitary pulmonary TB; (2) positive sputum AFB smears; (3) laryngeal involvement; (4) extensive pulmonary infection; or (5) congenital TB who are undergoing oropharyngeal procedures, such as endotracheal intubation.

When to Refer

- All patients suspected of active infection due to TB should be reported to the local health department according to state statute (1 working day).
- In many areas, young children with LTBI should be reported to the local health department, according to local regulations.
- Ideally, an experienced pediatric TB clinician should manage children with TB disease. If a specialist is not available, close and ongoing consultation with a pediatric TB expert should be established.

When to Admit

- Children with suspected tuberculous infection should be admitted to the hospital for culture collection. Early morning gastric aspirates have the highest yield when obtained from gastric secretions after a nasogastric tube was placed the night before and the child has not yet arisen or eaten.
- Patients with increased work of breathing, meningitis, or complicating simultaneous conditions should be admitted to the hospital for supportive and aggressive care.

Key Points

- In the United States, TB disproportionately affects immigrant, Hispanic, and black populations.
- Only children who have a new risk for TB exposure since the last TST or who have features suggestive of TB disease should undergo testing with the TST or IGRA.
- Interferon-γ assay testing is the recommended first line of testing in patients unlikely to return for skin test reading. However, the IGRA test may be indeterminant and thus not reliable in young children.
- All children diagnosed with latent TB infection should be treated and monitored for adherence and toxicity.
- Tuberculosis disease is diagnosed clinically and radiographically in children, often without the benefit of culture confirmation.

References

1. Walls T, Shingadia D. The epidemiology of tuberculosis in Europe. *Arch Dis Child.* 2007;92:726–729
2. Centers for Disease Control and Prevention. Trends in tuberculosis—United States, 2007. *MMWR Recomm Rep.* 2008;57(11):281–285
3. World Health Organization. *Multidrug and Extensively Drug-Resistant TB (M/XDR-TB): 2010 Global Report on Surveillance and Response.* Geneva, Switzerland: World Health Organization; 2010
4. Comstock GW. Epidemiology of tuberculosis. *Am Rev Respir Dis.* 1982;125:8
5. Rieder HL. Epidemiology of tuberculosis in children. *Ann Nestle.* 1997;55:1–9
6. Holt PG. Postnatal maturation of immune competence during infancy and childhood. *Pediatr Allergy Immunol.* 1995;6: 59–70
7. Beyers N, Gie RP, Schaaf HS, et al. A prospective evaluation of children under the age of 5 years living in the same household as adults with recently diagnosed pulmonary tuberculosis. *Int J Tuberc Lung Dis.* 1997;1:38–43
8. Marais BJ, Gie RP, Schaaf HS, et al. The clinical epidemiology of childhood pulmonary tuberculosis: a critical review of literature from the pre-chemotherapy era. *Int J Tuberc Lung Dis.* 2004;8:278–285
9. Cegielski JP, McMurray DN. The relationship between malnutrition and tuberculosis: evidence from studies in humans and experimental animals. *Int J Tuberc Lung Dis.* 2004;8:286–298
10. Colditz GA, Brewer TF, Berkey CS, et al. Efficacy of BCG vaccine in the prevention of tuberculosis. Meta-analysis of the published literature. *JAMA.* 1994;271:698–702
11. Barnes PF, Bloch AB, Davidson PT, Snider DE. Tuberculosis in patients with human immunodeficiency virus infection. *N Engl J Med.* 1991;324:1644–1650
12. American Academy of Pediatrics. Tuberculosis. In: Pickering LK, Baker CJ, Kimberlin DW, Long SS, eds. *Red Book: 2009 Report of the Committee on Infectious Diseases.* 28th ed. Elk Grove Village, IL: American Academy of Pediatrics; 2009:680
13. Menzies R, Vissandjee B. Effect of bacille Calmette-Guérin vaccination on tuberculin reactivity. *Am Rev Respir Dis.* 1992;145(3):621–625
14. Zar HJ, Hanslo D, Apolles P, Swingler G, Hussey G. Induced sputum versus gastric lavage for microbiological confirmation of pulmonary tuberculosis in infants and young children: a prospective study. *Lancet.* 2005;365:130–134
15. Moore DA, Evans CA, Gilman RH, et al. Microscopic-observation drug-susceptibility assay for the diagnosis of TB. *N Engl J Med.* 2006;355:1539–1550
16. Sarmiento OL, Weigle KA, Alexander J, Weber DJ, Miller WC. Assessment by meta-analysis of PCR for diagnosis of smear-negative pulmonary tuberculosis. *J Clin Microbiol.* 2003;41:3233–3240
17. Kalantri S, Pai M, Pascopella L, Riley L, Reingold A. Bacteriophage-based tests for the detection of *Mycobacterium tuberculosis* in clinical specimens: a systematic review and meta-analysis. *BMC Infect Dis.* 2005;5:59

18. Oberhelman RA, Soto-Castellares G, Caviedes L, et al. Improved recovery of *Mycobacterium tuberculosis* from children using the microscopic observation drug susceptibility method. *Pediatrics.* 2006;118:e100–e106
19. Ferrara G, Losi M, D'Amico R, et al. Use in routine clinical practice of two commercial blood tests for diagnosis of infection with *Mycobacterium tuberculosis:* a prospective study. *Lancet.* 2006;367:1328–1334
20. Pai M, Riley LW, Colford JM. Interferon-γ assays in the immunodiagnosis of tuberculosis: a systematic review. *Lancet Infect Dis.* 2004;4:761–776
21. Rangaka MX, Wilkinson KA, Seldon R, et al. Effect of HIV-1 infection on T-cell-based and skin test detection of tuberculosis infection. *Am J Respir Crit Care Med.* 2007;175:514–520
22. Liebeschuetz S, Bamber S, Ewer K, et al. Diagnosis of tuberculosis in South African children with a T-cell-based assay: a prospective cohort study. *Lancet.* 2004;364:2196–2203

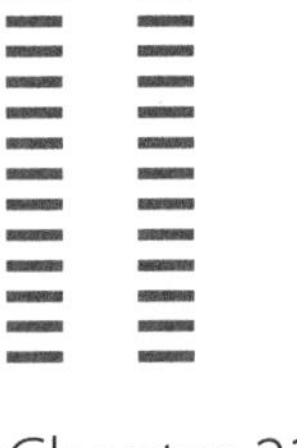

Chapter 23

Nontuberculous Mycobacteria

Alexandra F. Freeman, MD
Kenneth N. Olivier, MD, MPH

Case Report 23-1

A 14-year-old girl who has been followed in the cystic fibrosis (CF) center for several years underwent a computed tomography (CT) scan because of her failure to respond to the usual therapy for a pulmonary exacerbation. She reported recent weight loss and night sweats. The CT scan showed 2 cavities in the right upper lobe. She produced minimal sputum, so bronchoscopy was performed, which revealed bronchoalveolar lavage (BAL) with smear positive for acid-fast bacilli. *Mycobacterium abscessus* was cultured and she was treated with intravenous (IV) amikacin, imipenem, and an oral macrolide. Subsequent therapy will be decided based on response to treatment and sensitivity patterns.

Nontuberculous mycobacteria (NTM) are ubiquitous in the environment, commonly found in soil or water sources, and unlike *Mycobacterium tuberculosis* are not associated with person-to-person transmission. Nontuberculous mycobacteria have been associated with tap water sources of infection, including showerheads and faucets, and hospital outbreaks of nosocomial infections have been attributed to hospital water sources.[1,2] Symptoms of pulmonary NTM may include increased cough and sputum production; shortness of breath; weight loss; and less frequently fever and other systemic symptoms, such as night sweats.

The clinical presentation of NTM typically reflects the portal of entry. Oropharyngeal entry is thought to be the source of cervical lymphadenitis, the most common site of infection in children. The respiratory tract is thought to be the source for pulmonary disease associated with CF and other bronchiectasis syndromes, as well as endobronchial and mediastinal disease. Direct inoculation can occur through abrasions, as seen frequently with *Mycobacterium marinum* infection, and through surgical incisions and central catheters. The gastrointestinal tract can be associated with disseminated disease. Infection tends to remain localized to the site or organ of infection, but dissemination can occur, especially associated with HIV infection and in congenital immune defects of the interferon-γ/interleukin-12 (IFN-γ/IL-12) axis.

Clinical Manifestations

Nontuberculous mycobacteria infections most commonly manifest as isolated cervical lymphadenitis in otherwise healthy children, typically in the preschool age group. *Mycobacterium avium* complex (MAC) is a group of related *Mycobacterium* species that are the most common species identified in NTM infections.

Isolated thoracic node or endobronchial disease likely has a similar pathogenesis to the cervical node disease, and most commonly results from MAC. Presentation is typically within the first few years of life, often with persistent wheeze or stridor that is unresponsive to bronchodilator therapy. Systemic findings such as fever are reported, but are not always present, and these children often appear well. Presentation may also be incidental on chest imaging obtained as evaluation for a positive purified protein derivative, as cross-reactivity between MAC and tuberculosis may occur. Diagnosis is typically made after chest CT or bronchoscopy is performed for the persistent pulmonary findings. Biopsy of the node or endobronchial lesion shows granulomatous inflammation, and acid-fast bacteria may be seen on smears and grow in culture.[3,4]

Parenchymal pulmonary NTM disease is most commonly associated with CF or with other bronchiectasis syndromes. The prevalence of pulmonary NTM in children with CF increases with age; disease in the first decade of life is less common, with a prevalence of about 5% to 10%.[5,6] *Mycobacterium avium* complex is recovered most frequently, but rapid growers, typically *M abscessus*, are not uncommon. *Mycobacterium kansasii* is a rare pathogen in children and adolescents, being seen more frequently in older men. However, it can occur in individuals with underlying lung disease. *Mycobacterium kansasii* infection most closely mimics tuberculosis. Pulmonary NTM also are associated with other syndromes affecting the mucociliary clearance that lead to bronchiectasis, such as primary ciliary dyskinesia and certain immunodeficiencies, such as hyperimmunoglobulin E syndrome.[7,8] In these other disorders of mucociliary clearance, incidence of NTM disease increases with age and would be less likely in young children.

"Hot tub lung" is associated with diffuse pulmonary disease after exposure to aerosolized MAC droplets. This occurs typically with poorly drained indoor hot tubs and presents as a hypersensitivity-like pneumonitis with fever, dyspnea, and cough. Removal from the exposure source is indicated and additional treatment with corticosteroids or antimycobacterial drugs has frequently been used, but the additional role of these therapies is not well delineated.[9]

Disseminated NTM, which may present with pulmonary and extrapulmonary disease, is associated with immunodeficiency. Individuals typically present with fever, night sweats, and weight loss. Lymphadenopathy and hepatosplenomegaly may be present on physical examination. HIV should be excluded in individuals with disseminated NTM.[10] Primary immunodeficiencies consist of disorders of the IFN-γ/IL-12 pathway, such as defects of the IFN-γ receptor, defects of IL-12 or IL-12 receptor, and defects of nuclear factor-κB essential modulator operon.[11]

Etiology

Most human NTM pulmonary disease is caused by a limited number of NTM, and identifying the species helps determine whether the isolated species is pathogenic and guides therapy. Because NTM are ubiquitous, environmental contamination can occur in the laboratory, and interpreting single isolates of NTM needs to include the context of the clinical syndrome. Repeated positive cultures are often necessary to determine clinical significance.[12] For instance, *Mycobacterium gordonae* is typically an environmental contaminant, and treatment largely is not needed.

Nontuberculous mycobacteria are acid-fast bacteria and require special media to grow in the laboratory. Nontuberculous mycobacteria may be classified by their speed of growth. Those that grow rapidly (within 1 week) and are most commonly associated with lung disease are *M abscessus, Mycobacterium fortuitum,* and *Mycobacterium chelonae. Mycobacterium massiliense* and *Mycobacterium bolletii* are newly described rapid growers that previously were classified as *M abscessus.*[13]

The other *Mycobacteria,* including the typical pulmonary isolates of *M tuberculosis,* MAC (including *M avium, M intracellulare,* and "X" strains), and *M kansasii* typically take weeks to grow. Once growth is present, identification is preferentially performed using specific DNA probes, polymerase chain reaction techniques, or high-performance liquid chromatography.

Diagnosis of NTM Pulmonary Disease

Pulmonary NTM in children and adolescents occurs most frequently in the setting of underlying bronchiectasis from CF or other underlying diseases and should be considered in the setting of pulmonary exacerbations unresponsive to treatment of other CF pathogens or with clinical decline unassociated with more typical airway pathogens.[14] A low threshold to look for mycobacteria is necessary in the setting of underlying CF or primary ciliary dyskinesia because symptoms may not differ much from symptoms of pulmonary exacerbation from other pathogens.

Because NTM are environmental organisms, and thus environmental contamination can occur, diagnosis of disease requires clinical, radiographic, and microbiological evidence of disease. The American

Box 23-1. American Thoracic Society Criteria for Diagnosis of Nontuberculous Mycobacteria (NTM) Pulmonary Disease[a]

Clinical Criteria

1. Pulmonary symptoms with compatible chest imaging, including nodular or cavitary opacities on chest radiograph or multifocal bronchiectasis with small nodules on chest computed tomography
2. Exclusion of other diagnoses

Microbiological Criteria

1. Positive culture from at least 2 sputum samples
   or
2. Positive culture from at least one bronchial wash or lavage
   or
3. Transbronchial or lung biopsy with mycobacterial histopathologic features (granulomatous inflammation or acid-fast bacilli) and positive culture for NTM from biopsy, sputum, or bronchial washing

[a] Excerpted from Griffith DE, Aksamit T, Brown-Elliott BA, et al. An official ATS/IDSA statement: diagnosis, treatment, and prevention of nontuberculous mycobacterial diseases. *Am J Respir Crit Care Med.* 2007;175:367–416. Copyright © American Thoracic Society. Reprinted by permission.

Thoracic Society (ATS) and Infectious Diseases Society of America (IDSA) have compiled criteria for diagnosis of parenchymal NTM lung disease including these features (Box 23-1).[12] Although these guidelines have been developed for adults, they can likely be applied to children and adolescents who are capable of sputum production. Consultation with a pulmonologist or infectious diseases physician with experience diagnosing NTM disease is recommended. Evaluating pulmonary disease should include chest imaging (chest radiograph or chest CT if no cavitation or bronchiectasis on chest radiograph); at least 3 sputum samples for culture of acid-fast bacilli; and exclusion of other entities, such as tuberculosis. Because the presentation of NTM disease is largely subacute or chronic, there is typically time to collect this information before initiating therapy. In the setting of compatible chest imaging (nodular or cavitary opacities on chest imaging), consistent microbiological data include positive cultures from 2 or more sputa or positive cultures from BAL or lung biopsy with compatible granulomatous inflammation and positive mycobacterial culture from a respiratory source (biopsy, sputum, or BAL). The utility of gastric aspirates in children unable to produce sputum for diagnosing NTM pulmonary infection is not well delineated, and diagnosis by bronchoscopy or biopsy should be strongly considered.

In individuals with CF and other causes of underlying bronchiectasis, the diagnosis can be confounded by additional bacterial isolates (*Pseudomonas aeruginosa* may overgrow NTM) and by similar radiographic changes and symptoms from bacterial infections. To appropriately identify organisms in children with CF it is important to work with a knowledgeable microbiology laboratory that is adept at isolating these pathogens and at using proper isolation techniques.[15] Aggressively treating other isolated CF pathogens (eg, *P aeruginosa* or *Staphylococcus aureus*) may help determine the clinical significance of NTM disease. If the patient continues to have symptoms of a pulmonary exacerbation despite aggressive treatment, NTM should be considered and appropriate cultures obtained.

Diagnosis of nodal or endobronchial disease is through positive culture of a biopsy or needle aspirate in the context of a compatible clinical presentation.

Treating NTM Infections

Proper identification of the NTM infection assists antibiotic selection. Antibiotic sensitivity assays can be performed (usually at referral centers), but results can be unreliable, especially for certain commonly isolated NTM like MAC and *M abscessus*. With the exception of the macrolide class of antibiotics, there is little correlation between in vitro susceptibility tests and clinical response.[16–18] The ATS/IDSA guidelines recommend susceptibility testing for MAC isolates from patients previously treated for MAC lung disease, those who relapse or fail to respond after 6 months of a macrolide-containing regimen, and for isolates from patients with AIDS who develop bacteremia on macrolide prophylaxis or with positive blood cultures after 3 months on a macrolide-containing regimen. Rapidly growing *Mycobacteria* should be tested for susceptibility to amikacin, cefoxitin, ciprofloxacin, doxycycline, linezolid, sulfamethoxazole, and tobramycin.[12]

Treating pulmonary NTM disease requires combination antimycobacterial drug regimens to prevent resistance and, in general, should not be initiated until species identification is available (Table 23-1). Antimicrobial sensitivities usually require several weeks to obtain because of slow growth, and they are often unreliable. The choice of antibiotics requires knowledge of species-specific regimens as well as the antibiotic history of the individual patient. In addition, drug-drug interactions and adverse events need to be considered on an individual basis.[19] Given the complexity of these regimens, consultation with a pulmonologist or infectious disease specialist who is experienced in managing

Table 23-1. Treatment of Typical Nontuberculous Mycobacteria Infection (With Consultation of an Expert)

Organism	Antimicrobial Regimens
Mycobacterium avium complex	Azithromycin or clarithromycin, rifampin or rifabutin, and ethambutol For severe disease or if resistance suspected, addition of amikacin or a fluoroquinolone (ciprofloxacin or moxifloxacin)
Mycobacterium kansasii	Isoniazid, rifampin, ethambutol
Mycobacterium abscessus	Azithromycin or clarithromycin, and amikacin, imipenem, meropenem, or cefoxitin Consider linezolid or tigecycline (in adolescents)

NTM infections is recommended. The decision to treat and timing of treatment require a careful assessment of the morbidity of the illness and the patient's ability to commit to a prolonged, combination antimicrobial course. Because individuals with parenchymal NTM disease often have comorbidities (eg, bronchiectasis, concomitant pulmonary pathogens), objective data that can be tracked to assist in treatment response are necessary. Inflammatory markers, pulmonary function tests, semi-quantitative sputum acid-fast bacilli smears and cultures, and imaging studies may help assess response to therapy. In addition, in individuals with underlying bronchiectasis (such as CF), airway clearance measures, such as chest percussion/postural drainage, percussive vest, handheld oscillatory or resistive devices, and inhaled hypertonic saline treatments, should be initiated or continued.

The most common antibiotics used to treat pulmonary parenchymal MAC infection are macrolides (azithromycin or clarithromycin) and ethambutol. Three-drug therapy is thought to be superior to 2-drug therapy in preventing resistance, and the third drug is typically a rifamycin (rifampin or rifabutin).[12] If use of a rifamycin is not possible due to drug-drug interactions or poor tolerability, or in the setting of cavitary disease, an injected aminoglycoside (ie, amikacin) should be strongly encouraged. Fluoroquinolones are also used in combination therapy, but when combined solely with a macrolide, there may be an increased incidence of macrolide resistance compared with the combination of macrolides with ethambutol and a rifamycin.[16] As fluoroquinolones are largely not approved for children by the US Food and Drug Administration, consultation with an expert is recommended. Drug toxicities need to be considered if the patient has comorbidities (Table 23-2). The first treatment course has the best chance of response; therefore, multidrug therapy is very important. In addition, consideration has to be given to whether the patient has been on monotherapy with azithromycin, a common chronic therapy in CF, as the likelihood of macrolide resistance will be increased. Although antimicrobial sensitivity testing is largely unreliable, assessing macrolide resistance in individuals with a history of macrolide exposure or who fail an initial MAC treatment course is useful and can help in expanding the antibiotic regimen if macrolide resistance is present. Optimal length of therapy is not well defined, but a typical regimen is 12 months of therapy from the time of conversion to a negative sputum culture.[12] In adults, regimens for milder nodular bronchiectatic disease may be condensed

Table 23-2. Antimicrobial Toxicities and Monitoring

Drug	Major Side Effects	Monitoring
Azithromycin, clarithromycin	GI disturbance, decreased hearing, hepatitis	Clinical assessment, periodic hepatic enzymes
Ethambutol	Optic neuritis (loss of red/ green discrimination and acuity)	Ophthalmology at baseline and then monthly if dose 25 mg/kg or every 3 months if dose 15 mg/kg
Rifampin, rifabutin	Orange discoloration of body secretions, hepatitis, frequent drug interactions, leucopenia Thrombocytopenia In high dosages with rifabutin, uveitis, polyarthritis	Transaminase evaluation if symptomatic More frequent transaminase evaluation if underlying hepatic disease present
Aminoglycosides (amikacin)	Vestibular/ototoxicity, nephrotoxicity	Audiology at baseline and periodically (every 3 months) or if symptoms arise; periodic renal function monitoring (more frequent if renal insufficiency or other nephrotoxic medications), and aminoglycoside trough levels
Fluoroquinolones (eg, ciprofloxacin, moxifloxacin)	Tendinitis, GI disturbance, headache, dizziness	Clinical symptoms
Imipenem, meropenem	Hypersensitivity reactions, bone marrow suppression	Periodic CBC count and hepatic enzymes
Tigecycline	Tooth staining <8 years old, GI disturbance, pancreatitis	Clinical symptoms; very little data in children
Linezolid	Bone marrow suppression, peripheral neuropathy, optic neuritis	Weekly CBC count, ophthalmology at baseline and every 3 months, neurologic testing if symptoms develop Pyridoxine therapy may ameliorate toxicities.
Cefoxitin	Hypersensitivity reactions, bone marrow suppression	Periodic CBC count and hepatic enzymes
Isoniazid	Hepatotoxicity, peripheral neuropathy	Periodic hepatic enzymes in first 3 months of therapy when used in combination with other hepatotoxic agents or with clinical symptoms; pyridoxine supplementation recommended to decrease neurotoxicity

Abbreviations: CBC, complete blood cell; GI, gastrointestinal.

into thrice weekly dosages. However, little is known of the efficacy of these regimens for children.

Mycobacteria kansasii responds well to rifamycin-containing regimens, with a typical regimen, similar to tuberculosis, being with isoniazid, rifampin, and ethambutol. Treatment regimens are typically for 1 year after negative cultures.

Rapidly growing NTM are a common cause of NTM infection in children, and treatment guidelines are poorly defined for children and adolescents. Cure of rapidly growing NTM infections are often difficult, but symptoms may be managed with multidrug therapy. The most common pulmonary rapid grower is *M abscessus,* and compared with treatment of MAC, therapy typically requires IV agents. The most reliably effective antimicrobials are macrolides (azithromycin and clarithromycin), amikacin, carbapenems (imipenem and meropenem), and cefoxitin. Linezolid also has efficacy but requires close hematologic monitoring, due to bone marrow suppression, and neurologic monitoring, due to peripheral and optic neuropathy. Tigecycline has been efficacious in adults but is not approved for children. Tigecycline is in the tetracycline class of antibiotics; therefore, it should not be used in children younger than 8 years if other treatment options exist because of possible tooth and bone staining. For NTM infections, optimal drug dosage in children is not well described, and consultation with an expert is advised. In adults, lower dosages or less frequent dosing is often required compared with bacterial infections. For instance, tigecycline and linezolid both appear to be effective and better tolerated when administered once daily as opposed to typical twice-daily regimens. After initial improvement with IV therapy, or for initial treatment of milder disease, an oral regimen of a macrolide and linezolid combined with aerosolized amikacin may be considered, though there are no published data to support this approach.

Because the optimal drug dosages and schedules are not known for children, therapeutic drug monitoring can be very helpful, especially when second- or third-line medications are used or when a clinical response is not observed after 2 to 3 weeks of therapy (Table 23-2). In addition, obtaining drug levels can be helpful in individuals in whom malabsorption is present, as is the case for many children with CF.[20] Serum drug levels can be obtained at reference laboratories, such as the one at National Jewish Health (www.nationaljewish.org/research/clinical-labs/about/learn/infectious/idpl.aspx) or at the University of Florida (http://idpl.copwp.copdom.cop.ufl.edu).

Treating pulmonary NTM associated with defects in the IFN-γ/IL-12 axis (typically disseminated disease) may include immunomodulator therapy. If response to INF-γ is predicted by the defect, or documented in vitro, this therapy may augment antimicrobial therapy. Consultation with an immunologist or infectious disease expert is recommended.

Key Points

- Children with pulmonary NTM infections most likely have bronchiectasis, such as with CF.
- Nontuberculous mycobacteria are not transmitted from person to person.
- Rapid growers (eg, *M abscessus)* are cultured within 3 weeks, slow growers (eg, MAC) are cultured within 6 weeks.
- Not all patients with pulmonary NTM need to be treated
- Although sputum sensitivities are not very accurate they provide a basis for treatment approach, which will require multiple antibiotics.

Acknowledgment

This chapter has been funded in part by intramural funds of the National Institute of Allergy and Infectious Diseases. The content of this publication does not necessarily reflect the views or policies of the Department of Health and Human Services, nor does mention of trade names, commercial products, or organizations imply endorsement by the US government.

References

1. Feazel LM, Baumgartner LK, Peterson KL, Frank DN, Harris JK, Pace NR. Opportunistic pathogens enriched in showerhead biofilms. *Proc Natl Acad Sci USA*. 2009;106:16393–16399
2. Phillips MS, von Reyn CF. Nosocomial infections due to nontuberculous mycobacteria. *Clin Infect Dis*. 2001;33:1363–1374
3. Nolt D, Michaels MG, Wald ER. Intrathoracic disease from nontuberculous mycobacteria in children: two cases and a review of the literature. *Pediatrics*. 2003;112:e434

4. Freeman AF, Olivier KN, Rubio TT, et al. Intrathoracic nontuberculous mycobacterial infections in otherwise healthy children. *Pediatr Pulmonol.* 2009;44:1051–1056
5. Esther CR Jr, Henry MM, Molina PL, et al. Nontuberculous mycobacterial infection in young children with cystic fibrosis. *Pediatr Pulmonol.* 2005;40:39–44
6. Olivier KN, Weber DJ, Wallace RJ Jr, et al. Nontuberculous mycobacteria. I: multicenter prevalence study in cystic fibrosis. *Am J Respir Crit Care Med.* 2003;167:828–834
7. Noone PG, Leigh MW, Sannuti A, et al. Primary ciliary dyskinesia: diagnostic and phenotypic features. *Am J Respir Crit Care Med.* 2004;169:459–467
8. Melia E, Freeman AF, Shea YR, et al. Pulmonary nontuberculous mycobacterial infections in hyper-IgE syndrome. *J Allergy Clin Immunol.* 2009;124:617–618
9. Marras TK, Wallace RJ Jr, Koth LL, et al. Hypersensitivity pneumonitis reaction to mycobacterium avium in household water. *Chest.* 2005;127:664–671
10. Jones D, Havlir DV. Nontuberculous mycobacteria in the HIV infected patient. *Clin Chest Med.* 2002;23:665–674
11. Freeman AF, Holland SM. Persistent bacterial infections and primary immune disorders. *Curr Opin Microbiol.* 2007;10:70–75
12. Griffith DE, Aksamit T, Brown-Elliott BA, et al. An official ATS/IDSA statement: diagnosis, treatment, and prevention of nontuberculous mycobacterial diseases. *Am J Respir Crit Care Med.* 2007;175:367–416
13. Zelazny AM, Root JM, Shea YR, et al. Cohort study of molecular identification and typing of *Mycobacterium abscessus, Mycobacterium massiliense,* and *Mycobacterium bolletii. J Clin Microbiol.* 2009;47:1985–1995
14. Ebert DL, Olivier KN. Nontuberculous mycobacteria in the setting of cystic fibrosis. *Clin Chest Med.* 2002;23:655–663
15. Whittier S, Olivier K, Gilligan P, et al. Proficiency testing of clinical microbiology laboratories using modified decontamination procedures for detection of nontuberculous mycobacteria in sputum samples from cystic fibrosis patients. The nontuberculous mycobacteria in cystic fibrosis study group. *J Clin Microbiol.* 1997;35:2706–2708
16. Griffith DE, Brown-Elliott BA, Langsjoen B, et al. Clinical and molecular analysis of macrolide resistance in mycobacterium avium complex lung disease. *Am J Respir Crit Care Med.* 2006;174:928–934
17. Jeon K, Kwon OJ, Lee NY, et al. Antibiotic treatment of mycobacterium abscessus lung disease: a retrospective analysis of 65 patients. *Am J Respir Crit Care Med.* 2009;180:896–902
18. Kobashi Y, Yoshida K, Miyashita N, et al. Relationship between clinical efficacy of treatment of pulmonary mycobacterium avium complex disease and drug-sensitivity testing of mycobacterium avium complex isolates. *J Infect Chemother.* 2006;12:195–202

19. Ballarino GJ, Olivier KN, Claypool RJ, et al. Pulmonary nontuberculous mycobacterial infections: antibiotic treatment and associated costs. *Respir Med.* 2009;103:1448–1455
20. Gilljam M, Berning SE, Peloquin CA, et al. Therapeutic drug monitoring in patients with cystic fibrosis and mycobacterial disease. *Eur Respir J.* 1999;14:347–351

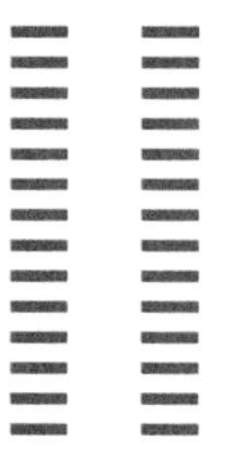

Chapter 24

Atelectasis

Girish D. Sharma, MD

Case Report 24-1

An 18-year-old boy with cystic fibrosis (CF), advanced lung disease, and a recent history of upper respiratory infection for 2 weeks presents with worsening respiratory distress and increased oxygen requirement. Physical examination is remarkable for few inspiratory crackles in the right middle zone posteriorly. A chest radiograph shows a triangular density corresponding to the right middle lobe. He is diagnosed with right middle lobe atelectasis.

Introduction

Atelectasis refers to a loss of lung volume due to collapse of part or the entire lung. Usually the magnitude of the collapsed alveolar spaces is severe enough to appear on a plain chest radiograph. Patients with conditions associated with increased and more viscid secretions, such as CF, are more likely to develop atelectasis. This may result in transient hypoxemia due to ventilation/perfusion ($\dot{V}/\dot{Q}$) mismatching. Secondary infection of the atelectatic lung and bronchiectasis in the atelectatic portion of a chronically infected lung may occur.

Epidemiology

Atelectasis is almost always a secondary phenomenon, occurring more frequently in young children because their airways are small and thus prone to blockage. No proclivity for gender or race has been reported. The incidence of atelectasis varies according to the cause and background conditions. The most common cause is asthma, but there are no incidence data in children. Patients with CF tend to develop atelectasis (up to 5%).[1] Much higher incidence is reported in postoperative cases (up to 23%)[2] and in patients with neuromuscular disorders (up to 85%).[3] In children with congenital heart disease, extrinsic compression of the airways due to enlarged heart chambers or dilated blood vessels can lead to atelectasis, especially in the postoperative period. The current emphasis on airway clearance in children with conditions such as primary ciliary dyskinesia,[4] neuromuscular disorders,[5,6] CF,[7] and postoperative cases after various surgeries[8] should result in a lower incidence of atelectasis. (See Chapter 46.)

Etiology

Atelectasis can result from either obstructive or non-obstructive causes (Box 24-1).

Obstructive Atelectasis

Obstructive atelectasis involves a loss of communication between alveoli and the trachea, resulting in reabsorption of the gas from the alveoli. There is lack of ventilation in the area distal to the obstruction and the air from the airways is absorbed by the circulating blood, leading to collapse of the corresponding alveoli. In the early stages, blood perfusion in this area continues, resulting in $\dot{V}/\dot{Q}$ mismatching and arterial hypoxemia.[9] The filling of alveolar spaces with secretions may occur, thereby preventing complete collapse of the atelectatic lung. There may be compensatory distension of the uninvolved surrounding lung tissue. When there is a large area of atelectasis, there can be a shift of the heart and the mediastinum toward the atelectasis, the diaphragm may be elevated, and the chest wall may flatten. These findings can appear within a short period of a few hours if there is an extensive area of atelectasis, and removal of the obstruction leads to return to normal state. In a protracted case of atelectasis, such as that caused by the viscid secretions in patients with CF, chronic aspiration, or undiagnosed foreign body, infection may occur. Persistent, untreated infection can lead to bronchiectasis.

The site of obstruction dictates the extent and distribution of atelectasis; for example, the obstruction of a lobar bronchus will cause lobar atelectasis. Intrinsic obstruction of the airways is the most common cause of atelectasis in children. Asthma is the most common underlying disorder predisposing children to atelectasis. Children with airway inflammation caused by asthma may have thicker secretions, which

Box 24-1. Causes of Atelectasis

Intrinsic Obstruction of the Airways

- Asthma
- Bronchiolitis
- Aspiration
- Endobronchial lesions (tuberculosis)
- Foreign body
- Cystic fibrosis (viscid secretions)

Extrinsic Compression of the Airways

- Enlarged lymph nodes
- Tumors
- Enlarged heart or vasculature

Compression of Lung Tissue

Decoupling of inward recoil of lung and outward recoil of chest wall due to presence of air, blood, pus, or chyle in the pleural space

- Pneumothorax
- Hemothorax
- Pyothorax
- Chylothorax

Compression due to causes other than pleural space

- Intrathoracic abdominal mass
- Chest wall mass
  - Enlarged heart
  - Over-distended adjacent lung tissue
  - Space-occupying lesions of the lung
  - Skeletal deformities of chest wall

Incomplete Expansion of the Alveoli and Collapse

- Hypoventilation due to muscle weakness in neuromuscular disorders
- Postoperative period
- Splinting of chest wall due to painful lesions resulting in hypoventilation
- Drug-induced hypoventilation
- Cicatrization atelectasis due to severe parenchymal scarring

Lack of Surfactant

- Lack of production (prematurity, acute respiratory distress syndrome)
- Inactivation (radiation pneumonitis, blunt trauma to the lung)
- Surfactant washout (drowning, pulmonary edema)

results in subsegmental or lobar atelectasis. This poses a diagnostic dilemma when children with asthma present with an exacerbation, an abnormal radiograph, and a possible diagnosis of pneumonia. Bronchiolitis; aspiration from any cause, including gastroesophageal reflux and oropharyngeal incompetence; foreign body aspiration; and airway obstruction due to viscid secretions (eg, CF) are some other common causes of obstruction.

Extrinsic compression of the airway from enlarged lymph nodes, or an enlarged heart compressing the left main or left lower lobe bronchus, as well as airway wall thickening caused by edema and inflammation, may be etiologic factors. The right middle lobe is particularly susceptible to atelectasis, and this is described as middle lobe syndrome or Brock syndrome. The right middle lobe bronchus is surrounded by lymph nodes that drain the right middle and lower lobes; the syndrome was originally described because of the frequency of compression by tuberculosis. Hypoventilation associated with neuromuscular disorders, splinting of the chest wall due to postoperative pain after thoracoabdominal surgery (Figure 24-1), medications (narcotics), and musculoskeletal deformities predispose to atelectasis if there is poor airway clearance and pooling of secretions in the airways.

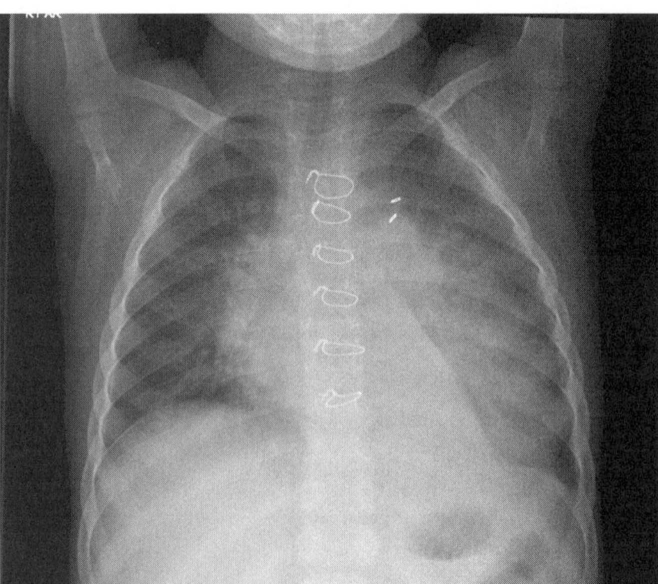

Figure 24-1. Left lower lobe atelectasis with volume loss and shift of the mediastinum.

Non-Obstructive Atelectasis

The loss of contact between the visceral and parietal pleura is the primary cause of non-obstructive atelectasis. Normally there is a balance between the factors responsible for inward and outward recoil of the chest wall to reduce the potential for lung or alveolar collapse. In addition, surfactant protein produced by type II alveolar epithelial cells lowers the surface tension in the alveoli and prevents alveoli from collapsing. As alveolar volume decreases with expiration, surface tension increases to the extent that, without surfactant, the alveolus will collapse completely. Surfactant deficiency can lead to adhesive atelectasis. Atelectasis is also caused by compression of lung tissue due to pleural effusion (pneumothorax, hemothorax, empyema, or chylothorax), space-occupying lesions of parenchyma, and hyperinflated adjacent lung parenchyma. Cicatrization atelectasis is due to severe parenchymal scarring.

Clinical Features

Small areas of atelectasis often are detected only when a chest radiograph is obtained for other reasons. Micro-atelectasis, common in patients with neuromuscular disorders, may not be visible on chest radiographs. With larger areas of atelectasis, there may be tachypnea as the patient tries to compensate for decreased tidal volume by increasing the frequency of respiration. Grunting may be heard as the child attempts to create an auto-positive end-expiratory pressure, and sudden hypoxia may develop as evidenced by a sudden or rapid fall in oxyhemoglobin saturation. Physical examination may not reveal any additional findings in children with small areas of atelectasis. In children with larger areas of involvement, such as lobar involvement or complete lung collapse, breath sounds are diminished, there is increased dullness on chest percussion, and a mediastinal shift may be present.

Diagnosis

Chest Radiography

Unrecognized atelectasis may be revealed by a chest radiograph. There may be a displacement of fissures and opacification of the collapsed lobe. The site of obstruction will dictate the portion or area of the atelectasis, which can be the entire lung or one or more lobes (Figure 24-2). Other indirect signs, such as hilar displacement, mediastinal shift toward the side of collapse, loss of volume in the corresponding area or ipsilateral hemithorax, crowding of the ribs, compensatory hyper-inflation of the adjacent area, or obliteration of the cardiac borders or diaphragm, may be visible on chest radiograph. Examination of air bronchograms on chest radiograph may help determine whether proximal or distal airways are obstructed.

Computed Tomography

Chest computed tomography may help evaluate airway compression, detect underlying pathology, and reveal diffuse disease undetected by chest radiograph.

Management

Some measures may prevent the formation of atelectasis (Table 24-1). These include aggressive and regular chest physical therapy and postural drainage in patients with CF[10] and primary ciliary dyskinesia.[4] Patients with neuromuscular disorders, such as Duchenne muscular dystrophy,[5,6] may benefit from breathing exercises and preventive

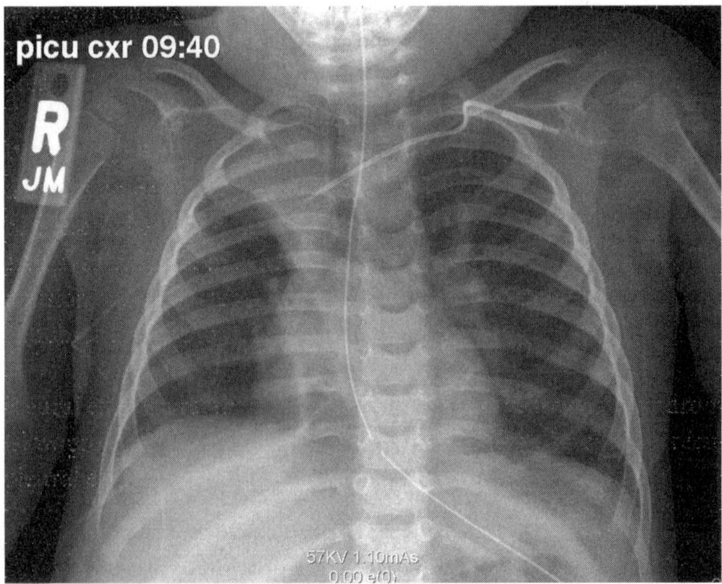

Figure 24-2. Right upper lobe atelectasis with volume loss.

airway clearance techniques. Adequate pain management, early ambulation, and frequent position changes in postoperative patients to prevent splinting of the chest may reduce the incidence of atelectasis. See Figure 24-3 for steps in managing suspected atelectasis.

Chest Physical Therapy

Though chest physical therapy (CPT) has traditionally been the first-line therapy to prevent atelectasis, the evidence for its efficacy is lacking.[11] Post-extubation chest physiotherapy in neonates did not prevent post-extubation atelectasis.[12]

Aggressive pulmonary toilet is the attempt to clear mucus and secretions from the trachea and bronchial tree and includes nebulized or inhaled bronchodilators (β_2-agonist such as albuterol) followed by CPT and postural drainage. Chest physical therapy may be provided by hand percussion and postural drainage or by using a mechanical method, the choice of which will depend on background disorder. For example, the CoughAssist Mechanical In-Exsufflator (Philips Respironics) recommended for patients with neuromuscular disorders[5] may not be appropriate for patients with CF who will be better served by a high-frequency chest wall oscillation device.[13,14] Other devices, such as the Flutter Mucus Clearing Device (Axcan Scandipharm Inc) or the Acapella Vibratory PEP Therapy System (Smiths Medical), may also be used for airway clearance. (See Chapter 46.)

Table 24-1. Preventive Measures to Reduce Atelectasis

Clinical Condition	Preventive Measures
Cystic fibrosis, primary ciliary dyskinesia	Chest physical therapy and postural drainage
Neuromuscular disorder	Use of "cough assist" device
Postoperative period	Chest physical therapy Pain control Early ambulation Frequent position changes

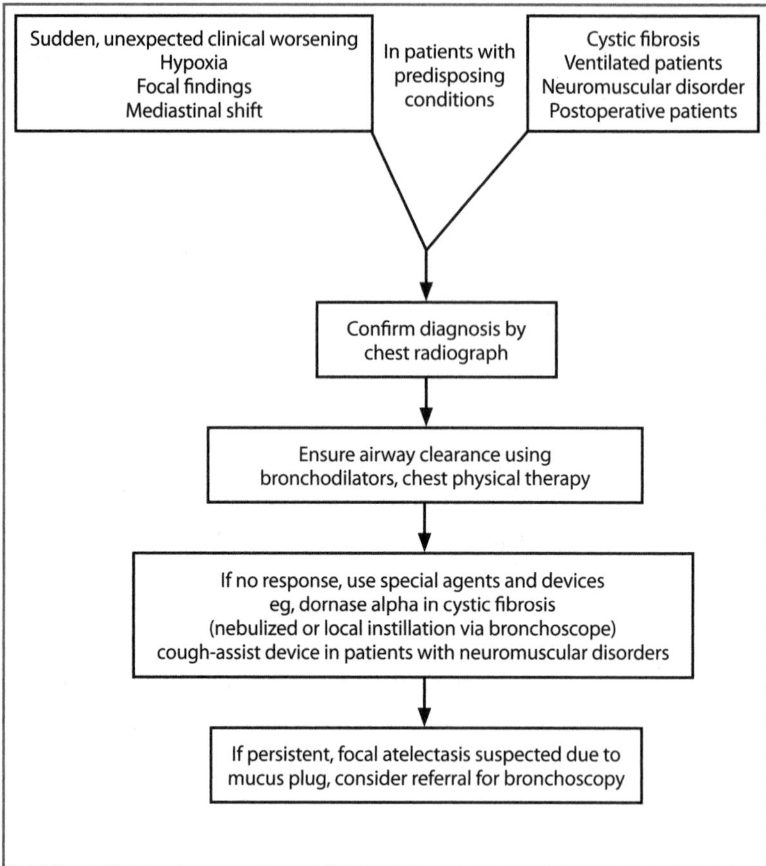

Figure 24-3. Management of suspected atelectasis.

Intrapulmonary Percussive Ventilation

Intrapulmonary percussive ventilation is a form of CPT delivered by a percussive pneumatic device that delivers high-flow jets of gas to the airways by a pneumatic flow interrupter at a rate of 100 to 300 cycles per minute. The duration of percussion is controlled by the patient or the therapist. The driving pressure and peak airway pressure are adjustable. Intrapulmonary percussive ventilation maintains lung volume in a state of partial inspiration while the airways are internally percussed. It has been used in patients with CF and neuromuscular disorders.[15,16]

Recombinant Human DNase

Dornase alfa is a recombinant human DNase that when nebulized or directly instilled into the airways reduces viscoelasticity of purulent secretions, especially in patients with CF. Regular use of dornase alfa by children with CF, 6 years or older, with moderate to severe lung disease is recommended.[14] There have been reports of successful use of bronchoscopically administered dornase alfa for the treatment of lobar atelectasis in patients with CF,[17] but the prospective controlled trials are lacking. (See Chapter 46).

Oximetry and Blood Gas Measurement

There may be a fall in oxyhemoglobin saturation or evidence of hypoxia on blood gas profile.

When to Refer

For bronchoscopy

- Bronchoscopy with therapeutic lavage should be considered when obstruction due to mucus plug is considered to be causing atelectasis and there is no response to noninvasive airway clearance.[5]
- Patients with CF with persistent lobar atelectasis may benefit from lavage with local administration of recombinant human DNase.[15]
- Atelectasis caused by a foreign body.

When to Admit

- Massive atelectasis
- Hypoxia
- Suspected foreign body

References

1. Stern RC, Wood RE, Ornestein DM, et al. Treatment and prognosis of lobar and segmental atelectasis in cystic fibrosis. *Am Rev Respir Dis.* 1978;118:821–826
2. Hasegawa S, Mori K, Inomata Y, et al. Factors associated with postoperative complications in pediatric liver transplantation from living donors. *Transplantation.* 1996;62(7):943–947
3. Schmidt-Nowara WW, Altman AR. Atelectasis and neuromuscular respiratory failure. *Chest.* 1984;85:792–795
4. Sharma GD. Primary ciliary dyskinesia. eMedicine from WebMD. http://www.emedicine.com/ped/topic1166.htm. Accessed November 1, 2008

5. Finder JD, Birnkrant D, Carl J, et al. Respiratory care of the patient with Duchenne muscular dystrophy: ATS consensus statement. *Am J Respir Crit Care Med.* 2004;170 (4):456–465
6. Miske LJ, Hickey EM, Kolb SM. Use of the mechanical in-exsufflator in pediatric patients with neuromuscular disease and impaired cough. *Chest.* 2004;125:1406–1412
7. Flume P, Robinson KA, O'Sullivan BP, et al. Cystic fibrosis pulmonary guidelines: airway clearance therapies. *Respir Care.* 2009;54(4):522–537
8. Birnkrant DJ, Panitch HB, Benditt JO, et al. American college of chest physicians consensus statement on the respiratory and related management of patients with Duchenne muscular dystrophy undergoing anesthesia and sedation. *Chest.* 2007;132:1–10
9. West JB. *Pulmonary Pathophysiology—The Essentials.* Baltimore, MD: Williams & Wilkins; 2008:165–167
10. Pryor JA, Main E, Agent P, Bradley JM. Physiotherapy. In: Cystic fibrosis in the 21st century. Bush A, Alton EWFW, Davies JC, Jaffe A, eds. *Progress in Respiratory Research.* Vol 34. Basel, Switzerland: Karger;2006:301–308
11. Alaiyan S, Dyer D, Khan B. Chest physiotherapy and post-extubation atelectasis in infants. *Pediatr Pulmonol.* 1996;21:227–230
12. Sharma GD. Cystic fibrosis. eMedicine from WebMD. http://www.emedicine.com/ped/TOPIC535.HTM. Accessed November 11, 2008
13. Schindler MB. Treatment of atelectasis; where is the evidence? *Crit Care.* 2005; 9:341–342. http://ccforum.com/content/9/4/341. Accessed November 10, 2008
14. Flume PA, O'Sullivan BP, Robinson KA, et al. Cystic fibrosis pulmonary guidelines: chronic medications for maintenance of lung health. *Am J Respir Crit Care Med.* 2007;176(10):957–969
15. Birnkrant DJ, Pope JF, Lewarski J, et al. Persistent pulmonary consolidation treated with intrapulmonary percussive ventilation: a preliminary report. *Pediatr Pulmonol.* 1996;21:246–249
16. Ha TKY, Bui TD, Tran AT, et al. Atelectatic children treated with intrapulmonary percussive ventilation via a face mask: clinical trial and literature review. *Pediatr Int.* 2007;49:502–507
17. Slattery DM, Waltz DA, Danham B, et al. Bronchoscopically administered recombinant human DNase for lobar atelectasis in cystic fibrosis. *Pediatr Pulmonol.* 2001;31:383–388

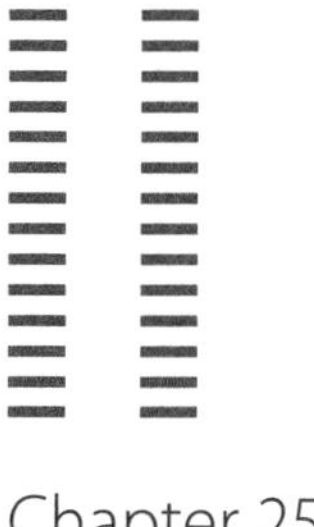

Chapter 25

Rheumatic and Granulomatous Diseases

Robyn Deterding, MD
Michael Henrickson, MD, MPH
Eli Sills, MD
Paul Stillwell, MD
Eric Zee, MD

Introduction

The lung has an enormous vascular network, both systemic and pulmonary. The lung also has an extensive immunologic network. Both are enmeshed in a vast matrix of connective tissue. Therefore, it is of little surprise that pulmonary involvement is common in systemic diseases with either a connective tissue component, a component of vasculitis, or an immunologic component. Because these systemic diseases are relatively infrequent in children, much of what we think we know about the lung involvement is extrapolated from information regarding adults from the medical literature. There is a growing body of literature regarding the pediatric experience, but often the reported series includes a small number of patients that are collected over a long period.

Rheumatic Diseases

The uncommon conditions of systemic sclerosis (scleroderma) and idiopathic inflammatory myositis (dermatomyositis and polymyositis) have a higher risk for pulmonary disease than the most frequently occurring pediatric rheumatic disease, juvenile idiopathic arthritis (JIA), which has relatively infrequent pulmonary disease (Table 25-1).[1–4] Systemic lupus erythematosus (SLE), a relatively common rheumatic disease, has frequent and diverse lung involvement (Table 25-2).

Table 25-1. Relative Frequency of Rheumatic Diseases and Associated Pulmonary Disease

Characteristic	Systemic JIA	SLE	JSS	JDM
Incidence (per 10^5)	1	0.3–0.9	Unknown	0.2–0.4
Age at onset (years)	Variable	Adolescence	Unknown	7
Antibody associations	None	ANA, anti-dsDNA	ANA, anti-Scl 70; anti-centromere (in CREST syndrome)	ANA, myositis-specific antibodies
Pulmonary involvement	+	+++	+++	++
Female to male ratio	1:1	4–5:1	Relation to age 8 y ≤: 1:1 >: 3:1	2–4:1
Ethnic predisposition	None	AA, Hispanic, Native American, Asian	AA, Native American	No

Abbreviations: +, occasional occurrence; ++, common or significant; +++, quite frequent or very significant; AA, African-American; anti-dsDNA, anti-double stranded deoxyribonucleic acid; ANA, antinuclear antibody; JDM, juvenile dermatomyositis; JIA, juvenile idiopathic arthritis; JSS, juvenile systemic sclerosis; SLE, systemic lupus erythematosus.

Table 25-2. Types of Lung Involvement in Rheumatic Diseases

Type of Lung Involvement	Systemic JIA	SLE	JSS	JDM
Pleural disease	+	++	+	–
Interstitial lung disease	+	++	+++	+
Alveolar hemorrhage	–	+	–	–
Abnormal pulmonary test	–	+++	++	++
Abnormal diffusion	–	++	++	++
Pneumonia	–	+++	++	++
Weakness	+	+	++	+++
Aspiration	–	–	+++	+++
Pulmonary hypertension	–	++	+++	–

Abbreviations: +, occasional occurrence; ++, common or significant; +++, quite frequent or very significant; JDM, juvenile dermatomyositis; JIA, juvenile idiopathic arthritis; JSS, juvenile systemic sclerosis; SLE, systemic lupus erythematosus.

Juvenile Idiopathic Arthritis

Formerly known as juvenile rheumatoid arthritis, JIA consists of several subtypes, including polyarthritis (≥5 joints affected) and systemic-onset JIA. Pulmonary involvement is most commonly seen with the systemic-onset JIA; it is rare in patients with polyarticular JIA.

Pulmonary function test abnormalities may precede the onset of arthritis.[5] The cause of pulmonary disease in JIA is not understood. The treatment of JIA with methotrexate may rarely result in the pulmonary complication of hypersensitivity pneumonitis independent of the underlying disease process.[6]

Pulmonary symptoms associated with JIA include cough, dyspnea, tachypnea, and chest pain. The presentations most commonly seen are pleurisy, with or without effusion; increased pulmonary infections; or interstitial lung disease. There may be an associated leukocytosis with neutrophils predominating. The presence of fever may indicate concomitant infectious pneumonia or a consequence of systemic-onset JIA.

The mainstay of acute treatment of JIA-associated pleuropulmonary disease remains systemic corticosteroids.

Systemic Lupus Erythematosus

Systemic lupus erythematosus in children is a multisystem autoimmune disease with great variability of symptoms. The most common organ systems affected include skin, the musculoskeletal system, and the kidney.[7] Diagnosis is based on the presence of at least 4 criteria from the American College of Rheumatology classification criteria used for children and adults in the absence of any other autoimmune disease that may explain symptoms.[8] Systemic lupus erythematosus rarely occurs before 5 years of age and its incidence varies between sex and ethnic groups; at-risk groups include females, Hispanics, African-Americans, Native Americans, and Asians.[9,10]

Clinical Manifestations

Initial constitutional symptoms include fever, hair loss, fatigue, weight loss, and other evidence of systemic inflammatory disease, such as lymphadenopathy and hepatosplenomegaly. Many systems can be involved in children with SLE from musculoskeletal (arthritis), skin (malar or photosensitive rash), neuropsychiatric (cognitive dysfunction, headaches), hematologic (cytopenia), cardiac (pericarditis, pericardial effusion, and premature atherosclerosis), renal (nephritis or nephrosis), and lung disease. Pulmonary symptoms can be seen in approximately 6% of children presenting with SLE, and overall these symptoms can occur in 25% to 75% of total cases.[10,11] Lung findings include pneumonitis, pleuritis, pulmonary hemorrhage, pulmonary fibrosis, and pneumothorax. Less common findings include diaphragmatic involvement (shrinking lung syndrome, phrenic nerve paralysis), vasculitis, and pulmonary embolus.[12] Simultaneous infectious pneumonia may complicate the clinical picture.

Pulmonary involvement has a wide range of clinical severity, from asymptomatic pulmonary function test abnormalities to severe life-threatening pulmonary hemorrhage. Clinically, patients most often have pleuritis, presenting as respiratory distress with chest pain, which can be unilateral.[11] Other pulmonary-related entities can accompany SLE. Chronic interstitial lung disease can present with cough, tachypnea, crackles, and nonproductive cough; imaging often reveals scattered nodular densities. Bronchiolitis obliterans with organizing pneumonia (BOOP) is a rare complication resulting in a chronic inflammatory and destructive process of the small airways. Pulmonary hypertension (PH) usually occurs late in the disease process; treatment with vasodilators (prostacyclins or inhaled nitric oxide) has not been shown to be effective. Pulmonary hypertension is associated with a poor prognosis.[13] Children may have more severe organ involvement than adults.[9]

Pulmonary Evaluation of a Patient With SLE

If pulmonary symptoms are present, including tachypnea with or without chest pain, imaging is indicated. Plain chest radiographs help to differentiate the clinical patterns that are seen: pleurisy with effusion, pleuropericarditis with diaphragm thickening or elevation, and fibrosing alveolitis.[13] A high-resolution computed tomography scan is indicated if the plain radiograph does not explain the symptoms and signs. Additional pulmonary investigations include early bronchoscopy with bronchoalveolar lavage as well as lung biopsy, especially to differentiate between SLE or infection.[10] Distinguishing lupus-induced pulmonary disease from infection can be a diagnostic challenge.

Pleural fluid should be obtained for culture and analysis. Generally, pleural fluid in active SLE is exudative (protein >3g/dL, pH >7.35), although it may be transudative on occasion. The fluid typically has an elevated white blood cell count (2,500–5,000 cells/mm^3) with mononuclear and lymphocyte predominance; LE cells may be present and the positive antinuclear antibody titer is usually greater than the patient's serum titer.[14] Pulmonary function tests are abnormal in two-thirds of patients, typically associated with small airways obstruction and decreased carbon dioxide diffusing capacity (DLCO).[15]

Management

The acute pulmonary management of patients with SLE and severe pulmonary involvement is corticosteroids, including high-dose pulse therapy. The specialist providing care should treat with a regimen of prednisone 2 mg/kg/d (not to exceed 80 mg/d) in divided doses, or intravenous (IV) pulse methylprednisolone therapy (3 days of high-dose IV corticosteroids) with continuation or tapering depending on response.[10] Failure to respond, typically due to persistent dyspnea and chest pain, may lead to a trial of an immunosuppressive agent or a biological response modifier, such as anti-CD19 monoclonal antibodies (rituximab).[16] Nonsteroidal anti-inflammatory drugs provide symptomatic relief for mild pleuritis if the patient is not at risk for hemorrhage or experiencing decreased renal function. Treatment may also be needed for specific processes, such as pulmonary hemorrhage and PH. Patients with SLE often are immunocompromised, increasing their risk for pulmonary infections. This immunocompromised state results from decreased complement or cell-mediated immunity consequent to inherent immune dysfunction and/or medication treatment, decreased airway clearance from lower respiratory tract inflammation, and neuromuscular weakness.[13]

Prognosis and When to Admit

Children with SLE experience more severe disease than adults, and they are at risk for a worse prognosis.[9] Recent 5-year survival has been as high as 100%, with 10-year survival rates as high as 86%. Survival is affected by socioeconomic status, access to health care, ethnic background, infection, and severity of renal or central nervous system disease. Earlier diagnosis and aggressive treatment lead to a more favorable prognosis than delayed, inadequate care. Patients with SLE require a multidisciplinary approach. The decision to hospitalize a patient depends on timing and complexity of making the diagnosis, noting that many patients can have an insidious, smoldering presentation. Organ involvement can be severe and life-threatening, potentially changing over time for a single patient.[16]

Systemic Sclerosis (Diffuse Scleroderma) and Juvenile Dermatomyositis

Systemic sclerosis (diffuse scleroderma) and juvenile dermatomyositis occur much less frequently than either JIA or SLE,[3,4] but both seem to have a high risk for pulmonary involvement.[16,17] Although extremely rare in localized scleroderma, cardiopulmonary disease occurs in 50% to 60% of children with systemic sclerosis. It is a primary cause of morbidity and mortality.[3] The pulmonary involvement includes interstitial fibrosis, reduced forced vital capacity, reduced diffusion capacity, and pulmonary hypertension. Dysphagia and esophageal dysmotility occur frequently with systemic sclerosis. Affected patients are at increased risk for aspiration, either during swallowing or after gastroesophageal reflux.

Juvenile idiopathic dermatomyositis also occurs infrequently. Musculoskeletal and cutaneous manifestations are usually present before there is any evidence of pulmonary involvement; however, as many as one-third of the patients will have pulmonary signs or symptoms sometime during the course of their disease.[16] Pulmonary disease in juvenile dermatomyositis may occur less often than in adult disease,[18] but this may reflect how frequently and intensively pulmonary involvement is sought, as well as how the progressive severity of weakness evolves. Interstitial lung disease, BOOP, restrictive pulmonary disease, and reduced diffusion capacity are the most common types of pulmonary disease. Serum KL-6 may be a useful marker for interstitial lung disease in dermatomyositis. Due to proximal weakness, patients with dermatomyositis may have impaired secretion control and increased susceptibility to pneumonia. They are also at risk for aspiration due to pharyngeal weakness. Anti-synthetase antibody-associated juvenile polymyositis may present initially with interstitial lung disease; weakness may ensue later.

Some children have a constellation of rheumatic and dermatologic problems that do not fit easily into a discrete diagnostic category. These diagnoses are termed mixed connective tissue diseases or overlap diseases; they comprise features of SLE, systemic sclerosis, and dermatomyositis. This group of patients seems to have a similar risk for pulmonary involvement with the same respiratory disease processes that occur in systemic sclerosis and dermatomyositis.

Vasculitic Diseases

Case Report 25-1

A 14-year-old girl presents with a year and a half history of symptoms of epistaxis, generalized edema, cough, dyspnea, hemoptysis, high blood pressure, and macroscopic hematuria. Chest radiography demonstrates the presence of a right lower lobe granuloma. Laboratory studies document thrombocytosis and elevated C-reactive protein (CRP). The diagnosis, a clinicopathologic one, is made by biopsy of appropriate lung tissue showing necrotizing granulomatous vasculitis. Following initial therapy with cyclophosphamide and prednisone therapy, she sustains remission at 5 years while treated with azathioprine.

Wegener Granulomatosis

Wegener granulomatosis (WG) is a rare necrotizing, granulomatous, small- to medium-sized vasculitis. Wegener granulomatosis has a pediatric incidence of 0.1 per 100,000 in the US population younger than 20 years. Although primarily manifesting in adults, WG occurs at all ages and has a clinical predilection for involvement of the upper airways, lungs, and kidneys, though any organ system can be affected. In children, WG is commonly associated with subglottic stenosis and nasal deformities.[18,19] Subglottic stenosis often occurs independently of other WG symptoms. Other clinical features of organ involvement are similar to adults. The cause of WG remains unknown. The presence of (1) granulomatous involvement of medium-sized vessels and (2) granulomas featuring acute and chronic inflammation (central necrosis, histiocytes, lymphocytes, and giant cells) suggest an autoimmune origin. In vitro studies show that cytoplasmic antineutrophil cytoplasmic antibodies (c-ANCA) interact with proteinase-3 (PR3) to activate pro-inflammatory pathways. Genetic factors play a role in the difference between varying phenotypes. The activity of the highly polymorphic alpha-1 antitrypsin, a natural inhibitor of PR3, plays a role in these varying phenotypes. Polymorphisms of interleukin-10 may contribute to disease susceptibility.

Clinical Manifestations

For the diagnosis of WG a patient should have at least 2 of 4 predefined criteria, per the American College of Rheumatology (Box 25-1). The presence of any 2 or more criteria yields a sensitivity of 88% and a specificity of 92%.[20] More than 90% of patients with WG initially seek medical attention for upper or lower airway symptoms.[21] Sinusitis is the most frequent presenting symptom, followed by fever, arthralgias, cough, rhinitis, hemoptysis, otitis, and ocular inflammation. Children are at high risk for subglottic stenosis and bronchial stenosis, which may require surgical intervention.

Necrotizing glomerulonephritis may occur more frequently in older children than in early infancy. Although present in 10% to 20% of patients at diagnosis, some studies describe renal involvement developing in 60% to 80% of patients during the disease course. Other findings include arthralgia of the knees, wrists, ankles, or hips occurring in almost half of patients. Additionally, skin involvement ranging from erythematous or purpuric macules to massive nodules and necrotizing ulcerations can be observed. Ocular and nervous system manifestations can also occur. In adults, nasal carriage of *Staphylococcus aureus* has been associated with a high risk of relapse.[21]

Box 25-1. 1990 Criteria for the Classification of Wegener Granulomatosis (WG)[a,b]

1. Nasal or oral inflammation
   Development of painful or painless oral ulcers or purulent or bloody nasal discharge
2. Abnormal-appearing chest radiograph
   Chest radiograph showing the presence of nodules, fixed infiltrates, or cavities
3. Abnormal urinary sediment
   Microhematuria (>5 red blood cells per high power field) or red cell casts
4. Granulomatous inflammation on biopsy
   Granulomatous inflammation within the wall of an artery or in the perivascular or extravascular area of an artery or arteriole

[a] Adapted from the American College of Rheumatology.
[b] For the purposes of classification, a patient should be diagnosed having WG if at least 2 of these 4 criteria are present.

Evaluation

Routine laboratory test results are generally nonspecific in WG. Common abnormalities include leukocytosis, thrombocytosis (>400,000/mL), marked elevation of the erythrocyte sedimentation rate (ESR) and CRP levels, and normochromic, normocytic anemia. Although nonspecific for necrotizing small vessel vasculitis, c-ANCA can be detected in 70% to 90% of patients with active WG.

Although one-third of chest radiographs in children are abnormal, these children do not have associated pulmonary symptoms. Common chest radiographic findings include densities, cavitation, and nodules. Less frequently atelectasis, pneumothorax, pleural effusion, pulmonary hemorrhage, and mediastinal or hilar lymphadenopathy are found.

Computed tomography of the sinuses and chest are useful in detecting airway stenosis and pulmonary granulomas. Bronchoscopy may be necessary to evaluate airway lesions fully. Pulmonary function testing reveals obstructive or restrictive lung disease as well as lower DLCO. Definitive diagnosis of WG is most often confirmed with a histopathologic demonstration of necrosis, vasculitis, and/or granulomatous inflammation.

Evaluation for WG can be involved. Children should be monitored and evaluated for signs of upper airway and lower airway obstruction. Pneumonia and sinusitis may also mask diagnosis and be found at initial time of diagnosis. Chronic renal failure is a major contributor to long-term morbidity.

Management

Initial treatment with glucocorticoids and cyclophosphamide induces remission in more than 90% of patients. Initially, children receive prednisone until symptoms improve; then it is gradually reduced. Cyclophosphamide may be continued for at least 1 year after disease control or remission and then is gradually reduced. Alternatively, methotrexate or azathioprine may be used after an initial 4- to 6-month tapering course of cyclophosphamide.[18] Unfortunately, subglottic stenosis related to WG does not frequently improve with systemic medical treatment. Serial intratracheal dilation and injection of long-acting glucocorticoids provide a safe and effective treatment, commonly mitigating the need for tracheostomy.

Complications

Treatment-related morbidity has also been noted. Cyclophosphamide-related malignancies have not been seen with childhood WG but have been seen in adults. Infections requiring hospitalization and IV therapy also have been reported. Prophylaxis against *Pneumocystis jiroveci* with trimethoprim-sulfamethoxazole is now commonplace with children undergoing treatment for WG.[22]

Churg-Strauss Syndrome

Churg-Strauss syndrome (CSS) involves multiple organ systems, including the sinopulmonary and gastrointestinal tracts, heart, nervous system, and skin. Churg-Strauss syndrome is characterized by development of eosinophilic vasculitis.[23] Churg-Strauss syndrome is defined by pulmonary eosinophilic granulomatous inflammation, necrotizing vasculitis with associated asthma, and blood eosinophilia. The histology of lung tissue shows granulomatous necrotizing vasculitis of the small- to medium-sized vessels and eosinophilic pneumonia.[24] The cause of CSS is unknown. The prominence of allergic features, such as elevated levels of serum immunoglobulin (Ig) E, and the presence of immune complexes, rheumatoid factor, and c-ANCA suggest an autoimmune origin.[25]

Clinical Manifestations

The American College of Rheumatology has established 7 criteria for the classification of CSS in patients with documented vasculitis (Box 25-2). The presence of 4 or more of these criteria yields a sensitivity of 85% and a specificity of 99.7% for CSS.[26] Similar to many eosinophilic syndromes, constitutional symptoms, including fever, weight loss, and generalized myalgias, are common. The prodromal phase occurs most commonly among

Box 25-2. 1990 Criteria for the Classification of Churg-Strauss Syndrome (CSS)[a,b]

1. Asthma
2. Eosinophilia >10% of white blood cell differential
3. History of seasonal allergy
4. Mono- or polyneuropathy
5. Pulmonary infiltrates, migratory or transitory
6. Paranasal sinus abnormality
7. Extravascular eosinophils

[a] Adapted from the American College of Rheumatology.
[b] For classification purposes, a patient shall be said to have CSS if at least 4 criteria are present.

individuals in the second and third decades of life, characterized by atopic disease, allergic rhinitis, and asthma. Features of the eosinophilic phase include peripheral blood eosinophilia and eosinophilic infiltration of multiple organs, especially the lung and gastrointestinal tract. In the third and fourth decades of life, a life-threatening systemic vasculitis of the medium and small vessels frequently occurs; this is often associated with vascular and extravascular granulomatosis. The vasculitic phase may be heralded by nonspecific constitutional symptoms and signs, especially fever, weight loss, malaise, and lassitude.

Diagnostic Evaluation

The diagnosis of CSS in childhood remains challenging. A strong clinical suspicion coupled with pathologic confirmation can expedite the diagnosis. Asthma is often associated with sinusitis and pulmonary symptoms, such as infiltrates and atelectasis. The diagnosis often is not made until abdomen, heart, and nervous systems become involved. Reports of CSS occurring in children are limited and generally consist of single case reports. The incidence of CSS in adults is estimated at 2.4 per million per year. Asthma is almost always present in CSS, but CSS is an extremely rare finding among children with asthma. Because of its rarity in children, the incidence of pediatric disease is unknown. A review of CSS in childhood from 1999 identified 10 published cases of children with an average age of 10.2 years and an age range of 4 to 16 years. However, an increasing number of reports have emerged in the last few years, suggesting either a rising incidence or, more likely, increased awareness of this entity in the pediatric community. Laboratory evaluation should include complete blood cell count with differential to detect eosinophilia, c-ANCA, and total IgE. Antineutrophil cytoplasmic antibodies are common but seem to have less specificity in children. Other nonspecific tests, including the ESR and immune complexes, have been used.

Radiographic findings are varied. Chest radiograph abnormalities are common and consist of bilateral, nonsegmental alveolar or interstitial infiltrates. Computed tomography chest findings include reticulonodular disease without cavitation (unlike WG), bronchial wall thickening, hyperinflation, interlobular septal thickening, lymphadenopathy, and pleural effusions. Because there are multiple organs involved with CSS, biopsy of the involved area should be done to evaluate for an eosinophilic inflammatory process or vasculitis.

Management

Corticosteroids are the mainstay of treatment in CSS, often with striking results. Recent data suggest early and aggressive treatment may lead to clinical remission in more than 90% of patients treated. In those not treated, there is a 50% survival rate within the first 3 months of diagnosis. Approximately 25% of all patients with CSS will relapse. Although cytotoxic agents, such as cyclophosphamide, do not improve survival rates, their use is associated with a reduced incidence of relapse. Other successful therapies have included intravenous Ig (IVIG) infusions, azathioprine, methotrexate, infliximab, or interferon-α.[27,28] Laboratory markers, such as serum eosinophils, often normalize within 2 weeks of treatment initiation. Clinical improvement can also be seen within 2 to 4 weeks, but often residual respiratory symptoms may require the continuation of low-dose prednisone therapy for longer periods. Cardiovascular disease occurs in approximately half of the patients with CSS irrespective of age. All patients with CSS should be screened for signs of cardiac involvement, which includes electrocardiogram and echocardiogram. Since immunosuppressive therapies increase the risk of opportunistic infection, prophylaxis with trimethoprim-sulfamethoxazole should be provided.[29]

Prognosis and When to Admit

Cerebral hemorrhage, renal failure, gastrointestinal bleeding, and heart failure are the most common acute causes of death associated with CSS. Pediatric case reports include combinations of asthma, polyarthralgia, myalgia, and neuropathies. Pulmonary manifestations are varied in severity, with most reporting pulmonary infiltrates responsive to corticosteroid therapy. Less common pulmonary symptoms include chest pain, hemoptysis, and pulmonary infarction. Prognosis is unknown with childhood CSS. Use of corticosteroids and associated immunomodulators control disease and minimize relapses. The decision for inpatient versus outpatient management should be made, in conjunction with rheumatology, cardiology, and/or pulmonary specialists, based on the patient's clinical presentation and cardiac function.

Pulmonary-Renal Syndromes, Alveolar Hemorrhage, and Small Vessel Vasculitis

Systemic vasculitis of the small-sized vessels often manifests as combined pulmonary and renal disease; WG, microscopic polyangiitis, and SLE are the most common, with Goodpasture's syndrome and CSS occurring less commonly.[30,31] Alveolar hemorrhage, often massive and life-threatening, can be a presenting manifestation of these syndromes or occur at various times during the course of the disease.[32] Specific antibodies are associated with each syndrome, which helps establish the correct diagnosis (Table 25-3). The renal involvement is often extensive at the time of diagnosis; response to treatment is often suboptimal, requiring dialysis for end-stage renal disease.

Granulomatous lung disease is defined by the presence of granulomas, which involve acute and chronic inflammation with central necrosis and histiocytes, lymphocytes, and giant cells, organized as a collection of mature mononuclear phagocytes. A wide range of pulmonary conditions may give rise to lung granulomas, including infectious and

Table 25-3. Most Common Alveolar Hemorrhage Syndromes

Characteristic	SLE	WG	MPA	Goodpasture's	CSS
Blood markers	ANA, anti-dsDNA	c-ANCA	p-ANCA	Anti-GBM	Eosinophilia
Renal disease	+++	+++	+++	+++	+
Skin involvement	+++	+	+	–	+
ENT involvement	+	+++	+	–	++
Arthritis	+++	++	+	–	–
Radiographic findings	ILD, hemorrhage	Nodules, cavities, hemorrhage	ILD, hemorrhage	Hemorrhage	Increased peribronchial markings

Abbreviations: +, occasional occurrence; ++, common or significant; +++, quite frequent or very significant; anti-GBM, anti-glomerular basement membrane antibody; ANA, antinuclear antibody; anti-dsDNA, anti-double stranded deoxyribonucleic acid; c-ANCA, antineutrophil cytoplasmic antibody (also anti-protease antibody); CSS, Churg-Strauss syndrome; ENT, ear nose and throat; ILD, interstitial lung disease; MPA, microscopic polyangiitis; p-ANCA, perinuclear antineutrophil cytoplasmic antibody; SLE, systemic lupus erythematosus; WG, Wegener granulomatosis.

noninfectious causes, and common lung pathology; a lung biopsy is confirmatory. Chronic granulomatous disease is presented in Chapter 44.

The initiating event in granuloma formation is believed to be the deposition within tissue of a relatively indigestible antigenic or inert foreign material that initiates a delayed type (Type IV) hypersensitivity reaction. These cell-mediated hypersensitivity reactions do not depend on antibodies. T lymphocyte proliferation and activation release lymphokines that recruit and activate macrophages and other lymphocytes. Infectious diseases account for a great many cases of granulomatous lung diseases in children. Infectious causes include bacterial, viral, fungal, protozoan, metazoan, and mycobacterial (Box 25-3).

Sarcoidosis

Sarcoidosis is a multisystem granulomatous disease that most commonly affects young adults and is relatively uncommon in children. Although the exact cause of sarcoidosis is unknown, a combination of environmental and host factors probably causes the characteristic granulomatous response. Infectious causes have been considered, including viral (Epstein-Barr virus, cytomegalovirus) and bacterial *(Mycobacterium tuberculosis, Propionibacterium acnes,* and *Propionibacterium granulosum),* but no conclusive evidence has been demonstrated.[33,34] The clinical presentation is widely variable and is due primarily to local tissue infiltration or injury by the mass effect of sarcoid lesions. Many organ systems can be involved in sarcoidosis, including skin, lymphatics, kidneys, bones, liver, spleen, heart, eyes parotid gland, and nervous and vascular systems.

Clinical Manifestations

Patients frequently present with hilar lymphadenopathy, pulmonary infiltration, ocular lesions, or cutaneous lesions. The lungs are affected in approximately 90% of patients, although much less so in children younger than 5 years. Pulmonary disease accounts for most of the morbidity and mortality associated with this disease.[35] Almost all childhood cases of sarcoidosis are symptomatic. Constitutional symptoms predominate, including weight loss, fatigue, lethargy, anorexia, and headache. Less common symptoms include dyspnea, chest pain,

Box 25-3. Differential Diagnosis of Granulomatous Lung Disease

Noninfectious Causes

- Autoimmune disease
  - Primary systemic vasculitides
    - Wegener granulomatosis
    - Churg-Strauss
  - Systemic lupus erythematosus
  - Crohn disease
  - Primary biliary cirrhosis
- Bronchocentric granulomatosis
- Immunodeficiencies
  - Chronic granulomatous disease (see Chapter 44)
  - Common variable immune deficiency
  - Hypogammaglobulinemia
- Histiocytosis X
- Hypersensitivity pneumonitis
  - Farmer's lung
  - Bird fancier's lung
- Neoplasms
  - Carcinomas
  - Sarcomas

Infectious Causes

- Viruses
  - Epstein-Barr virus
  - Herpes
  - Rubella
  - Cytomegalovirus
  - Measles
  - Coxsackie B
  - Parainfluenza
- Fungi
  - *Histoplasma*
  - *Aspergillus*
  - *Coccidioides immitis*
  - *Blastomycosis*
  - *Cryptococcus*
- Protozoa
  - *Toxoplasma*
  - *Leishmania*
- Metazoa *(Schistosoma)*
- Bacteria
  - *Yersinia*
  - *Borrelia*
  - *Brucella*
  - Mycobacteria
    - *Mycobacterium tuberculosis*
    - *Mycobacterium leprae*
    - Atypical mycobacteria

nausea, and prolonged fever. Children younger than 5 years uniquely present with a triad of rash, uveitis, and arthritis. In older children, involvement of the lungs, lymph nodes, and eyes predominate.

Pulmonary involvement is more common in older children. Symptoms are often limited to a dry, hacking cough without dyspnea or chest pain. Auscultation can reveal crackles and wheezing, but patients often have a quiet chest.

Diagnostic Evaluation

No definitive laboratory test diagnostic of sarcoidosis exists. In the absence of a known causative agent, sarcoidosis remains a diagnosis of exclusion, although a typical presentation may strongly suggest the diagnosis. Diagnosis depends on 3 factors: a suggestive clinical picture, histologic evidence of a typical non-caseating granuloma on a biopsy specimen, and exclusion of other conditions with similar findings.[34,35] Nonspecific laboratory findings include anemia, leukopenia, eosinophilia, hypergammaglobulinemia, and hypercalcemia. During the acute phase, an elevated ESR is common.

Angiotensin-converting enzyme (ACE) is often elevated in sarcoidosis (up to 80% of children). Angiotensin-converting enzyme is produced from the epithelioid cells of the granulomas and constitutes a potentially strong diagnostic factor. Although not pathognomonic, the activity of the sarcoid lesions is associated with an elevation of serum ACE. The use of routine ACE level monitoring in the follow-up care of children has not been clearly established. Serum lysozyme is also often elevated in sarcoidosis, serving as a marker of disease activity (up to 79% of children). Lysozyme can be elevated in 72% of children with sarcoidosis who have a normal ACE. Purified protein derivative tests should be done with control (tetanus, mumps, or candida) because anergy is classic in sarcoidosis and can contribute to the diagnosis. Because of difficulty in obtaining standardized test material and reports of varying sensitivity and specificity of the test, the Kveim test is not approved for general use by the US Food and Drug Administration.

Bilateral hilar adenopathy is the most common finding in children and occurs in almost all cases of sarcoidosis. Other radiographic findings include paratracheal and subcarinal adenopathy. Hilar lymphadenopathy typically is symmetrical, although it may appear unilaterally in rare instances. Pulmonary parenchymal involvement has also been described and predominantly appears radiographically as an interstitial pattern. Chest radiographs traditionally have been classified in 5 stages (0 through IV): stage 0 is normal chest radiograph, stage I is bilateral hilar lymphadenopathy alone, stage II is bilateral adenopathy with parenchymal infiltrates, stage III is parenchymal infiltrates without adenopathy, and stage IV is advanced pulmonary fibrosis.[34,35] Pulmonary function changes that occur with sarcoidosis are restrictive in nature, including a reduction in forced vital capacity, total lung capacity, and functional residual capacity. Obstruction is seen less often and can signify airway hyperreactivity, nodal compression, or endobronchial granuloma. Bronchoalveolar lavage (BAL) is significant for a nonspecific increase in the CD4/CD8 ratios and number of polymorphonuclear neutrophils. There is no association between histologic findings on BAL and the activity or prognosis of the disease. Although BAL yields a 3- to 5-fold increase in the number of lymphocytes and macrophages in children with sarcoidosis, BAL is not a routinely recommended diagnostic procedure.

Management

Management of children with sarcoidosis depends on presentation, clinical picture, and number and severity of organ systems involved. Asymptomatic children with hilar adenopathy may not need to be treated. Treatment should be considered for children with dyspnea, worsening lung function, and worsening radiologic findings. Severe neural, cardiac, ocular, and pulmonary involvement warrants immediate treatment. Corticosteroids are widely used and are often effective. Corticosteroids remain the therapy of choice for children with multisystem involvement, and pulse steroids can improve lung function. For pulmonary disease, 6 to 18 months of therapy may be a reasonable duration of therapy, but no time course has been well established for other organ systems. Additionally, inhaled corticosteroids are used in maintenance therapy with varying success. Corticosteroid-sparing agents include methotrexate, antimalarials, azathioprine, cyclophosphamide, and infliximab. Low-dose methotrexate administered orally in childhood sarcoidosis is effective and safe.[37]

Prognosis and When to Admit

Overall prognosis in children and adults is good. Spontaneous resolution occurs in two-thirds of patients, while 10% may have long-term symptoms. An increased risk of more severe disease in adults is associated with uveitis, chronic hypercalcemia, nephrocalcinosis, African American race, cystic bone lesions, neurosarcoidosis, and stage III or IV lung disease. Children who have eye, skin, and joint involvement when younger than 5 years often have a poorer prognosis than those without these features. Older children with lung involvement generally have a better prognosis. Hospitalization is indicated for severe dyspnea or chest pain, especially if hypoxia is present. Evaluation and diagnosis can be accomplished most efficiently through inpatient admission.

Histiocytosis X

Histiocytoses are a group of disorders resulting from a pathologic accumulation of monoclonal histiocytes, of which Langerhans cell histiocytosis (LCH) is the most common. There is broad spectrum of disease, from benign single-system disease (eosinophilic granuloma) to more severe, disseminated, and possibly fatal disease. These include entities known as histiocytosis X, Hand-Schuller Christian disease, and Letterer-Siwe disease.[38] Affected tissues are often infiltrated by large collections of unusual histiocytes organized into granulomas. Pulmonary involvement in LCH is rare in children and usually a less prominent factor in multisystem and disseminated disease. Pediatric cases are usually seen in young adult males, with a handful of case reports for children younger than 15 years. There are 2 possible reasons for the paucity of pediatric cases: pulmonary LCH is heavily associated with smoking and pulmonary LCH in children remains clinically occult.

Langerhans cells, alveolar macrophages, and lymphocytes are all thought to play a role in tissue damage in the lungs. Clinical symptoms include constitutional symptoms such as fever, malaise, and weight loss. Early symptoms include chronic cough and dyspnea. Exercise intolerance is also common. Spontaneous pneumothorax is also a common presenting symptom. Early radiologic findings consist of diffuse micronodular and reticular pattern. However, pulmonary progression to cystic lesions can cause multiple radiolucencies and a state aptly named "honeycomb lung." Treatment targets the underlying histiocytosis.

Common Variable Immunodeficiency

Common variable immunodeficiency is the most common symptomatic primary immunodeficiency and is characterized by hypogammaglobulinemia and recurrent infections, associated with a heterogeneous group of primary antibody deficiency disorders. As a group, they do not have a known genetic or molecular defect. Recurrent infections of the sino-pulmonary and gastrointestinal tract are most common. Lung involvement is primarily an interstitial lung disease, which includes lymphocytic non-caseating granulomas. Pathogens include *Streptococcus* and *Haemophilus influenzae*; pneumonia with *Pseudomonas* and *Pneumocystis jiroveci* is uncommon.[39] The diagnosis is made by reduction of multiple immunoglobulins in addition to failure to mount a specific antibody response to common antigens despite normal B-cell lymphocyte numbers. T-cell lymphocytes can be normal, but abnormalities have been seen in up to 60% of patients. Treatment lies with prophylactic IVIG and treatment of noninfectious complications.[39] Common variable immunodeficiency also has been implicated with certain malignancies.[40]

Bronchocentric Granulomatosis

Case Report 25-2

A 17-year-old girl presents with fever, cough, hemoptysis, intermittent fever, dyspnea on exertion, cyanosis, and weight loss. In addition to these clinical findings, there was a history of asthma, elevated serum eosinophilia, serum precipitins, and IgE antibodies to *Aspergillus fumigatus*. Persistent radiographic opacification in the left lower lung was also observed. Histologic examination of the specimen reveals bronchocentric granulomatosis. Noninvasive septate fungal hyphae compatible with *Aspergillus* were identified. Cultures from sputum and surgical specimens grew *Aspergillus*. The patient's condition is well controlled with prednisone and lobectomy.

Bronchocentric granulomatosis (BG) is a histologic finding characterized by necrotizing granulomas and inflammation of the bronchioles and bronchiolar epithelium. This inflammation can cause destruction and obliteration of the smaller airways. Bronchocentric granulomatosis is generally believed to represent a nonspecific response to various forms of airway injury. Most commonly, BG is associated with asthma and caused by allergic bronchopulmonary aspergillosis (ABPA).[41] Bronchocentric granulomatosis also has been implicated with a variety of other infections, such as Epstein-Barr virus and *Mycobacterium tuberculosis*.[42] Bronchocentric granulomatosis also has been implicated with WG, although whether BG is a manifestation or mimics WG is unclear. Some experts believe that BG is not a disease but a pathologic descriptive process and the term should be limited to a manifestation of ABPA or granulomatous process in non-asthmatics when other causes have been excluded.[41]

Crohn Disease

Crohn disease (CD) is a chronic inflammatory multisystem disorder involving the gastrointestinal tract and musculoskeletal, cutaneous, renal, vascular and hepatic systems. There have been case reports in adults and children in which latent granulomatous lung disease has been associated with CD. Speculation about etiology has focused on immunologic phenomenon as seen with sarcoidosis. Sarcoidosis and CD share pathologic features of non-caseating epithelioid granulomas. Crohn disease has also been found with granulomatous reactions seen outside the bowel.[43] Described treatments have included corticosteroids, immunosuppressive agents, and infliximab.[44]

References

1. Weiss JE, Ilowite NT. Juvenile idiopathic arthritis. *Pediatr Clin North Am.* 2005;52:413–442
2. Benseler SM, Silverman ED. Systemic lupus erythematosus. *Pediatr Clin North Am.* 2005;52:443–467
3. Zulian F. Scleroderma in children. *Pediatr Clin North Am.* 2005;52:521–545
4. Compeyrot-Lacassagne S, Feldman BM. Inflammatory myopathies in children. *Pediatr Clin North Am.* 2005;52:493–520
5. Wagener JS, Taussig LM, DeBenedetti C, et al. Pulmonary function in juvenile rheumatoid arthritis. *J Pediatr.* 1981;99:108–110
6. Cron RQ, Sherry DD, Wallace CA. Methotrexate-induced hypersensitivity pneumonitis in a child with juvenile rheumatoid arthritis. *J Pediatr.* 1998;132:901–902
7. Emery H. Clinical aspects of systemic lupus erythematosus in childhood. *Pediatr Clin North Am.* 1986;33:1177–1190
8. Tan EM, Fries JF, Masi AT, et al. The 1982 revised criteria for the classification of systemic lupus erythematosus. *Arthritis Rheum.* 1982;25:1271–1277
9. Sandborg CI. Childhood systemic lupus erythematosus and neonatal lupus syndrome. *Curr Opin Rheum.* 1998;10:481–487
10. Delgado EA, Malleson PN, Pirie GE, Petty RE. The pulmonary manifestations of childhood onset systemic lupus erythematosus. *Semin Arthritis Rheum.* 1990;19:285–293
11. Mochizuki T, Aotsuka S, Satoh T. Clinical and laboratory features of lupus patients with complicating pulmonary disease. *Respir Med.* 1999;93:95–101
12. Ferguson PJ, Weinberger M. Shrinking lung syndrome in a 14-year-old boy with systemic lupus erythematosus. *Pediatr Pulmonol.* 2006;41:194–197
13. Kamphuis S, Silverman ED. Prevalence and burden of pediatric-onset systemic lupus erythematosus. *Nat Rev Rheumatol.* 2010;6(9):538–546

14. Quismorio FP Jr. Pulmonary manifestations of systemic lupus erythematosus. In: Wallace DJ, Hahn BH, eds. *Dubois' Lupus Erythematosus*. 5th ed. Baltimore, MD: Williams & Wilkins; 1997
15. Morinishi Y, Oh-Ishi T, Kabuki T, Joh K. Juvenile dermatomyositis: clinical characteristics and the relatively high risk of interstitial lung disease. *Mod Rheumatol.* 2007;17:413–417
16. Terrier B, Amoura Z, Ravaud P, et al. Safety and efficacy of rituximab in systemic lupus erythematosus: results from 136 patients from the French AutoImmunity and Rituximab registry. *Arthritis Rheum.* 2010;62(8): 2458–2466
17. Misra R, Singh G, Aggarwal P, Aggarwal A. Juvenile onset systemic sclerosis: a single center experience of 23 cases from Asia. *Clin Rheumatol.* 2007; 26:1259–1262
18. Rottem M, Fauci AS, Hoffman GS, et al. Wegner granulomatosis in children and adolescents: clinical presentation and outcome. *J Pediatr.* 1993:122:26–31
19. Frosch M, Foell D. Wegener granulomatosis in childhood and adolescence. *Eur J Pediatr.* 2004;163:425–434
20. Leavitt RY, Fauci AS, Bloch DA, et al. The American College of Rheumatology 1990 criteria for the classification of Wegener's granulomatosis. *Arthritis Rheum.* 1990;33:1101–1107
21. Stegeman CA, Tervaert JW, Sluiter WJ, et al. Association of chronic nasal carriage of *Staphylococcus aureus* and high relapse rates in Wegener granulomatosis. *Ann Intern Med.* 1994;120:12–17
22. Grewal P, Brassard A. Fact or fiction: does the non-HIV/AIDS immunosuppressed patient need *Pneumocystis jiroveci* pneumonia prophylaxis? An updated literature review. *J Cutan Med Surg.* 2009;13(6):308–312
23. Wechsler ME. Pulmonary eosinophilic syndromes. *Immunol Allergy Clin North Am.* 2007;27:477–492
24. Boyer D, Vargas SO, Slattery D, et al. Churg-Strauss syndrome in children: a clinical and pathologic review. *Pediatrics.* 2006;118:e914–e920
25. Cottin V, Cordier JF. Churg-Strauss syndrome. *Allergy.* 1999;54:535–551
26. Masi AT, Hunder GG, Lie JT, et al. The American College of Rheumatology 1990 criteria for the classification of Churg-Strauss syndrome (allergic granulomatosis and angiitis). *Arthritis Rheum.* 1990;33:1094–1100
27. Gross WL. Churg-Strauss syndrome: update on recent developments. *Curr Opin Rheumatol.* 2002;14:11–14
28. Hellmich B, Gross WL. Recent progress in the pharmacotherapy of Churg-Strauss syndrome. *Expert Opin Pharmacother.* 2004;5:25–35
29. Noth I, Strek ME, Leff, AR. Churg-Strauss syndrome. *Lancet.* 2003;361: 587–594
30. Jennette JC, Falk RJ. Small-vessel vasculitis. *N Engl J Med.* 1997;337: 1512–1523
31. Brown KK. Pulmonary vasculitis. *Proc Am Thorac Soc.* 2006;3:48–57

32. Susaria SC, Fan LL. Diffuse alveolar hemorrhage syndromes in children. *Curr Opin Pediatr.* 2007;19:314–320
33. Fauroux, B, Clement A. Pediatric sarcoidosis. *Pediatr Respir Rev.* 2005;6: 128–133
34. Pattishall EN, Strope GL, Spinola SM, et al. Childhood sarcoidosis. *J Pediatr.* 1986;108:169–177
35. Baughman RP, Lower EE, du Bois RM. Sarcoidosis. *Lancet.* 2003;361:1111–1118
36. Tomita H, Sato S, Matsuda R, et al. Serum lysozyme levels and clinical features of sarcoidosis. *Lung.* 1999;177:161–167
37. Gedalia A, Molina JF, Ellis GS Jr, et al. Low-dose methotrexate therapy for childhood sarcoidosis. *J Pediatr.* 1997;130:25–29
38. Al-Trabolsi HA, Alshehri M, Al-Shomrani A, et al. "Primary" pulmonary Langerhans cell histiocytosis in a two year old child: case report and literature review. *J Pediatr Hematol Oncol.* 2006;28:79–81
39. Yong P, Tarzi M, Chua I, et al. Common variable immunodeficiency: an update on etiology and management. *Immunol Allergy Clin North Am.* 2008;20:367–386
40. Buckley RH. Pulmonary complications of primary immunodeficiencies. *Paediatr Respir Rev.* 2004;5(suppl A):S225–S233
41. Myers JL. Bronchocentric granulomatosis. Disease or diagnosis? *Chest.* 1989;96:3–4
42. Maguire GP, Rosen Y, Lyons HA. Pulmonary tuberculosis and bronchocentric granulomatosis. *Chest.* 1986;89;606–608
43. Puntis JW, Tarlow MJ, Raafat F, et al. Crohn disease of the lung. *Arch Dis Child.* 1990;65:1270–1271
44. Silbermintz A, Krishnan S, Banquet A, et al. Granulomatous pneumonitis, sclerosing cholangitis, and pancreatitis in a child with Crohn disease: response to infliximab. *J Pediatr Gastroenterol Nutr.* 2006;42:324–326

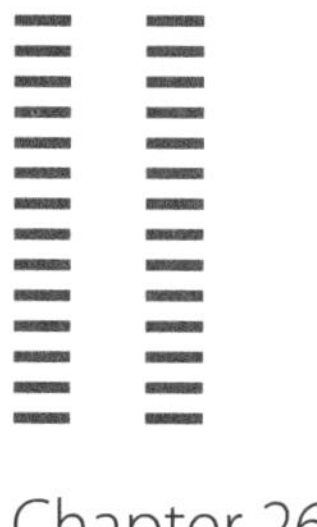

Chapter 26

Interstitial Lung Disease

Adrienne Prestridge, MD
Susanna A. McColley, MD

Introduction

The term interstitial lung disease (ILD) encompasses a group of rare, heterogeneous disorders characterized by diffuse pulmonary disease and disordered gas exchange. Interstitial lung disease includes any entity that results in derangement of the alveolar capillary interface, often characterized clinically with tachypnea, crackles, hypoxia, or diffuse infiltrates. Although a strict definition implies an abnormality of the interstitium, there are some diseases that have minimal interstitial defect but have pathologic abnormalities in the air spaces and distal airway that are considered under the broad term of ILD.[1] For this reason, some authors prefer the term diffuse lung disease. The estimated prevalence rate for ILD of unknown cause in immunocompetent children is 3.6 cases per million children from birth to age 16 years.[2] Increased awareness of ILD coupled with better definition of these diseases may increase the known prevalence.[3]

Much of what is known about ILD in children derives from case reports and small series. Interstitial lung disease in children differs from ILD in adults. For example, usual interstitial pneumonia (UIP) is a pathologic pattern of the clinical disease idiopathic pulmonary fibrosis or radiographic cryptogenic fibrosing alveolitis. Most adults with UIP die within 5 years of diagnosis; however, children with the same diagnosis live much longer and have a nonprogressive course. In more than 100 cases of UIP in the pediatric literature, none had the characteristic histopathology described in adults. This raises the question of whether UIP actually exists in children.[3] Trying to fit a pediatric disease into an adult classification scheme is not accurate and can lead to erroneous prognostic information. Two recent retrospective cohorts of patients, as well as other recent literature highlighting the underlying pathophysiology, have been published. The European Respiratory Society reported on 185 while the ChILD Research Co-operative from centers in North America reported on 187 cases.[4,5] Together, both provide a comprehensive description on the state of the clinical history, etiology, and prognosis of ILD in children. They offer differing perspectives on the pulmonology specialist and are recommended reading for those who have a special interest in this topic.

Interstitial lung disease encompasses 3 broad categories of disease, including those with known causes, those with unknown causes, and those with a presentation predominantly in infancy. Known causes of ILD include infection, aspiration, hypersensitivity pneumonitis, collagen vascular disease, environmental exposures, immunodeficiency, bronchopulmonary dysplasia, and lipid storage disease. Several disorders related to mutations in surfactant processing present as ILD in infancy: surfactant protein B (SP-B) deficiency, surfactant protein C (SP-C) deficiency,[6] and ABCA3 protein deficiency.[7] Other forms of ILD, such as pulmonary interstitial glycogenosis (PIG)[8] and neuroendocrine hyperplasia of infancy (NEHI)[9] present in infancy and have a less severe clinical, radiographic, and pathologic picture. The cause of many forms of pediatric ILD remains unknown.

Interstitial lung disease is characterized by a pathologic process affecting the interstitial space in the lung. In the normal lung, the interstitium, the area between the alveolar space and the capillary, is approximately one cell thick. However, in patients with ILD, this area becomes thickened. This likely occurs because inflammation leads to the deposition of connective tissue that forms areas of fibrosis. Inflammation is not the sole mechanism for ILD. In some forms of ILD, there is little or no inflammation visible on lung histopathologic studies, and treatment with anti-inflammatory agents does not consistently lead to clinical improvement. A second mechanism leading to an abnormal interstitium involves epithelial injury, leading to abnormal repair of the lung.[10] In children, the process of interstitial thickening is affected by age-specific lung growth and development. Genetic variations cannot be the only underlying cause but can modulate susceptibility and response to various injuries.[4] Epithelial injury, inflammation, and repair occur on a developing lung, leading to a distinct pathophysiology compared with adult ILD.

Diffusion of oxygen across the alveolus to the capillary is proportional to the thickness of the area. In patients with ILD, oxygen takes longer to diffuse across the thickened interstitium. This delay in diffusion leads to a compensatory increase in minute ventilation that is clinically manifest by tachypnea. Thus tachypnea without desaturation is often the earliest symptom of ILD, especially in infants. The diffusion impairment, when severe enough, cannot be overcome by increasing minute ventilation, and hypoxemia ensues.

Clinical Presentation

Case Report 26-1

An infant born at 37 weeks had tachypnea, retractions, and hypoxemia in the delivery room. She was treated for respiratory distress syndrome with intratracheal exogenous surfactant. She was extubated after therapy but continued to have tachypnea. A chest radiograph revealed diffuse infiltrates. Evaluation of all systems, including cardiac and gastrointestinal, was negative. She remained tachypneic but hypoxemia resolved, and she was discharged with a referral to a pediatric pulmonologist. A computed tomography (CT) scan of the chest showed ground-glass opacities and mosaic attenuation. Genetic studies for surfactant protein mutations were negative. A lung biopsy showed no evidence of significant inflammation and clusters of bombesin-positive cells in the bronchioles, consistent with neuroendocrine cell hyperplasia of infancy. Supportive therapy was provided.

The symptoms of ILD are variable, nonspecific, and sometimes subtle. Chronic dry cough, tachypnea, dyspnea, retractions, cyanosis, clubbing, and failure to thrive are all common presentations. The onset is insidious in the first year of life for 50% of the patients, making the diagnosis difficult.[1] Most symptoms occur in the first year of life.[4] Respiratory failure in a term or near-term infant who is not responsive to therapies, including mechanical ventilation and extracorporeal membrane oxygenation (ECMO), should raise suspicion of ILD, especially of surfactant protein abnormalities.[11] Pulmonary interstitial glycogenosis, NEHI, SP-B deficiency, SP-C deficiency, and ABCA3 protein deficiency usually present in infancy. Presentation in older children has a wider differential diagnosis, guided by history and clinical presentation. Additional symptoms include exercise intolerance and frequent respiratory infections. Crackles are not always present, wheezing is uncommon (~20%), and failure to thrive is found in up to two-thirds of patients.[4,5] Clubbing can be seen in about one-third of patients, whereas cyanosis is less common.[11] Other physical examination findings, such as joint disease and rashes, may provide clues to a systemic disease such as collagen vascular disease. Chronic dry cough, tachypnea, dyspnea, retractions, cyanosis, clubbing, and failure to thrive are all common presentations in children with ILD.

Diagnosis

One definition of chronic ILD is

- The presence of respiratory symptoms with or without diffuse infiltrates on chest radiograph
- Abnormal pulmonary function tests with evidence of restrictive ventilatory defect with or without impaired gas exchange
- Persistence of any of these findings for more than 3 months[4]

This definition delineates the components of a noninvasive evaluation of a child with presumed ILD. Invasive testing with bronchoscopy and lung biopsy should be performed only after a systematic evaluation with noninvasive tests is non-diagnostic.[12]

A systematic approach to evaluation is essential to the diagnosis to distinguish between primary pediatric ILD and that associated with systemic disease or other conditions, such as aspiration (Box 26-1). Specific tests are performed based on the patient's presentation (eg, respiratory failure at birth vs onset of exercise intolerance and abnormal pulmonary function studies in a school-aged child) and the severity of the respiratory disorder. A thorough medical history and physical examination will often provide clues to an underlying diagnosis. A family history is most likely to be positive in infants because many of the forms of ILD have a genetic basis.[11] In a retrospective analysis, 10% of case siblings were affected by similar diseases,[4] and up to 34% of patients have a family history of lung disease.[5] It is important to also obtain information about exposures, such as to radiation, birds, or toxins. In one report, only 25% of the clinicians' initial diagnoses based on patient history were correct except in cases where a history of a bird exposure led to a diagnosis of hypersensitivity pneumonitis.[1] A thorough review of systems, focusing on joints, skin, kidneys, sinuses, eyes, and nervous system, may raise suspicion of known causes of ILD, such as collagen vascular disease or Goodpasture syndrome (anti-glomerular basement membrane antibody disease).[11]

Box 26-1. Causes of Interstitial Lung Disease (ILD)

Disorders Prevalent in Infancy

Diffuse developmental disorders
- Acinar dysplasia
- Congenital alveolar dysplasia
- Alveolar capillary dysplasia with misalignment of pulmonary veins

Growth abnormalities reflecting deficiency
- Pulmonary hypoplasia
- Chronic neonatal lung disease/bronchopulmonary disease
- Disorders related to chromosomal defects
- Disorders related to congenital heart disease in chromosomally normal children

Specific conditions of undefined cause
- Neuroendocrine cell hyperplasia of infancy (also known as persistent tachypnea of infancy and chronic bronchiolitis)
- Pulmonary interstitial glycogenosis (also known as infantile cellular interstitial pneumonitis or histiocytoid pneumonia)

Surfactant dysfunction
- Surfactant protein B
- Surfactant protein C
- ABCA3 protein
- Congenital granulocyte macrophage colony-stimulating factor (GMCSF) receptor deficiency
- Lysinuric protein intolerance
- Disorders in which histology consistent with surfactant dysfunction disorder without a recognized genetic cause
  - Pulmonary alveolar proteinosis
  - Desquamative interstitial pneumonitis
  - Nonspecific interstitial pneumonia

Box 26-1. Causes of Interstitial Lung Disease (ILD) (continued)

Disorders Related to Systemic Disease Processes

Immune-mediated and collagen vascular disorders

- Disorders with specific pulmonary manifestations
  - Goodpasture syndrome
  - Acquired pulmonary alveolar proteinosis/autoantibody to GMCSF
  - Pulmonary vasculitis syndromes (ie, lupus erythematosus)
- Disorders with nonspecific pulmonary manifestations
  - Nonspecific interstitial pneumonia
  - Pulmonary hemorrhage syndromes
  - Lymphoproliferative disease
  - Organizing pneumonia
  - Nonspecific airway changes, including lymphocytic bronchiolitis, lymphoid hyperplasia, and mild constrictive changes
- Disorders with other manifestations of collagen-vascular disease
  - Storage disease
  - Sarcoidosis
  - Langerhans cell histiocytosis
  - Malignant infiltrates

Disorders of the Normal Host, Presumed Intact Immune System

Infectious or postinfectious processes

- Chronic airway changes with and without preceding history of viral respiratory infection
- Bronchiolitis obliterans/organizing pneumonia, also known as cryptogenic organizing pneumonia

Disorders related to environmental agents

- Hypersensitivity pneumonitis
- Toxic inhalation

Aspiration syndromes

Eosinophilic pneumonia

Acute interstitial pneumonia/Hamman-Rich syndrome/idiopathic diffuse alveolar damage

Nonspecific interstitial pneumonia

Idiopathic pulmonary hemosiderosis (bleeding in the lung)

Box 26-1. Causes of Interstitial Lung Disease (ILD) (continued)

Disorders of the Immunocompromised Host

Opportunistic infections

Related to therapeutic intervention—chemotherapeutic drug and radiation injury

- Chemotherapeutic drug injury
- Radiation injury
- Combined
- Drug hypersensitivity

Related to transplantation and rejection of lung and bone marrow transplantation and rejection syndromes

- Rejection
- Graft versus host disease
- Post-transplant lymphoproliferative disorder

Lymphoid infiltrates related to immune compromise (for non-transplanted patients)

- Nonspecific lymphoproliferation
- With lymphoid hyperplasia
- With poorly formed granulomas
- Malignant

Diffuse alveolar damage, unknown etiology

Disorders Masquerading as ILD

Arterial hypertensive vasculopathy

Congestive changes related to cardiac dysfunction

Veno-oclusive disease

Lymphatic disorders

- Lymphangiectasis
- Lymphangiomatosis

Pulmonary edema

Thromboembolic

ChILD (children with ILD) syndrome is diagnosed with the presence of 3 of the following, in absence of an identified cause: (1) symptoms of impaired respiratory function, (2) hypoxemia, (3) diffuse infiltrates, (4) presence of adventitious breath sounds, and (5) abnormal lung function[13] (Box 26-2).

Laboratory Testing

Laboratory tests to rule out immunodeficiencies, collagen vascular disease, and infectious etiologies can provide clues to the cause of ILD. Hypersensitivity panels to detect serum precipitins to various agents, such as bird antigens, should be considered and are essential if there is a history of a specific exposure. Pulmonary hypertension and congenital heart disease should be assessed with electrocardiography and echocardiography. Reflux and aspiration can be evaluated with a pH probe, barium esophagogram, and videofluoroscopic swallow study. Tests for more common diseases that cause similar symptoms should be considered, such as a sweat test to rule out cystic fibrosis or nasal ciliary biopsy for primary ciliary dyskinesia. Mutations in the genes involved in surfactant processing and production account for many neonatal ILD cases, thus genetic analysis (whole blood samples) for SP-B, SP-C, and *ABCA3* mutations (see below) can provide a diagnosis before more invasive investigations.

Box 26-2. ChILD (Children With Interstitial Lung Disease) Syndrome[14]

Presence of 3 of the following, in absence of an identified cause:

- Symptoms of impaired respiratory function
- Hypoxemia
- Diffuse infiltrates on chest radiograph
- Presence of adventitious breath sounds
- Abnormal lung function

Radiography

Radiographic evaluation of a child with suspected ILD should begin with a chest radiograph. Although 10% of chest radiographs in adults with ILD can be normal, chest radiographs are usually abnormal in children with ILD.[1,14] The chest radiograph of a child with ILD (Figure 26-1) reveals diffuse pulmonary infiltrates or specific patterns described as reticular, nodular, ground glass, or honeycombing.

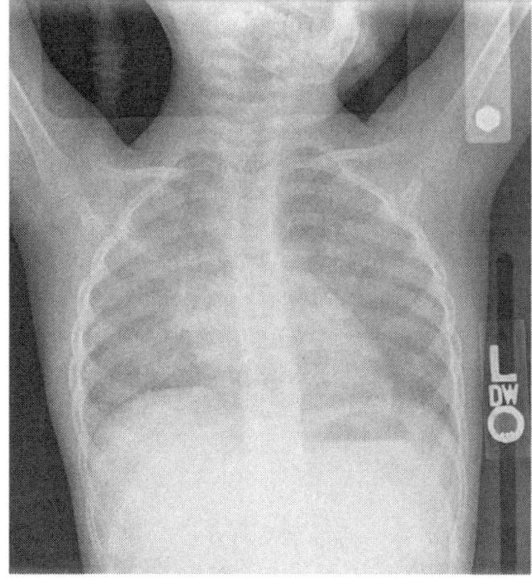

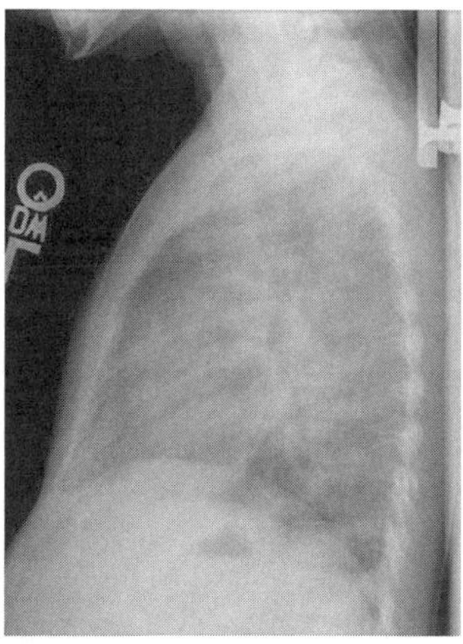

A

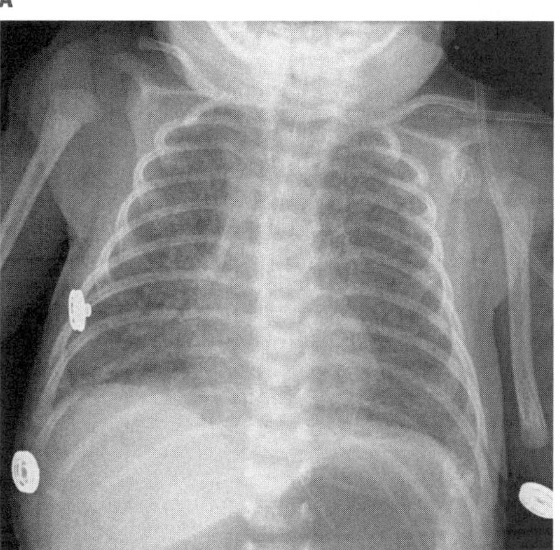

B

Figure 26-1. Chest radiograph. **A.** Bilateral interstitial and hazy alveolar opacities greater on the right than the left— patient with juvenile rheumatoid arthritis and biopsy diagnosed follicular bronchiolitis. **B.** Coarse infiltrates throughout both lungs, with hyperinflation— patient with genetic abnormality in *ABCA3* gene.

To further delineate parenchymal abnormalities, a high-resolution chest CT (HRCT) scan should be obtained (Figure 26-2). High-resolution chest CT scans can help evaluate the parenchyma of these children

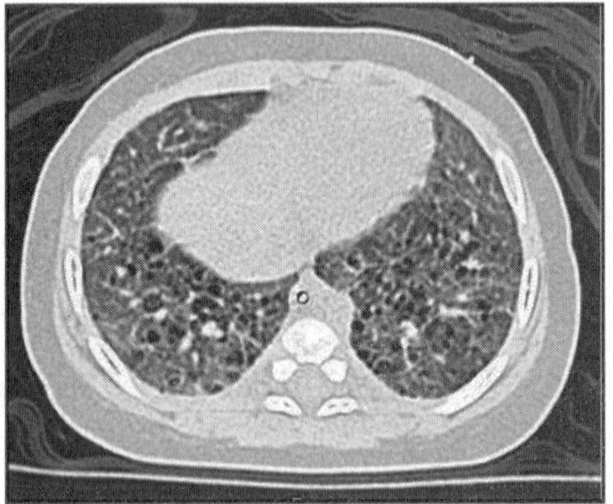

A

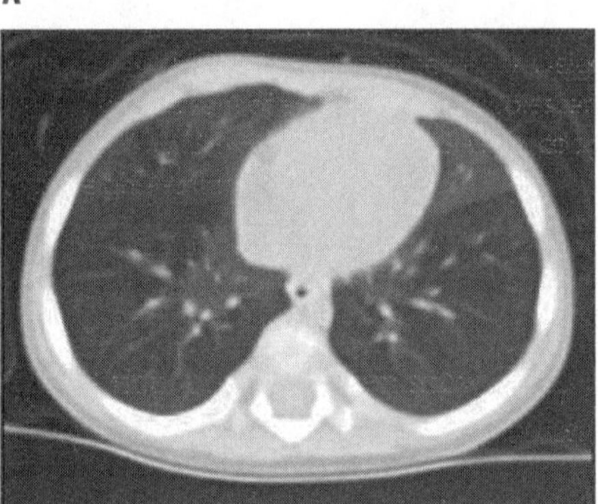

B

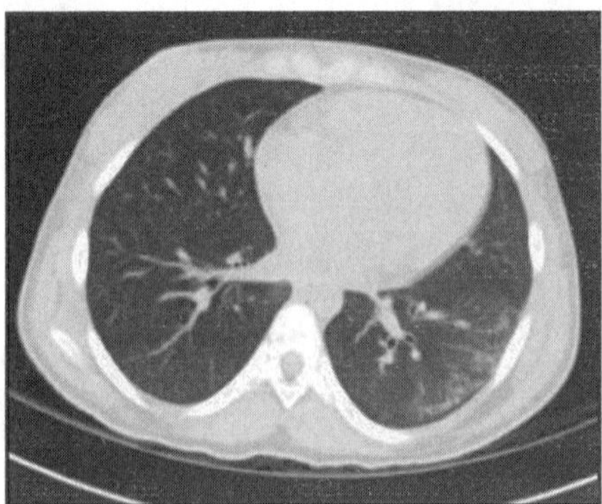

C

Figure 26-2. High-resolution computed tomography scan. **A.** Extensive diffuse ground-glass alveolar filling, with associated increased interstitial lung thickening. There are also multiple small- to moderate-sized cysts present within both lungs. **B.** Mosaic pattern with areas of denserand of more lucent lung in all lobes—patient found to have abnormality in *ABCA3* gene. **C.** Peripheral intralobular interstitial and interlobular septal thickening—patient with juvenile dermatomyositis

and help the surgeon determine the optimal site for biopsy. In adults and older children, patients perform a voluntary breath hold at full inspiration and expiration during the radiograph. However, infants and young children cannot cooperate with breathholding because respiratory motion produces motion artifacts that limit the quality of the imaging study.[15] The alternative is to use anesthesia with intubation to obtain acceptable images. Long and colleagues have developed a method that uses sedation combined with controlled ventilation, as used in infant pulmonary function tests, to provide a controlled pause in respiration.[15] During this procedure, hyperventilation of a child with a face mask produces a respiratory pause that is long enough (6–12 seconds) to scan the entire lung. Images can thus be obtained at full inspiration at 25 cm H_2O and at full expiration at 0 cm H_2O. It is very important to obtain high-quality scans, such as controlled ventilation HRCT, as there are cases of false-positives found with conventional scans.[15] Specific patterns on HRCT can be diagnostic. In a review of 20 children with ILD proven by biopsy, 56% of the confident first-choice diagnoses from HRCT were correct.[3,15]

Pulmonary Function Tests

Pulmonary function tests are sometimes able to identify functional patterns that aid in distinguishing different disorders and correlate with radiography and histologic findings.[3] Pulse oximetry and blood gas analysis are important to determine degree of hypoxia. Most patients will be normoxic, but may desaturate with sleep or exercise.[3] Exercise tolerance studies or evaluation of 6-minute walk distance may be of clinical utility. Spirometry will reveal a pattern of restrictive lung disease, with decreased lung volumes sometimes with an obstructive component of air trapping.[3] Diffusion capacity will be low, although may normalize when corrected for alveolar volume.[3]

Infant pulmonary function testing (iPFT) provides a physiological assessment and aids in diagnosis in some patients. Spirometry and plethysmography can now be obtained for infants at many major medical centers. Several reports show that iPFTs can distinguish disease, can correlate with radiographic and histologic findings, and can be used for assessment of therapy.[3,16] The utility of using iPFTs to aid in the diagnosis of ILD in infants is limited by the inability to perform this test routinely on patients who require ventilatory support and the limited number of centers that perform the test. To better classify the characteristics of the various forms of ILD, more iPFT data need to be obtained.

Bronchoalveolar Lavage

Pathologic evaluation with bronchoalveolar lavage (BAL) and lung biopsy is important to determine the diagnosis of ILD. The entire aspirate is recovered and sent for cell count, infectious studies (microbiology and polymerase chain reaction–based assays), and lipid and hemosiderin stains, which indicate processes such as infection, aspiration, and hemorrhage. In a prospective series of ILD cases, a specific diagnosis was made from the BAL in 17% of cases.[17] When evaluated retrospectively, the diagnosis was made in 30% of patients. One limitation of BAL in children is that techniques may be inconsistent,[14] and normal values from significant numbers of healthy children have not been established. While the usefulness of BAL is limited, it should be considered before obtaining a lung biopsy because BAL is less invasive. Bronchoalveolar lavage can also determine specific diagnosis in alveolar proteinosis, lysosomal storage disorders, and histiocytosis.[3]

Lung Biopsy

Lung biopsy is the gold standard in the diagnosis of ILD. Biopsy via video-assisted thoracoscopic surgery has become the standard approach, even in small infants, thereby dramatically reducing the morbidity associated with open thoracotomy.[7] A transthoracic procedure has a shorter operating time, a lower incidence of chest tube placement, and a short hospitalization,[18] although it requires a surgeon who is familiar with the technique. Current recommendations are to obtain biopsies from more than one lobe, including one area that is clearly affected and one area that is newly evolving or with an unaffected appearance on CT scan. In a review of a small series of cases, there was no increase in complications when more than one lobe was biopsied.[18] Once the specimen has been obtained, proper processing of the tissue is critical for a comprehensive diagnostic evaluation. Tissue should be obtained for culture, light microscopy, immunohistochemistry (for surfactant proteins), and electron microscopy. Stains that are useful include hematoxylin and eosin, trichrome, pentachrome, and periodic acid-Schiff with diastase.[19] Other immunostains, such as bombesin in NEHI and vimentin in PIG, have been described as diagnostic aids for specific causes of ILD. Electron microscopy shows distinctive type II cell abnormalities in specific surfactant gene mutations.[20] Other characteristic ultrastructural findings may indicate the presence of a metabolic disorder or PIG.[8]

Specific Diseases in Infancy

It is not possible to discuss all forms of ILD; however, a brief discussion of the newer entities of ILD, especially those with a presentation in infancy, is discussed here.

Surfactant is a mixture of proteins and phospholipids that prevent atelectasis at end expiration. Both SP-B and SP-C are important in lowering the surface tension in the alveoli.[21] The ABCA3 protein is believed to play a role in surfactant processing and transport within the alveolar type II cell.[7] Mutations in all 3 of these components can lead to ILD.

Surfactant protein B deficiency is a rare disorder, with clinical estimates of 1 per million live births.[21] These infants typically present within the first few hours of life with respiratory failure. The neonates are clinically similar to infants with respiratory distress syndrome (RDS), except that they are born at term and the RDS does not resolve. The only treatment for these patients is lung transplantation, without which the disease is fatal.[21]

Surfactant protein C deficiency has a variable presentation, and the onset of symptoms often occurs in term neonates who present with clinical symptoms similar to RDS but can be later in childhood and even in adulthood, when presentation is typical for later-onset ILD. Treatment is supportive, and many general ILD treatments have been used. Outcomes cover a wide spectrum, with some children going to lung transplantation and others improving enough over time that they no longer require supplemental oxygen.[21]

A deficiency of ABCA3 protein also has a varied presentation and clinical outcome. Similar to SP-B and SP-C deficiency, it can present in the newborn period with a clinical picture of RDS in a term infant. Infants can also present later with findings typical of ILD. Treatment is generally supportive. Outcome ranges from fatal in the newborn period to survival until adulthood.[7] Reports of children who have a milder course have led to the conclusion that some ABCA3 protein variants may lead to a milder course with prolonged survival.[7]

Pulmonary interstitial glycogenosis is a form of ILD that also presents in the neonatal period, and has been described in both term and preterm infants. The infants are typically tachypneic and hypoxic, and have crackles. Significantly they have hyperinflation on radiographic evaluation. It is postulated that this illness is due to a developmental disorder of pulmonary mesenchyme cells, not an inflammatory or reactive process. Experts believe this is the same entity as cellular interstitial pneumonitis of infants. Long-term outcome is quite favorable in most patients.[8]

Neuroendocrine cell hyperplasia of infancy was referred to as persistent tachypnea of infancy before the characteristic histopathology was described. Children with NEHI have an onset of symptoms usually in the first year of life, but sometimes later. They have persistent tachypnea, hypoxia, and crackles. Radiographic evaluation reveals hyperexpansion of the lungs. Treatment is mainly supportive. The duration of supplemental oxygen therapy may be several years, and most children improve slowly. This form of ILD has a favorable outcome with no associated mortality.[9]

Management

Treatment for ILD is limited. There is a significant mortality rate of 15%, determined from a retrospective review of 99 cases and a probability of survival of 83%, 72%, and 64% at 2, 3, and 4 years, respectively.[22]

The mainstay of treatment is supportive, specifically with oxygen. Most children have difficulty with diffusion of oxygen across the alveolar-capillary barrier and become tachypneic to maintain oxygen saturations. Administration of oxygen leads to less tachypnea. If the underlying disease is known, then treatment toward the specific cause should help the lung disease. Additional therapeutic recommendations include maintaining adequate nutrition, treatment of underlying gastroesophageal reflux or aspiration during feeding, immunizing against respiratory pathogens, aggressive treatment of intercurrent illnesses, and avoidance of environmental tobacco smoke and other pollutants.[10]

Beyond supportive care and disease-specific treatment, many modalities have been tried. Treatment effect can be judged by decreases in cough and dyspnea, and improvements in pulmonary function tests and saturation; however, radiographic changes do not occur quickly enough to follow frequently.[4] Immunomodulating agents have been reported as therapeutic agents for ILD, especially corticosteroids, which have a highly variable response. Various treatment regimens have been used, ranging from daily oral doses to monthly intravenous pulses of steroids. The optimal dose, frequency, and duration of therapy, as well as when to initiate or discontinue therapy and the relative harm compared with side effects, still remains unclear.[10] Hydroxychloroquine therapy has been successful in the treatment of some cases, but the clinical response is highly variable. Other steroid sparing agents have been tried, such as azathioprine, cyclophosphamide, methotrexate, cyclosporine, and IVIG.[3] Importantly, many of the reports of treatment are from case series that predate the current histologic classification of pediatric ILD.

Lung transplantation is an option for progressive ILD with respiratory failure. While the average survival rate for pediatric lung transplant recipients is about 4.5 years,[23] some children survive much longer. Complications from lung transplantation are common, with bronchiolitis obliterans being the most common but also including hypertension, renal dysfunction, diabetes mellitus, and hyperlipidemia. (See Chapter 33.) Infants who receive lung transplants for SP-B deficiency have similar outcomes to those infants who receive transplants for other reasons.[24] There are some anecdotal reports of recurrence of ILD in the transplanted lung.[10]

Close attention to growth parameters is important since failure to thrive is a common complication of ILD. Many children with ILD have increased calorie needs because of tachypnea and inflammation, and thus require close monitoring and, sometimes, interventions. In some cases, addition of supplemental oxygen will reduce tachypnea and improve weight gain, but many children need high-calorie formulas or supplemental feeding to augment caloric intake. Evaluation for supplemental enteral feeding via nasogastric or gastrostomy tube should be considered in addition to evaluation for other causes of failure to thrive, including aspiration and gastroesophageal reflux. Infants and children with ILD are at risk for respiratory decompensation caused by viral respiratory infections. Many will have limited respiratory reserve and will require hospitalization for monitoring, hydration, and management of supplemental oxygen during such illnesses. Some, especially those with more severe forms of ILD, may require mechanical ventilation. Good communication between the primary care provider and the pulmonologist provides optimal care.

Prognosis

Prognosis based on clinical symptoms at initial evaluation can be determined using the severity of illness classification. The score includes the following elements: presence of symptoms or not; saturations at rest, asleep, or with activity; and evidence of pulmonary hypertension. The higher the score, the higher the probability of decreased survival with each increase in score, increasing the risk of death by an estimated 140%.[3,22] Weight below fifth percentile for age, crackles, clubbing, family history of ILD, and symptom duration at initial evaluation did not influence survival.[11]

The outcome of a child with ILD depends on the disease that causes the ILD. The higher the severity of illness based on symptoms at initial presentation, the higher the probability of mortality.[3] Presence of pulmonary hypertension is the greatest predictor of mortality.[5] In a retrospective study of children younger than 2 years, only 30.2% died and 50% had ongoing pulmonary symptoms at follow-up; however, certain diseases, such as PIG and NEHI, had no mortality while children with diffuse developmental disorders of the lung had 100% mortality.[5] It is important to have an accurate diagnosis before prognosis is discussed with the family.

When to Refer

When to refer to a pulmonologist

- Hypoxia and tachypnea of unknown cause
- Radiographic findings of pulmonary ground-glass opacities
- Clubbing
- Chronic dry cough, tachypnea, dyspnea, retractions, cyanosis, clubbing, and failure to thrive in some combination
- Unexplained failure to thrive (found in two-thirds of children with ILD)[4,5]
- Unexplained exercise intolerance or frequent respiratory infections (Crackles may or may not be present.)

When to Admit

- Upper respiratory infection in a child with known ILD, especially with increasing hypoxia
- Prompt evaluation for any change in the patient's baseline respiratory health, such as increased tachypnea or dyspnea or a reduction from baseline oxyhemoglobin saturation

Key Points

- Interstitial lung disease is a rare, heterogeneous group of disorders, mainly pulmonary, and characterized by diffuse pulmonary disease with disordered gas exchange.
- Interstitial lung disease is any entity that results in derangement of the alveolar capillary interface often characterized clinically with tachypnea, crackles, hypoxia, or diffuse infiltrates.
- Diagnosis is one of exclusion of known causes. Lung biopsy is the gold standard.
- Treatment may include supportive therapy with oxygen supplementation, immunomodulating agents, or lung transplant depending on the severity of the symptoms.
- Close monitoring of nutritional status, with appropriate intervention, is important.
- Outcomes vary widely depending on the specific diagnosis, but are not uniformly fatal.

References

1. Fan LL, Langston C. Chronic interstitial lung disease in children. *Pediatr Pulmonol.* 1993;16(3):184–196
2. Dinwiddie R, Sharief N, Crawford O. Idiopathic interstitial pneumonitis in children: a national survey in the United Kingdom and Ireland. *Pediatr Pulmonol.* 2002;34(1):23–29
3. Fan LL, Deterding RR, Langston C. Pediatric interstitial lung disease revisited. *Pediatr Pulmonol.* 2004;38(5):369–378
4. Clement A. Task force on chronic interstitial lung disease in immunocompetent children. *Eur Respir J.* 2004;24(4):686–697
5. Deutsch GH, Young LR, Deterding RR, et al. Diffuse lung disease in young children: application of a novel classification scheme. *Am J Respir Crit Care Med.* 2007;176(11):1120–1128
6. Nogee LM, Dunbar AE III, Wert S, Askin F, Hamvas A, Whitsett JA. Mutations in the surfactant protein C gene associated with interstitial lung disease. *Chest.* 2002;121(3 suppl):20S–21S
7. Prestridge A, Wooldridge J, Deutsch G, et al. Persistent tachypnea and hypoxia in a 3-month-old term infant. *J Pediatr.* 2006;149(5):702–706
8. Canakis AM, Cutz E, Manson D, O'Brodovich H. Pulmonary interstitial glycogenosis: a new variant of neonatal interstitial lung disease. *Am J Respir Crit Care Med.* 2002;165(11):1557–1565

9. Deterding RR, Pye C, Fan LL, Langston C. Persistent tachypnea of infancy is associated with neuroendocrine cell hyperplasia. *Pediatr Pulmonol.* 2005;40(2):157–165
10. Clement A, Eber E. Interstitial lung diseases in infants and children. *Eur Respir J.* 2008;31(3):658–666
11. Fauroux B, Epaud R, Clement A. Clinical presentation of interstitial lung disease in children. *Paediatr Respir Rev.* 2004;5(2):98–100
12. Fan LL, Kozinetz CA, Deterding RR, Brugman SM. Evaluation of a diagnostic approach to pediatric interstitial lung disease. *Pediatrics.* 1998;101(1 pt 1):82–85
13. Deterding R, Fan LL. Surfactant dysfunction mutations in children's interstitial lung disease and beyond. *Am J Respir Crit Care Med.* 2005;172(8):940–941
14. Fan LL, Mullen AL, Brugman SM, Inscore SC, Parks DP, White CW. Clinical spectrum of chronic interstitial lung disease in children. *J Pediatr.* 1992;121(6):867–872
15. Brody AS. Imaging considerations: interstitial lung disease in children. *Radiol Clin North Am.* 2005;43(2):391–403
16. Kerby GW, SL, Heltshe SL, Accurso FJ, Deterding RR. Infant pulmonary function in pediatric interstitial lung disease. *Am J Respir Crit Care Med.* 2005;2:A474
17. Fan LL, Lung MC, Wagener JS. The diagnostic value of bronchoalveolar lavage in immunocompetent children with chronic diffuse pulmonary infiltrates. *Pediatr Pulmonol.* 1997;23(1):8–13
18. Fan LL, Kozinetz CA, Wojtczak HA, Chatfield BA, Cohen AH, Rothenberg SS. Diagnostic value of transbronchial, thoracoscopic, and open lung biopsy in immunocompetent children with chronic interstitial lung disease. *J Pediatr.* 1997;131(4):565–569
19. Langston C, Patterson K, Dishop MK, et al. A protocol for the handling of tissue obtained by operative lung biopsy: recommendations of the chILD pathology co-operative group. *Pediatr Dev Pathol.* 2006;9(3):173–180
20. Edwards V, Cutz E, Viero S, Moore AM, Nogee L. Ultrastructure of lamellar bodies in congenital surfactant deficiency. *Ultrastruct Pathol.* 2005;29(6):503–509
21. Hamvas A. Inherited surfactant protein-B deficiency and surfactant protein-C associated disease: clinical features and evaluation. *Semin Perinatol.* 2006;30(6):316–326
22. Fan LL, Kozinetz CA. Factors influencing survival in children with chronic interstitial lung disease. *Am J Respir Crit Care Med.* 1997;156(3 pt 1):939–942
23. Schecter MG, Elidemir O, Heinle JS, McKenzie ED, Mallory GB Jr. Pediatric lung transplantation: a therapy in its adolescence. *Semin Thorac Cardiovasc Surg Pediatr Card Surg Annu.* 2008:74–79
24. Palomar LM, Nogee LM, Sweet SC, Huddleston CB, Cole FS, Hamvas A. Long-term outcomes after infant lung transplantation for surfactant protein B deficiency related to other causes of respiratory failure. *J Pediatr.* 2006;149(4):548–553

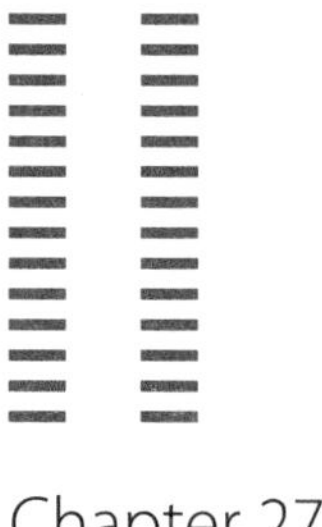

Chapter 27

Bronchopulmonary Dysplasia

Molly K. Ball, MD
Susanna A. McColley, MD

Introduction

Neonatal positive pressure ventilation (PPV), invented in the 1960s, dramatically increased the survival of preterm infants. However, infants who were mechanically ventilated developed bronchopulmonary dysplasia (BPD), a severe chronic lung disease of prematurity.[1] Initially, affected infants were those born between 30 to 34 weeks' gestation and treated with high-pressure ventilation and aggressive oxygen therapy.

Advances in the field of neonatology have led to further decreases in preterm mortality and permit the survival of increasingly premature neonates. These advances include regionalization of perinatal care, research and technology in neonatal critical care and ventilator techniques, antenatal steroid administration, and postnatal surfactant therapy. These combined interventions minimize significant lung injury in the late preterm population and allow the survival of increasingly premature infants.

Despite significant advances in perinatal and neonatal medicine, lung disease remains a major cause of morbidity and mortality in premature infants requiring mechanical ventilation.[2] Classically BPD was a disease of late preterm infants. Currently BPD is a chronic lung disease of extreme prematurity and lung immaturity. While the incidence of BPD in late preterm infants has decreased over the last 10 years, it has remained stable in the more premature population and affects more than 10,000 infants annually. Recent epidemiological studies report a 33% incidence of BPD in neonates with birth weights less than 1,000 g and an up to 46% incidence of birth weight less than 750 g,[3] although significant interhospital variability exists (reported incidences as high as 60%).[4] Disease mortality is estimated to be 10% to 20% within the first year.[2,4]

Infants most at risk for developing BPD are those who are premature, have low birth weight, and undergo prolonged mechanical ventilation. Data suggest neonates born at less than 26 weeks' gestation or with birth weights less than 1,100 g are at highest risk. Male sex, high initial inspired oxygen concentrations, and the need for multiple surfactant doses further increase the likelihood of developing BPD.[5] Infants with BPD, in addition to being affected by chronic respiratory disease, also experience multisystem comorbidities complicating their management. Furthermore, substantial evidence suggests poorer neurodevelopmental outcomes are associated with infants with BPD compared with infants born at the same gestational age who do not develop BPD.

Pathophysiology

Preterm lungs are highly susceptible to injury. In addition to being structurally and functionally immature, the preterm lung is deficient in surfactant production, and the chest wall is highly compliant and thus unable to provide resistance against overexpansion. This immaturity, coupled with the need for mechanical ventilation, supplemental oxygen therapy, and the resultant lung inflammatory response, initiates pulmonary developmental arrest with disordered lung repair.[6,7]

Much of what we understand about the pathogenesis of BPD comes from animal models, which permit controlled experimental settings for both physiological and histopathologic evaluation to identify mechanisms of lung injury. The currently accepted theory is that normal lung development, occurring via alveolarization, septation, and vascular capillary network formation, arrests and is replaced by premature maturation with maladaptive airway and vascular development.[8,9] Preterm animals with BPD demonstrate interrupted alveolarization, increased intra-airway inflammation, abnormal elastin distribution, and altered pulmonary vascular development with capillary hypoplasia.[7,10]

Ventilator-induced lung injury represents a significant causative factor in the development of BPD. Two specific injury mechanisms have been identified: volutrauma and atelectatrauma.[6] Volutrauma is a lung stretch injury resulting from localized overdistension. This occurs when preterm lungs, which exhibit heterogeneous compliance, are exposed to large tidal volumes, producing segmental overdistension with resultant stretch injury to airways and alveoli.[6,11,12] Atelectatrauma is a lung injury caused by alveolar collapse at end-expiration, seen in the setting of surfactant deficiency. This collapse results in alveolar de-recruitment and loss of functional residual volume, and is injurious to developing lungs.[6]

Oxygen therapy, while necessary in the treatment of chronic lung disease for tissue oxygen delivery, also induces lung injury. Oxygen-induced lung injury is mediated by reactive oxidant species, which cause damage to developing tissues through mechanisms including the inhibition of protein synthesis and surfactant formation. Because antioxidant activity largely develops at the end of gestation, premature lungs are uniquely vulnerable to free radical oxidant damage.[13] In preterm animals, hyperoxia exposure results in abnormal lung alveolarization independent of mechanical ventilation.[10] Infants receiving higher supplemental oxygen concentrations more often develop pneumonia and chronic lung disease, and more frequently require medical therapy for BPD.[14]

A third significant causative factor in BPD is an inflammatory response to lung injury leading to chronic pulmonary inflammation. Following the initiation of mechanical ventilation, inflammatory mediators, including inflammatory cells and pro-inflammatory cytokines, are increased in airways.[12] This lung inflammatory response is not transient, but rather persists as a marker of ongoing lung injury.[6–8] Animal studies have demonstrated that airway inflammation interferes with normal alveolar development.[15]

Further contributing to the issue of inflammatory response, chorioamnionitis before delivery and chronic colonization of the airway with *Ureaplasma* are both correlated with increased incidence of BPD.[15,16] Because chorioamnionitis is a major predisposing factor for preterm delivery, a significant number of fetuses are exposed in utero to pathogens that challenge their immature immune responses and initiate inflammatory cascades. While active research exists, the mechanistic link between prenatal exposure, lung inflammation, and bronchopulmonary dysplasia is not well understood.[15]

Multiple extrapulmonary factors exacerbate illness and are believed to contribute to the pathogenesis of BPD. Infection results in an increased disease risk. In addition to the inflammatory effects of prenatal exposures, postnatal infections may further amplify observed inflammatory responses.[17] The prolonged need for endotracheal tubes and indwelling lines in the very premature population increases the risk for recurrent infections. Poor nutrition with inadequate protein and caloric intake, variable fluid balance status, and increased pulmonary blood flow secondary to patent ductus arteriosus (PDA) are each believed to contribute to the development of BPD.[6,17]

Clinical Features

Historically, BPD was defined as the persistent need for supplemental oxygen at day of life 28. Current definitions improve diagnostic criteria and physiological classification, and incorporate historic criteria with gestational age stratification and severity categorization (Table 27-1).[8] Bronchopulmonary dysplasia is characterized by lung injury changes distinct from those originally described (Box 27-1). While classic BPD was characterized by fibrosis, hyperplasia, and alternating atelectasis/

Table 27-1. Diagnostic Criteria for New Bronchopulmonary Dysplasia[a]

Definition	Severity Classification	Gestational Age at Delivery	
		<32 Weeks	≥32 Weeks
Supplemental oxygen >21% for at least 28 days plus	**Mild**	Room air by 36 weeks' postnatal age or discharge to home, whichever comes first	Room air by 56 days' postnatal age or discharge to home, whichever comes first
	Moderate	Inspired oxygen 30% at 36 weeks' postnatal age or discharge to home, whichever comes first	Inspired oxygen 30% at 56 days' postnatal age or discharge to home, whichever comes first
	Severe	Inspired oxygen ≥30% or PPV/CPAP at 36 weeks' postnatal age or discharge to home, whichever comes first	Inspired oxygen ≥30% or PPV/CPAP at 56 days' postnatal age or discharge to home, whichever comes first

Abbreviations: CPAP, continuous positive airway pressure; PPV, positive pressure ventilation.

[a]Modified from Jobe AH, Bancalari E. Bronchopulmonary dysplasia. From NICHD/NHLBI/ORD Workshop Summary. *Am J Respir Crit Care Med.* 2001;163:1723–1729. Copyright © American Thoracic Society. Reprinted by permission.

Box 27-1. Pathophysiological Characteristics of Bronchopulmonary Dysplasia

- Increased lung fluid
- Diffuse airway inflammation
- Decreased alveolarization
- Altered pulmonary vascular development
- Minimal fibrosis
- Airway hyperreactivity

overinflation, currently described BPD exhibits more uniform inflammation and less fibrosis and smooth muscle hypertrophy. Key pathologic changes now seen are increased lung fluid; diffuse inflammatory infiltration; markedly fewer, larger alveoli from decreased alveolar septation; and altered vascular development with capillary hypoplasia.[8,18] Clinically, infants who develop BPD are extremely premature with low birth weight. They have respiratory distress syndrome treated with surfactant therapy, but often require only minimal initial ventilatory support and oxygen supplementation. However, these neonates develop increasing ventilator and oxygen requirements with the progression of respiratory disease. Chest radiographs may show diffuse haziness with segmental atelectasis.[18] In addition to hypoxia and chronic respiratory distress, these infants exhibit increased airway hyperreactivity as well as increased susceptibility to recurrent pulmonary infections.

Management

Prenatal

The current management of BPD has 2 major goals: disease prevention and symptomatic therapy. Management, therefore, begins in the prenatal period. At this stage efforts are focused on decreasing risks for premature delivery. Key interventions include maternal monitoring, interventions to decrease infection and preterm labor and delivery, and maximizing fetal growth and nutrition. The development of chorioamnionitis in the fetal period is highly associated with preterm delivery and is believed to be an independent contributing factor in BPD development.[15] If preterm delivery is anticipated, maternal steroids should be administered. Two regimens are currently accepted: betamethasone or dexamethasone, with current practice largely institutionally dependent.

Delivery Room and Neonatal Intensive Care Unit

At delivery, the fetus begins the transition from fetal to neonatal life and experiences significant changes in cardiorespiratory physiology. Most extremely preterm infants will undergo intubation in the delivery room for initiation of PPV; gentle ventilation should be established even during resuscitation.[6,12] In this setting, ventilation can be highly variable with the potential for large tidal volumes and expiratory collapse without readily available monitoring devices. Chest wall expansion is used as a measure of tidal volume; excessive expansion should be avoided to minimize lung stretch injury. Surfactant should be administered early, ideally before lung injury occurs. Surfactant improves lung compliance and uniformity of lung expansion, permits lower oxygen supplementation and ventilatory support, and protects against volutrauma in animal models.[11]

Mechanical Ventilation

The goal of ventilatory assistance should be to provide adequate gas exchange while minimizing lung injury. As discussed previously, ventilation should avoid both volutrauma and atelectatrauma. Current research supports a ventilation strategy that includes positive end-expiratory pressure to maintain lung recruitment and low tidal volume to achieve inflation but avoid overdistension.[6,11,12] Clinically, chest radiographs represent a noninvasive tool to assist in optimizing inflation. In addition to conventional mechanical ventilation, continuous positive airway pressure (CPAP), bubble CPAP, and high-frequency oscillatory or jet ventilation have been proposed as alternate methods with physiological benefit over conventional ventilation. In studies to date, however, no single ventilatory mode or strategy has proven superior in decreasing BPD incidence.[9,19] Permissive hypercapnia is a strategy used to minimize ventilatory settings and reduce the duration of mechanical ventilation. While research has shown mildly increased carbon dioxide levels to be safe in the developing preterm infant, studies have not demonstrated a clear outcome benefit.[20]

Drugs/Therapies

Supplemental oxygen represents both a treatment for and cause of lung disease in newborns. Therefore, management should focus on the avoidance of excessive supplementation to limit hyperoxia and free radical injury. Oxygen supplementation may be required throughout hospitalization and continued following discharge. While it is generally agreed that goal saturation limits for premature infants should be lower than for term infants, no universally accepted standards exist.

Diuretic therapy with the loop diuretic furosemide or thiazide hydrochlorothiazide is a long-standing medical treatment for established chronic lung disease that targets increased lung fluid. Diuretics decrease pulmonary edema and improve pulmonary compliance and gas exchange.[21] However, adverse effects include electrolyte imbalances, osteopenia, and nephrocalcinosis. While studies have shown symptomatic improvement, evidence to date fails to convincingly report long-term improvement and thus does not support their routine use.[21]

Systemic corticosteroids have been widely used as a treatment modality to decrease the chronic inflammation observed with BPD. Classically, high-dose dexamethasone was given in variable doses and duration for either the prevention or treatment of chronic lung disease. However, this therapy is associated with significant adverse effects, including hypertension, hyperglycemia, adrenocortical axis suppression, poor weight gain, gastrointestinal perforation and, more recently, adverse neurodevelopmental outcome.[8,22] Due to the severity of potential side effects and long-term developmental concerns, their routine use in extremely preterm infants is not recommended. The American Academy of Pediatrics (AAP) supports the use of postnatal high-dose systemic corticosteroids for extremely premature infants only in the setting of randomized controlled trials.[23]

Inhaled bronchodilators are commonly used to combat increased airway resistance and hyperreactivity. Medications including albuterol and ipratroprium are administered for bronchodilation in the setting of acute bronchospasm. While these medications can produce acute symptomatic improvement, their use does not affect long-term pulmonary outcomes.[24]

More recently, both vitamin A and caffeine have proven protective against the development of BPD. Vitamin A is essential for normal growth and maintenance of respiratory tract epithelium,[25] and its supplementation over the first month of life is associated with decreased BPD incidence.[26] Caffeine is a methylxanthine typically used for the treatment of prematurity-related apnea. Its use in extremely premature neonates during the first month of life also resulted in decreased BPD.[27]

Additional therapies have targeted the observed oxidant/antioxidant imbalance attributed to oxygen supplementation. Active research exists in this area, and preliminary clinical trials evaluating the antioxidant superoxide dismutase have been promising.[4]

Nitric oxide represents an emerging therapy for the prevention and treatment of BPD beyond its established use for pulmonary hypertension. Nitric oxide is released by vascular endothelium and functions to decrease pulmonary vascular tone. Therapeutically it is administered via continuous inhalation to induce pulmonary vasodilatation and improve ventilation/perfusion mismatch. Studies have shown improved oxygenation and pulmonary blood flow with decreased pulmonary artery pressure and airway inflammation,[5,28] yet have yielded conflicting results regarding both safety and efficacy.[5,28,29]

Additional Management

Excessive fluid administration should be avoided, particularly in the early postnatal period. Infants with less initial weight loss, attributable to fluid status, are at increased risk for lung disease.[17] Serial monitoring for the presence of a PDA should be performed and cardiac echocardiogram obtained if clinically indicated. Increased pulmonary vascular flow due to left-to-right shunting across a patent ductus has been implicated in the pathogenesis of BPD.[17] Efforts should be made to minimize nosocomial infection through hygiene practices, routine skin care, and limiting invasive procedures. Nutritional maximization plays an essential role in neonatal growth and development, and early undernutrition is linked with increased BPD. Early aggressive protein and calorie administration improves pulmonary outcomes.[25] Studies evaluating the beneficial pulmonary effects of intralipid supplementation, however, remain controversial.[8,25] Serial measurements of weight and growth parameters should be followed to monitor nutritional status.

Comorbidities

Infants with BPD experience numerous comorbidities, further challenging their management. Growth failure remains a significant concern in infants with BPD who demonstrate increased metabolic expenditure.[25] Caloric requirements may exceed 150 kcal/kg/day to achieve sustained growth.[25] Prolonged mechanical ventilation and enteral gavage feedings may result in oral aversion, making the transition to oral feeding difficult. Such infants require prolonged feeding by nasogastric tube while oromotor skills improve. In more severe cases, gastrostomy tube placement for gastric feeds may be required. Speech and occupational therapists should be involved as early as medically possible. Gastroesophageal reflux disease is a not uncommon problem that further contributes to the difficulty of maximizing nutritional status and may complicate chronic lung disease through increased risk of pulmonary aspiration and bronchospasm.[25] Symptomatic infants may benefit from medications to reduce gastric acidity or improve gastric motility. For severely affected infants, Nissen fundoplication with gastrostomy tube placement remains a surgical option.

Pulmonary hypertension most often develops in the setting of severe lung disease and is associated with significant increases in morbidity and mortality due to development of cor pulmonale. One study estimated a 2-year survival of only 50% for infants with BPD and pulmonary hypertension.[30] The abnormalities in pulmonary vascular development seen in BPD likely contribute to the development of pulmonary artery hypertension.[28,30] Currently electrocardiography and echocardiography are used to indirectly evaluate pulmonary artery and right ventricular pressures and are accepted noninvasive methods for the diagnosis and monitoring of pulmonary hypertension. Cardiac catheterization exists as an additional diagnostic modality, typically reserved for more severe disease. Catheterization permits evaluation for concomitant anatomical lesions and pulmonary vein stenosis or occlusion, as well as assessment of pulmonary hypertension and reactivity to oxygen or vasodilator therapy.[31] However, no universal screening guidelines exist. Treatment options for pulmonary hypertension include prolonged supplemental oxygen and inhaled nitric oxide; research for novel therapies is ongoing.

A second, often underappreciated, cardiovascular sequela of BPD is systemic hypertension with the potential for development of left ventricular hypertrophy. Blood pressure elevations may be severe enough to require long-term pharmacologic treatment.[31] The mechanisms involved in the development of systemic hypertension are not fully understood.

Perhaps the most concerning association is that of decreased functional and neurologic outcomes observed in BPD survivors. Infants with BPD display an increased prevalence of cerebral palsy and developmental delay, as well as poorer neurodevelopmental outcomes, which persist through school age.[32,33]

Post-Discharge

Lengthy hospital courses are expected for all infants born prematurely; lung disease only serves to increase the length of hospitalization. The transition to home can be a stressful adjustment for families and caregivers who must assume complete care of a medically complex child. Neonatal intensive care unit follow-up clinics or pediatric pulmonary clinics are well equipped to assist in tailoring therapeutic interventions and screening for pulmonary hypertension. Such clinics can also oversee and facilitate the multi-subspecialty involvement necessary for optimal care. Frequent pediatrician follow-up should be performed to monitor growth, weight gain, and developmental gains. Referral for speech, occupational, or developmental therapy evaluation should be made early if concerns are identified. In addition, blood pressure monitoring should be performed for infants with moderate to severe BPD at each outpatient visit.[31]

In cases of severe BPD, infants may remain dependent on respiratory support. Both oxygen therapy (see Chapter 51) and tracheostomy for mechanical ventilation (see Chapter 56) are available in home therapeutic options.

Rehospitalization risk is significant, particularly within the first 2 years, and is most often attributed to pulmonary infection or cardiorespiratory disease.[2,34] Therefore, current recommendations are for at-risk infants and children to receive annual influenza vaccinations as well as respiratory syncytial virus (RSV) prophylaxis through age 24 months during months of high risk. The AAP policy statement details criteria for RSV prophylaxis.[35] Measures to decrease transmission of upper and lower respiratory infection are critically important in this population, as is avoidance of environmental tobacco smoke. Infants presenting to medical attention with worsening respiratory symptoms should receive a complete physical examination with documentation of work of breathing, respiratory rate, and oxygen saturation level. A change in clinical status should prompt referral for possible hospitalization to permit continuous cardiorespiratory monitoring, provide therapeutic interventions, and optimize fluid and nutritional status during acute illness.

Many children with BPD exhibit ongoing airway hyperreactivity and are more likely to carry a diagnosis of asthma, although symptoms appear to improve over time.[36,37] Bronchodilator therapy can be an effective treatment; the addition of asthma controller therapy is indicated for persistent symptoms, consistent with published guidelines for asthma management (see Chapter 12). Several studies have also suggested persistent decrements in pulmonary function, although longitudinal data reflecting outcomes of the new BPD population is limited.[34,36] Pulmonary function tests, exercise testing, and chest computed tomography represent noninvasive modalities to follow lung function and appearance over time.[36] There is currently no consensus on which measures should be obtained, or how frequently.

Key Points

- Bronchopulmonary dysplasia remains a significant cause of neonatal morbidity and mortality.
- Key risk factors include gestational age less than 26 weeks, birth weight less than 1,100 g, male sex, high initial inspired oxygen concentrations, and the need for multiple surfactant doses.
- Oxygen toxicity, ventilator-induced lung injury, and chronic inflammation represent key causative factors.
- Long-term BPD sequelae include decreased pulmonary function, increased risk of respiratory infections, pulmonary hypertension, systemic hypertension, and poorer growth and neurodevelopmental outcomes.
- Current treatment is largely supportive; care of infants with BPD requires a multidisciplinary approach with frequent evaluation and monitoring.

References

1. Northway WH, Rosan RC, Porter DY. Pulmonary disease following respirator therapy of hyaline-membrane disease. Bronchopulmonary dysplasia. *N Engl J Med.* 1967;276:357–368
2. Furman L, Baley J, Borawski-Clark E, et al. Hospitalizations as a measure of morbidity among very low birth weight infants with chronic lung disease. *J Pediatr.* 1996;128:447–452
3. Fanaroff AA, Hack M, Walsh MC. The NICHD neonatal research network: changes in practice and outcomes during the first 15 years. *Semin Perinatol.* 2003;27(4):281–287
4. Davis JM, Parad RB, Michele T, et al for the North American Recombinant Human CuZnSOD Study Group. Pulmonary outcome at 1 year corrected age in premature infants treated at birth with recombinant human CuZn superoxide dismutase. *Pediatrics.* 2003;111(3):469–476
5. Ambalavanan N, van Meurs KP, Perritt R, et al. Predictors of death or bronchopulmonary dysplasia in preterm infants with respiratory failure. *J Perinatol.* 2008;28(6):420–426
6. Clark RH, Gertsmann DR, Jobe AH, et al. Lung injury in neonates: causes, strategies for prevention, and long-term consequences. *J Pediatr.* 2001;139(4):478–486
7. Coalson JJ, Winter VT, Siler-Khodr T, Yoder BA. Neonatal chronic lung disease in extremely immature baboons. *Am J Respir Crit Care Med.* 1999;160(4):1333–1346
8. Jobe AH, Bancalari E. Bronchopulmonary dysplasia. From NICHD/NHLBI/ORD Workshop summary. *Am J Respir Crit Care Med.* 2001;163(7):1723–1729
9. Ambalavanan N, Carlo WA. Bronchopulmonary dysplasia: new insights. *Clin Perinatol.* 2004;31(3):613–628
10. Coalson JJ, Winter V, deLemos RA. Decreased alveolarization in baboon survivors with bronchopulmonary dysplasia. *Am J Respir Crit Care Med.* 1995;152(2):640–646
11. Wada K, Jobe AH, Ikegami M. Tidal volume effects on surfactant treatment responses with the initiation of ventilation in preterm lambs. *J Appl Physiol.* 1997;83(4):1054–1061
12. Hillman NH, Moss TJ, Kallapur SG, et al. Brief, large tidal volume ventilation initiates lung injury and a systemic response in fetal sheep. *Am J Respir Crit Care Med.* 2007;176(6):575–581
13. Rogers S, Witz G, Anwar M, Hiatt M, Hegyi T. Antioxidant capacity and oxygen radical diseases in the preterm newborn. *Arch Pediatr Adolesc Med.* 2000;154(6):544–548
14. STOP-ROP Study Group. Supplemental therapeutic oxygen for prethreshold retinopathy of prematurity (STOP-ROP), a randomized, controlled trial. I: primary outcomes. *Pediatrics.* 2000;105(2):295–310

15. Jobe AH, Kallapur S, Moss TJM. Inflammation/infection: effects on the fetal/newborn lung. In: Bancalari E, Polin RA, eds. *The Newborn Lung: Neonatology Questions and Controversies.* Philadelphia, PA: Elsevier Health Sciences; 2008:119–140
16. Benstein BD, Crouse DT, Shanklin DR, Ourth DD. Ureaplasma in lung. 2. Association with bronchopulmonary dysplasia. *Exp Molec Pathol.* 2003;75(2):171–177
17. Marshall DD, Kotelchuck M, Young TE, et al. Risk factors for chronic lung disease in the surfactant era: a North Carolina population-based study of very low birth weight infants. North Carolina Neonatologists Association. *Pediatrics.* 1999;104(6):1345–1350
18. Bancalari E, Claure N. Definitions and diagnostic criteria for bronchopulmonary dysplasia. *Semin Perinatol.* 2006;30(4):164–170
19. Morley CJ, Davis PG, Doyle LW, et al. Nasal CPAP or intubation at birth for very preterm infants. *N Engl J Med.* 2008;358(14):700–708
20. Mariani G, Cifuentes J, Carlo WA. Randomized trial of permissive hypercapnia in preterm infants. *Pediatrics.* 1999;104(5 pt 1):1082–1088
21. Kao LC, Durand DJ, McCrea RC, et al. Randomized trial of long-term diuretic therapy for infants with oxygen-dependent bronchopulmonary dysplasia. *J Pediatr.* 1994;124(5 pt 1):772–781
22. Needelman H, Evans M, Roberts H, Sweney M, Bodensteiner JB. Effects of postnatal dexamethasone exposure on the developmental outcome of premature infants. *J Child Neurol.* 2008;23(4):421–424
23. American Academy of Pediatrics Committee on Fetus and Newborn. Postnatal corticosteroids to treat or prevent chronic lung disease in preterm infants. *Pediatrics.* 2002;109(2):330–338
24. Denjean A, Paris-Llado J, Zupan V, et al. Inhaled salbutamol and beclomethasone for preventing broncho-pulmonary dysplasia: a randomised double-blind study. *Eur J Pediatr.* 1998;157(11):926–931
25. Biniwale MA, Ehrenkranz RA. The role of nutrition in the prevention and management of bronchopulmonary dysplasia. *Semin Perinatol.* 2006;30(4):200–208
26. Tyson JE, Wright LL, Oh W, et al. Vitamin A supplementation for extremely-low-birth-weight infants: National Institute of Child Health and Human Development Neonatal Research Network. *N Engl J Med.* 1999;340(25):1962–1968
27. Schmidt B, Roberts RS, Davis P, et al. Caffeine therapy for apnea of prematurity. *N Engl J Med.* 2006; 354(20):2112–2121
28. Banks BA, Seri I, Ischiropoulos H, et al. Changes in oxygenation with inhaled nitric oxide in severe bronchopulmonary dysplasia. *Pediatrics.* 1999;103(3):610–618
29. Kinsella JP, Cutter GR, Walsh WF, et al. Early inhaled nitric oxide therapy in premature newborns with respiratory failure. *N Engl J Med.* 2006;355(4):354–364

30. Khemani E, McElhinney DB, Rhein L, et al. Pulmonary artery hypertension in formerly premature infants with bronchopulmonary dysplasia: clinical features and outcomes in the surfactant era. *Pediatrics.* 2007;120(6):1260–1269
31. Abman SH. Monitoring of cardiovascular function in infants with chronic lung disease of prematurity. *Arch Dis Child Fetal Neonatal Ed.* 2002;87(1):F15–F18
32. Palta M, Sadek-Badawi M, Evans M, Weinstein MR, McGuinnes G. Functional assessment of a multicenter very low birthweight cohort at age 5 years. Newborn Lung Project. *Arch Pediatr Adolesc Med.* 2000;154(1):23–30
33. Vohr BR, Wright LL, Dusick AM, et al. Neurodevelopmental and functional outcomes of extremely low birth weight infants in the National Institute of Child Health and Human Development Neonatal Research Network, 1993–1994. *Pediatrics.* 2000;105(6):1216–1226
34. Gross SJ, Iannuzzi DM, Kveselis DA, Anbar RD. Effect of preterm birth on pulmonary function at school-age: a prospective controlled study. *J Pediatr.* 1998;133(2):188–192
35. American Academy of Pediatrics Committee on Infectious Diseases. Modified recommendations for use of palivizumab for prevention of respiratory syncytal virus infections. *Pediatrics.* 2009;124:1694–1701
36. Bhandari A, Panitch HB. Pulmonary outcomes in bronchopulmonary dysplasia. *Semin Perinatol.* 2006;30(4):219–226
37. Ng DK, Lau WY, Lee SL. Pulmonary sequelae in long-term survivors of bronchopulmonary dysplasia. *Pediatr Int.* 2000;42(6):603–607

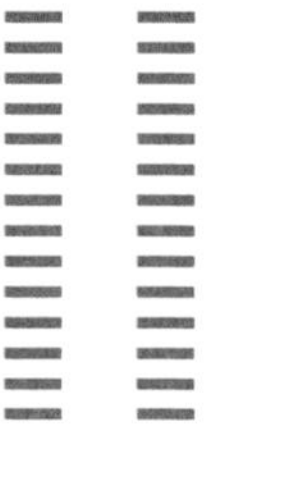

Chapter 28

Pleural Effusion (Nonbacterial)

Girish D. Sharma, MD

Case Report 28-1

A 4 -year-old boy with nephrotic syndrome developed sudden respiratory distress, hypoxia in room air, and abdominal distention. The laboratory investigations showed hyponatremia and anemia and the chest radiograph (Figure 28-1) shows density in the lower lobes. A pleural effusion is suspected.

Introduction

Pleural effusion is defined as the presence of an excessive amount (>10–20 mL) of fluid in the pleural space. This is the result of excessive filtration or defective absorption of accumulated fluid. Normally there

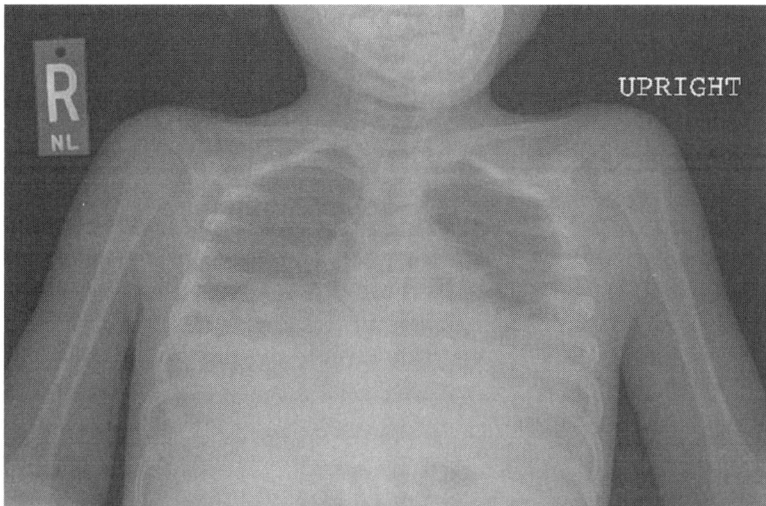

Figure 28-1. Bilateral pleural effusions in a 4-year-old boy with nephrotic syndrome, moderate on the left and smaller on the right side. (Courtesy: E. Comiskey, MD, Rush University Medical Center)

is a balance between the influx and outflow of fluid from the pleural space, resulting in a very small amount (0.1–0.2 mL/kg) of sterile, colorless fluid.[1] Nearly 90% of the amount of pleural fluid filtered out of the arterial end of the capillaries is reabsorbed at the venous end. The remaining 10% of the filtrate is returned via the lymphatic system. Final direction of fluid transport depends on the balance between filtration and absorption forces.[2]

The balance depends on several factors, including capillary filtration or hydrostatic pressure, capillary oncotic pressure (mainly due to albumin), pleural capillary hydrostatic pressure, and pleural fluid oncotic pressure. Normally capillary hydrostatic or driving pressure is higher than pleural hydrostatic pressure and pleural oncotic pressure lower than capillary oncotic pressure, which results, along with lymphatic drainage, in no net accumulation of pleural fluid. Alterations in fluid dynamics may occur with changes in hydrostatic or oncotic pressure in either compartment.

Fluid Characteristics

Pleural fluid can be transudative (due to congestive heart failure, atelectasis, or hypoalbuminemia) or exudative (due to pleuropulmonary infections, circulating toxins, systemic lupus erythematosus, rheumatoid arthritis, sarcoidosis, tumor, or pulmonary infarction) in nature. Fluid characteristics, such as protein concentration and the ratio of lactate dehydrogenase (LDH) between pleural fluid and plasma, can help determine if the pleural fluid is an exudate or a transudate (Table 28-1).[3]

Table 28-1. Pleural Fluid Characteristics to Differentiate Between Transudates and Exudates

Characteristic	Transudate	Exudate
Protein level	<3 g/dL	≥3 g/dL
Pleural fluid lactate dehydrogenase (LDH) vs serum LDH (upper level of serum LDH)	<2/3	>2/3
Pleural fluid: serum protein	<0.5	>0.5
Pleural fluid: serum LDH	<0.6	>0.6

Transudative Pleural Effusion

Disequilibrium between hydrostatic and oncotic forces results in ultrafiltration of plasma in the pleural space, causing transudative pleural effusion. Increased microvascular pressure is the mechanism in congestive heart failure, increased peri-microvascular pressure in atelectasis, and decreased oncotic pressure in hypoalbuminemia. (See Box 28-1 for a list of causes.) Due to the systemic nature of disorders causing transudative pleural effusion, pleural effusion tends to occur bilaterally.

Exudative Pleural Effusion

Exudative pleural effusion can be due to pleural or pulmonary inflammation, impaired lymphatic drainage from the pleural space, or transdiaphragmatic movement of inflammatory fluid from the peritoneal space. Infectious pleural effusions tend to occur unilaterally.

Hemorrhagic Pleural Effusion

Hemorrhagic pleural effusion can be due to trauma to the heart, the great vessels, and the chest wall; post-pericardiotomy syndrome;

Box 28-1. Causes of Pleural Effusion According to Type of Fluid

Causes of transudative pleural effusion	Causes of exudative pleural effusion
Hypoalbuminemia Congestive heart failure Atelectasis Nephrotic syndrome Cirrhosis Peritoneal dialysis Myxedema Constrictive pericarditis	Parapneumonic (most common cause in children) Pancreatitis Collagen vascular disorders (rheumatoid arthritis, systemic lupus erythematosus) Tuberculosis Sarcoidosis Trauma (esophageal perforation, post–cardiac surgery) Malignancy Pulmonary embolism Radiation pleuritis Meigs syndrome and pseudo-Meigs syndrome Yellow nail syndrome

hemorrhagic disorders such vitamin K deficiency; Henoch-Schönlein purpura; and malignancy. Hemothorax has been reported with congenital cystic adenomatoid malformation.[4] Patients with hemorrhagic pleural effusion, depending on the amount of bleeding, may have a reduced hematocrit. Hemothorax should be suspected if pleural fluid hematocrit is more than 50% of peripheral blood hematocrit.

Pleural Effusion Associated With Malignancies

In malignancies such as lymphomas and Hodgkin's disease, pleural effusion can be due to impaired pleural lymphatic flow secondary to pleural involvement and thoracic duct obstruction. Enlarged mediastinal lymph nodes, fibrosis, thickening of parietal pleura, and obstruction of the thoracic duct can result in exudative pleural effusion.[2] Pleural metastasis may result in increased permeability or obstruction of the pleural lymphatic vessels, resulting in pleural effusion. Post-radiation pleural fibrosis and malignancy-associated hypoproteinemia may also contribute to pleural effusion. Meigs syndrome is a triad of ascites, pleural effusion, and benign ovarian fibroma. It has been reported even in prepubertal children. Presence of an ovarian tumor other than a fibroma, ascites, and pleural effusion is called *pseudo-Meigs syndrome*. The prognosis in Meigs syndrome is good because most tumors are benign.

Chylous Pleural Effusion (Chylothorax)

Chyle is lymphatic fluid enriched with fat secreted by intestinal cells. In children, chylothorax is usually a postoperative complication of cardiac and thoracic surgery, other causes are thrombosis of the subclavian vein and malformation of pulmonary or thoracic lymphatic system as described in trisomy 21 and Noonan syndrome.[5]

Characteristics of chylous pleural fluid are milky appearance with triglycerides greater than 1.1 mmol/L (with minimal oral fat intake), total cell count greater than or equal to 1, 000 cells/µL, and lymphocytic fraction greater than 80%.[6] In cases that are due to postoperative complication there is a temporal relationship between the time of diagnosis of chylothorax and initiation of oral fat intake.

Clinical Presentation

The presentation of pleural effusion ranges from an incidental radiologic finding to symptoms of respiratory distress and hypoxia requiring urgent removal of fluid and treatment. Variants of pleural effusion include empyema or pyothorax, hemothorax, and chylothorax, which are due to collections of pus, blood, and lymph, respectively, in the pleural space. The degree of dysfunction and associated clinical picture is determined by the amount and rate of fluid collection, nature of underlying disorder, and patients' cardiopulmonary reserve. With a very small collection no obvious change may be apparent; larger collections will limit the lung inflation and may result in imbalance and decoupling of normally balanced inward recoil of lung and outward recoil of chest wall, which will further deflate the lung. This may result in compressive lung atelectasis; ventilation/perfusion mismatch; hypoxemia; and a clinical picture of the pleural space–occupying lesion, such as chest wall bulge, mediastinal shift, with corresponding radiologic changes. Inspiratory muscles are placed at a mechanical disadvantage, which may compromise inspiratory efforts.

The clinical picture of a patient with pleural effusion depends on the underlying disease, amount of pleural effusion, and rate at which the fluid accumulates in the pleural space. Many patients with pleural effusion may not have symptoms related to pleural effusion.

It is important to obtain history of the drugs that have been implicated in the etiology of pleural effusion. These include drugs that have been associated with lupus syndrome and other drugs that may cause pleural effusion (Box 28-2). Symptoms may include the following.

Box 28-2. Drugs Associated With Pleural Effusion

- Procainamide
- Procarbazine
- Hydralazine
- Bleomycin
- Quinidine
- Amiodarone
- Nitrofurantoin
- Mitomycin
- Dantrolene
- Methotrexate
- Methysergide

Chest Pain

Presence of transudative pleural effusion is not associated with chest pain as there is no inflammation of pleura in the disorders associated with transudates (Box 28-1). Involvement and inflammation of parietal pleura, since only parietal pleura has pain fibers, may result in pleuritic chest pain, which is present or gets worse during inspiration or coughing. Usually the pain is localized and coincides with the affected area of the pleura. The pain may be mild or severe and is stabbing or sharp in nature. At times, the pain may be referred to the abdomen or ipsilateral shoulder due to common nerve supply. The pain may decrease in severity as the quantity of pleural effusion increases since increased quantity of fluid between 2 layers of pleura prevent rubbing of the 2 surfaces against each other.

Dyspnea

Dyspnea, or shortness of breath, may be the most common presenting symptom. Mechanical inefficiency of respiratory muscles stretched by outward movement of the chest wall and downward movement of the diaphragm results in dyspnea. Presence of dyspnea indicates a large amount of pleural fluid collection. Underlying lung disease can also contribute to dyspnea.

Cough

Mild nonproductive cough is a less common symptom of pleural effusion. Distortion of the lung may cause cough; underlying lung disorder may also cause cough.

Physical Findings

Pleural rub may be the only finding in the early stages when the amount collected in the pleural space is very small. The pleural rub is present throughout the respiratory cycle loudest at end inspiration and early expiration. It will disappear when the patient holds his breath.

With increasing amounts of fluid, decreased breath sounds, increased dullness on percussion, decreased tactile fremitus, and egophony may be present. Large amounts will be associated with contralateral mediastinal shift. There may be fullness of intercostal spaces over the pleural effusion area. Ipsilateral mediastinal shift may be present when there is endobronchial obstruction by a foreign body or tumor.

Pleural effusion rarely may be associated with yellow nail syndrome (slow growing and discolored nails), lymphedema, or chronic recurrent pleural effusion.

Diagnostic Studies

Laboratory Studies

Conservative management with observation of the patient for the presence of complications may be reasonable in cases of pleural effusion associated with congestive heart failure, viral pleurisy, and postoperative pleural effusions. Thoracentesis should be considered in patients with unexplained pleural effusion when fluid quantity is sufficient to allow a safe procedure. Blood cell counts, erythrocyte sedimentation rate (ESR), and C-reactive protein estimation will help to confirm or rule out infective or inflammatory cause for pleural effusion. The results of pleural fluid analysis for pH, serum glucose, lactate dehydrogenase, protein, triglycerides, electrolyte levels, and microbiological studies are associated with different etiologies and used to differentiate between exudate and transudate[7] (Table 28-1).

Chest Radiograph

Chest radiograph confirms the diagnosis of pleural effusion. Radiographic features of pleural effusion are related to several factors,[4] including the amount of fluid, whether the fluid is free or loculated, presence of adjacent parenchymal lung disease, and the relative position of the patient with the radiograph beam. A small amount of fluid (<200 mL) may only be detected as blunting of costophrenic angle. A larger amount of fluid will show as homogeneous density with concave superior border on an upright posteroanterior (PA) view or lateral view. This meniscus sign may not be present when the radiograph is taken in supine position as in a portable radiograph and only a nonspecific haze over the affected hemithorax may be visible because of the fluid layers in the posterior area. In still larger fluid collection, whole hemithorax may be opacified and there may be evidence of mediastinal shift to the opposite side. The fluid may extend into major or minor fissures and appear as thickened fissures on chest radiograph (PA or lateral view). A subpulmonic pleural effusion with fluid between the inferior surface of the lung and superior margin of the diaphragm may appear as apparent elevation of the corresponding dome of the diaphragm. Lateral displacement of the apex of the diaphragm, increased space between the air bubble of gastric fundus and the superior margin of apparent diaphragm, absence of the lower lobe vessels normally visualized overlying the diaphragm on PA projection, and the sharp angulation of the anterior portion of the apparent diaphragm may also be seen.[8]

Ultrasonography

Ultrasonography is effective for visualization of effusion and to determine if the fluid is free flowing or loculated, and it may also be used to guide thoracentesis.[9] Ultrasonography can also differentiate between solid mass and effusion.

Computed Tomography (CT) Scan

Unless an underlying mass is a concern, CT of the chest may not be necessary to diagnose a simple pleural effusion. Nevertheless CT with contrast may provide additional information (underlying lung parenchymal information, necrotizing pneumonia, atelectasis, hilar adenopathy, and lung abscess). It may also have a role in cases of complicated effusion or the one unresponsive to therapy.

Management

Treatment of nonbacterial pleural effusion is primarily treatment of the primary disorder (Box 28-3). Refer to Chapter 20 for the management of bacterial pleural effusion, such as parapneumonic pleural effusion.

Thoracentesis

Thoracentesis may be considered therapeutic or diagnostic.

Therapeutic Thoracentesis

Thoracentesis is indicated to relieve dyspnea in patients with large effusions[8] and to prevent development of complicated parapneumonic effusions. As a general rule thoracentesis can be performed safely when the thickness of the pleural fluid layer on lateral decubitus chest radiograph is more than 10 mm or the loculated fluid is identified on ultrasound or chest CT. Hypoxemia as a complication of thoracentesis can be prevented by administration of supplemental oxygen during the procedure. It is important to withdraw enough fluid to improve the dyspnea without withdrawing too much fluid and too rapidly, which can cause reexpansion pulmonary edema and pneumothorax.[9] A small and clinically insignificant pneumothorax may be present after thoracentesis. The pneumothorax, if large, may present

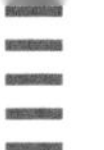

Box 28-3. Guidance to Manage a Patient With Nonbacterial Pleural Effusion in Pediatric Practice

- Document the presence of pleural effusion.
- Suspect pleural effusion in the presence of clinical disorders likely to be associated with it, such as nephrotic syndrome, hypoalbuminemia, congestive heart failure, and postoperative cardiothoracic cases.
- History and physical examination for symptoms such as chest pain, dyspnea, and cough and presence of physical signs such as pleural rub, decreased breath sounds, increased dullness, and mediastinal shift.
- Confirm the presence and estimate the quantity of pleural effusion by chest radiograph, ultrasound, or computed tomography.
- Investigate for possible causes of pleural effusion (blood counts, ESR, C-reactive protein).
- Employ thoracentesis to diagnose the type of fluid (transudate vs exudate) and possible cause.
- Employ thoracentesis when pleural effusion compromises the patient's respiratory status. Bacterial causes of pleural fluid, such as empyema, tuberculosis, and malignancy, may need thoracentesis for diagnostic and therapeutic reasons.[8]
- Apart from thoracentesis for diagnostic purposes and to relieve respiratory embarrassment, treatment of the underlying disorder should be the goal of therapy.

with increased respiratory distress, oxygen requirement, and clinical signs (see Chapter 29) and can be confirmed by chest radiograph.

Diagnostic Thoracentesis

Diagnostic thoracentesis is done in patients with effusion with no clear cause. The fluid can be tested to differentiate between transudates and exudates (Table 28-1). The fluid can be examined for physical characteristics, such as color, specific gravity, triglycerides, and chylomicrons. Other tests can be used to help diagnose a specific cause for pleural effusion, such as total and differential cell count, LDH, pH, protein levels, glucose level, Gram stain, mycobacterial studies, fungal stain and culture, and cytology.[8] Presence of levels of amylase more than twice the levels of serum amylase will suggest pancreatic pathology, such as acute pancreatitis, pancreatic pseudocyst, and malignancy. Esophageal rupture will also increase amylase levels in pleural fluid.

Management of Chylous Pleural Effusion

Usually initial therapy for postoperative chylothorax is pleural space drainage, use of medium chain triglyceride oil, fat-free oral feeds, or enteric rest with total parenteral nutrition. Chylous effusions often persist for a period of weeks. Surgery in the form of pleurodesis of leaking lymphatics and ligation of the thoracic duct is usually recommended if the effusion persists after more than 4 weeks of conservative treatment.[5]

Prognosis and When to Refer

Prognosis will depend on the cause of pleural effusion and the rate and the quantity of fluid collected. Small pleural effusions detected accidentally on chest radiographs and not associated with significant clinical findings may not require significant intervention, such as pleural drainage. Pleural effusions with a large amount of rapidly collecting fluid and clinical signs, especially respiratory distress, hypoxia, and mediastinal shift, will require more aggressive therapy and possible surgical intervention for drainage. Failure of conservative therapy and delay in initiation of specific therapy may result in complications, such as respiratory failure.

Key Points

- Nonbacterial pleural effusion should be suspected when a patient with underlying disorders, such as nephrotic syndrome, hypoalbuminemia, congestive heart failure, and postoperative cardiothoracic cases, develops respiratory distress, increased oxygen requirement, and clinical signs of effusion.
- Small pleural effusion may present as only an incidental finding on chest radiograph.
- Rapidly collecting large pleural effusions with respiratory embarrassment will require therapeutic thoracentesis.
- Pleural effusions with no obvious underlying cause need diagnostic workup, including diagnostic thoracentesis, investigations for possible underlying cause, and treatment according to the etiology.

References

1. Zocchi L. Physiology and pathophysiology of pleural fluid turnover. *Eur Respir Mon.* 2002;22:28–49
2. Montgomery M, Sigalet D. Air and liquid in the pleural space. In: Chernick V, Boat T, Wilmott R, Bush A, eds. *Kendig's Disorders of the Respiratory Tract in Children.* 7th ed. Philadelphia, PA: Saunders Elsevier; 2006:368–369
3. Light R, Macgregor M, Luchsinger P, Ball W. Pleural effusions: the diagnostic separation of transudates and exudates. *Ann Intern Med.* 1972;77 (4):507–513
4. Laberge JM, Puligandla P, Flageole H. Asymptomatic congenital lung malformations. *Semin Pediatr Surg.* 2005;14(1):16–33
5. Chernick V, Reed MH. Pneumothorax and chylothorax in the neonatal period. *J Pediatr.* 1970;76:625–632
6. Büttikar V, Fanconi S, Burger R. Chylothorax in children: guidelines for diagnosis and management. *Chest.* 1999;116:682–687
7. Light RW, ed. *Clinical Manifestations and Useful Tests in Pleural Diseases.* 5th ed. Baltimore, MD: Lippincott Williams and Wilkins; 2007:73
8. Jay JS. Diagnostic procedures for pleural disease. *Clin Chest Med.* 1985;6(1):33–48
9. Grogan DR, Irwin RS, Chernick R, et al. Complications associated with thoracentesis—a prospective randomized study comparing three different methods. *Arch Intern Med.* 1990;150:873–877

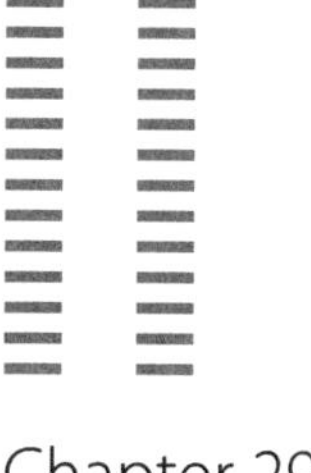

Chapter 29

Pneumothorax and Pneumomediastinum

Danna Tauber, MD

Pneumothorax

Pneumothorax is defined as the abnormal collection of air in the pleural space outside of the lung. Air can enter the pleural space by a leak in either the visceral or parietal pleura. Pneumothorax can be categorized as spontaneous or traumatic. Traumatic pneumothorax occurs as the result of blunt or penetrating trauma to the chest wall, or an injury from a diagnostic or therapeutic procedure. Spontaneous pneumothorax occurs without identified trauma and can further be subdivided into primary and secondary. In primary pneumothorax there is no identifiable lung disease that would lead to air leak. Many patients with primary pneumothorax have apical blebs of unknown etiology that may be recognized at the time of surgery or by computed tomography (CT).[1] Secondary pneumothorax occurs as a complication of underlying lung disease, such as cystic fibrosis. Incidence of primary spontaneous pneumothorax is highest between 15 and 34 years of age.[2] The peak incidence of secondary spontaneous pneumothorax occurs later in life due to its high association with chronic obstructive lung disease. Primary spontaneous pneumothorax typically occurs in tall, asthenic patients and more commonly in males in both the adult and pediatric populations.[3,4] Smoking increases the risk of pneumothorax.[5] Box 29-1 contains a complete list of causes of pneumothorax.

Box 29-1. Causes of Pneumothorax

Traumatic	Penetrating or blunt chest trauma
Iatrogenic	Mechanical ventilation (barotrauma) Central vein catheterization Procedures on airways: intubation, endoscopy, transbronchial biopsy Laparoscopic procedures Percutaneous biopsies
Primary spontaneous	Asthenic body habitus Idiopathic Cocaine or marijuana inhalation
Secondary spontaneous	Airway disease: asthma, cystic fibrosis Postinfection: measles, *Pneumocystis jiroveci,* tuberculosis, necrotizing pneumonia or abscess, parasitic (ecchinococcal) Interstitial lung disease: sarcoidosis, Langerhans cell granulomatosis Connective tissue disease: Marfan, Ehlers-Danlos, rheumatoid arthritis, systemic lupus erythematosus, polymyositis, dermatomyositis Malignancy: lymphoma, metastasis Aspiration: foreign body, other Catamenial pneumothorax
Congenital malformations	

Case Report 29-1

A 16-year-old African American male presented to the emergency department (ED) with a 2-day history of right chest pain. The only other symptom was shortness of breath on exertion. He has been in previously good health, is active, and participates in sports. The pain started when he was sitting quietly in the evening. His vital signs were normal except for a respiratory rate of 18. Oxygen saturation in room air was 97%. Physical examination revealed a tall and thin youth with normal chest configuration. The chest examination was normal, and auscultation of the heart and lungs negative. A chest radiograph revealed a small pneumothorax on the right. He was observed in the ED for 4 hours, during which time a CT scan was performed. The CT scan confirmed the pneumothorax and showed small apical blebs in both lungs. He was discharged home with no intervention and arrangements made for follow-up x-ray in 2 days.

Pathophysiology

Two causative mechanisms for pneumothorax may exist. The first mechanism suggests that large increases in transpulmonary pressure cause alveolar distention, and high pressure gradients cause the alveolus to rupture. Superficial alveoli can form subpleural blebs that rupture directly into the pleural space. In the second mechanism, direct injury to the visceral pleura secondary to underlying lung disease leads to pneumothorax. There is a negative pressure within the pleural space, relative to the alveoli, which helps to keep the pleural space intact. Spontaneous pneumothorax occurs when the visceral pleura is ruptured. A traumatic pneumothorax may involve either the parietal pleura (air entering from the outside) or visceral pleura (air entering from the lungs), or both. A tension pneumothorax develops when air enters the pleural space during inspiration but cannot exit during exhalation. This will lead to collapse of the affected lung and shift of the mediastinum away from the affected side. Tension pneumothorax is uncommon following a primary spontaneous pneumothorax, but is a potential risk following traumatic pneumothorax and secondary spontaneous pneumothorax, especially patients who are receiving positive-pressure assisted ventilation. Air enters the pleural space with each breath and is unable to escape, so that the mediastinum becomes shifted to the other side. Hypoxia results and there are hemodynamic changes that eventually lead to shock and death within a short period (sometimes minutes) if the pneumothorax is not treated.

Clinical Features

The cardinal manifestation of pneumothorax is the sudden onset of chest pain. Other common clinical manifestations include tachypnea, dyspnea, tachycardia, and cyanosis. The severity of symptoms depends on the volume of air in the pleural space, rapidity of onset, and the degree of respiratory compromise before the occurrence of the pneumothorax, which is influenced by the presence of underlying lung disease. Pain can range from localized acute retrosternal pain to overwhelming pleuritic pain, as well as ipsilateral shoulder pain. Physical examination findings include decreased breath sounds, decreased thoracic excursion, and hyperresonant percussion on the affected side. In cases of tension pneumothorax with shift of the mediastinum, the trachea will be displaced as will the point of maximal cardiac impulse. Subcutaneous emphysema results from air moving to areas of lower resistance and can reach the neck, upper extremities, abdominal wall, and peritoneum. In cases where the pneumothorax is small, the patient will frequently be asymptomatic and is usually an incidental finding on radiograph.

Diagnostic Tests

Diagnosis of a pneumothorax is accomplished by chest radiograph. Anteroposterior and lateral views will reveal the characteristic findings of air in the pleural space outlining the visceral pleura (pleural line) and hyperlucency and attenuation of vascular and lung markings on the affected side (Figure 29-1 and Figure 29-2). A CT of the chest is helpful to detect bullae and blebs in patients with recurrent pneumothorax and in cases where the radiograph is inconclusive.[6,7] Hypoxemia occurs due to collapse and poor ventilation. Hypercapnia is not usually seen in cases of pneumothorax without underlying chronic lung disease.[1] In cases of severe tension pneumothorax with mediastinal shift and cardiac displacement and rotation, electrocardiogram can reveal changes in the amplitude of the QRS complex and the cardiac axis.

Management

Treatment depends on the size and cause of the pneumothorax, the extent of respiratory distress, and the presence of underlying lung disease. The goals of treatment are removal of air from the pleural space and prevention of recurrence.[1,8] Treatment can range from observation and supplemental oxygen to simple needle aspiration or chest tube to pleurodesis, and in some cases more invasive surgery. Information on pediatric spontaneous pneumothorax is limited and management guidelines are based on published adult data.

Observation

In the case of a small pneumothorax (<15% of the involved hemithorax) when the patient is asymptomatic, simple observation can be instituted.[9,10] In a younger child, hospitalization is recommended. In the older child observation may be done on an outpatient basis. The exception to this is a traumatic pneumothorax because of the potential for tension pneumothorax. Most cases of traumatic pneumothorax should be treated with a chest tube, especially if positive pressure ventilation is used.

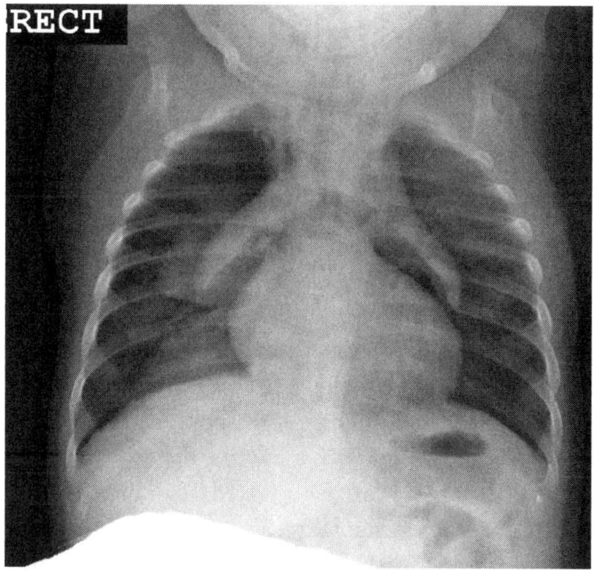

Figure 29-1. Spinnaker sail (angel wing) sign in a patient with pneumomediastinum and pneumothorax.

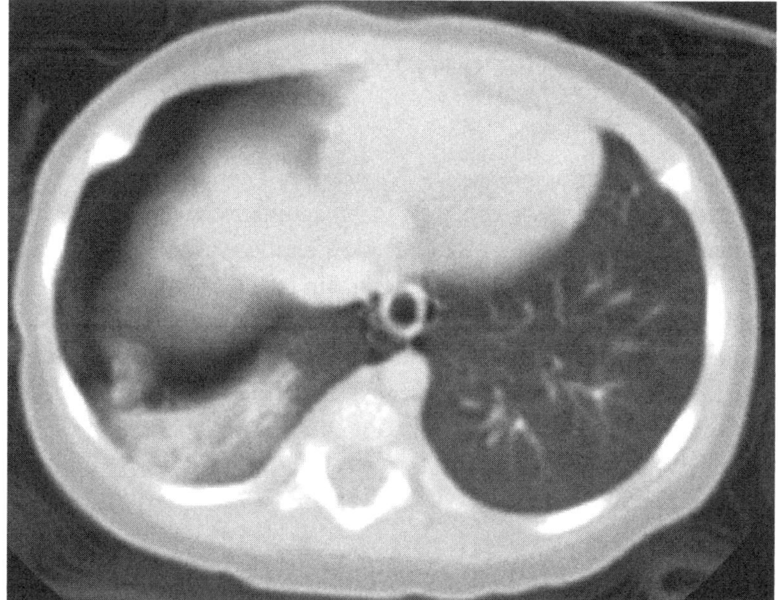

Figure 29-2. Computed tomography revealing both paratracheal air and pneumothorax in same patient seen in Figure 29-1.

Supplemental Oxygen

The rate of resorption of air from the pleural space is increased with the use of supplemental oxygen.[11] The increased alveolar oxygen tension creates a large gradient between capillary and pleural gas partial pressure of nitrogen, resulting in faster resorption of intrapleural air. Use of 100% oxygen via a non-rebreathing face mask has been suggested, although this should not be continued for a long period.

Needle Aspiration

Evacuation of air is required for symptomatic patients where the pneumothorax has been identified to occupy more than 15% of the involved hemithorax. Simple aspiration is done via a large-bore intravenous catheter connected to a large syringe with a 3-way stopcock. Air is withdrawn manually until no more can be aspirated. If air continues to be aspirated, this indicates a persistent air leak and a tube thoracostomy should be performed. If no further air can be aspirated, the stopcock is closed and the catheter is secured to the chest wall. A chest radiograph should be performed after 4 hours of observation; if adequate lung re-expansion is seen, the catheter can be removed and the patient observed. Published success rates vary and depend on whether the pneumothorax is primary or secondary.[8]

Thoracostomy Tube

This is indicated for patients who have large pneumothoraces, are clinically stable or unstable, or recurrent spontaneous pneumothorax.[12] This involves the use of a 1-way Heimlich valve or water seal device to prevent reaccumulation of air. In the American College of Chest Physicians guidelines, half of the panel members recommended clamping of the tube 4 hours after the last evidence of an air leak, the other half would never clamp a chest tube. A bubbling chest tube should never be clamped. A repeat chest radiograph should be taken 5 to 12 hours after the last evidence of an air leak in preparation for removal of the tube.

Pleurodesis

Pleurodesis is the procedure to manage recurrent pneumothoraces and can be chemical or surgical. In the pediatric population this is most likely necessary for recurrent pneumothorax as a result of cystic fibrosis. Chemical pleurodesis involves injection of a sclerosis agent, such as talc, tetracycline, doxycycline, autologous blood patches, or fibrin glue, at the time of thoracostomy tube placement. This method is less favored than surgical intervention for persistent air leak.[13] Mechanical pleurodesis by direct abrasion with gauze or laser, or chemical pleurodesis with talc or doxycycline at the time of surgery, has support in the literature to prevent recurrence.[12]

Surgical Intervention

This involves stapling or over-sewing ruptured blebs (bullectomy) or tears in the visceral pleura and resection of abnormal lung tissue. This can be done via video-assisted thorascopic surgery (VATS), mini-thoracotomy, and open thoracotomy, although many physicians prefer VATS. Surgery is indicated to treat persistent air leaks and to prevent recurrence. Surgery is recommended at the time of the first occurrence of a secondary spontaneous pneumothorax[12] and at the second occurrence of a primary spontaneous pneumothorax.[14]

Prognosis

Data regarding prognosis after spontaneous pneumothorax in children is limited. One reported series showed a 37% incidence of recurrent spontaneous pneumothorax.[15] In pediatric patients undergoing surgical management the reported risk of recurrence was 6% to 9%.[16,17] A recent study[18] evaluated primary versus delayed surgery for pediatric patients with primary spontaneous pneumothorax. The authors found that patients who had VATS-directed bullectomy and pleurodesis at the first presentation of spontaneous pneumothorax had 29% recurrence rate compared with 0% in the group of patients undergoing VATS on the second occurrence.

Pneumomediastinum

Pneumomediastinum is defined as the presence of air in the mediastinum. Cases of pneumomediastinum can be further subdivided into spontaneous or secondary pneumomediastinum. Spontaneous pneumomediastinum does not have an identifiable source. Secondary pneumomediastinum occurs in children with asthma and after chest trauma due to endotracheal or endoesophageal procedures, mechanical ventilation, cardiac catheterization, or thoracic surgery. Spontaneous pneumomediastinum is a rare condition in young children. However, due to respiratory infections, there is a first peak incidence between 6 months and 3 years of age.[19,20] Spontaneous pneumomediastinum is mostly seen in older children and adolescents, with reported incidences of 1 in 800 to 1 in 42,000 patients presenting to a hospital ED.[21] Stack and Caputo[19] found an incidence of spontaneous pneumomediastinum in 0.3% of 12,000 children presenting to a pediatric ED with asthma. Most studies report a slightly higher incidence in males.[21,22]

Pathophysiology

Alveolar rupture occurs due to excess pressure (from overdistention) in the alveolus compared with the surrounding tissue. The air leaks into the interstitial tissues toward the hilum along the peribronchial and perivascular sheaths. It then spreads toward the mediastinum, the cervical region, upper limbs and, in some cases, the retroperitoneum, peritoneum, spine, pericardium, and pleura.[21] In some cases of spontaneous pneumomediastinum a trigger can be found and often includes asthma, emesis, intense physical activity, inhalational drugs, and situations involving a strong Valsalva maneuver (ie, coughing, screaming).[22] Pneumothorax may accompany the pneumomedistinum.

Clinical Features

Patients typically present with retrosternal chest pain with radiation to the shoulders, back, and arms. The pain is worsened with deep inhalation. Other presenting symptoms include sore throat, dyspnea, swelling of the neck, torticollis, dysphagia, and abdominal pain. Physical examination findings include subcutaneous emphysema and the classic Hamman sign, which is a precordial systolic crepitation or crunching sound on auscultation of the chest. Esophageal perforation must be excluded in cases of spontaneous pneumomediastinum that occur after severe and violent emesis.[21]

Diagnostic Tests

The diagnosis of spontaneous pneumomediastinum can be confirmed on chest radiograph. There are a number of specific radiographic findings seen in pneumomediastinum.[21,23] The spinnaker sail sign or angel wing sign (Figure 29-1) is created by air lifting the thymus off the heart and major vessels. The continuous diaphragm sign is caused by air collecting between the diaphragm and the pericardium. The vertical lucent streak is seen on the left side of the heart due to air outlining the parietal pleura. Additional radiographic findings include thoracic and cervical subcutaneous emphysema and associated pneumothorax. If esophageal perforation is suspected then contrast radiography should be undertaken, which can be combined with computed tomography. Esophageal endoscopy can also be used to identify cases of perforation or radiotransparent foreign body. Electrocardiogram can show diffuse microvoltage, depressed ST interval, T-wave inversion, and axis deviation depending on the size and location of the pneumomediastinum.[21]

Management

In most cases spontaneous pneumomediastinum is benign and resolves in 3 to 15 days without further sequelae.[24] Management is usually supportive, including rest, analgesia, and treatment of the underlying condition if present. Patients are advised to avoid maneuvers that lead to forceful exhalation (measure of lung function, physical activity, and playing of wind instruments) for a few months after the episode. As with pneumothorax, one study proposed the idea of nitrogen washout with 100% inspired oxygen; however, efficacy was not conclusive.[25] Follow-up radiographs are not recommended.[21] Recurrence of spontaneous pneumomediastinum is rare but is likely linked to either the underlying diagnosis of asthma or a repeat of the causal situation (emesis, strong Valsalva) that led to the first pneumomediastinum.

Key Points

- Pneumothoraces present with the sudden onset of severe chest pain. Treatment depends on the size of the pneumothorax, with small pneumothoraces being treated with observation or supplemental oxygen to larger pneumothoraces requiring thoracotomy tube placement.
- Further evaluation with CT of the chest is indicated with recurrent pneumothorax.
- Most cases of pneumomediastinum in children are spontaneous and occur during an asthma exacerbation or after a strong Valsava maneuver. The course is typically benign and treatment is supportive.
- Tension pneumothorax is a potentially life-threatening emergency requiring immediate attention.

References

1. Sahn SA, Heffner JE. Spontaneous pneumothorax. *N Engl J Med.* 2000;342(12):868–874
2. Gupta D, Hansell A, Nichols T, et al. Epidemiology of pneumothorax in England. *Thorax.* 2000;55(8):666–671
3. Abolnik IZ, Lossos IS, Gillis D. Primary spontaneous pneumothorax in men. *Am J Med Sci.* 1993;305(5):297–303
4. Withers JN, Fishback CM, Kiehl PV, et al. Spontaneous pneumothorax. Suggested etiology and comparison of treatment methods. *Am J Surg.* 1964;108:772–776
5. Bense L, Eklund G, Wiman LG. Smoking and the increased risk of contracting spontaneous pneumothorax. *Chest.* 1987;92(6):1009–1012
6. Mitlehner W, Friedrich M, Dissmann W. Value of computer tomography in the detection of bullae and blebs in patients with primary spontaneous pneumothorax. *Respiration.* 1992;59(4):221–227
7. Choudhary AK, Sellars ME, Wallis C, et al. Primary spontaneous pneumothorax in children: the role of CT in guiding management. *Clin Radiol.* 2005;60(4):508–511
8. Baumann MH, Strange C. Treatment of spontaneous pneumothorax: a more aggressive approach? *Chest.* 1997;112(3):789–804
9. Kirby TJ, Ginsberg RJ. Management of the pneumothorax and barotrauma. *Clin Chest Med.* 1992;13(1):97–112
10. Paape K, Fry WA. Spontaneous pneumothorax. *Chest Surg Clin N Am.* 1994;4(3):517–538
11. Northfield TC. Oxygen therapy for spontaneous pneumothorax. *Br Med J.* 1971;4(779):86–88
12. Baumann MH, Strange C, Heffner JE, et al. Management of spontaneous pneumothorax: an American College of Chest Physicians Delphi consensus statement. *Chest.* 2001;119(2):590–602
13. Alfageme I, Moreno L, Huertas C, et al. Spontaneous pneumothorax. Long-term results with tetracycline pleurodesis. *Chest.* 1994;106(2):347–350
14. Baumann MH. Management of spontaneous pneumothorax. *Clin Chest Med.* 2006;27(2):369–381
15. Shaw KS, Prasil P, Nguyen LT, et al. Pediatric spontaneous pneumothorax. *Semin Pediatr Surg.* 2003;12(1):55–61
16. Poenaru D, Yazbeck S, Murphy S. Primary spontaneous pneumothorax in children. *J Pediatr Surg.* 1994;29(9):1183–1185
17. Cook CH, Melvin WS, Groner JI, et al. A cost-effective thoracoscopic treatment strategy for pediatric spontaneous pneumothorax. *Surg Endosc.* 1999;13(12):1208–1210
18. Qureshi FG, Sandulache VC, Richardson W, et al. Primary vs delayed surgery for spontaneous pneumothorax in children: which is better? *J Pediatr Surg.* 2005;40(1):166–169

19. Stack AM, Caputo GL. Pneumomediastinum in childhood asthma. *Pediatr Emerg Care.* 1996;12:98–101
20. Bierman CW. Pneumomediastinum and pneumothorax complicating asthma in children. *Am J Dis Child.* 1967;114:42–50
21. Chalumaeau M, Le Clainche L, Sayeg N, et al. Spontaneous pneumomediastinum in children. *Pediatr Pulmonol.* 2001;31:67–75
22. Caceres M, Ali SZ, Braud R, et al. Spontaneous pneumomediastinum: a comparative study and review of the literature. *Ann Thorac Surg.* 2008;86:962–966
23. Bullaro FM, Baroletti SC. Spontaneous pneumomediastinum in children: a literature review. *Pediatr Emerg Care.* 2007;23(1):28–30
24. Dekel B, Paret G, Szeinberg A, et al. Spontaneous pneumomediastinum in children: clinical and natural history. *Eur J Pediatr.* 1996;155:695–697
25. Tutor JD, Montgomery VL, Eid IN. A case of virus bronchiolitis complicated by pneumomediastinum and subcutaneous emphysema. *Pediatr Pulmonol.* 1995;19:393–395

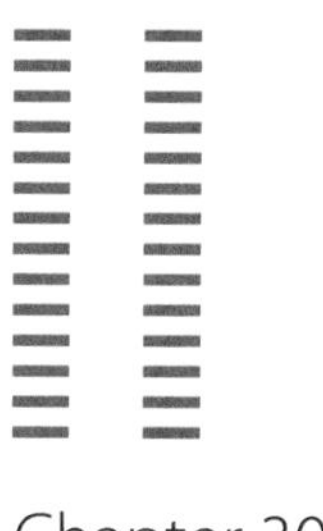

Chapter 30

Pulmonary Hemorrhage

Karen Z. Voter, MD
Clement L. Ren, MD

Introduction

Hemoptysis occurs uncommonly in children. While most episodes of hemoptysis are mild and short lived, they cause anxiety among parents and patients. Further, there is the possibility that the hemoptysis represents a severe underlying condition or a potential for life-threatening bleeding.

A report of "coughing up blood" may represent the presence of blood from the upper airway (nose and pharynx) or the lower airway, lung, or gastrointestinal tract, or it may be spurious and related to expectoration of saliva tinted with colored food or drink. A history sorting out the presence or absence of cough, possible foreign body exposure, underlying infection, nasal or pharyngeal trauma, and recent food consumption may help. Many people with pulmonary bleeding report the sensation of gurgling or bubbling in an area of the lung. A physical examination of the nose, pharynx, and mouth should be performed to look for signs of bleeding that would direct attention to the upper airway. Evidence of crackles, increased work of breathing, or localized wheezing would direct attention to causes of bleeding in the lower airways. Studies including a chest radiograph may help to localize the bleeding.

Etiology

Most cases of airway bleeding are from irritation of the airway mucosa (Box 30-1). Irritation of the airway mucosa from infection or trauma should trigger assessment for pneumonia, bronchitis, or foreign body

Box 30-1. Results of Select Studies of the Causes of Airway Bleeding

Godfrey Chart Review[a]

Upper airway bleeding—29%
Tracheotomy complications—18%
No cause—18%
Other causes—35%

Batra and Hollinger Chart Review[b]

Infectious causes—29%
Tracheotomy complications—14%
No cause—21%
Other causes—36%

Batra and Hollinger Bronchoscopy Studies[b]

Blood clots—37%
Purulence—21%
Mucosal inflammation—21%
Tracheal abrasion—11%
Granulation tissue—5%
Bronchial mass—5%

Coss-Bu Chart Review[c]

Cystic fibrosis—65%
Congenital heart disease, including ventricular septal defect, truncus arteriosus, complex cyanotic heart disease, transposition of the great arteries, arterioventricular canal, tetralogy of Fallot—16%
Other causes—18%

[a] Godfrey S. Pulmonary hemorrhage/hemoptysis in children. *Pediatr Pulmonol.* 2004;37:476–484.

[b] Batra PS and Hollinger LD. Etiology and management of pediatric hemoptysis. *Arch Otolaryngol Head Neck Surg.* 2001;127:377–382.

[c] Cross-Bu JA, Sachdeva RC, Bricker JT, Harrison GM, Jefferson LS. Hemoptysis: a 10-year restrospective study. *Pediatrics.* 1997;100(3).

aspiration. This is especially true in children with underlying conditions, such as cystic fibrosis (CF). Bleeding from a tracheotomy is characteristic of airway irritation, which can occur from dried secretions when there is inadequate humidification, minor suction trauma when a suction catheter is placed too deeply in the airway, or mechanical trauma from the tracheotomy tube itself. Airway bleeding from infection may also be related to mucosal irritation.

Increased pressure within the vasculature is another cause of bleeding (see Box 30-1). This is seen in children with congenital heart disease, or congenital vascular anomalies such as arterio-venous malformations. Pulmonary hypertension from any cause can increase the risk for bleeding. Bronchial arteries are under systemic pressure, and bleeding from these vessels may be massive. Hemorrhage into the alveoli is more unusual than other causes of airway bleeding. Alveolar hemorrhage is seen in children with autoimmune disorders, such as Wegener granulomatosis, Henoch-Schönlein purpura, or systemic lupus erythematosus. Fungal infections are more likely than bacterial infections to cause alveolar bleeding. Idiopathic bleeding can occur in pulmonary hemosiderosis.

General Evaluation of a Child With Pulmonary Hemorrhage and Hemoptysis

The first step in evaluating hemoptysis is to determine the site of bleeding. It is important to be aware that bleeding sources occur from the upper airway or gastrointestinal tract, though those processes will not be discussed here. It is helpful to estimate the amount of bleeding because children with large amounts of hemorrhage are likely to need hospitalization and rapid diagnostic and therapeutic intervention.

The physical examination should initially focus on the degree of respiratory distress that is present. This would include the presence of tachypnea or tachycardia as well as any increased work of breathing or fever. Regardless of the etiology of the bleeding, the most common finding on auscultation is crackles. These may be localized in the context of a single focus of bleeding, or can be diffuse if there is a non-focal process such as capillaritis.

It is important to differentiate between a single episode of hemoptysis and repeated, possibly undiagnosed, episodes. Aspects of the history that can be helpful would include evidence of other bleeding problems, recurrent or chronic respiratory symptoms, anemia, skin rash, jaundice, or renal disorders. Individuals with an acute episode of hemoptysis may have evidence of infection, such as fever, malaise, or cough. It is important to ask about foreign travel or use of medications (oral contraceptives, Coumadin, aspirin), which can affect the risk of thrombosis or bleeding. The environmental history may suggest exposures to floods and chronically water-damaged, moldy environments. The social history may suggest risk for abuse.

Imaging and Laboratory Evaluation

Individuals with known underlying processes such as a tracheotomy, bronchiectasis, or congenital heart disease may need only a focused evaluation (Table 30-1). Evaluating hemoptysis in children without underlying cardiorespiratory problems can be more involved (Table 30-2).

Table 30-1. Evaluation of Airway Bleeding in the Setting of a Preexisting Condition

Preexisting Condition	Probable Cause of Bleeding	Evaluation/Treatment
Tracheotomy	Dried secretions	Improve humidification
	Purulent secretions	Culture secretions, antibiotics
	Granulation tissue in airway Mucosal erosion	Ear, nose, throat or pulmonary referral Visualize airway Alter suction protocol Consider new tracheotomy tube size
Cystic fibrosis Bronchiectasis	Infection or exacerbation	Antibiotics, airway clearance
	Coagulopathy	Check clotting studies Vitamin K supplementation
	Central line clot Pulmonary embolism	Ultrasound or dye study to evaluate the line Remove central line Consider anticoagulation
	Massive hemorrhage (>300 mL/day)	Interventional radiology for dye study of the bronchial arteries Embolization of tortuous arteries Decreased airway clearance for a few days
Infection	Bacterial Fungal Tuberculosis Leptospirosis	Sputum culture Chest radiograph Consider bronchoscopy
	Foreign body	Chest radiograph Consider bronchoscopy
Congenital heart disease	Pulmonary hypertension Previous surgical repair Collateral vessels	Chest radiograph Cardiology evaluation, consider echocardiogram or catheterization

Table 30-2. Evaluation of Airway Bleeding in the Absence of Preexisting Conditions

Evaluation	Finding	Possible Diagnosis
History Physical examination	Fever	Infection, autoimmune process
	Weight loss	Autoimmune process
	Skin rash (butterfly, vasculitis)	Autoimmune process
	Skin rash (petechiae)	Infection
	Jaundice	Infection (leptospirosis)
	Nasal or sinus fullness or inflammation	Autoimmune process (Wegener granulomatosis)
	Arthralgias/arthritis	Autoimmune process (systemic lupus erythematosus, Wegener granulomatosis)
	Localized crackles	Can be any process, but may suggest focal infection, foreign body, or idiopathic
	Diffuse crackles	Autoimmune process
Sputum	Blood mixed with purulent sputum	Infection
Chest radiograph	Normal	Bleeding from a different site Foreign body Infection Cleared episode of idiopathic pulmonary hemosiderosis
	Focal	Foreign body Infection Autoimmune Idiopathic
	Diffuse	Autoimmune Idiopathic
Computed tomography scan (chest)	Vascular abnormalities	Arteriovenous abnormalities
	Interstitial prominence	Autoimmune process
	Alveolar filling	Infection Localization of blood
Computed tomography scan (sinus)	Mucosal thickening	Autoimmune process (Wegener granulomatosis)
Urinalysis	Blood or protein	Autoimmune process

Table 30-2. Evaluation of Airway Bleeding in the Absence of Preexisting Conditions (continued)

Evaluation	Finding	Possible Diagnosis
Complete blood cell count	Anemia	Severe or chronic process (autoimmune or idiopathic)
	Elevated white blood cell	Infection
Sedimentation rate, C-reactive protein, antinuclear antibodies, antineutrophil cytoplasmic antibody	Inflammation	Autoimmune process (systemic lupus erythematosus, Wegener granulomatosis, etc)
Bronchoscopy	Localization of bleeding	Infection Foreign body, or endobronchial lesion Mucosal erosion or inflammation Vascular abnormalities
	Bronchoalveolar lavage	Infection Hemosiderin-laden macrophages
	Biopsy of airway lesion	Pathologic diagnosis (care should be taken to be sure that bleeding can be controlled)
Lung biopsy	Capillaritis	Autoimmune processes
	Pulmonary hypertension	Chronic hypoxemia Cardiac disorders Arteriovenous malformation
	Hemosiderin-laden macrophages	Ongoing bleeding, Idiopathic hemosiderosis
Cardiology evaluation (echocardiogram, catheterization)	Congenital heart disease	Unsuspected findings such as cor triatriatum
	Pulmonary hypertension	Chronic hypoxemia Cardiac disorders Arteriovenous malformation

Laboratory evaluation may help determine the cause of bleeding. If the child can expectorate sputum, this can be analyzed for the presence of infection. The complete blood cell count (CBC) can help determine the amount of blood loss and the likelihood of infection. Significant anemia may suggest repeated episodes of bleeding or an acute, severe episode of bleeding. Clotting studies can be helpful to determine whether an underlying coagulopathy, vitamin K deficiency, or medication side effect is present. A chest radiograph may discriminate between focal or diffuse processes, and localize a particular site of bleeding. In some situations, a computed tomography (CT) scan may be helpful to determine whether a focal endobronchial lesion, diffuse interstitial process, or arteriovenous malformation is involved. A bronchoscopy may be important to localize the site of hemorrhage. Cardiac evaluation with either echocardiogram or catheterization may be indicated, especially if there is a history of previous cardiac disease. Ongoing bleeding from tortuous bronchial arteries can be localized and treated with dye studies and embolization of these vessels, usually by an interventional radiologist. In some cases lung biopsy is indicated to determine if there is evidence of capillaritis, immune complex deposition, or pulmonary hypertension. Susarla and Fan[1] suggest considering lung biopsy in any child with diffuse alveolar bleeding of unknown cause.

General Management

Minor amounts of bleeding from infection, airway dehydration, or trauma can often be managed on an outpatient basis if the cause of the bleeding is established and a treatment plan initiated. In the case of significant pneumonia or exacerbation of bronchiectasis, intravenous (IV) antibiotics may be indicated. If the cause of the hemoptysis is unknown, further evaluation with CT scan, bronchoscopy, cardiac assessment, or lung biopsy may be needed. It is important to consider the availability of the studies to determine whether admission or referral to specialists is indicated. Hemoptysis requires a prompt evaluation because of the risk of increased bleeding as well as the sometimes transient nature of the findings. If the cause of the bleeding is not known, it is important to consider the risk of additional, sometimes massive, bleeding in the decision about hospitalization.

Massive hemorrhage can be managed by endotracheal intubation and mechanical ventilation to raise the pressure in the airways. Transfusion of packed red blood cells may be indicated for stabilization of the patient. If tortuous vessels are suspected, embolization of the vessels can promptly stop the bleeding.

Causes of Hemoptysis

Infection

Infection is a frequent cause of hemoptysis. In otherwise healthy children, bacterial infections can cause irritation and friability of the airway mucosa. Bleeding is usually associated with sputum production and is small in volume.

Features of the history and physical examination that suggest an infection include fever, cough, diminished appetite or activity level, jaundice (leptospirosis), or exposure to other sick individuals. There may be localized or diffuse crackles, depending on the extent of the infection.

A CBC count may be helpful in determining the amount of blood loss and the likelihood of infection. A chest radiograph can be helpful in assessing if the lesion is focal, but it can be difficult to distinguish infection from blood in the lungs. A density on chest radiograph that resolves quickly is more likely to be blood than infection.

Treating the infection usually results in resolution of the bleeding. Worldwide, tuberculosis is probably the infection most associated with pulmonary bleeding. Bleeding results from either endobronchial infection or cavitary lesions.

Case Report 30-1

A 19-year-old woman with CF has evidence of moderate lung disease. She has needed IV antibiotics approximately twice yearly. She has been able to continue her daily routine with airway clearance, inhaled bronchodilators, inhaled DNase, and every other month inhaled antibiotics.

She was sitting quietly watching TV when she noticed the abrupt onset of a gurgling sensation in her right upper lung field. She coughed up approximately 1 cup of bright red blood. She was brought to the emergency department, where she had 2 more episodes of massive hemoptysis.

Evaluation included a chest radiograph with a new density in the right upper lobe. Her hematocrit was 29. Her coagulation studies were normal. She was started on bed rest and oxygen and given vitamin K. She was brought to interventional radiology, where an angiogram demonstrated tortuous bronchial arteries in both upper lobes. The radiologist embolized the tortuous vessels, and she was admitted for observation. She continued on bed rest, and airway clearance measures were stopped for 24 hours, then gradually resumed. She was discharged 3 days later with instructions to gradually resume her usual routine.

Cystic Fibrosis and Bronchiectasis

Clinical Features

Cystic fibrosis and non-CF bronchiectasis can be associated with either small or massive amounts of bleeding. Small volumes of blood are seen relatively frequently and are associated with infection and friability of the airway mucosa. As the infection progresses, there can be invasion into the airway with erosion into a bronchial artery. Massive hemoptysis

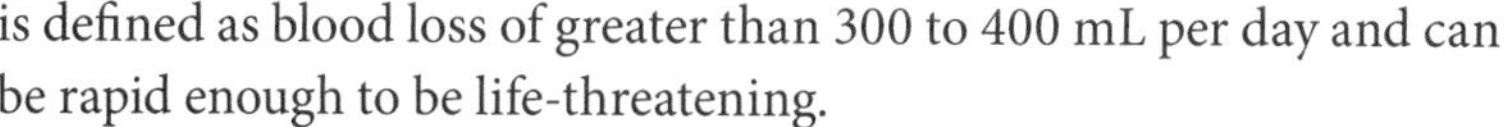

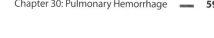

is defined as blood loss of greater than 300 to 400 mL per day and can be rapid enough to be life-threatening.

Evaluation and Imaging

Sputum can be cultured to determine the cause of the infection so appropriate antibiotics are initiated. A new infiltrate on the chest radiograph may help with localization of the bleeding and can help determine if pneumonia is present. Clotting studies can be helpful to determine whether an underlying coagulopathy, vitamin K deficiency, or medication side effect is present. Individuals with CF are at risk for vitamin K deficiency because of the malabsorption of fat-soluble vitamins and for a coagulopathy if there is associated liver disease.

Management

If there is significant bleeding in a child with CF, it may be worth stopping or using less vigorous methods of airway clearance treatments for a day or two to minimize the risk of massive hemoptysis. If a coagulopathy is determined, administering vitamin K can be helpful. If the patient has a central line or has been inactive, the possibility of a thrombus and pulmonary embolism must be considered.

Massive hemoptysis in this setting is usually related to erosion into a bronchial artery. The most definitive treatment of bleeding from tortuous vessels is embolization of the arteries. This is done under fluoroscopy by interventional radiologists. A catheter is introduced into the bronchial arteries from the aorta, and dye is infused to try to isolate the individual bleeding artery, which is then embolized. Many radiologists will embolize any bronchial artery that appears tortuous because of the risk of recurrent bleeding. Although most patients tolerate the procedure well, there are risks of embolizing vessels that may supply other organs, including the spinal cord.

Trauma and Tracheotomy

Clinical Features

Trauma to the airway is a common cause of bleeding. This is particularly true in patients with a tracheotomy. Abrasion of the airway mucosa with either the tip of the tracheotomy tube or suction catheter can cause small amounts of bleeding. Repeated episodes of these abrasions can stimulate the formation of granulation tissue, which can be friable. Bleeding is worsened with dry secretions, and maintaining adequate humidity is critical to controlling bleeding. Humidification of secretions in children with a tracheotomy can be increased with use of a mist collar, Humid-Vent, or frequent nebulized saline treatments. The incidence of massive bleeding in the presence of a tracheotomy may indicate erosion into the mucosa. Rarely, erosion into an anterior innominate artery has caused massive hemoptysis.

Southall et al[2] found evidence of bleeding from the nose or mouth in infants who had been under covert surveillance for evaluation of an apparent life-threatening event that was suspected to be caused by non-accidental suffocation. Child abuse should be considered as a cause of reported hemoptysis in infants in whom no other cause is discovered.

Evaluation and Imaging

Children with a tracheotomy are likely to have localized bleeding in the central airways. If there are small amounts of blood, consider the characteristics of the airway secretions. Thick or discolored secretions may indicate an infection. A chest radiograph may be helpful in determining whether pneumonia is present. Secretions can be cultured to determine the possible role of infection. More massive hemorrhage is often associated with mucosal disruption. Large amounts of blood or persistent bleeding should be evaluated by visualizing the airway mucosa by bronchoscopy. This will identify areas of mucosal disruption, granulation tissue, or erosion into the airway.

Management

Bleeding caused by airway infection will usually respond to antibiotics. Small amounts of blood with suctioning are likely to be related to dehydration of the secretions. It is important to review the humidification and suctioning techniques. The tracheotomy should always have some source of humidification. Acute management of dehydrated secretions can include nebulized or instilled saline. If the child is also on a ventilator, the temperature of the humidification system may need to be adjusted to allow for maximal humidification. Suctioning of the airway should be performed primarily to clear the tracheotomy tube, not the lower airways. Limiting the depth of the suctioning will minimize the risk of damage to the airway mucosa. If granulation tissue has already become established, the child may need surgical evaluation.

Cardiac Abnormalities

Clinical Features

Bleeding related to cardiovascular problems can arise in several situations. A thrombus or pulmonary embolism may occur, especially in the settings of a clotting disorder or the use of oral contraceptives in women. Pulmonary hypertension can be associated with pulmonary hemorrhage, especially if the vessels have become tortuous or collateral vessels have developed.[3] Those who have had surgical repair of congenital heart disease may have leak from aneurysms at the site of the previous repair. In some cases, such as cor triatriatum, the congenital anomaly was not suspected before the hemoptysis.[4] Arteriovenous malformations in the lungs can be a cause of hemorrhage as well.

Evaluation and Imaging

Individuals with known congenital heart disease or pulmonary hypertension require reassessment of the pulmonary vasculature. Chest radiography or CT scan may help localize areas of aneurysms or arteriovenous malformations. These patients are usually seen by a cardiologist, who should be involved in the evaluation and management of the bleeding. Many of these patients will need echocardiogram or catheterization of the vessels to identify possible sites of bleeding.

Management

Medications to decrease the pulmonary hypertension may be helpful, but in some cases surgical intervention is required to stop the bleeding. If pulmonary hypertension is identified in the absence of congenital heart disease, more evaluation to determine possible underlying causes is indicated.

Autoimmune Pulmonary Hemorrhage

Clinical Features

Diffuse alveolar hemorrhage is less common than other forms of pulmonary hemorrhage but can be life-threatening. It can be seen in association with pulmonary capillaritis in such processes as Wegener granulomatosis, microscopic polyangiitis, Goodpasture syndrome, and systemic lupus erythematosus. Other rare causes of capillaritis have included autoimmune hepatitis, Crohn disease, and drug reactions. The cause of disrupted capillaries is frequently autoimmune in nature.

Evidence that the process is chronic includes poor growth and pallor. The presence of a rash suggesting one of the collagen vascular diseases should prompt further autoimmune evaluation, whereas the presence of petechiae leads to evaluation of bleeding disorders or infection. Several of the collagen vascular disorders, which can be associated with pulmonary hemorrhage, especially Wegener granulomatosis and microscopic polyangiitis, are noted for involvement of the nose and sinuses, as well as swelling and inflammation of characteristic joints.[5] Joint involvement is also prominent in children with systemic lupus erythematosus.

Evaluation and Imaging

Evaluation of these autoimmune causes of pulmonary bleeding includes tests to find evidence of autoimmune dysfunction, including CBC count (to look for evidence of chronic anemia), Coombs test (to look for evidence of hemolysis), screening for evidence of renal involvement, and levels of antineutrophil cytoplasmic antibodies (ANCAs). If the bleeding is occult, bronchoalveolar lavage can be used to evaluate for the presence of hemosiderin-laden alveolar macrophages, which would indicate the presence of blood in the airways or alveoli. Many of the collagen vascular disorders have associated renal involvement, so a urinalysis may aid in the diagnosis. Other laboratory evaluations that are useful in diagnosing collagen vascular diseases include sedimentation rate, C-reactive protein, antinuclear antibody, and ANCA (which can be either perinuclear or cytoplasmic patterns). Final diagnosis may require a lung biopsy to confirm disruption of the pulmonary capillaries.[1]

Management

Most of the autoimmune disorders and idiopathic pulmonary hemosiderosis respond to anti-inflammatory medications, though the treatment course may be months or years in duration. These medications may include corticosteroids, cyclophosphamide, azathiaprine, methotrexate, hydroxychloroquin, and IV immunoglobulin. Initial therapy of alveolar hemorrhage with high doses of IV methylprednisolone is usually successful in controlling the bleeding. Susarla and Fan[1] describe

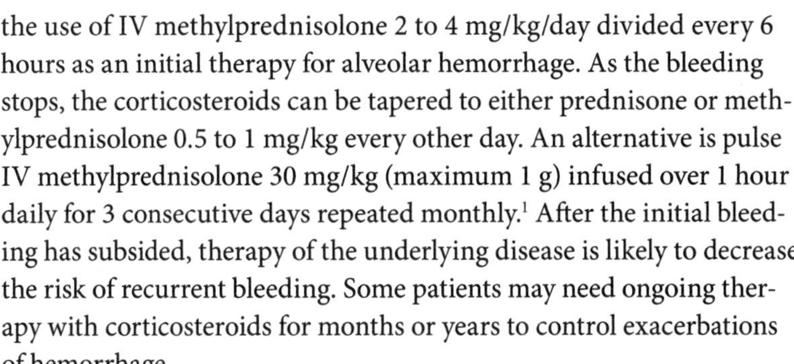

the use of IV methylprednisolone 2 to 4 mg/kg/day divided every 6 hours as an initial therapy for alveolar hemorrhage. As the bleeding stops, the corticosteroids can be tapered to either prednisone or methylprednisolone 0.5 to 1 mg/kg every other day. An alternative is pulse IV methylprednisolone 30 mg/kg (maximum 1 g) infused over 1 hour daily for 3 consecutive days repeated monthly.[1] After the initial bleeding has subsided, therapy of the underlying disease is likely to decrease the risk of recurrent bleeding. Some patients may need ongoing therapy with corticosteroids for months or years to control exacerbations of hemorrhage.

Case Report 30-2

A 10-year-old boy presents with respiratory distress. He was born at 26 weeks' gestation and subsequently diagnosed with bronchopulmonary dysplasia. Although he was discharged from the neonatal intensive care unit at 3 months of age, he developed hypoxemia requiring chronic oxygen therapy at 7 months of age. At the age of 14 months, he had an acute deterioration with respiratory distress and hypoxemia and was admitted to the hospital for evaluation and treatment. Evaluation included

1. Cardiac catheterization, which revealed suprasystemic pulmonary hypertension, right ventricular diastolic dysfunction, significant right pulmonary vein desaturation, atrial septal defect (right-to-left shunting), and diffuse pulmonary interstitial disease.
2. Bronchoscopy, which revealed diffusely hemorrhagic and friable bronchial tissue.

He was treated with intubation and mechanical ventilation. He developed bright red blood from the endotracheal tube and was treated with increased pressure on the ventilator. Lung biopsy revealed changes consistent with pulmonary hemosiderosis. Allergy testing revealed sensitivity to milk, eggs, and peanuts.

He was treated with high-dose IV solumedrol and inhaled nitric oxide. He required numerous transfusions to maintain his hemoglobin. He gradually improved, tapered off inhaled nitric oxide, and was ready for discharge 2 months after admission. Prednisone was tapered over approximately 2 years, and was increased with subsequent viral infections. He has maintained a milk-, egg-, and peanut-free diet. He continues on nighttime oxygen and sildenafil to treat his pulmonary hypertension, but is able to attend school and participate in activities including physical education. He had one episode of subsequent pulmonary hemorrhage, approximately 6 months after his admission, but otherwise has not had evidence of further bleeding.

Idiopathic Pulmonary Hemorrhage and Hemosiderosis

Clinical Features

Idiopathic pulmonary hemorrhage is characterized by alveolar bleeding without the presence of capillaritis. This bleeding tends to be recurrent, and the diagnosis is by exclusion of other causes. Lung biopsy in these patients generally demonstrates erythrocytes and hemosiderin-laden alveolar macrophages, but no inflammation of the capillaries. A subset of children with idiopathic pulmonary hemosiderosis is thought to have cow's milk hypersensitivity (Heiner syndrome).[6] Acute idiopathic pulmonary hemorrhage (AIPH) of infancy is a more acute variation of pulmonary bleeding that was first described in Cleveland associated with indoor exposure to molds, including *Stachybotrys chartarum*.[7] Young infants often present without frank hemoptysis, and the diagnosis can be suspected in the presence of respiratory distress, densities on chest radiographs, and anemia. Although the causal association between exposure to mold and AIPH in infants has not been firmly established, the Cleveland study, additional case series, case reports from independent sources, and basic scientific studies in animal models have provided some evidence of plausibility. Epidemiologic studies suggest that exposure to secondhand cigarette smoke may be an additional risk factor.[8]

Evaluation and Imaging

The appearance of an acute episode of pulmonary hemorrhage on a chest radiograph is similar to pneumonia. However, the infiltrates are more transient and tend to resolve in 1 to 2 days. Repeated testing of hemoglobin and hematocrit can be useful in determining the severity of the bleeding. Many of these children will need bronchoscopy and bronchoalveolar lavage to document the presence of alveolar bleeding. Care should be taken in children with active bleeding because there is some risk of accelerated bleeding after bronchoscopy.

Management

Idiopathic pulmonary hemosiderosis has been associated with a poor prognosis in the past, but aggressive anti-inflammatory therapy has improved this, with recent 5-year survival rates greater than 80%.[1] Milk allergy should be considered and tested for. If present, the children should be instructed to avoid milk protein.

The American Academy of Pediatrics recommends that parents of infants with AIPH try to find and eliminate sources of chronic moisture and mold growth before the child returns to the home. Avoidance of exposure to secondhand cigarette smoke is always recommended, but especially in cases of AIPH.[9]

Other Causes of Hemoptysis

Clinical Features

Malignancy is a common cause of airway bleeding in adults. Although the incidence of airway tumors is much lower in children, between 2% and 6% of children with hemoptysis are found to have masses.[1,10] These include endobronchial lesions such as carcinoid, adenoma, mucoepidermoid tumor, metastases, teratoma, carcinoma, and pseudotumor.[11,12] Some airway lesions, such as carcinoid and hemangioma, are highly vascularized, and caution should be used when obtaining biopsy samples, especially through a flexible bronchoscope.

Obstruction of an airway by an endobronchial lesion will usually produce atelectasis visible on chest radiograph. It is important to differentiate atelectasis from infiltrate by radiography to determine the appropriate evaluation. The presence of an airway obstruction will need further evaluation by CT scan or bronchoscopy. Bronchoscopy will allow differentiation of a foreign body from an airway mass. Determining the cause of the mass will require pathologic evaluation.

The location and pathology of the airway mass will determine the management. Some lesions can be removed through the bronchoscope, but other lesions may require surgical removal of the affected lobe.

Summary

Pulmonary bleeding can arise from a number of causes, ranging in significance from minor irritations and infections to life-threatening hemorrhage. In many cases, the bleeding is related to an underlying condition of the patient and can easily be evaluated and treated. Other times the cause is more elusive and will need careful radiologic, bronchoscopic, and pathologic evaluation to determine the etiology of the bleeding. Evaluation of the child's home is sometimes indicated to assess if it is a water-damaged environment.[13] Treatment begins with stabilization of the patient if necessary. Specific treatment will depend on the cause of the bleeding and may include antibiotics, humidification, cardiac or thoracic surgery, or long-term anti-inflammatory medications.

Key Points

- Stabilize the patient (intubation, transfusion if necessary).
- Identify the location of bleeding.
- Evaluate expected complications of known problems.
  - Tracheotomy, CF, bronchiectasis, congenital heart disease
- Consider new problems.
  - Acute or chronic infection, foreign body aspiration, pulmonary hypertension, pulmonary embolism, or thrombosis
  - Arteriovenous malformation, autoimmune disorder, idiopathic diffuse alveolar hemorrhage
- Diligently work to establish the diagnosis.
  - Evaluate coagulation status, imaging, sputum culture, bronchoscopy, echocardiogram or cardiac catheterization, lung biopsy, autoimmune evaluation
- Treat the underlying condition.
  - Embolization of bronchial arteries for massive bleeding
  - Anti-inflammatory therapy for autoimmune disease

References

1. Susarla SC, Fan LL. Diffuse alveolar hemorrhage syndromes in children. *Curr Opin Pediatr.* 2007;19:314–320
2. Southall DP, Plunkett MCB, Banks MW, Falkov AF, Samuels MP. Covert video recordings of life-threatening child abuse: lessons for child protection. *Pediatrics.* 1997;100:735–760
3. Haroutunian LM, Neill CA. Pulmonary complications of congenital heart disease: hemoptysis. *Am Heart J.* 1972;84:540–549
4. Sritippayawan S, Margetis MF, MacLaughlin EF, et al. Cor triatriatum: a cause of hemoptysis. *Pediatr Pulmonol.* 2002;34:405–408
5. O'Sullivan BP, Erickson LA, Niles JL. Case records of The Massachusetts General Hospital. Weekly clinicopathological exercises. Case 30-2002. An eight-year-old girl with fever, hemoptysis, and pulmonary consolidation. *N Engl J Med.* 2002;347:1009–1017

6. Boat TF, Polmar SH, Whitman V, Kleinerman JI, Stern RC, Doershuk CF. Hyperreactivity to cow milk in young children with pulmonary hemosiderosis and cor pulmonale secondary to nasopharyngeal obstruction. *J Pediatr.* 1975;87:23–29
7. Centers for Disease Control and Prevention. Acute pulmonary hemorrhage/hemosiderosis among infants—Cleveland, January 1993–November 1994. *MMWR Morb Mortal Wkly Rep.* 1994;43:881–883
8. Mazur LJ, Kim J; American Academy of Pediatrics Committee on Environmental Health. Technical report: spectrum of noninfectious health effects from molds. *Pediatrics.* 2006;118:e1909–e1926
9. American Academy of Pediatrics Committee on Environmental Health. Policy statement: spectrum of noninfectious health effects from molds. *Pediatrics.* 2006;118:2582–2586
10. Godfrey S. Hemoptysis in children. *Pediatr Pulmonol Suppl.* 2004;26:177–179
11. Al-Qahtani AR, Di Lorenzo M, Yazbeck S. Endobronchial tumors in children: institutional experience and literature review. *J Pediatr Surg.* 2003;38:733–736
12. Eggli KD, Newman B. Nodules, masses, and pseudomasses in the pediatric lung. *Radiol Clin North Am.* 1993;31:651–666
13. *World Health Organization Guidelines for Indoor Air Quality: Dampness and Mold.* Copenhagen, Denmark: World Health Organization; 2009

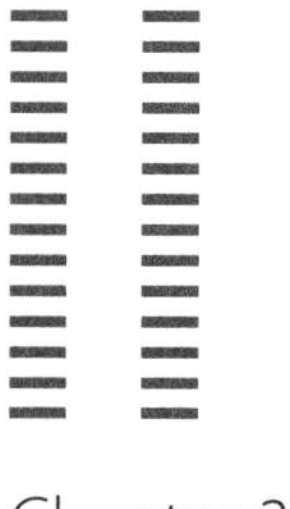

Chapter 31

Apparent Life-Threatening Events

Keyvan Rafei, MD
Carol J. Blaisdell, MD

Case Report 31-1

A 5-month-old infant with cyanosis and hypotonia born at 24 weeks' gestation was on a home cardiorespiratory monitor for apnea and bradycardia of prematurity. A download was ordered by the child's pediatrician and reviewed by a pediatric pulmonologist (Figure 31-1). The tracing demonstrated bradycardia to 48 beats/min (QRS and heart rate signal) that follows shallow breathing on the impedance tracing. This suggested hypoxemia as the cause of the bradycardia, but the finding was not specific, so a polysomnogram was requested by the specialist. The polysomnogram (Figure 31-2) demonstrated a mixed apnea (central for the first 5 seconds, then obstructive apnea) leading to hypoxemia (pulse oximeter dropped to 54%) and bradycardia (rate was 42 beats/min, and electrocardiogram shows slowing of the RR interval). The baby was prescribed supplemental oxygen by the specialist and the bradycardic and obstructive episodes resolved on follow-up review of the cardiorespiratory monitor and by repeat polysomnogram.

Introduction

Apparent life-threatening events (ALTEs) are common and frequently challenging diagnostic dilemmas. Although most evaluations of these patients usually take place in a hospital, primary care physicians will be frequently asked to contribute to various stages of the management of these cases, from initial evaluation of the patient to decisions about long-term monitoring.[1]

The management of a child with an ALTE requires an understanding of commonly accepted definitions, the various potential causes, and

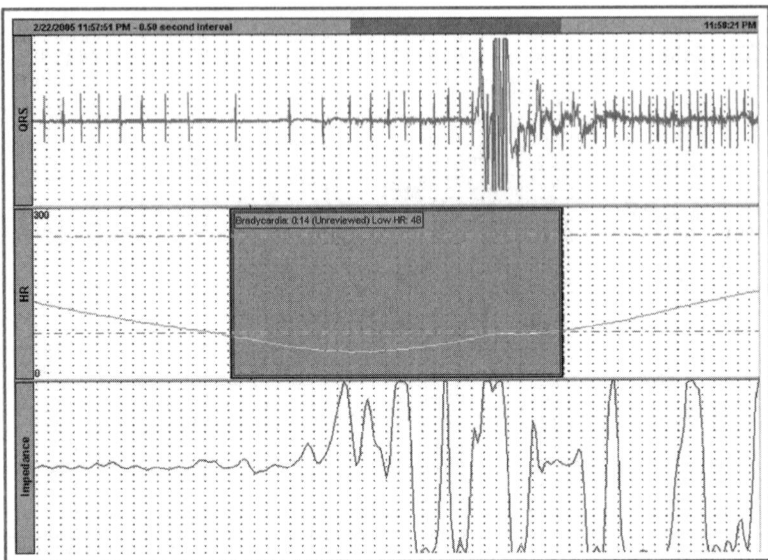

Figure 31-1. Cardiorespiratory monitor tracing from a 5-month-old premature infant with cyanosis and hypotonia. Note QRS tracing, which demonstrates slowing of the RR interval, and bradycardia of 40 beats/min on the heart rate tracing, which follows shallow breathing on the impedance tracing. This tracing suggests hypoxemia as the cause of the bradycardia, but the finding is not specific; thus a polysomnogram was requested.

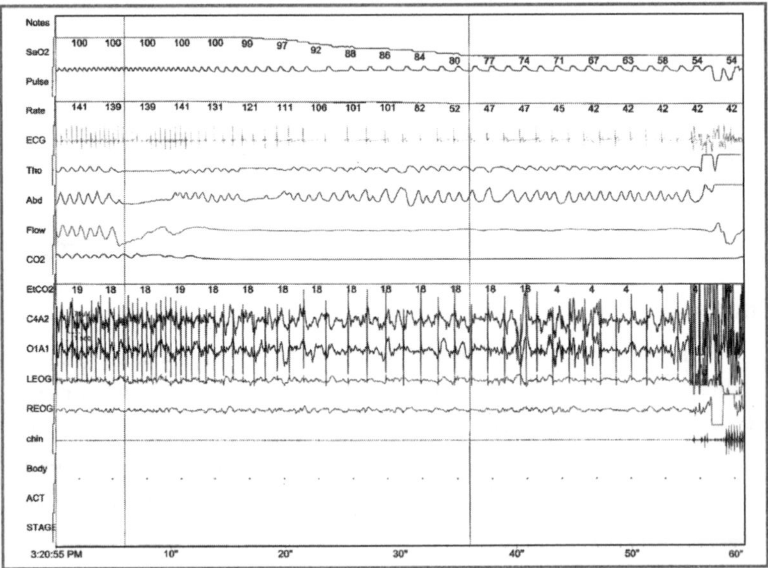

Figure 31-2. Polysomnographic tracing of the same infant as in Figure 31-1 demonstrating a mixed apnea leading to hypoxemia and bradycardia. At the end of this 60-second period, an adult intervenes; note motion artifact, particularly the electroencepalogram channels C4A2 and O1A1 and chin electromyogram channels.

the most appropriate management strategies. In a 1986 National Institutes of Health consensus document,[2] an ALTE was defined as "an episode that is frightening to the observer and is characterized by some combination of apnea, color change, marked change in muscle tone, choking, or gagging" in which, "in some cases, the observer fears that the infant has died."[2] This definition was intended to replace the term aborted crib death or near-miss sudden infant death syndrome (SIDS), which misleadingly implied an association between ALTE and SIDS.[2] Other important definitions of concepts related to ALTE are listed in Box 31-1. Most notably, pathologic apnea is defined as "a respiratory pause that is prolonged, lasting 20 seconds or longer, or is associated with cyanosis, pallor, hypotonia or bradycardia."[2] In contrast, periodic breathing, which is commonly noted in young infants, is "a breathing pattern in which there are 3 or more respiratory pauses of greater than 3 seconds' duration with less than 20 seconds of respiration between pauses."[2]

Box 31-1. Definitions of Breathing Patterns and Concepts Related to Apparent Life-Threatening Events (ALTEs)

Periodic Breathing
A breathing pattern in which there are 3 or more respiratory pauses of >3 seconds' duration with <20 seconds of respiration between pauses

Apnea
Cessation of respiratory airflow. Apnea may be central, obstructive, or mixed.

Pathologic Apnea
Respiratory pause that is prolonged (20 seconds) or associated with cyanosis, pallor, hypotonia, or bradycardia.

Apnea of Infancy
Unexplained episodes of pathologic apnea with onset at >37 weeks' gestational age in infants for whom no specific cause of ALTE can be identified.

Apnea of prematurity
Periodic breathing with pathologic apnea in a premature infant.

Sudden Infant Death Syndrome
Sudden death of any infant that is unexplained by history and by postmortem and death scene examination.

From National Institutes of Health.[2]

Case Report 31-2

A distraught mother brings her 3-month-old son for evaluation. She describes an episode in which her son turned blue and became limp. A health care worker by training, she relates how she provided rescue breathing before coming to the hospital. A similar episode occurred twice before and required the infant to be hospitalized once. The infant is again hospitalized for further evaluation. Initial diagnostic studies, including a complete blood count, urinalysis, chest radiograph, electrocardiogram, and upper gastrointestinal series, are all normal. A computed tomography scan of the head is obtained and reveals a left temporoparietal subdural hematoma. A subsequent skeletal survey reveals multiple healing rib fractures with callus formation. Child abuse was suspected, and child protective services was contacted for further investigation.

Prevalence

The exact frequency and prevalence of ALTEs are unknown due to difficulties in classifying the subjective and heterogeneous nature of presenting symptoms and discharge diagnosis.[3] Rates have been estimated as 0.21% of all children and 0.6% of all patients younger than 1 year seeking care at an emergency department (ED) or as 9.4 per 1,000 live births.[4–6] Recurrence rates for ALTEs vary from 0% to 24%.[7]

The median age of presentation of infants with an ALTE ranges between 7 and 8 weeks of age; sex distribution is relatively equal.[4,5,8] Approximately one-third of patients with an ALTE had a history of prematurity, and 19% had a history of a previous ALTE. The morbidity and mortality resulting from an ALTE vary by the underlying diagnosis; the mortality of infants with apnea of infancy ranges between 0% and 6%.[2,7]

ALTE and SIDS

Strong epidemiologic evidence suggests that ALTEs and SIDS are not related.[1,3,9] The average age of patients with an ALTE is 1 to 3 months younger than infants who die of SIDS, and ALTEs generally occur during the day and while sleeping supine. Moreover, while SIDS mortality rates markedly decreased between 1986 and 1994, the incidence for ALTEs did not change significantly.[6]

Despite the lack of an epidemiologic association between SIDS and ALTEs, it is important to note that a very small minority of ALTEs do go on to have SIDS and that a small minority of SIDS deaths had a preceding ALTE.[2,10]

Diagnosis

Because an ALTE describes a subjective report of a clinical syndrome rather than a specific diagnosis, a variety of different disorders can lead to an episode.[1,2] The most common types of problems associated with an ALTE are gastrointestinal, neurologic, respiratory, cardiovascular, metabolic, and endocrine in nature.[3] Most common specific diagnoses associated with ALTEs include gastroesophageal reflux (31%), seizures (11%), and lower respiratory tract infections (8%), although many different diagnoses have been recorded.[7] Up to 50% of cases of ALTEs remain unexplained and are considered idiopathic.[2,3]

Although gastroesophageal reflux (GER) is the diagnosis most often associated with an ALTE, its precise role in these cases is debated. A relationship between apnea and GER disease (GERD) has been posited, but a definite causal relationship has not been demonstrated.[11,12] Although GERD can lead to an ALTE in certain infants, the frequency of GERD in the general population should caution the clinician in assuming a causal relationship when it is discovered in an infant with a history of an ALTE.[13]

Neurologic and respiratory disorders are the second and third most commonly associated diagnoses in patients with an ALTE. The most common specific diagnoses are seizures in the former category, and pertussis and respiratory syncytial virus infection in the latter group.[4,7] Other important but less common diagnoses in infants with an ALTE include urinary tract infections, inborn errors of metabolism, cardiac arrhythmias, brain tumor, persistent ductus arteriosus, and opioid-related apnea.[4,7]

Child abuse (non-accidental trauma and suffocation) and factitious illness (Munchausen syndrome by proxy) may account for up to 11% of unexplained ALTEs.[14] (See Box 31-2.) All pediatric providers should be aware of the potential relationship, trained to recognize the historical features and physical examination findings, and have a systematic approach to screen all ALTE patients for abuse.[15]

Box 31-2: Signs of Intentional Suffocation

When a death occurs in an infant with a prior history of apparent life-threatening event (ALTE), the following circumstances should indicate the possibility of intentional suffocation:

- Previous recurrent cyanosis, apnea, or ALTE while in the care of the same person
- Age at death older than 6 months
- Previous unexpected or unexplained deaths of one or more siblings
- Simultaneous or nearly simultaneous death of twins
- Previous death of infants under the care of the same unrelated person
- Discovery of blood on the infant's nose or mouth in association with ALTEs

From Stirling J; American Academy of Pediatrics Committee on Child Abuse and Neglect.[15]

Evaluation

Most patients will be discharged from the ED or hospital without a *specific* diagnosis or with a self-limited condition not requiring treatment. However a minority may have one of a vast array of occult disorders that can lead to significant morbidity or mortality if not identified. No single accepted standard exists for evaluating these events, but a stepwise approach beginning with a detailed history and physical examination is most prudent.[4,5,7,8] A thorough clinical assessment is more likely than an array of diagnostic studies to lead to a diagnosis of the underlying problem.[8] The selection of any diagnostic studies and the extent and duration of observation should be based on the findings of the clinical assessment and not on an undirected battery of tests.[16,17]

Seeking a detailed history and description of the infant at the time of the ALTE is particularly important because most infants appear normal by the time of the evaluation.[4,5,8] Important historical questions to address are listed in Box 31-3. A complete history should include a review of the patient's medical and family history, a description of the patient's living conditions, descriptions of events immediately before and during the ALTE, and prior history or family history of SIDs or ALTEs.[3] All patients should be screened for risk factors for child abuse.

Even though most infants with an ALTE are found to be normal at the time of the initial evaluation, a detailed physical examination is essential to uncover any clues to the underlying cause. The clinician should pay particular attention to neurologic, respiratory, and cardiac abnormalities that may account for the infant's symptoms, noting any

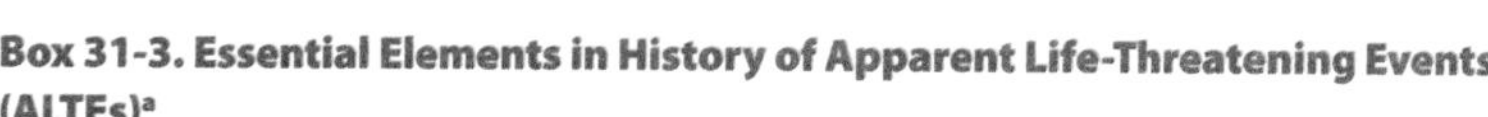

Box 31-3. Essential Elements in History of Apparent Life-Threatening Events (ALTEs)[a]

Personal and Family History

- Perinatal history
  - Full-term or premature birth
  - Pregnancy or perinatal complications
- Medical and surgical history
  - Previous evaluations and treatments
  - Prior hospitalizations
  - Medications
- Sleep and feeding habits
  - Breastfeeding vs bottle feeding
  - Usual amount and frequency of feedings
  - Usual behavior and temperament
- Family history
  - Siblings with ALTE, sudden infant death syndrome, or early death
  - Family history of genetic, metabolic, cardiac, or neurologic problems
- Parental/caretaker history
  - Smoking or drinking habits
  - Recent medical problems and treatments

Daily Life Conditions

- Usual sleep conditions
  - Sleep position when placed down for sleep and when found
  - Sleeping attire
  - Bedding materials
- Other conditions
  - Clothing
  - Room temperature
  - Use of pacifiers

Events Immediately Preceding the ALTE

- Recent fever or illness
- Medications of the infant and others in the home
- Immunizations
- Sleep deprivation
- Change in daily life routine

Box 31-3. Essential Elements in History of Apparent Life-Threatening Events (ALTEs)[a] (continued)

Description of the ALTE

- Place and time
  - Exact place in which ALTE occurred (eg, child's bed, parent's bed, parent's arms, bathroom, sofa, car)
  - Time of event
  - Time since last feeding
  - The estimated time to recover from the ALTE
  - Estimated duration of event
- Witnesses and interventions
  - Who discovered and/or witnessed the ALTE
  - Reason that led to the discovery of the ALTE (noise, unusual cry)
  - Any interventions performed (gentle stimulation, shaking, cardiopulmonary resuscitation)
  - Child's response to the intervention
- Description of infant during ALTE
  - State of infant when event began—asleep or awake
  - If asleep
    - ≈ Child's body position
    - ≈ Type of bedding
    - ≈ Face covered or free
  - If awake
    - ≈ Was child being fed, handled, crying, being bathed?
  - Child's appearance when found
    - ≈ Consciousness
    - ≈ Muscle tone
    - ≈ Color
    - ≈ Respiratory effort
    - ≈ Choking
    - ≈ Gasping
    - ≈ Emesis
    - ≈ Sweating
    - ≈ Limb or eye movements
    - ≈ Pupil size
    - ≈ Skin or rectal temperature

[a] Adapted from Kahn A. Recommended clinical evaluation of infants with an apparent life-threatening event. Consensus document of the European Society for the Study and Prevention of Infant Death, 2003. *Eur J Pediatr.* 2004;163(2):108–115, with permission from Springer Science + Business Media.

evidence for physiological compromise (eg, mental status changes, cyanosis, apnea).[3–5] Physical examination features for child abuse, such as unexplained bruising, bleeding, or petechiae of the face, should be noted.[7,13,15] No minimal standard set of diagnostic studies to evaluate infants with an ALTE have been developed.[3,8] Although a detailed history of the event and the physical examination of the infant frequently result in finding a suspected cause for the ALTE, laboratory testing may be a useful adjunct to confirm the diagnosis.[8] In infants younger than 12 months the basis of the diagnosis can be found in 21% of patients by only history and physical examination.[8] With no additional information gained from laboratory testing, the yield of diagnostic testing can be low (only 2.5%).[5] Therefore, using the findings of the history and physical examination is important to direct appropriate diagnostic testing.[8]

A greater challenge is presented by infants without suggestive findings at the initial history and physical examination. When selecting diagnostic studies for this group, an important point to remember is that the yield of most studies is low, and even if a positive result is found, the question of a causal relationship still remains.[7,8]

To evaluate infants with an ALTE the focus must first be on identifying emergent and life-threatening causes, then extending the evaluation to additional studies if no answers are found. Box 31-4 lists the

Box 31-4: Evaluating an Infant Who Experienced an ALTE

The initial basic set of tests that might be considered in infants with no identified cause after initial clinical assessment includes

- Complete blood count
- Urinalysis
- Electrocardiogram
- Chest radiograph
- Blood culture
- Urine culture

Additional studies that might be considered after an initial period of observation[3,4,7,8] include

- Polysomnogram or pneumogram
- Esophogram and gastroesophageal reflux study
- Modified barium swallow study
- Neuroimaging
- Metabolic studies
- Tests for respiratory pathogens as indicated

evaluations that may be considered. These studies may not be available in all hospitals, and a pediatric specialist may need to be consulted to interpret the results of the tests.

More than half of the time, when evaluating the ALTE, the result leads to the diagnosis of GERD.[8] However, this diagnosis likely includes common choking episodes following emesis or reflux of stomach contents. Such an event is a mixed obstructive event, which is self-limited and does not require further workup or treatment. Further evaluation may be indicated in less common events of "silent" reflux followed by central apnea or aspiration requiring intervention. The upper gastrointestinal (UGI) series is not recommended to diagnose GERD because GER is present in most infants.[18] In rare circumstances a UGI series may be used to identify intestinal obstruction (eg, volvulus, gastric outlet obstruction) or congenital esophageal abnormalities (eg, tracheoesophageal fistula, vascular rings) that contribute to GERD. If GERD is the suspected cause for an ALTE, then a 24-hour pH probe or milk scan by technicum-99m is preferable; however, up to 89% of infants with an ALTE may have a positive milk scan but only 41% of these infants have a correlating clinical diagnosis.[4] This circumstance highlights the problem of exhaustively testing all infants if the clinical history or physical examination is not suggestive of a diagnosis. If enough tests are performed, especially when the index of suspicion is low, then the increasing likelihood of false-positive results will diminish the diagnostic use of these studies and unnecessarily increase the risk for iatrogenic complications.

When the history and physical examination do not suggest a probable diagnosis for an ALTE, the following studies or interventions are often considered: white blood cell count and blood culture, urinalysis and culture, cerebral spinal fluid analysis and culture, viral antigen and pertussis testing, chest radiograph, neuroimaging, and polysomnography (PSG). The risk compared to the benefit of routine testing in this population is unknown. However, a single center study looking at hospitalized patients showed that for many tests the likelihood of a positive result was low and the likelihood of a contributory result was even lower.[19] Routine testing may be warranted in higher-risk groups. For example, a single center study of infants younger than 2 months and with a history of prematurity does suggest occult urinary tract infection (UTI), bacteremia, and pertussis of 2.7%.[20]

Because many patients with child abuse can present with ALTE, a high index of suspicion should be maintained, especially when the history and physical examination do not indicate a likely cause. Although there is little evidence to suggest routine testing in this population, the clinician should judiciously consider a dilated fundoscopic examination, neuroimaging, toxicology screen, and skeletal survey.

Seizures may account for 5% of ALTEs, and one 5-year follow-up study showed that up to 3.6% of all patients with an ATLE will go on to develop epilepsy; however, routine neurology workup is not indicated in these patients unless traumatic brain injury is suspected.[14,21] Without suggestive findings in the history or physical examination, the results of tests of chemistries, cerebrospinal fluid, nasopharyngeal aspirates, echocardiogram, and electrocardiogram will likely be unrevealing.[19]

Management

There is no evidence to support routine hospitalization of all patients with ALTEs. The decision to hospitalize infants should be guided by the findings of the initial assessment along with some special consideration for higher-risk groups (including whether or not there is a responsible adult in the home who has CPR training). One study from a tertiary care pediatric hospital showed little benefit in routine hospital admission in patients older than 1 month and where there is no clear etiology and the infant is well appearing after ED evaluation.[3] In another study from an ED, 2.7% of afebrile infants younger than 2 months with a history of prematurity had bacteremia, UTI, or pertussis.[20] However, if it is not the first episode, it requires intense stimulation from a reliable provider, or when the initial physical examination reveals something abnormal, then hospitalization with continuous cardiorespiratory (CR) monitoring and further evaluation are more likely to be beneficial.[3,7] The hospital environment may help document recurrent ALTEs, provide time for test results to return, and reveal social concerns indicative of child abuse. For example, continuous CR monitoring with pulse oximetry may detect apnea, bradycardia, and hypoxemia. It is important to note that typical apnea settings of 20 seconds on a CR monitor may miss clinically relevant respiratory pauses (<20 sec), obstructive and mixed apnea events that lead to hypoxemia, and/or bradycardia. Documentation of apnea, bradycardia, and hypoxemia events in the hospital setting should warrant further evaluation and consultation with a pulmonary specialist. The benefit to hospitalization must also be weighed against unintended consequences, such as increasing parental anxiety, risk for nosocomial infections, and unnecessary testing or use of hospital resources. If the witnessed event or a review of the history suggests severe CR compromise, then the infant should be admitted to an intensive care unit. Treatment directed at the underlying diagnosis determined by the evaluation should be started—for example, antibiotics for suspected bacterial infection, anticonvulsants for an infant with seizures, and medications for GERD.

Routine PSG is unnecessary but may contribute to a diagnosis in cases where there was significant respiratory compromise, concern for central apnea, and anatomical abnormalities of the head and neck, or when there has been more than one ALTE. At institutions where PSG is not available, home equipment companies may arrange for the data acquisition of respiratory and cardiac events by using a pneumogram, which an outside consultant reviews. Pneumograms are unattended studies that collect data on respiratory effort by using a thoracic impedance monitor, nasal flow, oxygenation, and cardiac rhythm but not sleep staging, carbon dioxide signal, or abdominal effort. More technical artifacts exist from pneumograms because no technician adjusts the leads and maintains adequate signal quality. Because the PSG is more informative, pneumograms should be limited to medical centers where PSG is unavailable.

In preparation for discharge home, parents and other caregivers should be taught safe sleeping tips and counseled on CPR. While parents are often anxious after witnessing an ALTE, the American Academy of Pediatrics (AAP) policy on SIDS stresses the hazards of adults sleeping with an infant in the same bed due to the potential for accidental suffocation.[10] Co-sleeping should be discouraged because the safest place for an infant to sleep is in a crib in the parents' room for the first 6 months of life. In severe cases requiring CPR or where apneas were demonstrated during hospitalization, especially where there is not a clear etiology, home cardiorespiratory monitoring may help determine when the events have resolved and provide reassurance for the family. The AAP policy statement on apnea, SIDS, and home monitoring notes that an indication for home monitoring may include infants who have had an ALTE.[9] An important point to remember is that episodes of periodic breathing and obstructive apnea events will not be captured on home CR monitoring unless a secondary effect of these events on heart rate occurs (Figure 31-3). The CR monitor results should be reviewed by a practitioner or specialist who is trained in their review, and the physician should establish a specific plan for periodic review. In most cases, results should be reviewed monthly if the guardian has no concerns about the baby or sooner if the guardian reports one or more significant events. The Collaborative Home Infant Monitoring Evaluation study group suggested that healthy term and premature infants may have apnea events and that these events become rare by 43 weeks' postmenstrual age.[16] Monitoring may be discontinued once no further physiologically significant events have occurred and home monitoring shows no further objective evidence of pathologic events for at least 6 weeks. If obstructive apnea is identified as a cause for an ALTE, then repeat PSG may be necessary to determine when and if intervention is needed.

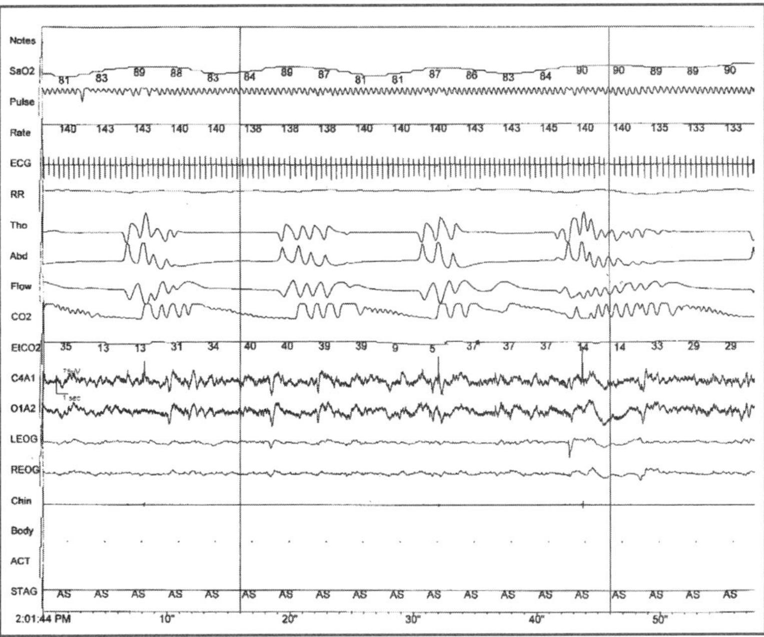

Figure 31-3. Polysomnographic tracing of a 3-month-old infant with hypoxemia. This infant has brief pauses in series (periodic breathing) that lead to hypoxemia.

Long-term outcomes for infants with an unexplained ALTE are unpredictable. Infants with a severe event who require resuscitation and experience a recurrent ALTE or a seizure disorder have a more than 25% risk of death.[17] However, other studies have reported normal cognitive and behavior outcomes up to 10 years after an ALTE.[19]

When to Refer

- When home CR monitoring is considered after a severe event requiring CPR
- Suspected seizure disorder
- Suspected hypoxemia or hypercarbia
- Suspected central, obstructive, or mixed apnea
- Suspected cardiac dysrhythmia
- Vascular ring identified
- Congenital craniofacial anomalies with suspected obstructive apnea
- Evidence of child abuse
- Atypical manifestation

When to Admit

- History of prematurity
- Witnessed apnea and oxygen desaturation and/or bradycardia by medical staff
- Age younger than 2 months
- Family history of SIDS
- Suspected child abuse
- Multiple ALTEs
- Suspicion for central apnea

Key Points

- An ALTE is a common, nonspecific disorder of the young infant that is usually self-limited, although rarely it is a symptom of a potentially serious and life-threatening disorder.
- By understanding the definition, and by eliciting a complete history and performing a thorough physical examination, the physician can focus on determining the best laboratory and imaging studies to diagnose the underlying cause of the event.
- A period of observation with CR monitoring in the hospital may be beneficial to gather additional information and direct appropriate diagnostic studies if a benign cause is not evident.
- Education and guidance should be provided to the guardian, with monitoring in the home setting after hospitalization to detect the infrequent recurrence of ALTEs.
- Providers should have a high index of suspicion of child abuse.

AAP Policy Statements

American Academy of Pediatrics Committee on Fetus and Newborn. Apnea, sudden infant death syndrome, and home monitoring. *Pediatrics.* 2003;111(4):914–917. http://www.aappolicy.aappublications.org/cgi/content/full/pediatrics;111/4/914

Hymel KP; American Academy of Pediatrics Committee on Child Abuse and Neglect; National Association of Medical Examiners. Distinguishing sudden infant death syndrome from child abuse fatalities. *Pediatrics.* 2006;118(1):421–427. http://aappolicy.aappublications.org/cgi/content/ full/pediatrics;118/1/421

Suggested Resources

American Academy of Pediatrics Committee on Fetus and Newborn. Apnea, sudden infant death syndrome, and home monitoring. *Pediatrics.* 2003;111(4 pt 1):914–917

National Institutes of Health. Consensus Development Conference on Infantile Apnea and Home Monitoring, September 29 to October 1, 1986. *Pediatrics.* 1987;79(2):292–299

Ramanathan R, Corwin MJ, Hunt CE, et al. Cardiorespiratory events recorded on home monitors: comparison of healthy infants with those at increased risk for SIDS. *JAMA.* 2001;285(17):2199–2207

References

1. American Academy of Pediatrics Task Force on Prolonged Infantile Apnea. Prolonged infantile apnea: 1985. *Pediatrics.* 1985;76(1):129–131
2. National Institutes of Health. Infantile apnea and home monitoring. *Natl Inst Health Consens Dev Conf Consens Statement.* 1986;6(6):1–10
3. Kahn A. Recommended clinical evaluation of infants with an apparent life-threatening event. Consensus document of the European Society for the Study and Prevention of Infant Death, 2003. *Eur J Pediatr.* 2004;163(2): 108–115
4. Davies F, Gupta R. Apparent life threatening events in infants presenting to an emergency department. *Emerg Med J.* 2002;19(1):11–16
5. De Piero AD, Teach SJ, Chamberlain JM. ED evaluation of infants after an apparent life-threatening event. *Am J Emerg Med.* 2004;22(2):83–86
6. Mitchell EA, Thompson JM. Parental reported apnea, admissions to hospital and sudden infant death syndrome. *Acta Paediatr.* 2001;90(4):417–422
7. McGovern MC, Smith MB. Causes of apparent life threatening events in infants: a systematic review. *Arch Dis Child.* 2004;89(11):1043–1048
8. Brand DA, Altman RL, Purtill K, et al. Yield of diagnostic testing in infants who have had an apparent life-threatening event. *Pediatrics.* 2005;115(4):885–893
9. American Academy of Pediatrics Committee on Fetus and Newborn. Apnea, sudden infant death syndrome, and home monitoring. *Pediatrics.* 2003;111(4 pt 1):914–917
10. American Academy of Pediatrics Task Force on Sudden Infant Death Syndrome. The changing concept of sudden infant death syndrome: diagnostic coding shifts, controversies regarding the sleeping environment, and new variables to consider in reducing risk. *Pediatrics.* 2005;116(5):1245–1255
11. Ariagno RL, Guilleminault C, Baldwin R, et al. Movement and gastroesophageal reflux in awake term infants with "near miss" SIDS, unrelated to apnea. *J Pediatr.* 1982;100(6):894–897
12. Mousa H, Woodley FW, Metheney M, et al. Testing the association between gastroesophageal reflux and apnea in infants. *J Pediatr Gastroenterol Nutr.* 2005;41(2):169–177
13. Arad-Cohen N, Cohen A, Tirosh E. The relationship between gastroesophageal reflux and apnea in infants. *J Pediatr.* 2000;137(3):321–326

14. Bonkowsky JL, Guenther E, Filloux FM, Srivastava R. Death, child abuse, and adverse neurological outcome of infants after an apparent life-threatening event. *Pediatrics.* 2008;122:125–131
15. Stirling J; American Academy of Pediatrics Committee on Child Abuse and Neglect. Beyond Munchausen syndrome by proxy: identification and treatment of child abuse in a medical setting. *Pediatrics.* 2007;119(5):1026
16. Altman RL, Li KI, Brand DA. Infections and apparent life-threatening events. *Clin Pediatr (Phila).* 2008;47(4):372–378
17. Genizi J, Pillar G, Ravid S, Shahar E. Apparent life-threatening events: neurological correlates and the mandatory work-up. *J Child Neurol.* 2008;23(11):1305–1307
18. Vandenplas Y, Rudolph CD, DiLorenzo C, et al. Pediatric gastroesophageal reflux clinical practice guidelines: joint recommendations of the North American Society for Pediatric Gastroenterology, Hepatology, and Nutrition (NASPGHAN) and the European Society for Pediatric Gastroenterology, Hepatology, and Nutrition (ESPGHAN). *J Pediatr Gastroenterol Nutr.* 2009;49:498–547
19. Brand DA, Altman RL, Purtill K, et al. Yield of diagnostic testing in infants who have had an apparent life-threatening event. *Pediatrics.* 2005;115(4):885–893 [erratum in: *Pediatrics.* 2005;116(3):802–803]
20. Zuckerbraun NS, Zomorrodi A, Pitetti RD. Occurrence of serious bacterial infection in infants aged 60 days or younger with an apparent life-threatening event. *Pediatr Emerg Care.* 2009;25:19–25
21. Bonkowsky JL, Guenther E, Srivastava R, Filloux FM. Seizures in children following an apparent life-threatening event. *J Child Neurol.* 2009;24:709–713

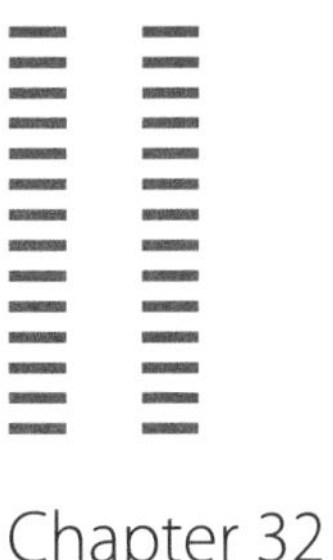

Chapter 32

Aspiration (Foreign Body, Food, Chemical)

John Colombo, MD
Paul H. Sammut, MD

Introduction

Aspiration of materials that are foreign to the lower respiratory tract is associated with considerable illness seen in the typical pediatric practice, both in terms of prevalence and severity of illness. Aspiration may also occur in healthy children and adults, and may be clinically undetectable. Aspiration often produces acute life-threatening situations, including massive aspiration of gastric contents, hydrocarbons, or foreign bodies. Dysphagia with aspiration is reportedly the most common cause of recurrent pneumonia, resulting in hospitalization of children with this condition.[1] The 3 major types of aspiration lung disease are (1) airway foreign body, (2) massive aspiration, and (3) recurrent small volume aspiration. While infectious consequences may develop secondary to any of the above events, infectious pneumonias will be discussed elsewhere in this manual.

Airway Foreign Body—Mechanical Obstruction

Aspiration of foreign bodies is a relatively common event in children, most commonly in those aged 1 to 3 years, but it occurs in all age groups. The incidence is up to 2-fold higher in boys. Food is the most commonly aspirated material in toddlers, whereas small nonedible objects are more common in older children (Box 32-1). Most children who aspirate a foreign body have a sudden onset of symptoms, and in a significant proportion (≥25%) the parents are not aware of any aspiration or choking event.[2,3] There is often an asymptomatic period after the choking spell once the foreign body becomes lodged in the lower tracheobronchial tree.

Case Report 32-1

A 20-month-old boy had a sudden onset of choking and coughing while his mother was on the telephone in the next room. The cough continued throughout the next 24 hours, and he developed intermittent wheezing for which she took him to the pediatrician. He had a prior history of wheezing with respiratory syncytial virus (RSV) at age 6 months. She was not aware of any potential foreign bodies in his environment. On examination he was afebrile with a respiratory rate of 36 breaths/min, mild suprasternal retractions, and an oxygen saturation of 98%. Lung auscultation revealed a monophonic expiratory wheeze, which was transmitted equally throughout the chest. Chest radiograph showed mild bilateral hyperinflation without infiltrates. He was referred to surgery for evaluation for rigid bronchoscopy. Tracheal foreign body was suspected from the history and physical examination.

Clinical Presentation

The most common presentation of a child who has aspirated is a history that includes a choking event followed by acute cough, but parents will often not associate an acute short coughing event with a foreign body. A careful history should attempt to elicit the details surrounding the beginning of a cough. Transient or persistent cough is the primary symptom in approximately 75% of children with airway foreign bodies. Physical findings may reveal observation of asymmetrical chest expansion, decreased breath sounds over the affected lung, and localized wheezing, but may be normal. However, a tracheal foreign body is more likely associated with bilateral wheezing, usually monophonic in nature.

Box 32-1. Foreign Bodies Commonly Aspirated by Children

Food
- Peanuts
- Popcorn
- Seeds
- Hot dogs
- Vegetable material

Nonorganic
- Toy parts
- Pen pieces
- Pins
- Crayons
- Tacks
- Nails
- Screws

Diagnosis

A plain chest radiograph, carefully reviewed, is often highly indicative of either radiopaque or radiolucent foreign bodies (Figure 32-1). Most foreign bodies are radiolucent, thus indirect evidence must usually be relied on. An expiratory film is particularly helpful in demonstrating air trapping on the affected side from a ball-valve effect, although tracheal or bilateral foreign bodies will not likely cause asymmetrical findings (Figure 32-2). Atelectasis may be a later finding. However, a normal chest radiograph does not exclude an airway foreign body. A normal radiograph is particularly common for tracheal; laryngeal; and smaller, more distal foreign bodies.[2] If the physical examination and a plain radiograph are not diagnostic, fluoroscopy, inspiratory and expiratory films, or bilateral decubitus films (particularly in the uncooperative young child) may be helpful, although recent reviews of a decubitus radiograph and fluoroscopy found them of limited predictive value for airway foreign body.[3,4]

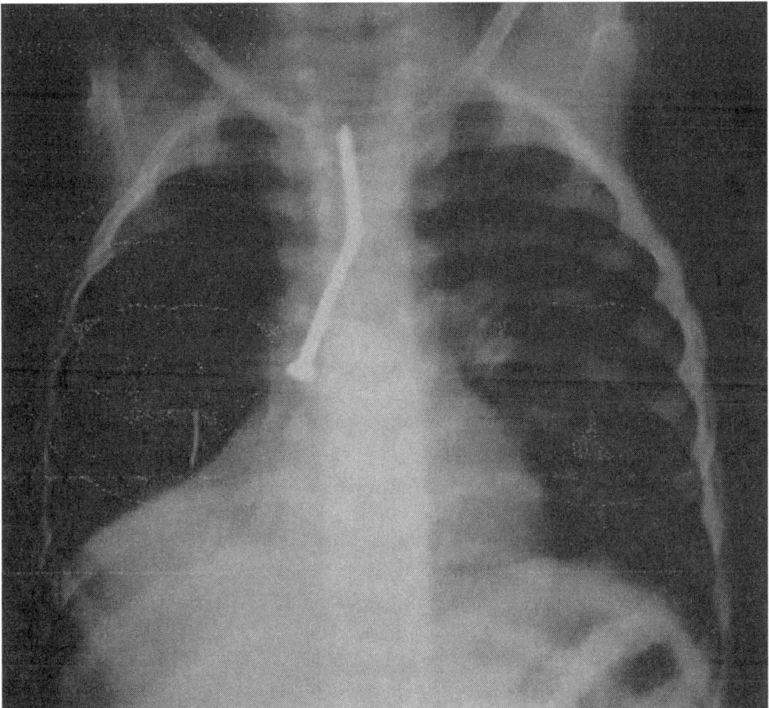

Figure 32-1. Nail lodged in the trachea and right mainstem bronchus.

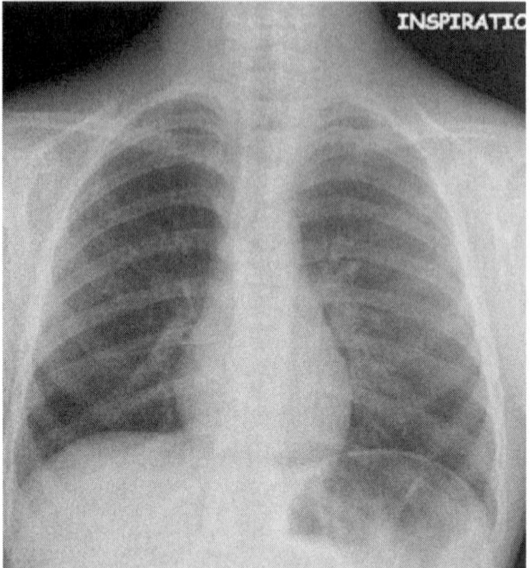

A

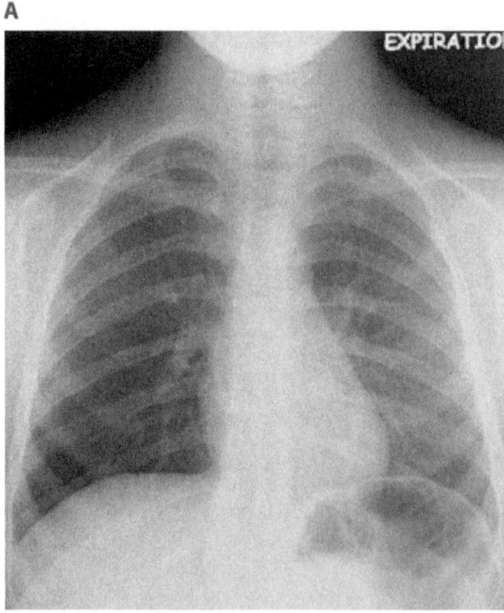

B

Figure 32-2. (A) Inspiratory and **(B)** expiratory chest radiographs with right bronchus intermedius foreign body, demonstrating ball-valve effect with right-sided air trapping on expiratory film.

Low-dose multidetector computed tomography (CT) and virtual bronchoscopy have been used to investigate suspected foreign body aspirations[5]; however, these are probably more useful in detecting residual foreign bodies after bronchoscopies[6] (Figure 32-3.)

Management

If complete airway obstruction occurs with a witnessed choking event, abdominal thrusts (Heimlich maneuver) are indicated for children older than 1 year. For infants younger than 1 year, chest thrusts and back blows in the head-down position are recommended. If a foreign body is likely based on the history, examination, or radiographs, rigid bronchoscopy should be performed as soon as safely possible to prevent possible dislodgement into a more central and potentially life-threatening position in the airway; reduce local inflammation making the foreign body more difficult to remove; and reduce parenchymal lung complications, including pneumothorax, atelectasis, and bronchiectasis. Small distal foreign bodies may require special instrumentation and sometimes fiberoptic bronchoscopy. If the diagnosis is unlikely to be foreign body, flexible bronchoscopy can confirm this, provide another diagnosis, and sometimes avoid the need for more invasive rigid bronchoscopy. Rarely a thoracotomy with bronchotomy may be necessary to remove a highly embedded foreign body.

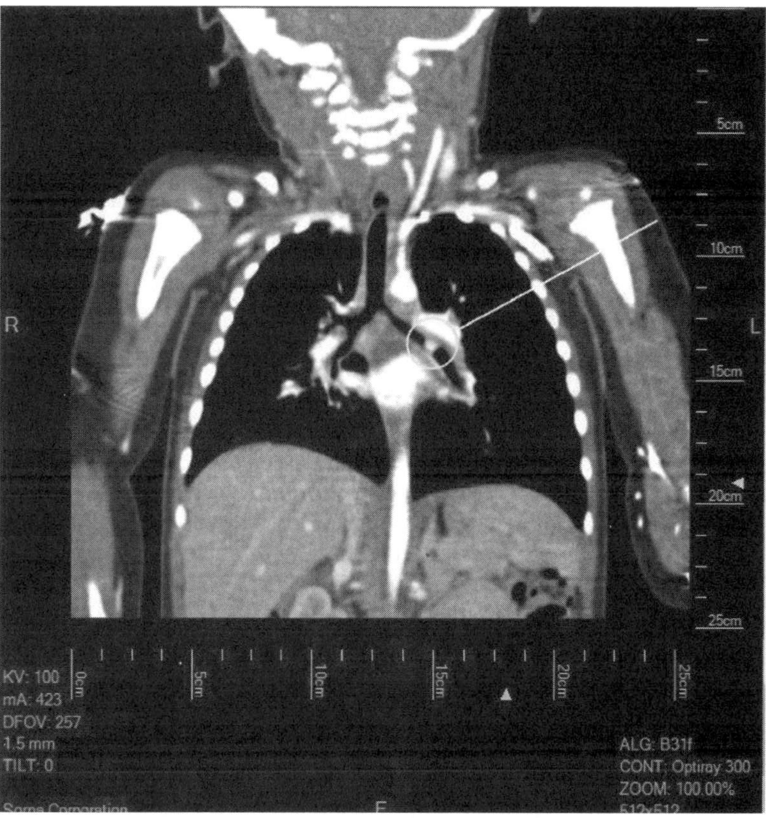

Figure 32-3. Coronal view of computed tomography scan showing foreign body at the takeoff of the left upper lobe bronchus.

Preemptive education for parents of infants and toddlers should be standard in pediatric practice. This includes advising that commonly aspirated foods, such as peanuts or similar-sized foods and other objects, be kept out of reach; food should be cut into small pieces; and latex-type balloons should not be allowed in the home.

When to Refer/Admit

Any child with a sudden onset of choking followed by coughing or wheezing should be suspected to have an airway foreign body. Those children should be referred to an ear, nose, and throat specialist or pediatric surgeon for evaluation via rigid bronchoscopy. A child with a choking event but who has no further symptoms, such as cough, dyspnea, or fever, and has a normal physical examination or chest radiographic findings may not require bronchoscopy.[7] If the diagnosis is in question, consultation from a pediatric pulmonologist is warranted. Follow-up is important to monitor for late-onset signs or symptoms, and repeat radiographs if these develop. A history of acute choking should never be ignored. Also, suspicion of foreign body should exist in a child with chronic problems, such as persistent chest radiograph abnormalities, wheezing or cough unresponsive to asthma therapy, or recurrent pneumonias regardless of no history for choking. Flexible bronchoscopy should be considered in these cases.

Massive Aspiration

Large volume aspiration is typically associated with vomiting, particularly with an altered level of consciousness state during which upper airway protective reflexes are diminished. It may occur in children with trauma, in children with seizures, during general anesthesia, or with significant underlying neuromotor disorders. Animal studies have shown that volumes greater than 1 mL/kg or pH less than 2.5 are associated with the most severe outcomes, although aspiration of particulate material also contributes to significant lung injury.[8] When acute massive aspiration is suspected, immediate management is paramount.

Case Report 32-2

An 8-year-old boy with developmental delay developed fever and upper airway congestion. He subsequently began vomiting and appeared to become dyspneic. Given his history of aspiration, his mother took him to their local hospital. His blood oxygen saturation was 83% while receiving high-flow supplemental oxygen. Inspiratory crackles were audible in both lower lobes. While his evaluation was underway, he became increasingly tachypneic, dyspneic, and more dusky. He was intubated and mechanically ventilated and, because of his rapid decline, he was airlifted to a children's hospital. His chest radiograph showed complete opacification of his right lower lobe and streaky infiltrates and haziness in his right upper and left lower lobes. He required intensive management with mechanical ventilation for 2 weeks and supplemental oxygen for several days. Subsequent discussions center around the need for tracheostomy placement or other procedures to reduce morbidity from future aspiration events.

Clinical Presentation

There is no difficulty in making the diagnosis of acute aspiration when the patient is observed to vomit and choke immediately afterward. Whether witnessed or not, the patient typically presents with dyspnea and, possibly, cyanosis. Clinical observation frequently reveals accessory muscle use and retractions. Inspiratory coarse crackles are usually auscultated throughout the chest. Wheezes of varying pitch can usually also be found. If the child has a tracheostomy tube, suctioning of the tube may return some formula or stomach contents. Evidence of vomitus may still be present in the oropharynx of the patient. In severe cases, the patient may have lost consciousness or have suffered respiratory arrest. Generalized seizures may occur secondary to associated hypoxic encephalopathy.

Diagnosis

If it is suspected that a child has inhaled substances with significant particulate matter, bronchoscopy may be warranted. Identification and removal of large airway particles are of diagnostic as well as potential therapeutic value. If no large particles are seen in the airways, bronchoalveolar lavage may still reveal diagnostic foreign material, such as meat or vegetable fibers. If lipid is aspirated, lipid-laden macrophages may be observed within a few hours after aspiration.[9] The classic findings are "asthma-like" as described by Mendelson,[10] whose original description was of complications of aspiration during obstetric anesthesia. These findings typically include coughing, wheezing, tachypnea, and possibly cyanosis. After a latent period of 1 to a few hours, fever and crackles may develop. Initial radiograph findings typically show bilateral multi-lobar infiltrates, which then worsen over the next 24 to 36 hours secondary to the inflammatory response (Figure 32-4).

Management

Bronchoscopy may play a role in some cases of massive aspiration. There is no value in attempting to neutralize acid aspiration, as this occurs endogenously within seconds after the event. Corticosteroids have not been shown to be beneficial and are not recommended. Sukumaran et al[11] showed that if they can be given immediately, essentially simultaneously, with an aspiration event there may be some benefit. Antibiotics are generally reserved for suspected infectious complications of a chemical pneumonitis. If antibiotics are deemed necessary due to a severely compromised patient or for other reasons, they

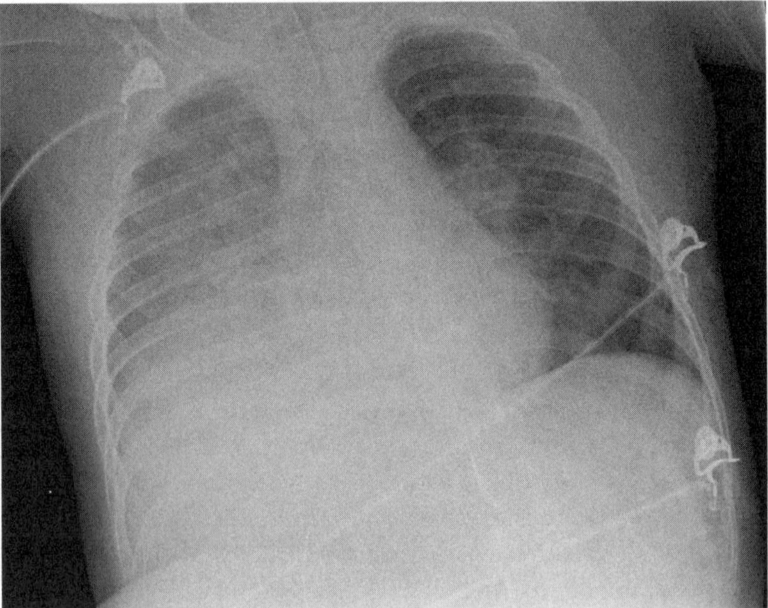

Figure 32-4. Chest radiograph taken a few hours after patient vomited and aspirated a large volume of gastric material.

should be individualized depending on the clinical situation. For example, if the patient has been institutionalized, more broad-spectrum antibiotics would be warranted, including coverage for gram-negative bacteria as well as methicillin-resistant *Staphylococcus aureus* and anaerobes. However, in the immediate treatment for most cases of large-volume aspiration, antibiotics are not indicated. General supportive measures, including supplemental oxygen, bronchodilators, and mechanical ventilation, are the mainstays of acute treatment.

For patients at risk for vomiting and aspiration, gastric volume should be minimized. Whenever possible, gastric acid should be suppressed. If vomiting is witnessed in a patient with a poorly protected airway or artificial airway, immediate suctioning of the airway is critical. Elevation of the head of the bed to 30 to 45 degrees, avoiding excess sedation (if possible), and monitoring gastric residual volumes during enteral feedings all may be helpful preventive measures.

When to Refer/Admit

All patients who become rapidly dyspneic from large-volume aspiration should be admitted to a hospital. In fact, unless the physical examination, oxygen saturation, and chest radiograph are normal, all patients suspected to have suffered large-volume aspiration ought to be admitted for close observation. If a patient is able to maintain near-normal blood oxygen levels with reasonable amounts of supplemental oxygen (fraction of inspired oxygen <0.6), is only mildly or moderately dyspneic, is not in an altered neurologic state, and can be monitored by experienced staff, it is reasonable that he or she is cared for in a community hospital. The patient should be observed closely for a minimum of 48 hours, however, as late-onset deterioration can occur. A child who deteriorates rapidly, requires increasing oxygen supplementation, becomes obtunded, or requires intubation and assisted ventilation should be transferred to a center with pediatric pulmonary and critical care specialists. It is very likely that, in these situations, the patient will require prolonged and intensive treatment and will require extended follow-up in specialty clinics.

Recurrent Small-Volume Aspiration

Recurrent aspiration of small volumes of food, gastric, oral, or nasal contents leads to acute and chronic respiratory problems. Risk factors for chronic recurrent aspiration are listed in Box 32-2. Aspiration of feedings has been reported as a significant complication of RSV bronchiolitis.[12] However, chronic aspiration with isolated swallowing dysfunction occurs in otherwise apparently healthy young children.[13] The most common underlying problem associated with recurrent pneumonia causing hospitalization has been reported to be oropharyngeal incoordination.[1] However, in patients with multisystem disease, the effect of oropharyngeal dyscoordination on the development of pneumonia appears to be reduced when other factors, such as Down syndrome, asthma, tube feeding, oral care, and GER disease, are taken into account.[14,15] Gastroesophageal reflux may be associated with respiratory symptoms, such as hypersecretion and wheezing, without causing aspiration. This likely occurs through vagally mediated reflexes.

Box 32-2 Risk Factors for Recurrent Aspiration

- Neurologic impairment
- Congenital anomalies of the airways (such as laryngeal cleft, vascular ring, and tracheoesophageal fistula)
- Craniofacial anomalies
- Muscular diseases
- Dysautonomia
- Poor oral hygiene
- Poor feeding techniques
- Gastroesophageal reflux
- Swallowing immaturity

Case Report 32-3

A 9-month-old boy presents with a recurrent cough that is present more days than not for the past 6 months. His newborn screen for cystic fibrosis was normal. He spits up after most feedings, more than his older siblings did. His cough seems to have no particular pattern, but with specific questioning, the mother states it may be more common toward the end of and after feedings. His physical examination was normal except for transient inspiratory and expiratory wheezes after a feeding. A chest radiograph showed patchy infiltrates predominantly in the posterior right upper lobe and to a lesser extent apical left upper lobe and right lower lobe with mild-to-moderate hyperinflation. He has had intermittent low-grade fever. His cough did not improve significantly with a course of amoxicillin. He was referred for a videofluoroscopic swallow study (VFSS), which showed tracheal aspiration with thin barium and mild laryngeal penetration with nectar consistency barium.

Clinical Presentation

Clinical respiratory findings include tachypnea, chronic cough, recurrent wheeze, stridor, rattly breathing, and apnea with presentations, including recurrent bronchitis or bronchiolitis, recurrent pneumonia, and atelectasis. Although choking or coughing with feedings is common with aspiration from dysphagia, silent aspiration occurs, especially in neurologically impaired patients. Chronic aspiration can also be a coincident finding in patients with other chronic conditions, such as cystic fibrosis, primary ciliary dyskinesia, and asthma.

Diagnosis

Because of the intermittent nature and small volumes involved with chronic recurrent aspiration (microaspiration), combined with the fact that aspiration and GER may be seen in healthy children without causing disease, proving a cause-effect association of recurrent small-volume aspiration and lower respiratory tract disease is difficult. Considerable clinical judgment is required. The evaluation begins with a careful history and physical examination. Caregivers should be asked about the timing of symptoms and relationship to feedings, positional changes, spitting, vomiting, or arching. In older children gastric discomfort or increased nocturnal symptoms of coughing or wheezing may be reported. The value of observing a feeding cannot be overemphasized. A child who presents with repeated gagging, coughing, wheezing, or crackles after feeding or after visible regurgitation may need very little further evaluation. Other findings may include difficulty with sucking, nasopharyngeal reflux, decreased or significantly increased gag reflex, drooling or pooling of oral secretions, as well as development of postprandial crackles or wheezes.

The initial study for a child suspected of recurrent aspiration is a plain chest radiograph. However, there are no findings specific to aspiration, and the results may range from normal to classically described consolidations in dependent lobes or segments. A CT scan may show infiltrates with decreased attenuation, suggestive of lipoid pneumonia, particularly in dependent areas. Depending on clinical suspicion, the next evaluation may include either a simple barium esophagram and upper gastrointestinal series or a modified barium swallow with videofluoroscopic evaluation of swallowing. The former can detect gross anatomical abnormalities, such as hiatal hernia, tracheoesophageal fistula, vascular ring, and gross aspiration or GER.

The VFSS is generally considered the gold standard for evaluating swallowing and oropharyngeal aspiration (Figure 32-5). It should be performed with the assistance of a pediatric feeding specialist and a parent. The purpose of this evaluation is to assess pharyngeal function and define motility problems in the oral cavity, pharynx, and upper esophagus. It is usually performed with the child seated in a normal eating position using various consistencies of barium or food soaked in barium. While very sensitive for oropharyngeal aspiration, it does not evaluate lower esophageal motility or GER. It is possible for this study to have false-positives, as at times aspiration (particularly with thin

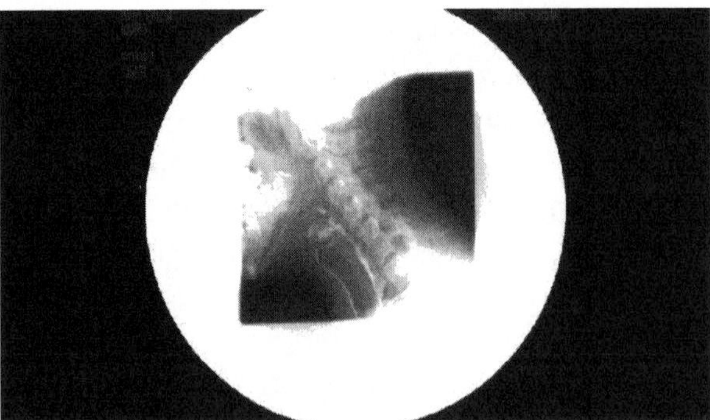

Figure 32-5. Videofluoroscopic swallow study showing tracheal aspiration of a large volume of thin barium.

barium) is seen and does not correlate with the respiratory status of the patient. The VFSS has also been shown to have a significant false-negative rate in predicting if oropharyngeal aspiration will progress to produce pneumonias.

Gastroesophageal scintigraphy (milk scan), although offering theoretical advantages of being more physiological and giving a longer window of viewing than the barium esophagram for detecting GER or aspiration, is quite insensitive for detection of aspiration. Another radionuclide scan, termed the salivagram, has also been used to assess aspiration of oropharyngeal contents. With this test, a small of amount of radionuclide is given orally to mimic the amount of saliva in the mouth, and scanning is performed to look for tracheal or pulmonary aspiration. It is probably more sensitive than the gastroesophageal scintiscan, and is of approximately the same sensitivity to the VFSS.[16]

Fiberoptic endoscopic evaluation of swallowing (FEES) has utility in children, and is shown to be of similar sensitivity to VFSS without the radiation.[17] With this test, the endoscopist views with a small nasopharyngoscope the tip just above the supraglottic area and watches multiple swallows of various food consistencies. This allows both anatomical and functional evaluation of swallowing, except that nothing can be viewed during pharyngeal contraction due to airway closure. It can sometimes be used in children with an oral aversion, although some level of cooperation, or at least tolerance, is necessary. Fiberoptic endoscopic evaluation of swallowing and VFSS assess only one brief period, which can lead to both false-positive and false-negative results. An advantage to both VFSS and FEES is that they can assist with providing treatment recommendations, such as thickening of feeds or special positioning.

In patients with a tracheostomy or endotracheal tube, a small amount of dye can be placed on the tongue or mixed in feeds followed by suctioning to look for stained tracheal secretions. This is a useful and simple test that can be repeated multiple times, although reports of sensitivity and specificity are quite varied. It is not recommended to add dye to large volumes of tube feedings. This is highly insensitive for detecting aspiration and also has potential toxicity.

Gastroesophageal reflux may produce respiratory symptoms with or without aspiration. The gold standard for diagnosing acid reflux from the stomach has been 24-hour esophageal pH monitoring. More recently esophageal impedance monitoring has allowed detection of nonacid GER.[18] A cause-effect relationship between GER and respiratory symptoms is difficult to prove. It is important to recognize that even if studies for GER, including esophageal pH or impedance monitoring, indicate results are within the normal range, if episodes of GER result in aspiration or respiratory symptoms in a susceptible host (such as a child with asthma), the normal GER results are pathologic. It is for primarily this reason that an empirical trial of conservative and medical treatment for GER is often the best and most cost-effective diagnostic test.[19]

Examination of tracheobronchial aspirates obtained at bronchoscopy or deep samples from artificial airways can yield valuable information regarding aspiration, including analysis for glucose, pepsin, vegetable or meat fibers, and lipid-laden macrophages. Other limited studies have looked at various substances added to foods, such as carbon or polystyrene microspheres. Pepsin[20] analysis appears promising in some studies, but it can only detect aspiration occurring from GER, not from dysphagia. The sighting of lipid-laden macrophages is nonspecific to aspiration, but when these cells are semi-quantitated, this has been shown to have a high correlation with other tests for aspiration. Using proper histological technique, the absence of lipid-laden macrophages highly suggests that lipid aspiration is not occurring.[21]

It is critically important to consider diagnoses other than aspiration as the cause of respiratory disease. Children with cystic fibrosis, asthma, interstitial pneumonitis, and primary ciliary dyskinesia, among other conditions, may present with an abnormal history or study indicating aspiration, thus significantly delaying diagnosis of their primary problem.

Management

Treatment should be directed at the underlying condition that contributes to aspiration, if known. Other treatment will depend on the severity of respiratory problems and whether the aspiration is caused by a swallowing dysfunction or GER. Conservative measures to improve aspiration during swallowing include thickening of feeds, pacing feedings, swallow stimulation, and change of feeding position. Thickening feeds, upright positioning, avoidance of bottle propping and smoke exposure, and weight loss (if indicated) all can be helpful in reducing GER. Medical treatment with proton pump inhibitors can reduce acid reflux, but has not been shown to reduce nonacid reflux. Prokinetic agents available in the United States include metaclopramide and erythromycin. The efficacy of either drug is not well substantiated, and side effects are common with metaclopramide. A trial of nasogastric feedings can be used while waiting for temporary swallowing dysfunction to improve. With significant GER, post-pyloric feedings may be considered. Surgical treatment is reserved for patients with more severe problems, such as recurrent hospitalization for pneumonia or evidence of progressive lung injury. Fundoplication is usually successful in eliminating GER. This should be performed in conjunction with a gastrostomy tube placement in children with significant GER. Judgment must be used to decide if this should be performed at the time of a gastrostomy in children without significant GER demonstrated preoperatively. A significant number of patients develop GER after gastrostomy tube placement. Recurrent pneumonias may continue even after both fundoplication and gastrostomy due to continued aspiration of oral secretions, especially in neurologically impaired children. Anticholinergic agents, such as glycopyrrolate and scopolamine, may reduce excess salivation, but tolerance can develop and adverse side effects may occur, such as blurred vision and difficulty urinating.[22] Salivary gland injection of botulinum toxin[22] has been shown to reduce salivation, but the effects are usually short term. Surgical intervention with salivary gland removal, ductal ligation, or laryngotracheal separation may be considered in children not responsive to more conservative therapy.[22] Tracheostomy, although often associated with an increase in aspiration, can be considered in a patient with chronic aspiration and poor ability to clear their airway due to underlying conditions, such as poor cough, and as a means to improve pulmonary hygiene and ability to provide ventilatory assistance and oxygen delivery. Management of children with chronic aspiration is difficult. There are many variables of diagnosis and treatment that are best individualized for the patient by close collaboration between the primary physician, pulmonologist, family, and surgical subspecialties.

When to Refer/Admit

A child with recurrent pneumonia or persistent chest radiograph abnormality, dysphagia, coughing or choking with feedings, or recurrent wheezing not responsive to routine asthma therapy should be referred for further evaluation. Hospital admission would be indicated if there is significant dyspnea, hypoxemia, progressive pulmonary signs or symptoms, equivocal history, and acute life-threatening event. Any of these may indicate acute or cumulative effect of chronic aspiration.

Key Points

- Oropharyngeal aspiration from swallowing dysfunction is reportedly the most common cause of recurrent pneumonia in children.
- A high index of suspicion is necessary for airway foreign body because the history, physical examination, and radiographs may be normal. The ultimate diagnosis can often only be made by bronchoscopy. Choking episodes should never be ignored.
- There is no test for aspiration that is both highly sensitive and specific. Clinical judgment is always necessary to determine if aspiration is a likely cause of existing respiratory disease.
- Esophageal monitoring of pH will not detect nonacid reflux (eg, post-prandial), which is likely to be the major culprit in chronic pulmonary aspiration.
- Though esophageal impedance monitoring detects nonacid reflux, it does not indicate if reflux, even a normal amount, leads to pulmonary aspiration.
- Oropharyngeal aspiration is more likely to be associated with recurrent pneumonia than GER, the latter being more likely associated with respiratory symptoms such as wheezing and cough.
- Acid suppression therapy cannot be expected to significantly improve recurrent aspiration if aspiration is related to nonacid GER or swallowing dysfunction.

References

1. Owayed AF, Campbell DM, Wang EL. Underlying causes of recurrent pneumonia in children. *Arch Pediatr Adolesc Med.* 2000;154:190–194
2. Sevval E, Akin E, Dikici B, Mehmet D, Mehmet N. Foreign body aspiration in children: experience of 1160 cases. *Ann Trop Paediatr.* 2003;23(1):31–37
3. Lea E, Nawaf H, Yoav T, Samet E, Zonis Z, Kugelman A. Diagnostic evaluation of foreign body aspiration in children: a prospective study. *J Pediatr Surg.* 2005;40:1122–1127

4. Asseffa D, Amin N, Stringel G, Dozor A. Use of decubitus radiographs in the diagnosis of foreign body aspiration in young children. *Pediatr Emerg Care.* 2007;23(3):154–157
5. Adaletli I, Kurugoglu S, Ulus S, et al. Utilization of low-dose multidetector CT and virtual bronchoscopy in children with suspected foreign body aspiration. *Pediatr Radiol.* 2007;37(1):33–40
6. Shin SM, Kim WS, Cheon JE, et al. CT in children with suspected residual foreign body in airway after bronchoscopy. *AJR Am J Roentgenol.* 2009;192:1744–1751
7. Cohen S, Avital A, Godfrey S, Gross M, Derem E, Springer C. Suspected foreign body inhalation in children: what are the indications for bronchoscopy? *J Pediatr.* 2009;155(2):276–280
8. Hamelberg W, Bosomworth PP. Aspiration pneumonitis: experimental studies and clinical observations. *Anesth Analg.* 1964;43(6):669–677
9. Colombo J, Hallberg T, Sammut P. Time course of lipid-laden pulmonary macrophages with acute and recurrent milk aspiration in rabbits. *Pediatr Pulmonol.* 1992;12:95–98
10. Mendelson C. The aspiration of stomach contents into the lungs during obstetric anesthesia. *Am J Obstet Gynecol.* 1946;52:191–205
11. Sukumaran M, Granada MJ, Berger HW, Lee M, Reilly TA. Evaluation of corticosteroid treatment in aspiration of gastric contents: a controlled clinical trial. *Mt Sinai J Med.* 1980;47(4):335–340
12. Hernandez E, Khoshoo V, Thoppil D, Edell D, Ross G. Aspiration: a factor in rapidly deteriorating bronchiolitis in previously healthy infants. *Pediatr Pulmonol.* 2002;33:30–31
13. Lefton-Greif M, Carroll J, Loughlin G. Long-term follow-up of oropharyngeal dysphagia in children without apparent risk factors. *Pediatr Pulmonol.* 2006;41(11):1040–1048
14. Weir K, McMahon S, Barry L, Ware R, Masters B, Chang A. Oropharyngeal aspiration and pneumonia in children. *Pediatr Pulmonol.* 2007;42:1024–311
15. Langmore S, Terpenning M, Schork A, et al. Predictors of aspiration pneumonia: how important is dysphagia? *Dysphagia.* 1998;13(2):69–81
16. Baikie G, South M, Reddihough D, et al. Agreement of aspiration tests using barium videofluoroscopy, salivagram, and milk scan in children with cerebral palsy. *Dev Med Child Neurol.* 2005;47:86–93
17. Willging JP, Thompson DM. Pediatric FEESST: fiberoptic endoscopic evaluation of swallowing with sensory testing. *Curr Gastroenterol Rep.* 2005;7(3):240–243
18. Vandenplas Y, Salvatore S, Devreker T, Hauser B. Gastro-esophageal reflux disease: oesophageal impedance versus pH monitoring. *Acta Paediatr.* 2007;96:956–962
19. Koshoo V, Le T, Haydel R Jr, Landry L, Nelson C. Role of gastroesophageal reflux in older children with persistent asthma. *Chest.* 2003;123:1008–1013

20. Starosta V, Kitz R, Hartl D, Marcos V, Reinhardt D, Griese M. Bronchial pepsin, bile acids, oxidation, and inflammation in children with gastroesophageal reflux disease. *Chest.* 2007;132;1557–1564
21. Colombo J, Hallberg T. Pulmonary aspiration and lipid-laden macrophages: in search of gold (standards). *Pediatr Pulmonol.* 1999;28(2):79–82
22. Little SA, Kubba H, Hussain SSM. An evidence-based approach to the child who drools saliva. *Clin Otolaryngol.* 2009;34:236–239

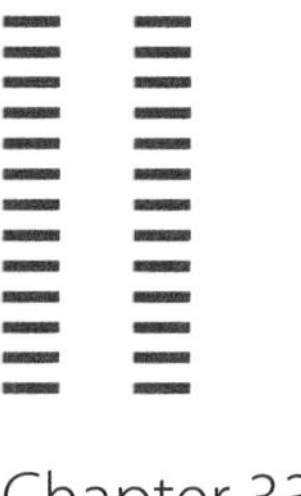

Chapter 33

Lung Transplantation

Carol Conrad, MD

Introduction

The first pediatric lung transplant was performed in 1986. Lung and heart-lung transplants are still rare in children, especially when compared with adults. As of 2005 there were 32 centers performing 77 lung transplants within the United States. In that same year, 5 children received a heart-lung transplant. Most centers perform fewer than 5 transplants in children per year.

Survival after a lung or heart-lung transplant is lower in both children and adults than that for any other solid organ, because chronic graft rejection is not readily controlled. For all recipients of lungs between the years of 1990 and 2005, the average half-life of the transplanted organs was 4.3 and 4.8 years, respectively. For recipients of heart-lung transplants, the survival appears to be slightly worse. The average survival of children with lung transplants varies by age group (Figure 33-1). While the first year mortality is much higher for infants younger than 1 year at the time of transplant, the mortality rate for all age groups is similar (Figure 33-2).

The most life-limiting factor for lung and heart-lung transplant recipients is chronic graft rejection that manifests histologically as obliterative bronchiolitis (OB). Its clinical equivalent is bronchiolitis obliterans syndrome (BOS). Obliterative bronchiolitis describes luminal obliteration of the bronchioles with fibrous tissue and, if not controlled, leads to respiratory failure. Obliterative bronchiolitis is thought to be the final common pathway occurring as a result of various forms of postoperative lung injury, including ischemia-reperfusion injury, primary graft dysfunction, immunologic phenomena, rejection episodes, and infection.

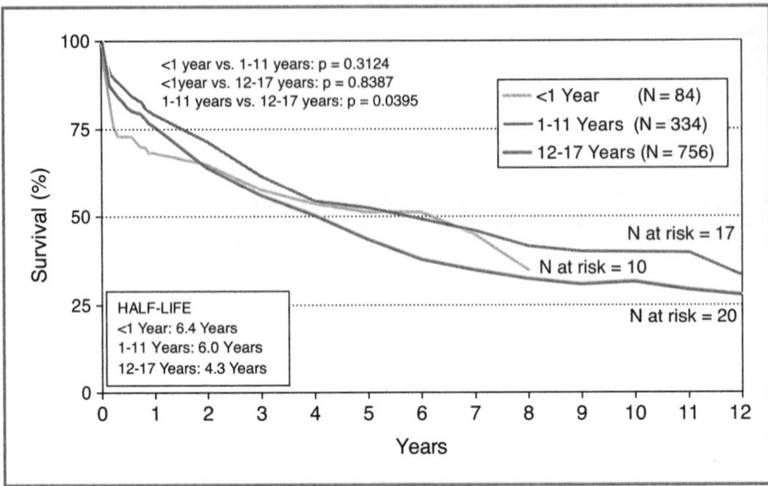

Figure 33-1. Pediatric lung transplantation. Kaplan-Meier survival by age group (Transplants: January 1990–June 2008). (From Aurora P, Edwards LB, Kucheryavaya A, et al. Registry of the International Society for Heart and Lung Transplantation: eleventh official pediatric lung and heart/lung transplantation report—2010. *J Heart Lung Transplant.* 2010;29:1129–1141.)

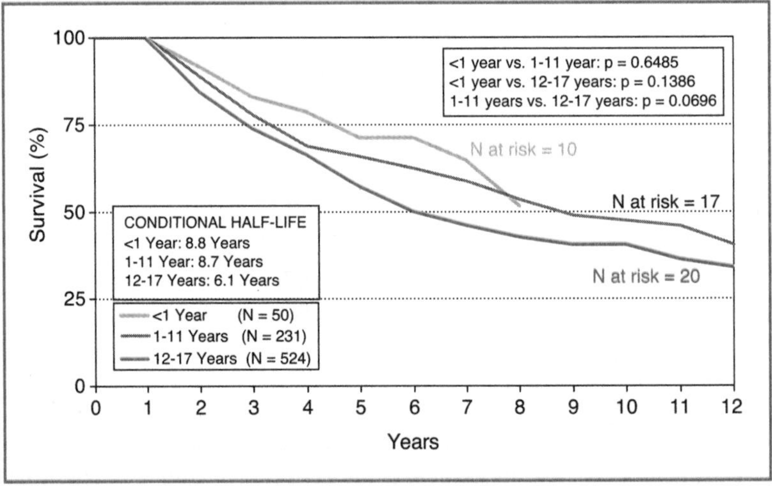

Figure 33-2. Conditional half-life survival by age group of children with a lung transplant. Data censored to include only survivors beyond the first year (Transplants: January 1990–June 2008). (From Aurora P, Edwards LB, Kucheryavaya A, et al. Registry of the International Society for Heart and Lung Transplantation: thirteenth official pediatric lung and heart/lung transplantation report—2010. *J Heart Lung Transplant.* 2010;29:1129–1141.)

Types of Lung Transplantation

There are 4 major types of lung transplantation: unilobar, bilateral, heart-lung, and living donor transplants. Unilobar lung transplants are rarely performed in children because of extremely high mortality. Unilobar lung transplants are commonly performed in adults with non-suppurative chronic obstructive pulmonary disease and pulmonary fibrosis, which rarely are diagnosed in children.

Bilateral lung transplantation is the most common type of lung transplant performed in children. The most recent surgical technique for bilateral lung transplantation is to transplant each lung individually. This allows many bilateral transplant recipients to undergo the surgery without requiring cardiopulmonary bypass and avoid many of its perioperative complications.

The number of pediatric heart-lung transplants performed per year has fallen to fewer than 20 worldwide. Because this type of graft may use up to 3 donor organs, it is reserved for children who have advanced pulmonary vascular disease, lung disease associated with poor left ventricular function, or complex congenital cardiac anomalies and Eisenmenger syndrome who are not amenable to bilateral isolated lung transplant with intracardiac repair.[1] Patients with severe right ventricular dysfunction secondary to pulmonary hypertension but with preserved left ventricular function almost always do well with isolated bilateral or unilateral lung grafts. The right side of the heart is generally able to remodel and repair once the stress of the pulmonary arterial pressures is relieved.[2]

Several transplantation programs now include living donor procedures. In the most common approach, 2 donors are used. A right lower lobe is removed from one donor and a left lower lobe from the other. The recipient has both diseased lungs removed, and the right lobe is transplanted in the right side and the left in the left side. This approach was sought since, intuitively, if the donors were related, relatively good tissue human leukocyte antigen (HLA) matches were achievable, and ischemic times could be minimized. The ethical issues regarding the risk to the donors have been explored and were not found to be a greater barrier than those faced by potential kidney donors. No donor deaths were recorded in a report from the largest living donor program.[3,4]

General Clinical Indications

Guidelines for adult transplantation have been firmly established, but the issues and the challenges regarding lung transplantation for children are distinctly different than those for adults. The International Pediatric Lung Transplantation Collaborative published guidelines for selection of pediatric candidates for lung transplantation in 2007.[5] These vary by age group, but in general, lung or heart-lung transplantation should be considered in children with end-stage or progressive lung disease or life-threatening pulmonary vascular disease for which there is no other medical or surgical therapy (Table 33-1) and life

Table 33-1. Indications for Lung Transplant in Children (January 1991–June 2006)[a]

Indication	Age <1 y (%)	Age 1–5 y (%)	Age 6–11 y (%)	Age 12–17 y (%)
Cystic fibrosis	-	3.7	54.9	69
Primary pulmonary hypertension	16.1	22.2	11.8	8.3
Re-transplant (OB)	-	7.4	4.1	3.4
Congenital heart disease	30.6	9.9	1.0	0.8
Idiopathic pulmonary fibrosis	-	8.6	3.1	3.6
OB (non-transplant)	-	6.2	4.6	3.3
Re-transplant: not OB	4.8	1.2	3.6	2.5
Interstitial pneumonitis	9.7	13.6	0.5	0.8
Pulmonary vascular disease	11.3	4.9	3.1	0.2
Eisenmenger syndrome	1.6	6.2	2.6	0.9
Surfactant protein B deficiency	14.5	2.5	-	-
COPD/emphysema	-	1.2	1.0	0.8
Bronchopulmonary dysplasia	1.6	2.5	3.1	-
Bronchiectasis	-	-	1.5	0.6
Other	8.1	8.6	3.1	4.1

Abbreviations: COPD, chronic obstructive pulmonary disease; OB, obliterative bronchiolitis.
[a]Adapted from Aurora P, Edwards LB, Christie J, et al. Registry of the International Society for Heart and Lung Transplantation: eleventh official pediatric lung and heart/lung transplantation report—2008. *J Heart Lung Transplant.* 2008;27:978–983.

expectancy is severely limited. For infants, congenital heart disease is the most common indication and accounts for about 30% of transplants in this age group. Infants with primary pulmonary hypertension and pulmonary hypertension secondary to pulmonary vascular disease (eg, pulmonary venous obstruction or Eisenmenger syndrome) comprise the next largest groups, and surfactant protein B deficiency and interstitial pneumonitis account for most of the remainder of indications for infants. Primary pulmonary hypertension and interstitial pneumonitis remain as predominant reasons for transplants for 1- to 5-year-olds. The primary reason for lung transplant in 6- to 17-year-olds is complications of cystic fibrosis (CF), and primary pulmonary hypertension is the second most common reason.

The characteristics of lung transplant candidates that are associated with good outcomes are listed in Box 33-1. Commonly accepted absolute and relative contraindications to lung transplantation are listed in Box 33-2.

Timing of Referral

There are no guidelines that determine the most appropriate time to refer a patient for a lung or heart-lung transplant. Before 2005 all lung transplant candidates were prioritized according to the length of time they had been waiting to receive organs. This led to long waiting lists filled with candidates who had varying degrees of lung dysfunction and a high mortality rate among the most severely ill patients. The United Network of Organ Sharing devised a Lung Allocation Score (LAS) that took effect in 2005. The LAS applies to patients 12 years and older. It uses a complex formula that takes into account aspects of the

Box 33-1. Characteristics of Lung Transplant Candidates Associated With the Best Outcomes

1. A well-defined diagnosis or projected trajectory of illness that puts the child at risk of dying without a lung transplant despite optimal medical therapy
2. Adequate caregivers to provide support
3. Satisfactory network of resources that ensure consistent access to transplant services and medications after transplant
4. Sufficient evidence of motivation and demonstration of the ability on the part of patient and parent to adhere to the rigorous therapy, daily monitoring, and reevaluation schedule after transplant

Box 33-2. Absolute and Relative Contraindications to Lung Transplantation[a,b]

Absolute
- Active malignancy
- Sepsis
- Active tuberculosis
- Severe neuromuscular disease
- Documented, refractory non-adherence
- Multiple organ dysfunction
- Immune deficiencies, including hypogammaglobulinemia
- Hepatitis C with histologic liver disease
- Infection with HIV

Relative
- Pleurodesis
- Renal insufficiency
- Markedly abnormal body mass index (overweight or underweight)
- Mechanical ventilation
- Severe scoliosis or kyphosis
- Poorly controlled diabetes mellitus
- Osteoporosis
- Chronic airway infection with multiple resistant organisms
- Fungal infection/colonization
- Hepatitis B surface antigen positive
- Chronic steroid usage (eg, prednisone ≥10 mg daily)
- Abuse of illicit drugs

[a] These contraindications have been derived primarily from adults and vary from center to center.

[b] From Faro A, Mallory GB, Visner GA, et al. American Society of Transplantation executive summary on pediatric lung transplantation. *Am J Transplant.* 2007;7:285–292.

candidate's health, diagnosis, and lung function to assign a level of severity of illness that calculates the survival benefit and targets the neediest patients for organ allocation at a time when they can benefit most. Donor lungs for children younger than 12 years continue to be allocated by time accrued on the waiting list, though the new policy also prioritizes the transplant of lungs from pediatric donors into children. Other factors that are considered include ABO blood type, HLA (major histocompatibility tissue antigen) sensitization, and the distance between the donor and transplant centers.

Selection of Candidates for Transplantation

The single most important aspect of successful outcome in lung or heart-lung transplantation is selection of appropriate candidates for the procedure. Candidates for transplant should have generally good medical health. Candidates may have comorbid medical conditions that are well-controlled and should not have significant end-organ damage (other than their lung disease). Acceptable medical conditions include systemic hypertension, diabetes mellitus, and peptic ulcer disease. Relative and absolute contraindications to lung transplant are listed in Box 33-2.

Transplant Candidate Selection Guidelines for Those With Specific Diseases

Cystic Fibrosis

Criteria for referral of patients with CF for a lung transplant are based primarily on the longitudinal study of Kerem and coworkers,[6] who evaluated predictors for mortality in a large, single-center population of patients with CF. This early study was a retrospective analysis that found that patients with a forced expiratory volume at 1 second (FEV_1) of less than 30% predicted, partial pressure of oxygen less than 55 mm Hg, or partial pressure of carbon dioxide more than 50 mm Hg have a 2-year mortality rate above 50%. In this investigation, the FEV_1 was the most significant predictor of mortality and was the basis for the guidelines published in 1998 for patient referral for lung transplant.[4] Since then, several new models for selection of appropriate transplant candidates with CF have been proposed (Table 33-2).

The criteria used to recommend referral are more liberal than those used to recommend transplantation. Patients with CF will usually be considered for lung transplantation if (1) there is a less than 50% 2-year predicted survival, (2) quality of life (QOL) is likely to be improved by transplantation, (3) there are no absolute contraindications to transplantation, and (4) the patient is fully informed and committed to proceeding. Most pediatric transplant centers assess QOL qualitatively and take into account the ability of the child to participate in daily activities, exercise tolerance, time spent in hospital, and requirement for oxygen and intravenous antibiotic therapy. Functional status can be quantitated with the New York Heart Association's (NYHA) Functionality Classification System (Table 33-3).

Predicted life expectancy is taken into consideration so that life expectancy following the transplant exceeds life expectancy without the procedure (including the likely waiting time for an appropriate

Table 33-2. Factors That Affect Prognosis of Lung Transplant of Children With Cystic Fibrosis

Factor	Measurement
Spirometry	FEV_1, FVC
Poor exercise tolerance	Decreased 6-minute walk distance Desaturation on exercise Decreased maximal oxygen consumption
Abnormal blood gas	Resting hypercarbia Resting hypoxemia
$\dot{V}/\dot{Q}$ mismatch	$\dot{V}/\dot{Q}$ scan
Pulmonary hypertension	Cardiac catheterization, pulmonary arterial pressure >30 mm Hg
Poor nutrition	Hypoalbuminemia Anemia Short stature Poor weight for height Low body mass index
Rapid decline	Rapid rate of fall of FEV_1 Frequent exacerbations Young age
Female	
Increased energy expenditure	Resting tachycardia
Multisystem involvement	Liver disease Diabetes mellitus

Abbreviations: FEV_1, forced expiratory volume at 1 second; FVC, forced vital capacity; $\dot{V}/\dot{Q}$, ventilation/perfusion.

Table 33-3. New York Heart Association (NYHA) Functional Classification

NYHA Class	Symptoms
I	No symptoms and no limitation in ordinary physical activity (eg, shortness of breath when walking, climbing stairs, etc).
II	Mild symptoms (mild shortness of breath or angina) and slight limitation during ordinary activity.
III	Marked limitation in activity due to symptoms, even during less-than-ordinary activity (eg, walking short distances [20–100 m]). Comfortable only at rest.
IV	Severe limitations. Experiences symptoms even while at rest. Mostly bedbound patients.

organ to become available). Early referral for transplant assessment allows the evaluation to proceed in an organized manner, for treatment to be optimized through a thorough evaluation and multidisciplinary discussion, and for patient education to proceed. It also provides adequate time for the patient (and also the referring center) to develop a good working relationship with the transplant center. For some patients, this is the first occasion that the possibility of their death from lung disease has been fully discussed. This can be a traumatic experience, especially for children, and it may take some time before parents and caregivers can give an informed decision regarding transplantation.

Microbiological Issues in Patients With Cystic Fibrosis

Most patients are colonized with organisms that have developed resistance to many classes of antibiotics. Pre-transplant colonization with multidrug-resistant organisms does not preclude transplantation and is often successfully treated with antibiotic therapy. In the era of routine use of inhaled antibiotics (aminoglycosides or colistimethate) and current development of others (eg, amikacin, aztreonam, ciprofloxacin, levofloxacin), CF sputum flora commonly includes *Staphylococcus aureus,* both methicillin-resistant and methicillin-sensitive; *Pseudomonas aeruginosa; Xanthomonas (Stenotrophomonas) maltophilia;* and *Achromobacter (Alcaligenes) xylosoxidans.* The latter 2 organisms are innately resistant to most classes of antibiotics. However, in vitro panresistance is now considered a relative contraindication because in vitro sensitivities do not necessarily correspond to in vivo sensitivities. It is recommended that microbiological review of sputum be performed on a periodic basis, usually at 3-month intervals during the pre-transplantation waiting period.

Few data are available from pediatric transplant centers regarding the effect colonizing organisms that are present pre-transplant have on survival and other outcomes in pediatric transplantation. Data that follow are culled from studies on adult transplant recipients, unless otherwise noted.

Burkholderia cenocepacia Complex

Colonization with *B cenocepacia* (formerly *B cepacia* genomovar III) has a negative effect on post-transplant survival that has yet to be mitigated by modified surgical technique or tailored antibacterial therapy.[7–10] A recent study using data from patients referred for transplant in the United States suggests that the risk of poor outcome is limited to patients colonized with non-epidemic strains of *B cenocepacia.* The authors also found that post-transplant mortality was increased in patients infected with *Burkholderia gladioli.*[11] It is thus considered a strong relative, if not an absolute, contraindication to lung transplantation internationally.

Fungus and Molds

A retrospective analysis in pediatric lung transplant recipients demonstrated an increased risk of mortality from pulmonary fungal infections the first year after lung transplant. Risk factors for pulmonary fungal infection included pre-transplant colonization.[12] Known fungal colonization should prompt secondary prophylaxis in the perioperative period.

Nontuberculous Mycobacteria (NTM)

Data regarding mortality associated with mycobacterial infection or colonization in adult transplant patients with CF are limited and mostly anecdotal. Studies indicate that while NTM disease caused significant morbidity in a small number of patients after transplantation, it was successfully treated and did not influence the post-transplant course of the disease.[13,14] The isolation of NTM before transplantation in patients with CF should not be an exclusion criterion for lung transplantation, but it may alert the clinician to patients at risk of recurrence after transplantation. Thus centers vary in their acceptance of patients colonized with NTM.

Surfactant Deficiencies

Infants diagnosed with surfactant protein B deficiency should be referred immediately on diagnosis, because mortality is nearly 100% during the perinatal period. Surfactant protein B deficiency presents with unrelenting respiratory failure or progressive interstitial lung disease with respiratory insufficiency, unresponsive to medical interventions. However, if treatment with extracorporeal membrane oxygenation is required, this may be a contraindication to transplant, particularly if there is other organ insufficiency, such as a comorbidity, or if cerebral hemorrhage has occurred.

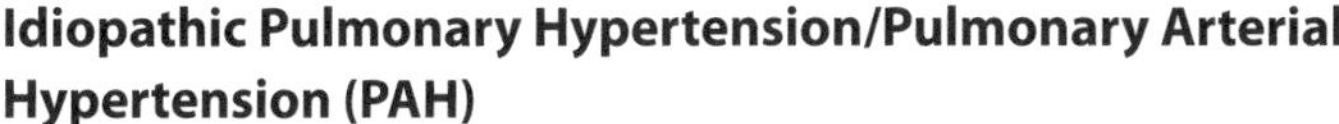

Idiopathic Pulmonary Hypertension/Pulmonary Arterial Hypertension (PAH)

Patients with idiopathic pulmonary hypertension or PAH should be referred to a lung transplant center if they are considered to be NYHA or World Health Organization functional class III or IV despite treatment with intravenous, oral, or inhalation vasodilator therapy or if they have a low exercise tolerance with a 6-minute walk test of less than 350 m, symptoms of uncontrolled syncope, hemoptysis, or right-sided heart failure. The primary indications for referral are an irreversibly severe condition or failure to respond adequately to vasodilator therapy. Some patients present to medical care with these symptoms, and they should be referred for lung transplant (or heart-lung transplant for those with cor pulmonale) at the same time they begin treatment for PAH. Major comorbidities are a contraindication for transplant and include renal failure and liver failure with hyperbilirubinemia. Identifiable causes for the PAH must be ruled out or confirmed. These include collagen vascular disease, primary pulmonary pathology, chronic thromboembolism, and surgically remediable causes of pulmonary venous obstruction.

Eisenmenger Syndrome

Children with Eisenmenger syndrome should be referred to a transplant center if they have profound hypoxemia despite therapy aimed at avoiding polycythemia, iron deficiency, and dehydration. Contraindications for lung transplant in these children include the presence of major comorbidities, left ventricular failure, irreparable congenital heart defect (heart-lung transplantation should be considered), or recurrent thoracotomies, because the scarring from previous surgeries can increase the intraoperative mortality dramatically. Patients with Eisenmenger syndrome should be referred when the trajectory of pulmonary hypertension appears to be worsening and they have impaired exercise tolerance and worsening quality of life.

Other Pulmonary Vascular Disorders

Patients with other pulmonary vascular disorders should be referred urgently since they typically do not respond to medical management. Additionally, infants born with total or partial anomalous pulmonary venous return who undergo surgical repair and have recurrence of obstruction soon thereafter should be urgently referred.

Bronchopulmonary Dysplasia

Consideration for lung transplantation for infants with bronchopulmonary dysplasia should begin if the infant requires extended time with ventilator support without clinical improvement, or if the infant experiences prolonged or repeated episodes of respiratory failure or evidence of pulmonary hypertension that is unresponsive to oxygen therapy. Contraindications for transplantation include the presence of significant irreversible comorbidities or a history of cerebral hemorrhage with severe developmental delay.

Diffuse Parenchymal Lung Disease

Diffuse parenchymal lung diseases have heterogeneous etiologies, and include surfactant deficiency due to *ABCA3* gene mutations and idiopathic interstitial lung diseases that demonstrate unremitting progression despite optimal medical management. Contraindications for transplantation of patients with diffuse parenchymal lung disease include the presence of systemic disease that might affect the allograft. Candidates for transplant should be referred early.

Evaluation of the Donor

Criteria to assess the acceptability of lung donors have been developed. Box 33-3 describes the criteria used to define an ideal donor. These criteria have been developed largely from clinical experience instead of from large multicenter trials. Specific criteria for donors to children

Box 33-3. Features of the Ideal Donor

- Age <55 years
- ABO compatibility
- No HLA antibody sensitization by recipient
- Clear chest radiograph
- PaO_2 >300 on FiO_2 = 1.0, PEEP = 5 cm H_2O
- Nonsmoker (never smoked)
- Absence of chest trauma
- No evidence of aspiration/sepsis
- No prior cardiopulmonary surgery
- Absence of organism and polymorphonuclear cells on sputum Gram stain
- Absence of purulent secretions at bronchoscopy

Abbreviations: FiO_2, fraction of inspired oxygen; HLA, human leukocyte antigen; PaO_2, partial pressure of oxygen; PEEP, positive end-expiratory pressure.

have not been established. However, it is generally accepted that the ideal lung donor for children should be a nonsmoker of the same size (particularly of chest dimension from the diaphragm to the apex of the lung) and blood type, or ABO-compatible. The donor should have no significant history of lung disease, including asthma. There should be no pulmonary trauma or infections, gas exchange should not be impaired, and ischemic time should be minimal. Some pediatric lung transplant centers may apply more stringent criteria if the candidate in question is reasonably stable. Donor offers from younger donors may be more desirable in some cases.

Depending on the need of the candidate, nonideal donors, also called extended or marginal donors, may be accepted. There are limited data to either support or prohibit the use of lungs from a nonideal donor. There is no evidence that a marginal donor will have any effect on either immediate or long-term morbidity or mortality, except in egregious cases of the diagnosis of bronchopneumonia or presence of purulent lower airways disease in the donor. It is believed, but has not been demonstrated, that lungs obtained from donors older than 55 years who have a significant smoking history are at risk for developing malignancy in the setting of immune suppression.

Post-Transplant Management of the Pediatric Lung Transplant Recipient

Postoperative Management

Immunosuppression

One of the major hurdles to successful lung transplantation is to prevent both acute and chronic allograft rejection by the recipient immune system. Transplanted lungs still contain bronchus-associated lymphoid tissue, which is intimately associated with the bronchi and, thus, cannot be completely removed at the time of donor organ harvesting nor at the time of transplantation. This, along with increased immunogenicity of the lungs compared with other solid organ transplants and frequent infectious insults with suppressed defense mechanisms, are possibly the main reasons for the higher rate of acute cellular rejection in the transplanted lung. Aggressive strategies to prevent rejection will often result in infection, and the reverse can be true as well if immune suppression must be diminished in order to allow for recovery from infection, or Epstein-Barr virus (EBV)–associated post-transplant lymphoproliferative disorder (PTLD).

Induction Therapy

Both acute and chronic rejections occur frequently in lung transplant recipients. Recurrent acute rejection episodes contribute to the development of chronic airway rejection, a morbidity that affects most lung transplant recipients. Many transplant centers, both pediatric and adult, use induction immunotherapy at the time of transplant to decrease the risk of rejection, though debate continues as to the efficacy of these drugs in achieving this goal. Aside from demonstrating a decrease in the incidence of acute rejection in the first year after transplant when an induction agent was used, there are no data to indicate that induction therapy is associated with an improvement in BOS-free survival, or with survival overall.

Maintenance Immunosuppression

Based on side effects in children and efficacy, the International Pediatric Lung Transplant Collaborative has adopted a standard immunosuppressive protocol consisting of tacrolimus, mycophenolate mofetil (MMF), and prednisone as the cornerstone of maintenance immunosuppression.[4] The most widely accepted regimens still rely on a calcineurin phosphatase inhibitor (CNI), together with a cell cycle inhibitor and a corticosteroid preparation. The 2 main CNIs currently in use are cyclosporine (CsA) and tacrolimus with approximately 24% of patients receiving CsA and 76% receiving tacrolimus. Both work via similar mechanisms, and both have significant but not identical systemic side effects. There is no clear benefit of one over another in preventing OB or affecting survival. Adverse events associated with tacrolimus treatment include hyperglycemia, alopecia, and possibly PTLD, while an increased incidence of hypercholesterolemia, hirsutism, gingival hyperplasia, and hypertension are associated with CsA-based regimens.

In addition to a combination of calcineurin inhibitors and corticosteroids, approximately 61% of pediatric lung transplant recipients are now prescribed MMF, a cell-cycle inhibitor. Despite a number of trials in adult lung transplant recipients comparing azathioprine and MMF, no clear benefit of one versus the other has emerged.[15,16]

Virtually all pediatric lung transplant programs include steroids as part of a triple drug immunosuppression regimen.[1] The steroid dose is weaned to reduce potential complications, including osteopenia and hyperglycemia. Although virtually all lung transplant recipients at 1- and 5-year follow-up still receive prednisone, these protocols continue to be center-specific.

Long-term Follow-up After Transplant

The prognosis after a successful lung transplant is guarded. Mortality due to complications is 10% to 15% in the first year, with most complications occurring in the first 6 months post-transplant.[1] Early graft dysfunction occurs as a result of ischemia and reperfusion injury (IRI), and accounts for most deaths in the first 30 days after transplant. Most lung transplant recipients demonstrate some clinical expression of primary graft dysfunction (PGD) caused by IRI postoperatively, typically within the first 72 hours after the transplant. The syndrome manifests as various levels of severity of graft dysfunction, from mild hypoxemia to fulminant graft failure. Primary graft dysfunction is noted histologically with neutrophil infiltration. The incidence of higher grades of PGD has decreased dramatically with improvements in organ preservation techniques at the time of organ harvesting.

Ischemia and reperfusion injury that progresses to severe primary graft dysfunction is highly associated with chronic graft dysfunction or BOS.

Long-term Monitoring

Care for children with a lung transplant is complex. Monitoring the patient and graft health requires the coordination of care among many services. The transplant team components include the patient and their family; a pulmonary function laboratory that is familiar with working with children; and ancillary services, including radiology, interventional radiology, pharmacy, laboratory, social work, specialty nursing, and committed primary care and pulmonary physicians. Most transplant centers monitor patients routinely with laboratory tests, surveillance bronchoscopy for assessment of rejection and infection, spirometry and other pulmonary function tests, and x-rays. Because of the limitations of infant pulmonary function testing and the fact that sedation is required for many diagnostic procedures, follow-up of infant lung transplant recipients presents additional challenges. Transbronchial biopsies can be performed safely by well-trained personnel and are the primary means by which acute cellular rejection is diagnosed.

Rejection

Children who have received lung transplants may experience 1 or more of 4 types of rejection. See Box 33-4.

Hyperacute Rejection

Hyperacute rejection is rare, but can cause complete rejection of the lungs within 24 hours. Hyperacute rejection is caused by antibodies to the allograft formed by the recipient after a sensitizing event (blood transfusion, pregnancy, connective tissue disease, or previous transplantation). The exact mechanism of hyperacute rejection appears to involve preformed antibodies against major allograft antigens, usually HLA or ABO. Hyperacute rejection is manifest clinically as severe graft dysfunction with worsening oxygenation, a decrease in lung function, fever, pleural effusions, pulmonary edema, and diffuse parenchymal infiltrates and can present as diffuse alveolar damage.[17–19]

Acute Cellular Rejection

Acute cellular rejection occurs when T lymphocytes identify foreign proteins on the surface of cells in the transplanted lung and cause injury to those cells. This is a normal function of the immune system and is important as a response to control the growth of tumors and viral infections.

Box 33-4. Types of Lung Transplant Rejection

1. Hyperacute rejection (immediately after transplant)—This is a rare event and occurs if human leukocyte antigen sensitization to the donor antigens is present.
2. Acute rejection (most common in the first 6–12 months)—This is the most common type of rejection and occurs with highest frequency in the first year after transplantation.
3. Humoral rejection—Antibody-mediated rejection that occurs if donor-specific antibody develops.
4. Chronic airway rejection—The process begins in all lung recipients within the first or second year, and progression depends on host factors as well as immunologic factors related to the graft. Chronic vascular rejection occurs in the cardiac graft in heart and lung transplants, and is the equivalent of chronic airway rejection.

Acute rejection usually occurs in the first 6 to 12 months and is usually detected at a mild stage, because of increased surveillance with bronchoscopy and biopsy during the first 6 months after transplant. Transplant centers differ in their protocols for transbronchial biopsy surveillance, but on average, bronchoscopy and biopsy are performed monthly for the first 3 months, at the sixth month, the ninth month, and then again at 12 months. There is controversy as to when or if transbronchial biopsies should be done after the first year, but many centers will perform surveillance bronchoscopy annually thereafter, and obtain biopsies if clinically indicated. Biopsies are performed if there is suspicion of acute rejection or in the case of suspected cytomegalovirus infection. Indications will likely broaden, especially in efforts to detect evidence of antibody-mediated rejection in case of BOS and high-specificity donor-specific antibody formation.

Acute rejection is graded depending on how far the lymphocytes extend into the tissue surrounding the blood vessels (Figure 33-3A–D). Acute rejection can occur with or without outward symptoms. If symptoms are present, they are similar to a lung infection and include fever, cough, dyspnea on exertion, decrease in pulmonary function tests (forced vital capacity [FVC] and FEV_1), elevated white blood cell count, and an abnormal chest radiograph (pleural effusion or pneumonia-like changes).

Most initial episodes of acute rejection respond to treatment with high doses of steroids and do not significantly affect lung function once treated. If the pathology is classified as grade A2 or worse, treatment is initiated with a pulse of intravenous corticosteroid once a day for 3 days. A follow-up bronchoscopy and transbronchial biopsy are performed 2 to 4 weeks after completing treatment to confirm response. If rejection is still present on the follow-up biopsy, and it is not grade A1 or improved, anti-lymphocytic antibody (rabbit antithymocyte globulin [rATG] or daclizumab) treatment may be initiated and immunosuppressive agents may be altered or increased.

Most patients have at least one episode of acute rejection in the first year, though the risk may be lower in children younger than 1 year. If rejection is detected early and is low-grade (A2 or better), allograft dysfunction can be avoided with the use of pulsed immune suppression therapy. In most patients, mild acute rejection resolves after treatment.

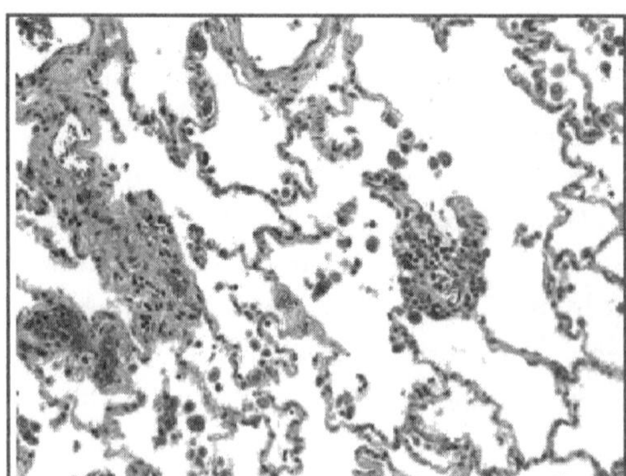

A

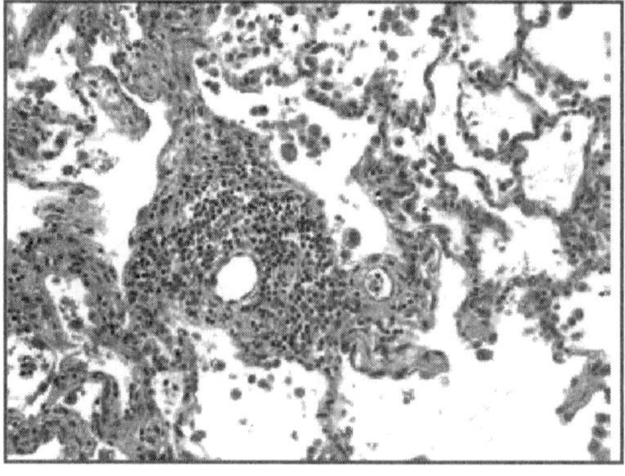

B

Figure 33-3. Hisotpathology of acute cellular rejection and grades of severity. **(A)** Grade A1: minimal acute cellular rejection, **(B)** grade A2: mild acute cellular rejection.

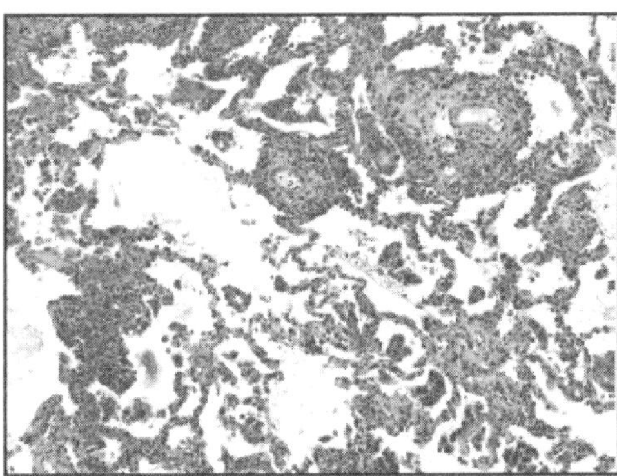

C

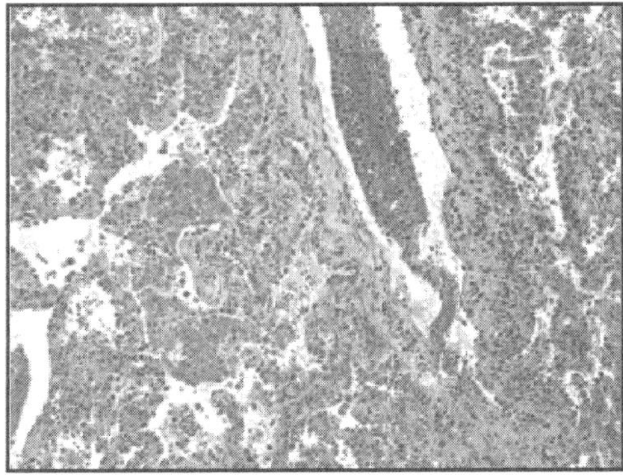

D

Figure 33-3. Hisotpathology of acute cellular rejection and grades of severity. **(C)** grade A3: moderate acute cellular rejection, **(D)** grade A4: severe acute cellular rejection.

Bronchiolitis Obliterans

Rejection is a persistent threat to graft and patient survival throughout the rest of the recipient's life. In the case of chronic graft rejection (ie, long-standing), the chance of reversing the rejection process is low, and mortality (death) is high since the lungs cannot function normally. Bronchiolitis obliterans is the most important life-limiting complication to restrict long-term survival after lung transplantation. It is also the most common complication occurring more than a year after lung transplant. There are different names for bronchiolitis obliterans: OB, chronic airway rejection, chronic lung rejection, and chronic graft rejection. The term bronchiolitis obliterans refers specifically to the pathology seen on biopsy. Bronchioles are the smallest airways in the lungs and these are the parts damaged in OB. Initially, they show T lymphocytes in the airway walls, and as damage progresses, scars form. Chronic rejection is manifest by fibrous scarring, which is often dense and eosinophilic, involving the bronchioles and sometimes associated with accelerated fibrointimal changes affecting pulmonary arteries and veins (Figure 33-4).

There is no specific prevention or cure for OB. Obliterative bronchiolitis likely represents a common lesion in which different inflammatory insults, such as ischemia-reperfusion injury,[20] microvascular injury,[21] rejection,[13,22–25] and infection[14,26] lead to a similar histologic and clinical outcome.

The symptoms of BOS include shortness of breath and low oxygen saturation levels. Patients who develop OB may have chest cold symptoms

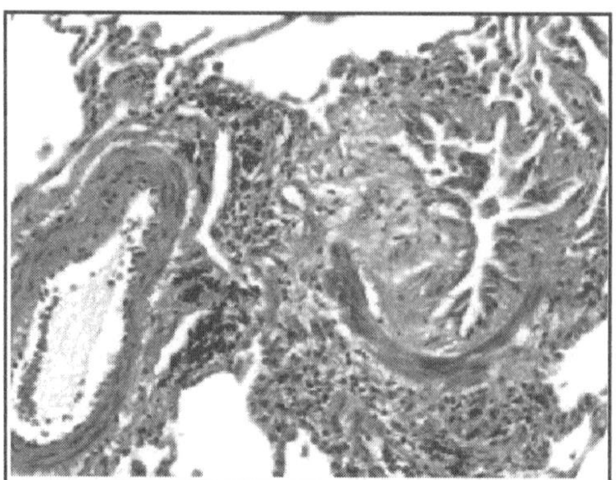

Figure 33-4. Obliterative bronchiolitis.

or initially may have no symptoms at all. It is detected clinically with the use of pulmonary function testing.

The most useful early indicator of OB is a drop in lung function, specifically, the FEV_1 and the forced expiratory flow from 25% to 75% of FVC that is not otherwise explained. See Table 33-4 for grading criteria of BOS. The potential-BOS stage alerts the physician to the need for close functional monitoring and assessment. Symptoms of more severe OB include a dry cough or productive cough that is not related to an infection, a new onset of shortness of breath with or without exercise, and a decrease in lung function (FEV_1) that is otherwise unexplained. A decrease in oxygen saturation measure will eventually occur but is a late sign.

The diagnosis of OB is difficult clinically, particularly in children who cannot consistently perform pulmonary function testing. A ventilation/perfusion scan and a computed tomography scan are helpful in the workup to assess for evidence of maldistribution of ventilation and air trapping. An open lung biopsy may be necessary to confirm the diagnosis.

Obliterative bronchiolitis/BOS cannot be cured, but the progression of lung damage can often be halted or slowed if the cause is treatable (eg, infection or aspiration of gastric acid). The treatment is variable

Table 33-4. Classification and Staging of Bronchiolitis Obliterans Syndrome (BOS)

BOS Stage	Definition
0	FEV_1 >90% of baseline and FEF_{25-75} >75% of baseline
0-p	FEV_1 81%–90% of baseline and/or FEF_{25-75} ≤75% of baseline
1	FEV_1 66%–80% of baseline
2	FEV_1 51%–65% of baseline
3	FEV_1 ≤50% of baseline

Abbreviations: FEF_{25-75}, forced expiratory flow from 25% to 75% of forced vital capacity; FEV_1, forced expiratory volume at 1 second; O-p, potential BOS.

and depends on previous complications or infections that occurred after transplant. In the absence of infection or other treatable medical condition, treatment with rATG or daclizumab and a change in the regular immunosuppression medicines may be initiated. If the cause of BOS is humoral rejection, plasmapheresis, intravenous immunoglobulin, and rituximab (anti–B-cell therapy) are initiated.

Post-Transplant Lymphoproliferative Disease

All transplant patients are at risk of developing PTLD because of the immunosuppression treatment that is required to maintain good graft function, avoid rejection, and avoid BOS. Post-transplant lymphoproliferative disease is a form of cancer that occurs most often in children who were not exposed to EBV before transplantation, but who are exposed after the transplant. It can also develop in children who were previously infected with EBV. The virus lies dormant in the B lymphocyte cells, and the EBV might reactivate because the child is immunosuppressed. When this happens, the B cells can multiply so rapidly that they resemble a cancer tumor.

Post-transplant lymphoproliferative disease occurs in about 10% to 15% of pediatric lung transplant recipients. It most commonly occurs in the first 2 to 3 months following transplantation at the time of highest immune suppression, but may occur many years after transplant. Some patients do not have symptoms at all and the tumor is found during a routine physical examination. Other patients have flu-like symptoms, and some patients have problems associated with the location of the tumor (diarrhea, pharyngitis, hepatitis, cough, etc). The prognosis depends on the amount and location of tumor formation and the response to treatment. In a small number of cases PTLD is fatal.

There are several types of treatment options for PTLD. Most often, the doses of the immunosuppressive medicines will be decreased. This may cause the tumor to shrink or even disappear. The risk of rejection is then increased, so the children are monitored more closely for rejection. In some cases surgery is necessary to remove large, bulky tumors and, on rarer occasions, chemotherapy is required.

Survival

Bronchiolitis obliterans syndrome is the most significant reason for poor long-term survival for lung and heart-lung transplant recipients. Children who survive 1 year after transplant have good functionality of the allograft, though approximately 13% have OB and the incidence increases over time.[1] The prevalence of OB is greater than 50% in both adults and children who survive 5 years after transplantation. For those who receive transplants from a diseased donor, OB is the most common cause of death beyond the first year. Living donor lobar transplant recipients generally die from complications of infection.[27] Overall survival is equivalent regardless of the source of the transplant.

Children with lung transplants are subject to similar complications as adults, though growth and developmental issues are unique. In addition, non-adherence is a more frequent problem for adolescents. The 5-year survival rate after lung transplant in children is about 50% (Figure 33-1).[1] Survival among children with noninfectious lung disease (other than CF) is better than patients with pulmonary vascular disease or CF.[28] Infants have a higher 1-year mortality, although long-term survival in infants is similar to other pediatric recipients. Pediatric re-transplantation has much lower first-year and long-term survival compared with primary transplants in children and adults.[1,29,30] Risk factors for mortality after lung transplant include repeat transplant, mechanical ventilation at transplant, and diagnosis of congenital heart disease.

Key Points

- Lung and heart-lung transplantation is indicated in children who have developed end-stage lung disease who have no other medical or surgical treatment options, and life expectancy is less than 2 years.
- Children and adolescents are most frequently referred for transplant because of end-stage diseases of CF and pulmonary arterial hypertension.
- Lung transplantation is elected as an option after careful consideration and extensive education and does not occur emergently.
- Postoperative care is complex and requires the close interaction between the primary care practitioner and the transplant team for the rest of the life of the recipient.
- The immune suppression regimen consists of a triple-drug regimen, including a calcineurin inhibitor, a T lymphocyte anti-proliferative medication, and corticosteroid therapy. These are continued for the rest of the patient's life.
- The maintenance medication regimen is dosed carefully to maintain a balance between preventing rejection and preventing infection.
- The most important life-limiting complication that restricts long-term survival of lung and heart-lung transplant recipients after the first year is OB, chronic graft rejection.
- Lung and heart-lung transplantation extend and improve the quality of life, but because of the occurrence of OB, they are not a likely means to extend life beyond approximately 7 to 10 years.

References

1. Spray TL, Mallory GB, Cantor CB, et al. Pediatric lung transplantation: indications, techniques and early results. *J Thorac Cardiovasc Surg.* 1994;107:990–1000
2. Gammie JS, Keenan RJ, Pham SM, et al. Single versus double-lung transplantation for pulmonary hypertension. *J Thorac Cardiovasc Surg.* 1998;115:397–402
3. Cohen RG, Starnes VA. Living donor lung transplantation. *World J Surg.* 2001;25:244–250

4. International guidelines for the selection of lung transplant candidates. The American Society for Transplant Physicians (ASTP)/American Thoracic Society(ATS)/European Respiratory Society (ERS)/International Society for Heart and Lung Transplantation (ISHLT). *Am J Respir Crit Care Med.* 1998;158:335–339
5. Faro A, Mallory GB, Visner GA, et al. American Society of Transplantation Executive Summary on Pediatric Lung Transplantation. *Am J Transplant.* 2007;7:285–292
6. Kerem H, Reisman J, Corey M, et al. Prediction of mortality in patients with cystic fibrosis. *N Engl J Med.* 1992;326:1187–1191
7. Aris RM, Routh JC, LiPuma JJ, et al. Lung transplantation for cystic fibrosis patients with *Burkholderia cepacia* complex. Survival linked to genomovar type. *Am J Respir Crit Care Med.* 2001;164:2102–2106
8. De Soyza A, McDowell A, Archer L, et al. *Burkholderia cepacia* complex genomovars and pulmonary transplantation outcomes in patients with cystic fibrosis. *Lancet.* 2001;358:1780–1781
9. Boussaud V, Guillemain R, Grenet D, et al. Clinical outcome following lung transplantation in patients with cystic fibrosis colonised with *Burkholderia cepacia* complex: results from the French centres. *Thorax.* 2008;63:732–737
10. Alexander BD, Petzold EW, Reller LB, et al. Survival after lung transplantation of cystic fibrosis patients infected with *Burkholderia cepacia* complex. *Am J Transplant.* 2008;8:1025–1030
11. Murray S, Charbeneau J, Marshall BC, LiPuma JJ. Impact of burkholderia infection on lung transplantation in cystic fibrosis. *Am J Respir Crit Care Med.* 2008;178:363–371
12. Danziger-Isakov LA, Worley S, Arrigain S, et al. Increased mortality after pulmonary fungal infection within the first year after pediatric lung transplantation. *J Heart Lung Transplant.* 2008;27(6):655–661
13. Bando K, Paradis IL, Simiol S, et al. Obliterative bronchiolitis after lung and heart–lung transplantation: an analysis of risk factors and management. *J Thorac Cardiovasc Surg.* 1995;110:4–13
14. Levy RD, Estenne M, Weder W, Cosio MG. Post-transplant bronchiolitis obliterans. *Eur Respir J.* 2003;22:1007–1018
15. McNeil K, Glanville AR, Wahlers T, et al. Comparison of mycophenolate mofetil and azathioprine for prevention of bronchiolitis obliterans syndrome in de novo lung transplant recipients. *Transplantation.* 2006;81(7):998–1003
16. Palmer SM, Baz MA, Sanders L, et al. Results of a randomized, prospective, multicenter trial of mycophenolate mofetil versus azathioprine in the prevention of acute lung allograft rejection. *Transplantation.* 2001;71(12):1772–1776
17. Choi J, Kearns J, Palevsky HI, et al. Hyperacute rejection of a pulmonary allograft. Immediate clinical and pathologic findings. *Am J Respir Crit Care Med.* 1999;160:1015–1018

18. Lau A, Palmer SM, Posther KE, et al. Influence of panel-reactive antibodies on posttransplant outcomes in lung transplant recipients. *Ann Thorac Surg.* 2000;69:1520–1524
19. Masson E, Stern M, Chabod J, et al. Hyperacute rejection after lung transplantation caused by undetected low titer anti-HLA antibodies. *J Heart Lung Transplant.* 2007;26:642–645
20. Fiser SM, Tribble CG, Long SM, et al. Ischemia-reperfusion injury after lung transplantation increases risk of late bronchiolitis obliterans syndrome. *Ann Thorac Surg.* 2002;73:1041–1047
21. Babu AN, Murakawa T, Thurman JM, et al. Microvascular destruction identifies murine allografts that cannot be rescued from airway fibrosis. *J Clin Invest.* 2007;117:3774–3785
22. Date J, Lynch JP, Sundaresan S, Patterson GA, Trulock EP. The impact of cytolytic therapy on bronchiolitis obliterans syndrome. *J Heart Lung Transplant.* 1998;17:869–875
23. Tikkanen JM, Lemstrom KB, Koskinen PK. Blockade of CD28/B7-2 costimulation inhibits experimental obliterative bronchiolitis in rat tracheal allografts: suppression of helper T cell type 1-dominated immune response *Am J Respir Crit Care Med.* 2002;165:724–729
24. Duncan SR, Leonard C, Theodore J, et al. Oligoclonal CD4(+) T cell expansions in lung transplant recipients with obliterative bronchiolitis. *Am J Respir Crit Care Med.* 2002;165:1439–1444
25. Duncan SR, Valentine V, Roglic M, et al. T cell receptor biases and clonal proliferations among lung transplant recipients with obliterative bronchiolitis. *J Clin Invest.* 1996;97:2642–5260
26. Vos R, Vanaudenaerde BM, Geudens N, et al. Pseudomonal airway colonization: risk factor for bronchiolitis obliterans syndrome after lung transplantation. *Eur Respir J.* 2008;31:1037–1045
27. Woo MS, MacLaughlin EF, Horn MV, Szmuszkovicz JR, Barr ML, Starnes VA. Bronchiolitis obliterans is not the primary cause of death in pediatric living donor lobar lung transplant recipients. *J Heart Lung Transplant.* 2001;20(5):491–496
28. Sweet SC. Pediatric lung transplantation: update 2003. *Pediatr Clin North Am.* 2003;50(6):1393–1417
29. Huddleston CB, Mendeloff EN, Cohen AH, Sweet SC, Balzer DT, Mallory GB Jr. Lung retransplantation in children. *Ann Thorac Surg.* 1998;66(1):199–203; discussion 203–204
30. Novick RJ, Stitt LW, Al-Kattan K, et al. Pulmonary retransplantation: predictors of graft function and survival in 230 patients. Pulmonary Retransplant Registry. *Ann Thorac Surg.* 1998;65(1):227–234

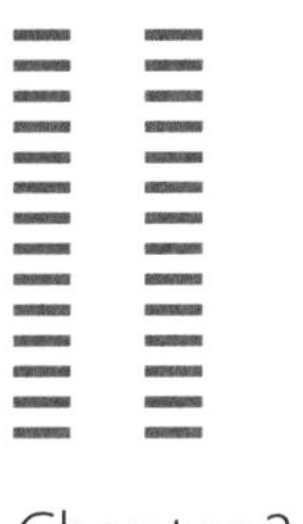

Chapter 34

Respiratory Disorders Associated With Obesity

Douglas N. Homnick, MD, MPH

Case Report 34-1
T.A. is a 14-year-old African American girl who arrives in the office with complaints that she "can't catch her breath" with exertion, including running laps in gym class and climbing stairs. She also occasionally wakes at night with shortness of breath and feels more comfortable sleeping with 2 pillows. Her examination in the clinic reveals an obese young female with a body mass index (BMI) of 38 (>97th percentile) but is otherwise normal. Spirometry done in the clinic shows a forced vital capacity of 72% predicted and forced expiratory volume over 1 second (FEV_1) of 70% predicted. She does not respond to a bronchodilator.

Introduction

Overweight and obesity remain significant public health problems, with increases in the prevalence in both adults and children over the last 2 decades (Figure 34-1). In the United States, 65% of adults 20 years or older are overweight or obese (defined by BMI ≥30 kg/m^2) and 16% of children are overweight (obese defined by BMI ≥95th percentile).[1] Overweight carries significant health risks, including cardiovascular disease, type II diabetes, orthopedic problems, dermatologic conditions, psychosocial issues, and reduced life expectancy, among others. Childhood obesity is a strong risk factor for adult obesity and its associated disabilities.[2]

The upper and lower respiratory tracts are affected significantly by obesity. Increases in body weight lead to upper airway obstruction during sleep and decreased lung function. An increase in body mass is negatively associated with FEV_1 both in children and adults.[3–5]

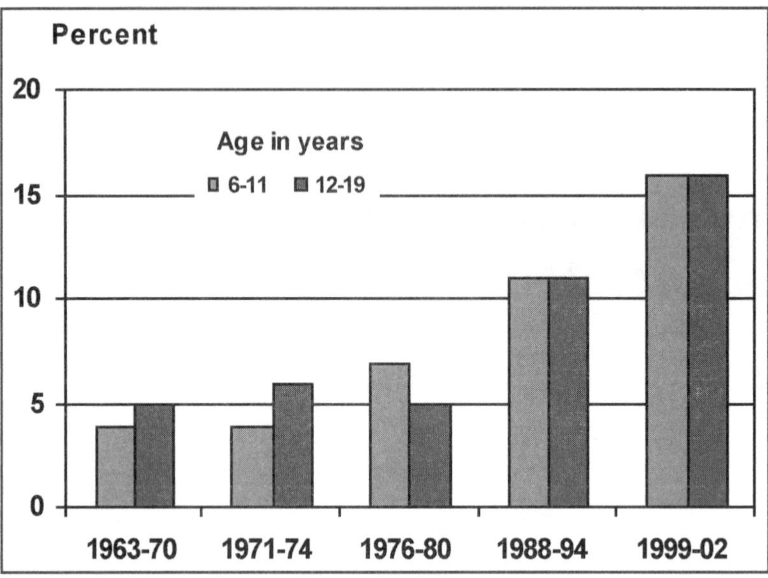

Figure 34-1. Increasing prevalence of overweight among children and adolescents aged 6–19 (percent of all children and adolescents in the United States). (Adapted from CDC/NHCS, NHES, and NHANES, www.cdc.gov/nchs/data/hestat/overweight/overweight99.htm.)

In addition, obese children show decreased static lung volumes similar to adults, as well as diffusion impairments[6] (Box 34-1).

In overweight individuals, wheezing and breathlessness (dyspnea) are the predominant respiratory symptoms. There are multiple factors that are responsible for this, including deconditioning, systemic inflammation, and disturbed chest wall mechanics. Both aerobic and anaerobic work capacity increase with training (regular physical exercise), as measured by increased oxygen consumption and decreased lactate production for a given workload. In childhood obesity, deconditioning often occurs with a sedentary lifestyle (eg, excess television viewing). When overweight children attempt to exercise there is a higher oxygen cost of breathing that leads to dyspnea and early cessation of activity.

Mechanically, excess weight compressing the chest wall and abdomen leads to inefficient ventilation because of decreased respiratory compliance. This is due to reduced lung volumes from decreased chest wall and diaphragm movement, fatty infiltration of the chest wall, and an

Box 34-1. Effects of Obesity on the Respiratory Tract

Clinical Presentation

Increased upper airway resistance and obstructive sleep apnea due to tonsillar hypertrophy or increased hypopharyngeal tissue

Wheezing due to airway inflammation

Dyspnea due to poor conditioning and increased work of breathing

Gastroesophageal reflux with possible aspiration causing airway inflammation or secondary to obesity and lung hyperinflation

Pulmonary Function Abnormalities

Decreased spirometry (forced vital capacity, forced expiratory volume over 1 second, forced expiratory flows between 25% and 75% of the forced vital capacity)

Decreased lung volumes

Increased oxygen consumption/decreased work capacity

increase in blood volume.[7] Compression also leads to inefficient respiratory muscle function, which increases both work of breathing and oxygen consumption. Systemic inflammation possibly leading to airway inflammation and increased airway hyperresponsiveness (AHR) may also contribute to this airway narrowing (see Clinical Features on page 668 for in-depth discussion). In addition to the physical restrictions on activity posed by obesity, the psychosocial cost is significant, and feelings of helplessness and despair can also affect behaviors that continue the obesity-inactivity-deconditioning cycle.

Obesity, Wheezing, and Asthma

Although the literature on the association of asthma and obesity is more extensive in adults, prospective studies in children suggest but do not consistently prove a similar relationship. For example, several large longitudinal studies have shown conflicting data with risk of asthma increased in obese boys only or obese girls only.[8,9] Whether increased BMI in early childhood predicts asthma in later years is likewise unknown. The Tucson Children's Respiratory Study[10] found no association with BMI at 6 years of age and wheezing at any age, but obese girls at 11 years of age were more likely to have increased bronchial hyperreactivity during early teen years. Contrary to this, a meta-analysis of 12 prospective studies of early childhood overweight on subsequent asthma risk showed a 50% greater risk of subsequent asthma occurring in those children with increased body weight at infancy through early childhood.[11] Many studies have not controlled for physical activity, and therefore it is unclear the exact relationship between deconditioning, wheezing, and asthma.[12] Whether asthma is more severe in the obese child is also unknown, as the relative contribution of inactivity because of poorly controlled asthma and increasing obesity as a result of oral corticosteroid use may confound the data.

Clinical Features

Asthma is defined as AHR or an exaggerated response to a stimulus (eg, asthma trigger, such as dust mites) associated with chronic inflammation and bronchoconstriction, leading to reversible airway obstruction. The degree of airway obstruction is measured by spirometry and static lung volumes, and AHR is measured by spirometry following bronchial challenge with methacholine, histamine, hypertonic saline, cold air, etc. Studies on the relationship of BMI and AHR have been inconsistent. Obesity was associated with increased inhaler use and asthma symptoms but not AHR in a large study of 5,984 children.[13] Other studies have shown an association of obesity with AHR similar to normal weight children and in some cases even less than non-obese peers.[14] If rates of AHR are similar to normal weight children, what accounts for increased dyspnea and wheezing, and increased severity of asthma symptoms, in obese youth? Several mechanisms are likely and include the following:

1. Abdominal and chest restriction due to excess weight on the abdominal and chest walls leads to reduction in lung volume and associated decreased airway caliber. Obese individuals breathe with a lower tidal volume and higher rate to maintain adequate minute ventilation.[15] There is some evidence to suggest that increased airway hyperreactivity can occur when airway smooth muscle is not at its optimal length.[14] Closure of peripheral airways can occur, particularly when patients are supine, leading to increased work of breathing and atelectasis.
2. Airway inflammation may occur secondary to the increased systemic inflammation in obesity. Increases in circulating inflammatory mediators are well documented in studies of obese adults and in some pediatric studies. Increased visceral fat is associated with higher circulating levels of tumor necrosis factor α, interleukin 6, and the acute phase reactant C-reactive protein (CRP).[7,12] Leptin,

an appetite suppressing hormone released from adipose tissue, increases in inflammation while adiponectin, which is involved in the prevention of insulin resistance and is an anti-inflammatory protein, decreases in obesity.[7] The role that circulating proinflammatory molecules have in promoting asthma and wheezing in obese individuals is generally unknown, but with weight loss and increased pulmonary function, serum concentrations of these are reduced.

3. Evidence suggests that response to therapy may be suboptimal in obese adults and children with asthma. Obese patients may have difficulty achieving asthma control with an inhaled corticosteroid or with a long-acting β-agonist/inhaled corticosteroid (LABA/ICS) combination.[16] In addition, obese adults presenting to the emergency department are more likely to be admitted, and overweight children with asthma have longer intensive care unit and hospital lengths of stay due to slower response to therapy.[17] The mechanism of suboptimal response to therapy is unknown but may be aggravated by reduced baseline airway caliber.

Clinical Presentation

Acutely, wheezing and dyspnea are the presenting symptoms and indicate need for a trial of rescue therapy (systemic corticosteroids, short-acting β-agonist [SABA]). Chronically, patients will present with history of wheezing and dyspnea with even minor exertion. A physical examination will often, but not always, reveal symmetrical wheezing, which is exacerbated in a supine position and with exertion. Rational therapy must be based on lung function evaluation. Managing asthma without spirometry is akin to managing diabetes without blood sugars. Response to bronchodilators can be determined in the office with a bronchodilator challenge (ie, measure baseline spirometry, administer a SABA, repeat spirometry in 20 minutes). A 12% increase in FEV_1 indicates reversible airway obstruction, and likely the child will benefit from a trial of a LABA/ICS combination. Persistent obstruction despite a bronchodilator challenge indicates potential response to anti-inflammatory therapy (see Management on page 670). One can also quantify AHR with bronchial challenge using methacholine, histamine, hypertonic saline, cold air, etc. Methacholine is commonly used, and a 20% drop in FEV_1 during administration of drug dilutions indicates the presence of AHR. Obese children are no more likely than their normal weight peers to have exercise-induced asthma.[18] A discussion of the use of bronchial challenge to guide rational use of asthma medications can be found in Chapter 12.

Management

Optimal control of wheezing and dyspnea in obese children is multifold. Defining the degree of airway obstruction and response to therapy with spirometry and the physical examination is important. Asthma should be treated according to the National Heart, Lung, and Blood Institute National Asthma Education and Prevention Program guidelines,[19] taking into account the patient's current level of asthma control, which is a function of both degree of impairment and risk of exacerbations. Patients are then treated with daily inhaled corticosteroids alone or, if incompletely controlled, in combination therapy with an added LABA or leukotriene receptor antagonist, plus a SABA for rescue intervention. This is extensively discussed in Chapter 12. However, because of the mechanical and systemic inflammatory effects of obesity, reversal of airway obstruction is often incomplete, and overtreatment with corticosteroids is possible. Additional reversal of airway obstruction and reversal of wheezing depends on overcoming these mechanical effects with weight loss and conditioning. Weight loss leads to reduced symptoms, improvements in lung function, decreased indicators of systemic inflammation, and improved quality of life.[20,21] Weight loss is unlikely to occur without an increase in physical activity. Conditioning improves asthma symptoms and quality of life in children, whether overweight or not.[22] Therefore, a supervised exercise program must be included in any serious intervention.

Prognosis and When to Refer

The prognosis of asthma in obese children and adolescents varies with their ability to adhere to a rational drug regimen, undertake environmental controls, psychological intervention, and regular follow-up. Weight loss is the ideal goal, but it is hard to achieve even with an organized, supervised program of calorie restriction and increased physical activity. Referral to a pediatric pulmonologist or allergist can help establish that asthma is the definitive diagnosis and, if so, help develop a good asthma intervention plan, provide for regular asthma follow-up, reinforce primary care recommendations, and provide for interpretation of specialized pulmonary function testing.

Obesity and Obstructive Sleep Apnea Syndrome

Obesity is a well-documented risk factor for sleep-disordered breathing (SDB), including obstructive sleep apnea syndrome (OSAS). However, adenotonsillar hypertrophy/hyperplasia (discussed in detail in Chapter 36) remains the single most important cause in children. Obesity is definitely associated with OSAS in adults, and increasing numbers of studies have shown its importance in children as well. Obese children are at increased risk of SDB, including OSAS (defined as recurrent episodes of partial or complete upper airway obstruction during sleep associated with a disruption of normal gas exchange and sleep fragmentation), which appears to be proportional to the degree of obesity.[23] In fact, obese children aged 2 to 18 years have a 4- to 5-fold increased risk of SDB compared with normal weight peers, with sleep study (polysomnographic) abnormalities occurring in 24% to 66% of individuals.[24,25]

The consequences of untreated SDB, including OSAS, are substantial. Neurobehavioral effects are well documented and include aggressiveness, agitation, daytime somnolence, and poor school performance.[26] Although the mechanisms remain unclear, cases of attention-deficit/hyperactivity disorder have been attributed to SDB. Systemic hypertension has also been reported in children with OSAS as well as elevated CRP, a predictor of future cardiovascular problems.[27,28]

Clinical Features

Most children with OSAS are not obese but, as noted previously, a disproportionate percentage of obese children have this condition. Also, most children with OSAS have enlarged tonsils and adenoids, including those who are overweight. However, it has been pointed out that adenotonsillar enlargement is not always the only contributing factor to OSAS.[29] Like adults, fatty infiltration of the upper airway and anterior neck may contribute to airway collapse during sleep. Also increased adipose tissue infiltrating the chest wall leads to decreased ventilation, through increased work of breathing and decreased lung volumes.

Peripheral and central leptin resistance occurs in obesity. Leptin is an adipose tissue derived hormone that is responsible for the sense of satiety.[30] It is also a potent respiratory stimulant and has central chemoreceptor modulatory properties; decreased activity of which leads to reduced responses to hypercapnia and reduced ventilatory drive.[31] This may contribute to SDB in children.

Clinical Presentation

Snoring is the sine qua non of OSAS risk and indicates increased upper airway resistance. Snoring is estimated to occur in up to 27% of children.[32] Clinical presentation is no different in the obese child, but polysomnographic abnormalities occur more frequently and, therefore, signs and symptoms of SDB must be carefully sought through history and physical examination.[29] Polysomnography is the gold standard of objective SDB evaluation, and it is particularly important to document abnormalities before undergoing surgical therapy. Further information on polysomnography can be found in Chapter 36.

Management

After polysomnographic documentation of SDB, the first line of therapy is adenotonsillectomy (T&A), which is curative in up to 75% of patients, including those who are overweight.[33] Specifically in obese children, T&A results in improved respiratory disturbance indices and resolution of OSAS (46%).[34] Because of pathophysiological considerations other than increased upper airway resistance due to adenotonsillar hypertrophy, T&A may only partially resolve the problem. Frequency of residual OSAS after T&A is higher in obese children and, therefore, postoperative polysomnography is important in these patients to define these residua.[29] Because of increased postoperative complications in obese children, hospitalization and monitoring after T&A is important.[35]

Weight loss improves SDB in children as well as adults and must be a component of a therapeutic plan. Programs simply promoting dietary management are often unsuccessful and a combined approach, including psychological evaluation and counseling, increased physical activity, and dietary modification, has the best chance to succeed. Bariatric surgery has been used in the case of extreme obesity in adolescent patients, with complete resolution of OSAS in many.[36]

Prognosis and When to Refer

Prognosis is generally very good after T&A, with complete resolution of symptoms in most cases. Referral to a pediatric sleep specialist for evaluation and polysomnography helps not only detect the severity of preoperative sleep disturbance but allows for postoperative evaluation to detect and manage residual problems. Because of the higher risk of postoperative complications, pediatric pulmonary or critical care consultation before surgery is prudent.

Other Conditions in Which Obesity Affects the Respiratory Tract

Gastroesophageal Reflux Disease (GERD)

Symptoms associated with GERD, including regurgitation and heart burn, are increased in both overweight children and adults, and in patients with asthma. However, the contribution of each condition to GERD is unclear. Additionally in the case of asthma, the onset of GERD in relationship to the onset of asthma symptoms is likewise unclear. It appears that overweight and asthma are both independent risk factors for development of GERD and controlling both conditions, as well as reducing GERD symptoms, is prudent.[37] Weight loss plus anti-secretory medications and bariatric surgery for morbid obesity have been shown to reduce GERD symptoms.[38] Referral to a pediatric gastroenterologist is recommended when symptoms are not controlled with dietary measures and medications.

Neuromuscular Disease (NMD)

Excess weight gain in children with NMDs, such as Duchenne muscular dystrophy, is due to a combination of factors, including inactivity, overfeeding, and use of corticosteroids. Fatty loading of the chest wall can contribute to low lung volumes and associated decreased airway caliber, compromising the already weakened respiratory musculature and, ultimately, ventilation. In one study, metabolic syndrome (obesity, hypertension, dyslipidemia, insulin resistance) occurred in a high percentage (55%) of patients with slowly progressive types of NMD, putting these patients at risk for future cardiovascular events.[39] Sleep-disordered breathing also occurs to a higher degree in patients with NMD, especially preceding respiratory failure.[40] Obesity is a risk factor for increased upper airway resistance and OSAS and low lung volumes and increased work of breathing for hypoxemia, and can contribute to early development of SDB and, ultimately, respiratory failure. Referral to a sleep specialist and pediatric pulmonologist for pulmonary function evaluation and polysomnography is important to detect and manage the degree of respiratory compromise caused by NMD and provide for early intervention in emerging respiratory failure.

Prader-Willi Syndrome (PWS)

Prader-Willi syndrome is a genetic disorder causing hypotonia, developmental delay, behavioral problems, growth hormone deficiency with short stature, hypogonadism, and obesity, stemming from hyperphagia. The hyperphagia appears to be due at least in part to high circulating levels of ghrelin, an orexigenic hormone.[41]

Children with PWS often exhibit excess daytime sleepiness associated with a variety of breathing abnormalities during sleep. These include primary abnormal ventilatory responses to hypercapnea and hypoxia and other forms of SDB, including OSAS, central apneas, and nocturnal alveolar hypoventilation. Obesity may aggravate these primary conditions, and a comprehensive treatment plan should include weight control through behavioral modification, T&A, and ventilatory support for those who develop respiratory insufficiency. Referral to sleep a specialist and pediatric pulmonologist can help with evaluation and management of these children, especially where ventilatory support is needed.

Obesity Hypoventilation Syndrome (OHS)

Also known as Pickwickian syndrome, OHS involves obesity and awake hypercapnia. Presentation is similar to OSAS, with daytime somnolence, morning headaches, and fatigue. Chronic hypoxemia and hypercapnia may eventually lead to right-sided heart failure (cor pulmonale) secondary to pulmonary hypertension and polycythemia.[28] It has been rarely described in children in the absence of neurologic disease but is likely to become more common with increasing rates of childhood obesity. The hallmark is decreased ventilatory responses to hypercapnia and hypoxemia both during awake periods and sleep, which is quantified during polysomnography. It is thought to be due to mechanical loading of the respiratory tract and genetically determined abnormal responses to chemoreceptor stimulation during both hypoxemia and hypercapnia. As discussed previously, leptin is a central respiratory stimulant that appears to be deficient in those with this condition.

Therapy for OHS is initially T&A and requires close postoperative observation in the hospital, as these patients tend to experience respiratory failure in the immediate postsurgical period.[28] Patients will benefit from preoperative positive pressure therapy to stabilize their cardiopulmonary status and reverse daytime hypoventilation. Initiating this therapy prior to surgery reduces the risk of respiratory failure in the immediate postoperative period. Weight loss, although difficult to accomplish, will improve daytime hypercapnia, as well as increase lung volumes, and is an essential component of long-term management. Prognosis is guarded, with some individuals requiring long-term noninvasive ventilation with bilevel positive airway pressure, especially if T&A is not effective and weight control cannot be achieved. Referral to a pediatric pulmonologist is helpful, especially where long-term ventilatory support is needed.

Key Points

- The respiratory tract and cardiorespiratory physiology are significantly disturbed in many obese patients. Weight loss and control of weight are still the most important and potentially curative interventions. This is difficult to achieve without a supervised exercise program, attention to depression and other psychological barriers, a strong family support system, and dietary intervention.
- Overweight children and adolescents have more postoperative complications and should be monitored in the hospital following T&A and other procedures.
- Children with NMD benefit from early evaluation in consultation with a pediatric pulmonologist because obesity impacts the respiratory status. Polysomnography will detect early compromise of ventilation and provide for intervention with mechanical support. Prevention of obesity in patients with NMD will prolong the ability to self-ventilate.
- Symptomatic GERD not responding to usual dietary and medical therapies is a cause for referral to a pediatric gastroenterologist. Obesity aggravates this condition, and weight reduction combined with medical therapy produces clinical improvement.
- Establishing definitively the diagnosis of asthma is important as respiratory symptoms due to other causes, such as dyspnea due to deconditioning and GERD, may be confused. Pulmonary function testing along with referral for pediatric pulmonary consultation will help establish the diagnosis and provide for sound intervention.

References

1. Hedley AA, Ogden CL, Johnson CL, Carroll MD, Curtin LR, Flegal KM. Prevalence of overweight and obesity among US children, adolescents and adults, 1999–2002. *JAMA.* 2004;291(23):2847–2850
2. World Health Organization. Obesity and overweight. Fact Sheet no. 311. September 2006. http:www.who.int/mediacentre/factsheets/fs311/en.index.html
3. Carey IM, Cook DG, Strachman DP. The effects of adiposity and weight change on forced expiratory volume decline in a longitudinal study of adults. *Int J Obes Relat Metab Disord.* 1999;23:979–985
4. Lazarus R, Colditz G, Berkey CS, et al. Effects of body fat on ventilatory function in children and adolescents: cross-sectional findings from a random population sample of school children. *Pediatr Pulmonol.* 1997;24:187–194
5. Camargo CA Jr, Weiss ST, Zhang S, et al. Prospective study of body mass index, weight change, and risk of adult-onset asthma in women. *Arch Intern Med.* 1999;159:2582–2588
6. Li AM, Chan D, Wong E, et al. The effects of obesity on pulmonary function. *Arch Dis Child.* 2003;88:361–363
7. Beuther DA, Weiss ST, Sutherland ER. Obesity and asthma. *Am J Crit Care Med.* 2006;174:112–119
8. Gilliland FD, Berhane K, Islam T, Mcconnel R, Gauderman WJ, Gilliland SS. Obesity and the risk of newly diagnosed asthma in school-age children. *Am J Epidemiol.* 2003;158:406–415
9. Gold DR, Damokosh AI, Dockery DW, Berkey CS. Body-mass index as a predictor of incident asthma in a prospective cohort of children. *Pediatr Pulmonol.* 2004;36:514–521
10. Castro-Rodriguez JA, Holberg CJ, Morgan WJ, Wright AL, Martinez FD. Increased incidence of asthma-like symptoms in girls who become overweight or obese during the school years. *Am J Respir Crit Care Med.* 2001;163:1344–1349
11. Flaherman V, Rutherford GW. A meta-analysis of the effect of high weight on asthma. *Arch Dis Child.* 2006;91:334–339
12. Lucas SR, Platts-Mills TAE. Pediatric asthma and obesity. *Paediatr Respir Rev.* 2006;7:233–238
13. Bibi H, Shoseyov D, Feigenbaum D, et al. The relationship between asthma and obesity in children: is it real or a case of over diagnosis? *J Asthma.* 2004;41:403–410
14. Shore SA, Fredberg JJ. Obesity, smooth muscle, and airway hyperresponsiveness. *J Allergy Clin Immunol.* 2005;115:921–924
15. Sampson MG, Grassino AE. Load compensation in obese patients during quiet tidal breathing. *J Appl Physiol.* 1983;55:1269–1276
16. Boulet LP, Franssen E. Influence of obesity on response to fluticasone with or without salmeterol in moderate asthma. *Respir Med.* 2007;101(11):2240–2247

17. Carroll CL, Bhandari A, Zucker AR, Schramm CM. Childhood obesity increases duration of therapy during severe asthma exacerbations. *Pediatr Crit Care Med.* 2006;7(6):527–531
18. Joyner BL, Fiorino EK, Mmatta-Arroyo E, Needleman JP. Cardiopulmonary exercise testing in children and adolescents who report symptoms of exercise-induced asthma. *J Asthma.* 2006;43:675–678
19. National Heart, Lung, and Blood Institute. *Expert Panel Report 3: Guidelines for the Diagnosis and Management of Asthma,* Bethesda, MD: US Department of Health and Human Services, National Institutes of Health; 2007
20. Hakala K, Stenius-Aarniala B, Sovijarvi A. Effects of weight loss on peak flow variability, airways obstruction, and lung volumes in obese patients with asthma. *Chest.* 2000;118:1315–1321
21. Johnson JB, Summer W, Cutler RG et al. Alternate day calorie restriction improves clinical findings and reduces markers of oxidative stress and inflammation in overweight adults with moderate asthma. *Free Radic Biol Med.* 2007;42:665–674
22. Fanelli A, Barros Cabral AL, Neder JA, Martins MA, Fenandes Carvalho CR. Exercise training on disease control and quality of life in asthmatic children. *Med Sci Sports Exerc.* 2007;39(9):1474–1480
23. Tauman R, Gozal D. Obesity and obstructive sleep apnea in children. *Paediatr Respir Rev.* 2006;7:247–259
24. Mallory GB Jr, Fiser DH, Jackson R. Sleep-associated breathing disorders in morbidly obese children and adolescents. *J Pediatr.* 1989;115:892–897
25. Silvestri JM, Weese-Mayer DE, Bass MT, Kenny AS, Hauptman SA, Pearsall SM. Polysomnography in obese children with a history of sleep-associated breathing disorders. *Pediatr Pulmonol.* 1993;16:124–129
26. Weissbluth M, Davis AT, Poncher J, Reiff J. Signs of airway obstruction during sleep and behavioral, developmental, and academic problems. *J Dev Behav Pediatr.* 1983;4:119–121
27. Marcus CL, Greene MG, Carroll JL. Blood pressure in children with obstructive sleep apnea. *Am J Respir Crit Care Med.* 1998;157:1098–1103
28. Tauman R, Ivanenko A, O'Brien LM, Gozal D. Plasma C-reactive protein levels among children with sleep-disordered breathing. *Pediatrics.* 2004;113:e564–e569
29. Marcus CL, Curtis S, Koener CB, Joffe A, Serwint JR, Loughlin GM. Evaluation of pulmonary function and polysomnography in obese children and adolescents. *Pediatr Pulmonol.* 1996;21:176–183
30. Shore SA. Obesity and asthma: possible mechanisms. *J Allergy Clin Immunol.* 2008;21(5):1087–1093
31. Polotsky VY, Smaldone MC, Scharf MT, et al. Impact of interrupted leptin pathways on ventilatory control. *J Appl Physiol.* 2004;96:991–998
32. Owen GO, Canter RJ, Robinson A. Snoring, apnea, and ENT symptoms in the pediatric community. *Clin Otolaryngol Allied Sci.* 1996;21:130–134

33. Schecter MS; American Academy of Pediatrics Section on Pediatric Pulmonology, Subcommittee on Obstructive Sleep Apnea Syndrome. Technical report: diagnosis and management of childhood obstructive sleep apnea syndrome. *Pediatrics.* 2002;109:e69
34. Mitchell RB, Kelly J. Adenotonsillectomy for obstructive sleep apnea in obese children. *Otolaryngol Head Neck Surg.* 2004;131:104–108
35. American Academy of Pediatrics Section on Pediatric Pulmonology, Subcommittee on Obstructive Sleep Apnea Syndrome. Clinical practice guideline: diagnosis and management of childhood obstructive sleep apnea syndrome. *Pediatrics.* 2002;109:704–712
36. Kalra M, Inge T. Effect of bariatric surgery on obstructive sleep apnea in adolescents. *Pediatr Respir Rev.* 2006;7:260–267
37. Stordal K, Johannesdottir GB, Bentsen BS, Carlsen KC, Sandvik L. Asthma and overweight are associated with symptoms of gastro-esophageal reflux. *Acta Pediatr.* 2006;95(10):1197–1201
38. Sise A, Friedenberg FK. A comprehensive review of gastroesophageal reflux disease and obesity. *Obes Rev.* 2008;9(3):194–203
39. Aitkens S, Kilmer DD, Wright NC, McCrory MA. Metabolic syndrome in neuromuscular disease. *Arch Phys Med Rehabil.* 2005;86(5):1030–1036
40. Piper A. Sleep abnormalities associated with neuromuscular disease: pathophysiology and evaluation. *Semin Respir Crit Care Med.* 2002;23(3):211–219
41. Delparigi A, Tschop M, Heiman ML, et al. High circulating ghrelin: a potential cause for hyperphagia and obesity in Prader-Willi syndrome. *J Clin Endocrinol Metab.* 2002;87(12):5461–5464

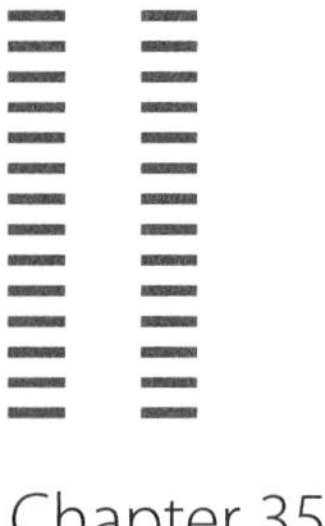

Chapter 35

Functional Respiratory Disorders

Douglas N. Homnick, MD, MPH

Introduction

Functional respiratory disorders are diagnoses of exclusion made after detectable "organic" disease is ruled out through history, physical examination, and specific testing. The variations of symptoms probably represent a spectrum of psychologically driven disorders that have a common origin in anxiety rather than specific, individual etiologies. Common clinical signs and symptoms of functional disease include heavy breathing or dyspnea; cough, sighing, or sneezing; various breathing sounds; tightness of the throat or chest; pain; and fear.[1] A characteristic feature includes the disappearance of symptoms with sleep and with distraction. Many of the disorders discussed herein contain features of both a conversion disorder and panic attacks; the diagnostic criteria for each are found in Box 35-1 and Box 35-2. However, these disorders are real and disabling, and delay in diagnosis can lead to greater resistance to therapy as well as potentially dangerous overtreatment.[2] There is also the risk of missing serious pulmonary disease; therefore, primary care pediatricians must balance their suspicions with a careful history and medical examination, judicious testing, careful medication trials and, often, pulmonology specialty referral before committing patients to behavioral evaluation and therapy. Several common presentations of functional respiratory disorders include habit or psychogenic cough, vocal cord dysfunction, hyperventilation, sighing dyspnea, and the functional aspects of asthma. These are not necessarily mutually exclusive, and features of several may occur simultaneously or over time in any one patient.

Box 35-1. Diagnostic Criteria for Panic Attack[a,b]

A discrete period of intense fear or discomfort, in which 4 (or more) of the following symptoms developed abruptly and reached a peak within 10 minutes:

1. Palpitations, pounding heart, or accelerated heart rate
2. Sweating
3. Trembling or shaking
4. Sensations of shortness of breath or smothering
5. Feeling of choking
6. Chest pain or discomfort
7. Nausea or abdominal distress
8. Feeling dizzy, unsteady, lightheaded, or faint
9. Derealization (feelings of unreality) or depersonalization (being detached from oneself)
10. Fear of losing control or going crazy
11. Fear of dying
12. Paresthesias (numbness or tingling sensations)
13. Chills or hot flashes

[a] A panic attack is not a codable disorder. Code the specific diagnosis in which the panic attack occurs (eg, 300.21 panic disorder with agoraphobia [page 441]).
[b] From *Diagnostic and Statistical Manual of Mental Disorders.* Fourth Edition. Text Revision. Washington, DC: American Psychiatric Association; 2000:432. Reprinted with permission.

Box 35-2. Diagnostic Criteria for Conversion Disorder (300.11)[a]

A. One or more symptoms or deficits affecting voluntary motor or sensory function that suggest a neurologic or other general medical condition.
B. Psychological factors are judged to be associated with the symptom or deficit because the initiation or exacerbation of the symptom or deficit is preceded by conflicts or other stressors.
C. The symptom or deficit is not intentionally produced or feigned (as in factitious disorder or malingering).
D. The symptom of deficit cannot, after appropriate investigation, be fully explained by a general medical condition, or by the direct effects of a substance, or as a culturally sanctioned behavior or experience.
E. The symptom or deficit causes clinically significant distress or impairment in social, occupational, or other important areas of functioning or warrants medical evaluation.
F. The symptom or deficit is not limited to pain or sexual dysfunction, does not occur exclusively during the course of somatization disorder, and is not better accounted for by another mental disorder.

Specify type of symptom or deficit
- With motor symptom or deficit
- With sensory symptom or deficit
- With seizures or convulsions
- With mixed presentation

[a] From *Diagnostic and Statistical Manual of Mental Disorders.* Fourth Edition. Text Revision. Washington, DC: American Psychiatric Association; 2000:498. Reprinted with permission.

Habit Cough

Chronic cough is defined in pediatrics as lasting more than 3 weeks. It has multiple causes as outlined in Box 35-3. In this chapter, the 2 most common terms, habit cough and psychogenic cough, may be substituted interchangeably as the differences, if any, in clinical characteristics have never been studied prospectively.[3] Other synonyms used in the literature include habit cough syndrome, cough tic, psychogenic cough tic, and involuntary cough. However, parents may be more willing to accept the term habit cough (HC) rather than psychogenic because of the perceived stigma of a psychological disorder.

Case Report 35-1

D.J. is a 14-year-old boy who is brought to your office by his mother with a complaint of cough for 3 months without systemic symptoms. A trial of inhaled corticosteroid and a short-acting bronchodilator have not produced improvement. The cough is dry to slightly productive with thin, white mucus and does not change with activity, nor is it present during sleep. It is disruptive of activities, including school, from which he has been sent home multiple times. Your examination is normal except for a dry, harsh, "honking" cough that seems to increase in intensity and frequency during your discussions with the mother and the patient. Subsequent workup, including chest radiography, sinus radiography, and spirometry, are all normal. The parent and youngster return for further evaluation and therapy.

Box 35-3. Causes of Chronic Cough[a]

Upper Airway	Postnasal drip/nasal allergy Sinusitis Foreign body in external auditory canal
Lower Airway	Asthma Infectious (tuberculosis, mycoplasma, chlamydia, pertussis) Cystic fibrosis Primary ciliary dyskinesia Irritative (primary smoking, secondhand smoke, indoor pollution)
Other	Gastroesophageal reflux disease Psychogenic Aspiration

[a] Adapted from Homnick DN, Pratt HD. Respiratory diseases with a psychosomatic component in adolescents. *Adolesc Med.* 2000;11(3):547–565, with permission from Elsevier.

The cough may start spontaneously or may occur following an upper respiratory tract infection and persist for weeks or months before parents or patient seek medical care. Because cough variant asthma is a common presentation of asthma leading to persistent cough, many patients will have had a trial of anti-inflammatory medications and short-acting bronchodilators with a history of little benefit.

Habit cough has many of the features of a conversion disorder, with secondary gain of school avoidance and attention-seeking. It is not a conscious or voluntary activity but does result in an often unconsciously desired effect of withdrawal from social interaction. In about 25% of cases the cough follows an upper respiratory infection, although the pathophysiological significance of this is unknown.

Clinical Presentation

The cough is characteristic and described as honking, loud, repetitive, and disruptive to social interaction (eg, during history taking with a parent in the room). It occurs typically in late childhood and early adolescence and is quite common. In one series of children and adolescents with cough for longer than 4 weeks, HC represented 32% of cases.[4] There are usually no physical consequences of HC except for mild erythema of the airway noted with bronchoscopy, but it may be severe enough in rare cases to produce rib fracture.[5] A careful history and physical examination will reveal only the characteristic cough, and distracting the youth will often produce its transient decrease or disappearance. As in most other functional disorders, the cough does not occur during sleep. Questions regarding any history of primary smoking or secondhand smoke exposure are essential in all older children and adolescents with chronic cough.

Diagnosis

The diagnosis of HC is often apparent based on the typical hollow sounding, repetitive honking cough that is absent during sleep. Extensive testing is usually not necessary; however, the differential diagnosis of HC includes cough variant asthma, gastroesophageal reflux disease (GERD), postnasal drip, and other infectious or postinfectious causes of persistent cough. Appropriate testing and therapy for these conditions may be done as indicated. If cough variant asthma is a consideration as a primary cause or comorbid condition, a short course of oral corticosteroid or a trial of inhaled corticosteroid and a short-acting bronchodilator or leukotriene modifier may be undertaken. If there is no response to these therapies, then HC is a consideration. Although cough tic has sometimes been included synonymously with HC, it is usually thought to be a manifestation of Tourette disorder, which presents with a spectrum of neurobehavioral problems, including attention-deficit and obsessive-compulsive disorders.[3] Other vocalizations, such as grunting, throat clearing, barking, sniffing, etc, often accompany the cough in Tourette disorder.

Because HC has a psychological genesis, a history of anxiety, obsessive-compulsive behavior, and other proven somatoform disorders (eg, chronic abdominal pain or headache) often helps point to the diagnosis. Children may also display relative indifference to HC with much less anxiety concerning its persistence than their parents. This indifference is commonly found in the other somatoform disorders discussed here.[6]

Although a history of anxiety, lack of nighttime symptoms, and the characteristic cough may point strongly to the diagnosis of HC, a basic workup for other causes of chronic cough is prudent. As indicated, this may include a sweat test for cystic fibrosis, pulmonary function testing with and without a bronchodilator, bronchoprovocation testing (eg, with methacholine), an upper gastrointestinal series, an otolaryngology examination and, occasionally, bronchoscopy.

Management

Once other causes of chronic cough have been ruled out, the treatment of HC is primarily behavioral. Effective behavioral therapies include simple suggestion, reassurance, patient and parental monitoring of the cough with social and material rewards for cough reduction, biofeedback, breathing exercises, and relaxation techniques.[7–10] An example of this is to (1) self-monitor the cough, (2) increase awareness of the initial sensations that trigger coughing, (3) learn how to interrupt the coughing at successively earlier stages in the cough sequence, and (4) substitute gentle laryngeal cough or laughter for the harsh cough of HC.[6] Another example of a successful method using suggestion therapy is presented in Box 35-4. This method involves a 15-minute session with the goal of convincing the patient that they have the ability to resist the urge to cough and thereby break the cough cycle that irritates the airways and perpetuates the cough.[9] Another reinforced suggestion technique includes wrapping the chest with a bed sheet after informing the youth that weak chest muscles are the cause of the cough. He or she is told that supporting the chest muscles for a few days will strengthen the muscles and resolve the cough. Cohlan and Stone[11] state that this technique resolved HC in 31 of 33 pediatric patients aged 5 to 14 years. Family and patient issues with anxiety or other emotional stress may require individual or family psychotherapy.

Prognosis and When to Refer/Admit

The prognosis for HC with behavioral therapy is good, with long-term remission in most cases. However, even when habit or psychogenic cough is recognized and correctly diagnosed, absence of a specific treatment plan can result in prolonged symptoms. In one study,[12]

Box 35-4. A Technique of Suggestion for the Treatment of Habit Cough[a]

- Express confidence, communicated verbally and behaviorally, that the therapist will be able to show the patient how to stop the cough.
- Explain the cough as a vicious cycle of an initial irritant, now gone, that had set up a pattern of coughing that caused irritation and further symptoms.
- Encourage suppression of the cough in order to break the cycle. The therapist closely observes for the initiation of the muscular movement preceding coughing and immediately exhorts the patient to hold the cough back, emphasizing that each second the cough is delayed makes further inhibition of cough easier.
- An alternative behavior to coughing is offered in the form of inhaling a generated mist or sipping body-temperature water with encouragement to inhale the mist or sip the water every time they begin to feel the urge to cough.
- Repeat expressions of confidence that the patient is developing the ability to resist the urge to cough.
- When some ability to suppress cough is observed (usually after about 10 minutes), ask in a rhetorical manner if they are beginning to feel that they can resist the urge to cough, eg, "You're beginning to feel that you can resist the urge to cough, aren't you?"
- Discontinue the session when the patient can repeatedly answer positively to the question, "Do you feel that you can now resist the urge to cough on your own?" This question is only asked after the patient has gone 5 minutes without coughing.

[a] Adapted from Lokshin B, Lindgren S, Weinberger M, Koviach J. Outcome of habit cough in children treated with a brief session of suggestion therapy. *Ann Allergy.* 1991;67:579–582, with permission from Elsevier.

44 of 60 patients required an average of 6 months beyond the diagnosis for resolution and 16 continued to be symptomatic for a mean duration of 5.9 years. When the diagnosis is unclear, the parents are resistant to a psychological diagnosis, or there are other suspected comorbid respiratory conditions, such as asthma, referral to a pediatric pulmonologist may help reinforce the suspected diagnosis or clarify another confounding pulmonary condition. Specific testing, such as bronchoprovocation or bronchoscopy, may be indicated. Referral to a child psychologist or psychiatrist is indicated when simple measures, such as suggestion and reassurance, do not resolve the HC. Hospitalization is rarely indicated for psychogenic cough unless serious psychiatric problems are also present.

Vocal Cord Dysfunction (VCD)

Case Report 35-2

T. S. is a 13–year-old female who comes with her mother to the pediatrician's office with a complaint of shortness of breath when playing soccer. The symptoms occur most severely during league games, less with practices, and rarely at other times. It is described as sudden onset of "wheezing" described by her mother as crowing during inspiration accompanied with dry cough and complaints of throat tightness. Her mother has also noted that T. S. has difficulty talking during the episodes and has a hoarse, quiet voice. The symptoms resolve over a couple of minutes with rest but may recur during the same sports event. She has never lost consciousness. A trial of a short-acting β-adrenergic agent given to the patient during an emergency department (ED) visit did not help the symptoms.

Vocal cord dysfunction (also known as paradoxical vocal cord motion, laryngeal dyskinesia, functional stridor, Munchausen stridor, psychosomatic stridor, and factitious asthma) is a psychologically driven disorder often underrecognized and most often mistaken for resistant asthma.[13] As a result, many youngsters are overtreated with asthma medications with underresponse to therapy that is frustrating to the family and physician. Because 30% to 50% of patients with VCD also have coexisting asthma, the diagnosis and relative contribution of each condition can be confusing. Frequently, VCD is associated with sports activities, particularly in adolescents, and may mimic exercise-induced asthma, although significant differences are evident as outlined in Table 35-1. As a more unusual variant, it may also occur at rest with persistent adduction of the vocal cords, often prompting a trip to the ED where spontaneous remission occurs regardless of specific therapy.[14] Like other functional respiratory disorders, VCD has features of a conversion disorder.

Clinical Presentation

A typical episode of VCD consists of the sudden onset of inspiratory stridor with accompanying complaints of throat tightness, hoarse voice, dry cough and, occasionally, wheezing. As with the other psychosomatic respiratory disorders, VCD rarely, if ever, occurs during sleep. Triggers are most often unknown except when VCD occurs during exercise and, even then, symptoms may only occur during the high stress of competition and not during regular practice sessions. The physical examination during a VCD episode will reveal, on auscultation, inspiratory stridor localized over the glottis without

Table 35-1. Vocal Cord Dysfunction (VCD) and Exercise-Induced Asthma (EIA)[a]

Characteristic	VCD	EIA[b]
Women > men	+	–
Associated psychiatric diagnosis	+	±
Exercise-induced	+	+
Very short duration of symptoms	+	–
Improves with bronchodilator	–	+
Eosinophilia	–	±
Hypoxia	–	+
Syncope	–	+
Dyspnea	+	+
Stridor	+	–
Wheeze	Inspiration	Expiration > inspiration
Spirometry	Blunted inspiration portion of flow-volume loop	Normal inspiration portion of flow-volume loop
Laryngoscopy	Tonic adduction of cords during inspiration or inspiration/expiration	Abduction during inspiration
Chest x-ray	Normal	Hyperinflation

Key: +, present; –, absent; ±, sometimes present.

[a] Adapted from Homnick D, Marks J. Exercise and sports in the adolescent with chronic pulmonary disease. *Adolesc Med.* 1998;9:467–481, with permission from Elsevier.
[b] Without coexistent VCD.

hypoxia. Patients are able to hold their breath and to vocalize despite the sensation of respiratory distress. This ability to vocalize and the lack of hypoxia differentiate this condition from laryngospasm.

Diagnosis

Direct visualization of the vocal cords during a VCD episode is diagnostic but presents a rare opportunity. The laryngoscopic appearance is that of paradoxical motion of the vocal cords with anterior apposition and a small posterior, diamond-shaped opening, also termed posterior glottic "chink" (Figure 35-1). Even without acute symptoms, direct visualization at some point in the workup is important to rule out other laryngeal problems, such as erythema from GERD, papillomas, hemangiomas, and laryngeal cysts and webs. Direct visualization by a trained speech therapist will often reveal subacute paradoxical vocal cord motion and confirm the diagnosis prior to initiating specific therapy. Spirometry is characteristic, with flattening of the inspiratory portion of the flow-volume loop (Figure 35-2).[14,15] Bronchoprovocation with methacholine or exercise may also bring out the pattern of this extrathoracic airway obstruction as well as defining coexisting asthma.[16]

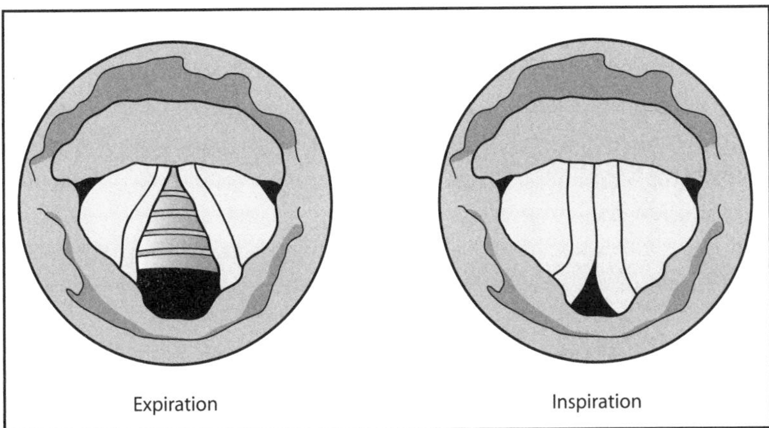

Figure 35-1. Laryngoscopic appearance of the vocal cords in vocal cord dysfunction.

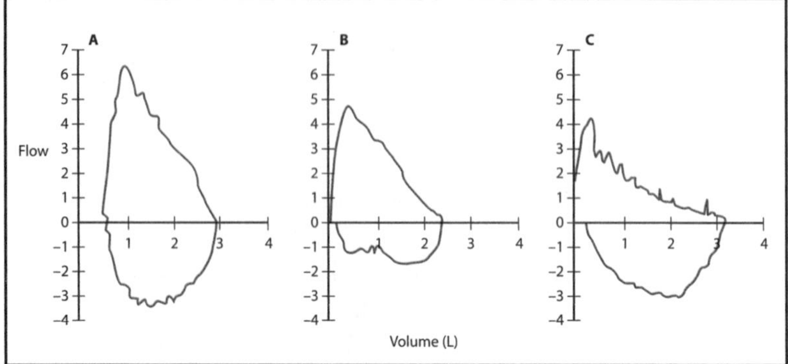

Figure 35-2. Flow-volume loop in vocal cord dysfunction. **A.** Normal flow-volume loop. **B.** Flattened inspiratory loop during vocal cord dysfunction. **C.** Scooped expiratory curve during acute asthma. (Adapted from Landwehr LP, Wood RP II. Vocal cord dysfunction mimicking exercise-induced bronchospasm in adolescents. *Pediatrics.* 1996;98:971–974.)

Management

Underlying coexisting asthma must be controlled with appropriate measures (see Chapter 12). Vocal cord dysfunction is a functional disorder, the mechanism for which is unknown. The typical adolescent experiencing VCD is described as highly competitive and success oriented and often comes from a family with similar characteristics.[6] Therapy for stress disorders, including relaxation techniques such as use of relaxing imagery, self-hypnosis, and posthypnotic suggestion, have proved successful in some cases of VCD.[16] Other behavioral therapies include speech therapy for hyperfunctional voice disorders by a therapist skilled in this treatment and biofeedback; short-term intervention is often successful in the receptive patient.[16–20] For exercise-induced VCD, some have recommended pretreatment with an aerosolized anticholinergic agent (ipratropium) to help prevent symptoms.[21]

Prognosis and When to Refer/Admit

As in other functional respiratory disorders, if serious psychopathology is suspected, referral for a psychological or psychiatric evaluation and therapy is important. A pediatric pulmonologist can help sort out comorbid symptoms, such as asthma, and help confirm a suspected diagnosis with pulmonary function evaluation and provocative testing, such as with exercise, as well as reinforce the diagnosis with a parent resistant to a psychological diagnosis and intervention. As noted previously, referral to a speech therapist with skill in dealing with VCD will provide the tools important for the youth to achieve rapid resolution of his or her symptoms and resume normal activities, making the prognosis in this condition good. A serious underlying psychiatric disorder may require hospitalization.

Hyperventilation

Case Report 35-3

Z.L. is a 12-year-old brought to your primary care office by her parents with complaints of inability to catch her breath, which is often associated with her school basketball team activities but has also occurred at rest while watching TV or during other random activities. During these episodes she often experiences light-headedness, sweating, chest pressure, and occasional tingling in her hands and feet. She has never lost consciousness but must stop activities when the symptoms occur. Z.L. is a top student, participates in multiple school clubs, is the editor of the school paper, and plays team and individual sports in all seasons. She's had no wheezing, persistent cough, or other systemic symptoms.

Hyperventilation (HV), or overbreathing, is most common in the early adolescent years. It is defined as respiration in excess of metabolic needs that may lead to hypocapnia and respiratory alkalosis. However, the symptoms do not depend on this metabolic dysfunction because experimental isocapnic HV (maintaining normal partial pressure of carbon dioxide by adding it to inspired gases) produces the same symptoms.[22] Although the HV syndrome has been promulgated as a distinct and separate syndrome from other psychosomatic conditions, it likely is a feature of panic attacks (Box 35-1).

Clinical Presentation

Sudden onset of dyspnea (rapid, labored breathing) is the presenting feature of HV. Because this is also the presenting feature of many acute cardiorespiratory conditions, care must be taken in diagnosing HV, especially with the first episode. It is a diagnosis of exclusion, and other causes of organic respiratory disease must be eliminated. Other complaints include those also found in panic attacks and include dizziness, light-headedness, weakness, palpitations, sweating, numbness or tingling of the hands, headache, and feelings of being cold or hot. Tetany as a complication is rare.[23] Attacks range in duration from a few minutes up to several hours and tend to begin in the early teen years.

Hyperventilation during competitive activities is not rare and is one of the causes of exercise-induced dyspnea.[24] It is particularly troublesome when it puts the youngster at risk of harm, such as during swimming. This most often occurs in youth who are highly competitive with a similar profile to those experiencing VCD. Psychological disturbance, including anxiety disorder, depression, conversion reaction, and psychosis, have all been associated with hyperventilation; therefore, treatment must be directed specifically at these various conditions.[25]

Diagnosis

The possibility of serious underlying metabolic or cardiopulmonary disease, such as cardiac dysrhythmia or hypoglycemia, dictates that a judicious evaluation be undertaken before making the diagnosis of HV. This would include an electrocardiogram with rhythm strip, pulmonary function testing, electrolytes, blood glucose, serum pH, thyroid screen, and chest radiography. Provocation tests, such as the HV provocation test, have been used to reproduce symptoms associated with HV. This involves 3 minutes of rest followed by 3 minutes of voluntary overbreathing followed by a 3-minute recovery period. The validity of this test has been questioned because similar symptoms may be produced by a stressful mental task alone or 3 minutes of isocapnic overventilation.[22,26] Although symptoms of HV can occur without hypocapnia and elevated pH, these findings on a blood gas taken during an attack can help with the diagnosis.[22]

Management

Therapies for HV must be individualized, especially considering the range of possible underlying psychological conditions. These include reassurance, relaxation and breathing control, biofeedback, group therapy, cognitive-behavioral therapy, and psychotherapy.[27–30] Until sufficient resolution of symptoms has occurred, patients undertaking sports and other activities where trauma may be a risk need to temporarily stop or modify their activities.

Prognosis and When to Refer/Admit

Referral to a pediatric pulmonologist may be helpful where the diagnosis is unclear, to reinforce a psychological diagnosis, or where comorbid disease occurs, such as asthma.[31,32] Asthma and HV often occur together, leading to a circle of HV, increasing asthma symptoms, and increasing anxiety, leading to persistence or worsening of HV.[33] Early referral to a psychologist/psychiatrist for evaluation and appropriate therapy is important, as long-term established HV is harder to alleviate. Rarely, patients with serious psychological disturbance will need to be hospitalized. Unfortunately, the prognosis in HV is guarded. Approximately 40% of youth with HV continued to experience this problem into adulthood, along with other signs and symptoms of chronic anxiety.[29,34]

Sighing Dyspnea (SD)

Case report 35-4
R.H. is a 15-year-old male brought to your office by his parents with complaints of inability to catch his breath. This occurs suddenly at rest accompanied by deep sighing respirations and anxious agitation. R.H. finds some relief by going to an open window and forcibly taking deep breaths, and at school he has been forced to leave the classroom. The episodes occur over a few minutes and resolve quickly, but can recur several times a day. Parents note that this has never occurred at night.

Sighing is a normal daily function to reduce microatelectasis and maintain physiological lung volumes. It is also a normal consequence of emotional states, such as anxiety. Some children may experience intermittent episodes of recurrent benign sighing as an apparent habit that concerns the parents but not the child and does not disrupt activities. However, when sighing becomes excessive and disruptive of activities, it may come to the attention of the pediatrician. Sighing dyspnea is distinctly rarer than HV but probably related and associated with the same anxiety disorders as the other functional respiratory conditions. Limited published reports suggest a female predominance most common between the second and fourth decade, but the disorder does occur in older children and in males.[35,36]

Clinical Presentation

A typical patient with SD reports difficulty getting a complete breath ("I can't seem to get enough air."), often with a feeling of chest heaviness or constriction. Deep sighing respirations, generally without an increase in respiratory rate, are noted, which become more pronounced with increasing anxiety and often end with a long sigh or with some type of environmental manipulation, such as opening a window. Patients may also use accessory muscles of respiration during deep sighing, and physical examination is necessary to eliminate other acute causes of dyspnea, such as asthma. As in other functional respiratory disorders, a distracted patient may show transient elimination or reduction in symptoms, and symptoms do not occur during sleep.

Diagnosis

After a complete history and physical examination, evaluation is similar to the other functional disorders and includes pulmonary function testing, bronchoprovocation testing, serum pH, glucose, electrolytes, chest radiography, and thyroid screen. This condition is most often a result of an anxiety disorder and, after a normal physical examination and testing, psychological evaluation and intervention are necessary.

Management

As in the other functional disorders, effective interventions for SD have included reassurance, relaxation and breathing training, anxiolytic drugs, and psychotherapy.[37,38]

Prognosis and When to Refer/Admit

Because there are few studies of long-term intervention in SD, long-term prognosis is unknown. Early diagnosis and psychological intervention are likely important, and hospitalization is reserved only for those with significant psychopathology. Referral to a pediatric pulmonologist can be helpful when other causes of dyspnea are suspected or there are coexisting comorbid conditions, such as asthma.

Functional Aspects of Asthma

Most clinicians who treat asthma note patients may have acute worsening of symptoms when anxious or stressed. Anxiety is considered a non-immunologic trigger and has been shown to contribute to airway lability.[39] Additionally, increased morbidity and mortality in patients with asthma have been shown to be associated with psychiatric disturbance when non-adherence to therapy and delay in seeking emergency treatment are large contributors.[40] The increase in airflow obstruction and resistance to emergency therapy in those with panic-anxiety is likely due to psychogenic-based vagal stimulation mediated through cholinergic (and perhaps non-adrenergic, non-cholinergic) neural pathways and is responsible for acute bronchoconstriction and hypersecretion.[41] The phenomenon that psychological state can be responsible for acute asthma symptoms is demonstrated by response to suggestion. When subjects with asthma were told that a physiological saline aerosol was an allergen, 50% responded with increased airway resistance.[41] Simple recall of stressful situations may trigger bronchoconstriction. When asthmatic children were asked to recall events associated with intense anger or fear, decreases in airflow measured by spirometry were consistently recorded.[42]

Clinical Manifestations

Many patients with anxiety and other psychological disorders will display evidence of poor asthma control with frequent exacerbations and episodes requiring emergency intervention. This poor control may often be due to non-adherence or exacerbations associated with recurrent stressful situations, such as family conflict. The signs and symptoms of asthma exacerbations and the determinants of severity are discussed in the Chapter 12.

Diagnosis

Since any chronic disease can lead to anxiety and depression, both the underlying disease and psychological disturbance must be treated simultaneously (see Chapter 12).

As in the other functional respiratory disorders, treatment for panic-anxiety includes relaxation, breathing control, psychoactive medications, hypnosis, and psychotherapy. Asthma must also be vigorously and systematically controlled using severity grading and appropriate intervention and monitoring as outlined in Chapter 12. Elimination of confounding medical conditions, including GERD; substance abuse problems, including tobacco; and severe environmental trigger exposure must also be done.

Prognosis and When to Refer/Admit

The severity of an asthma episode and its response to rescue therapy will determine hospitalization. Referral to a pediatric pulmonologist to help develop and monitor a therapeutic plan, especially for patients with moderate to severe asthma, is helpful. Referral to a psychologist/psychiatrist to evaluate and treat the underlying anxiety disorder will help with asthma management and should be an integral part of a therapeutic plan for patients with asthma exacerbated by emotional state.

Key Points

- Anxiety disorders are the common denominator of functional respiratory disorders, and an effective treatment strategy is summarized in Box 35-4.
- Early intervention for functional respiratory disorders, after careful history, physical examination, and judicious testing, is important to lessen resistance to therapy.
- Many patients with functional respiratory disorders have coexisting asthma, which must be defined and treated.
- The treatment of functional disorders is behavioral not pharmacologic. See Table 35-2. Overtreatment of anxiety-related functional disorders is common, and response to specific therapy should be monitored as much for signs of improvement as its lack.
- Functional respiratory disorders are diagnoses of exclusion requiring the elimination of other pulmonary disease before accepting a functional diagnosis.

Table 35-2. Therapy Options for Functional Disorders[a,b]

Therapy Option	Habit Cough	Vocal Cord Dysfunction	Hyperventi-lation	Sighing Dyspnea	Asthma	Panic Disorder	Conversion Disorder
Behavior therapy							
Reinforcement suggestion therapy	+						+
Breathing exercises and control	+	+	+	+	+	+	
Relaxation techniques	+	+	+		+	+	+
Social/material rewards	+						+
Biofeedback	+	+	+		+	+	+
Psychoeducation	+	+	+	+	+	+	+
Simple reassurance	+		+	+		+	+
Bedsheet	+						
Hypnosis	+	+	+	+	+	+	+
Cognitive-behavioral therapy	+		+		+	+	+
Psychotherapy							
Individual			+	+	+	+	+
Group			+		+	+	+

[a]Adapted from Homnick DN, Pratt HD. Respiratory diseases with a psychosomatic component in adolescents. *Adolesc Med.* 2000;11(3):547–565.
[b]Treatment interventions may be effective independently or in conjunction with selective pharmacotherapy, with permission from Elsevier.

References

1. Niggeman B. Functional symptoms confused with allergic disorders in children and adolescents. *Pediatr Allergy Immunol.* 2002;13:312–318
2. Hayes J, Nolan M, Brennan N, et al. Three cases of paradoxical vocal cord adduction followed up over a 10-year period. *Chest.* 1993;104:678–680
3. Irwin RS, Glomb WB, Chang AB. Habit cough, tic cough, and psychogenic cough in adult and pediatric populations: ACCP evidence-based clinical practice guidelines. *Chest.* 2006;129:174–179
4. Holinger JB, Fanurik D, Hanna DE, et al. Chronic cough in infants and children: an update. *Laryngoscope.* 1991;101:596–604
5. Lorin MI, Slovis TL, Haller JO. Fracture of ribs in psychogenic cough. *NY State J Med.* 1978;2078–2079
6. Homnick DN, Pratt HD. Respiratory diseases with a psychosomatic component in adolescents. *Adolesc Med.* 2000;11(3):547–565
7. Gay M, Blager F, Bartsch, et al. Psychogenic habit cough: review and case reports. *J Clin Psychiatry.* 1987;48:483–486
8. LaVigne JV, Davis AT, Fauber R. Behavioral management of psychogenic cough. *Pediatrics.* 1996;98:971–974
9. Lokshin B, Lindgren S, Weinberger M, et al. Outcome of habit cough in children treated with a brief session of suggestion therapy. *Ann Allergy.* 1991;76:579–582
10. Riegel B, Warmonth JE, Midbaugh SJ, et al. Psychogenic cough treated with biofeedback and psychotherapy. *Am J Phys Med Rehabil.* 1995;74:55–58
11. Cohlan SQ, Stone SM. The cough and the bedsheet. *Pediatrics.* 1984;74:11–15
12. Rojas AR, Sachs MI, Yunginger JW, et al. Childhood involuntary cough syndrome: a long-term follow up study. *Ann Allergy.* 1991;66:106
13. Christopher KL, Wood RP II, Eckert RC, et al. Vocal-cord dysfunction presenting as asthma. *N Engl J Med.* 1983;308:1566–1570
14. Newman KB, Mason UG III, Schmaling KB. Clinical features of vocal cord dysfunction. *Am J Respir Crit Care Med.* 1995;152:1382–1386
15. Wood PW, Milgrom H. Vocal cord dysfunction. *J Allergy Clin Immunol.* 1996;98:481–485
16. Smith MS. Acute psychogenic stridor in an adolescent treated with hypnosis. *Pediatrics.* 1983;2:247–248
17. McFadden ER, Zawadski DK. Vocal cord dysfunction masquerading as exercise-induced asthma: a physiologic cause for "choking" during athletic activities. *Am J Respir Crit Care Med.* 1996:942–947
18. Blager FB, Gay MS, Wood RP. Voice therapy techniques adapted to treatment of habit cough: a pilot study. *J Commun Disord.* 1988;21:393–400
19. Goldman J, Muers M. Vocal cord dysfunction and wheezing (editorial). *Thorax.* 1991;46:401–404
20. Kayani M, Ben-Ziv Z. Stridor caused by vocal cord dysfunction associated with exercise in adolescent girls. *Chest.* 1998;113:540–542

21. Doshi D, Weinberger M. Long-term outcome of vocal cord dysfunction. *Ann Allergy Asthma Immunol.* 2006;96:794–799
22. Hornsveld H, Garssen B, Fiedeldij Dop M, et al. Symptom reporting during voluntary hyperventilation and mental load: implications for diagnosing hyperventilation syndrome. *J Psychosom Res.* 1990;34:687–697
23. Joorbachi B. Expressions of the hyperventilation syndrome in childhood. *Clin Pediatr.* 1977;16:1110–1115
24. Hammo AH, Weinberger M. Exercise induced hyperventilation: a pseudo-asthma syndrome. *Ann Allergy Asthma Immunol.* 1999;82:574–578
25. Enzer NB, Walker PA. Hyperventilation syndrome in childhood. *J Pediatr.* 1967;521–532
26. Hornsveld HK, Garssen B, Fiedeldij Dop M, et al. Double-blind placebo-controlled study of the hyperventilation provocation test and the validity of the hyperventilation syndrome. *J Psychosom Res.* 1996;348:154–158
27. Bass C. Hyperventilation syndrome: a chimera. *J Psychosom Res.* 1997;42:421–426
28. Grossman P, de Swart JCG, Defares PB, et al. A controlled study of breathing therapy for treatment of hyperventilation syndrome. *J Psychosom Res.* 1985;29:49–58
29. Hodgens JB, Fanurik D, Hanna DE, et al. Adolescent hyperventilation syndrome. *Ala J Med Sci.* 1988;25:423–426
30. Holinger LD, Sanders AD. Chronic cough in infants and children: an update. *Laryngoscope.* 1991;101:596–604
31. Keely D, Osman L. Dysfunctional breathing and asthma. *BMJ.* 2001;322:1075–1076
32. Stoop A, De Boo T, Lemmens W, Folgering H. Hyperventilation syndrome: measurement of objective symptoms and subjective complaints. *Respiration.* 1986;49:37–44
33. Gardner WN, Bass C, Moxham J. Recurrent hyperventilation tetany due to mild asthma. *Respir Med.* 1992;86:349–351
34. Herman SP, Stickler GB, Lucas AR. Hyperventilation syndrome in children and adolescents: long-term follow up. *Pediatrics.* 1981;67:183–187
35. Butani J, O'Connel EJ. Functional respiratory disorders. *Ann Allergy Asthma Immunol.* 1997;79:91–101
36. White P, Hahn R. The symptom of sighing in cardiovascular diagnosis: with spirographic observations. *Am J Med Sci.* 1929;177:179–188
37. Perin PV, Perin RJ. When a sigh is not just a sigh and not asthma. *Ann Allergy.* 1993;71:478–480
38. Soley MH, Shock NW. The etiology of effort syndrome. *Am J Med Sci.* 1938;196:840–851
39. Harrison BDW. Psychological aspects of asthma. *Thorax.* 1998;53:519–525
40. Nouwen A, Freestone MH, Labbe R, et al. Psychological factors associated with emergency room visits among asthmatic patients. *Behav Modif.* 1999;23:217–233

41. McFadden ER, Luparello T, Lyons HA, et al. The mechanism of action of suggestion in the inducement of acute asthma attacks. *Psychosom Med.* 1969;31:134–143
42. Tal A, Miklich DR. Emotionally induced decreases in pulmonary flow rates in asthmatic children. *Psychosom Res.* 1976;38:190–200

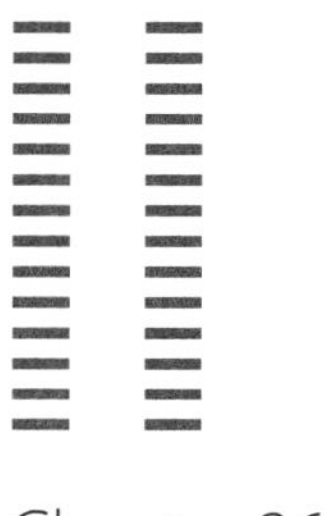

Chapter 36

Sleep-Disordered Breathing

John Norman Schuen, MD
Karen Kay Thompson, MD

Introduction

Sleep-disordered breathing (SDB) in children encompasses a broad range of breathing-related diagnoses, including primary snoring, obstructive sleep apnea (OSA), obstructive hypoventilation, and upper airway resistance syndrome. Except for the role obesity plays in disordered breathing, nearly every aspect of childhood sleep disorders differs from SDB in adults, including the clinical presentation, diagnosis, and treatment.

Pediatric clinical guidelines provide a structured and systematic approach for primary care providers and sleep specialists to screen, diagnose, and manage sleep-related disorders in young people. The number of US pediatric sleep centers has increased significantly since the 1990s to help facilitate better access to diagnostic and management guidance.

Epidemiology of SDB, Primary Snoring, and OSA

Epidemiologic studies throughout the world shed light on the incidence of SDB diagnoses and highlight risk based on age, pediatric syndromes, and craniofacial structure. The incidence of primary snoring ranges from 12% to 20%, in contrast to OSA syndrome (OSAS), where the incidence is approximately 2% to 3%.[1–5] Although seen in infants and toddlers, OSAS is most common in children between the ages of 2 and 15 years, with a peak between 3 to 6 years. An epidemiologic study by Redline and colleagues[6] identified risk factors for OSA that included family history, obesity, African-American race, sinus disease, and "persistent wheeze." Prematurity also increases the risk for the broad continuum of SDB in children ages 8 to 11 years, although the significance in adolescent years is yet unclear.

Diagnosis

Screening Evaluation During Health Supervision Visits

During routine health supervision visits, children should be screened regularly for habitual snoring. Although virtually all children snore on occasion, most frequently during an upper respiratory tract infection or due to seasonal allergic rhinitis, habitual snoring occurs nightly or almost every night. The nature of the snoring may lead parents to either a false sense of security or excessive concern. Additionally, perceptions of parents vary widely. A study in the 1990s identified that a child with a reliable history of loud, habitual snoring may only have primary snoring, whereas a child with an unimpressive history of quiet snoring may actually have severe OSAS.[7] Therefore, the diagnosis of OSAS cannot be made reliably by clinical history and physical examination alone.[8]

If habitual snoring is present in the review of systems and history or physical examination suggests possible OSAS, the clinician must decide the appropriate next step for evaluation. Physical examination findings consistent with an increased risk of OSAS are noted in Box 36-1; however, it is important to remember that a child with OSAS may have no physical abnormalities on examination. A thorough history may reveal some of the sequelae of OSAS as listed in Box 36-2. If neither history nor examination suggests OSAS in a patient with habitual snoring, the patient should be screened again at the next health supervision visit.

If there is concern for OSAS and the patient has a high-risk condition, such as a craniofacial, genetic, metabolic, or neuromuscular disorder, then referral to a specialist is recommended. Also considered high risk are infants or children with a history of chronic lung disease or those who have evidence of cardiac or respiratory compromise. Appropriate specialist referral could include a pediatric pulmonologist, neurologist, otolaryngologist, or intensivist with board certification in sleep medicine.

Box 36-1. Physical Examination Findings in Obstructive Sleep Apnea[a]

General
- Sleepiness
- Obesity
- Failure to thrive

Cardiovascular
- Hypertension
- Loud P2 (heart sound)

Extremities
- Edema
- Clubbing (rare)

Head
- Swollen mucous membranes
- Deviated septum
- Adenoidal facies: intraorbital darkening, elongated face, mouth breathing
- Tonsillar hypertrophy
- High-arched palate
- Overbite
- Crowded oropharynx
- Macroglossia
- Midfacial hypoplasia
- Micrognathia/retrognathia
- Intermittent runny nose, nasal congestion
- Hyponasal speech

[a] Modified from Katz E, Marcus C. Diagnosis of obstructive sleep apnea syndrome in infants and children. In: Sheldon S, Feber R, Kryger M, eds. *Principles and Practice of Pediatric Sleep Medicine*. Philadelphia, PA: Elsevier/Saunders; 2005:197–210, with permission from Elsevier.

Even when the child is not considered high risk by the evaluating clinician, the sleep study remains today's gold standard for evaluation. However, in cases where a sleep laboratory is not readily available, there are alternatives that may be considered. One such alternative, the overnight pulse oximetry study, offers a cost-effective alternative. An abnormal pulse oximetry study consisting of frequent oxyhemoglobin desaturations during a night's sleep indicates a high diagnostic sensitivity for OSAS in an otherwise normal child.[9] However, a normal pulse oximetry study is completely compatible with OSAS and should not reassure the provider. Therefore, the patient with a normal overnight pulse oximetry study may still require an overnight sleep study. Review of an audiotape or videotape of the child sleeping can also help the clinician decide on the likelihood of OSAS. When the gold

Box 36-2. Sequelae of Obstructive Sleep Apnea Syndrome by System

Cardiovascular
- Cor pulmonale, pulmonary hypertension
- Heart failure (primarily right-sided)
- Polycythemia

Behavioral
- Developmental delay
- Behavioral and/or academic problems
- Excessive daytime sleepiness

Growth
- Failure to thrive
- Short stature

Neurologic
- Morning headache
- Increased intracranial pressure
- Lethargy, dull affect
- Nocturnal enuresis (defective arousal mechanisms)
- Hypoxic seizures

Gastrointestinal
- Difficulty swallowing (dysphagia)
- Gastroesophageal reflux

Surgical
- Intraoperative death
- Postoperative death (rare and underreported)
- Postoperative respiratory compromise

standard (the sleep study) is not used, then extra care should be exercised to assess the child for right ventricular hypertrophy, cor pulmonale, and other potential high-risk factors that would complicate surgical intervention.

Diagnostic Approach to SDB

Given the importance of an accurate diagnosis and operative risk assessment, pediatric sleep laboratories provide a bounty of valuable sleep information. The primary goal of a pediatric sleep laboratory study is to obtain objective data on a child's sleep, including breathing during sleep, sleep quality, severity of gas exchange abnormalities, and severity of sleep disturbance. A night in the sleep laboratory helps to correlate a history from the parents as well.

Case Report 36-1

Emma is a 6-year-old female who is brought to her primary care physician for a health supervision visit. She is healthy with the exception of allergic rhinitis, for which she takes loratidine as needed. She began the first grade 3 months ago. The teacher reports concerns about Emma's ability to sit still in her seat, poor attention span, and impulsivity. She is struggling to keep up with her peers with reading skills. A sleep diary reveals that she gets about 10 to 11 hours of sleep per night. History reveals habitual snoring, and examination is consistent with tonsillar hypertrophy as well as mildly boggy nasal mucosa. There is no locally available pediatric sleep laboratory available, therefore the physician orders an overnight pulse oximeter study. This study reveals frequent desaturations at least 1 to 2 times per hour with a nadir of 75%. The provider orders an electrocardiogram, venous blood gas, and complete blood cell count, which are all normal. She refers the child to a local ear, nose, and throat (ENT) physician who performs an adenotonsillectomy. She is admitted for observation postoperatively and does well without further desaturations. When her mother returns with her for follow-up, her impulsivity and hyperactivity have improved dramatically and she is doing much better in school.

Over the years, the American Academy of Sleep Medicine, American Academy of Pediatrics (AAP) and American Thoracic Society (ATS) have established specific recommendations for optimal channels for diagnostic monitoring and diagnosis. In 1996 the ATS set the standards and indications for pediatric sleep studies.[10] The AAP provides a detailed algorithm for the diagnosis and management of childhood OSAS as well.[11] The experience of the physician reviewing the sleep study and the criteria she or he uses to diagnose OSAS in children is important in making an accurate diagnosis. In the 1990s a study revealed that when practitioners applied adult criteria to pediatric polysomnographic interpretation, the diagnosis of 80% of pediatric OSAS was missed.[12] This supports appropriate use of pediatric criteria as provided by experienced pediatric sleep medicine providers.

Understanding Polysomnogram Results

The primary care physician receives a copy of the sleep study report. The obstructive index (OI) represents the total number of complete obstructive apneas per hours of total sleep time. An OI greater than 1 is considered pathologic. The apnea-hypopnea index (AHI) denotes the sum of the complete obstructive events plus partial obstructive events (also called hypopneas) per hour of total sleep time. The *International Classification of Sleep Disorders: Diagnostic and Coding Manual, Second Edition,* identifies an AHI greater than 1 as pathologic; however, some pediatric sleep laboratories use an AHI greater than 5 to reflect pathologic SDB.[13]

Obstructive sleep apnea, upper airway resistance syndrome, and obstructive hypoventilation (OH) represent different but similar subtypes of obstructed breathing that occur during sleep. If episodes of snoring are present due to greater than one partial or complete upper airway obstructive event per hour during sleep, it is called OSA. These events are often associated with gas exchange abnormalities. When frequent and prolonged periods of elevated end-tidal carbon dioxide ($EtCO_2$) occurs in association with increased airway resistance during sleep or paradoxical inward rib cage motion, it is referred to as OH. Although this can occur in healthy children, it is often associated with obesity, hypotonia, or muscle weakness syndromes. Upper airway resistance syndrome refers to the presence of numerous discrete periods of increased work of breathing during sleep, which results in significant arousal throughout the night's sleep without significant obstructive hypoventilation.[14,15] When snoring is not associated with apnea, gas exchange abnormalities, sleep disturbance, or associated daytime symptoms, it is referred to as primary snoring. Normative data have recently been published in children who do not snore.[16]

Medical and Financial Impact of OSAS

Obstructive sleep apnea syndrome significantly and negatively impacts our youth from a medical perspective, and can result in multi-organ system dysfunction when left untreated. Obstructive sleep apnea syndrome often results in, or contributes to, many childhood problems seen in primary care, including failure to thrive, developmental delay, behavioral and academic problems, headaches, and reflux. Research in the 1990s uncovered that the increased work of breathing associated with OSAS in children resulted in increased caloric expenditure and helped explain poor growth and even failure to thrive.[17] Research has begun to unravel the cost of OSAS in terms of cognitive and behavioral problems as well. Gozal and Pope[18] revealed that the lowest quartile in an urban elementary classroom had a disproportionately high incidence of OSAS. This article also hypothesized that a learning debt may occur in these children if their OSAS is left undiagnosed or untreated. Another recent study of children diagnosed with attention-deficit/hyperactivity disorder (ADHD) reveals significant pathology with an AHI greater than 1 and subsequent improvement in behavioral symptoms with adenotonsillectomy.[19] Gas exchange abnormalities, along with large, regular and recurrent swings in intrathoracic pressure, may explain cognitive as well as cardiac problems that can occur in children with OSAS. Box 36-2 provides, by system, a more complete list of the short-term and long-term sequelae of untreated OSAS.

In adults with OSA, significant morbidity and mortality occur with great economic impact. Much less is known about the financial impact of childhood OSAS; however, an Israeli study found children with untreated OSA incurred significantly more health care expenses related primarily to upper airway tract infections.[20] Treatment of OSAS with adenotonsillectomy led to a substantial decrease in health care use in this population.

Sequelae of Primary Snoring

Historically, most pediatric sleep physicians generally considered primary snoring in childhood to be a benign condition that did not require treatment. However, a number of studies now suggest that persistent snoring is associated with poor school performance, behavioral difficulties, higher likelihood of health care use, impaired growth, cardiac-related issues, and IQ deficits.[21–23] One investigator team examined 5- to 7-year-olds with snoring and a group of controls (who didn't snore). More than 11,000 questionnaires were sent out and a random subset of 118 full sleep studies were performed.[22] Compared with the controls, the primary snoring group demonstrated decreased attention measures, more social problems, more anxious/depressive symptoms, lesser cognitive abilities, and decreased language and visual-spatial functions. More recently, Chervin et al[23] examined approximately 100 children, ages 5 to 13 years, with SDB (but no OSAS) and normal controls. The groups were studied with overnight polysomnograms. At baseline, the SDB group had more problems with sleepiness and were more likely to have ADHD and inattentiveness on cognitive testing.

One year following adenotonsillectomy, the difference between the SDB and control group disappeared. Another recent prospective study also demonstrated significant improvement in symptoms in children with SDB (not necessarily OSAS) status post-adenotonsillectomy.[23] Thus treating selected individuals who have primary snoring with adenotonsillectomy should be considered in those with significant daytime behavioral problems or nighttime disrupted sleep due to loud snoring.

Pathophysiology

Although tonsils and adenoids represent the most common reason for SDB in childhood, a classic triad of features can also contribute to this problem. Large tonsils and/or adenoids clearly represent only one factor influencing whether or not a child develops OSAS. One recent study discovered that large adenoid size alone does not accurately predict whether a child will have OSAS, contradicting the long-held view that large adenoids or tonsils are highly associated with OSAS.[24] Yet the study also revealed that when large adenoids and OSAS coexisted, the combination predicted significant and marked gas exchange abnormalities. Then why does OSAS and clinically significant SDB occur in children? A Venn diagram depicting the classic triad reveals the complex interaction of various upper airway influences that lead to significant SDB (Figure 36-1).[25] Intrinsic abnormality of upper airway neuromotor control during sleep; anatomical abnormalities; and genetic, hormonal, and other factors combine in varying degrees to result in the presence or absence of OSAS.

Common Medical Conditions Contributing to SDB

Although tonsils and adenoids represent the most common underlying etiology for OSAS, several other significant and common clinical disorders result in increased upper airway resistance. The swollen nasal passages and increased secretions caused by allergic rhinitis commonly result in snoring that may last for days, weeks, or months. Perennial allergic rhinitis causes year-round persistent snoring, increased upper airway resistance, and intermittent obstruction.[26] Similarly, sinusitis, whether acute or chronic in nature, results in swollen nasal passages and purulent nasal drainage that may disrupt sleep. Finally, the epidemic of obesity in childhood also contributes to the increased incidence of

SDB.[27] Pickwickian syndrome applies to the morbidly obese and results in both restrictive lung disease and circumferential upper airway narrowing that contribute to OSAS in pediatric as well as adult populations.

Syndromes Contributing to OSAS

Down syndrome, achondroplasia, and other craniofacial syndromes embody the most common syndromes that carry a high incidence of SDB difficulties. The incidence of OSAS in children with Down syndrome ranges from 60% to 100% depending on the study examined.[28,29] These children present a particular challenge to clinicians due to macroglossia, low motor tone, and a high propensity toward obesity. Given these physiological features, it is no surprise that children with Down syndrome may not resolve their OSAS following adenotonsillectomy or that they require additional medical therapies in future years. This group also poses a challenge when surgical therapies fail and positive airway pressure (PAP) devices or tracheostomy must be considered.

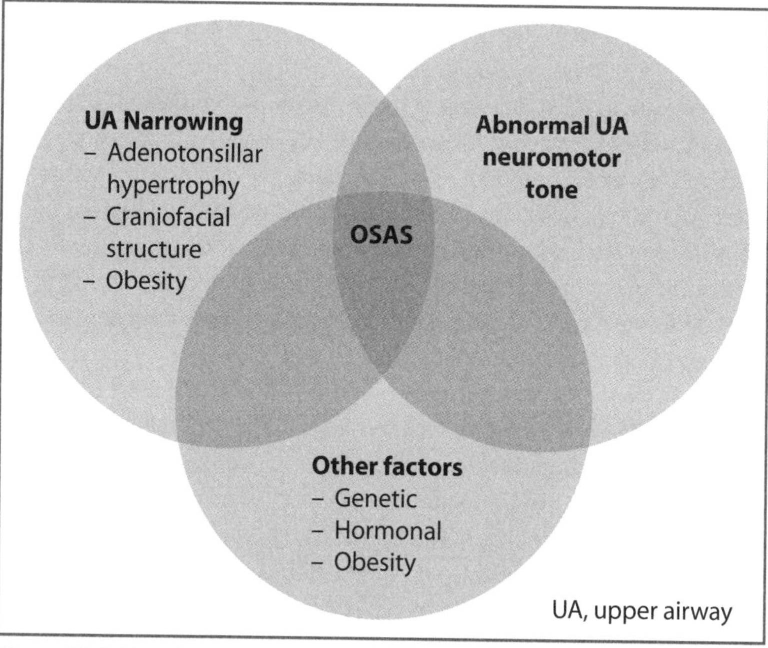

Figure 36-1. Venn diagram of factors contributing to obstructive sleep apnea syndrome (OSAS). (From Sheldon S, Feber R, Kryger M, eds. *Principles and Practice of Pediatric Sleep Medicine*. Philadelphia, PA: Elsevier/Saunders; 2005: 223–229, with permission from Elsevier.)

Box 36-3. Congenital Conditions Associated With Sleep-Disordered Breathing

- Achondroplasia
- Congenital muscular dystrophy
- Spinal muscular atrophy
- Nemaline rod myopathy
- Cruzon syndrome
- Apert syndrome
- Down syndrome
- Pierre-Robin sequence
- Duchene muscular dystrophy
- Prader-Willi syndrome

In contrast, children with achondroplasia find themselves at a much higher risk for OSA due to midfacial hypoplasia, narrow nasal passages and, in some cases, hypotonia. Children with achondroplasia may also present with other sleep-related breathing problems, such as central apnea or periodic breathing related to foramen magnum stenosis.[30,31] Therefore, a polysomnogram is vitally important to fully evaluate this population for surgical risk as well. Other syndromes associated with OSAS are listed in Box 36-3.

Management

Medical Preoperative Evaluation Following Sleep Study

Following a sleep study diagnostic for OSAS, the clinician should evaluate the patient for the next step in treatment, which should proceed irrespective of the type of OSAS diagnosed. In the child diagnosed with OSAS, evaluation with an otolaryngologist is typically the first step. Adenotonsillectomy, as opposed to isolated adenoidectomy or tonsillectomy, represents the most common initial treatment for OSAS, and is the preferred operation (when applicable) to avoid 2 separate surgeries over time. For children older than 3 years with generous tonsils and/or adenoids and no other medical problems, the sleep study results guide the next step in preoperative planning. In most uncomplicated cases with mild and selected cases with moderate OSAS in children 3 years and older, consideration of an outpatient operation is quite reasonable. Children with moderate to severe OSAS and severe gas exchange abnormalities should undergo preoperative evaluation that includes a 12-lead electrocardiogram or echocardiogram to identify right ventricular hypertrophy and/or cor pulmonale, a hemoglobin/hematocrit count to evaluate for polycythemia, a bicarbonate test to evaluate for hypercarbia, and a first morning venous or capillary gas to look for gas exchange abnormalities. Additional preoperative recommendations may follow from the pediatric pulmonologist regarding chronic respiratory-related conditions, such as asthma, cystic fibrosis,

Case Report 36-2

Darren is a 15-year-old male who comes in for health supervision visit. He is having trouble keeping up in school and had "Cs" and "Ds" on his last report card. Mom reports that he always appears tired, and Darren admits that he sometimes falls asleep in class because his "classes are boring." His sleep diary reveals that he is getting an average of 8.5 hours of sleep per night. He sleeps alone upstairs, and his mom is unsure if any snoring is present. His medical history is negative with the exception of recurrent tonsillar infections and an adenotonsillectomy at age 10. On examination, he is modestly overweight but there are no other abnormalities. Referral to local ENT reveals that there has been no regrowth of his tonsils or adenoids. He is referred to a pulmonary and sleep specialist, who orders a sleep study. He is found to have an AHI of 12 and oxygen desaturations with nadir of 82%. Bi-level PAP (BiPAP) therapy is ordered, and the BiPAP titration study reveals resolution of his OSAS with settings of 10/4 cwp (centimeters of water pressure). He has some difficulty tolerating the BiPAP initially; however, he eventually adapts fairly well, wearing it on school nights only. He no longer falls asleep in class and on his next report card, he receives "Bs" and an occasional "C."

chronic lung disease of infancy, chronic bronchiectasis, primary ciliary dyskinesia, and the muscular weakness syndromes.

Postoperative Management

Children with moderate to severe OSAS and/or severe gas exchange abnormalities should undergo close postoperative monitoring. This consists of an admission to the pediatric intensive care unit or a step-down unit that is able to closely monitor for possible respiratory compromise. Two studies from the 1990s identified characteristics of patients undergoing adenotonsillectomy that represent high risk for respiratory compromise or failure and are summarized in Box 36-4.[32–34] Children younger than 3 years are at a substantially increased risk for respiratory compromise regardless of other risk factors and also merit close observation. Those with severe OSAS or patients that meet risk factor criteria elaborated in Box 36-4 also should undergo more intensive monitoring following adenotonsillectomy. Most patients can be safely discharged within 24 hours following adenotonsillectomy; however, some may require home supplemental oxygen or even continuous PAP (CPAP)/BiPAP postoperatively if postoperative inflammation and edema cause continued obstruction. Figure 36-2 is an algorithm for the treatment of severe OSAS in children.

Box 36-4. Risk Factors for Respiratory Compromise Following Adenotonsillectomy

Children or adolescents with the following complicating medical conditions:

- Neuromuscular disorders
- Pulmonary hypertension
- Dwarfism
- Craniofacial abnormalities
- Marked obesity
- Hypotonia and related syndromes (eg, Down syndrome and Prader-Willi syndrome)
- Severe obstructive sleep apnea syndrome
- Obstructive index >10
- Apnea-hypopnea index >15
- Oxyhemoglobin saturation nadir ≤75%
- Age <3 years

Although adenotonsillectomy represents the best initial therapy in cases of severe OSAS, a follow-up sleep study is mandatory to determine whether further medical or alternative surgical options are necessary. The patient with severe OSAS often experiences incomplete resolution from adenotonsillectomy alone, necessitating further medical or surgical intervention. In children with moderate to severe OSAS, a follow-up sleep study at least 8 weeks after tonsillectomy/adenoidectomy will determine whether resolution of the immediate postoperative changes also results in resolution or improvement of SDB. The success rate of an adenotonsillectomy in the patient with OSAS has been reported in a recent meta-analysis of 14 peer-reviewed articles as 82.8% with a range of 52.9% to 100%.[35] However, these studies reflect short-term studies, and longitudinal studies have not been conducted. Given that family history of OSAS increases the likelihood of said disease in the offspring, the long-term risk is distinctly possible, and these patients may require repeat sleep study.[36] Rapid growth of tonsils and adenoids occurs between the ages of 3 to 6 years; therefore, the 3-year-old that undergoes tonsillectomy may present to the primary provider in the future with recurrent snoring or SDB due to generous adenoidal tissue.

Approach to Treatment in Infancy

Obstructive sleep apnea syndrome in infancy is rare, and there are no epidemiologic studies documenting its incidence in this age group. However, our experience suggests that infancy represents a signifi-

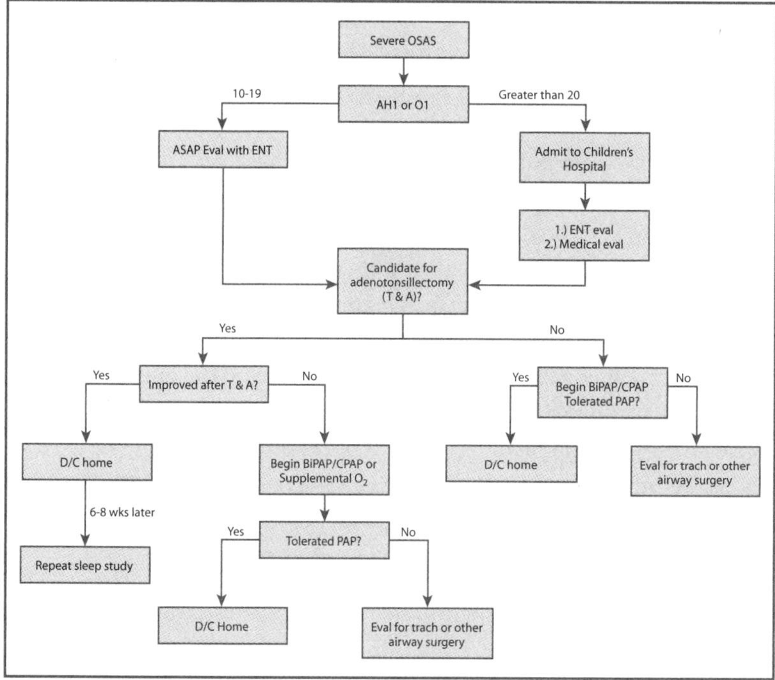

Figure 36-2. Algorithm for the treatment of severe obstructive sleep apnea in children.

cantly different group. Craniofacial and congenital neurologic syndromes form most SDB problems in this age (Box 36-3). This group requires overnight polysomnography and consideration of supplemental oxygen in the case of mild to moderate OSAS. In the case of severe OSAS, therapies such as PAP devices (CPAP/BiPAP), craniofacial reconstruction, and/or tracheostomy may be required in combination over time.

Medical Management of OSAS

In the 21st century, medical management of OSAS now offers a variety of scientifically validated, effective strategies to treat children. In children where surgery is not an option, supplemental oxygen, nasal steroids, montelukast, and PAP devices provide a variety of realistic short-term and long-term therapeutic options for SDB.

Supplemental Oxygen

Nocturnal supplemental oxygen represents one of the oldest medical therapies, which is effective in many individuals. Supplemental oxygen certainly fails to treat the underlying cause of OSAS, but minimizes or eliminates oxyhemoglobin desaturations during sleep in some cases. Children with severe OSAS may respond abnormally to supplemental oxygen due to a blunted upper neuromotor airway response, which improves following adenotonsillectomy.[37] A blunted partial pressure of CO_2 drive, which can occur in the presence of severe OSAS, leaves the child only their hypoxic drive intact to adjust minute ventilation during sleep. Once placed on supplemental oxygen, the hypoxic drive is suppressed and respiratory depression or even respiratory arrest may ensue during the course of the night. Caution must therefore be used when starting supplemental oxygen to avoid respiratory depression or arrest.[38] A sleep study in a pediatric laboratory that tracks $EtCO_2$ trends helps identify those individuals at risk when oxygen is considered as treatment.

Nasal Steroids

Nasal steroids, such as fluticasone and budesonide, significantly reduce the obstructive index in children with mild OSAS in several different studies. The most recent studies are small in number, but are double-blind, placebo-controlled trials that monitor responses with pretreatment and posttreatment polysomnogram over 6 weeks.[39] Kheirandish-Gozal and Gozal[40] reported that in children with mild OSAS, AHI normalized and sleep architecture, such as percent REM time, significantly improved. Eight weeks following treatment with nasal budesonide had stopped, the improvement in sleep architecture and AHI still remained. It is hypothesized that nasal steroids shrink adenoidal tissues, which was noted in at least one of the clinical trials. Subsequently, this therapy represents a reasonable and effective medical therapy for mild OSAS.

Montelukast

Montelukast, a leukotriene receptor antagonist, represents a possible emerging medical therapy for the treatment of mild OSAS. In a peer-reviewed journal, one team reported their open-label study of 24 children (10 boys) who were given montelukast for 16 weeks.[41] Pretreatment and posttreatment polysomnogram revealed significant improvement in obstructive index as well as improved adenoid-pharyngeal ratio (Figure 36-3), which was not related to atopy. The mechanism for this improvement likely relates to increased expression of leukotriene receptors in upper airway lymphoid tissue in children with SDB.[42] Although this work is encouraging, this reflects only one clinical study and requires further study with a larger population.

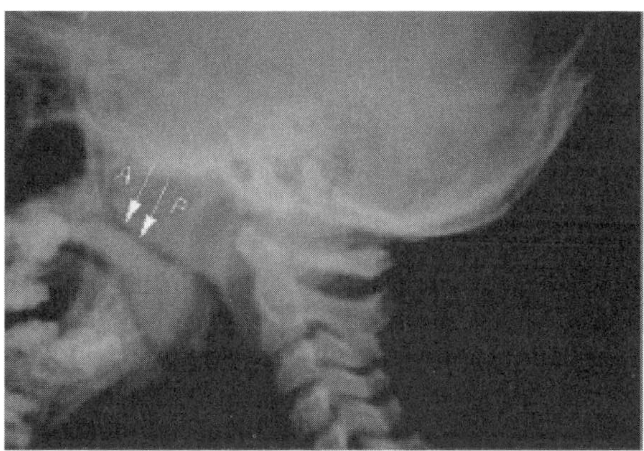

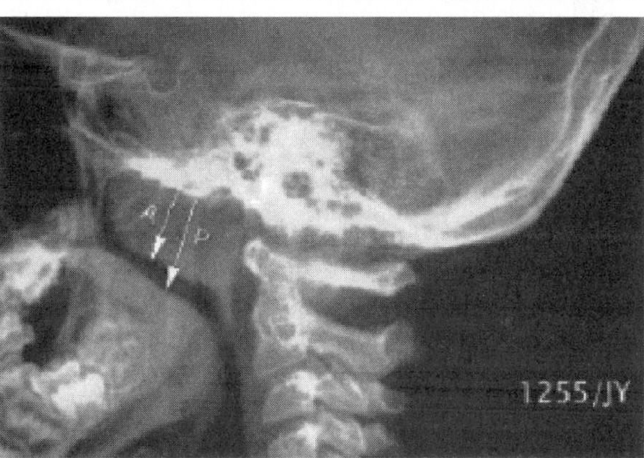

Figure 36-3. Lateral neck films demonstrate montelukast effect on adenoidal-nasopharyngeal ratio. (Goldbart A, Goldman G, Li R, et al. Differential expression of cysteinyl leukotriene receptors 1 and 2 in tonsils of children with obstructive sleep apnea and recurrent infection. *Chest.* 2004;126:13–18. Copyright © American Thoracic Society. Reprinted by permission.)

PAP Devices

Positive airway pressure devices include CPAP or BiPAP modes that represent a validated treatment for children with OSAS. Currently at least one PAP device with a mask is approved by the US Food and Drug Administration for children weighing more than 30 kg. The most frequent use for PAP is in children who are obese after adenotonsillectomy. Adherence represents the most difficult issue in chronic PAP use, and parents are counseled on helping children adapt and wear the device reliably throughout the night. Some providers present desensitization protocols to help their families adapt to the CPAP/BiPAP device in a structured fashion. Once the child has acclimated and is using the PAP device regularly throughout the night, then a CPAP or BiPAP titration study will fine-tune the amount of positive airway support required to eliminate obstructive events. Potential side effects of PAP therapy include nasal congestion, epistaxis, pressure ulcers over the nasal bridge, zygomatic prominences, and forehead prominence. In the case of a full face mask, the risk of aspiration is also increased, at least theoretically. In rare circumstances, long-term use may result in midface hypoplasia related to many years of continuous pressure in a single location.[43] We have also observed central apneic events while children wear BiPAP. This can be relieved with the addition of a backup rate.

Other Treatment Options for SDB

In the presence of OSAS following adenotonsillectomy, or when adenotonsillectomy is not indicated, other options exist for the patient with SDB. If significant time has passed after adenotonsillectomy, a reevaluation with the otolaryngologist will rule out regrowth of adenoids that contribute to a reappearance of OSAS in children. However, in children with severe OSAS that is refractory to other surgical options, tracheostomy is extremely effective in resolving significant upper-airway resistance. Fortunately, other surgical and dental alternatives also exist to effectively treat OSAS. These innovative craniofacial and minimally invasive dental treatments increase the breadth of proven alternatives available to providers today.

Key Points

- In children, SDB encompasses a broad range of breathing-related diagnoses, including primary snoring, OSA, OH, and upper-airway resistance syndrome.
- The incidence of primary snoring ranges from 12% to 20% in contrast to OSAS, where the incidence is approximately 2% to 3%.
- Future research is needed to improve our understanding of the cognitive sequelae of SDB.
- Although the gold standard for diagnosis of OSAS is the sleep study, alternatives are available.
- Adenotonsillectomy is the most common initial treatment for OSAS.
- Children with moderate to severe OSAS or severe gas exchange abnormalities should undergo close postoperative monitoring. Other high-risk conditions have been identified.
- In cases of severe OSAS, a follow-up sleep study is mandatory to determine whether further medical or alternative surgical options are necessary.
- Other treatments for OSAS are available, including medications, CPAP or BiPAP, and surgical and dental options.

Acknowledgment

We would like to thank Ms Sarah VanElderen, who provided significant assistance in the preparation of this chapter.

References

1. Owen G, Canter R, Robinson A. Snoring, apnoea and ENT symptoms in the paediatric community. *Clin Otolaryngol.* 1996;21:130–134
2. Corbo GM, Forastiere F, Agabiti N, et al. Snoring in 9- to 15-year-old children: risk factors and clinical relevance. *Pediatrics.* 2001;108:1149–1154
3. Ferreira AM, Clemente V, Gozal D, et al. Snoring in Portuguese primary school children. *Pediatrics.* 2000;106:e64
4. Ali N, Pitson D, Stradling J. Snoring, sleep disturbance, and behaviour in 4–5 year olds. *Arch Dis Child.* 1993;68:360–366
5. Brunetti L, Rana S, Lospalluti M, et al. Prevalence of obstructive sleep apnea syndrome in a cohort of 1,207 children of southern Italy. *Chest.* 2001;120:1930–1935

6. Redline S, Tishler P, Schluchter M, et al. Risk factors for disordered breathing in children: associations with obesity, race, and respiratory problems. *Am J Respir Crit Care Med.* 1999;159:1527–1532
7. Carroll J, McColley S, Marcus C, et al. Inability of clinical history to distinguish primary snoring from obstructive sleep apnea syndrome in children. *Chest.* 1995;108:610–618
8. Brietzke S, Katz E, Roberson D. Can history and physical examination reliably diagnose pediatric obstructive sleep apnea/hypopnea syndrome? A systemic review of the literature. *Otolaryngol Head Neck Surg.* 2004;131:827–832
9. Brouillette R, Morielli A, Leimanis A, et al. Nocturnal pulse oximetry as an abbreviated testing modality for pediatric obstructive sleep apnea. *Pediatrics.* 2000;105:405–412
10. American Thoracic Society. ATS consensus statement: standards and indications for cardiopulmonary sleep studies in children. *Am J Respir Crit Care Med.* 1996;153:866–878
11. American Academy of Pediatrics Section of Pediatric Pulmonology, Subcommittee of Obstructive Sleep Apnea syndrome. Clinical practice guideline: diagnosis and management of childhood obstructive sleep apnea syndrome. *Pediatrics.* 2002;109:704–712
12. Rosen C, D'Andrea L, Haddad G. Adult criteria for obstructive sleep apnea do not identify children with serious obstruction. *Am Rev Respir Dis.* 1992;146:1231–1234
13. American Academy of Sleep Medicine. *The International Classification of Sleep Disorders: Diagnostic and Coding Manual.* 2nd ed. Westchester, IL: American Academy of Sleep Medicine; 2005:56–59
14. Katz E, Marcus C. Diagnosis of obstructive sleep apnea syndrome in infants and children. In: Sheldon S, Feber R, Kryger M, eds. *Principles and Practice of Pediatric Sleep Medicine.* Philadelphia, PA: Elsevier/Saunders; 2005:197–210
15. Guilleminault C, Stoohs R, Clerk A, et al. A cause of excessive daytime sleepiness: the upper airway resistance syndrome. *Chest.* 1993;104:781–787
16. Uliel S, Tauman R, Greenfeld M, et al. Normal polysomnographic respiratory values in children and adolescents. *Chest.* 2004;125:872–878
17. Marcus C, Carroll J, Koerner C, et al. Determinants of growth in children with obstructive sleep apnea syndrome. *J Pediatr.* 1994;125:556–562
18. Gozal D, Pope D. Snoring during early childhood and academic performance at ages thirteen to fourteen years. *Pediatrics.* 2001;107:1394–1999
19. Huang Y, Guilleminault C, Li H, et al. Attention-deficit/hyperactivity disorder with obstructive sleep apnea: a treatment outcome study. *Sleep Med.* 2007;8:18–30
20. Reuveni H, Simon T, Tal A, et al. Health care services utilization in children with obstructive sleep apnea syndrome. *Pediatrics.* 2002;110:68–72
21. Halbower A, Ishman S, McGinley B. Childhood obstructive sleep-disordered breathing: a clinical update and discussion of technological innovations and challenges. *Chest.* 2007;132:2030–2041

22. O'Brien L, Mervis C, Holbrook CR, et al. Neurobehavioral implications of habitual snoring in children. *Pediatrics.* 2004;114:44–49
23. Chervin R, Ruzicka D, Giordani B, et al. Sleep disordered breathing, behavior, and cognition in children before and after adenotonsillectomy. *Pediatrics.* 2006;117:e769–e778
24. Brooks L, Stephens B, Bacevice A. Adenoid size is related to severity but not the number of episodes of obstructive apnea in children. *J Pediatr.* 1998;132:682–686
25. Brooks LJ. Obstructive sleep apnea syndrome in infants and children: clinical features and pathophysiology. In: Sheldon S, Feber R, Kryger M, eds. *Principles and Practice of Pediatric Sleep Medicine.* Philadelphia, PA: Elsevier/Saunders; 2005:223–229
26. McColley S, Carroll JL, Curtis S, et al. High prevalence of allergic sensitization in children with habitual snoring and obstructive sleep apnea. *Chest.* 1997;111:170–173
27. Levers-Landis C, Redline S. Pediatric sleep apnea: implications of the epidemic of childhood overweight. *Am J Respir Crit Care Med.* 2007;175:436–441
28. Shott S, Amin R, Chini B, et al. Obstructive sleep apnea: should all children with Down syndrome be tested? *Arch Otolaryngol Head Neck Surg.* 2006;132:432–436
29. Levanon A, Tarasiuk A, Tal A. Sleep characteristics in children with Down syndrome. *J Pediatr.* 1999;134:755–760
30. William O, Collins M, Sukgi S. Otolaryngologic manifestations of achondroplasia. *Arch Otolaryngol Head Neck Surg.* 2007;133:237–244
31. Mogayzel P, Carroll J, Loughlin G, et al. Sleep-disordered breathing in children with achondroplasia. *J Pediatr.* 1998;132:667–671
32. McColley SA, April MM, Carroll JL, et al. Respiratory compromise after adenotonsillectomy in children with obstructive sleep apnea. *Arch Otolaryngol Head Neck Surg.* 1992;118:940–943
33. Rosen GM, Muckle RP, Mahowald MW, et al. Postoperative respiratory compromise in children with obstructive sleep apnea syndrome: can it be anticipated? *Pediatrics.* 1994;93:784–788
34. Lipton A, Gozal D. Treatment of obstructive sleep apnea in children: do we really know how? *Sleep Med Rev.* 2003;7:61–80
35. Brietzke S, Gallagher D. The effectiveness of tonsillectomy and adenoidectomy in the treatment of pediatric obstructive sleep apnea/hypopnea syndrome: a meta-analysis. *Otolaryngol Head Neck Surg.* 2006;134:979–984
36. Buxbaum SG, Elston RC, Tishler PV, Redline S. Genetics of the apnea hypopnea index in Caucasians and African Americans: I. Segregation analysis. *Genet Epidemiol.* 2002;22:243–253
37. Marcus C, Katz E, Lutz J, et al. Upper airway dynamic responses in children with the obstructive sleep apnea syndrome. *Pediatr Res.* 2005;57:99–107

38. Marcus C, Carroll J, Bamford O, et al. Supplemental oxygen during sleep in children with sleep-disordered breathing. *Am J Respir Crit Care Med.* 1995;152:1297–1301
39. Brouillette R, Manoukian J, Ducharme F, et al. Efficacy of fluticasone nasal spray for pediatric obstructive sleep apnea. *J Pediatr.* 2001;138:838–844
40. Kheirandish-Gozal L, Gozal D. Intranasal budesonide treatment for children with mild obstructive sleep apnea syndrome. *Pediatrics.* 2008;122:e149–e155
41. Goldbart A, Goldman J, Veling M, et al. Leukotriene modifier therapy for mild sleep-disordered breathing in children. *Am J Respir Crit Care Med.* 2005;172:364–370
42. Goldbart A, Goldman G, Li R, et al. Differential expression of cysteinyl leukotriene receptors 1 and 2 in tonsils of children with obstructive sleep apnea and recurrent infection. *Chest.* 2004;126:13–18
43. Li K, Riley R, Guilleminault C. An unreported risk in the use of home nasal continuous positive airway pressure and home nasal ventilation in children: mid-face hypoplasia. *Chest.* 2000;117:916–918

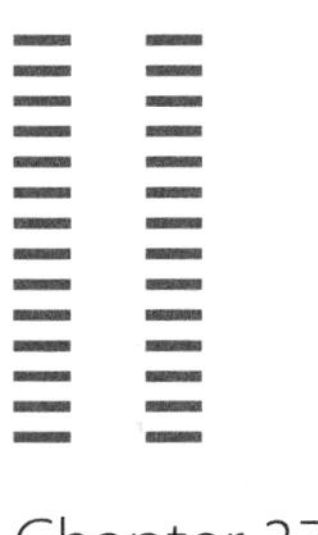

Chapter 37

Cystic Fibrosis

Michael S. Schechter, MD, MPH
Brian P. O'Sullivan, MD

Introduction

Cystic fibrosis (CF) was, in the past, typically described as the most common lethal genetic disease in the white population, but the outlook for people diagnosed with CF has improved dramatically in the past 10 to 20 years. The US Cystic Fibrosis Foundation (CFF) projected life expectancy for patients has increased from 31 to 37 years over the past decade[1] (Figure 37-1), and a United Kingdom model predicts that a child born with CF today can expect to live past 50 years of age.[2] Birth prevalence varies from country to country and with ethnic background; CF occurs in approximately 1 in 3,000 white Americans, 1 in 4,000 to 10,000 Hispanic Americans, and 1 in 15,000 to 20,000 African Americans. The prevalence is quite low among Africans, Asians, and Native Americans.[3]

Pathogenesis

Genetics

Cystic fibrosis is an autosomal recessive disease caused by an abnormal gene on the long arm of chromosome 7. The gene product, called cystic fibrosis transmembrane conductance regulator (CFTR), localizes to the apical cell membrane and regulates ion transport by a blend of Na^+ absorption and Cl^- secretion.[4] While there have been more than 1,500 CFTR mutations identified, 50% of CF patients with a Northern European background are homozygous for the ΔF508 mutation (involving the deletion of phenylalanine, which is normally the 508th amino acid in the protein), and 35% are compound heterozygotes with one ΔF508 allele. Although *CFTR* mutation frequency varies from population to population, worldwide no single mutation other than ΔF508 occurs in a frequency greater than approximately 5%.[3]

Case Report 37-1

J. W. is a 12-year-old girl with CF diagnosed at age 3 months after prolonged respiratory symptoms following a viral respiratory infection in association with abnormal stools. She is in seventh grade, is a good student, and is an avid soccer player. Her height and weight are both at about the 50th percentile and her forced expiratory volume in 1 second (FEV_1) was 108% predicted at her last CF clinic visit. Her airway cultures (obtained by throat swab because she does not expectorate sputum) have grown methicillin-resistant *Staphylococcus aureus* (MRSA) for the past few years but no *Pseudomonas.* Her current treatment regimen consists of airway clearance augmentation with high-frequency chest wall oscillation (the Vest) twice a day, dornase alfa (Pulmozyme) by nebulization once a day, ibuprofen 500 mg twice a day, pancreatic enzymes, and vitamins. She recently developed a cough in association with a viral respiratory infection that the family members also experienced. She was seen at her pediatrician's office, with negative physical findings other than rhinorrhea, but after consultation with her CF doctor she was started on trimethoprim/sulfamethoxazole (to which her MRSA was susceptible). At follow-up in the CF clinic, her cough was better but her FEV_1 was 95% predicted. She was prescribed linezolid and advised to increase airway clearance therapy to 3 or 4 times a day. Three weeks later, on return to the CF clinic, she reported an occasional cough at night, her FEV_1 was 92% predicted, and she had normal findings on chest examination. Her chest radiograph showed slightly increased markings in the right upper lobe.She was hospitalized and underwent bronchoscopy with bronchoalveolar lavage, which grew non-mucoid *Pseudomonas aeruginosa.* After 2 weeks of intravenous (IV) ceftazidime and tobramycin, she was asymptomatic and her FEV_1 had returned to 106% predicted. She was discharged on inhaled tobramycin 300 mg twice a day to be followed up at the CF clinic in a month to verify eradication of *Pseudomonas* and to discuss how long the inhaled tobramycin should be continued.

Different classes of gene mutation lead to different types of abnormality in the CFTR protein (defective CFTR production, defective CFTR processing within the cytoplasm, defective regulation, and defective ion conduction). These, in turn, may be associated with different degrees of functional compromise in CFTR.[5] Certain mutations are associated with enough residual CFTR activity to allow for normal pancreatic function, and patients with pancreatic sufficiency tend to have milder pulmonary disease. However, in any given individual, CFTR mutation is a much better predictor of pancreatic function than of lung involvement. This is because lung disease is also influenced by

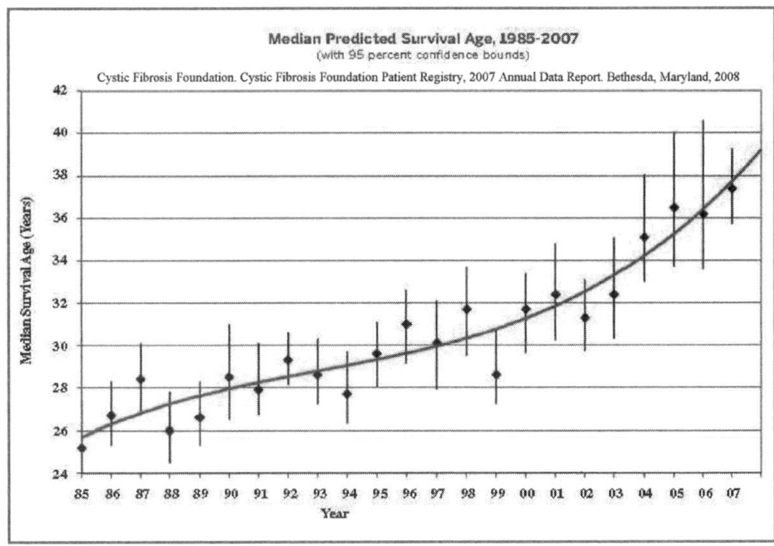

Figure 37-1. Median predicted survival age for those with cystic fibrosis. (From Cystic Fibrosis Foundation Patient Registry, 2007 Annual Data Report. Bethesda, Maryland © 2008 Cystic Fibrosis Foundation. Reprinted by permission.)

nutritional status, sociodemographic and environmental factors, and variations in health care interventions, to an extent that blurs distinct genotype-phenotype associations in lung disease.[6] In addition, the presence of gene modifiers (polymorphisms in non-*CFTR* genes that control the inflammatory response, such as mannose-binding lectin, tumor necrosis factor, and alpha-1 antitrypsin) may also affect severity of CF lung disease.

Pathophysiology

There are several hypotheses regarding how CFTR dysfunction leads to the phenotypic disease known as CF, but the most well-accepted is the so-called low volume hypothesis, which holds that a combination of excessive reabsorption of sodium and deficient chloride secretion, along with passive movement of water, result in dehydration of airway surface materials and low airway surface water volume.[4] This in turn leads to a reduction in the lubricating layer between epithelium and mucus, with compression of cilia and inhibition of normal ciliary and cough clearance (Figure 37-2). Mucus adherent to the underlying epithelium forms plaques with hypoxic niches that can harbor bacteria,

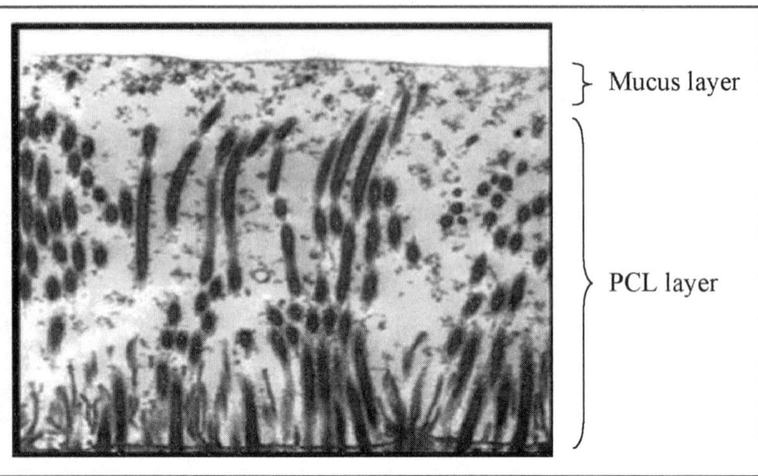

Figure 37-2A. Mechanical clearance via mucus transport provides the primary innate defense against inhaled bacteria. The promotion of efficient mucus transport: the maintenance of a well-defined periciliary liquid (PCL) layer that exhibits an optimal height (ie, the height of extended cilia) and viscosity for effective ciliary beating and cell surface lubrication to clear inhaled organisms. Cystic fibrosis transmembrane conductance regulator (CFTR) is key to this process.

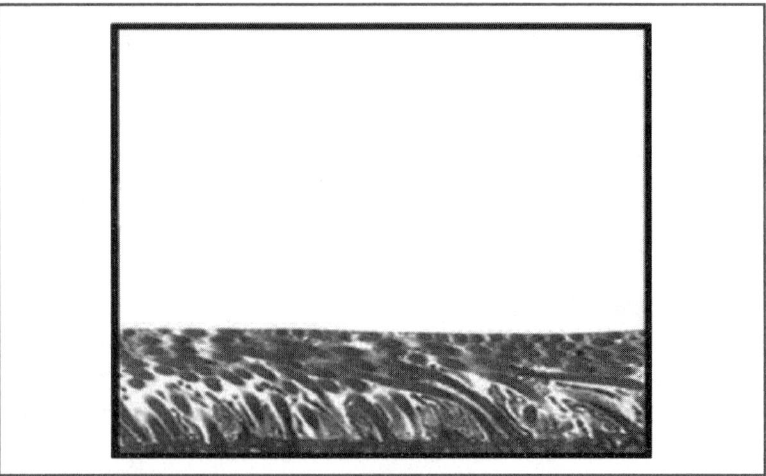

Figure 37-2B. Absence of CFTR leads to isotonic reduction in the airway surface liquid, depleting the PCL layer and compromising ciliary function and the system of mucociliary clearance.

particularly *P aeruginosa*. There is also some evidence of intrinsic dysregulation of the host inflammatory response. Lung lavage studies show that inflammation is present in children as young as 4 weeks who are apparently free of infection.[7] It remains unclear if the degree of inflammation seen in patients with CF is a primary manifestation of the basic defect, a reaction to the chronic infection permitted by this defect, or a combination of the two.[8]

Cystic fibrosis transmembrane conductance regulator dysfunction in the airways thus leads to susceptibility to bronchial infection. Persistent infection leads to elaboration of chemotactic cytokines, which recruit large numbers of polymorphonuclear (PMN) cells into the airways that necrose and release DNA, leading to increased sputum viscosity.[9] Thereafter, bacterial exotoxins and products of the damaged neutrophils spur further PMN recruitment, more inflammation, and increased tissue damage. This "vicious cycle" of cellular events leads to obstruction and bronchiectasis, persistence of infection and inflammation, and eventual respiratory failure (Figure 37-3). Outside of the

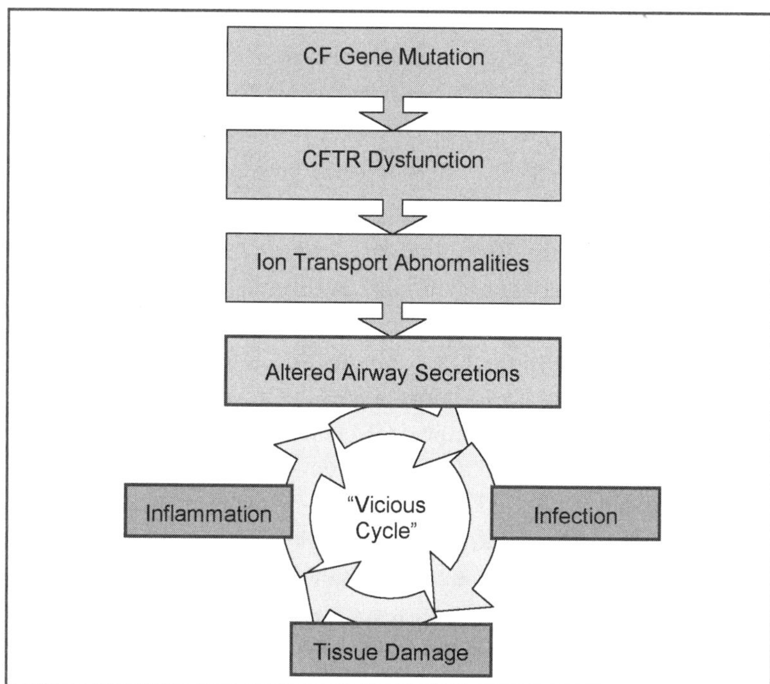

Figure 37-3. Pathogenesis of cystic fibrosis.

airway, abnormalities in ion transport lead to excessive salt content of the sweat and decreased water in pancreatic and male reproductive tract secretions, leading to ductal obstruction, pancreatic insufficiency, and congenital bilateral absence of the vas deferens.

Clinical Features

Diagnosis

For all patients currently cared for at CF centers in the United States, the median age at diagnosis is 6 months, but the mean age at diagnosis is 3 years because many patients were diagnosed later in childhood or even in adulthood. The most common features leading to evaluation and diagnosis were respiratory symptoms (50%), failure to thrive/malnutrition (34%), steatorrhea/abnormal stools (26%), and meconium ileus (21%). Family history in a first-degree relative led to the diagnosis in 16% of patients. However, with the widespread adoption of newborn screening over the last few years, an increasing number of asymptomatic infants are diagnosed in the first month of life. In 2008, 43% of new diagnoses were made by newborn screening.

The diagnosis of CF requires a combination of specific clinical characteristics with biochemical or genetic markers of CFTR dysfunction.

The sweat test remains the most readily available and clinically useful approach to making the diagnosis of CF, provided it is performed at a laboratory that adheres to strict guidelines using pilocarpine iontophoresis and a quantitative determination of chloride concentration.[10] A sweat chloride greater than 60 mmol/L is almost always diagnostic of CF. Patients with a sweat chloride in the so-called intermediate range (30–59 for infants younger than 6 months, 40–59 for older patients) will often be found to have abnormalities in CFTR function and should be referred to an accredited CF center for further evaluation. Sweat testing is feasible and reliable by 3 days of age, although it might be more difficult to obtain adequate sweat in young infants, especially those with low birth weight.[11] There are limited causes of false-negative or false-positive sweat tests, and most of these will be clinically apparent (Box 37-1). In practice, the most common cause of incorrect sweat test results is poor laboratory proficiency, which is common in laboratories that are not associated with CFF-accredited care centers.[12]

Box 37-1. Conditions Associated With a False-Positive or False-Negative Sweat Test

False-Positive	False-Negative
Atopic dermatitis (eczema)	Dilution of sample
Malnutrition	Malnutrition
Congenital adrenal hyperplasia	Peripheral edema
Mauriac syndrome	Low sweat rate (quantity not sufficient)
Fucosidosis	Hypoproteinemia
Ectodermal dysplasia	Dehydration
Klinefelter syndrome	Cystic fibrosis transmembrane conductance regulator mutations with preserved sweat duct function (eg, 3849+10kb C→T; R117H-7T)
Nephrogenic diabetes insipidus	
Adrenal insufficiency	
Hypothyroidism	
Autonomic dysfunction	
Environmental deprivation	
Munchausen by proxy	

As already noted, CF may be diagnosed by identifying 2 disease-causing mutations, and a number of analytical methods for CFTR mutation detection are commercially available. In general, use of a discrete panel of mutations is faster and less costly than expanded mutation analysis, and incorporation of approximately 40 of the most frequent disease-associated mutations will detect more than 90% of affected individuals in most populations. However, the diagnosis will be missed if the subject is affected by a mutation that is not included on the panel in use. Full sequence analysis will detect virtually all CFTR mutations, but its interpretation is sometimes difficult because it often uncovers polymorphisms and novel mutations whose significance is not known.[13]

Nasal transepithelial potential difference (NPD) measurement is sometimes used to assess patients who may have CF but do not meet classical diagnostic criteria. Unfortunately, NPD is labor intensive and technically difficult and is only available at a relatively small number of CF research centers. It is primarily a research tool for evaluation of the ability of pharmaceutical agents to alter chloride channel function, and it has had limited validation as a diagnostic tool.[13]

Although most patients with CF have the classic triad of lung disease, pancreatic insufficiency, and a high sweat chloride, there is a growing number of people recognized as having milder problems possibly associated with CFTR dysfunction. These problems include male infertility, recurrent pancreatitis, chronic sinusitis, and primary sclerosing cholangitis.[14] Patients displaying characteristics suggestive of atypical CF should have CFTR mutation analysis performed. Sweat testing alone is not sufficient in this population since it is likely that the sweat chloride will be borderline or normal. There is an analogous group of infants who are found through newborn screening to have elevated immunoreactive trypsinogen (IRT) and borderline or normal sweat chlorides and CF mutations that are not clearly disease causing. The term CF-related metabolic syndrome has been suggested for use with this group,[15] allowing appropriate follow-up for complications without labeling them as clearly having CF. These patients should be evaluated at CF centers with expertise and experience with this clinical presentation.

Newborn Screening

Newborn screening is performed by measuring IRT in blood spots taken from newborns. A very high IRT concentration implies pancreatic injury consistent with (but not specific for) CF. This marker is elevated even in infants with milder genotypes associated with pancreatic sufficiency. Those infants who have an elevated IRT on initial testing then have further evaluation via a repeat IRT 1 to 3 weeks later (IRT/IRT) or by analysis of the initial blood spot for a specified panel of CFTR mutations (IRT/DNA). The advantage of IRT/IRT screening is that it avoids the problems associated with detecting mutations of uncertain clinical significance and of having to counsel families in regard to carrier status or non-paternity. However, the IRT/IRT algorithm requires obtaining a second blood spot 1 to 3 weeks after the first one, which may be a major logistical problem in some populations, whereas the IRT/DNA method allows complete testing on one blood specimen. The IRT/DNA method uses a panel of the most common CF mutations that is applied to infant blood spots with high IRT levels. Because this does not evaluate all CFTR mutations, the finding of just one mutation is considered to be screen-positive and leads to referral for sweat test (an alternative protocol being evaluated in California performs DNA sequencing on these infants). A positive screening result by either IRT/IRT or IRT/DNA method only indicates that a child is at increased risk for CF; a sweat test must still be done to confirm the diagnosis.[16]

Multiple studies have shown that early diagnosis associated with CF newborn screening leads to improved nutritional outcomes.[17] Given that weight for age in infancy correlates with lung function at 6 years of age,[18] it is reasonable to infer that newborn screening will lead to improved pulmonary function later in life and, in fact, there are data supporting this hypothesis.[19] In 2006 the Centers for Disease Control and Prevention issued a statement supporting adoption of CF newborn screening throughout the United States,[20] and as a result virtually all states have initiated programs in the last several years.

Clinical Manifestations

Cystic fibrosis is a multisystem disorder that primarily affects the respiratory tract, gastrointestinal tract, sweat glands, and reproductive tract (Box 37-2). The appearance of CF-related symptoms occurs throughout life, with great overlap and variability from patient to patient.

Respiratory Tract Disease

Upper respiratory tract disease, especially chronic sinusitis, is universal in children with CF and often a cause of considerable morbidity. Extensive polyposis may be an additional cause of severe nasal obstruction. The pathogenesis, as in other organ systems, is inspissation of abnormal secretions due to CFTR dysfunction. Some children with CF require repeated surgical procedures for this problem because, unfortunately, sinus disease and polyps almost invariably recur.

The lungs of children with CF are normal at birth, but airways quickly become infected, inflamed, and obstructed in a self-perpetuating cycle (Figure 37-3). Infection rarely spreads beyond the respiratory tract. Chronic airway infection is typically established within the first year of life and can be controlled but not eradicated. Chronic bronchitis progressing to obstructive lung disease and bronchiectasis is the hallmark of CF lung disease. Complications of this process include atelectasis due to plugging of segmental and subsegmental bronchi; pneumothorax due to the development of subpleural blebs and cysts, which then rupture; and hemoptysis due to bleeding from hypertro-

Box 37-2. Systems Possibly Involved in Cystic Fibrosis[a]

Respiratory Tract
- Sinusitis
- Nasal polyps (3% require surgery)
- Chronic bronchitis
  - Bronchiectasis
  - Atelectasis
  - Pneumothorax (1%)
  - Hemoptysis (massive in 2%)
  - Respiratory failure

Gastrointestinal Tract
- Pancreatic insufficiency (92%)
- Meconium ileus (21%)
- Distal ileal obstruction syndrome (3%)
- Rectal prolapse (4%)
- Biliary obstruction, cirrhosis (6%)

Other
- Diabetes mellitus (21% of patients ≥14 years of age)
- Osteoporosis (12% of 18- to 24-year-olds)

Reproductive Tract
- Congenital bilateral absence of the vas deferens

Sweat Glands
- Increased chloride content of sweat (99.3%)

[a] The prevalence of involvement, when provided, is from the 2007 Cystic Fibrosis Foundation Patient Registry.

phied bronchial vessels. Pulmonary insufficiency is responsible for the most CF-related deaths.

The microbiology of infection in patients with CF follows a fairly typical course. Most infants initially harbor *Haemophilus influenzae* and/or *Staphylococcus aureus;* without specific intervention, *P aeruginosa* eventually becomes the predominant organism found in the airways.[1] Figure 37-4 shows the frequency of different organisms by age. Organisms that play a significant role include

- ***Haemophilus influenzae***—Typically found in infancy, and less often with increasing age.
- ***Staphylococcus aureus***—Also typically found in infancy, but often persists throughout life. Methicillin-resistant *S aureus* is becoming increasingly prevalent in the CF population as in others; there are conflicting data regarding whether its acquisition is associated with worsening lung disease.

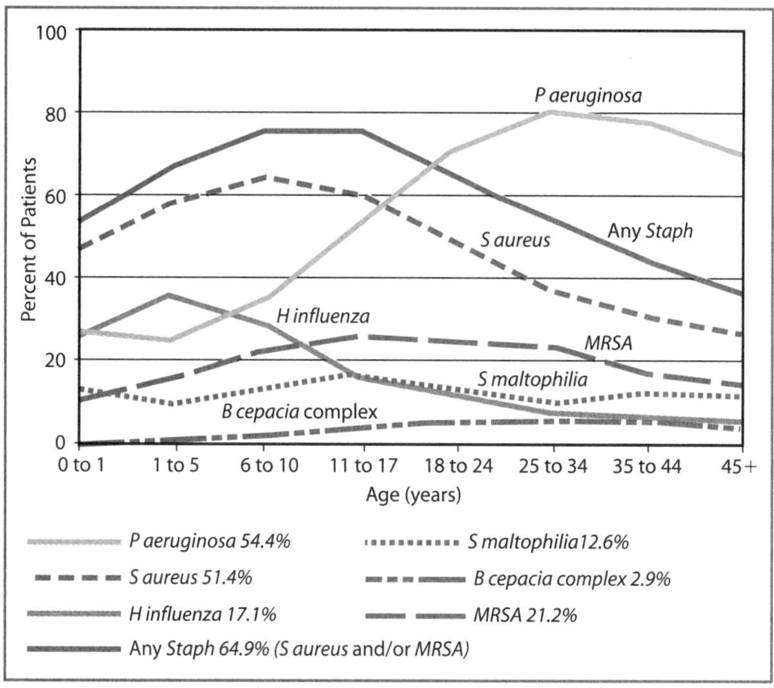

Figure 37-4. Age-specific prevalence of respiratory pathogens in patients with cystic fibrosis. (From Cystic Fibrosis Foundation Patient Registry, 2007 Annual Data Report. Bethesda, Maryland © 2008 Cystic Fibrosis Foundation. Reprinted by permission.)

- ***Pseudomonas aeruginosa***—Acquisition of *P aeruginosa* becomes increasingly prevalent as patients get older. Initially, *P aeruginosa* grows as a non-mucoid strain that can be cleared by the host or eradicated with aggressive antibiotic therapy.[21] Over time, *P aeruginosa* colonies elaborate an alginate coat and form biofilms.[22] These biofilms, once established, are difficult if not impossible to clear with standard antibiotic therapy. There is a pronounced survival benefit for those patients who remain free of *Pseudomonas* infection, and for this reason, heightened surveillance for *P aeruginosa* has become common practice, combined with strategies to eradicate early *Pseudomonas* infection (see below).[23]
- ***Stenotrophomonas maltophilia***—A relatively resistant organism that has not been associated with acceleration of lung disease.[24]
- ***Achromobacter xylosoxidans* (formerly *Alcaligenes xylosoxidans*)**—Another relatively resistant organism whose prognosis is less clear.

- ***Burkholderia cenocepacia***—An uncommon organism that uniquely infects patients with CF and has worrisome implications, as it is innately multiresistant, can cause fulminant disease, and is transmissible. Infection with *B cenocepacia* can cause a rapid decline in pulmonary function and increased mortality in patients with CF. Occasionally, infection with *B cenocepacia* can cause an invasive, fatal bacteremia, the so-called cepacia syndrome. *Burkholderia cenocepacia* is particularly transmissible and is associated with a striking deterioration in health, perhaps due to its ability to elicit a more robust inflammatory response from host cells. However, other *B cenocepacia* strains can also be transmitted from person to person and lead to acute deterioration, highlighting the need for effective infection control at all CF centers.[25]
- **Nontuberculous mycobacteria**—*Mycobacterium avium* complex (72%) and *Mycobacterium abscessus* (16%) were the most common species found in a survey of US CF centers.[26] It is not always clear whether recovery of these organisms from a patient's sputum represents true infection or only saprophytic colonization, but patients with persistently positive sputum smears or cultures should be monitored closely for development of worsening disease and treated as described in recommended protocols. For more information on the diagnosis and treatment of nontuberculous mycobacteria, see Chapter 23.
- ***Aspergillus fumigatus***—An intense hypersensitivity response to *A fumigatus,* known as allergic bronchopulmonary aspergillosis (ABPA), is seen in 1% to 15% of patients with CF, the incidence varying with geography. Allergic bronchopulmonary aspergillosis classically manifests with wheezing, pulmonary infiltrates, and central bronchiectasis, but these clues might be obscured by the background of more typical CF lung disease. Diagnostic criteria for ABPA include acute or subacute clinical deterioration; total serum immunoglobulin (Ig) E concentraton greater than 500 IU/mL (1200 ng/mL); immediate cutaneous reactivity to *Aspergillus;* and one of the following: (a) precipitins to *A fumigatus* or IgG antibody to *A fumigatus* or (b) abnormalities on chest radiography or computed tomography scan that have not cleared with standard antibiotic therapy.[27] For more information on the diagnosis and treatment of ABPA, see Chapter 9.

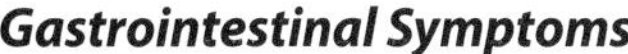

Gastrointestinal Symptoms

Approximately 21% of infants with CF are born with meconium ileus, an obstructive phenomenon secondary to inspissated material in the small and large bowels. More than 90% of people with CF develop pancreatic insufficiency (PI), which is usually present at birth but may evolve during the first year of life. Pancreatic dysfunction is due to obstruction of intra-pancreatic ducts with thickened secretions. Typical signs of PI are steatorrhea, flatulence, abdominal bloating, and poor weight gain. Pancreatic insufficiency leads to fat-soluble vitamin deficiency and malnutrition. Abnormal intestinal secretions, malabsorption, and decreased gut motility can lead to distal intestinal obstruction syndrome and chronic constipation in older patients.[28] Poor absorption of fat-soluble vitamins (A, D, E, and K) can lead to acrodermatitis, anemia, neuropathy, night blindness, osteoporosis, and bleeding disorders.

Patients with CF are at risk for focal biliary cirrhosis due to obstruction of intrahepatic bile ducts. Clinically apparent cirrhosis is seen in about 5% of patients with CF; it may present in infancy and usually is noted by age 15 years.[28]

Reproductive Tract

The vas deferens is exquisitely sensitive to CFTR dysfunction. Virtually all men with classical CF have azoospermia and are infertile due to congenital bilateral absence of the vas deferens (CBAVD), and CBAVD may be seen in men with only one CFTR mutation and no other manifestations of CF.[14] Women with CF have cervical mucus abnormalities, but the primary determinant of fertility is their overall health and nutritional status. Older studies suggested that pregnancy led to worsening lung disease in women with CF, but more recent studies show that women who have adequate nutritional and pulmonary reserve can do quite well with pregnancy, although they are more likely to develop diabetes.[29]

Other Common Disorders

As patients with CF age, the pancreas undergoes autolysis and fatty replacement with loss of insulin-producing islet cells. When a sufficient proportion of islet cells are no longer functional, the patient will develop insulin insufficiency and carbohydrate intolerance. Cystic fibrosis–related diabetes mellitus (CFRD) is not the same as typical type 1 or type 2 diabetes mellitus. Several factors unique to CF affect glucose metabolism, including elevated energy expenditure, acute and chronic infection, glucagon deficiency, liver dysfunction, decreased intestinal transit time, and increased work of breathing. Clinically apparent CFRD is increasingly common after the first decade of life; the prevalence is more than 30% in adults.[1] The onset of CFRD seems to lead to worsening of both nutritional status and lung disease, and female patients with diabetes have poorer survival than males.[30] Annual screening with fasting blood sugars and oral glucose tolerance tests should be performed in all patients with CF 10 years of age and older.[31]

Osteoporosis secondary to vitamin D deficiency, chronic systemic inflammation, and intermittent corticosteroid usage is increasingly being recognized as a complication of CF. Osteopenia starts in childhood but generally manifests in adulthood. Bone resorption exceeds bone formation even in well-nourished, clinically stable patients with CF.[32]

Management

While several novel therapies have become available in the last 15 years, the dramatic improvements in life expectancy and quality of life that have been seen for people with CF have come about largely because of an increased appreciation of the importance of maintaining adequate nutrition and an anticipatory and aggressive approach to the control of chronic airway infection. The benefit of a proactive approach to CF care has been borne out by the observation that CF centers, where patients have the best average lung function, monitor their patients more frequently with clinic visits and respiratory tract cultures, and use more antibiotics (oral and IV) than do lower-performing centers.[33,34]

Nutritional Therapies

The benefits of maintaining good nutrition in regard to long-term survival and lung health are well established,[18] making nutritional support an integral component of disease management from early infancy. Pancreatic enzyme therapy should be prescribed to patients demonstrating pancreatic insufficiency either on clinical grounds (steatorrhea, failure to thrive) or as documented by low human pancreatic fecal elastase-1 levels.[35] Dosing is titrated to minimize fat malabsorption and is standardized according to the lipase activity of the enzyme preparation. The typical dose is between 1,500 and 2,500 units of lipase per kilogram at each meal and snack. Very high doses (>6,000 units/kg) have been associated with a rare complication, fibrosing colonopathy. Pancreatic enzyme preparations are not completely acid stable, and patients who appear to need relatively high doses will also commonly use a proton-pump inhibitor or histamine-2 antagonist to suppress gastric acidity. Fat-soluble vitamin supplementation is recommended for all patients with PI.[35] Vitamin D deficiency in particular is common. Infants with CF can be safely breastfed, and this form of feeding may confer lifelong benefits.[36] Determination of height, weight, and body mass index (BMI) should be obtained at every CF clinic visit, and patients showing a decline in these parameters should receive nutritional counseling and other interventions. Given the strong correlation between nutritional status and pulmonary function, attention to nutritional well-being should be considered one of the cornerstones of good lung health in CF, and enteral supplements (given orally or via gastrostomy tube) should be strongly considered in any patient demonstrating less than optimal growth. Patients with CF can and should be expected to maintain BMI near the 50th percentile for age. For more information regarding nutrition in patients with CF, see Chapter 50.

Pulmonary Therapies

Airway infection and inflammation generally begin in the first year of life, often in the absence of any signs or symptoms. Pulmonary function testing is not sensitive to these early changes, and the average FEV_1 at 5 years of age is 100% predicted. The early institution of a number of preventive and aggressive therapeutic strategies slows the progression of symptomatic lung disease. These interventions can be associated with each of the pathophysiological steps shown in Figure 37-1.

Abnormal Gene, Abnormal CFTR, Abnormal Ion Transport

Interventions directed against these early pathogenic steps are the subject of intense research at the moment, but none are currently available for general use. See below for further discussion.

Bronchial Obstruction

Airway clearance augmentation techniques (ACT)—Modalities used by patients with CF to augment clearance of tenacious airway secretions include percussion and postural drainage; positive expiratory pressure (PEP) devices; oscillatory PEP devices; high-frequency chest wall oscillation devices (the Vest, etc); and controlled breathing techniques, such as autogenic drainage and active cycle of breathing. Recent CFF-sponsored guidelines recommend the use of twice daily ACT for all patients beginning in infancy.[37] As there is no clear evidence of superiority of one technique over the others, convenience, ease of administration, and patient satisfaction are the primary driving forces for choosing a mode of airway clearance. Exercise has many beneficial effects on cardiovascular fitness and sense of well-being. A number of studies show that aerobic and anaerobic exercise improve quality of life in patients with CF and may stabilize lung function to some degree, but exercise should complement and not supplant ACT.[38] For a complete discussion of airway clearance techniques, see Chapter 46.

Bronchodilators—About 25% of patients with CF have consistent bronchodilator responsiveness, and most have it intermittently. The routine use of bronchodilators (such as albuterol) has been recommended by the CFF consensus guideline on pulmonary therapies for patients who demonstrate a response on pulmonary function testing.[39]

Dornase alfa (recombinant human DNAse, Pulmozyme)—Neutrophils participating in the inflammatory response undergo necrosis, releasing DNA that increases viscoelasticity and adhesiveness of CF sputum. Dornase alfa breaks down extracellular DNA, improving mucus clearability. The dose is 2.5 mg once a day, by inhalation. The CFF consensus guidelines recommend its use for patients older than 5 years[39]; it is often used in younger patients but there is less evidence of benefit in this group.

Hypertonic (7%) saline—Acting as an hyperosmolar agent, hypertonic saline is thought to draw water into the airways, rehydrating the periciliary layer and improving mucociliary clearance. Twice daily administration as an aerosol has been shown to be beneficial in clinical trials.[40] If hypertonic saline can correct the basic hydration defect in

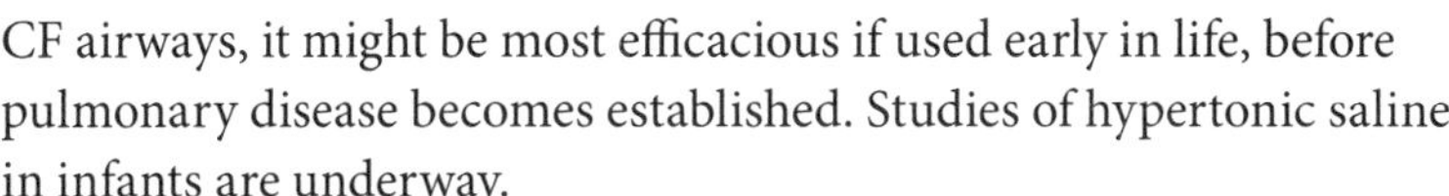

CF airways, it might be most efficacious if used early in life, before pulmonary disease becomes established. Studies of hypertonic saline in infants are underway.

Infection

Patients who have chronic persistent airway infection with *P aeruginosa* benefit from the use of inhaled antibiotics (tobramycin and aztreonam are currently available though others are in development). Aerosolized antibiotics achieve high concentration in the airway, so they are potentially effective even when the organism is resistant to levels of antibiotic that might be attainable through systemic administration. However, aerosols do not penetrate into airways that are obstructed, so they don't reach the most involved areas of the lung and are probably less effective during pulmonary exacerbations.

The benefit of using chronic prophylactic antibiotics (especially systemic) in children uninfected with *P aeruginosa* is not clear. The US CFF recommends against the use of prophylactic anti-staphylococcal agents because of fears that it increases the likelihood of acquiring *P aeruginosa,*[39] but there is not universal agreement regarding this issue.[41]

At initial acquisition, *P aeruginosa* can often be eliminated. Thus frequent surveillance airway cultures are performed, and at initial detection, inhaled, oral, or IV antibiotics are prescribed to eradicate *P aeruginosa* (even in asymptomatic individuals). The most effective approach to eliminating *P aeruginosa* is unclear and the subject of active investigation.[23]

Pulmonary Exacerbations and Their Treatment

Intermittent flare-ups of infection periodically occur in patients with CF, which are associated with increased inflammation and airway obstruction, and are identified by the development of new respiratory signs and symptoms. Increased cough, change in sputum color or quantity, decreased appetite or weight, and change in respiratory rate and examination are particularly important features (Box 37-3).

Box 37-3. Signs and Symptoms of a Pulmonary Exacerbation

Symptoms
- Cough
- Dyspnea
- Chest tightness
- Hemoptysis
- Increased Sputum
- Anorexia

Signs
- New wheezes or crackles
- Weight loss

Laboratory
- Decreased forced expiratory volume at 1 second
- Chest radiograph changes

These episodes are termed pulmonary exacerbations and treated with discrete courses of systemic antibiotic therapy, which are chosen based on previous cultures of airway secretions. Typically, treatment with oral antibiotics is initially attempted, and if this does not successfully return the patient to baseline status, IV antibiotics are used.

There are currently no uniformly accepted defining criteria for what constitutes a pulmonary exacerbation of CF.[42] An aggressive approach to treatment with oral antibiotics, even in patients whose symptoms may be mild, or primarily viral in etiology, with the addition of IV antibiotics when baseline is not promptly reattained, leads to better long-term pulmonary outcomes in patients with CF.[33]

Once identified, therapy for a pulmonary exacerbation of CF generally includes antibiotics (oral, inhaled, or IV), increased use of airway clearance techniques, and improved nutrition. Combination antibiotic therapy with 2 or more agents displaying different modes of action is preferred to avoid emergence of resistant strains, and therapy is generally given for at least 14 days.[43] Domiciliary treatment with IV antibiotics is feasible, but may not be as efficacious as hospital-based therapy.[44] Box 37-4 lists typical orders for inpatient admission and treatment of a pulmonary exacerbation of CF.

Box 37-4. Routine Orders for Patients With Cystic Fibrosis Admitted With Pulmonary Exacerbation

Diagnosis: Cystic Fibrosis Exacerbation
Condition: Good/Fair/Poor
Vitals: As per floor routine
Pulse oximetry overnight X 1 then prn
Allergies:____________________
Activity ad lib—encourage exercise
Diet: high-calorie diet with snacks, supplements as per nutritionist
Consults
- Nutrition
- Respiratory therapy (airway clearance assistance qid—Chest physiotherapy, PEP valve, Vest, etc)
- Physical Therapy (to facilitate activity and exercise)
- Teachers, child life specialist (for prolonged stays)
- Endocrinology (for patients with CF-related diabetes)
- Gastroenterology (for patients with GI issues)

IV to heparin or saline lock in between antibiotic administrations (to facilitate activity)
Arrange PICC line insertion (except for patients with implanted central catheter)
Laboratory testing
- Initial blood work may be done with first aminoglycoside level
  - CBC, electrolytes, glucose, creatinine, U/A, liver enzymes, albumin, PT, PTT
  - Total IgE (a screen for allergic bronchopulmonary aspergillosis)
  - Prealbumin [a screen for nutritional status]
  - Vitamin A , 25-OH D, and E levels
  - HgbA1C (if >10 years old)
  - Chest x-ray (if not done just prior to admission)
  - Spirometry (simple) in PFT lab (if not done just prior to admission)
  - Sputum culture (CF protocol)
    - Bacterial culture
    - Fungal culture
    - AFB smear and culture
- Aminoglycoside levels
- Audiometry on admission (if >6 years and receiving aminoglycosides)
- Oral glucose tolerance test—fasting and 2 hours after 1.75 g/kg of glucose solution
- 72-hour stool fat collection

[a] The dose of antibiotics for cystic fibrosis exacerbations is not uniformly agreed on. Consultation with your hospital pharmacist is appropriate; the highest acceptable dose of each antibiotic should be prescribed.

Box 37-4. Routine Orders for Patients With Cystic Fibrosis Admitted With Pulmonary Exacerbation (continued)

Medications

ADEK vitamins (tabs or drops)

Vitamin K 5 mg PO

Pancreatic enzymes (as per home routine)

Ursodeoxycholic acid

Insulin: ____________________

Pulmozyme (rhDNAse) 2.5mg by aerosol qd

Albuterol

Hypertonic saline (7%) 4 cc by aerosol bid

Tobi 300 mg by aerosol bid

Antibiotics (usually a combination of aminoglycoside and β-lactam) based on sensitivities of most recent sputum culture.

Key:

Applies to all patients

Applies to some patients

Inflammation

A number of anti-inflammatory agents have been shown to be beneficial in CF, but there is some controversy regarding their use. Box 37-5 describes the use of anti-inflammatory agents.

Box 37-5. Use of Anti-inflammatory Agents

- Systemic steroids may be used in selected patients acutely or chronically. They improve airway function when used chronically, but are associated with the expected significant side effects, such as glucose intolerance and cataracts.[45]
- Inhaled corticosteroids are used commonly, particularly in patients with apparent airway reactivity, but their benefit has not been clearly demonstrated.[39]
- Ibuprofen, when given in high doses (20–30 mg/kg twice daily to a maximum 1,600 mg/dose), leads to long-term benefits in lung function, particularly in children between 5 and 13 years of age. There are concerns regarding gastrointestinal and renal toxicity, but experience has shown these to be unusual.[46]
- Macrolide antibiotics (alternate day azithromycin 250 mg if weight <40 kg or 500 mg if weight ≥40 kg) improve lung function.[47] It is unclear whether macrolides work via an influence on *Pseudomonas aeruginosa* virulence factors or an anti-inflammatory effect.[48]

Tissue Damage

The end result of long-standing infection and inflammation is irreversible bronchiectasis and eventual respiratory failure. At that point, the only remaining option is bilateral lung transplant, which is generally offered when predictive models (which consider current FEV_1, age, gender, lung microbiology, and rate of decline of FEV_1) suggest that death is likely to be imminent (ie, within 2 years). How best to select patients, especially children, for this high-risk procedure is being vigorously debated.[49] The 5-year survival following lung transplantation is approximately 50%, with bronchiolitis obliterans due to chronic rejection an ongoing problem. Use of nocturnal noninvasive ventilation can improve chest symptoms, sleep-associated hypoventilation, and quality of life in patients with awake hypercapnia who are awaiting transplantation.[50]

The Role of the General Pediatrician in the Care of Patients With CF

Diagnosis

Cystic fibrosis newborn screening occurs throughout the United States. However, the approach to newborn screening varies greatly from state to state. To appropriately counsel the families of patients with a positive newborn screen, the general pediatrician should understand the local state screening process and help facilitate it. For example, many (but not all) states rely on the pediatrician to arrange for sweat testing of infants who screen positive. In states that use the IRT/DNA approach, many infants with a positive screen do not have CF but are carriers whose families then need genetic counseling. Furthermore, the sensitivity of the CF newborn screening process is no better than 95%, so there will always be patients who will be diagnosed symptomatically at a later age. Thus the pediatrician still needs to consider CF in the differential diagnosis of children with chronic or recurrent respiratory symptoms and gastrointestinal complaints.

Immunizations/Prophylaxis

All infants and children, particularly those with CF, should receive all recommended immunizations. Special attention should be given to the annual influenza vaccines for all patients with CF and their immediate contacts. The American Academy of Pediatrics recommends the following: "Limited studies suggest that some patients with CF may be at increased risk of respiratory syncytial virus (RSV) infection. Whether RSV infection exacerbates the chronic lung disease of CF is not known. In addition, insufficient data exist to determine the effectiveness of palivizumab use in this patient population. Therefore, a recommendation for routine prophylaxis in patients with CF cannot be made."[51] The Cystic Fibrosis Foundation has recommended: "for infants with CF under 2 years of age that the use of palivizumab be considered for prophylaxis of respiratory syncytial virus."[52] Physicians must take into account individual circumstances relative to the care of children with CF.

Evaluation and Treatment of Apparently Viral Respiratory Tract Infections

Aggressive antibiotic treatment of respiratory tract symptoms is key to attaining better disease outcomes. When children with CF are seen in the general pediatric setting for what appears to be a mild viral respiratory tract infection, it would be advisable to contact the CF center to discuss criteria for antimicrobial treatment as well as the optimal choice of antibiotic based on previous airway cultures. Secondary bacterial infection following a viral infection is a common cause of CF exacerbations.

Psychosocial Issues

The emphasis on good weight gain that begins early in the course of treatment may sometimes lead to behavioral feeding problems that can cause significant family dysfunction. Problems are often easily alleviated by appropriate referral to a psychologist with experience in this area. Psychological problems, especially anxiety and depression, are prevalent in children with CF, as well as in their caregivers,[53] and can affect adherence and long-term outcomes of disease. They should be carefully sought and, when found, the family should be referred for appropriate mental health services. The teenage years of patients with CF can be tumultuous, with significant medical challenges caused by treatment non-adherence and participation in other risk-taking behaviors including smoking, alcohol, and illicit drugs.[54]

Future Therapies

The marked improvement in life expectancy for patients with CF over the last 2 decades is largely the result of improvements in the application of previous available therapies, primarily more aggressive nutritional management and antimicrobial use. Application of data gleaned from national patient registries and implementation by the CFF of quality improvement programs have changed practice for the better.[33,34,55] Many recent advances in the understanding of CF pathophysiology have not yet had time to result in dramatic improvements in clinical care, but there is great hope for the future that therapies treating the basic defect will normalize life expectancy for those born with *CFTR* mutations. Gene therapy, with replacement of the abnormal gene using a viral or liposomal vector, is being actively investigated but does not appear to be a therapeutic option for the near future. Furthermore, several therapies that potentiate or correct mutant CFTR are undergoing early clinical trials.

When to Refer

- Any child with an abnormal or borderline abnormal sweat test should be referred to a CFF-accredited care center for evaluation and treatment.
- The CF center should be consulted if a CF patient has
  - Persistent cough or congestion (>1 week)
  - Wheezing or new crackles on chest examination
  - Any new abnormality on chest radiograph
  - Acute dyspnea or hemoptysis
  - Any respiratory infection requiring antibiotics
  - Poor weight gain or weight loss
  - Change in stools: decrease in number, increased steatorrhea
  - Abdominal pain

When to Admit

- It is generally ideal for patients with CF, when hospitalized, to be cared for by CF center physicians. There are exceptions; if hospitalization is considered by the primary care pediatrician, the CF center should be contacted to discuss this.

Key Points

- Cystic fibrosis is a multisystem disease that requires close attention to pulmonary and nutritional parameters.
- In the near future, most patients with CF in the United States will be diagnosed by newborn screening. Infants who screen positive should be promptly evaluated with a sweat test performed by a laboratory associated with an accredited CF center.
- Patients should be cared for in centers with experience caring for individuals with CF and that offer expertise in a broad range of areas. A multidisciplinary team, including nurses, pharmacists, nutritionists, respiratory therapists, social workers, and others, is necessary to achieve the best outcomes. Good communication between the primary care pediatrician and CF care center is key to ensuring optimal care.
- Successful treatment philosophy combines an aggressive approach with high expectations and active participation by patients and family, with the goal of maintaining good (ie, normal) nutrition and respiratory status.

References

1. Cystic Fibrosis Foundation. *Cystic Fibrosis Foundation Patient Registry, 2007 Annual Data Report.* Bethesda, MD: Cystic Fibrosis Foundation; 2008
2. Dodge JA, Lewis PA, Stanton M, Wilsher J. Cystic fibrosis mortality and survival in the UK: 1947–2003. *Eur Respir J.* 2007;29(3):522–526
3. Walters S, Mehta A. Epidemiology of cystic fibrosis. In: Hodson M, Geddes DM, Bush A, eds. *Cystic Fibrosis.* London: Edward Arnold, Ltd; 2007:21–45
4. Boucher RC. Airway surface dehydration in cystic fibrosis: pathogenesis and therapy. *Annu Rev Med.* 2007;58:157–170
5. de Gracia J, Mata F, Alvarez A, et al. Genotype-phenotype correlation for pulmonary function in cystic fibrosis. *Thorax.* 2005;60(7):558–563
6. Collaco JM, Cutting GR. Update on gene modifiers in cystic fibrosis. *Curr Opin Pulm Med.* 2008;14(6):559–566
7. Khan TZ, Wagener JS, Bost T, Martinez J, Accurso FJ, Riches DW. Early pulmonary inflammation in infants with cystic fibrosis. *Am J Respir Crit Care Med.* 1995;151:1075–1082
8. Hoiby N. Inflammation and infection in cystic fibrosis—hen or egg? *Eur Respir J.* 2001;17(1):4–5

9. Henke MO, Ratjen F. Mucolytics in cystic fibrosis. *Paediatr Respir Rev.* 2007;8(1):24–29
10. LeGrys VA, Yankaskas JR, Quittell LM, Marshall BC, Mogayzel PJ Jr. Diagnostic sweat testing: the Cystic Fibrosis Foundation guidelines. *J Pediatr.* 2007;151(1):85–89
11. Eng W, LeGrys VA, Schechter MS, Laughon MM, Barker PM. Sweat-testing in preterm and full-term infants less than 6 weeks of age. *Pediatr Pulmonol.* 2005;40(1):64–67
12. LeGrys VA. Assessment of sweat-testing practices for the diagnosis of cystic fibrosis. *Arch Pathol Lab Med.* 2001;125(11):1420–1424
13. Farrell PM, Rosenstein BJ, White TB, et al. Guidelines for diagnosis of cystic fibrosis in newborns through older adults: Cystic Fibrosis Foundation consensus report. *J Pediatr.* 2008;153(2):S4–S14
14. Boyle MP. Nonclassic cystic fibrosis and CFTR-related diseases. *Curr Opin Pulm Med.* 2003;9(6):498–503
15. Borowitz D, Parad RB, Sharp JK, et al. Cystic Fibrosis Foundation practice guidelines for the management of infants with cystic fibrosis transmembrane conductance regulator-related metabolic syndrome during the first two years of life and beyond. *J Pediatr.* 2009;155(6 suppl):S106–S116
16. Comeau AM, Accurso FJ, White TB, et al. Guidelines for implementation of cystic fibrosis newborn screening programs: Cystic Fibrosis Foundation workshop report. *Pediatrics.* 2007;119(2):e495–e518
17. Farrell PM, Kosorok MR, Rock MJ, et al. Early diagnosis of cystic fibrosis through neonatal screening prevents severe malnutrition and improves long-term growth. Wisconsin Cystic Fibrosis Neonatal Screening Study Group. *Pediatrics.* 2001;107(1):1–13
18. Konstan MW, Butler SM, Wohl ME, et al. Growth and nutritional indexes in early life predict pulmonary function in cystic fibrosis. *J Pediatr.* 2003;142(6):624–630
19. McKay KO, Waters DL, Gaskin KJ. The influence of newborn screening for cystic fibrosis on pulmonary outcomes in new South Wales. *J Pediatr.* 2005;147(3 suppl):S47–S50
20. Grosse SD, Boyle CA, Botkin JR, et al. Newborn screening for cystic fibrosis: evaluation of benefits and risks and recommendations for state newborn screening programs. *MMWR Recomm Rep.* 2004;53(RR-13):1–36
21. Hoiby N, Frederiksen B, Pressler T. Eradication of early *Pseudomonas aeruginosa* infection. *J Cyst Fibros.* 2005;4 (suppl 2):49–54
22. Campodonico VL, Gadjeva M, Paradis-Bleau C, Uluer A, Pier GB. Airway epithelial control of *Pseudomonas aeruginosa* infection in cystic fibrosis. *Trends Mol Med.* 2008;14(3):120–133
23. Treggiari MM, Rosenfeld M, Retsch-Bogart G, Gibson R, Ramsey B. Approach to eradication of initial *Pseudomonas aeruginosa* infection in children with cystic fibrosis. *Pediatr Pulmonol.* 2007;42(9):751–756

24. Goss CH, Mayer-Hamblett N, Aitken ML, Rubenfeld GD, Ramsey BW. Association between *Stenotrophomonas maltophilia* and lung function in cystic fibrosis. *Thorax.* 2004;59(11):955–959
25. Kalish LA, Waltz DA, Dovey M, et al. Impact of *Burkholderia dolosa* on lung function and survival in cystic fibrosis. *Am J Respir Crit Care Med.* 2006;173(4):421–425
26. Olivier KN, Weber DJ, Wallace RJ Jr, et al. Nontuberculous mycobacteria. I: multicenter prevalence study in cystic fibrosis. *Am J Respir Crit Care Med.* 2003;167(6):828–834
27. Stevens DA, Moss RB, Kurup VP, et al. Allergic bronchopulmonary aspergillosis in cystic fibrosis—state of the art: Cystic Fibrosis Foundation Consensus Conference. *Clin Infect Dis.* 2003;37 (suppl 3):S225–S264
28. Wilschanski M, Durie PR. Patterns of GI disease in adulthood associated with mutations in the *CFTR* gene. *Gut.* 2007;56(8):1153–1163
29. McMullen AH, Pasta DJ, Frederick PD, et al. Impact of pregnancy on women with cystic fibrosis. *Chest.* 2006;129(3):706–711
30. Milla CE, Billings J, Moran A. Diabetes is associated with dramatically decreased survival in female but not male subjects with cystic fibrosis. *Diabetes Care.* 2005;28(9):2141–2144
31. O'Riordan SM, Robinson PD, Donaghue KC, Moran A. Management of cystic fibrosis-related diabetes. *Pediatr Diabetes.* 2008;9(4 pt 1):338–344
32. Aris RM, Merkel PA, Bachrach LK, et al. Guide to bone health and disease in cystic fibrosis. *J Clin Endocrinol Metab.* 2005;90(3):1888–1896
33. Johnson C, Butler SM, Konstan MW, Morgan W, Wohl ME. Factors influencing outcomes in cystic fibrosis: a center-based analysis. *Chest.* 2003;123(1):20–27
34. Padman R, McColley SA, Miller DP, et al. Infant care patterns at epidemiologic study of cystic fibrosis sites that achieve superior childhood lung function. *Pediatrics.* 2007;119(3):e531–e537
35. Borowitz D, Baker RD, Stallings V. Consensus report on nutrition for pediatric patients with cystic fibrosis. *J Pediatr Gastroenterol Nutr.* 2002;35(3):246–259
36. Parker EM, O'Sullivan BP, Shea JC, Regan MM, Freedman SD. Survey of breast-feeding practices and outcomes in the cystic fibrosis population. *Pediatr Pulmonol.* 2004;37(4):362–367
37. Flume PA, Robinson KA, O'Sullivan BP, et al. Cystic fibrosis pulmonary guidelines: airway clearance therapies. *Respir Care.* 2009;54(4):522–537
38. Bradley J, Moran F. Physical training for cystic fibrosis. *Cochrane Database Syst Rev.* 2008(1):CD002768
39. Flume PA, O'Sullivan BP, Robinson KA, et al. Cystic fibrosis pulmonary guidelines: chronic medications for maintenance of lung health. *Am J Respir Crit Care Med.* 2007;176(10):957–969

40. Elkins MR, Robinson M, Rose BR, et al. A controlled trial of long-term inhaled hypertonic saline in patients with cystic fibrosis. *N Engl J Med.* 2006;354(3):229–240
41. Smyth A. Prophylactic antibiotics in cystic fibrosis: a conviction without evidence? *Pediatr Pulmonol.* 2005;40(6):471–476
42. Goss CH, Burns JL. Exacerbations in cystic fibrosis. 1: epidemiology and pathogenesis. *Thorax.* 2007;62(4):360–367
43. Doring G, Conway SP, Heijerman HG, et al. Antibiotic therapy against *Pseudomonas aeruginosa* in cystic fibrosis: a European consensus. *Eur Respir J.* 2000;16(4):749–767
44. Nazer D, Abdulhamid I, Thomas R, Pendleton S. Home versus hospital intravenous antibiotic therapy for acute pulmonary exacerbations in children with cystic fibrosis. *Pediatr Pulmonol.* 2006;41(8):744–749
45. Eigen H, Rosenstein BJ, FitzSimmons S, Schidlow DV. A multicenter study of alternate-day prednisone therapy in patients with cystic fibrosis. Cystic Fibrosis Foundation Prednisone Trial Group. *J Pediatr.* 1995;126(4):515–523
46. Konstan MW. Ibuprofen therapy for cystic fibrosis lung disease: revisited. *Curr Opin Pulm Med.* 2008;14(6):567–573
47. Saiman L, Marshall BC, Mayer-Hamblett N, et al. Azithromycin in patients with cystic fibrosis chronically infected with *Pseudomonas aeruginosa:* a randomized controlled trial. *JAMA.* 2003;290(13):1749–1756
48. Schultz MJ. Macrolide activities beyond their antimicrobial effects: macrolides in diffuse panbronchiolitis and cystic fibrosis. *J Antimicrob Chemother.* 2004;54(1):21–28
49. Aurora P, Carby M, Sweet S. Selection of cystic fibrosis patients for lung transplantation. *Curr Opin Pulm Med.* 2008;14(6):589–594
50. Young AC, Wilson JW, Kotsimbos TC, Naughton MT. Randomised placebo controlled trial of non-invasive ventilation for hypercapnia in cystic fibrosis. *Thorax.* 2008;63(1):72–77
51. American Academy of Pediatrics. Respiratory syncytial virus. In: Pickering LK, Baker CJ, Kimberlin DW, Long SS, eds. *Red Book: 2009 Report of the Committee on Infectious Diseases.* 28th ed. Elk Grove Village, IL: American Academy of Pediatrics; 2009:568
52. Borowitz D, Robinson KA, Rosenfeld M, et al. Cystic Fibrosis Foundation evidence-based guidelines for management of infants with cystic fibrosis. *J Pediatr.* 2009;155:S73–S93
53. Cruz I, Marciel KK, Quittner AL, Schechter MS. Anxiety and depression in cystic fibrosis. *Semin Respir Crit Care Med.* 2009;30(5):569–578
54. Britto MT, Garrett JM, Dugliss MA, et al. Risky behavior in teens with cystic fibrosis or sickle cell disease: a multicenter study. *Pediatrics.* 1998;101(2):250–256
55. Schechter MS, Margolis P. Improving subspecialty healthcare: lessons from cystic fibrosis. *J Pediatr.* 2005;147(3):295–301

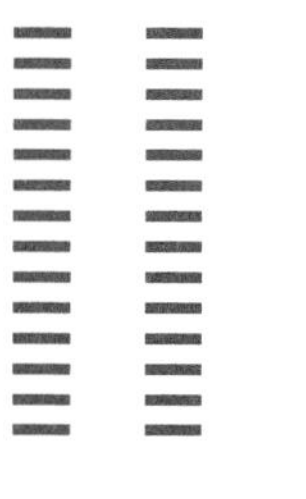

Chapter 38

Primary Ciliary Dyskinesia and Other Genetic Lung Diseases

Madhuri Penugonda, MD
Dawn M. Simon, MD
Michael Light, MD

Introduction

Several respiratory disorders in children have a genetic predisposition; however, some of these disorders may not manifest in infancy. Recognizing the clinical presentations will aid in early diagnosis. Specific therapies can then be offered, which can decrease the severity of the lung disease or delay progression. Chronicity of respiratory symptoms is a better indication of a genetic defect than severity. An inherited component should be suspected when chronic lung disease presents with other disease syndromes, such as pancreatic insufficiency, heat intolerance, male sterility, situs inversus, and emphysema at a young age. Referral to a genetic counselor should be considered when a genetic disorder is identified or suspected to assist in discussions of prognosis and risk to future pregnancies.

Respiratory Defenses

The respiratory system is constantly exposed to inhaled pathogens. Several defense mechanisms normally protect the respiratory system. The oropharynx and nasal passages warm and humidify the air, thus preventing drying of the airway epithelium. Turbinates in the nasal passages trap large particles. The epiglottis closes over the larynx during swallowing to prevent food from entering the lungs. Inside the lungs, mucus is secreted into the airways, where it traps particles that are then removed by the mucociliary transport system. Immunologic defenses include macrophages, neutrophils, and lymphocytes that help remove pathogens. The middle ear, nares, paranasal sinuses, and large airways are lined with ciliated pseudostratified columnar epithelial cells, each of which are covered by approximately 200 cilia on their apical surface (Figure 38-1). Normal cilia have an array of longitudinal microtubules, which are anchored by a basal body in the apical cytoplasm of the cell (Figure 38-2). There are 9 doublets arranged in an outer circle around a central pair of single tubules.[1] This structure is maintained by a network of various proteins. Tubulin is the main protein of the microtubules. Nexin protein links the outer doublets together, creating a circumferential network, and the radial spokes connect the outer doublets to the central pair. Dynein is attached to the microtubules as inner and outer arms. Each dynein arm has heavy, intermediate, and light chains. The heavy chains have adenosine triphosphatase, which provides energy for ciliary movement. There are 2 phases of ciliary motion that occurs within an aqueous layer of airway surface liquids.[1,2] A stroke phase, which is forward movement, and a

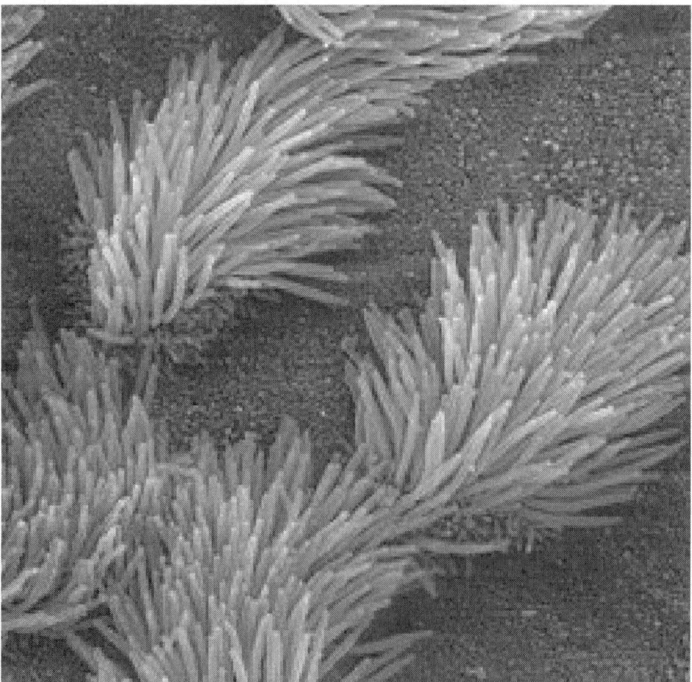

Figure 38-1. Scanning electron microscope image of a lung trachea epithelium with both ciliated and non-ciliated cells. (Source: http://remf.dartmouth.edu/imagesindex.html.)

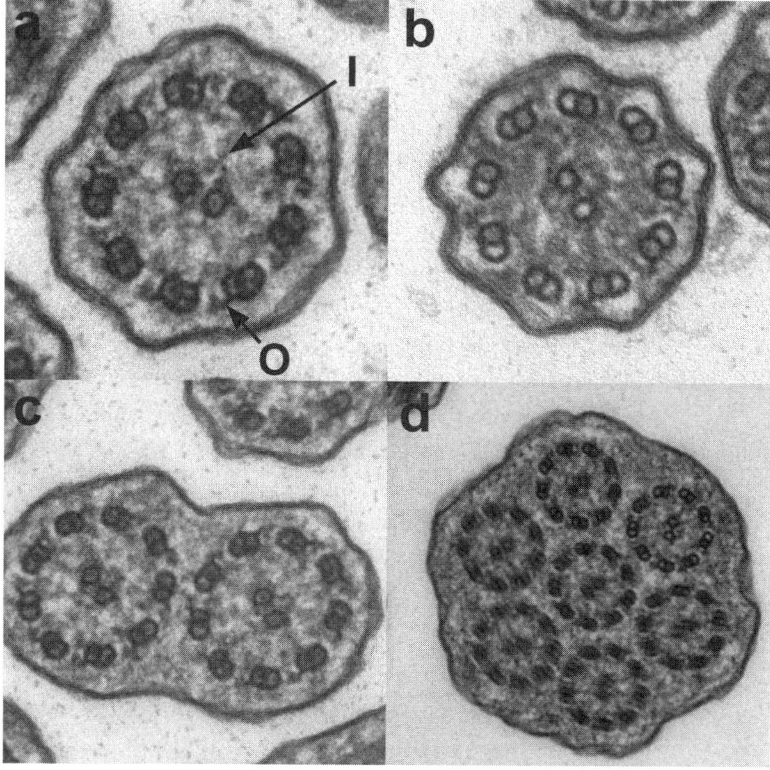

Figure 38-2. Normal ciliary ultrastructure: **A.** Cross-section of normal cilium showing a central pair of microtubules and a ring of 9 outer tubules that are connected to the central pair by spokes (I) and to each other by dynein arms (O). A spectrum of abnormal ciliary ultrastructures found in ciliary dyskinesia: **B.** Cross-section of cilium showing absence of spokes and dynein arms. **C.** Fusion of cilia showing 2 axonemes within a single membrane. **D.** Fusion of 7 axonemes within a single membrane. (Courtesy of Bahig M. Shehata, MD, Medical Director of Pathology, Children's Healthcare of Atlanta, Atlanta, Georgia.)

recovery phase, which is backward movement. Cilia bend in a rapid, rhythmic, synchronized wave-like motion to propel mucus from the distal airways to the oropharynx. The frequency of movement is faster in children than adults and is faster in the proximal airways than distal airways.[2] Cells are generally aligned such that the central pair of tubules in adjacent cells are in a parallel orientation, and ciliary motility is maintained in the same plane.[1] In addition to the respiratory system, ciliated cells are found in the ventricular ependyma of the brain and the fallopian tubes. Cilia share a similar core structure and motility as spermatozoa flagella.[3,4]

Primary Ciliary Dyskinesia

Primary ciliary dyskinesia (PCD) is a group of inherited disorders that involve defects in ciliated cells that line the sinuses, middle ear, and airways. Previously, it was believed that patients had immotile cilia, hence the term immotile-cilia syndrome was used, though subsequent studies have demonstrated a wide range of ciliary dysmotility.[1] Therefore, the more comprehensive term is PCD. The resultant defect is impaired ciliary motion and mucociliary clearance leading to recurrent sinopulmonary infections and chronic otitis media. Inheritance is mostly autosomal recessive but there have been some rare cases of autosomal dominant or x-linked inheritance. The incidence is 1 in 15,000 births. Fifty percent of patients have situs inversus, where the major organs are reversed from their normal positions, though this appears to be random and not genetically predetermined. Kartagener syndrome is a triad of chronic sinusitis, bronchiectasis, and situs inversus resulting from ciliary dyskinesia.[1] The recurrence rate for the recessive disorder is approximately 25%.

Pathophysiology and Genetics

Primary ciliary dyskinesia is characterized by an ultrastructural defect in the cilia, most commonly in the dynein arms, though PCD can involve a defect in or malalignment of any portion of the structure.[5] This causes disorganized ciliary movement with impaired mucociliary transport and ineffective clearance of mucus and inhaled particles and pathogens. Secondary ciliary defects, including ultrastructural defects, may be seen following injury to the respiratory epithelium as a result of viral infection or pollutant exposure and are distinguished from PCD by the fact that these are usually transient, and normal cilia structures can be found in adjacent sections of a biopsy sample.[6] The spectrum of ciliary dysfunction and the numerous ultrastructural phenotypes suggest that PCD has genetic heterogeneity.[7] To date, 3 outer dynein arm gene mutations have been identified: *DNAH5*, *DNAI1*, and *DNAH11*.[8–10] There is ongoing research into other genes involved in regulating ciliary structure and function. Clinical molecular genetic testing for PCD is available for the most common mutations.

Clinical Features

The clinical features of PCD are variable and include chronic otitis media, sinusitis, and chronic cough. Neonates with PCD frequently develop respiratory distress due to the role of cilia in fetal lung fluid absorption.[11] Unfortunately, this diagnosis is rarely considered unless there is situs inversus or a family history of PCD. Instead, these infants are usually incorrectly diagnosed with neonatal pneumonia, transient tachypnea of the newborn, or aspiration pneumonitis. Signs and symptoms beyond the neonatal period include chronic nasal congestion with mucopurulent drainage without seasonal variation, chronic otitis media, sinusitis, chronic productive cough, wheeze, recurrent pneumonia, and bronchiectasis[1,11] (Box 38-1). Thirty-three percent of patients may have nasal polyps.[1] Cough is the most consistent, albeit nonspecific, feature and is frequently productive of mucoid or purulent sputum in older children and usually most apparent in the morning. In children with PCD, the cough reflex is preserved and is a compensatory clearance mechanism. Due to poor mucociliary clearance, bacteria colonize the respiratory tract. The more common bacterial infections in patients with PCD are *Haemophilus influenzae* (non-

Box 38-1. When to Consider a Diagnosis of Primary Ciliary Dyskinesia (PCD)

- Family history of PCD
- Situs inversus
- Chronic productive cough
- Chronic nasal congestion with mucopurulent drainage without seasonal variation
- Chronic otitis media
- Sinusitis
- Nasal polyposis
- Wheeze
- Recurrent pneumonia
- Bronchiectasis
- Respiratory distress in term neonates
- Male infertility
- Hydrocephalus (rare)

typable), *Staphylococcus aureus, Streptococcus viridans, Streptococcus pneumoniae,* and *Pseudomonas aeruginosa,* though the latter is usually found in older patients who develop bronchiectasis.[1] All of these bacteria bind to the mucus, release toxins, and cause further inflammation. Chronic infections and mucus obstruction of the airways can lead to repeated infections, bronchiectasis (dilation of the airways), and scarring of the lung. Progressive obstructive airway disease (typically not bronchodilator responsive) can lead to dyspnea and exercise intolerance.

In males with PCD, infertility is common because of defective sperm flagellae, which share a nearly identical internal structure as cilia.[3] While the fallopian tubes are lined with ciliated epithelial cells, there is no consistent evidence that female fertility is affected although ectopic pregnancy has been reported.[3] Situs inversus occurs in approximately 50% of patients, including transposition of the left and right lungs, presumably because of the role of cilia in normal visceral rotation during embryogenesis.[12] When cilia are dysfunctional, rotation becomes a chance occurrence. While not common in children with PCD, there have also been a few cases of hydrocephalus described with defects in the ventricular ependymal cilia.[4]

On physical examination, children may have nasal congestion, nasal polyps, and tympanic membrane inflammation. Lung auscultation can be variable from localized crackles to wheezing, though the latter is less common. Older patients may have digital clubbing, suggesting bronchiectasis. There may be situs inversus with prominent heart tones in the right chest and the liver palpable in the left abdomen.

Chest radiographs and computed tomography (CT) scans of children with PCD may show hyperinflation, bronchial wall thickening, segmental atelectasis, bronchiectasis, and situs inversus. Lung abnormalities tend to exist in the middle lobe and lingula as opposed to cystic fibrosis (CF), where the apices are most involved[13] (Figure 38-3 and Figure 38-4). Pulmonary function test results may be normal earlier in life and then may show a progressive obstructive pattern with variable bronchodilator response.

Bronchiectasis in a child should prompt evaluation by a pulmonary specialist and referral for genetic counseling.

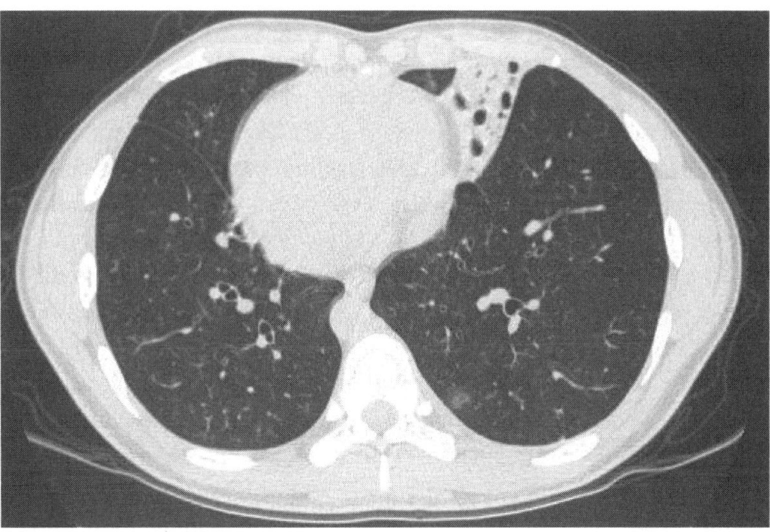

Figure 38-3. Chest computed tomography (CT) scan of a 13-year-old child with primary ciliary dyskinesia. The CT shows tree-in-bud densities with scattered bronchiectasis. (Image and interpretation courtesy of Stephen Simoneaux, MD, Children's Healthcare of Atlanta, Atlanta, Georgia.)

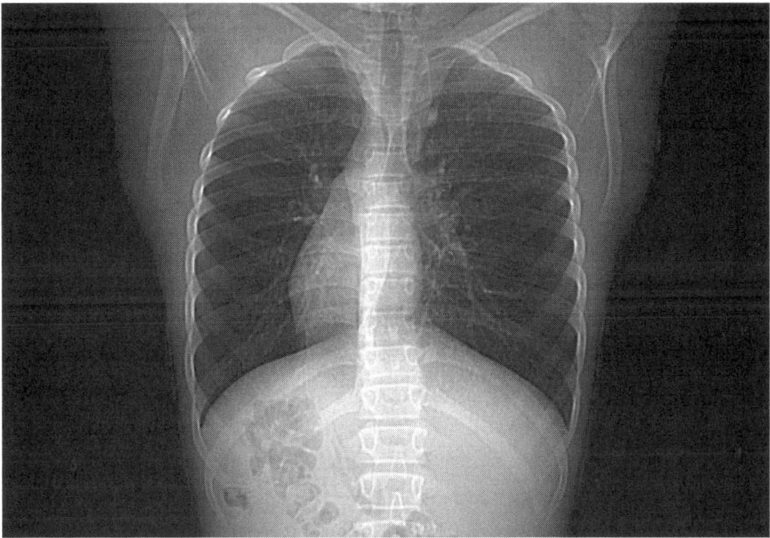

Figure 38-4. Chest radiograph of an 18-year-old adolescent with situs inversus as seen in primary ciliary dyskinesia. The imaging demonstrates situs inversus totalis, including dextrocardia and intra-abdominal organ reversal and lingular bronchiectasis. (Image and interpretation courtesy of Stephen Simoneaux, MD, Children's Healthcare of Atlanta, Atlanta, Georgia.)

Diagnosis

Managing PCD begins with an accurate diagnosis, which is not always easy and generally is by exclusion. In the differential diagnosis are CF (intestinal malabsorption, positive sweat test, and positive gene mutation), allergies (positive skin allergen test, increased immunoglobulin E, seasonal), and immunodeficiencies (abnormal immunoglobulin levels). The diagnosis of PCD is made by demonstrating abnormal ciliary ultrastructure and motility in nasal brush biopsy or bronchial biopsy. Analysis should be done by an experienced electron microscopist because skilled processing of the tissue and interpretation are key to making the diagnosis. Identifying impaired motility and a specific ultrastructural abnormality in a patient with a history and physical examination consistent with PCD should be diagnostic. However, there is significant clinical overlap with other diseases, and the motility and ultrastructural analysis may be inconclusive in distinguishing primary from secondary defects. Studies have shown that nasal nitric oxide levels are very low in PCD and may be a useful screening tool or serve as an adjunctive diagnostic test in individuals with uncertain pathologic diagnosis, although this tool is not available in most centers.[14] Additionally, the effectiveness of ciliary beat may be evaluated by measuring mucociliary clearance of saccharin applied to the anterior nares or by rate of removal of inhaled radiolabeled particles.[15,16] These studies as well are generally used in research and are not available for clinical use. With the discovery of dynein arm mutations, there is anticipation that genetic analysis will become available as well.

Treatment

Treatment is aimed at enhancing mucociliary clearance, preventing respiratory infections, and treating bacterial infections. Approaches to augment the normal mucociliary clearance mechanisms through aggressive airway clearance are similar to those used in CF and include chest percussion, Vest (Hill-Rom) or Acapella (Smiths Medical) therapy, postural drainage, and regular exercise. Because cough remains effective in PCD, patients are encouraged to cough, and they should avoid cough suppressants. Bronchodilators may be helpful in those who have a clinical response by signs, symptoms, or pulmonary function testing. Pulmozyme (DNAse) and other anti-inflammation agents may also help, but their use has not been well defined in PCD.[17]

Aggressive measures to prevent respiratory infections include routine vaccination for pertussis, measles, *H influenzae* type b, *S pneumoniae*, and yearly influenza virus. At times of acute bacterial infection, patients with PCD should be treated with sputum or throat culture–directed antibiotics early. Bronchoscopy and bronchoalveolar lavage may be indicated for cultures if sputum for bacterial cultures is difficult to obtain or if the patient is not clinically improving on current therapy. Patients may need extended treatment to eradicate infections or even remain on prophylactic antibiotics for recurrent or chronic infections. Surgical interventions that may be needed are tympanostomy with ventilation tube placement for recurrent otitis media, nasal polypectomy for nasal polyps, sinus drainage surgery for chronic sinusitis, partial lung resection, and lung transplant for end-stage lung disease. Finally, since exposure to pollutants or irritants, such as tobacco smoke, can further impair mucus clearance, preventing exposure is crucial (see Chapter 52).

Prognosis

Prognosis is variable, though most children do slowly develop chronic lung disease with bronchiectasis and some degree of pulmonary disability. Further studies are necessary to know if early and aggressive intervention as described previously will affect the course of the disease.

Other Genetic Lung Diseases

Mounier-Kuhn Syndrome

Mounier-Kuhn syndrome is a rare congenital disorder characterized by tracheobronchomegaly.[18] Eighty-two cases have been reported until 1988, with ages ranging from 18 months to 76 years.[18,19] A familial form has been described but no specific gene has been identified.[18]

Although the root cause is unclear, the disease is caused by a congenital deficiency (absence or atrophy) of large airway smooth muscle and elastic fibers.[18] This leads to enlargement of the trachea and segmental bronchi, resulting in retention of airway secretions. It has been associated with Ehlers-Danlos syndrome, cutis laxa, and Kenny-Caffey syndrome.[20] Mounier-Kuhn syndrome is generally diagnosed in the third to fifth decade of life and may be more common in males.[18]

Patients commonly present with recurrent pneumonia, though may have hemoptysis, pneumothoraces, bronchiectasis, emphysema, pulmonary fibrosis, and respiratory failure. A CT scan of the chest would show dilation of the trachea and bronchi[21] (Figure 38-5).

Treatment is supportive with chest physiotherapy, antibiotics, and possibly the use of positive end-expiratory pressure and stenting of the trachea.[18]

Williams-Campbell Syndrome

Williams-Campbell syndrome is a rare congenital disorder characterized by diffuse bronchomalacia initially described in 1960 as a rare form of bronchiectasis.[22] As of 1993, 22 cases had been reported.[23]

Bronchial cartilage maintains airway patency during expiration. These cartilage C-rings are normally present in the trachea, and large- and medium-sized airways. Williams-Campbell syndrome is a rare congenital disorder of diffuse bronchomalacia caused by congenital absence of cartilage in the second to seventh divisions of bronchi. This leads to airway instability with airway collapse, retention of secretions, and ultimately bronchiectasis.[22]

Patients often present early with recurrent pneumonia, fever, failure to thrive, and chronic productive cough. A CT scan of the chest would show extensive peripheral bronchiectasis[24] (Figure 38-6).

Treatment is supportive with chest physiotherapy, airway clearance, and antibiotics.

Pulmonary Lymphangiomyomatosis

Pulmonary lymphangiomyomatosis (LAM) is a rare condition that mainly affects postpubertal females.[25] There have been rare cases in prepubertal girls and males.[26,27]

The disease is characterized by proliferation of neoplastic cells resembling smooth muscle cells within the lung, kidney, and lymphatics. Within the lung, these cells proliferate around the bronchi causing luminal narrowing. This leads to air trapping and formation of cysts, resulting in lung parenchyma destruction and risk of pneumothoraces. With disease progression, blood vessels can also become affected, leading to impaired diffusion, hemosiderosis, and hemoptysis.

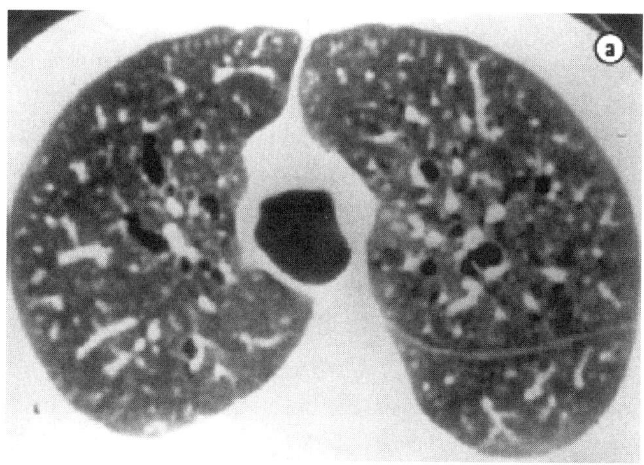

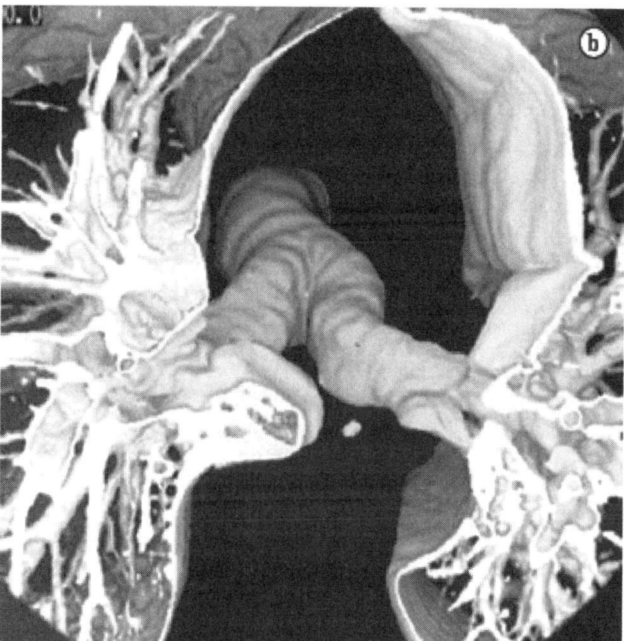

Figure 38-5. Tracheobronchomegaly in Mounier-Kuhn syndrome. **A.** Computed tomography scan demonstrates irregular diffuse dilation of the trachea with bronchiectasis. **B.** Three-dimensional reconstruction demonstrates marked dilation of trachea and main bronchi. (Reprinted with permission from Marchiori E, Pozes AS, Souza AS Jr, et al. Diffuse abnormalities of the trachea: computed tomography findings [in Portuguese]. *J Bras Pneumol.* 2008;34[1]:47–54.)

Additionally, lymphatics may become involved, leading to chylothorax. Female hormones may contribute to the disease pathogenesis. It is largely limited to postpubertal, premenopausal females with reports of exacerbations with pregnancy, menstruation, and estrogen use.[25] It has also been associated with the neurocutaneous syndrome tuberous sclerosis, suggesting a genetic component. There are 2 forms of LAM: tuberous sclerosis complex (TSC)-associated LAM and a sporadic type. Harmatin and tuberin proteins, which are encoded on *TSC 1* gene and *TSC 2* gene, respectively, are absent.[25]

Presenting symptoms vary: dyspnea, chronic dry cough, wheeze, hemoptysis, pneumothorax, cyanosis, cor pulmonale, and respiratory failure. Pulmonary function tests show variable patterns from normal, obstructive, restrictive, to mixed.[25] Diffusion capacity for carbon monoxide is generally decreased. Chest radiographs may show normal lung tissue to reticulonodular interstitial infiltrate to end-stage honeycombing. Additionally, pneumothorax and pleural effusions may be seen on radiographs. A CT scan of the chest shows diffuse, thin-walled cysts, which are classic signs of LAM (Figure 38-6).

Diagnosis can often be made on classic CT appearance and associated findings of LAM. If diagnosis remains uncertain, histologic diagnosis from lung biopsy or transbronchial biopsy may be necessary. Treatment is symptomatic, primarily reversing complications such as pneumothorax, ascites, and hemorrhage. General pulmonary support includes supplemental oxygen as needed, routine vaccination, and rehabilitation. There have been some studies using hormonal therapy with variable results.[25–27] Currently, clinical trials using anti-angiogenic, anti-inflammatory, and anti-proliferative medications are ongoing. A lung transplant may be an option in end-stage disease. Survival is about 8 to 10 years, with most children succumbing to progressive respiratory failure.[25]

Alpha-1 Antitrypsin Deficiency

Alpha-1 antitrypsin (AAT) deficiency is an autosomal recessive disorder that was first recognized in 1963. It is mainly a disease of adults characterized by severe emphysema, but it can rarely show manifestations in children, who largely present with liver disease.[28] Prevalence is 1 in 2,500.

Alpha-1 antitrypsin is a 394 amino acid glycoprotein that inhibits the activity of certain proteolytic enzymes. It is a serine protease inhibitor encoded by *SERPINA 1* gene (also known as *PI)* that is located on the long arm of chromosome 14 and is mainly synthesized by hepatocytes. More than 100 alleles have been identified, and the Z allele is most frequently associated with lung disease.[28] Normal lung homeostasis and repair requires a balance between protease inhibitors and proteolytic enzymes. Neutrophil elastase is the main protease in the lung where it degrades elastin, collagen, proteoglycan, and other proteins in the alveolar wall, which if left unchecked can lead to alveolar destruction. Alpha-1 antitrypsin is the main anti-neutrophil elastase and prevents degradation of the lung architecture. An imbalance between protease

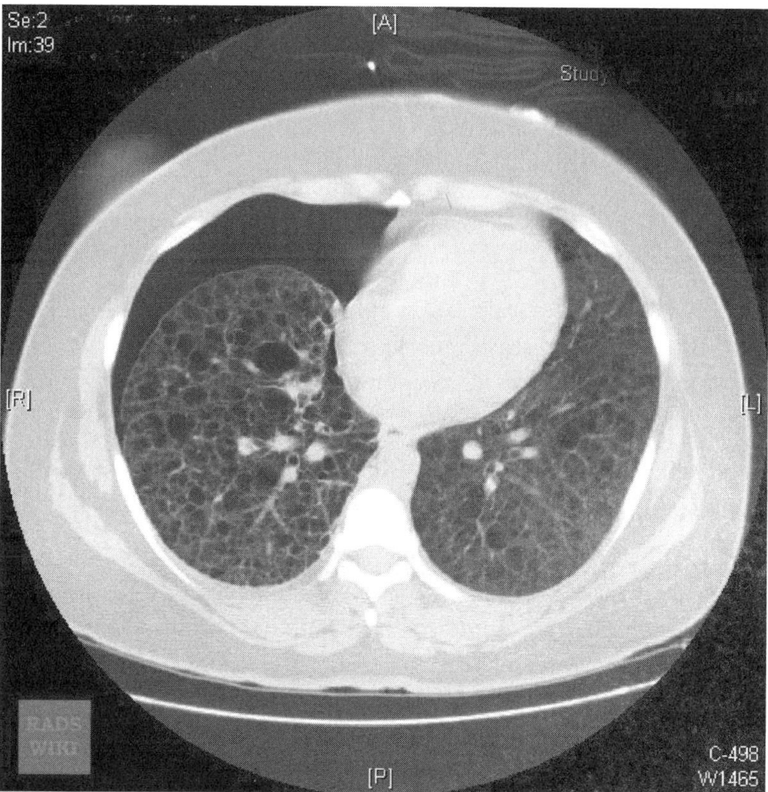

Figure 38-6. Chest computed tomography scan findings in pulmonary lymphangiomyomatosis. Note bilateral diffuse thin-walled cysts with right-sided pneumothorax. (Image reprinted with permission from http://www.radswiki.net/main/index.php?title=Lymphangioleiomyomatosis.)

inhibitors and proteolytic enzymes can lead to lung damage such as that seen in emphysema. Smoking is an independent risk factor for emphysema, though in AAT deficient individuals it can hasten the development of disease secondary to the accumulation of lung inflammatory cells, release of proteases from inflammatory cells, and release of smoke-associated oxidants that inhibit antitrypsin.[29] Together these further contribute to protease-antiprotease imbalance and ultimately lung damage.

Clinical Features

Most people with AAT deficiency do not present with respiratory complaints until the third or fourth decade of life, or a decade earlier in those that smoke.[29] There are a few rare cases of emphysema in children with severe AAT deficiency.[28,29] However, pulmonary function abnormalities, complaints of wheezing, and diagnosis of asthma are not uncommon in the second decade of life, especially if firsthand or secondhand smoking is present.[29] Children may have wheezing, chronic cough, or dyspnea on exertion. Liver disease, such as jaundice, hepatitis, and cirrhosis, is associated with lung disease in children. In adults, AAT deficiency usually presents as progressive dyspnea and panacinar emphysema.

The results of this physical examination are usually normal, though with advanced lung disease, growth retardation, and digital clubbing, and signs of chronic obstructive pulmonary disease, such as dyspnea, tachypnea, hyperexpansion, or barrel chest, may be present.

Chest radiographs may show hyperinflation with bibasilar hyperlucency. High-resolution chest CT is more sensitive than plain radiography and may demonstrate emphysema and bronchiectasis.

Pulmonary function testing may be normal, though as the disease progresses, evidence of chronic obstructive pulmonary disease develops with an obstructive pattern on spirometry, air trapping on lung volume measurements, and diffusion impairment.

Diagnosis

Alpha-1 antitrypsin deficiency should be considered in cases of prolonged neonatal jaundice; liver disease in any age group; and adults with emphysema, bronchitis, and late-onset asthma. The differential diagnosis should include asthma, CF, and immunodeficiencies. Serum AAT levels can be measured and the risk of disease predicted from the relative deficiency, as 100% of individuals with no detectable AAT develop emphysema and 60% to 85% of those with severe deficiency develop disease.[30] Alpha-1 antitrypsin is an acute phase reactant, and levels may be falsely elevated with any acute or chronic inflammation, such as infection, stress, or pregnancy. Currently there is no routinely available method for prenatal diagnosis, but protein phenotyping and genotyping are available to confirm the diagnosis, aid in genetic counseling for families, and predict the disease course.[28]

Treatment

The clinical course of the lung disease in AAT deficiency is variable, suggesting a prominent role for environmental or genetic modifiers.[30] Smoke exposure seems to be the most important risk factor. Therefore, avoiding smoke exposure is paramount in prevention of lung disease in patients known to be AAT deficient. Augmentation therapy, which consists of weekly intravenous infusions of AAT, is proving to be safe and effective at raising AAT levels, may retard the progression of lung disease, and should be considered in consultation with a pulmonary specialist.[31] Supportive therapies include early antibiotics for bacterial infections, bronchodilators, nutritional support, and oxygen as needed for desaturation. Patients are recommended to receive routine vaccinations (yearly influenza and lifetime pneumococcal). Surgical options, such as bullectomy and ultimately lung transplant, may be needed in cases of severe disease.

Pulmonary Complications of Other Congenital Disorders

Achondroplasia

Achondroplasia is the most common form of short-limb dwarfism. It is classified as a chondrodysplasia and is autosomal dominant. It is caused by mutations in the fibroblast growth factor receptor-3 *(FGFR3)*, which is on chromosome 4. The average adult height is 131 cm (51.5 inches) for males and 123 cm (48.5 inches) for females. The prevalence is 1 in 25,000. Intelligence is in the normal range.

Clinical Features

The major features of achondroplasia are hypotonia, megalencephaly (large head) with frontal bossing, and short stature and other skeletal abnormalities, including a small thoracic cavity. The large head and abnormality at the craniocervical junction contribute to significant mortality in the first year of life. The risk for sudden death is 2% to 5%, with the major cause of death being spinal cord compression. Central apnea may result from arterial compression at the foramen magnum or brain stem compression, and obstructive apnea may result from midface hypoplasia.

Respiratory difficulty is commonly seen in achondroplasia as follows:

- Restrictive lung disease secondary to small chest cavity
- As many as 75% have significant apnea both central and obstructive
- Obstructive sleep apnea

Tasker et al[32] studied 14 boys and 3 girls with achondroplasia starting before age 1 year and identified 3 groups. The first group had mild obstructive sleep apnea, the second group had more significant apnea with hypdrocephalus and a small foramen magnum, and the third group developed cor pulmonale, with 3 of 5 subjects dying of cardiorespiratory failure. The third group also had significant gastroesophageal reflux, and the respiratory failure resulted from severe upper airway obstruction resulting from hypoglossal canal stenosis.

Stokes et al[33] evaluated 12 healthy subjects with achondroplasia and concluded that there is a reduction in vital capacity (restrictive lung disease) out of proportion of what would be expected if these subjects had normal limb size. In addition they found that while the lungs are small they and the airways are functionally normal.

Management

Caregivers must be aware of the risk of craniocervical compression, which in extreme form may result in atlantoaxial dislocation. Endotracheal intubation is difficult because of the midface hypoplasia and the necessity of avoiding extension of the head (backward). Fiberoptic bronchoscopy assistance may be the safest way to intubate, particularly during infancy and early childhood. Referral to pulmonology and neurology specialists in the first year is important to diagnose respiratory disorders as described and assess the craniocervical area of the spinal column.

Arthrogryposis Multiplex Congenita

The feature of arthrogryposis multiplex congenita (AMC) is multiple contractures that are present at birth. During embryogenesis there is motion of the limbs, which aids development of joints. Decreased fetal movement causes extra connective tissue to develop around joints, which results in fixation of the joint, leading to contractures. Decreased fetal movement may result from multiple fetal disorders, including neurologic, muscular, or connective tissue disorders. Other causes include maternal issues, such as misshapen uterus, infection, and drugs. The earlier in pregnancy that the fetal movement is reduced the more severe the joint abnormalities. Although a genetic cause may be identified in 30% of cases, most cases are of undetermined etiology.

Clinical Features

The deformities are present at birth and the condition is not progressive. The condition that causes AMC (eg, muscular dystrophy) may progress.

Classic arthrogryposis is also known as amyoplasia with symmetrical involvement of limb deformity and normal intelligence. This form is sporadic. Various subtypes of distal arthrogryposis have been described involving hands and feet. The pulmonary complications tend to be related to the size and shape of the chest wall, which may result in a restrictive defect. Williams et al[34] reported significant pulmonary findings in children with distal arthrogryposis type 5 (DA5). Although this report is from Salt Lake City, UT (altitude 7,000 feet) and refers to DA5, the conclusions apply to children at other altitudes, including sea level and other variants of DA. These conclusions include pulmonary function tests showing severe chest restriction (forced vital capacity 30% predicted; total lung capacity 51% predicted) and reduction of maximal inspiratory and expiratory pressures. Arterial blood gases documented alveolar hypoventilation. Restrictive chest disease is a component of DA5. This implies involvement of the skeletal and respiratory muscles. They recommend pulmonary evaluation of children with distal arthrogryposis because of these findings. Additional respiratory complications include tracheal and laryngeal clefts or stenosis. The respiratory muscles as well as the diaphragm may be weak.

Scoliosis is common. Early onset respiratory failure has a poor prognosis for long-term survival.

Management

The respiratory manifestations may be severe and require assisted ventilation. Endotracheal intubation may be difficult because those affected tend to have a small, immobile jaw. Also the airway may be compromised so that a tracheostomy may be necessary.

Box 38-2. Pulmonary Complications of Down Syndrome

- **Sleep-disordered breathing**
  - Laryngomalacia
  - Large tongue
  - Lax pharynx
  - Adenotonsillar hypertrophy
  - Obesity
- **Airway abnormalities**
  - Laryngomalacia
  - Tracheomalacia
  - Bronchomalacia
  - Tracheal bronchus
- **Parenchymal lung disease**
  - Subpleural cysts
  - Interstitial lung disease
- **Pneumonia**
  - Immune deficiency
  - Aspiration
- **Pulmonary Vascular Problems**
  - Pulmonary artery hypertension
  - Pulmonary hemorrhage
  - Pulmonary edema
- **Asthma**

Down Syndrome

Trisomy 21, which results in Down syndrome, is the most common chromosomal abnormality, affecting 1 in every 600 to 800 live births. Pulmonary complications of Down syndrome are multiple, and pneumonia is the most common indication for hospital admission. Despite being multiple, the pulmonary features are often underappreciated.[35] There are several categories of pulmonary problems as shown in Box 38-2.

Sleep-Disordered Breathing

Sleep-disordered breathing (SDB) during infancy is common in those with Down syndrome and also occurs in older children with Down syndrome. It is reported to be as high as 30% to 75% compared with 2% to 3% in the general population. In infancy the most usual cause is related to laryngotracheomalacia and after infancy secondary to adenoidal or tonsillar hypertrophy. Obesity also is often a contributing factor. The symptoms of sleep apnea include snoring, restless sleep, difficulty awaking, and daytime sleepiness with behavioral changes, including school problems. Evaluation of SDB, including polysomnography, should be considered in infancy and later because early recognition will reduce the likelihood of developing pulmonary hypertension.

Upper airway obstruction may result from the small size of the midface, small nasal airways, micrognathia, increased collapsibility (laxness) of the oropharynx and nasopharynx, and enlargement of the tongue.

Sleep-disordered breathing is so common that the American Academy of Pediatrics recommends referral to a specialist as early as the first year for evaluation.[36] The parents are often unaware of problems even though 97% of children with Down syndrome who snore have SDB confirmed by polysomnography.

Airway Abnormalities

Laryngomalacia and tracheomalacia are common in those with Down syndrome and should be evaluated with flexible bronchoscopy. Large tonsils and adenoids, lingual tonsils, large tongue, and lax pharyngeal tissue all contribute to the potential for upper airway obstruction. This can lead to otitis media and alveolar hypoventilation with resulting hypoxemia, which may lead to pulmonary hypertension. Subglottic stenosis and tracheal stenosis are also common. Tracheal bronchus, also known as pig bronchus, where the right upper lobe bronchus originates from the trachea above the carina, is not uncommon. Tracheal bronchus should be considered if there is persistent right upper lobe infection or consolidation.

Parenchymal Lung Disease

Pathologists have long been aware of the presence of subpleural cysts in patients with Down syndrome. The cysts are not visible on chest radiograph but are prominently visible in CT scan. They are seen in 20% to 36% of children with Down syndrome and are more common in children with Down syndrome who have congenital heart disease. The presence of cysts confers an increased risk for pneumothorax.

Children with Down syndrome studied at autopsy have shown a decrease in the number of alveoli with increase in alveolar size. The number of alveoli are decreased by 58% to 83% regardless of the presence of heart disease. In addition, pulmonary hypoplasia, pulmonary lymphangiectasia, and interstitial lung disease occur more in children with Down syndrome than in children who do not have Down syndrome.

Pneumonia

Pneumonia is the most common cause for hospital admission, and of these patients 10% require admission to the intensive care unit (ICU). The presence of congenital heart defect (CHD) did not influence admission rates to the hospital, but those with CHD seem to have more severe illness with more ICU admissions and longer length of stay.[37] The causes of recurrent pneumonia are multiple and include pharyngeal incoordination with aspiration as well as immune deficiency. Airway abnormalities include laryngomalacia and tracheomalacia, and tracheal bronchus may be found on CT scan or bronchoscopy.

Pulmonary Vascular Problems

Pulmonary vascular problems of children and adolescents with Down syndrome include pulmonary hypertension, pulmonary edema, and pulmonary hemorrhage. Congenital heart defects are common, with various abnormalities occurring in 43% of 482 children with trisomy 21 in the review by Weijerman et al.[38] They reported atrioventricular (AV) septal defect (includes AV canal) in 54% of cases, ventricular septal defect in 33.3%, and patent ductus arteriosus in 5.8%. Their incidence of primary pulmonary hypertension was 5.2%, considerably higher than that seen in the general population. Pulmonary hypertension in children with Down syndrome has various etiologies, including polycythemia (35%), asphyxia (12%), hemangioendothelioma (6%), and unknown (47%). Children with Down syndrome who have a large left-to-right shunt typically develop pulmonary artery hypertension (PAH), but whereas some die in the first few months, others do not develop PAH despite having a large shunt.

Pulmonary artery hypertension also develops in children with Down syndrome who have SDB with resultant hypoxia. The problem of PAH may even occur in Down syndrome without any obvious reason for its occurrence.

Chronic pulmonary hemorrhage is a not uncommon complication of Down syndrome. It is a complication of children who have large left-to-right shunt, increased pulmonary venous pressure from mitral valve dysfunction, or pulmonary venous obstruction. Even in the absence of cardiac abnormalities it occurs with recurrent pneumonia or aspiration. The clinical features vary from frank hemoptysis to a drop in hemoglobin with minimal symptoms.

Pulmonary edema is also common and is especially seen following relief of upper airway obstruction either intraoperatively or postoperatively. Non-cardiogenic pulmonary edema is also seen associated with acute lung injury in children with Down syndrome with pneumonia and postoperatively following cardiac surgery. High altitude pulmonary edema is more common in children with Down syndrome than in children who do not have Down syndrome.

Asthma

Most studies concerning asthma in children with Down syndrome have reported a lower incidence of asthma than in the general population. There is an increased risk for severe respiratory syncytial virus infection, including bronchiolitis, but the long-term risk for recurrent wheezing is decreased.

Hermansky-Pudlak Syndrome

Hermansky-Pudlak syndrome (HPS) is a rare group of autosomal recessive disorders caused by defects in lysosome function.[39,40]

Pathophysiology

The lysosomal dysfunction causes the accumulation of ceroid deposition in various tissues. In the lungs, this causes pulmonary fibrosis in approximately 50% of patients with HPS.[39] There is a high prevalence in Puerto Rico (1:1,800 births), particularly the northwestern quarter, consistent with the genetics of the disorder.[41] The gene mutation has been identified, and there are 8 known human subtypes. The HPS 1 mutation is the most common, and it is a 16 bp duplication. The HPS 1 and HPS 4 subtypes are at risk for developing pulmonary fibrosis.[42]

Clinical Features

There have been cases described in children as young as 3 years; however, pulmonary fibrosis does not develop until adulthood.[39] Patients with HPS have tyrosinase-positive oculocutaneous albinism with related ocular findings, bleeding caused by poor platelet aggregation, pulmonary fibrosis, granulomatous enteropathic disease, and renal failure.[39] Pulmonary function testing may demonstrate a restrictive defect with reduced total lung capacity and impaired diffusion capacity consistent with pulmonary fibrosis. High-resolution chest CT scans are abnormal in most patients (up to 85%)[40] (Figure 38-7).

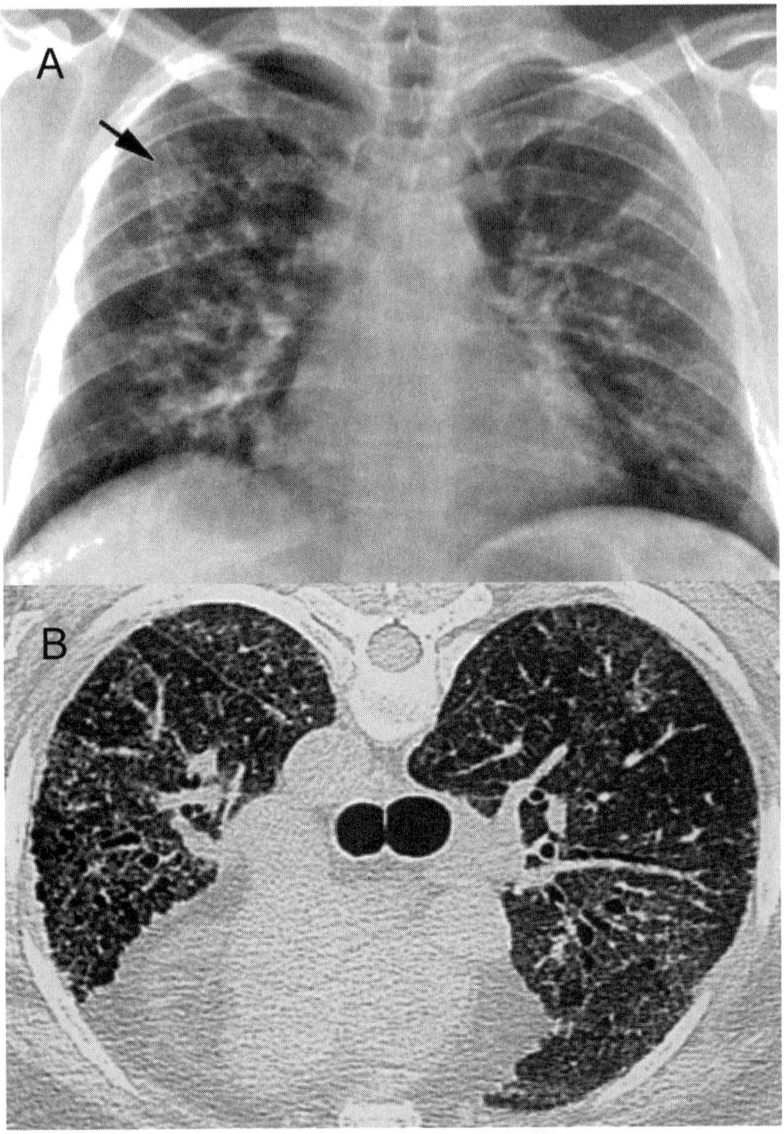

Figure 38-7. Radiographic findings in Hermansky-Pudlak syndrome. **A.** Posteroanterior chest radiograph shows patchy areas of interstitial infiltrates (arrow). **B.** High-resolution computed tomography scan shows ground-glass opacities, bronchiectasis, peribronchovascular thickening, septal lines, and reticulation. (Images from Avila NA, Brantly M, Premkumar A, et al. Hermansky-Pudlak syndrome: radiography and CT of the chest compared with pulmonary function tests and genetic studies. *AJR Am J Roentgenol.* 2002;179:887–892, with permission.)

Management

Diagnosis can be made by careful ophthalmologic examination and confirming tyrosinase-positive oculocutaneous albinism via hair bulb analysis.[39] Patients generally survive to 30 to 50 years and die of complications from organ damage.[39] There is high mortality related to pulmonary complications. Patients should be referred to a pulmonologist in early adulthood or sooner if respiratory symptoms develop. Therapy is generally supportive, with the goal being to reduce bleeding risks and improve pulmonary quality of life.

Mucopolysaccharidosis

Mucopolysaccharidoses (MPS) are a group of lysosomal storage diseases caused by a deficiency of an enzyme involved in the degradation of acid mucopolysaccharides, now called glycosaminoglycans (GAG). They are inherited as autosomal recessive disorders except for MPS type II (Hunter syndrome), which is an X-linked disorder. Mucopolysaccharidoses type I-H is the most severe form (formerly known as Hurler syndrome), and MPS type I-S (Scheie syndrome) is milder and used to be classified as MPS type 5. Mucopolysaccharidoses type I-H, MPS type I-S, and MPS type I-H/S have varying degrees of deficiency of α-L-iduronidase.

Glycosaminoglycans is an important constituent of the extracellular matrix, joint fluid, and connective tissue throughout the body. Accumulation of GAG within the cells of various organs causes the change in appearance and alters function of those organs.

Clinical Features

Children born with Hurler syndrome appear normal at birth and develop the characteristic appearance during the first years of life. It was also known as gargoylism because of the gargoyle-like facies. There is progressive deterioration in the most severe form, with mental retardation and life span less than 10 years. Progressive skeletal dysplasia (dysostosis multiplex) affects all bones, and linear growth ceases by 3 years of age. There are frequent upper and lower airway infections, and the most common cause of death is a consequence of airway obstruction. Respiratory obstruction results from a large tongue and adenotonsillar hypertrophy. The trachea and bronchi tend to be narrow and abnormally shaped. Sleep apnea is a common complication. The lower airways tend to be further obstructed by tracheobronchomalacia, and recurrent pneumonia is common. Scheie and Hurler/Scheie are milder forms that are typically associated with normal intelligence and life spans up to 70 years.

The severe form of Hunter syndrome is diagnosed between 2 to 4 years of age, with progressive neurologic disorder and somatic effects. The somatic effects include coarse facial features, short stature, skeletal deformities, and mental retardation. Progressive airway obstruction is also a common finding in Hunter syndrome, and complications of this are the most common cause of death.[43]

Management

The more severe forms of MPS require tracheostomy and continuous positive airway pressure, and may require assisted ventilation to maintain airway patency.

Pseudohypoaldosteronism

Pseudohypoaldosteronism (PHA) is a hereditary salt-wasting disorder characterized by renal unresponsiveness or resistance to aldosterone. Pseudohypoaldosteronism has been classified into a type I (PHA-I) and type II (PHA-II). Recently, PHA-I has been described to have 2 forms, with either renal or multi-target organ disorder (MTOD).[44] The renal form or classic PHA of infancy is inherited as an autosomal dominant trait, and patients have normal to mildly abnormal electrolyte values. The severe form of PHA, which involves other organs, including the lung, is inherited as an autosomal recessive trait and causes severe salt loss secondary to a mutation in the epithelial sodium channel.[45] This defect leads to defective sodium transport in organs such as the kidney, lung, colon, and sweat and salivary glands. Pulmonary symptoms are common in MTOD PHA-I, where increased airway sodium chloride concentration impairs bacterial killing.

Patients with MTOD PHA-I have clinical signs and symptoms similar to those with CF, including recurrent pneumonia secondary to impaired bacterial killing.[44] They may have periods of dyspnea, fever, tachypnea, and increased work of breathing with crackles auscultated on examination. These individuals also have severe salt-wasting episodes and are prone to periods of dehydration. Pseudohypoaldosteronism is recognized as a cause of a false-positive sweat test, where sweat sodium and chloride values are elevated secondary to defective electrolyte transport.[44] Chest radiography can demonstrate thickened airways caused by failure to absorb liquid from the airway surface.[46] This can also appear similar to radiographs in early CF. The diagnosis of PHA is clinical with the identification of elevated urinary sodium. Treatment is similar to CF, with aggressive management of dehydration and electrolyte imbalance as well as early antibiotics for pulmonary infections. Supplemental oxygen may be needed during times of active infection. Dietary modification with high sodium, low potassium foods is generally recommended. Other therapies, such as diuretics, potassium-binding resins, and alkalinizing agents, may be indicated. Prognosis is guarded, with potential mortality in infancy due to the severe metabolic/electrolyte derangements. Additionally, MTOD PHA-I does not improve with advancing age. Treatment and monitoring is lifelong.

Key Points

Primary Ciliary Dyskinesia

- Primary ciliary dyskinesia is an autosomal recessive inherited disorder involving defects in ciliated cells of the respiratory tract and middle ear, spermatozoa, fallopian tubes, and ciliated cells of the ventricular ependyma of the brain.
- Kartagener syndrome is a triad of chronic sinusitis, bronchiectasis, and situs inversus (50% of patients).
- Infertility is common in men.
- Mimics of PCD include viral infections and pollutant exposure, but these cause secondary ciliary defects, which are transient.
- Clinical features are variable from acute otitis media, sinusitis, bronchitis, and pneumonia.
- Treatment is to enhance mucociliary clearance with cough, chest percussion, and drainage to prevent and treat respiratory infections.
- Referral to a pulmonologist should be considered early when the diagnosis is suspected to confirm and closely manage their lung disease.
- Genetic counseling is recommended for subsequent pregnancies.

Key Points (continued)

Mounier-Kuhn Syndrome

- Mounier-Kuhn syndrome is a rare congenital disease caused by absence or atrophy of large airway smooth muscles and elastic fibers that results in tracheobronchomegaly.
- Patients clinically present with recurrent pneumonia, bronchiectasis, pneumothoraces, hemoptysis, emphysema, pulmonary fibrosis, and respiratory failure.
- Treatment is supportive care with chest physiotherapy, antibiotics, and positive end-expiratory pressure.
- Referral to a pulmonologist should be considered early when the diagnosis is suspected to confirm and closely manage their lung disease.

Williams-Campbell Syndrome

- Williams-Campbell syndrome is a rare congenital disorder involving absence of cartilage in the second to seventh divisions of bronchi leading to diffuse bronchomalacia.
- Patients present with recurrent pneumonias, fever, failure to thrive, and chronic productive cough.
- Treatment is supportive with airway clearance and antibiotics.
- Referral to a pulmonologist should be considered early when the diagnosis is suspected to confirm and closely manage lung disease.

Pulmonary Lymphangiomyomatosis

- Pulmonary lymphangiomyomatosis is a rare condition affecting postpubertal females.
- Neoplastic cells proliferate in the lung, kidney, and lymphatics causing airway narrowing, impaired diffusion, cyst formation, and chylothorax in the respiratory system.
- Symptoms vary from chronic dry cough, wheeze, hemoptysis, cyanosis, cor pulmonale, and respiratory failure.
- Treatment is supportive.
- Referral to a pulmonologist should be considered early when the diagnosis is suspected to confirm and closely manage lung disease.

Key Points

Alpha-1 Antitrypsin Deficiency

- Alpha-1 antitrypsin deficiency is an autosomal dominant inherited disorder caused by the imbalance of protease-antiprotease enzymes in the lung.
- Clinically patients present with symptoms later in life with rare cases of emphysema in children.
- Smoke exposure is an independent risk factor for emphysema in these patients.
- Treatment is supportive with avoidance of tobacco exposure, early antibiotics, bronchodilators, oxygen as needed, and nutrition.
- Genetic counseling is recommended when the diagnosis is suspected.
- Referral to a pulmonologist should be considered when the diagnosis is confirmed to closely monitor and manage progression of lung disease.

Achondroplasia

- The first year of life is important because prevention of complications related to craniocervical compression.
- Obstructive sleep apnea is common, and symptoms of snoring and other SDB should be evaluated by a sleep specialist.

Arthrogryposis Multiplex Congenita

- The condition is caused by decreased fetal movement, with 30% having a genetic component.
- The most common form is peripheral arthrogryposis.
- Pulmonary complications result from restrictive lung disease and airway anomalies.
- Pulmonary management is supportive and may require assisted ventilation.

Key Points (continued)

Down Syndrome

- Airway and pulmonary complications of Down syndrome may be underappreciated.
- Sleep-disordered breathing is very common in Down syndrome. Infants and children should be evaluated by a sleep specialist.
- Pneumonia is the most common cause for admission and 10% require ICU admission.

Hermansky-Pudlak Syndrome

- Hermansky-Pudlak syndrome is a rare autosomal recessive disorder characterized by tyrosinase-positive oculocutaneous albinism, bleeding diathesis, and pulmonary fibrosis.
- Treatment is supportive.
- Referral to a pulmonologist should be considered when the diagnosis is confirmed to closely monitor and manage progression of lung disease.

Mucopolysaccharidosis

- Hurler and Hunter syndromes have a broad spectrum of symptomatology.
- Airway problems are the most problematic and have the most potential for morbidity and mortality.
- The airway abnormalities may require tracheostomy.

Pseudohypoaldosteronism

- Pseudohypoaldosteronism is a hereditary salt-wasting disorder caused by renal unresponsiveness or resistance to aldosterone.
- The severe form is inherited as an autosomal recessive trait that involves a defect in sodium transport in various organs, including the lungs.
- Clinical features are similar to CF with recurrent pneumonias.
- Patients may have false-positive sweat test.
- Treatment is rehydration, early antibiotics, oxygen as needed, and dietary modification.
- Referral to a pulmonologist should be considered when the diagnosis is confirmed to closely monitor and manage progression of lung disease.

References

1. Leigh MW. Primary ciliary dyskinesia. *Semin Respir Crit Care Med.* 2003;24:653–662
2. Chilvers MA, Rutman A, O'Callaghan C. Functional analysis of cilia and ciliated epithelial ultrastructure in healthy children and young adults. *Thorax.* 2003;58:333–338
3. Afzelius BA, Eliasson R. Male and female infertility problems in the immotile-cilia syndrome. *Eur J Respir Dis Suppl.* 1983;127:144–147
4. Greenstone MA, Jones RW, Dewar A, et al. Hydrocephalus and primary ciliary dyskinesia. *Arch Dis Child.* 1984;59:481–482
5. Fliegauf M, Benzing T, Omran, H. When cilia go bad: cilia defects and celiopathies. *Nat Rev Mol Cell Biol.* 2007;8:880–893
6. Pedersen M. Ciliary activity and pollution. *Lung.* 1990;168S:368–376
7. Zariwala MA, Knowles MR, Omran H. Genetic defects in ciliary structure and function. *Annu Rev Physiol.* 2007;69:423–450
8. Schwabe GC, Hoffmann K, Loges NT, et al. Primary ciliary dyskinesia associated with normal axoneme ultrastructure is caused by DNAH11 mutations. *Hum Mutat.* 2008;29:289–298
9. Zariwala MA, Leigh MW, Ceppa F, et al. Mutations of DNAI1 in primary ciliary dyskinesia: evidence of founder effect in a common mutation. *Am J Respir Crit Care Med.* 2006;174:858–866
10. Hornef N, Olbrich H, Horvath J, et al. DNAH5 mutations are a common cause of primary ciliary dyskinesia with outer dynein arm defects. *Am J Respir Crit Care Med.* 2006;174:120–126
11. Ferkol T, Leigh M. Primary ciliary dyskinesia and newborn respiratory distress. *Semin Perinatol.* 2006;30:335–340
12. Kennedy MP, Omran H, Leigh MW, et al. Congenital heart disease and other heterotaxic defects in a large cohort of patients with primary ciliary dyskinesia. *Circulation.* 2007;115:2814–2821
13. Santamaria F, Montella S, Tiddens HA, et al. Structural and functional lung disease in primary ciliary dyskinesia. *Chest.* 2008;134:351–357
14. Corbelli R, Bringolf-Isler B, Amacher A, et al. Nasal nitric oxide measurements to screen children for primary ciliary dyskinesia. *Chest.* 2004;126:1054–1059
15. Trindade SH, de Mello JF Jr, Mion Ode G, et al. Methods for studying mucociliary transport. *Braz J Otorhinolaryngol.* 2007;73:704–712
16. Canciani M, Barlocco EG, Mastella G, et al. The saccharin method for testing mucociliary function in patients suspected of having primary ciliary dyskinesia. *Pediatr Pulmonol.* 1988;5:210–214
17. Lie H, Ferkol T. Primary ciliary dyskinesia: recent advances in pathogenesis, diagnosis and treatment. *Drugs.* 2007;67:1883–1892
18. Menon B, Aggarwal B, Iqbal A. Mounier-Kuhn syndrome: report of 8 cases of tracheobronchomegaly with associated complications. *South Med J.* 2008;101:83–87

19. Shin MS, Jackson RM, Ho KJ. Tracheobronchomegaly (Mounier-Kuhn syndrome): CT diagnosis. *AJR Am J Roentgenol.* 1988;150:777–779
20. Sane AC, Effmann EL, Brown SD. Tracheobronchiomegaly. The Mounier-Kuhn syndrome in a patient with the Kenny-Caffey syndrome. *Chest.* 1992;102:618–619
21. Marchiori E, Pozes AS, Souza AS Jr, et al. Diffuse abnormalities of the trachea: computed tomography findings [in Portuguese]. *J Bras Pneumol.* 2008;34(1):47–54
22. Williams H, Campbell P. Generalized bronchiectasis associated with deficiency of cartilage in the bronchial tree. *Arch Dis Child.* 1960;35182–191
23. Jones VF, Eid NS, Franco SM, et al. Familial congenital bronchiectasis: Williams-Campbell syndrome. *Pediatr Pulmonol.* 1993;16:263–267
24. George J, Jain R, Tariq SM. CT bronchoscopy in the diagnosis of Williams-Campbell syndrome. *Respirology.* 2006;11:117–119
25. Hancock E, Osborne J. Lymphangioleiomyomatosis: a review of the literature. *Respir Med.* 2002;96:1–6
26. Nussbaum E, Groncy P, Finklestein J, et al. Early onset of childhood pulmonary lymphangiomyomatosis. *Clin Pediatr (Phila).* 1988;27(6):279–284
27. Duckett JG, Lazarus A, White KM. Cutaneous masses, rib lesions, and chylous pleural effusion in a 20-year-old man. *Chest.* 1990;97:1227–1228
28. Kohnlein T, Welte T. Alpha-1 antitrypsin deficiency: pathogenesis, clinical presentation, diagnosis, and treatment. *Am J Med.* 1008;121:3–9
29. von Ehrenstein OS, von Mutius E, Maier E, et al. Lung function of school children with low levels of alpha1-antitrypsin and tobacco smoke exposure. *Eur Respir J.* 2002;19:1099–1106
30. Coakley RJ, Taggart C, O'Neill S, et al. Alpha1-antitrypsin deficiency: biological answers to clinical questions. *Am J Med Sci.* 2001;321:33–41
31. Hubbard RC, Sellers S, Czerski D, et al. Biochemical efficacy and safety of monthly augmentation therapy for alpha 1-antitrypsin deficiency. *JAMA.* 1988;260:1259–1264
32. Tasker RC, Dundas I, Laverty A, et al. Distinct patterns of respiratory difficulty in young children with achondroplasia: a clinical, sleep, and lung function study. *Arch Dis Child.* 1998;79(2):99–108
33. Stokes DC, Wohl ME, Wise RA, et al. The lungs and airways in achondroplasia. Do little people have little lungs? *Chest.* 1990;98(1):145–152
34. Williams MS, Elliott CG, Bamshad MJ. Pulmonary disease is a component of distal arthrogryposis type 5. *Am J Med Genet A.* 2007;143(7):752–756
35. McDowell KM, Craven DI. Pulmonary complications of Down syndrome during childhood. *J Pediatr.* 2010;158(2):319–325
36. American Academy of Pediatrics Committee on Genetics. Health supervision for children with Down syndrome. *Pediatrics.* 2001;107:442–449
37. Hilton JM, Fitzgerald DA, Cooper DM. Respiratory morbidity of hospitalized children with Trisomy 21. *J Paediatr Child Health.* 1999;35(4):383–386

38. Weijerman ME, Furth AM, Vonk Noordegraaf A, et al. Prevalence of congenital heart defects and persistent pulmonary hypertension of the neonate with Down syndrome. *Eur J Pediatr.* 2010;169(10):1195–1199
39. Pierson DM, Ionescu D, Qing G, et al. Pulmonary fibrosis in Hermansky-Pudlak syndrome. a case report and review. *Respiration.* 2006;73:382–395
40. Avila NA, Brantly M, Premkumar A, et al. Hermansky-Pudlak syndrome: radiography and CT of the chest compared with pulmonary function tests and genetic studies. *AJR Am J Roentgenol.* 2002;179:887–892
41. Witkop CJ, Almadovar C, Pineiro B, et al. Hermansky-Pudlak syndrome (HPS). An epidemiologic study. *Ophthalmic Paediatr Genet.* 1990;11:245–250
42. Wei ML. Hermansky-Pudlak syndrome: a disease of protein trafficking and organelle function. *Pigment Cell Res.* 2006;19:19–42
43. Martin R, Beck M, Eng C, et al. Recognition and diagnosis of mucopolysaccharidosis II (Hunter syndrome). *Pediatrics.* 2008;121(2):e377–e386
44. Hanukoglu A, Bistritzer T, Rakover Y, et al. Pseudohypoaldosteronism with increased sweat and saliva electrolyte values and frequent lower respiratory tract infections mimicking cystic fibrosis. *J Pediatr.* 1994;125:752–755
45. Edelheit O, Hanukoglu I, Gizewska M, et al. Novel mutations in epithelial sodium channel (ENaC) subunit genes and phenotypic expression of multisystem pseudohypoaldosteronism. *Clin Endocrinol (Oxf).* 2005;62:547–553
46. Kerem E, Bistritzer T, Hanukoglu A, et al. Pulmonary epithelial sodium-channel dysfunction and excess airway liquid in pseudohypoaldosteronism. *N Engl J Med.* 1999;341:156–162

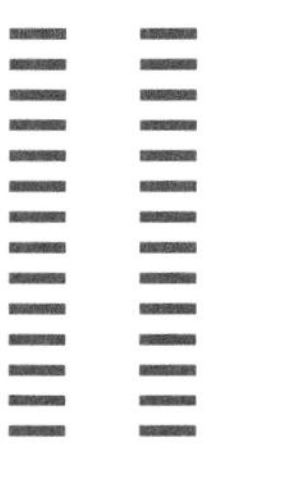

Chapter 39

Respiratory Considerations in Children With Cardiac Disease

Robert W. Morrow, MD
Nandini Madan, MD
Daniel V. Schidlow, MD

Introduction

The heart and the lungs function as a connected single unit; they share the same physical space. The pulmonary and systemic circulation represent a series circuit. Abnormalities in the pulmonary vascular bed can cause cardiac alterations and, conversely, changes in blood flow and pressures in the great vessels and pulmonary vascular bed can cause serious airway and lung changes.

Symptoms referable to the pulmonary system are often the initial and sometimes the only manifestation of cardiac disease, especially in the infant. The first symptom of congestive heart failure is often tachypnea, initially comfortable, which progresses if untreated to dyspnea with intercostal and subcostal retractions. Tachypnea is initially due to increased pulmonary venous pressure or volume. Later in the clinical course, bronchial compression, either due to enlarged pulmonary arteries or left atrium, leads to hyperinflation and atelactasis. In some patients the clinical picture is dominated by pulmonary symptoms such as chest discomfort, dyspnea, wheezing, and cough, leading to the eponym "cardiac asthma." Additional symptoms of airway compression, including dysphagia, recurrent respiratory infections, and stridor, leading to acute respiratory distress or "dying spells" may occur in patients with vascular anomalies (vascular ring, vascular sling).[1]

This chapter examines the interactions between these systems and, more specifically, will highlight the pathophysiology and clinical manifestations attributable to the respiratory system often present in children with congenital heart diseases.

Physiology/Pathophysiology

Distribution of Pulmonary Blood Flow

Pulmonary blood flow depends on the interaction between cardiac output and pulmonary vascular resistance. Alterations in pulmonary vascular resistance occur due to passive and active changes to pulmonary vessel caliber. Gravity-dependent and gravity-independent factors may alter distribution of pulmonary blood flow. Gravity-dependent variations in pulmonary blood flow occur due to the net differences in 3 intrapulmonary pressures: intra-alveolar pulmonary capillary pressure, alveolar pressure, and venous pressure. Gravity-independent determinants of passive pulmonary blood flow are affected by changes in lung volumes causing changes in pulmonary vessel caliber.

Active changes in pulmonary vascular resistance due to changing caliber of the resistance vessels in the pulmonary vascular bed lead to changes in pulmonary blood flow. A variety of physiological and pharmacologic stimuli can cause alterations in the pulmonary resistance. The most important of these factors is alveolar hypoxia. Alveolar hypoxia causes localized pulmonary vasoconstriction referred to as hypoxic pulmonary vasoconstriction. Regional alveolar hypoxia causes localized increased vascular resistance and shunts blood toward normal lung, which improves ventilation/perfusion ($\dot{V}/\dot{Q}$) mismatch. Increased pulmonary blood flow in children with congenital heart defects (left-to-right shunts) and in children with systemic arteriovenous malformations leads to pulmonary vasoconstriction and can ultimately lead to irreversible changes in the pulmonary vascular bed and progressive pulmonary vascular disease.

Alterations in Respiratory Physiology in Congenital Heart Disease

Increased pulmonary blood flow is the physiological sequela of congenital cardiac lesions associated with left-to-right intracardiac shunts. These left-to-right shunts are most commonly seen in non-cyanotic defects (ventricular septal defect, patent ductus arteriosus, atrioventricular canal defects, atrial septal defect). However, certain cyanotic defects may have increased pulmonary blood flow as well as right-to-left shunt (truncus arteriosus, transposition, total anomalous pulmonary venous return, single ventricle with unrestricted pulmonary blood flow). The respiratory derangements seen in these patients are secondary to a combination of excessive pulmonary blood volume and increased pulmonary vascular pressures. Systemic arteriovenous malformations are a special case of a non-cardiac congenital defect that produces increased pulmonary blood flow and pulmonary hypertension, particularly in neonates.

Increased pulmonary blood volume results in perfusion in excess of ventilation and a $\dot{V}/\dot{Q}$ inequality. When alveolar ventilation is inadequate for pulmonary blood flow, partial pressure of oxygen (Pao_2) falls and hypoxia occurs. Increased pulmonary blood volume also causes increased lung weight leading to alterations in pulmonary mechanics. Increased lung weight and hypertensive pulmonary arteries lead to decreased lung compliance. Increased pulmonary blood flow increases pulmonary arteriolar, capillary, and venous pressures. These conditions favor the development of increased extravascular fluid. This along with alveolar atelectasis, often seen due to the concomitant cardiomegaly, causes a loss of lung volume, a reduction in lung compliance, and a decrease in tidal volume and a compensatory increase in respiratory frequency.

With spontaneous respiration the hypertensive pulmonary arteries in patients with left-to-right shunts, in combination with less compliant pulmonary parenchyma, results in stenting of the lungs, which in turn requires more respiratory effort to produce an effective lung inflation. A secondary effect of this reduction in pulmonary compliance is the need for increased airway pressure to generate adequate lung volume in patients on mechanical ventilation.

Clinical and Laboratory Findings

Lesions Associated With Decreased Pulmonary Blood Flow

Right-to-left shunts due to cyanotic heart disease associated with decreased pulmonary blood flow have almost diametrically opposite effects on respiratory mechanics when compared with lesions with increased pulmonary blood flow. Cyanosis in certain cyanotic defects (pulmonary atresia, critical pulmonary stenosis, tetralogy of Fallot, single ventricle with pulmonary stenosis) results from a combination of obstruction to pulmonary blood flow and an intracardiac defect that permits right-to-left shunting. Decreased pulmonary flow results in a decreased lung weight, improved lung compliance, and alterations in $\dot{V}/\dot{Q}$ matching.[2] Physiological dead space increases due to ventilation of underperfused lung. The extent of the $\dot{V}/\dot{Q}$ mismatch directly correlates with the level of hypoxia.[3] The increase in dead space leads to compensatory mechanisms, which include an increase in minute ventilation and a reduction in arterial carbon dioxide. The magnitude of the increase in minute ventilation correlates inversely with the magnitude of the reduction in Pao_2. Thus the acutely hypoxic newborn with decreased pulmonary blood flow typically has effortless tachypnea and cyanosis both due to increased physiological dead space and stimulation of hypoxia pulmonary drive.[4]

In contrast, it is well known that chronic hypoxia as seen in children with palliated or uncorrected cyanotic heart disease blunts the respiratory responses to acute hypoxia. These findings may explain the further oxygen desaturation seen during sleep in some of these patients.[5] Loss of normal compensatory responses to hypoxic stimuli may also account for the devastating effects of pulmonary infection in these patients.

Airway Compression With Congenital Heart Disease

Vascular compression of the airway in children is usually caused either by congenital anomalies of the great vessels (vascular rings, vascular slings) or enlargement of otherwise normal structures (see Chapter 14). Both large and small airway obstruction can occur in patients with increased pulmonary blood flow. Small airway obstruction results either from intrinsic narrowing of the airways due to fluid collecting in the lumen or extrinsic obstruction from either interstitial edema or dilatation of the pulmonary vessels.[2]

Increased pulmonary blood flow combined with pulmonary arterial hypertension causes dilatation of the pulmonary arteries and the left atrium, which predisposes to large airway compression and, consequently, air trapping[6] or atelectasis. The latter is most commonly observed in the left lower lobe, followed by the left upper lobe bronchus as the left main bronchus is entrapped and compressed between an enlarged, hypertensive left pulmonary artery and the left atrium. The left bronchus is normally hyparterial (ie, located below the pulmonary artery) while the right is eparterial and courses above the artery, thus being much less prone to compression.

Large airway obstruction results in restriction to airflow, primarily during expiration. When obstruction is severe inspiration may also be compromised. Gas trapping occurs, chest radiographs demonstrate increased lung volumes, and studies of respiratory mechanics show abnormalities of expiratory flow and increased airway resistance. A rare variant of tetralogy of Fallot, tetralogy of Fallot with absent pulmonary valve, produces airway obstruction of both large and small airways leading to lobar collapse, bronchial obstruction with air trapping, and often severe distress. Paradoxically, symptoms related to the congenital heart defect in these infants are uncommon.

A combination of imaging techniques is usually required for a full assessment of airway compression in a child with congenital heart disease. The historical approach was to perform chest radiography and a barium esophagram to evaluate children with suspected extrinsic compression of the airway. These investigations, while sufficient for diagnosis and treatment in the past, do not delineate precise anatomical details and in most centers have been replaced by multi-slice computed tomography or magnetic resonance imaging. These can also be used to demonstrate not only vascular anomaly but also the relationship of vascular structures to the airway and airway caliber.

Often the abnormalities of pulmonary function and respiratory mechanics can be reversed with surgical correction of the vascular anomalies and other cardiac causes of airway compression. However, long-standing extrinsic airway compression may lead to tracheobronchomalacia, which may persist even after correction of the cardiac defect. Therapy should be directed at reversing the underlying cardiac lesion, as surgical interventions aimed at the airway, such as aortopexy and stenting of airways, offer temporary relief or are often unsuccessful.

Eisenmenger Syndrome and Pulmonary Vascular Disease

Heath and Edwards[7] described pulmonary vascular disease, which when progressive and severe leads to pulmonary hypertension and ultimately right ventricular failure. One of the most common causes of pulmonary vascular disease is the result of prolonged left-to-right shunting. This usually follows a period of decreased resistance and high pulmonary blood flow but may rarely occur in patients who never have clinical features associated with a large left-to-right shunt, namely tachypnea, tachycardia, poor feeding, and failure to thrive. Paradoxically, clinical signs of congestive heart failure improve with increasing pulmonary vascular resistance. This is followed by the appearance of cyanosis and progressively oligemic lung fields. Although now rare due to early diagnosis and treatment of congenital heart disease, Eisenmenger syndrome results when an unrestricted and large left-to-right shunt leads to irreversible pulmonary vascular disease and subsequent right-to-left shunt.[8]

Pulmonary vascular disease may also develop due to congenital heart defects causing increased pulmonary venous pressure, such as congenital mitral stenosis, cor triatriatum, and pulmonary venous stenosis. Lastly, there are certain cyanotic congenital cardiac defects associated with pulmonary hypertension and, if uncorrected, with pulmonary vascular disease. These include pulmonary atresia with ventricular septal defect and unrestricted flow through aortopulmonary collaterals, as well as truncus arteriosus.

Pulmonary Artery Hypertension

Pulmonary artery hypertension (PAH) is defined as an elevated mean pulmonary arterial pressure of greater than 25 mm Hg at rest or 30 mm Hg during exercise.[9] Pulmonary artery hypertension may occur in the absence of congenital heart disease and has been traditionally classified according to the presence or absence of an identifiable underlying cause into primary or secondary PAH. It is now recommended that PAH be classified as idiopathic, familial, or PAH related to risk factors and associated conditions.

Idiopathic Pulmonary Artery Hypertension

Idiopathic PAH previously was referred to as primary pulmonary hypertension. The World Health Organization conference in 2003 reclassified pulmonary hypertension as shown in Box 39-1.[10] Signs and symptoms appear late in the clinical course of patients with pulmonary hypertension complicating congenital heart disease. As mentioned previously, when pulmonary vascular disease complicates pulmonary overcirculation, signs of congestive heart failure improve as the degree of left-to-right shunt diminishes. Months to years later, poor growth and cyanosis become apparent. The symptoms are nonspecific and listed in Box 39-2.

Box 39-1. Classification of Pulmonary Hypertension[a]

(Group 1) Pulmonary Artery Hypertension

(1.1) Idiopathic pulmonary hypertension
(1.2) Familial
(1.3) Pulmonary hypertension associated with the following:
- (a) Collagen vascular disease
- (b) Congenital heart disease with left-to-right shunt
- (c) Portal hypertension
- (d) Human immunodeficiency virus infection
- (e) Drugs (anorexigens or other toxins)
- (f) Thyroid disorders
- (g) Other entities (Gaucher disease, hereditary hemorrhagic telangiectasia, hemoglobinopathies)

(1.4) Persistent pulmonary hypertension of the newborn
(1.5) Pulmonary veno-occlusive disease

(Group 2) Pulmonary Hypertension With Left Heart Disease

(2.1) Left atrial or left ventricular disease
(2.2) Left-sided valvular disease

(Group 3) Pulmonary Hypertension Associated With Respiratory Disorders and/or Hypoxemia

(3.1) Chronic obstructive lung disease
(3.2) Interstitial lung disease
(3.3) Sleep-disordered breathing
(3.4) Alveolar hypoventilation
(3.5) Chronic exposure to high altitude
(3.6) Neonatal lung disease
(3.7) Alveolar-capillary dysplasia
(3.8) Other

(Group 4) Pulmonary Hypertension Due to Chronic Thrombotic/Embolic Disease

(4.1) Thrombotic obstruction of proximal pulmonary arteries
(4.2) Obstruction of distal pulmonary arteries
Pulmonary embolism (thrombus, tumor, parasites)
In situ thrombosis

(Group 5) Miscellaneous (eg, sarcoid)

[a]Adapted from Simonneau G, Galié N, Rubin LJ, et al. Clinical classification of pulmonary hypertension. *J Am Coll Cardiol.* 2004;43(12 suppl S): 5S–12S, with permission from Elsevier.

Box 39-2. Symptoms of Idiopathic Pulmonary Artery Hypertension

Poor appetite	Nausea	Lethargy	Tachypnea
Poor growth	Vomiting	Sweating	Tachycardia

Typically the pulmonic component of the second heart sound is accentuated. A right ventricular heave with or without chest wall distortion may be noted as a result of right ventricular hypertrophy and/or dysfunction. Tricuspid regurgitation is common. If infants have a patent foramen ovale, they may also present with cyanosis either at rest or with exercise because of a concomitant right-to-left shunt. In infants and children without the atrial level "pop-off," syncope can be a presenting symptom that is somewhat ominous. Older children and adolescents tend to present with exertional dyspnea and chest pain. Clinical signs of right heart failure, such as hepatomegaly, peripheral edema, and acrocyanosis, are rare in infants but can be observed in older children and adults.

Electrocardiographic features of right ventricular hypertrophy, which accompanies progressive pulmonary vascular disease, may be difficult to recognize in the presence of preexisting electrocardiographic changes.

Initially, the chest radiographs of patients with large ventricular septal defects and congestive heart failure demonstrate a large heart with increased pulmonary vascular markings. A decrease in vascular engorgement and decrease in cardiomegaly occur as pulmonary vascular disease worsens. Severe pulmonary hypertension is characterized by an enlarged main pulmonary artery segment and diminished pulmonary vascularity. Echocardiography can be used to confirm a clinical suspicion of pulmonary hypertension and evaluate right ventricular function. The most direct estimate of pulmonary artery pressure is obtained by the velocity of the tricuspid regurgitation jet. The peak velocity of the tricuspid regurgitation jet is proportional to the right ventricular to right atrial pressure. In addition there are other indirect observations that can suggest the presence of pulmonary hypertension, such as flattening of the interventricular septum and right ventricular hypertrophy.

The definitive test for evaluation of a patient with advanced pulmonary hypertension is cardiac catheterization. Cardiac catheterization can be used to determine the severity of pulmonary hypertension and test the response to vasodilators. Though cardiac catheterization is regarded as the gold standard, presence of sedation, hypoventilation, and hypoxia may change the pulmonary vascular resistance. Thus measurements obtained in the cardiac catheterization laboratory may not reflect the pulmonary vascular resistance in actual circumstances. Lastly, cardiac catheterization in the presence of advanced pulmonary vascular disease is associated with a higher risk of morbidity and mortality.

Evaluation of pulmonary vascular structure in lung biopsy specimens can provide important information, especially in preoperative patients. The Heath–Edwards Classification describes 6 grades of changes seen in patients with pulmonary hypertension.[7] These changes range from medial hypertrophy in stage I to formation of angiomatoid lesions and fibrinoid necrosis in stage VI, which convert the lung to a stiff mesh-like organ. It is believed that pulmonary vascular changes of grades I and II severity are reversible, whereas more advanced changes indicate that pulmonary vascular disease will persist or worsen following correction of the underlying lesion. However, in practice, biopsy is rarely performed, in part due to the nonuniform nature of pulmonary vascular disease and in part due to lack of widespread expertise in preparing and interpreting pulmonary vascular changes. Catheterization with assessment of pulmonary vascular reactivity is the procedure of choice in assessing the potential reversibility of pulmonary vascular disease.

Pulmonary Hypertension Secondary to Pulmonary Disease

The major causes of secondary PAH associated with pulmonary disease are cystic fibrosis; chronic obstructive pulmonary diseases, including bronchopulmonary dysplasia; and interstitial lung diseases. The pathophysiology varies, but the common factors include chronic hypoxia with resulting vasoconstrition and muscular arteriolar hypertrophy. The hypertrophy is initially reversible if the underlying condition, especially the hypoxia related to this condition, is remediable. Nighttime-induced hypoxia may be unrecognized in the above-mentioned conditions and adds an additional etiology that is obstructive sleep apnea.

Prognosis

The prognosis for patients with all forms of pulmonary hypertension has improved in the era of targeted medical therapy. In the most recent report from the UK Pulmonary Hypertension Service, survival rates for secondary forms of pulmonary hypertension were 92.3%, 83.8%, and 56.9% at 1, 3, and 5 years, respectively.[11] The best outcomes were seen with Eisenmenger syndrome, with a 5-year predicted survival of 95.3%, while the worst were patients with postoperative congenital heart disease, of whom 23% died.

Surgical Treatment of Pulmonary Hypertension

The recognition and management of pulmonary hypertension is important both preoperatively and postoperatively. In most cases, early repair of the underlying lesion will prevent development of pulmonary vascular disease; however, in some cases pulmonary hypertension may persist and progress to pulmonary vascular disease despite appropriate and timely interventions. This process seems to be accelerated at high altitudes and in patients with Down syndrome. The timing and selection of patients for surgical repair is of utmost importance, as intervention may be futile and counterproductive if advanced vascular disease is present. The availability of medical therapy, including epoprostenol, bosentan, sildenafil, and others, increases the possibility for surgical repair of defects in children who previously would not have been candidates for surgery.

Medical Treatment of Pulmonary Hypertension

The histopathologic and pathobiological changes seen in patients with pulmonary hypertension associated with congenital heart disease are similar to those seen in idiopathic or secondary forms of pulmonary hypertension. Thus similar treatment strategies have empirically been adopted and are only recently being validated by clinical trials.[4] General measures include recommendations for limitation of physical activity, prevention of pregnancy, and aggressive treatment of infections.

Phlebotomies are only recommended when symptomatic hyperviscosity occurs, usually in the presence of a hematocrit greater than 65%. The use of supplemental oxygen is controversial and it should only be used when consistent improvement in arterial saturations has been demonstrated. Oral anticoagulation with warfarin is cautiously used in patients with careful monitoring for hemoptysis. For patients who demonstrate reactivity at catheterization, the use of calcium channel blocking agents and other agents discussed below may be effective in lowering pulmonary artery pressure.

Three classes of drugs targeting the endothelial dysfunction of the pulmonary vasculature are currently approved for use in this patient population: (1) prostacyclin analogs, (2) endothelin receptors antagonists, and (3) phosphodiesterase inhibitors. The efficacy and safety of these drugs have been demonstrated in small nonrandomized uncontrolled studies.[8,9,12] Patients being treated for pulmonary hypertension should be followed by specialists in cardiology or pulmonology. Finally, in patients unresponsive to medical management who have less than 50% predicted 2-year survival, the option of last resort is lung or heart-lung transplantation combined with repair of the heart defect.

Special Considerations for Children With Congenital Heart Disease

Children with congenital heart disease represent a high-risk group for viral respiratory infections. The complex risk factors include altered cardiorespiratory status at baseline, altered pulmonary mechanics, potential cyanosis with or without pulmonary hypertension, and $\dot{V}/\dot{Q}$ mismatch, which have been discussed previously. All of these factors exacerbate the adverse effects of respiratory disease and blunt normal compensatory mechanisms. A recent epidemiological review of respiratory infections in children younger than 24 months with significant congenital heart disease demonstrated a 10.4% incidence of hospitalization.[13] Risk factors for hospitalization (in order of decreasing odds ratio) include presence of 22q11 deletion, weight below the 10th percentile for age, previous respiratory infections, incomplete prophylaxis against respiratory syncytial virus (RSV), recent cardiopulmonary bypass, trisomy 21, and siblings younger than 11 years. In the first report of children with congenital heart disease and RSV, a 37% mortality was noted, with a 73% mortality in patients with pulmonary hypertension.[14] More recent studies have noted an improvement in survival, with mortality rates of 2.5% to 3.6%.[15,16] Morbidity remains high, with about 30% requiring intensive care unit admission and prolonged mechanical ventilation. Improved outcomes have been attributed to early repair of hemodynamically significant lesions and, more recently, use of palivizumab for immunoprophylaxis. A large, multicenter, international clinical trial of immunoprophylaxis in infants with congenital heart disease demonstrated a reduction in hospitalization by 45% when compared with the placebo group.[17] The investigators concluded that monthly palivizumab prophylaxis is safe and effective in children with serious congenital heart disease. The current American Academy of Pediatrics (AAP) guidelines recommend that monthly palivizumab prophylaxis is indicated for children younger than 24 months with significant heart disease.[18] Patients most likely to benefit are those with moderate to severe pulmonary hypertension, congestive heart failure, and cyanosis. Other anti-RSV antibodies, subunit, live–attenuated and recombinant virus, and polypeptide vaccines are in clinical trials and have the potential for increasing protection in this vulnerable patient population.[19]

The only antiviral agent approved for treatment of RSV infection is ribavirin.[20] It is expensive and cumbersome to deliver in a spontaneously breathing patient and has potential health risks for caregivers, therefore its use is restricted to the highest-risk patients. Moreover, studies have documented marginal benefit, if any, for most patients. Nevertheless, the AAP recommends that ribavirin may be considered for use in highly selected situations involving documented RSV bronchiolitis with severe disease or in those who are at risk for severe disease (eg, immunocompromised or hemodynamically significant cardiopulmonary disease).[21] Other respiratory infections, even if trivial, should be treated symptomatically with close follow-up and early hospitalization if indicated in this patient population.

Key Points

- The cardiac and respiratory system function as one unit, and pulmonary manifestations occur in most patients with congenital heart disease.
- Pulmonary blood flow is dependent on both cardiac output and pulmonary vascular resistance.
- Increased pulmonary blood flow and pulmonary hypertension are seen in many forms of congenital heart disease with left-to-right shunts and are a cause of impairment of lung mechanics.
- Pulmonary vascular disease is the end result of severe pulmonary hypertension and carries a high mortality and morbidity.
- Newer treatment strategies for pulmonary hypertension, such as prostacyclin analogues, endothelial receptor antagonists, and phosphodiesterase inhibitors, have shown good short-term results.
- Infections with respiratory viruses, especially RSV, can be devastating in children with congenital heart disease; appropriate prophylaxis with palivizumab is important in this patient population to reduce morbidity and mortality.

References

1. Morrow WR. Aortic arch and pulmonary artery anomalies. In: Oski FA, DeAngelis C, Feigin RD, eds. *Principals and Practice of Pediatrics.* 4th ed. Philadelphia, PA: Lippincott Company; 2006
2. Davies CJ, Cooper SG, Fletcher ME, et al. Total respiratory compliance in infants and children with congenital heart disease. *Pediatr Pulmonol.* 1990;9:196
3. Fletcher R. Relationship between alveolar dead space and arterial oxygenation in children with congenital cardiac disease. *Br J Anesth.* 1989;62:168–176
4. Tissot C, Ivy DD, Beghetti M. Medical therapy for pediatric pulmonary arterial hypertension. *J Pediatr.* 2010;157(4):528–532
5. Hiatt PW, Mahoney L, Tepper RS. Oxygen desaturation during sleep in infants and young children with congenital heart disease. *J Pediatr.* 1992;121:226–232
6. Wetzel RC, Herold CJ, Zerhouni EA, Robotham JL. Intravascular volume loading reversibly decreases airway cross-sectional area. *Chest.* 1993;103:865–870
7. Heath D, Edwards JE. The pathology of hypertensive pulmonary vascular disease. *Circulation.* 1958;18:533–537
8. Barst RJ, Maislin G, Fishman AP. Vasodilator therapy for primary pulmonary hypertension in children. *Circulation.* 1999;99:1197–1208
9. Humpl T, Reyes JT, Holtby H, Stephens D, Adatia I. Beneficial effect of oral sildenafil therapy on childhood pulmonary arterial hypertension: twelve-month clinical trial of a single drug, open-label, pilot study. *Circulation.* 2005;111:3274–3280
10. Simonneau G, Galié N, Rubin LJ, et al. Clinical classification of pulmonary hypertension. *J Am Coll Cardiol.* 2004;43(12 suppl S): 5S–12S
11. Haworth SG, Hislop AA. Treatment and survival in children with pulmonary arterial hypertension: The UK Pulmonary Hypertension Service for Children 2001–2006. *Heart.* 2009;95:312–317
12. Barst RJ, Ivy D, Dingemanse J, et al. Pharmacokinetics, safety, and efficacy of bosentan in pediatric patients with pulmonary arterial hypertension. *Clin Pharmacol Ther.* 2003;73:372–382
13. Medrano C, Garcia-Guereta L, Grueso J, et al. Respiratory infection in congenital cardiac disease. Hospitalizations in young children in Spain during 2004 and 2005: the CIVIC Epidemiologic Study. *Cardiol Young.* 2007;17:360–371
14. MacDonald NE, Hall CB, Suffin SC Alexson C, Harris PJ, Manning JA. Respiratory syncytial virus infection in infants with congenital heart disease. *N Engl J Med.* 1982;307:397–400

15. Wang EE, Law BJ, Stephens D. Pediatric Investigator Collaborative Network on Infections in Canada (PICNIC) prospective study of risk factors and outcomes in patients hospitalized with respiratory syncytial viral lower respiratory tract infection. *J Pediatr.* 1995;26:212–219
16. Navas L, Wang E, de Carvalho V, Robinson J. Improved outcome of respiratory syncytial virus in high-risk hospitalized population of Canadian children. *J Pediatr.* 1992;121:348–354
17. Feltes TF, Cabalka AK, Meissner HC, et al. Palivizumab prophylaxis reduces hospitalizations due to respiratory syncytial virus in young children with hemodynamically significant congenital heart disease. *J Pediatr.* 2003;143:532–540
18. American Academy of Pediatrics Subcommittee on Diagnosis and Management of Bronchiolitis. Diagnosis and management of bronchiolitis. *Pediatrics.* 2006;118:1774–1793
19. Venkatesh MP, Weisman LE. Prevention and treatment of respiratory syncytial virus infection in infants: an update. *Expert Rev Vaccines.* 2006;5(2):261–268
20. Chen CH, Lin YT, Yang YH, et al. Ribavirin for respiratory syncytial virus bronchiolitis reduced the risk of asthma and allergen sensitization. *Pediatr Allergy Immunol.* 2008;19:166–172
21. American Academy of Pediatrics. Respiratory syncytial virus. In: Pickering LK, Baker CJ, Kimberlin DW, Long SS, eds. *Red Book: 2009 Report of the Committee on Infectious Diseases.* 28th ed. Elk Grove Village, IL: American Academy of Pediatrics; 2009:562

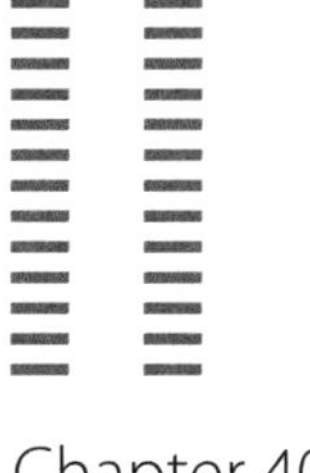

Chapter 40

Lung Disease Associated With Endocrine Disorders

Martin B. Draznin, MD

Case Report 40-1

A 14-year-old female with a 5-year history of type 1 diabetes mellitus is evaluated in the office for shortness of breath with exercise that has worsened over the last year and is beginning to interfere with her sports activities. A trial of a short-acting bronchodilator before exercise has been only partially helpful. Complete pulmonary function testing (PFT) is ordered and the girl is referred to the pediatric pulmonologist for evaluation. Findings on PFT include a slight reduction in forced vital capacity (FVC) and forced expiratory volume in 1 second (FEV_1) (minimally reversed with a short-acting bronchodilator), increased residual volume, and slightly decreased single breath carbon monoxide (CO) diffusion capacity when corrected for alveolar volume. The parents ask several questions, including, "Is this common in kids with diabetes? Is this progressive? Can her shortness of breath be improved with better control of blood glucose?"

Introduction

Endocrine disorders may lead to pulmonary disease (Table 40-1). Thyroid disorders may affect pulmonary function at the level of respiratory drive; parathyroid disorders may lead either to tetany with attendant laryngospasm or to muscle weakness from hypercalcemia. Diabetes has considerable effect on lung structure and function, although pituitary, adrenal, and reproductive disorders have little effect on lung function.[1]

Table 40-1. Examples of Pulmonary Effects of Endocrine Disorders

Endocrine Disorder	Pulmonary Effect	Clinical Significance
Hypothyroidism	Diminished respiratory drive	Usually subclinical, reversible with treatment
	Pleural or pericardial effusion	Usually subclinical and reversible, can be severe
Hyperthyroidism	Increased respiratory drive	Usually subclinical, reversible with treatment
Thiourea drugs for hyperthyroidism	Diffuse alveolar hemorrhage	Life-threatening, prolonged supportive care needed
Hypercalcemia due to hyperparathyroidism	Pulmonary calcinosis with respiratory failure	Can be severe, symptoms reversible, lung changes partly reversible
Hypocalcemia	Stridor due to tetany	Reversible with therapy
Growth hormone deficiency	Diminished lung volumes and respiratory pressures	Treatable with appropriate dose of growth hormone for appropriate duration
Diabetes	Restrictive lung disease Vascular disease Autonomic nerve function Oxidative stress	All are subclinical, may be present at diagnosis, might manifest at high altitude, in presence of chronic lung disease

Thyroid Diseases

A pair-controlled study of hyperthyroid adults, in which various respiratory parameters were measured, provides a comparison between function in the hyperthyroid state versus that posttreatment in the euthyroid state. The authors concluded that there is a significant and direct relationship between thyroid hormone levels and both an increase in the central inspiratory drive and responsivity to carbon dioxide (CO_2) levels.[2] Clinically, what is seen more often in children is rapid breathing with complaints of shortness of breath and exercise intolerance. The usual assumption is that the exercise intolerance is related to tachycardia due to enhanced adrenergic sensitivity. Associated findings are myopathic weakening of respiratory muscles, increased oxygen uptake in the hyperthyroid state, and lower resting arterial CO_2 tension. These changes may not have clinical significance for hyperthyroid children and youth as they are routinely advised to avoid strenuous exercise until their thyroid hormone levels have normalized, resting heart rates are normal, and beta-blocking agents are no longer needed.

In hypothyroidism there is reduced respiratory drive[3]; however, the clinical risk seems mostly theoretical as hypothyroid children tend to be much less active than euthyroid children, and do not push their physical limits. While pediatric endocrinologists routinely see hypothyroid patients present with subcutaneous myxedema, pleural or pericardial effusion is uncommon in the pediatric population. Even when the physical findings are very evident, with diminished breath or heart sounds, the children are, for the most part, asymptomatic.

A report of hypothyroidism leading to severe pericardial tamponade presenting with respiratory distress and anasarca shows that severe compromise is indeed possible.[4] Permanent changes in pulmonary function and structure do not seem to be a consequence of thyroid disorders because treatment results in clearance of the effusion with return to full exercise capacity. Common agents used to treat hyperthyroidism also carry potential pulmonary and cardiovascular risk. Diffuse alveolar hemorrhage due to antineutrophil cytoplasmic antibody positive vasculitis, while uncommon, is a reported complication of antithyroid agent treatment for hyperthyroidism. A recent report notes that this complication seems to be a function of the thiouracil class of agents because it occurs in patients treated with propylthiouracil as well as the patient treated with benzylthiouracil in the report.[5] The case was that of an 8-year-old girl who presented with rapidly worsening dyspnea, more than the exercise intolerance often seen in hyperthyroidism. She required intensive care, ventilator support, and potent glucocorticoid drugs, with the illness resolving after a long course.

Parathyroid Disorders

Hypercalcemia due to primary hyperparathyroidism is uncommon in infants and children. A 2-month-old infant with pulmonary calcinosis due to hyperparathyroidism presented with respiratory distress and failure to thrive.[6] Chest radiograph and radionuclide scanning demonstrated calcium deposits within lung tissue. The respiratory distress resolved when calcium levels were normalized, yet the pulmonary calcinosis did not fully resolve. Reversible respiratory muscle weakness due to the hypercalcemia would be an expected finding, anatomical changes, though, are less likely. A more severe case of pulmonary calcification from hyperparathyroidism was reported in which respiratory failure ensued requiring 40 days of ventilator support.[7] The severity was such that the patient had only partial clearing of the lung abnormalities over a 1-year period.

The respiratory disorder one would expect to be associated with hypocalcemia would be tetany leading to increased respiratory muscle tone and stridor due to vocal cord spasm. The lungs in children with rickets seem to be affected most by chest wall deformity as reported in a series of 30 infants and children from Iran. In the oldest 3 children, the findings were mild. However, in the rest, lobar or segmental atelectasis and compression atelectasis under the costochondral junctions, where the "rachitic rosary" is seen, was described. The deformity of the chest wall and resultant restrictive defect together with malnutrition results in diminished reserve and in some cases interstitial pneumonitis.[8] Treatment for chronic hypocalcemic states is routinely monitored for induction of nephrocalcinosis; it may be prudent to assess pulmonary changes.

Pituitary Disorders

Lung volume and respiratory muscle strength are diminished in those with growth hormone deficiency, which may simply be a function of small size in children. A study comparing subjects with adult onset growth hormone deficiency, adults with childhood onset growth hormone deficiency, and healthy adults showed a reduction of maximal inspiratory and expiratory mouth pressures as well as a reduction of total lung capacity, vital capacity, and functional residual capacity in those with childhood onset.[9] These findings were in a setting where the subjects had an average of 9 years of growth hormone treatment during childhood and the studies were done an average of 4 years after cessation of treatment. The adult onset of growth hormone deficiency was not associated with deficiencies of lung volume, and only the expiratory pressure was diminished prior to treatment with growth hormone. While the volumes did not change on treatment in the adult subjects, the pressures did normalize. After 12 months of treatment, the childhood onset subjects had improvement in pressures and volumes such that they were no longer statistically different from controls. One explanation given for these findings is the possibility that patients with childhood onset had received insufficient growth hormone replacement. At the time of the study, the dose of human growth hormone used for children in most of Europe was considerably lower than that used in the United States.

Acromegaly is a disease of adults, and pituitary gigantism in children is quite rare. Contemporary information about pulmonary function in children with growth hormone excess is lacking.

Cushing syndrome is a consequence of excess exposure to exogenous or endogenous corticosteroids. Patients with Cushing syndrome were studied for lung volumes.[10] In the adults suffering from endogenous hypercortisolism there were no disturbances of lung volume or ventilatory performance. This is in contrast to the myopathic changes in ventilatory muscles seen in experimental animals and adult humans treated with high doses of corticosteroids for chronic obstructive pulmonary disease. Current pediatric studies are not available.

Diabetes Mellitus

Children with diabetes are encouraged to be physically active. In those with type 2 diabetes, increased activity helps reduce insulin resistance and weight and so directly assists in the diabetes management. In children with type 1 diabetes, exercise and physical activity are encouraged to achieve fitness and maintain cardiovascular health. Diabetes clinicians do not usually hear complaints of respiratory problems other than those associated with acute infectious illnesses or chronic processes such as asthma. There are professional athletes and many more amateur athletes with diabetes who seem to have no difficulties in performing at an elite level, including a champion Olympic swimmer and a successful mountaineer who climbed the tallest peak on each of 7 continents.

There have been numerous reports of compromise of lung function due to diabetes. One study from the Netherlands, done in anticipation of safety and efficacy trials for an inhaled form of insulin, showed increased airway resistance and no correlation with duration of disease or age of the children.[11] A subsequent brief review in the diabetes literature also suggested that there were no reports of functional limitations in daily activities, yet it listed diminished lung elasticity and lung transfer of CO as findings from several studies.[12] The concern was that the studies had been small and that more systematic studies might be helpful, but the conclusion is that the lung is definitely a target organ for damage from diabetes with both microvascular and other tissue changes being likely. An Italian study of children with type 1 diabetes found FVC, FEV_1, and transfer factor for CO to be diminished compared with age-matched controls.[13] Of interest was that changes in these indices were noted at the time of diagnosis in the subset studied from onset and that, counter to expectations, the duration of diabetes and level of blood glucose control or presence of associated complications did not correlate with the degree of the changes. Again, the subjects had no clinical complaints.

A more recent review summarizes changes in pulmonary physiology from the standpoint of lung mechanics, gas exchange, autonomic function, and a newer area of interest: the pulmonary effects of oxidative stress.[14] The interesting idea that some of the changes could occur years before diabetes is diagnosed, as is true in adult type 2 diabetes, is important in children as the incidence of type 2 diabetes in youth is increasing rapidly; they are reported to accrue the other complications at a more rapid rate than adults. This larger review again notes that the changes are subclinical until unmasked by intercurrent illness, high altitude, aging, or onset of primary lung disease. Obesity, which is a nearly universal finding in type 2 diabetes when diagnosed in children and adolescents, also impacts pulmonary function. (See Chapter 34.)

When to Refer

The disorders of lung function that have been outlined are uncommon accompaniments of less than common conditions, with the exception of diabetes mellitus and hypothyroidism. It would not seem cost effective to investigate each case of dyspnea for an underlying endocrine disease. However, there are many examples of when a combined evaluation by a pediatric endocrinologist and pulmonologist would be valuable. Although rickets is less common in more well-developed countries, it is important to evaluate a stridorous, afebrile patient without an anatomical airway disorder for tetany. The changes from diabetes may not be preventable if indeed they occur prior to diagnosis, even in type 1 diabetes, and monitoring of lung function with the help of a pediatric pulmonologist is appropriate.

When to Admit

The need to hospitalize flows from the level of lung function and the necessity to treat the underlying endocrine disorder as an inpatient. The changes from lung calcification seen in hyperparathyroidism are the most severe, while the changes from diabetes seem to be subclinical in children.

Key Points

- Although not always clinically evident, endocrine disorders potentially have an effect on lung function and physiology.
- Hyper- and hypothyroidism can lead to reduced exercise tolerance, which normalizes with treatment.
- Pulmonary hemorrhage may be a complication of treatment of hyperthyroidism with thiouracil agents.
- Hypocalcemia is a non-pulmonary cause of stridor in infants.
- Diabetes can cause early changes in lung structure and function and, therefore, lung function monitoring in diabetes should be studied further to assess its value to patients.

References

1. Brüssel T, Matthay M, Chernow B. Pulmonary manifestations of endocrine and metabolic disorders. *Clin Chest Med.* 1989;10(4):645–653
2. Pino-Garcia JM, Garcia-Rio F, Díez JJ, et al. Regulation of breathing in hyperthyroidism: relationship to hormonal and metabolic changes. *Eur Respir J.* 1998;12:400–407
3. Cakmak G, Saler T, Sağlam ZA, et al. Spirometry in patients with clinical and subclinical hypothyroidism. *Tuberk Toraks.* 2007;55(3):266–270
4. Shastry RM, Shastry CC. Primary hypothyroidism with pericardial tamponade. *Indian J Pediatr.* 2007;74(6):580–581
5. Thabet F, Sghiri R, Tabarki B, et al. ANCA-associated diffuse alveolar hemorrhage due to benzylthiouracil. *Eur J Pediatr.* 2006;165:435–436
6. Topalaglu A, Yuksel B, Tuncer R, et al. Primary hyperparathyroidism in an infant with three parathyroid glands and pulmonary calcinosis. *J Pediatr Endocrinol Metab.* 2001;14:1173–1175
7. Poddar B, Bharti S, Parmar VR, et al. Images in pediatrics: respiratory failure due to pulmonary calcification in primary hyperparathyroidism. *Arch Dis Child.* 2002;87:257
8. Khajavi A, Amirhakimi MD. The rachitic lung. *Clin Pediatr.* 1977;16(1):36–38

9. Merola B, Longobardi S, Sofia M, et al. Lung volumes and respiratory muscle strength in adult patients with childhood- or adult-onset growth hormone deficiency: effect of 12 months' growth hormone replacement therapy. *Eur J Endocrinol.* 1996;135:553–558
10. Azezli AD, Bayraktaroglu T, Ece T, et al. Static lung volumes in patients with Cushing's disease. *Exp Clin Endocrinol Diabetes.* 2008;116(1):53–57
11. Van Gent R, Brackel HJL, De Vroede M, et al. Lung function abnormalities in children with type I diabetes. *Respir Med.* 2000;96:976–978
12. Goldman M. Lung dysfunction in diabetes. *Diabetes Care.* 2003;6:1915–1918
13. Cazzato S, Bernard F, Salardi S, et al. Lung function in children with diabetes mellitus. *Pediatr Pulmonol.* 2004;37:17–23
14. Kaparianos A, Argyropoulou E, Sampsonas F, et al. Pulmonary complications in diabetes mellitus. *Chron Respir Dis.* 2008;5:101–108

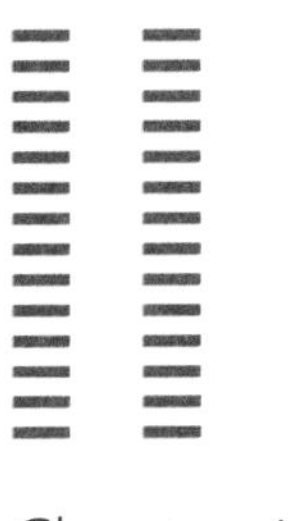

Chapter 41

Pulmonary Complications of Gastrointestinal Diseases

Sebnem Ozdogan, MD
Edward Fong, MD

Introduction

The interactions between the different organ systems in the body usually occur very smoothly, allowing the body to function without any problems. However, these interactions can be very complex and what starts out as a minor problem in a seemingly unrelated organ system may blossom into a major morbidity in another organ system. The interaction of the gastrointestinal (GI) system does have a role, sometimes controversial to its extent, in causing morbidity in the pulmonary system. The role the GI system can have on the pulmonary system will be discussed in this chapter. Aspiration syndromes are presented in Chapter 31.

Gastroesophageal Reflux (GER)

Pathogenesis of GER

Despite a strong association between GER and chronic respiratory disease, the mechanism by which GER precipitates respiratory illness remains incompletely understood. Gastroesophageal reflux is usually caused by transient lower esophageal sphincter (LES) relaxation. Other mechanisms include a low resting LES pressure and increased intragastric pressure. Increased intra-abdominal pressure due to coughing raises the gastroesophageal pressure gradient and increases the risk of reflux; the presence of a hiatal hernia will also increase the risk of reflux.

Clinical Manifestations

The most common respiratory symptoms of GER are wheezing and nighttime coughing (Box 41-1). However, the particular presenting symptoms may be age dependent.[1]

Infants

Gastroesophageal reflux is common in infants and is usually not pathological. Regurgitation is present in 50% to 70% of all infants, peaks at age 4 months, and typically resolves by 1 year of age (physiological GER), and there is a weak association with later development of GER disease (GERD). Infants and children with an absent or blunted cough reflex may present with silent aspiration and have findings of only increased respiratory mucus, chronic wheeze, recurrent bronchitis, or recurrent pneumonia. Others with an active cough reflex may present with cough associated with meals or sometimes only with chronic cough. A small group of infants may develop other symptoms, including feeding refusal, irritability, hematemesis, anemia, and failure to thrive.

Box 41-1. Clinical Findings in Gastroesophageal Reflux[a]

Frequent	Common	Uncommon
Cough (nocturnal)	Apnea	Hoarseness
Gagging	Acute life-threatening event	Hematemesis
Emesis	Failure to thrive	Anemia
Feeding resistance	Stridor	Pulmonary fibrosis
Wheezing	Abnormal head, neck, and thorax positioning (Sandifer syndrome)	
Recurrent bronchitis/ pneumonia		

Preschool

Preschool-aged children with GERD may present with intermittent regurgitation and less commonly with respiratory complications, including persistent wheezing. Abnormal hyperextension of the neck from torticollis (Sandifer syndrome) also has been described in developmentally delayed children with more severe GERD. Young children with GERD and swallowing difficulty may present with only decreased food intake without any other complaints.

Older Children and Adolescents

After infancy and preschool age, more classic symptoms of esophagitis, including chronic heartburn, nausea, dysphagia, odynophagia, and/or epigastric pain, predominate. Complications of GERD, including esophagitis, strictures, Barrett esophagus, and hoarseness due to reflux laryngitis, also may be seen.

Pulmonary Disorders Associated With GER

Apnea or Apparent Life-threatening Event (ALTE)

In patients with ALTEs, recurrent regurgitation or emesis is common. However, investigations in patients with ALTEs have not demonstrated a convincing relationship between GER and apnea or bradycardia. However, in patients with frequent ALTE episodes in which the role of GER is uncertain, esophageal pH or impedance monitoring with simultaneous measurement of respiration and chest wall movement may be useful to determine if there is a temporal association of acid or nonacid reflux with ALTE. The North American Society for Pediatric Gastroenterology and Nutrition recommends that infants with ALTE and GER may be more likely to respond to anti-reflux therapy when there is gross emesis or oral regurgitation at the time of the ALTE than when episodes occur in the awake infant, and when the ALTE is characterized by obstructive apnea.[1]

Asthma

Symptoms of GER are common in asthma. Its prevalence is estimated to range between 34% to 89%. However, it is not entirely clear which condition causes the other or whether they are both due to common factors. In patients where symptoms of asthma and GER coexist as well as those individuals with chronic vomiting or regurgitation and recurrent episodes of cough or wheezing, a 3-month empiric trial of vigorous acid suppressant therapy for GER has been recommended.[2] In patients with nocturnal asthma symptoms more than once a week; radiographic evidence of recurrent pneumonia; requiring either continuous oral corticosteroids, high-dose inhaled corticosteroids, frequent bursts of oral corticosteroids (>2 per year); or those with persistent asthma unable to wean their medical management despite the absence of GER symptoms, esophageal pH or impedance monitoring is recommended. If esophageal or pH impedance monitoring demonstrates an increased frequency or duration of esophageal acid exposure or nonacid reflux, a trial of prolonged medical therapy for GER is recommended.

Diagnosis

Establishing the diagnosis of GER presents a very difficult task in many cases. In most infants with vomiting, and in most older children with regurgitation and heartburn, a history and physical examination are sufficient to reliably diagnose GER, recognize complications, and initiate empiric medical management.

Empiric Medical Therapy

A trial of time-limited medical therapy for GER is useful to determine if GER is causing specific symptoms. Empiric therapy is widely used but has not been validated for any symptom presentation in pediatric patients.

Upper Gastrointestinal (UGI) Series and Modified Barium Swallow (MBS) Study

The UGI series and MBS study are used to evaluate for anatomical or physiological abnormalities of the upper GI tract, to quantify the degree of aspiration during swallowing, and to assess texture-specific food swallowing. These tests are neither sensitive nor specific in the diagnosis of GER. Since these tests only capture a particular time, a negative test does not necessarily mean that the patient does not have aspiration or GER.

Gastroesophageal Scintigraphy

Gastroesophageal scintigraphy, also referred to as a milk scan, is a radionuclide study that involves the ingestion of technetium-labeled food or formula followed by scanning to detect the distribution of the isotope in the stomach, esophagus, and lungs. If isotope is seen in the lungs this is indicative of aspiration. Unlike esophageal pH monitoring, scintigraphy can detect postprandial reflux of both acidic and nonacidic gastric contents and measure gastric emptying time. It can also assist in distinguishing between indirect versus direct aspiration, as well as demonstrating nighttime and salivary aspiration. Radiation exposure is minimal (using technetium 99m), and the test is noninvasive.

24-hour Esophageal pH Probe and Impedance Monitoring

This is considered the gold standard test for the diagnosis of GER. The test is performed by the gastroenterologist, usually in an inpatient setting. The probe is placed through the nasal cavity, and using fluoroscopy, the tip is positioned approximately at 87% of the distance from the alae to the lower esophageal sphincter. Activities, meals, position, and symptoms are recorded while the probe remains in place. Acid reflux is defined as a decrease in pH to less than or equal to 4. The frequency, overall time of esophageal exposure to acid, and longest reflux episode are recorded. It should be remembered that asymptomatic episodes of acid reflux can occur in healthy infants and children. On the other hand, esophageal pH monitoring results may be normal in some patients with GERD, particularly those with respiratory complications. Since esophageal pH monitoring does not detect nonacidic reflux, but nonacid reflux material can be aspirated and cause lung disease, multichannel intraluminal impedance and pH monitoring may be a better diagnostic evaluation. Multichannel intraluminal impedance and pH monitoring have been increasingly studied for the ability to detect anterograde and retrograde passage of acid, nonacid, and gaseous material. These studies have found that in contrast to adults, infants with GER have a much greater proportion of nonacid reflux than acid reflux.[3]

Endoscopy and Biopsy

Endoscopy with biopsy allows the advantage of directly visualizing lesions or anatomical anomalies. It can assess the presence and severity of esophagitis, strictures, and Barrett esophagus, as well as exclude other disorders, such as Crohn disease and eosinophilic or infectious esophagitis. A normal appearance of the esophagus does not exclude histopathological esophagitis since subtle mucosal changes, such as erythema and pallor, may be observed in the absence of esophagitis.

Treatment of GERD

Conservative Measures

The first line of therapy is non-medicinal. It includes smaller, more frequent meals and dietary modifications with formulas composed of medium-chain triglycerides, whey-hydrolysate, soy, or low osmolality formulas. It also includes positioning maneuvers, such as keeping the child in the 30- to 45-degree position for at least 30 minutes after feeding and placing the child horizontally in the prone position. It is not recommended that children sit at 90 degrees after feeding as studies have shown that GER worsens when sitting up after meals. This is a result of increased intra-abdominal pressure generated from bending at the waist. Milk-thickening agents do not improve acid reflux index scores but do decrease the number of episodes of vomiting.

Medical Therapy

The second line of therapy for the treatment of GERD involves medication. Cryoprotective agents, prokinetic agents, histamine-2 (H_2) receptor blockers, and proton pump inhibitors (PPIs) are all used in the control of GER.

Antacids work by neutralizing gastric acid and provide quick, short-term relief of intermittent symptoms in older children. It has been shown that if given in high doses, aluminum hydroxide is as effective as cimetidine (an H_2 blocker) for the treatment of peptic esophagitis in children 2 to 42 months of age but has toxicity at high levels.[4] Gaviscon, an over-the-counter antacid preparation of alginic acid, does not contain aluminum and may be of some benefit in infants.

The H_2 blockers work by inhibiting the histamine receptor of the parietal cells that affect acid production and have been shown to be safe and effective in treating children with GERD. They are often the first-line medical treatment in GERD.

Proton pump inhibitors are the mainstay of medical treatment of GERD. The PPIs effectively inhibit acid production by antagonizing the proton pump. Compared to H_2 blockers, PPIs decrease acid production and have longer duration of action. Because of limited experience with the use of these agents in children, PPIs are usually used after a therapeutic failure of H_2 blockers.

Adult studies have shown that PPI therapy, particularly with long-term or high-dose administration, is associated with several potential adverse effects, including enteric infections (eg, *Clostridium difficile)* and community-acquired pneumonia.[5,6]

Prokinetic agents act to increase lower esophageal sphincter pressures. However, the number of reflux episodes remains largely unchanged in patients on prokinetic agents because of transient relaxations of the lower esophageal sphincter. Metoclopramide is probably the most commonly used prokinetic agent that works as a cholinergic agonist and dopamine antagonist. Erythromycin stimulates the motilin receptor on intestinal smooth muscle cells, but is not approved by the US Food and Drug Administration as a prokinetic agent. Cisapride showed marginal improvement over placebo; however, secondary to the problems with cardiac arrhythmias and life-threatening events, cisapride was removed from the US market. The efficacy of the other prokinetic agents in children has not been proven.

The surface agents sodium alginate and sucralfate protect the mucosa of the esophagus and stomach from the damaging effects of gastric acid by forming a surface gel. There is not sufficient evidence regarding safety and efficacy of surface agents in the treatment of GERD in children.

Surgery

Surgery is the treatment of choice in children who fail maximal medical therapy. Nissen fundoplication is the most commonly used procedure by pediatric surgeons. Both open and laparoscopic techniques appear to be equally effective. Success rates vary by study but are around 75%. The most common complications include breakdown of the fundoplication, small bowel obstruction, infection, pneumonia, perforation, esophageal stricture, and obstruction. Mortality varies from 0% to 4.7%. Reoperation rates vary from 3 to 18%.[7]

Inflammatory Bowel Disease

Bronchopulmonary manifestations of inflammatory bowel disease (IBD) have been rarely described in children. Only isolated cases have been reported in the literature.[8–11] The pulmonary involvement in IBD may include airway inflammation involving both pulmonary parenchymal disease and small and large airways.

Pulmonary Parenchymal Disease

The most common lung parenchymal involvement that has been described in IBD is bronchiolitis obliterans with organizing pneumonia and interstitial lung disease. Pulmonary function testing in patients with airway involvement usually reveals an obstructive respiratory pattern. Munck et al[11] showed that 26 children with acute or quiescent Crohn disease (CD) all had normal chest radiographs. Even though no significant differences were found between acute and quiescent CD for pulmonary volumes and expiratory flows, carbon monoxide diffusing capacity was significantly decreased during the active phase of the disease as compared with remission (15%–53% versus 19%–81% predicted). This may indicate an early interstitial disease process.[12] Although pediatric reports are sparse, isolated or diffuse lung granulomas have also been noted to be associated with IBD. (See Chapter 25.) In addition, pulmonary infiltrates in the setting of immunosuppression present a diagnostic dilemma because it is not clear if the abnormalities are secondary to the immunosuppression or the underlying disease. Krishnan et al[9] reported 3 children with CD who presented with lung lesions that were unresponsive to antimicrobial therapies but responded quickly to infliximab therapy. Although an empiric trial of medication may help with diagnosis, usually a definitive diagnosis requires a lung biopsy.

Airway Inflammation

Bronchial involvement is the most common, but inflammation of the trachea and bronchioles can also occur in IBD. Patients with bronchial involvement due to IBD may have bronchiolitis, unexplained chronic bronchitis, or bronchiectasis. The pathogenesis of the pulmonary disease associated with IBD is not known. A common systemic mechanism affecting both the bronchial and colonic epithelium may be responsible. It has been reported that the incidence of respiratory changes is greater in ulcerative colitis than in CD.[13] Mansi et al[13] showed that bronchial hyperresponsiveness (BHR) occurs in 71% of children and adolescents with CD even in the absence of clinical, radiologic, and functional evidence of airway disease. This indicates that BHR may be the only representation of subclinical airway inflammation, which in turn is most likely responsible for the development of the various pulmonary manifestations in CD.[14]

Histologic similarities between the inflammatory infiltrate of the airways and that of the colon suggest that the bronchial disease may result from a common abnormality in immune regulation that affects both the bowel and the bronchial tree.[15]

Diagnosis and Treatment

Drug-induced lung disease and superimposed bacterial infection should be considered in patients with IBD who have lung involvement. If drug toxicity is suspected, the offending drug should be discontinued. In those patients with signs of airway disease and chronic purulent sputum production, superimposed bacterial infection must be ruled out. When drug toxicity and bacterial infection have been ruled out, traditional therapies for IBD, including mesalamine and other immunosuppressive agents, may be effective depending on the type of pulmonary complications.

Alpha-1 Antitrypsin Deficiency

Alpha-1 antitrypsin (AAT) deficiency is one of the most common inherited disorders among Caucasians. It is a recessively inherited condition that can cause cirrhosis, usually in childhood, and chronic obstructive pulmonary disease, which usually doesn't present until adulthood. Pulmonary symptoms typically begin in the third to fourth decade of life, but children as young as 18 months can have respiratory manifestations.[16–19]

Diagnosis

Initially, a serum AAT level is performed if this disease is suspected. If the level is low, then a confirmatory genetic test is obtained. Occasionally, in patients with both the clinical manifestations and a family history of AAT deficiency, the genetic testing is performed outright. At least 100 alleles of AAT have been identified, all of which are categorized into 4 basic groups.[20]

1. Normal—There are normal levels and functioning of AAT; genotype is MM.
2. Deficient—Plasma AAT levels are less than 35% of the average normal level. The most common deficient allele associated with emphysema is the Z allele, which is carried by 2% to 3% of the Caucasian population in the United States. This genotype is MZ.

3. Null—No detectable AAT levels in plasma; individuals are rare and have the most severe form of the disease. This genotype is ZZ.
4. Dysfunctional—Normal quantity of AAT protein, but it does not function properly.

Population studies suggest a minimum plasma threshold of 11 µmol/L (corresponding to 50–80 mg/dL, depending on the assay used) is required for proper functioning. Below this level there is insufficient AAT to protect the lung, leading to a risk of developing emphysema.

Clinical Manifestations

Symptoms include asthma, which is more severe in individuals with PI*MZ; bronchitis; panacinar emphysema, occurring primarily in the lung bases; chronic obstructive lung disease; and bronchiectasis.[21] Pulmonary disease is very rare in children.

Treatment

Treatment focuses on controlling and slowing the progression of the clinical symptoms of lung and liver disease. Weekly or monthly intravenous infusion of purified human AAT can normalize plasma and lung AAT levels, inhibit protease activity, and diminish airway reactivity. However, it has no effect on intracellular aggregation of the protein in hepatocytes. Lung and liver transplantation are end-stage measures for terminal organ dysfunction.

Alcohol and Its Effect on Lungs

Underage drinking is one of the leading public health and social problems in the United States and is the third leading cause of death among youths.[22] It has been reported that alcohol, in particular wine, appears to be a trigger for asthmatic responses. Sensitivity to the sulfite additives in wine is the likely reason for many of these reactions.[23] In addition, chronic alcohol consumption increases the risk of developing pulmonary tuberculosis, chronic bronchitis, aspiration pneumonitis, lung abscess, pulmonary complications of alcoholic cirrhosis, and pulmonary problems from alcoholic cardiomyopathy. The effects of alcohol on the respiratory system include diminished ciliary motion, decreased migration of alveolar macrophages, interference with surfactant production, and increased prevalence of oropharyngeal gram-negative bacilli. Acute respiratory distress syndrome (ARDS) is reported to occur with higher frequency in patients with a history of alcohol abuse. Recent studies showed that alcohol dependence is independently associated with sepsis, septic shock, and hospital mortality among patients in the intensive care unit.[24,25]

Pulmonary Involvement in Liver Disease

Hepatic disease may cause or be associated with pulmonary disorders without a clear understanding of etiology[26] (Table 41-1). However, acute hepatic disease associated with lung complications can result from infections, medications, and toxins. Also, chronic hepatic disease can cause pulmonary disorders through mechanisms that result in cirrhosis and liver failure, which in turn cause chronic pulmonary infection. Systemic disorders, such as AAT deficiency, chronic granulomatous disease of childhood, cystic fibrosis, hereditary hemorrhagic telangiectasia, Langerhans cell histiocytosis, and sarcoidosis, can also be associated with hepatopulmonary disease.

Hepatopulmonary syndrome (HPS), which consists of liver disease, abnormal pulmonary vascular tone, and arterial hypoxemia, is associated with chronic liver disease, most commonly cirrhosis of the liver regardless of cause. The disease mechanisms include the imbalance of vasoactive substances caused by the diseased liver, which leads to pulmonary vascular dilatations resulting in ventilation/perfusion mismatch, hypoxemia, and loss of hypoxic pulmonary vasoconstriction. As the hepatic damage progresses, the alveolar-capillary disequilibrium worsens and leads to intrapulmonary venoarterial shunting and serious limitation of oxygen diffusion and, finally, severe respiratory failure. Portopulmonary anastomoses and pulmonary arterial hypertension may also occur.[27,28] Liver transplantation for HPS in children may be appropriate even in the absence of cirrhosis.[29]

Table 41-1. Pulmonary Disorders Associated With Hepatic Disorders

Hepatic Disease	Pulmonary Disorder
Infections	Hilar adenopathy, pneumonia tracheobronchitis, pleural effusions
Primary sclerosing cholangitis	Bronchitis, bronchiectasis
Chronic active hepatitis	Pneumonia, atelectasis, interstitial pneumonitis, interstitial fibrosis, fibrosing alveolitis, pleural effusion, pulmonary hypertension, pulmonary hemorrhage
Cirrhosis (alcoholic, postnecrotic, cryptogenic)	Pneumonia, pleural effusion, pulmonary angiodysplasia, pleural vasodilatations, pulmonary hypertension
Primary biliary cirrhosis	Hyperreactive airway disease, interstitial pneumonitis, interstitial fibrosis, fibrosing alveolitis, pulmonary hypertension

Pulmonary Involvement in Pancreatic Disease

Pulmonary disorders associated with acute and chronic pancreatitis are listed in Box 41-2.[30]

Clinical Manifestations

Pleural Effusion

Although pleuropulmonary complications of pancreatitis have been described most commonly in adults due to alcoholism, trauma, and

Box 41-2. Pulmonary Disorders Associated With Pancreatitis

Acute Pancreatitis	Chronic Pancreatitis
Pleural effusion	Pancreatopleural fistula
Hemidiaphragm elevation	Pancreatobronchopleural fistula
Atelectasis: left lower lobe	Recurrent pleural effusion
Pneumonia: left lower lobe	Recurrent lobar pneumonia
Pulmonary embolism	
Pulmonary infarction	
Acute respiratory distress syndrome	
Pulmonary edema	

cholelithiasis, the presence of pleural effusions has also been reported in children with pancreatitis. Most pleural effusions are left-sided, but may be right-sided or bilateral.[30] Pleural effusions usually occur shortly after the onset of acute pancreatitis and are characterized by small, serous, serosanguineous, or hemorrhagic exudate with high amylase levels. Fluid resorption correlates with the resolution of intra-abdominal etiology. However, chronic pancreatic disease, such as a pseudocyst, abscess, or pancreatopleural fistula, may result in a chronic pleural effusion. The etiology and pathogenesis of the fluid have not been defined. Transdiaphragmatic lymphatic blockade, pancreatopleural fistulae, and disruption of the pancreatic duct or pseudocyst have been speculated.[30,31] Treatment of pancreatic pleural effusion is usually conservative, but may require thoracentesis and further treatment when symptomatic.

Acute Respiratory Distress Syndrome

Acute respiratory distress syndrome is the most serious complication of pancreatitis. The mechanism of pancreatitis-induced ARDS is very complex and has not been completely elucidated yet. It is thought to occur secondary to the release of active enzymes and vasoactive substances, including leukotrienes and pancreatic elastase, from the pancreas. These chemical mediators increase vascular permeability and decrease pulmonary surfactant production, which promotes the development of ARDS.[31]

Atelectasis

Decrease in pulmonary surfactant increases alveolar surface tension and promotes lung collapse. This results from release of phospholipid A2 (lecithinase) that hydrolyzes lecithinase, the main component of the phospholipids in surfactant.

Diagnosis and Therapy

Because pancreatitis-associated acute lung injury has a wide spectrum of presentation, the diagnosis of pancreatopulmonary complications rely on a thorough history, physical examination, and radiographic and laboratory studies.

Therapy includes standard supportive measures; antibiotics for pneumonia; thoracentesis or chest tube drainage for an effusion causing respiratory distress; chest physical therapy, if tolerated, for atelectasis; anticoagulants for pulmonary emboli; and lung protective ventilation strategies.

Key Points

- Because the pulmonary and GI systems are interconnected, disorders that are primarily GI in etiology can cause serious sequelae in the pulmonary system.
- The role of GERD in asthma is controversial, but treatment of GERD may improve a patient's asthma.
- Inflammatory bowel disease may directly affect the lung parenchyma with disease or indirectly cause lung disease secondary to the immunosuppression used to treat IBD.
- Alpha-1 antitrypsin deficiency rarely causes pulmonary disease in children, but should be considered if there is a family history of early onset (<45 years old) of emphysema.

References

1. Rudolph CD, Mazur LJ, Liptak GS, et al. Guidelines for evaluation and treatment of gastroesophageal reflux in infants and children: recommendations of the North American Society for Pediatric Gastroenterology and Nutrition. *J Pediatr Gastroenterol Nutr.* 2001;32(suppl 2):S1–S31

2. Skopnik H, Silny J, Heiber O, et al. Gastroesophageal reflux in infants: evaluation of a new intraluminal impedance technique. *J Pediatr Gastroenterol Nutr.* 1996;23:591–598
3. Cucchiara S, Staiano A, Romaniello G, et al. Antacids and cimetidine treatment for gastro-oesophageal reflux and peptic oesophagitis. *Arch Dis Child.* 1984;59(9):842–847
4. Dial S, Delaney JAC, Barkun AN, Suissa S. Use of gastric acid suppressive agents and the risk of community-acquired *Clostridium difficile*-associated disease. *JAMA.* 2005;294:2989–2995
5. Gulmez SE, Holm A, Frederiksen H, et al. Use of proton pump inhibitors and the risk of community-acquired pneumonia. *Arch Intern Med.* 2007;167(9):950–955
6. Lopez M, Kalfa N, Forque D, et al. Laparoscopic redo fundoplication in children: failure causes and feasibility. *J Pediatr Surg.* 2008;43(10):1885–1890
7. Calder CJ, Lacy D, Raafat F, et al. Crohn's disease with pulmonary involvement in a 3 year old child. *Gut.* 1993;34:1636–1638
8. Carvalho RS, Wilson L, Cuffari C. Pulmonary manifestations in a pediatric patient with ulcerative colitis: a case report. *J Med Case Reports.* 2008;2:59
9. Krishnan S, Banquet A, Newman L, et al. Lung lesions in children with Crohn's disease presenting as nonresolving pneumonias and response to infliximab therapy. *Pediatrics.* 2006;117:1440–1443
10. Valletta E, Bertini M, Sette L, et al. Early bronchopulmonary involvement in Crohn disease: a case report. BMC *Gastroenterol.* 2001;1:13
11. Munck A, Murciano D, Pariente R, et al. Latent pulmonary function abnormalities in children with Crohn's disease. *Eur Respir J.* 1995;8:377–380
12. Higenbottam T, Cochrane GM, Clark TJH, et al. Bronchial disease in ulcerative colitis. *Thorax.* 1980;35:581
13. Mansi A, Cucchiara S, Greco L, et al. Bronchial hyperresponsiveness in children and adolescents with Crohn's disease. *Am J Respir Crit Care Med.* 2000;161:1051–1054
14. Camus P, Colby TV. The lung in inflammatory bowel disease. *Eur Respir J.* 2000;15:5–10
15. Perlmutter DH. Liver injury in alpha1-antitrypsin deficiency. *Clin Liver Dis.* 2000;4(2):387–408
16. Perlmutter DH. Alpha1-antitrypsin deficiency. *Semin Liver Dis.* 1998;18(3):217–225
17. Needham M, Stockley RA. Alpha1-antitrypsin deficiency. 3: clinical manifestations and natural history. *Thorax.* 2004;59:441
18. Teckman JH. Alpha1-antitrypsin deficiency in childhood. *Semin Liver Dis.* 2007;27(3):274–281
19. American Thoracic Society/European Respiratory Society Statement: standards for the diagnosis and management of individuals with alpha1-antitrypsin deficiency. *Am J Respir Crit Care Med.* 2003;168:818–900

20. Wall M, Moe E, Arborelius M Jr, et al. Long-term follow-up of a cohort of children with alpha1-antitrypsin deficiency. *J Pediatr.* 1990;116:248
21. Miller JW, Naimi TS, Brewer RD, et al. Binge drinking and associated health risk behaviors among high school students. *Pediatrics.* 2007;119:76–85
22. Vally H, de Klerk N, Thompson PJ. Alcoholic drinks: important triggers for asthma. *J Allergy Clin Immunol.* 2000;105(3);462–467
23. Moss M, Burnham EL. Chronic alcohol abuse, ARDS and multiple organ dysfunction. *Crit Care Med.* 2003;31(4):5207–5212
24. O'Brein JM Jr, Lu B, Ali NA, et al. Alcohol dependence is independently associated with sepsis, septic shock, and hospital mortality among adult intensive care unit patients. *Crit Care Med.* 2007;35(2):345–350
25. Baum GL, Crapo DJ, Celli BR, et al. *Textbook of Pulmonary Diseases.* 6th ed. Philadelphia, PA: Lippincott-Raven; 1998:1133–1155
26. Rodriguez-Roisin R, Krowka MJ, Herve P, et al. Pulmonary-hepatic vascular disorder. *Eur Respir J.* 2004;24:861–880
27. Tumgor G, Arikan C, Yuksekkaya HA, et al. Childhood cirrhosis, hepatopulmonary syndrome and liver transplantation. *Pediatr Transplant.* 2008;12(3):353–357
28. Gupta NA, Abramowsky C, Pillen T, et al. Pediatric hepatopulmonary syndrome is seen with polysplenia/interrupted inferior vena cava and without cirrhosis. *Liver Transpl.* 2007;13(5):680–686
29. Taussing LM, Landau LI, Le Souef PN, et al. *Pediatric Respiratory Medicine.* 2nd ed. China: Elsevier; 2008:1053–1079
30. Browne GW, Pitchumoni CS. Pathophysiology of pulmonary complications of acute pancreatitis. *World J Gastroenterol.* 2006;12(44):7087–7096
31. Lipsett P, Cameron J. *Treatment of Ascites and Fistulas.* Oxford, UK: Blackwell Science Ltd; 1998

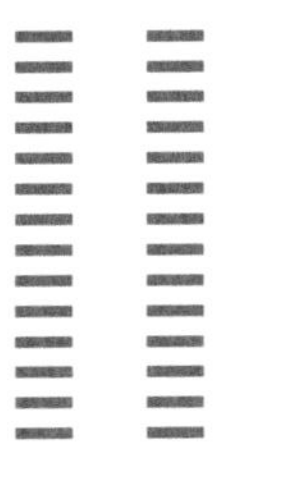

Chapter 42

The Pulmonary Complications of Sickle Cell Disease

Robyn T. Cohen, MD, MPH
Robert C. Strunk, MD

Introduction

Sickle cell disease (SCD) affects more than 70,000 individuals in the United States and is the most common inherited disorder among African Americans.[1] Despite advances in recent decades regarding diagnosis, preventive management, and treatment, the median life expectancy is 42 years for males and 48 years for females.[2] Median life expectancies may improve with more common use of hydroxyurea. The pulmonary complications of SCD are numerous and have been associated with an increased risk of early death.[2–4] A recent study of sudden deaths among sickle cell patients showed that 71% of patients had significant pulmonary pathology at the time of death.[5]

Acute Chest Syndrome

Acute chest syndrome (ACS) is a new infiltrate on chest radiograph in individuals with a sickle hemoglobinopathy (HbSS, HbSC, HbS-thalassemia), and is associated with one or more of the following: fever, cough, tachypnea, chest pain, wheezing, and hypoxemia.[6] Despite advances in diagnosis and treatment, ACS remains a leading cause of hospitalization and early death in individuals with SCD.[2,7]

Case Report 42-1

A.J. is a 7-year-old boy with sickle cell anemia (HbSS), steady-state hemoglobin (Hb) of 8.5 g/dL, and 3 to 4 admissions for painful episodes per year. He was admitted with a 2-day history of nasal congestion and cough, and a 1-day history of head and back pain not controlled on oral pain medications. On admission he was febrile to 38.2°C, with a heart rate of 140 beats per minute, respiratory rate of 24 breaths per minute, and an oxygen saturation of 96% on room air. His Hb at admission was 7.9 g/dL. His chest radiograph at admission was clear. He was started on intravenous (IV) morphine and ketorolac, IV ampicillin/sulbactam, and IV fluids, and received an incentive spirometer, which he used sporadically during his first hospital day. On his second hospital day A.J. became increasingly tachypneic with wheezing, intercostal retractions, and hypoxia, and required 2 L/minute of oxygen by nasal cannula to maintain an oxygen saturation above 92%. Repeat Hb was 5.2 g/dL. A repeat chest radiograph showed right upper lobe and left lower lobe opacities. Azithromycin and albuterol were added, and he received a packed red blood cell transfusion. By hospital day 3 his Hb was 7.0 g/dL, his oxygen requirement had decreased to 1 L/minute, and he was able to use the incentive spirometer more consistently. By hospital day 5 A.J. was no longer febrile, he did not require supplemental oxygen, his pain was well controlled on oral analgesia, and he was discharged home.

Pathophysiology

The National Acute Chest Syndrome Study Group reviewed 671 episodes of ACS in 538 patients. Community-acquired infection was the most common identifiable cause (most commonly chlamydia, mycoplasma, and respiratory syncytial virus), followed by fat embolism in association with severe vaso-occlusive pain crisis. Oil red O staining of lipid-laden macrophages was considered diagnostic for the fat-emboli syndrome. Pulmonary infarction was presumed to be the cause of ACS in 16% of cases in which no cause could be identified.[6]

Infection, fat embolism, and in-situ vaso-occlusion likely initiate a complex process that involves increased expression of adhesion molecules on sickled erythrocytes (integrin α4β1) and endothelial cells (VCAM-1).[8] Combined with the elevated granulocyte counts seen in SCD[2] and in ACS specifically,[6] adherence of sickled red blood cells to granulocytes and to vascular endothelium leads to increased transit time, more extensive polymerization of sickled erythrocytes, and obstruction of microvascular flow.[9] In addition to pulmonary vaso-occlusion, increased pulmonary vasoactivity contributes to ACS pathogenesis, secondary to increased levels of the pulmonary vasoconstrictor endothelin-1, and decreased production and increased consumption of the potent pulmonary vasodilator nitric oxide.[10,11]

Clinical Features

In 2 large clinical studies of ACS, fever and cough were the most common presenting symptoms, with tachypnea, rales, and wheeze the most common physical findings among younger children. Chest and rib pain were more commonly seen in adolescents and adults.[6,12] Varying degrees of hypoxemia can be seen with ACS, although the best way to measure oxyhemoglobin saturation has been controversial.[13,14] If there is any question about the accuracy of pulse oximetry or routine blood gas analysis in a particular clinical situation, blood gas analysis with co-oximetry should be the method of choice, because all forms of Hb, including the carboxyhemoglobin produced during hemolysis, are accounted for.[15]

Chest radiographic findings may include segmental, lobar, or multilobar consolidation. Lower lobe involvement is the most common finding at all ages, though young children are more likely to have upper lobe involvement than adults, and pleural effusions—both at presentation and developing during the course of the hospitalization—are more often seen in adolescents and adults. The mean erythrocyte count is typically decreased from steady-state value, and mean white blood cell count at presentation is often greater than 20,000.

Acute chest syndrome can progress to respiratory failure requiring mechanical ventilation (22% of adults vs 10% of children and adolescents in one study) and death (9% of adults vs <1% of children and 2% of adolescents).[6]

Management

One of the main goals of overall treatment of SCD should be prevention of ACS. Prophylactic penicillin and vaccination against *Streptococcus pneumoniae, Haemophilus influenzae,* and seasonal influenza vaccination may have a role in the improved survival among children with SCD because of a reduced frequency of pulmonary infection. Incentive spirometry has been shown to reduce the incidence of ACS among patients hospitalized with chest and back pain and a clear chest radiograph.[16]

Treatment of ACS is primarily supportive. The immediate goals of treatment of an episode of ACS include prevention of alveolar collapse, maintenance of gas exchange, and prevention of further lung injury.[17] Careful pain management is essential, with a careful balance to control chest wall pain[18] and avoid the associated rapid, shallow breathing without promoting the hypoventilation associated with overuse of narcotic agents or IV diphenhydramine.[19,20] Incentive spirometry devices should be used to prevent atelectasis.[21] Supplemental oxygen should be administered to patients with oxygen saturation in Hb (Sao_2) less than 92% to 95% (depending on their baseline Sao_2) or oxygen partial pressure in arterial blood less than 70 to 80 mmHg.[22] Epidemiologic data suggest that broad-spectrum antibiotics, including a macrolide, should be initiated.[6,23] Given the prevalence of airway lability among patients with SCD[24,25] and the frequency of wheezing associated with ACS,[6] bronchodilators have become important empiric therapy. Although vaso-occlusive pain crises are often treated with aggressive IV fluid regimens (1.5–2 times maintenance), once ACS develops this should be reduced in order to avoid worsening pulmonary edema that develops from the increased vascular permeability from damaged lung tissue.[26] Red blood cell transfusion early in the course of ACS serves 2 purposes: to increase oxygen carrying capacity and to reduce the percentage of sickled erythrocytes. This can be accomplished by either simple red blood cell transfusion[27] (with phenotypically matched, sickle negative, leukocyte-depleted packed red blood cells with extended crossmatching[21]) or by exchange transfusion, which does not have the associated risks of iron overload or hyperviscosity but carries the risk for the development of catheter-associated deep venous thrombosis.[28] The use of steroids to treat ACS remains controversial. Although one clinical trial showed a beneficial effect from IV dexamethasone in children with ACS,[29] other studies have shown an increased risk of readmission and pain following the use of systemic corticosteroids.[30,31]

Because recurrent vaso-occlusive and ACS episodes are associated with progressive cardiopulmonary morbidity and mortality,[32] long-term preventive strategies must be considered. Given the prevalence of viral-induced wheeze and the frequency of wheeze as a presenting symptom of ACS in young children, a trial of preventive asthma therapy may benefit some children—particularly in the setting of a history of eczema and a positive family history of asthma. Hydroxyurea, which increases the concentration of HbF, thus causing a decrease in the proportion of

HbS, has been shown to reduce the incidence of new ACS episodes in adults with frequent pain crises; however, the data are less definitive for infants and children.[33] Chronic transfusions have been shown to reduce the incidence of ACS in children.[34,35] Because neither option is risk-free, hematologists should be involved in the decision to implement hydroxyurea or chronic transfusion regimens for patients with SCD.

Asthma

The pathophysiology, clinical features, and management of asthma in the general pediatric population are discussed in detail in Chapter 12. This section discusses asthma as it relates specifically to SCD.

Asthma is the most common chronic disease in childhood, with African Americans disproportionally affected.[36] Because SCD is the most common inherited genetic disorder among African Americans,[1] a certain number of children will be affected with both SCD and asthma. Several studies have reported an association between asthma and complications of SCD, such as ACS and painful crises,[37–39] and increased risk of mortality.[4] It is not known whether asthma exists as a comorbid condition with SCD and acts synergistically to worsen SCD outcomes, if SCD pathogenesis contributes to an obstructive pulmonary process in children causing clinical features similar to asthma, or both.

Pathophysiology

Very little is known about the pathophysiological mechanisms, or the causal direction, between SCD and its complications and asthma; however, using an experimental asthma model, Nandedkar and colleagues[40] assessed inflammatory responses to ovalbumin sensitization in SCD transgenic mice. Sensitized SCD mice had exaggerated inflammatory responses (including higher serum immunoglobulin E levels and more peribronchial thickening) compared with sensitized wild-type murine HbS mice and transgenic human HbA mice.[40]

Clinical Features

If the diagnosis of asthma is made, it seems to have a strong contributory effect toward the incidence of ACS in children with SCD. Among 291 children with HbSS in a prospective cohort that began in infancy, those with a comorbid diagnosis of asthma were younger at the time of their first episode of ACS, had twice as many episodes of ACS and had more frequent vaso-occlusive crises than the children without asthma.[37] Among 80 children with SCD in Jamaica, asthma and atopy were more common among those with a history of recurrent ACS (≥4 episodes) compared to those with 1 or fewer episodes of ACS (53% vs 12%, $P<.001$).[38]

Determining which children with SCD have asthma is difficult. Many children with SCD and ACS present with wheezing on physical examination.[6] However, whether these children have partially reversible airway obstruction or reproducible symptoms in response to known triggers—in other words, meet clinical criteria for asthma—at steady-state is not always clear. Children with SCD may be more prone to airway obstruction and airway hyperresponsiveness.[41] Some data show a high prevalence of airway hyperresponsiveness to methacholine.[25] In one study of pulmonary function of 20 infants and toddlers (age 3–30 months) with SCD, all subjects had evidence of lower airway obstruction and hyperinflation regardless of history of ACS, suggesting that SCD has pulmonary sequelae as early as infancy.[42]

Management

Management of chronic asthma in children with SCD should follow guidelines established by the National Asthma Education Prevention Program.[43] Regarding acute asthma exacerbations, there are data regarding the increased risk of vaso-occlusive episodes following courses of systemic corticosteroids given during episodes of ACS.[30,31] This finding suggests that a prolonged taper following a course of oral steroids might be beneficial, but there are no data to support this recommendation.

To date there are no published studies on the effect of improved asthma management on sickle cell outcomes. However, the consequences of asthma exacerbations, including ventilation/perfusion mismatch and local pulmonary tissue hypoxia, on patients with sickle cell are serious. The use of evidence-based asthma guidelines[43] in the treatment of children with both SCD and asthma is crucial. Referral to a pediatric pulmonologist should be made for all children with SCD who meet criteria for persistent asthma.

Sleep-Disordered Breathing

Pathophysiology

Children with SCD are at increased risk of nocturnal desaturation compared with children without SCD.[44–46] Some have attributed this finding to upper airway obstruction from compensatory adenotonsillar hypertrophy after splenic infarction or resection.[47,48] Others suggest that abnormalities in gas exchange—specifically decreased oxyhemoglobin affinity, are the cause of nocturnal desaturation, given the finding that nocturnal desaturation is most commonly seen in SCD patients with low daytime Sao_2.[44,45] In one study of 20 patients with nocturnal desaturation (defined as Sao_2 <92% for ≥5% of total sleep time), 12 patients had no obstructive apnea events.[44] In another study of patients referred for polysomnography (PSG) because of a one-time daytime Sao_2 measurement of less than 94%, all had nocturnal desaturations (average Sao_2 89% for the entire cohort) but only 35% had documented obstructive sleep apnea syndrome (OSAS).[45]

Clinical Features

Although there are no large cohort studies on the prevalence and severity of sleep-disordered breathing (SDB) in children in the general population, smaller studies suggest that children with SCD and OSAS may have more severe SDB than children without SCD. Kaleyias and colleagues[49] reviewed the PSG results of 19 children with SCD and a clinical history suspicious for SDB (snoring, snorting, gasping, or pauses in breathing while asleep) and found 12 children had OSAS. They then compared the PSGs of the 12 children with SCD and OSAS to 10 age, sex, ethnicity, and apnea-hypopnea index–matched controls (termed "uncomplicated OSAS") and found that the children with SCD had lower Sao_2 nadirs (81% in the SCD group vs 89% in the uncomplicated OSAS group), higher peak end-tidal carbon dioxide measurements (58 mm Hg vs 52 mm Hg), and a higher percentage of total sleep time with Sao_2 less than 92%.[49] Needleman et al[44] studied 20 children with SCD (18 with HbSS and 2 with HbS β-thalassemia) and nocturnal desaturation and found that 20% of those children spent more than 80% of total sleep time with Sao_2 less than 92%.

Data show an association between SDB and SCD morbidity. In a study of 95 children with SCD and no history of stroke, nocturnal desaturation (but not obstructive events) was an independent risk factor for central nervous system events (seizure, stroke, or transient ischemic attack).[50] In the same cohort, nocturnal desaturation was highly associated with rates of pain (every increase of Sao_2 percentage point was associated with 0.83 fewer days of pain per year, $P<.0001$).[46]

Management

All children with SCD should be screened for clinical signs and symptoms of SDB. If a history of snoring, disturbed sleep, poor school performance, daytime somnolence, or hyperactivity is elicited, or if daytime oxyhemoglobin desaturation (Sao_2) is 94% or less[45] or tonsillar enlargement is detected on physical examination, patients should be referred for nocturnal PSG. In contrast to the children without SCD in which adenotonsillectomy is often curative, children with SCD frequently have residual PSG abnormalities following adenotonsillectomy. Positive airway pressure (PAP) therapy could be considered.[51] We recommend that children with SCD and abnormal sleep studies who undergo adenotonsillectomy should have follow-up PSG 6 to 8 weeks postoperatively to assess the potential need for PAP.

Sickle Cell Chronic Lung Disease

Case Report 42-2

M.T. is an 18-year-old adolescent with severe sickle cell anemia characterized by 5 to 6 admissions for pain per year, recurrent priapism, nocturnal hypoxemia, and chronic dyspnea. His steady-state Hb averages 5 to 6 mg/dL. He has had spirometry annually that has revealed long-standing, partially reversible airway obstruction, though for the past 2 years he has also developed a restrictive defect on box plethysmography, with a recent total lung capacity of 72% of predicted. A recent 6-minute walk test demonstrated a resting oxygen saturation of 94% on room air, but he became hypoxic to 88% after 2 minutes of walking. His 6-minute walk distance was 390 m (median for healthy adult males = 580 m).[52] Fortunately, a transthoracic echocardiogram 1 month ago did not show any evidence of pulmonary hypertension (PHTN). After many years of reluctance, M.T. and his family agreed to start hydroxyurea therapy 6 months ago. After an initial period of noncompliance, he now uses a bi-level positive airway pressure ventilation device routinely during sleep. The frequency of painful episodes and priapism have decreased over the past 6 months; however, he continues to report significant dyspnea when walking across the campus of his community college. He has reluctantly agreed to a trial of portable, supplemental oxygen when he knows he has to walk long distances.

Pathophysiology

There is a wide range of pathophysiological processes leading to chronic pulmonary dysfunction in patients with SCD. Many of these processes are similar to those implicated in ACS, including a propensity toward inflammation with elevated neutrophil counts and circulating proinflammatory cytokines[53]; increased expression of adhesion molecules on red blood cells, endothelium, and granulocytes[54]; chronic, multifactorial hypoxemia with sickling of red blood cells and chronic microvessel occlusion; and repeated injury from chronic intravascular hemolysis and oxidant stress.[55] In addition to these processes that take place at the molecular level, other factors are implicated in SCD patients with reduced pulmonary function. Miller and Serjeant[56] and Stevens et al[57] have suggested that growth pattern abnormalities due to chronic anemia, bone infarction, and timing of epiphyseal closure lead to reduced chest size relative to limb size and height in patients with SCD. Although initially the conventional wisdom was that repeated episodes of ACS put patients at increased risk for sickle cell chronic lung disease,[32] more recent studies have not found this to be the case.[58,59]

Clinical Features

Sickle cell chronic lung disease (SCLD) has been described as permanent lung disease with hypoxia, abnormal pulmonary function, radiographic evidence of diffuse interstitial fibrosis, and eventual cor pulmonale with right ventricular hypertrophy.[32] Chronic dyspnea is commonly reported among adults with SCD. Miller and Serjeant[56] found 17 of 25 adults with HbSS (68%, mean age 28 years) reported dyspnea with severity ranging from mild to severe. Delclaux and colleagues[60] found that 34 of 49 adults with HbSS (69%, mean age 29 years for women and 31 years for men) reported moderate to severe dyspnea on validated symptom scales. Baseline tachypnea was also common, with mean respiratory rates of 23 for women and 19 for men.[60] After reviewing 28 cases of SCLD, Powars et al[32] outlined a staging system that is summarized in Table 42-1. They found that abnormal pulmonary function tests were the earliest marker of SCLD, with the onset of disease occurring at approximately 24 years of age.[32] In contrast to the obstructive defects often noted in children with SCD, several studies have shown the development of a restrictive pattern on pulmonary function tests among adults with SCD (Table 42-2), characterized by reductions in total lung capacity, forced vital capacity (FVC),

Table 42-1. Classification of Sickle Cell Chronic Lung Disease[a]

Assessment	Stage 1	Stage 2	Stage 3	Stage 4
ABG	Normal Sao_2	Normal Sao_2	Mild hypoxia (Po_2≈70)	Hypoxia (Po_2<60)
PFTs	Mild restriction	Moderate restriction	Severe restriction	Patient unable to do PFTs
EKG/Echo	LV predominance	Biventricular hypertrophy	RVH, RA enlargement	Severe RV/RA hypertrophy, cor pulmonale
Pulmonary artery pressure	Normal	Normal	Borderline ↑	Markedly ↑

Abbreviations: ABG, arterial blood gas; Echo, echocardiogram; EKG, electrocardiogram; LV, left ventricle; PFT, pulmonary function test; RA, right atrium; RV, right ventricle; RVH, right ventricular hypertrophy; Sao_2, oxygen saturation in hemoglobin.

[a] Adapted from Powars D, Weidman JA, Odom-Maryon T, Niland JC, Johnson C. Sickle cell chronic lung disease: prior morbidity and the risk of pulmonary failure. *Medicine (Baltimore)*. 1988;67(1):66–76, with permission from Wolters Kluwer Health.

Table 42-2. Comparison of Pulmonary Function Testing Results Across Studies of Adults With Sickle Cell Disease

Study Details	Klings, 2006[58]	Sylvester, 2006[61]	Field, 2008[59]	Anthi, 2007[62]	
				Without PHTN	With PHTN
Number of subjects	310	33	92	15	24
Mean Age (years)	30.7	36	36	41	43
TLC (% predicted)	70	83	87	85	80
FVC (% predicted)	84	82	71	82	70
FEV_1 (% predicted)	83	83	79	85	71
FEV_1/FVC	99	85	85	.80	.78
DLCO (% predicted)	62	75		91	72
Classification of Pulmonary Function Abnormalities					
Obstructive (%)	1	14	36		
Restrictive (%)	74	26	19		
Mixed (%)	2	11			

Abbreviations: DLCO, diffusion capacity for carbon monoxide; FEV_1, forced expiratory volume in 1 second; FVC, forced vital capacity; PHTN, pulmonary hypertension; TLC, total lung capacity.

and forced expiratory volume in 1 second (FEV_1) with a normal FEV_1/FVC ratio.[58,59,61] Many patients also have abnormalities in the diffusion capacity for carbon monoxide,[58,60,61] which worsen with age[58] and correlate with the level of dyspnea, independent of the degree of anemia.[60] Radiographic abnormalities appear to correlate with abnormal pulmonary function. Powars et al[32] found progression of interstitial fibrosis on chest radiographs among the patients in their cohort, and others have found abnormalities on high-resolution computed tomography (HRCT), including a reticular pattern and ground-glass opacification with lobar volume loss[61]and thickened interalveolar septa.[62] However, the clinical utility of HRCT in screening for more advanced complications of SCD, including PHTN, is unclear. While Anthi et al[62] found that the extent of pulmonary fibrosis seen on HRCT was associated with increased pulmonary artery pressures, another study comparing HRCT findings between 16 adults with SCD and PHTN with 35 adults with SCD and no PHTN found no differences in extent of HRCT abnormalities between the 2 groups.[63]

Management

Once identified, there are no specific management strategies for SCLD other than optimizing the care for the other sickle cell–associated pulmonary conditions, including asthma and SDB. Referral to a cardiologist for routine screening for PHTN is essential. Supplemental oxygen may offer some relief of daytime dyspnea, especially if a 6-minute walk test reveals a tendency toward oxygen desaturation with exertion. Reducing the severity of the patient's underlying SCD with hydroxyurea or chronic red cell transfusion should be considered, in collaboration with the patient's hematologist.

Pulmonary Hypertension

Pathophysiology

Gladwin and Vichinsky[9] have proposed 2 overlapping subtypes of SCD complications: (1) microvessel occlusion in patients with high steady-state Hb and leukocyte counts (resulting in vaso-occlusive pain episodes and ACS)[9] and (2) increased intravascular hemolysis resulting in progressive vasculopathy from endothelial dysfunction (resulting in priapism, stroke, and PHTN).[9] Chronic hemolysis leads to a deficiency in nitric oxide, causing increased vasoconstriction and increased intravascular adhesion due to impaired down-regulation of endothelial adhesion molecules.[8] Intravascular hemolysis also leads to platelet activation and a hypercoagulable state.[64] Several autopsy studies have shown the presence of in situ thrombosis in patients who had PHTN at the time of death.[5,65]

Clinical Features

The threshold values that define PHTN in children with sickle cell (mean pulmonary artery pressures of ≥30 mm Hg or a tricuspid regurgitant jet velocity [TRV] of at least 2.5 to 3 m/sec)[3,66] are lower than values seen in symptomatic patients with other forms of PHTN. This is because patients with SCD are more likely to develop clinical manifestations at less elevated pulmonary pressures due to decreased oxygen-carrying capacity from chronic anemia as well as diffuse end-organ damage due to chronic microvessel dysfunction.[67]

The most common symptom of PHTN is exertional dyspnea, which is also common in those with chronic anemia without PHTN. Individuals with SCD and PHTN had a significantly shorter mean 6-minute walk test distance compared with those without PHTN in a recently published study (320 m vs 435 m).[62] In looking specifically at children with SCD, the prevalence of PHTN as assessed by screening steady-state echocardiogram has been estimated at 25% to 46% in school-aged children.[68-70] Most studies indicate that HbSS genotype and a lower steady-state Hb are associated with increased risk of PHTN. Some have shown markers of hemolysis, such as reticulocyte count,[70] serum lactate dehydrogenase, and bilirubin[69] are also associated with increased risk. While the development of PHTN in adulthood has clearly been associated with mortality in adults with SCD,[3,68] the significance and progression of this finding in children is less clear. In a retrospective chart review of 61 children with screening echocardiograms, the 3 deaths that occurred were not in children meeting echocardiography criteria for PHTN.[68]

Management

The management of SCD-related PHTN is complicated because of the lack of SCD-specific data on the safety and efficacy of pharmacologic agents used for PHTN in other populations. To date, there is only one small (n=12) published study of a therapeutic agent for SCD-associated PHTN.[71] Each category of medications is associated with adverse effects that would be particularly undesirable in patients with SCD.

Prostanoids (such as epoprostenol) are associated with thrombosis and increases in cardiac output. Endothelin-1 receptor antagonists (such as Bosentan) are associated with hepatotoxicity and decreases in Hb. Prostaglandin inhibitors (such as sildenafil) increase the risk of priapism.[71] Data suggest that PHTN in children may be reversible, especially with improved management of underlying SCD-associated complications. In a study of 18 children with echocardiography diagnosed PHTN, 8 had normalization of TRV at a 2-year follow-up echocardiogram. Improvement was seen in children who were treated with hydroxyurea and who were screened and treated for associated asthma and SDB. The children with persistently elevated TRV had higher TRV at baseline (3.0 vs 2.7 m/sec), lower steady-state Hb (7.7vs 8.9 mg/dL), and lower oxygen saturation (93% vs 98%) compared with the children whose TRV normalized over time.[72]

Key Points

- Pulmonary complications of SCD are a common feature of the disease and lead to significant morbidity and mortality.
- Management of ACS includes careful pain management, supplemental oxygen, antibiotics, bronchodilators, incentive spirometry, and frequently red blood cell transfusion.
- Children with SCD should be screened for asthma and, when indicated, be managed according to guidelines established by the National Asthma Education Prevention Program.
- Children with SCD should be screened for SDB.
- Patients with SCD should have routine pulmonary function testing. Reversible airway obstruction suggests the need for a trial of asthma therapy. A restrictive pattern may be the earliest indication of sickle cell chronic lung disease and may be associated with PHTN.
- Children with signs or symptoms of persistent asthma, SDB, recurrent ACS, or chronic dyspnea should be referred to a pediatric pulmonologist.
- More research is needed regarding the optimal management strategy for SCD-associated PHTN.

References

1. National Heart, Lung, and Blood Institute. *Sickle Cell Research for Treatment and Cure*. Bethesda, MD: National Institutes of Health; 2002
2. Platt OS, Brambilla DJ, Rosse WF, et al. Mortality in sickle cell disease. Life expectancy and risk factors for early death. *N Engl J Med*. 1994;330(23):1639–1644
3. Gladwin MT, Sachdev V, Jison ML, et al. Pulmonary hypertension as a risk factor for death in patients with sickle cell disease. *N Engl J Med*. 2004;350(9):886–895
4. Boyd JH, Macklin EA, Strunk RC, DeBaun MR. Asthma is associated with increased mortality in individuals with sickle cell anemia. *Haematologica*. 2007;92(8):1115–1118
5. Graham JK, Mosunjac M, Hanzlick RL. Sickle cell lung disease and sudden death: a retrospective/prospective study of 21 autopsy cases and literature review. *Am J Forensic Med Pathol*. 2007;28(2):168–172
6. Vichinsky EP, Neumayr LD, Earles AN, et al. Causes and outcomes of the acute chest syndrome in sickle cell disease. National Acute Chest Syndrome Study Group. *N Engl J Med*. 2000;342(25):1855–1865
7. Steinberg MH, Barton F, Castro O, et al. Effect of hydroxyurea on mortality and morbidity in adult sickle cell anemia: risks and benefits up to 9 years of treatment. *JAMA*. 2003;289(13):1645–1651
8. Setty BN, Stuart MJ. Vascular cell adhesion molecule-1 is involved in mediating hypoxia-induced sickle red blood cell adherence to endothelium: potential role in sickle cell disease. *Blood*. 1996;88(6):2311–2320
9. Gladwin MT, Vichinsky E. Pulmonary complications of sickle cell disease. *N Engl J Med*. 2008;359(21):2254–2265
10. Stuart MJ, Setty BN. Sickle cell acute chest syndrome: pathogenesis and rationale for treatment. *Blood*. 1999;94(5):1555–1560
11. Gladwin MT, Rodgers GP. Pathogenesis and treatment of acute chest syndrome of sickle-cell anaemia. *Lancet*. 2000;355(9214):1476–1478
12. Vichinsky EP, Styles LA, Colangelo LH, Wright EC, Castro O, Nickerson B. Acute chest syndrome in sickle cell disease: clinical presentation and course. Cooperative Study of Sickle Cell Disease. *Blood*. 1997;89(5):1787–1792
13. Blaisdell CJ, Goodman S, Clark K, Casella JF, Loughlin GM. Pulse oximetry is a poor predictor of hypoxemia in stable children with sickle cell disease. *Arch Pediatr Adolesc Med*. 2000;154(9):900–903
14. Ortiz FO, Aldrich TK, Nagel RL, Benjamin LJ. Accuracy of pulse oximetry in sickle cell disease. *Am J Respir Crit Care Med*. 1999;159(2):447–451
15. Needleman JP, Setty BN, Varlotta L, Dampier C, Allen JL. Measurement of hemoglobin saturation by oxygen in children and adolescents with sickle cell disease. *Pediatr Pulmonol*. 1999;28(6):423–428
16. Bellet PS, Kalinyak KA, Shukla R, Gelfand MJ, Rucknagel DL. Incentive spirometry to prevent acute pulmonary complications in sickle cell diseases. *N Engl J Med*. 1995;333(11):699–703

17. Johnson CS. The acute chest syndrome. *Hematol Oncol Clin North Am.* 2005;19(5):857–879, vi–vii
18. Needleman JP, Benjamin LJ, Sykes JA, Aldrich TK. Breathing patterns during vaso-occlusive crisis of sickle cell disease. *Chest.* 2002;122(1):43–46
19. O'Sullivan B. Respiratory complications of sickle cell disease. In: Schidlow D, Smith D, eds. *A Practical Guide to Pediatric Respiratory Diseases.* Philadelphia, PA: Hanley & Belfus; 1994:192–194
20. van Beers EJ, van Tuijn CF, Nieuwkerk PT, Friederich PW, Vranken JH, Biemond BJ. Patient-controlled analgesia versus continuous infusion of morphine during vaso-occlusive crisis in sickle cell disease, a randomized controlled trial. *Am J Hematol.* 2007;82(11):955–960
21. Melton CW, Haynes J Jr. Sickle acute lung injury: role of prevention and early aggressive intervention strategies on outcome. *Clin Chest Med.* 2006;27(3):487–502, vii
22. National Heart, Blood, and Lung Institute. Acute chest syndrome and other pulmonary complications. In: *The Management of Sickle Cell Disease.* 4th ed. 2002:103-110. NIH Publication 02-2117
23. Neumayr L, Lennette E, Kelly D, et al. Mycoplasma disease and acute chest syndrome in sickle cell disease. *Pediatrics.* 2003;112(1 pt 1):87–95
24. Leong MA, Dampier C, Varlotta L, Allen JL. Airway hyperreactivity in children with sickle cell disease. *J Pediatr.* 1997;131(2):278–283
25. Strunk RC, Brown MS, Boyd JH, Bates P, Field JJ, DeBaun MR. Methacholine challenge in children with sickle cell disease: a case series. *Pediatr Pulmonol.* 2008;43(9):924–929
26. Dampier C. Commentary: respiratory complications of sickle-cell disease. In: Schidlow D, Smith D, eds. *A Practical Guide to Pediatric Respiratory Diseases.* Philadelphia, PA: Hanley & Belfus; 1994:195–196
27. Emre U, Miller ST, Gutierez M, Steiner P, Rao SP, Rao M. Effect of transfusion in acute chest syndrome of sickle cell disease. *J Pediatr.* 1995;127(6):901–904
28. Liem RI, O'Gorman MR, Brown DL. Effect of red cell exchange transfusion on plasma levels of inflammatory mediators in sickle cell patients with acute chest syndrome. *Am J Hematol.* 2004;76(1):19–25
29. Bernini JC, Rogers ZR, Sandler ES, Reisch JS, Quinn CT, Buchanan GR. Beneficial effect of intravenous dexamethasone in children with mild to moderately severe acute chest syndrome complicating sickle cell disease. *Blood.* 1998;92(9):3082–3089
30. Strouse JJ, Takemoto CM, Keefer JR, Kato GJ, Casella JF. Corticosteroids and increased risk of readmission after acute chest syndrome in children with sickle cell disease. *Pediatr Blood Cancer.* 2008;50(5):1006–1012
31. Darbari DS, Castro O, Taylor JG, et al. Severe vaso-occlusive episodes associated with use of systemic corticosteroids in patients with sickle cell disease. *J Natl Med Assoc.* 2008;100(8):948–951

32. Powars D, Weidman JA, Odom-Maryon T, Niland JC, Johnson C. Sickle cell chronic lung disease: prior morbidity and the risk of pulmonary failure. *Medicine (Baltimore).* 1988;67(1):66–76
33. Brawley OW, Cornelius LJ, Edwards LR, et al. National Institutes of Health Consensus Development Conference statement: hydroxyurea treatment for sickle cell disease. *Ann Intern Med.* 2008;148(12):932–938
34. Hankins J, Jeng M, Harris S, Li CS, Liu T, Wang W. Chronic transfusion therapy for children with sickle cell disease and recurrent acute chest syndrome. *J Pediatr Hematol Oncol.* 2005;27(3):158–161
35. Miller ST, Wright E, Abboud M, et al. Impact of chronic transfusion on incidence of pain and acute chest syndrome during the Stroke Prevention Trial (STOP) in sickle-cell anemia. *J Pediatr.* 2001;139(6):785–789
36. Akinbami LJ, Schoendorf KC. Trends in childhood asthma: prevalence, health care utilization, and mortality. *Pediatrics.* 2002;110(2 pt 1):315–322
37. Boyd JH, Macklin EA, Strunk RC, DeBaun MR. Asthma is associated with acute chest syndrome and pain in children with sickle cell anemia. *Blood.* 2006;108(9):2923–2927
38. Knight-Madden JM, Forrester TS, Lewis NA, Greenough A. Asthma in children with sickle cell disease and its association with acute chest syndrome. *Thorax.* 2005;60(3):206–210
39. Sylvester KP, Patey RA, Broughton S, et al. Temporal relationship of asthma to acute chest syndrome in sickle cell disease. *Pediatr Pulmonol.* 2007;42(2):103–106
40. Nandedkar SD, Feroah TR, Hutchins W, et al. Histopathology of experimentally induced asthma in a murine model of sickle cell disease. *Blood.* 2008;112(6):2529–2538
41. Koumbourlis AC, Zar HJ, Hurlet-Jensen A, Goldberg MR. Prevalence and reversibility of lower airway obstruction in children with sickle cell disease. *J Pediatr.* 2001;138(2):188–192
42. Koumbourlis AC, Hurlet-Jensen A, Bye MR. Lung function in infants with sickle cell disease. *Pediatr Pulmonol.* 1997;24(4):277–281
43. Expert Panel Report 3 (EPR-3): Guidelines for the Diagnosis and Management of Asthma-Summary Report 2007. *J Allergy Clin Immunol.* 2007;120(5 suppl):S94–S138
44. Needleman JP, Franco ME, Varlotta L, et al. Mechanisms of nocturnal oxyhemoglobin desaturation in children and adolescents with sickle cell disease. *Pediatr Pulmonol.* 1999;28(6):418–422
45. Spivey JF, Uong EC, Strunk R, Boslaugh SE, DeBaun MR. Low daytime pulse oximetry reading is associated with nocturnal desaturation and obstructive sleep apnea in children with sickle cell anemia. *Pediatr Blood Cancer.* 2008;50(2):359–362
46. Hargrave DR, Wade A, Evans JP, Hewes DK, Kirkham FJ. Nocturnal oxygen saturation and painful sickle cell crises in children. *Blood.* 2003;101(3):846–848

47. Samuels MP, Stebbens VA, Davies SC, Picton-Jones E, Southall DP. Sleep related upper airway obstruction and hypoxaemia in sickle cell disease. *Arch Dis Child.* 1992;67(7):925–929
48. Maddern BR, Reed HT, Ohene-Frempong K, Beckerman RC. Obstructive sleep apnea syndrome in sickle cell disease. *Ann Otol Rhinol Laryngol.* 1989;98(3):174–178
49. Kaleyias J, Mostofi N, Grant M, et al. Severity of obstructive sleep apnea in children with sickle cell disease. *J Pediatr Hematol Oncol.* 2008;30(9):659–665
50. Kirkham FJ, Hewes DK, Prengler M, Wade A, Lane R, Evans JP. Nocturnal hypoxaemia and central-nervous-system events in sickle-cell disease. *Lancet.* 2001;357(9269):1656–1659
51. Massa F, Gonsalez S, Laverty A, Wallis C, Lane R. The use of nasal continuous positive airway pressure to treat obstructive sleep apnoea. *Arch Dis Child.* 2002;87(5):438–443
52. Stevens D, Elpern E, Sharma K, Szidon P, Ankin M, Kesten S. Comparison of hallway and treadmill six-minute walk tests. *Am J Respir Crit Care Med.* 1999;160(5 pt 1):1540–1543
53. Platt OS. Sickle cell anemia as an inflammatory disease. *J Clin Invest.* 2000;106(3):337–338
54. Okpala I, Daniel Y, Haynes R, Odoemene D, Goldman J. Relationship between the clinical manifestations of sickle cell disease and the expression of adhesion molecules on white blood cells. *Eur J Haematol.* 2002;69(3):135–144
55. Akohoue SA, Shankar S, Milne GL, et al. Energy expenditure, inflammation, and oxidative stress in steady-state adolescents with sickle cell anemia. *Pediatr Res.* 2007;61(2):233–238
56. Miller GJ, Serjeant GR. An assessment of lung volumes and gas transfer in sickle-cell anaemia. *Thorax.* 1971;26(3):309–315
57. Stevens MC, Hayes RJ, Serjeant GR. Body shape in young children with homozygous sickle cell disease. *Pediatrics.* 1983;71(4):610–614
58. Klings ES, Wyszynski DF, Nolan VG, Steinberg MH. Abnormal pulmonary function in adults with sickle cell anemia. *Am J Respir Crit Care Med.* 2006;173(11):1264–1269
59. Field JJ, Glassberg J, Gilmore A, et al. Longitudinal analysis of pulmonary function in adults with sickle cell disease. *Am J Hematol.* 2008;83(7):574–576
60. Delclaux C, Zerah-Lancner F, Bachir D, et al. Factors associated with dyspnea in adult patients with sickle cell disease. *Chest.* 2005;128(5):3336–3344
61. Sylvester KP, Desai SR, Wells AU, et al. Computed tomography and pulmonary function abnormalities in sickle cell disease. *Eur Respir J.* 2006;28(4):832–838
62. Anthi A, Machado RF, Jison ML, et al. Hemodynamic and functional assessment of patients with sickle cell disease and pulmonary hypertension. *Am J Respir Crit Care Med.* 2007;175(12):1272–1279

63. van Beers EJ, Nur E, Schaefer-Prokop CM, et al. Cardiopulmonary imaging, functional and laboratory studies in sickle cell disease associated pulmonary hypertension. *Am J Hematol.* 2008;83(11):850–854
64. Villagra J, Shiva S, Hunter LA, Machado RF, Gladwin MT, Kato GJ. Platelet activation in patients with sickle disease, hemolysis-associated pulmonary hypertension, and nitric oxide scavenging by cell-free hemoglobin. *Blood.* 2007;110(6):2166–2172
65. Haque AK, Gokhale S, Rampy BA, Adegboyega P, Duarte A, Saldana MJ. Pulmonary hypertension in sickle cell hemoglobinopathy: a clinicopathologic study of 20 cases. *Hum Pathol.* 2002;33(10):1037–1043
66. Bunn HF, Nathan DG, Dover GJ, et al. Pulmonary hypertension and nitric oxide depletion in sickle cell disease. *Blood.* 2010;116(5):687–692
67. Machado RF, Gladwin MT. Chronic sickle cell lung disease: new insights into the diagnosis, pathogenesis and treatment of pulmonary hypertension. *Br J Haematol.* 2005;129(4):449–464
68. Hagar RW, Michlitsch JG, Gardner J, Vichinsky EP, Morris CR. Clinical differences between children and adults with pulmonary hypertension and sickle cell disease. *Br J Haematol.* 2008;140(1):104–112
69. Onyekwere OC, Campbell A, Teshome M, et al. Pulmonary hypertension in children and adolescents with sickle cell disease. *Pediatr Cardiol.* 2008;29(2):309–312
70. Pashankar FD, Carbonella J, Bazzy-Asaad A, Friedman A. Prevalence and risk factors of elevated pulmonary artery pressures in children with sickle cell disease. *Pediatrics.* 2008;121(4):777–782
71. Machado RF, Martyr S, Kato GJ, et al. Sildenafil therapy in patients with sickle cell disease and pulmonary hypertension. *Br J Haematol.* 2005;130(3):445–453
72. Pashankar FD, Carbonella J, Bazzy-Asaad A, Friedman A. Longitudinal follow up of elevated pulmonary artery pressures in children with sickle cell disease. *Br J Haematol.* 2009;144(5):736–741

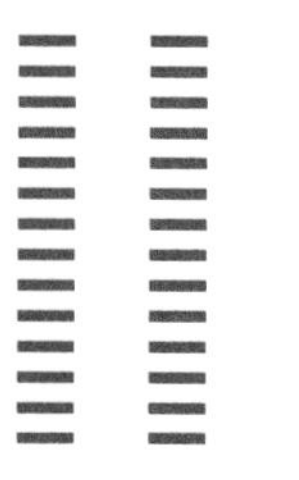

Chapter 43

Pulmonary Manifestations of Oncologic Disease and Treatment

Theresa D. Pattugalan, MD
Mark E. Dovey, MD

Introduction

In children, pulmonary oncologic disease can be divided into primary tumors, tumors metastatic to the lung, and systemic malignancies involving the lung. This chapter provides an overview of these disease categories. Pulmonary disease associated with cancer therapies for children will also be discussed.

Thoracic Tumors

Pulmonary neoplasms in the pediatric age group are relatively uncommon. The true incidence and etiologic predisposing factors are unknown. Disordered pulmonary development may play a role in some tumors.[1] The identification of thoracic tumors sometimes occurs incidentally when a chest x-ray is obtained for unrelated reasons. The diagnosis and surgical intervention are often delayed because of the paucity of specific symptoms. They may also present at any age. An overview of benign and malignant pediatric thoracic tumors is provided in Table 43-1. The lesions are grouped according to their anatomical location.

Airway Tumors

Tumors arising from the conducting airways often manifest with nonspecific signs and symptoms of bronchial obstruction, such as chronic

Table 43-1. Malignant and Benign Pediatric Thoracic Tumors

Anatomical Region	Malignant	Benign
Airways	Bronchial adenomas • Bronchial carcinoids • Adenoid cystic/cylindroma • Mucoepidermoid Bronchogenic carcinoma	Capillary hemangioma Pulmonary inflammatory pseudotumor/plasma cell granuloma Mucus gland adenomas Leiomyomas Benign hamartomas Myoblastomas
Anterior mediastinum	Lymphoma or leukemia Germ cell tumors • Teratoma • Non-teratoma	Normal thymus Teratoma Lymphangioma Bronchogenic cyst Cystic hygroma
Posterior mediastinum	Ganglion cell • Neuroblastoma • Ganglioneuroma • Ganglioneuroblastoma Lymphoma	Ganglioneuroma Bronchogenic cyst Thoracic meningocele Cystic hygroma Neurofibroma
Parenchymal	Primary tumors • Bronchoalveolar carcinoma • Pleuropulmonary blastoma Metastatic solid tumors Lymphoma • Non-Hodgkin's • Hodgkin's • Posttransplantation Lymphoproliferative disease	Granulomatous disease (histoplasmosis; tuberculosis) Round pneumonia Inflammatory pseudotumor Hamartoma Radiation pneumonitis
Chest wall origin	Ewing sarcoma family of tumors (Askin tumor) Rhabdomyosarcoma Lymphoma	Lipoma Hemangioma Osteochondroma Neurofibroma

cough and wheezing. They may present with chest pain, hemoptysis, and recurrent or persistent localized pulmonary infections.[2] An obstructive airflow pattern will be present on pulmonary function tests. Poor response to medical intervention with bronchodilators, corticosteroids, or antibiotics warrants further investigation. In addition to a plain chest radiograph, helpful diagnostic studies include computed tomography (CT) scans and bronchoscopy. If an airway tumor is seen, definitive confirmation is through histopathologic studies of biopsies of resected lesions.

Benign Airway Tumors

The most common of the benign tumors is the inflammatory pseudotumor, or plasma cell granuloma, an inflammatory reactive lesion to a previous pulmonary insult. Capillary hemangiomas are developmental proliferations of tightly packed, trabeculated blood vessels that may arise along the surface of the conducting airways.[3] Pulmonary hamartomas consist largely of cartilage and variable quantities of epithelium, fat, and muscle. They are usually located in the periphery of the lung but involvement of primary and intermediate bronchi has been reported. Other benign airway tumors include mucus gland adenomas, leiomyomas, and myoblastomas. Most of these lesions are benign and amenable to complete surgical resection.

Malignant Airway Tumors

Bronchial Adenomas

The most common of the malignant tumors are the bronchial adenomas, which are endobronchial tumors arising from the airway epithelium with glandular histologic features. Most are slow-growing tumors with potential for malignant transformation but generally associated with excellent prognosis in childhood.[4] Treatment is focused on complete surgical resection.

Bronchial carcinoid is the most common endobronchial tumor in children and adolescents. It accounts for nearly half of all malignant pediatric primary lung tumors.[2] These tumors arise from neuroendocrine cells within the bronchial epithelium, and often appear as polypoid projections into the airway lumen. The more common are the well-differentiated carcinoids, which are less invasive and have favorable prognosis. The poorly differentiated carcinoids are more aggressive, often with invasive lesions at the time of presentation.[5] The excessive secretion of vasoactive peptides from carcinoid tumors, referred to as carcinoid syndrome, is rare in pediatric tumors.

Tracheobronchial mucoepidermoid tumors originate from mucus glands within the bronchial submucosa. These may be locally invasive, but low-grade histology favors long-term survival. Adenoid cystic carcinoma is more associated with local infiltration and metastasis.

Bronchogenic Carcinomas

Although considered rare in children, bronchogenic carcinoma is the second most frequent malignant pulmonary tumor of childhood. In a review of 230 cases of primary pulmonary tumors in childhood, 47 cases of bronchogenic carcinoma were reported in children younger than 16 years.[6] Most bronchogenic carcinomas are adenocarcinoma or undifferentiated small cell carcinoma variety. Similar to adults, these tumors are aggressive, often with metastatic lesions at the time of diagnosis. Prognosis is generally poor.

Mediastinal Tumors

Most lesions in the mediastinum remain asymptomatic and are found incidentally on a routine chest radiograph. Symptoms arise when pressure is exerted on sensitive structures of the mediastinum or when structures are displaced. Respiratory symptoms are the result of direct pressure on structures, specifically narrowing of the trachea or bronchi and compression of the lung parenchyma. Nonspecific symptoms include dry cough, stridor, localized wheezing, distal obstructive emphysema or atelectasis, hemoptysis, pneumonitis, or chronic recurrent lower respiratory tract infections with fever and leukocytosis. Hoarseness and brassy cough result when a lesion exerts pressure on the recurrent laryngeal nerve. Progressive dyspnea and life-threatening airway compression may be present depending on the mass size.[7]

Physical examination findings are nonspecific and may include wheeze, rales or rhonchi, dullness to percussion over the area of mediastinal enlargement and, occasionally, tenderness over the chest wall, especially when the tumor exerts pressure on the parietal pleura.

The mediastinum is conventionally divided into anterior, middle, and posterior compartments. Most of the malignant mediastinal tumors arise from anterior and posterior compartments as described in this section.[8]

Anterior Mediastinum

The anterior mediastinum is posterior to the sternum and anterior to the heart and contains the thymus, lymphatic tissue, extrapericardial aorta and its branches, and the great veins. Masses in the anterior compartment are more likely to be malignant than those found in other mediastinal compartments.[8] The most important tumors in this area are lymphomas and germ cell tumors. Very large lymphomas may present with superior vena cava syndrome—dilatation of veins in the upper extremity, head, and neck.

Both Hodgkin's and non-Hodgkin's lymphomas frequently present with a primary mass and adenopathy in the anterior mediastinum, and a contrast CT scan provides the best characterization of the mass. With recent therapeutic advancement of combined radiation and chemotherapy, 5-year survival rates have improved to 95% for Hodgkin's and 81% for non-Hodgkin's lymphoma.[9]

Germ cell tumors represent 24% of anterior mediastinal tumors in children.[10] Germ cells migrate from the urogenital ridge to the gonads during embryogenesis, and primary germ cell tumor appears from these cells that failed to complete migration. Germ cell tumors have varied histology, with the most common being mixed cellularity. The group includes the benign teratomas; seminomas; and embryonal tumors such as embryonal carcinomas, choriocarcinomas, yolk sac tumors, and teratocarcinomas.[10] Computed tomography images may distinguish the attenuation of fluid, soft tissue, calcium, and fat, which can be suggestive of the diagnosis. Surgical resection and adjuvant chemotherapy have improved survival.

Posterior Mediastinum

The posterior mediastinum is the area posterior to the heart and trachea to the thoracic vertebral margins, and encompasses the thoracic aorta, esophagus, azygos veins, autonomic ganglia and nerves, thoracic duct, and lymph nodes. Tumors in this region account for 30% to 40% of pediatric mediastinal tumors, and 90% are neurogenic in origin.[4]

Ganglion cell tumors include neuroblastomas, ganglioneuromas, and ganglioneuroblastomas. A neuroblastoma is a malignant tumor arising from the adrenal medulla and occasionally from ganglia of the sympathetic nervous system. Ganglioneuroma is a benign tumor made of mature ganglion cells in a stroma of nerve fibers. Ganglioneuroblastoma is a tumor composed of various portions of neuroblastoma and ganglioneuroma.[11] One differentiating feature is the median age of occurrence. Neuroblastoma frequently occurs before the age of 2 years and 95% by age 10 years, while ganglioneuroma and ganglioneuroblastoma are more likely to occur after the age of 2 years.

More often, the benign type of neurogenic tumors are asymptomatic. Symptoms that may suggest malignancy include radicular pain, paraplegia, motor disturbances, Horner syndrome, upper respiratory tract infections, dyspnea, elevated temperature, weight loss, and asthenia.

Parenchymal Tumors

Most of the parenchymal nodules seen in pediatric radiographs represent a granulomatous infection. Etiologies of benign nodules include histoplasmosis, round pneumonia, round atelectasis, inflammatory pseudotumor, hamartoma, and radiation pneumonitis.[12]

Secondary metastatic nodules or masses are much more common than are primary tumors. Patients with parenchymal malignancies are usually asymptomatic or have nonspecific complaints until masses become large (advanced stages) to cause pressure symptoms and present as respiratory distress.

Helpful in the diagnosis are history of malignancy and radiation exposure, and radiographic information. If previous radiographs show pulmonary nodules that did not change in size over 2 years, there is high probability that the nodule is benign. High-resolution CT scan provides additional findings suggestive of benign lesions: calcifications within a nodule, a laminated pattern consistent with granuloma, or evidence of intranodular fat suggestive of hamartoma.[13] Surgical removal and histopathologic evaluation are necessary for lesions that carry a high probability for malignancy.

Pulmonary blastoma is a rare tumor primarily seen in adults; however, increasing numbers of cases are being reported in children. This is a very aggressive tumor, with mesenchymal metastasis in 20% with associated mortality of 32.1%.[2]

Chest Wall Tumors

The chest wall is a critical component of the respiratory pump, and diseases that alter its structure result in respiratory compromise and failure. Primary chest wall tumors are not common in children; most are malignant. These are aggressive tumors that primarily arise from the soft tissues of the chest wall or as extensions from bony structures or the mediastinum. Neoplastic chest wall lesions may present as a painful, palpable chest wall mass; cough; and dyspnea. Benign lesions tend to be asymptomatic.[14]

The most common chest wall tumors are a group of tumors from the Ewing sarcoma family of tumors or malignant small round cell tumor.[14] This group includes primitive neuroectodermal tumors of the chest wall known as Askin tumors, Ewing sarcoma of bone, and extraosseus Ewing. These are aggressive tumors with a poor prognosis and high rate of recurrence, and complete resection offers the best possibility of a cure.

Rhabdomyosarcomas are the second most common group of chest wall tumors. These tumors present as large heterogenous masses with rib destruction and occasionally a pleural effusion. Less common malignant chest wall tumors are congenital fibrosarcoma, chondrosarcomas, and primary osteosarcomas.[14]

Pulmonary Metastatic Lesions

Malignant tumors from other parts of the body may present with pulmonary metastases that are sufficiently widespread to be symptomatic at diagnosis. Table 43-2 provides a summary of pediatric tumors that are known to metastasize to the lungs.

Metastatic masses or nodules can be solitary or multiple, and may be found at the time of diagnosis of the malignancy or as a recurrence of the disease. The diagnosis of pulmonary metastasis can be inferred when multiple pulmonary nodules are present in a child with cancer that is known to metastasize in the lungs.[15] However, the presence of a single pulmonary nodule in a child with cancer cannot be assumed to be a pulmonary metastasis as many of these solitary nodules are benign even in a child with known malignancy.[12]

The most common childhood tumor to present with pulmonary metastases is Wilms tumor, where pulmonary nodules may be numerous enough to give the appearance of pulmonary consolidation. Osteosarcoma has a high recurrence rate in the lung. Trophoblastic choriocarcinomas may present in female adolescents as multiple pulmonary nodules without an obvious primary site.

Computed tomography has been a trusted modality for detection of pulmonary metastases, as much in children as in adults. A lobulated contour, which implies uneven growth and an irregular or speculated margin with distortion of adjacent vessels, often described as sunburst or corona radiata appearance, is a typical morphologic feature associated with malignancy.[13]

Table 43-2. Summary of Pediatric Tumors That Metastasize to the Lungs

Primary Site	Specific Tumors
Skeletal system	Osteosarcoma Ewing sarcoma Chondrosarcoma Ameloblastoma
Musculoskeletal system	Rhabdomyosarcoma Soft-tissue sarcomas Synovial cell sarcoma Malignant fibrous histiocytoma Chondrosarcoma Fibrosarcoma Liposarcoma Malignant neurilemoma
Gastrointestinal tract	Hepatoblastoma Hepatocellular carcinoma Embryonal sarcoma of liver Leiomyosarcoma Adenocarcinoma of colon
Genitourinary tract	Wilms tumor Malignant rhabdoid tumor of the kidney Clear cell sarcoma of the kidney Gonadal germ cell tumor Trophoblastic choriocarcinoma
Endocrine system	Differentiated thyroid carcinoma Adrenocortical carcinoma

The primary treatment for lung metastases is resection, if possible. In general, the indications for resection of metastatic pulmonary disease should be based on unilateral pulmonary involvement and evidence of local control of the primary malignancy for a period of 1 year before pulmonary resection.[13]

Adjuvant therapies include chemotherapy and whole-lung irradiation. Wilms tumors with pulmonary metastases (Stage IV) have good response to preoperative chemotherapy followed by pulmonary metastasectomy with a 5-year recurrence-free rate of 83%.[16]

Whole-lung irradiation is associated with a subsequent 12% rate of diffuse interstitial pneumonitis; hence, it is usually reserved for inoperable metastases.

Systemic Neoplasms Affecting the Lung

Systemic malignant disease is an infrequent cause of pulmonary pathology in children but when it occurs, early recognition is of great importance. This discussion focuses on lung involvement in systemic malignancies of childhood, specifically leukemias and lymphomas.

Pulmonary oncologic diseases in childhood that present as diffuse pulmonary infiltrates usually are leukemic infiltration, non-Hodgkin's lymphoma, or Langerhans cell histiocytosis.[15] Myeloid and lymphocytic leukemia and Hodgkin's disease may involve the lung during the course of the disease, but isolated pulmonary disease has not been reported.[17]

Langerhans cell histiocytosis is an important but very rare lesion that most pediatricians will never encounter in practice. Details of this lesion are found in textbooks of pediatric hematology/oncology and provided references.

Leukemias

Acute lymphoblastic leukemia (ALL) is the most common malignancy of childhood. It is a malignant disorder of lymphocyte development and regulation. Acute myelogenous leukemia (AML), on the other hand, affects the myeloid differentiation. Both types have genetic predisposition and are multifactorial in etiology. There is increased risk in children with Down syndrome and Fanconi anemia. The peak incidence of ALL is between 2 and 6 years of age. Signs and symptoms include pallor, fatigue, fever, bruising, petechiae, mucosal bleeding, epistaxis, lymphadenopathy, hepatosplenomegaly, leukopenia, thrombocytopenia, and anemia.

Diffuse pulmonary involvement is a relatively common finding at autopsy in patients dying of leukemia; however, diffuse interstitial pneumonia in children during the course of treatment for leukemia and other oncologic diseases is usually due to an infectious agent. In one series of patients with diffuse interstitial pneumonia, leukemic pulmonary infiltrates were responsible for 9% of the cases.[18] Early bronchoscopy and open lung biopsy are recommended for such cases. Patients with AML or chronic myelocytic leukemia who present with hyperleukocytosis (white blood cell counts >100,000) are at risk for pulmonary leukostasis. Patients with pulmonary leukostasis may develop tachypnea, fever, and pulmonary infiltrates and, later on, hypoxia, hemorrhage, and infarction secondary to the intravascular clumping of leukemic blast cells.[19] This is a medical emergency that requires early institution of cytoreductive therapy, including chemotherapy and leukapheresis. Leukapheresis or exchange transfusion aims to lower the leukocyte count in patients with hyperleukocytosis. Packed red blood cell transfusion should be withheld or given with caution to prevent an increase in blood viscosity prior to lowering of the leukocyte count.[15]

In addition to pulmonary leukostasis, the release of enzymes and intracellular contents of blast cells following leukemic cell lysis causes pulmonary tissue damage and edema, which may lead to respiratory failure, a condition called leukemic cell pneumonopathy.[15]

Aggressive multiagent chemotherapy is successful in inducing remission in about 80% of patients with AML. Most children with ALL have a survival rate of greater than 80% at 5 years from the time of diagnosis. Bone marrow or stem cell transplantation after remission has been shown to achieve long-term disease-free survival in 60% to 70% of leukemia patients who fail sustained remission.[20]

Lymphomas

Lymphomas are neoplastic transformations of normal lymphoid cells, which reside predominantly in lymphoid tissues. They are morphologically subdivided into 2 major categories: non-Hodgkin's lymphoma and Hodgkin's lymphoma.[21] Non-Hodgkin's lymphoma is further categorized into indolent, aggressive, and highly aggressive lymphomas. Hodgkin's lymphoma comprises 2 disease entities: classical Hodgkin's lymphoma and nodular lymphocyte predominant Hodgkin's lymphoma.

Patients with non-Hodgkin's lymphoma typically present with Stage B symptoms of fever, weight loss, and night sweats. These systemic symptoms are compatible with the widespread nature of the disease. About 80% to 90% have nonspecific respiratory symptoms. The most frequently described radiographic appearances of parenchymal non-Hodgkin's lymphoma are multiple nodular densities, masses, and diffuse interstitial infiltrates. Pleural effusions and involvement of the intrathoracic nodes are also common.

The distinguishing epidemiologic feature of Hodgkin's lymphoma is its bimodal age distribution curve: one peak in young adults and one in older age groups. The disease is histopathologically defined by the presence of clonal malignant Hodgkin/Reed-Sternberg cells. Presenting symptoms in children include painless lymphadenopathy, hepatosplenomegaly, and nonspecific symptoms such as fatigue, anorexia, and weight loss. Between 17% and 40% of children with Hodgkin's lymphoma have a mediastinal mass at the time of presentation. The bulky mediastinal mass may cause dysphagia, dyspnea, cough, stridor, or superior vena cava syndrome.[22]

Diagnosis of lymphoma is established by histopathologic examination, usually excision biopsy of an enlarged lymph node or, as in some cases of parenchymal lymphoma, open lung biopsy. Imaging studies are used to establish the extent of the disease. Management depends on the staging of the disease and may include high-dose radiation therapy and/or combination chemotherapy.

Tracheal compression and superior vena cava syndrome in a child are almost always caused by Hodgkin's lymphoma and non-Hodgkin's lymphoma. Symptoms are usually alleviated by therapy with radiation (50–100 cGy to the midplane for 3 days), corticosteroids (2 mg/kg every 6 hours), or both.[15]

Pulmonary Complications of Cancer Therapies

Patients with malignancies who are treated with chemotherapeutic drugs or radiation, or recipients of hematopoietic stem cell transplants, may develop myriad of infectious and noninfectious pulmonary manifestations. This can either be a complication of the disease or the multimodality treatments used to address the disease.

With the advent of newer antimicrobial agents and effective prophylaxis, the incidence of infectious complications has decreased while noninfectious and iatrogenic pulmonary complications have emerged as major causes of early and late morbidity and mortality.[23]

Drug-Induced Pulmonary Injury

Drug-induced reactions should always be considered as a cause of pulmonary complications in immunocompromised hosts. About one-third of such reactions are due to chemotherapeutic agents used

Box 43-1. Cytotoxic Drugs Affecting the Lungs

Antibiotics
- Bleomycin
- Mitomycin

Alkylating Agents
- Cyclophosphamide
- Chlorambucil
- Busulfan (Myleran)
- Melphalan

Nitrosoureas
- Carmustine (bis-chloronitrosourea)

Antimetabolites
- Methotrexate
- Azathioprine
- 6-Mercaptopurine
- Cytosine arabinoside

Other Cytotoxic Agents
- Procarbazine
- Teniposide (VM-26)
- Vinca alkaloids

in treatment of childhood neoplasms (Box 43-1).

The incidence of pulmonary toxicity varies between 3% and 30%, and the risk may be dose-related (carmustine, bleomycin, cyclophosphamide) or not dose-dependent (methotrexate).[24] Some drug-induced pulmonary damage is reversible, but persistent and potentially fatal injury may occur. The most frequent clinical syndrome is diffuse interstitial pneumonitis and fibrosis. Hypersensitivity lung disease, noncardiogenic pulmonary edema, pleural effusion, bronchiolitis obliterans, and alveolar hemorrhage are also encountered.[25–30]

Two main mechanisms of drug-induced injury are implicated: direct toxicity to lung cells, mediated by reactive oxygen metabolites (which damage the DNA, particularly of type II pneumocytes), or interference with collagen metabolism, which is a dose-independent reaction with features suggesting a hypersensitivity reaction.[24]

The diagnosis of drug-induced lung injury is often complicated by the following factors: (1) patients may be exposed to several cytotoxic drugs concurrently or in sequence; (2) the time to onset of pulmonary toxicity may vary among drugs, making it difficult to ascertain which agent is responsible for a particular reaction; (3) the combination of drugs may lead to drug interactions producing enhanced toxicity; and (4) presence of concurrent infections.[23]

The clinical presentation often includes fever, malaise, dyspnea, and a nonproductive cough. Radiologic studies demonstrate diffuse alveolar and/or interstitial involvement. Computed tomography scan provides early evidence of parenchymal abnormalities. Pathologic features consist of interstitial thickening with chronic inflammatory cell infiltrate in the interstitial or alveolar compartment, fibroblast proliferation, fibrosis, and hyperplasia of type II pneumocytes.[25] Treatment usually entails withdrawal of the offending agent, systemic corticosteroids, and supportive care.

Radiation-Induced Pulmonary Injury

Radiation therapy plays a major role in the curative or palliative treatment of many intrathoracic and chest wall malignancies. Radiation therapy produces dramatic effects in the lung. Most patients remain asymptomatic with subclinical manifestations of radiation-related changes. As the number of new invasive cancers and numbers of survivors increase, several late and unusual effects of radiation are becoming evident.[31]

Ionizing radiation causes the localized release of energy sufficient to break strong chemical bonds and generate reactive free radicals. Radiation-induced lung injury results from the combination of (1) direct cytotoxicity on normal lung tissue, where there is DNA damage that causes clonogenic death and apoptotic pathways for lung epithelial cells, and (2) the development of fibrosis triggered by radiation-induced cellular signal transduction and mediated by a number of different cytokines.

Two distinct clinical stages are recognized in radiation-induced lung disease: the early stage, radiation pneumonitis, usually occurs about 4 to 12 weeks after treatment; the late stage, chronic radiation fibrosis, occurs later and becomes stable 12 to 15 months after completion of radiation therapy.[32]

The risk of radiation pneumonitis depends on the dose delivered to the lung, which includes previous radiation, the daily fractionation of the dose, coadministration of chemotherapeutic agents or oxygen, and individual susceptibility.[23] Radiologic changes are variably present after a total dose of 30 to 40 Gy (to part of the lung) and universally seen after more than 40 Gy.[32] The International System of Units of radiation dose is expressed in terms of absorbed energy per unit mass of tissue. The gray (Gy) is the unit of absorbed dose and has replaced the rad (1 Gy equals 1 joule/kilogram and also equals 1 rad).

Radiation pneumonitis has an insidious onset and may present as a productive cough, dyspnea on exertion, low-grade fever, pleuritic or substernal chest pain, malaise, and weight loss. Physical examination may reveal crackles or a pleural rub, dullness to percussion if with effusion, and skin erythema outlining the radiation port. Tachypnea, cyanosis, and signs of pulmonary hypertension may be seen in advanced cases. Pulmonary function testing reveals a reduction in lung volumes, diffusing capacity, and lung compliance.

Radiographic changes are generally confined to the field of irradiation. Initially, there is a diffuse haze in the irradiated region with obscuring of vascular outlines. Patchy consolidations appear then coalesce to form a relatively sharp edge that conforms to the treatment portals. These changes may clear gradually and disappear completely, but may lead to fibrous changes in case of severe injury.[33]

Fibrous changes take 6 to 24 months to evolve but usually remain stable after 2 years.[33] Chronic radiation fibrosis is indicated by findings of a well-defined area of atelectasis with parenchymal distortion, traction bronchiectasis, mediastinal shift, or pleural thickening.

For treatment, there are reports of improvement with the use of corticosteroids for patients with subacute onset of radiation-induced lung injury. Corticosteroids (60 mg/day) are generally given for 2 weeks and a gradual taper over 3 to 12 weeks.[34] Significant improvements in the perfusion and ventilation of injured lung tissue may be noted from 3 to 18 months after radiation therapy. After 18 months, however, further improvement appears unusual.

Pulmonary Complications of Stem Cell Transplantation

Hematopoietic stem cell transplantation (HSCT) has made a great deal of progress as salvage therapy after chemotherapy and radiation for several hematologic and non-hematologic malignancies. Hematopoietic stem cell transplantation is a general term that covers transplantation of progenitor cells from any source, such as bone marrow, peripheral blood or umbilical cord, either an autologous (self) or allogeneic (non-self) stem cell source.

Significant pulmonary complications have been described with these procedures and are the leading cause of mortality and morbidity following HSCT. Pulmonary complications are reported in 30% to 60%

of all recipients and represent a major cause of mortality.[35] A major proportion of these pulmonary complications are the direct result of infection; however, noninfectious complications are also common and severe.

Acute Lung Injury After HSCT

This discussion focuses on early, noninfectious causes of acute lung injury in the HSCT recipient. Early complications are usually defined as those occurring in the first 100 to 120 days after transplantation.[36]

Oropharyngeal Mucositis

Oropharyngeal mucositis generally occurs in almost all patients receiving HSCT, especially following high-dose chemotherapy, and total body irradiation. It typically peaks on days 6 to 12 post-transplant and begins to resolve by days 14 to 18.[36] Severe oral mucositis may cause some upper airway obstruction, which typically responds to corticosteroids.

Idiopathic Pneumonia Syndrome

Idiopathic pneumonia syndrome (IPS) is a clinical syndrome of widespread alveolar injury in the absence of lower respiratory tract infection. Criteria for alveolar injury include the presence of acute, multilobar pulmonary infiltrates; associated symptoms of pneumonia, such as cough, dyspnea, and crackles; and physiological impairment, such as hypoxemia and restrictive physiology. Absence of infection is evidenced by negative bronchoalveolar lavage or lung biopsy samples, ideally followed by a second negative test within 2 weeks.[37] Idiopathic pneumonia syndrome encompasses 2 entities: peri-engraftment respiratory distress syndrome and diffuse alveolar hemorrhage.

The incidence of IPS ranges from 2% to 5%, with median onset of 42 to 49 days and a relative peak in the first 2 weeks. Overall mortality rate is 70% to 80%.[37] Risk factors associated with IPS are acute graft-versus-host-disease (GVHD), conventional induction therapy, methotrexate use, and greater patient age.[2] The pathogenesis of IPS is not fully understood but it is thought to reflect multiple pathways of diffuse acute lung injury, which involves humoral and cellular mediators of both host and donor origin. Contributing to direct lung injury are complement activation, leukocyte recruitment, neutrophilic alveolitis, and release of inflammatory mediators such as lipopolysaccharide, interferon-γ, and tumor necrosis factor α.[38]

Management is typically supportive, such as supplemental oxygen and positive pressure ventilation. Many patients receive anti-infective agents if infection cannot be excluded with certainty. There are reports of response to high-dose corticosteroids.

Peri-engraftment Respiratory Distress Syndrome

The clinical features of engraftment syndrome seen in autologous HSCT recipients overlap with acute GVHD: fever, skin rash, generalized edema, weight gain, diarrhea, hypoalbuminemia, and noninfectious pulmonary infiltrates, often with interstitial edema and pleural effusion on chest imaging.[36]

Peri-engraftment respiratory distress syndrome defines a subset of patients presenting with features compatible with IPS in the setting of engraftment.[39] Peri-engraftment respiratory distress syndrome was identified in 19 of 416 autologous HSCT recipients (4.6%), with median time to onset of 11 days after transplantation, and occurred within 5 days of neutrophil recovery. This subset of patients has better overall outcome compared with diffuse alveolar hemorrhage, with reported good response to corticosteroids.

Diffuse Alveolar Hemorrhage

Diffuse alveolar hemorrhage (DAH) defines another subset of IPS that has an incidence of approximately 5%, less common with allogeneic than autologous HSCT. This entity is usually seen in the first 2 weeks after HSCT. Criteria for DAH after HSCT are (1) signs and symptoms of pneumonitis (hypoxemia, restrictive ventilatory defects, and radiographic evidence of widespread alveolar injury); (2) absence of infection; and (3) bronchoalveolar lavage with progressively bloodier return from separate subsegmental bronchi, more than 20% hemosiderin-laden macrophages in lavage fluid, or blood in at least 30% of the alveolar surfaces on biopsy.[40]

Patients may present with dyspnea, fever, cough and, in some instances, hemoptysis (20%). Radiographs reveal alveolar and interstitial infiltrates involving middle and lower lung zones. Computed tomography scan may show ground-glass infiltrates or areas of consolidation. Bronchoscopy with bronchoalveolar lavage studies confirms the diagnosis. Reported mortality approximates 70% to 75% despite high-dose corticosteroid therapy.[40]

Chronic Lung Disease After HSCT

Pulmonary Function Abnormalities

Frequent long-term sequelae, particularly after allogeneic transplantation, include restrictive and obstructive ventilatory defects and gas transfer abnormalities such as decreased carbon monoxide diffusing capacity (DLCO).[41]

Identified risk factors for the development of pulmonary function test abnormalities after HSCT include smoking, pretransplantation pulmonary infection, chemotherapy and conditioning regimen, viral infection in the early posttransplantation period, GVHD, and human leukocyte antigen mismatch.[42] Respiratory muscle weakness caused by GVHD-associated myositis may also be a contributing factor to restrictive pulmonary function abnormalities.[43]

Bronchiolitis Obliterans

Bronchiolitis obliterans is a nonspecific inflammatory injury primarily affecting the small airways, often sparing the interstitium, and results in airflow limitation.[44] Philit and colleagues[45] recommended the term *post-transplant obstructive lung disease* instead of bronchiolitis obliterans, for it takes into account both the functional definition and the clinical context of the syndrome.[45]

In most cases of HSCT recipients, bronchiolitis obliterans is considered a severe manifestation of chronic GVHD. The strong association between the 2 entities suggests that host bronchiolar epithelial cells serve as targets for donor cytotoxic T lymphocytes.[45]

Bronchiolitis obliterans can occur 2 months to 9 years after transplantation. Most patients present insidiously with dry cough and dyspnea, 40% develop wheezing, and 20% have cold symptoms; fever is notably absent. Pulmonary function testing reveals irreversible airflow obstruction in clinically significant disease. Chest radiograph is usually normal or may show hyperinflation. The most common finding on CT scan is decreased lung attenuation, which is more extensive in the lower lobes. Other findings include segmental or subsegmental bronchial dilatation, diminution of peripheral vascularity, centrilobular nodules, and expiratory air trapping.[46]

Therapy consists of empiric corticosteroids and augmented immunosuppression. Macrolide antibiotics are known to have anti-inflammatory properties and have been shown to improve symptoms, lung function, and mortality in patients who have panbronchiolitis.[47]

Bronchiolitis Obliterans Organizing Pneumonia

Bronchiolitis obliterans organizing pneumonia (BOOP) is characterized by the presence of granulation tissue within the terminal and respiratory bronchioles, alveolar ducts, and alveoli. It can be either idiopathic or associated with other conditions, such as infections, drugs, radiation, or connective tissue diseases. Idiopathic BOOP is an inflammatory lung disease of unknown cause. It occurs almost exclusively in allogeneic HSCT recipients who have GVHD, suggesting that it may represent a form of alloimmune injury to the lung by the transplanted stem cell.[48] Onset is usually 1 month to 2 years after transplantation. Patients may present with dry cough, dyspnea, fever, and inspiratory crackles on physical examination. Pulmonary function tests usually show a restrictive defect, decreased DLCO, and normal flow rates. Imaging shows patchy air space consolidation, ground-glass attenuation, and nodular opacities.[49]

The diagnostic histology from lung biopsy is patchy intraluminal fibrosis consisting of polypoid plugs of immature fibroblast tissue resembling granulation tissue obliterating the distal airways, alveolar ducts, and peribronchial alveolar space.[50] About 80% of HSCT recipients with BOOP favorably respond to corticosteroids.[48]

Pulmonary Cytolytic Thrombi

Pulmonary cytolytic thrombi (PCT) is a noninfectious pulmonary complication seen exclusively after allogeneic procedures in the setting of GVHD.[49] Pathogenesis is unknown but hypothesized to be a manifestation of GVHD targeting the endothelium of the pulmonary vasculature.

The onset of PCT is between 8 to 343 days, with median of 72 days, after transplantation. Most patients have fever and cough at the time of presentation. Abnormal chest radiograph findings include nodules, interstitial prominence, and atelectasis. Chest CT shows multiple peripheral pulmonary nodules.[51] Bronchoalveolar lavage studies exclude infection. Patients usually are treated with anti-infectives and corticosteroids if an infectious cause of pulmonary nodules cannot be ruled out.

Pulmonary Veno-Occlusive Disease

Pulmonary veno-occlusive disease (PVOD) is a rare cause of pulmonary hypertension associated with HSCT. There is intimal fibrosis obstructing the pulmonary veins and venules.[48] Infection, radiation, and chemotherapeutic agents such as bis-chloronitrosourea, mitomycin, and bleomycin are implicated as contributing factors for the development of vascular injury.

Patients initially present with nonspecific dyspnea, lethargy, and chronic cough. As pulmonary hypertension progresses, orthopnea, cyanosis, chest pain, abdominal pain, and exertional syncope may be evident.[52] Physical examination reveals bibasilar crackles and findings indicative of pulmonary hypertension, such as right ventricular heave, loud pulmonic heart sound, lower extremity edema, and elevated jugular venous pressure.

Imaging shows evidence of pulmonary edema, such as Kerley B lines, prominent central pulmonary arteries, scattered patchy opacities, and pleural effusion.[52] Pulmonary function test shows decreased DLCO and restrictive ventilator defect. Echocardiogram and catheterization show elevated pulmonary artery pressure. Surgical lung biopsy studies confirm the diagnosis. With the progressive nature of the disease and, to date, no proven therapy for PVOD, most patients die within 2 years from the time of diagnosis.[52]

Key Points

- Malignant disease is an infrequent cause of pulmonary pathology in the pediatric population.
- Primary tumors of the airways, mediastinum, and lung parenchyma usually present with nonspecific symptoms, such as cough, wheezing, dyspnea, and chest pain.
- A variety of pediatric tumors may metastasize to the lung, often seen radiographically as pulmonary nodules.
- Langerhans cell histiocytosis, leukemias, and lymphomas are the major systemic malignancies with pulmonary involvement in children.
- Pediatric cancer therapies, including chemotherapy, radiation therapy, and bone marrow transplantation, are all associated with significant pulmonary morbidities.
- Monitoring of pulmonary function can be useful in identifying early changes resulting from such therapy.

References

1. Manivel JC, Priest JR, Watterson J, et al. Pleuropulmonary blastoma: the so-called pulmonary blastoma of childhood. *Cancer.* 1998;62:1516–1526
2. Hancock BJ, Di Lorenzo M, Youssef S, et al. Childhood primary pulmonary neoplasms. *J Pediatr Surg.* 1993;28:1133–1136
3. Al-Qahtani AR, Di Lorenzo M, Yasbeck S. Endobronchial tumors in children: institutional experience and literature review. *J Pediatr Surg.* 2003;38(5):733–736
4. Deterding R, Montgomery G. Thoracic tumors. In: Taussig L, Lindall L et al. *Pediatric Respiratory Medicine.* 2nd ed. St Louis, MO: Mosby; 2008:1025–1030
5. Fauroux B, Aynie V, Larroquet M, et al. Carcinoid and mucoepidermoid bronchial tumours in children. *Eur J Pediatr.* 2005;164:748–752
6. Hartman GE, Shochat SJ. Primary pulmonary neoplasms of childhood: a review. *Ann Thorac Surg.* 1983;36:108–119
7. Brooks J, Krummel T. Tumors of the chest. In: Chernick V, Boat T, eds. *Kendig's Disorders of the Respiratory Tract in Children.* 6th ed. Philadelphia, PA: WB Saunders Co; 1998:754–787
8. Davis RD Jr, Oldham HN Jr, Sabiston DC Jr. Primary cysts and neoplasms of the mediastinum: recent changes in clinical presentation, methods of diagnosis, management and results. *Ann Thorac Surg.* 1987;44:229
9. Schwartz CL. Prognostic factors in pediatric Hodgkin disease. *Curr Oncol Rep.* 2003;5:498–504

10. Luna MA, Valenquela-Tamariz J. Germ cell tumors of the mediastinum: postmortem findings. *Am J Clin Pathol.* 1976;65:450
11. Simpson I, Campbell PE. Mediastinal masses in childhood: a review from a paediatric pathologist's point of view. *Prog Pediatr Surg.* 1991;27:92–126
12. Cohen M, Smith WL, Weetman R, Provisor A. Pulmonary pseudometastases in children with malignant tumors. *Radiology.* 1981;141:371–374
13. Erasmus JJ, Connolly JE, McAdams HP, et al. Solitary pulmonary nodules: part I. Morphologic evaluation for differentiation of benign and malignant lesions. *Radiographics.* 2000;20:43–58
14. Fefferman NR, Pinkney LP. Imaging evaluation of chest wall disorders in children. *Radiol Clin North Am.* 2005;43:355–370
15. Rackoff W, Weetman R. Hematologic and oncologic disorders. In: Loughlin G, Eigen H. *Respiratory Disease in Children: Diagnosis and Management.* Baltimore, MD: Williams & Wilkins; 1994:621–638
16. Kayton ML. Pulmonary metastasectomy in pediatric patients. *Thorac Surg Clinic.* 2006;16:167–183
17. Kobrinsky NL, Gritter, HL, Shuckett B. Langerhans cell histiocytosis. In: Chernick V, Boat T, eds. *Kendig's Disorders of the Respiratory Tract in Children.* 6th ed. Philadelphia, PA: WB Saunder's Co; 1998:1058–1071
18. Wells RJ, Weetman RM, Ballantine T, Grosfeld JL, Baehner RL. Pulmonary leukemia in children presenting as diffuse interstitial pneumonia. *J Pediatr.* 1980;96:262–264
19. Lange B, D'Angio G, Ross AJ, O'Neill JA, Packer RJ. Oncologic emergencies. In: Pizzo PA, Poplack DG, eds. *Principles and Practice of Pediatric Oncology.* 2nd ed. Philadelphia, PA: JB Lippincott; 1993:951–972
20. Tubergen DG, Bleyer A. The leukemias. In: Kliegman RM, Behrman RE, Jenson HB, and Stanton BF, eds. *Nelson Textbook of Pediatrics.* 18th ed. Philadelphia, PA: Saunders; 2007:2116–2122
21. Morton LM, Turner JJ, Cerhan JR, et al. Proposed classification of lymphoid neoplasms for epidemiologic research from the Pathology Working Group of the International Lymphoma Epidemiology Consortium (Interlymp). *Blood.* 2007;110:695
22. Sandoval C, Venkateswaran L, Billups C, et al. Lymphocyte-predominant Hodgkin disease in children. *J Pediatr Hematol Oncol.* 2002;24:269
23. Camus P, Caostabel U. Drug-induced respiratory disease in patients with hematological diseases. *Semin Respir Crit Care Med.* 2005;26(5):458–481
24. Poletti V, Salvucci M, Zanchini R, et al. The lung as a target organ in patients with hematologic disorders. *Haematologica.* 2000;85(8):855–864
25. Henry MM, Noah TL. Lung injury caused by pharmacologic agents. In: Chernick V, Boats T eds. *Kendig's Disorders of the Respiratory Tract in Children.* 6th ed. Philadelphia, PA: WB Saunders Co; 1998:1123–1136
26. Zhang K, Gharaee-Kermani M, Jones ML, et al. Lung monocyte chemoattractant protein-1 gene expression in bleomycin-induced pulmonary fibrosis. *J Immunol.* 1994;153:4733–4741

27. Wolley J, Collett J, Goldstein D. Diffuse alveolar damage following a single administration of a cyclophosphamide containing chemotherapy regimen. *Aust NZ J Med.* 1997;27:605–606
28. Cole SR, Myers TJ, Klatsky AU. Pulmonary disease with chlorambucil therapy. *Cancer.* 1978;41:455
29. Aronin PA, Mahaley MSJ, Rudnick SA, et al. Prediction of BNCU pulmonary toxicity in patients with malignant gliomas: an assessment of risk factors. *N Engl J Med.* 1980;303:183–188
30. Rivera MP, Kris MG, Gralla RJ, White DA. Syndrome of acute dyspnea related to combined mitomycin plus vinca alkaloid therapy. *Am J Clin Oncol.* 1995;18:245–250
31. Mesurolle B, Qanadli SD, Merad M, et al. Unusual radiologic findings in the thorax after radiation therapy. *Radiographics.* 2000;20:67–81
32. Logan PM. Thoracic manifestations of external beam radiotherapy. *AJR Am J Roentgenol.* 1998;171:569–577
33. Park KJ, Chung JY, Chun MS, Suh JH. Radiation-induced lung disease and the impact of radiation methods on imaging features. *Radiographics.* 2000;20:83–98
34. Arbetter KR, Prakash UBS, Tazelaar HD, Douglas WW. Radiation-induced pneumonitis in the nonirradiated lung. *Mayo Clin Proc.* 1999;74:27
35. Cordonnier CJ, Bernaudin F, Bierling P, et al. Pulmonary complications occurring after allogeneic bone marrow transplantation. A study of 130 consecutive transplanted patients. *Cancer.* 1986;58:1047–1054
36. Peters SG, Afessa B. Acute lung injury after hematopoietic stem cell transplantation. *Clin Chest Med.* 2005;26:561–569
37. Clark JG, Hansen JA, Hertz MI, et al. NHLBI workshop summary. Idiopathic pneumonia syndrome after bone marrow transplantation. *Am Rev Respir Dis.* 1993;147:1601–1606
38. Gerbitz A, Nickoloff BJ, Olkiewicz K, et al. A role for tumor necrosis factor-alpha mediated endothelial apoptosis in the development of experimental idiopathic pneumonia syndrome. *Transplantation.* 2004;78:494–502
39. Capizzi SA, Kumar S, Huneke NE, et al. Periengraftment respiratory distress syndrome during autologous hematopoietic stem cell transplantation. *Bone Marrow Transplant.* 2001;27:1299–1303
40. Afessa BA, Tefferi MR, Litzow MJ, et al. Diffuse alveolar hemorrhage in hematopoietic stem cell transplant recipients. *Am J Respir Crit Care Med.* 2002;166:641–645
41. Griese M, Rampf U, Hofmann D, et al. Pulmonary complications after bone marrow transplantation in children: twenty-four years of experience in a single pediatric center. *Pediatr Pulmonol.* 2000;30(5):393–401
42. Marras TK, Chan CK, Lipton JH, et al. Long term pulmonary function abnormalities and survival after allogeneic marrow transplantation. *Bone Marrow Transplant.* 2004;33(5):509–517

43. Stephenson AL, Mackenzie IR, Levy RD, et al. Myositis associated graft-versus-host-disease presenting as respiratory muscle weakness. *Thorax.* 2001;56(1):82–84
44. King TE Jr. Overview of bronchiolitis. *Clin Chest Med.* 1993;14(4):607–610
45. Philit F, Wisendanger T, Archimbaud E, et al. Post-transplant obstructive lung disease ("bronchiolitis obliterans"): a clinical comparative study of bone marrow and lung transplant patients. *Eur Respir J.* 1995;8(4):551–558
46. Jung JI, Jung WS, Hahn ST, et al. Bronchiolitis obliterans after allogenic bone marrow transplantation: HRCT findings. *Korean J Radiol.* 2004;5(2):107–113
47. Kanazawa S, Nomura S, Muramatsu M, et al. Azithromycin and bronchiolitis obliterans. *Am J Respir Crit Care Med.* 2004;169(5):654–655
48. Epler GR. Bronchiolitis obliterans organizing pneumonia. *Arch Intern Med.* 2001;161(2):158–164
49. Afessa B, Peters SG. Chronic lung disease after hematopoietic stem cell transplantation. *Clin Chest Med.* 2005;26:571–586
50. Myers JL, Colby TV. Pathologic manifestations of bronchiolitis, constrictive bronchiolitis, cryptogenic organizing pneumonia and diffuse panbrochiolitis. *Clin Chest Med.* 1993;14(4):611–622
51. Wodard JP, Gulbahce E, Shreve M, et al. Pulmonary cytolytic thrombi: a newly recognized complication of stem cell transplantation. *Bone Marrow Transplant.* 2000;25(3):293–300
52. Mandel J, Mark EJ, Hales CA. Pulmonary veno-occlusive disease. *Am J Respir Crit Care Med.* 2000;162(5):1964–1973

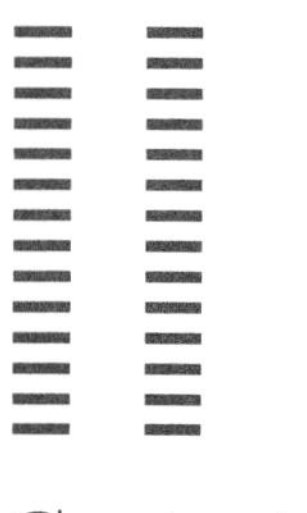

Chapter 44

Pulmonary Complications of Immunologic Disorders

Clement L. Ren, MD

Introduction

The respiratory tract is continuously exposed to pathogens through inhalation. To protect against infection, the lungs have a variety of defense mechanisms, including a mucociliary barrier, the innate immune system, and the adaptive immune system. This chapter focuses on pulmonary complications arising from defects in adaptive immunity.

Each component of the immune system serves a specific role in host defense. A deficiency in any one element of the immune system renders individuals susceptible to specific groups of pathogens. Table 44-1 summarizes the pattern of infections seen in children with different immunodeficiency syndromes.

Infectious Complications of Immunodeficiency

Complications of Neutrophil Defects

Polymorphonuclear neutrophils (PMNs) are the primary phagocytic cells of the immune system. They play a key role in eliminating opsonized bacterial and fungal pathogens through release of proteolytic enzymes and reactive oxidant species. This function may be impaired through abnormalities in cell adhesion, cell signaling, cell number, granule function or formation, and intracellular killing.[1]

Table 44-1. Typical Pathogens Associated With Specific Immunodeficiencies

Element of the Immune System Affected	Example Diseases	Typical Pulmonary Pathogens
Neutrophils	Chronic granulomatous disease	*Staphylococcus aureus, Aspergillus fumigatus*
B lymphocytes	X-linked (Bruton) agammaglobulinemia Common variable immunodeficiency	*Streptococcus pneumoniae, Haemophilus influenzae*
T lymphocytes	Severe: severe combined immunodeficiency Less severe: ataxia-telangiectasia, Wiskott-Aldrich syndrome	*Pneumocystis jiroveci* pneumonia, viruses, fungi Bacterial pneumonia

Chronic Granulomatous Disease

The most common PMN disorder is chronic granulomatous disease (CGD), with an estimated prevalence of 1 in 200,000 in the United States.[1,2] The primary defect in CGD is a loss of nicotinamide adenine dinucleotide phosphate (NADPH) oxidase function. Chronic granulomatous disease exists in X-linked and autosomal recessive forms, depending on which gene coding for the NADPH oxidase complex is mutated; the X-linked form is more common. Loss of NADPH oxidase activity leads to a markedly reduced oxidative burst following phagocytosis. Polymorphonuclear neutrophils from patients with CGD can phagocytose bacteria but cannot kill them. The most common organisms that cause pulmonary infections in CGD are *Aspergillus* species, *Staphylococcus aureus, Burkholderia cepacia* complex, *Nocardia* species, and *Serratia marcescens.*[1]

Patients with CGD present with atypical or unusually severe lymphadenitis, skin abscesses, pneumonia, or osteomyleitis secondary to infections with the aforementioned agents. Hepatosplenomegaly due to non-cirrhotic portal hypertension is common as well. In addition, patients with CGD often develop granulomas involving a number of different organs, including the bladder, gastrointestinal tract, and lungs. Chronic granulomatous disease colitis can be mistaken for Crohn disease. Data from a national registry of 368 patients with CGD in the United States provide considerable insight into the pulmonary complications of CGD.[3] Eighty percent of the patients in the registry have had pneumonia at least once. *Aspergillus* was the most common causative organism, responsible for 41% of pneumonias in the days before oral antifungals were used as prophylaxis. *Aspergillus* pneumonia with or without dissemination was the most common cause of death in patients with CGD, causing 35% of deaths. *Staphylococcus* species caused 12% of pneumonias. *Burkholderia cepacia* is the third most common cause of pneumonia (8%), but the second most common cause of death (18%). Other pathogens reported to cause pneumonia in these patients include *Nocardia,* mycobacteria, and gram-negative bacteria. It should be noted, however, that this registry was published prior to a large study showing that antifungal prophylaxis is effective, and thus leading to widespread use of azoles for *Aspergillus* prophylaxis.[4]

Trimethoprim-sulfamethoxazole (TMP-SMX) prophylaxis was introduced in 1990 and has been effective in reducing the frequency of serious bacterial infections.[1] Itraconazole prophylaxis has been used since its availability, and a randomized prospective blinded study showed strong activity in the prevention of all fungal infections in CGD.[4] Determination of the infecting microbe is of great importance, as most patients are on prophylaxis so antimicrobial sensitivity patterns are needed to assist in the proper treatment of infection.

Pulmonary abscesses also occur frequently in patients with CGD. Sixteen percent of patients in the registry had a lung abscess. Of those, the most common organism isolated was *Aspergillus* (23%), although *Nocardia* species, *B cepacia,* and *Staphylococcus* species can also cause abscesses.[3]

Other Neutrophil Disorders

Other PMN disorders include hyper-immunoglobulin (Ig) E syndrome (also known as Job syndrome) and Chediak-Higashi syndrome (CHS).[1] Hyper-IgE syndrome (HIES) is a rare disorder caused by heterozygous mutations in an intracellular signaling protein (STAT3). Patients typically present with characteristic facial features, recurrent skin infections, and extremely high serum IgE levels. A hallmark feature of pulmonary infection associated with the hyper-IgE syndrome is the formation of pneumatoceles and bronchiectasis. Although *S aureus* is the most common organism causing pneumonia in those with HIES initially, after pneumatoceles and bronchiectasis are present, these patients are predisposed to gram-negative pulmonary infections (frequently *Pseudomonas),* mold infection (typically *Aspergillus),* and nontuberculous mycobacteria. These infections are the main source of morbidity and mortality for these individuals. Chediak-Higashi syndrome is an autosomal recessive disorder resulting from mutations in a lysosomal protein transport gene. Patients with CHS have multiple abnormalities, including reduced PMN phagocytosis and chemotaxis. In general, pulmonary complications in these disorders are pneumonias but not pneumatoceles or bronchiectasis.

Complications of B Lymphocyte Disorders

B lymphocytes are the only source of Ig, or antibody.[5] There are 5 different Ig isotypes: IgM, IgG, IgA, IgD, and IgE. B cells initially express only surface IgM and IgD, but with appropriate T lymphocyte help they will switch to making other isotypes. Immunoglobulins play a key role in the opsonization and clearance of encapsulated bacterial organisms. Thus patients with B cell deficiencies are prone to infection with these organisms, primarily *Streptococcus pneumoniae* (pneumococcus) and *Haemophilus influenzae*. In contrast, because T-cell function is intact, patients tend to have normal defenses against viruses, fungi, and mycobacteria. Because maternal IgG crosses the placental barrier, infants with B cell disorders receive passive protection from infection for the first 6 to 9 months of life. After this age, patients will present with recurrent bacterial infections of the middle ear, sinuses, and lungs. Complications such as mastoiditis are common. Sepsis and osteomyelitis may also be seen.[5]

The most severe forms of B cell disorders arise from defects in B cell development, leading to virtual absence of circulating B cells. Of this group, X-linked (Bruton) agammaglobulinemia (XLA) is the most common. The molecular defect in XLA is due to mutations in the Bruton tyrosine kinase (BTK) gene.[5] Absence of BTK results in a block in B cell maturation at the pre–B cell stage. Thus patients with XLA have essentially no circulating B cells and make no antibody to antigenic stimulation (immunization). Pulmonary infections are very common in XLA, mainly due to *S pneumoniae* and *H influenzae*.[6] In contrast to other B cell disorders, patients with XLA can develop *Pneumocystis jiroveci* pneumonia (PCP).[5] The reason for this is unclear, although it may be related to the role of B cells as antigen-presenting cells. Alternatively, it may be that loss of BTK function leads to subtle defects in cellular immunity.

Common Variable Immunodeficiency

Common variable immunodeficiency (CVID) is the name given to a heterogeneous group of disorders characterized by varying degrees of hypogammaglobulinemia with or without other abnormalities of T cell function.[5] The prevalence of CVID is estimated to be 1 per 50,000 to 200,000 individuals.[7] Patients with CVID usually have normal numbers of B cells, but the function of these cells is impaired. Other immunologic abnormalities that can be seen in CVID include impaired lymphocyte proliferative response to antigens, deficiency of antigen-primed T cells, increased macrophage activation, and reduced production or expression of cytokines. Common variable immunodeficiency can frequently occur in older children or adults following a viral infection, and it is sometimes referred to as acquired hypogammaglobulinemia. Although patients with CVID may have subtle defects in T cell function, they usually do not develop opportunistic infections. More commonly, patients with CVID are prone to recurrent bacterial infections, generally of the sinopulmonary tract. Because the condition may present in later childhood and the diagnosis may be delayed, many of these patients have bronchiectasis at the time of presentation.[7,8]

IgA Deficiency

Immunoglobulin A deficiency is the most common antibody deficiency, with an approximate incidence of 1 in 400 to 3,000 individuals depending on the ethnicity of the population.[5] Most patients with IgA deficiency are asymptomatic, perhaps because of compensatory protection by IgG. Those who are symptomatic are at increased risk of gastrointestinal and sinopulmonary infections. Symptomatic IgA deficiency is often seen in association with IgG subclass deficiency.

The introduction of intravenous Ig (IVIG) replacement therapy has had a significant effect on the morbidity and mortality of B cell immunodeficiencies.[5,9,10] Intravenous Ig and the more recently introduced subcutaneous IgG (SCIG) are prepared from pooled plasma collected from a large number of donors. As a blood product, IVIG does carry a potential risk for pathogen transmission. However, improved purification protocols have rendered this risk extremely small.[10] Intravenous IG/SCIG therapy significantly reduces the incidence and severity of pneumonia and other respiratory tract infections in patients with

XLA, CVID, and other antibody deficiency syndromes.[9] However, bronchiectasis can still develop in some patients in spite of IVIG/SCIG therapy[8,9] (Figure 44-1).

Pulmonary Infections Associated With T Lymphocyte Disorders

T lymphocytes play important roles in coordinating the adaptive immune system and actively eliminating foreign pathogens.[11] Because of the multiple roles that T cells play in the immune system, impairment of their function may have profound consequences for immunity. T cells can be divided into multiple subclasses based on their cell sur-

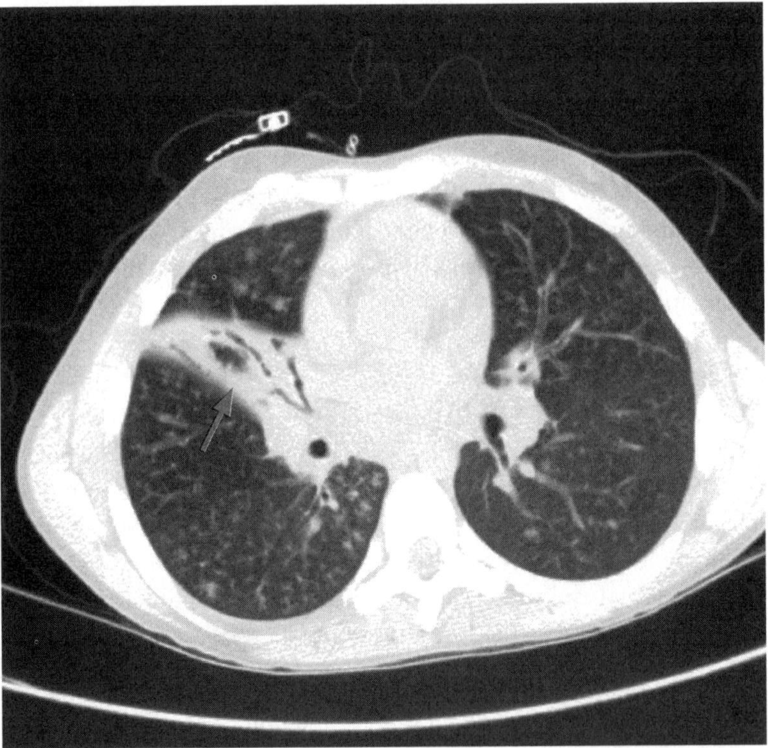

Figure 44-1. Chest computed tomogram (CT) from an 11-year-old girl with common variable immunodeficiency (CVID). This child was diagnosed with CVID at 3 years of age when she presented with chronic respiratory infections. Intravenous immunoglobulin therapy was started at that time. In the intervening years, she did not have acute episodes of pneumonia, but she was seen by a pulmonologist because of a 1-year history of increasing cough. A chest CT was obtained. Consolidation and bronchiectasis of the right middle lobe can be seen (blue arrow).

face protein expression, gene expression, and function. Cytotoxic T lymphocytes (CTLs) usually express CD8 and are responsible for cell-mediated immune responses. Helper T (Th) cells usually express the cell surface receptor CD4 and are critical for B cell activation and optimal antibody production. Helper T cells also coordinate the activity of CTLs. Regulatory T cells (Tregs) express CD4, CD25 (the alpha chain of the interleukin-2 receptor), and FOXP3, a forkhead transcription factor. Tregs are thought to play a vital role in autoimmune and allergic disease.[12] FOXP3 is critical for the development of Tregs, and loss of FOXP3 function results in immune dysregulation, polyendocrinopathy, enteropathy, and X-linked syndrome.[13] There are many other T cell subsets that have recently been defined, but their role in primary immunodeficiency is not well defined at this time.

Severe Combined Immunodeficiency

Severe combined immunodeficiency (SCID) is the term used to identify the most severe forms of T cell disorders. Severe combined immunodeficiency can result from a diverse array of genetic mutations that affect lymphocyte production, development, metabolism, or cell signaling.[11] Regardless of the underlying genetic defect, the immunologic consequence is that there is near total loss of T cell number or function. Because B and T lymphocytes develop from a single lymphoid lineage, many cases of SCID are also associated with absent B cells. In those cases with residual circulating B cells, the lack of T cell help renders them nonfunctional.

The loss of T cell function in patients with SCID leads to their being susceptible to opportunistic infections such as *P jiroveci,* fungi, and viruses. Patients with SCID tend to present early in infancy because of the severe loss of immune function. Pulmonary infections are a common initial presenting sign in SCID, and up to 67% of patients with SCID present with pulmonary disease at diagnosis.[14] In patients with pulmonary complaints at presentation, 60% present with a persistent pulmonary infiltrate and chronic cough, while the other 40% present with more acute symptoms of respiratory distress secondary to pneumonia. *Pneumocystis jiroveci* is the most common cause of pneumonia and is associated with significant mortality (43%). Bacterial pneumonia can also occur, with *Klebsiella pneumoniae, S pneumoniae,* and *S aureus* being the most common pathogens isolated. Viral infections contribute to morbidity and mortality in these patients and can include parainfluenza, cytomegalovirus (CMV), adenovirus, and respiratory syncytial virus (RSV). In patients not treated with immune reconstitution, pulmonary disease together with failure to thrive are significant causes of morbidity and mortality. Subsequent pulmonary infection occurs in 80% to 100% of patients after initial diagnosis.[14]

Besides SCID, immunodeficiency can also arise from other, less severe, defects in T cell function. Because some degree of residual T cell function persists in these other conditions, the severity of disease tends to be less than that of SCID. Pulmonary complications, however, continue to be common in this group of patients.

Other T Cell Disorders

DiGeorge Syndrome

DiGeorge syndrome results from errors in the formation of the third and fourth pharyngeal pouches during embryogenesis, resulting in hypoplasia or complete absence of the thymus and parathyroid glands.[11] Other midline structures may also be affected, such as the heart and great vessels, craniofacial bones and tissues, and upper limbs. The immunologic defect is due to thymic dysplasia and ranges from a severe depression of T cell function in patients with no thymus, to near normal function in patients with mild thymic hypoplasia. In contrast to SCID, patients with DiGeorge syndrome are not commonly infected with *P jiroveci.* Bacterial pneumonia with gram-negative organisms is more commonly seen. Severe RSV infections have also been reported.

Wiskott-Aldrich Syndrome

Wiskott-Aldrich syndrome (WAS) is an X-linked recessive T cell disorder caused by mutations in the Wiskott-Aldrich syndrome protein (WASP) gene.[15] The classic clinical triad of WAS is thrombocytopenia, eczema, and recurrent bacterial infection. Although the exact function of WASP is still undetermined, loss of WASP function results in an inability to generate antibody to polysaccharide antigens. Patients with WAS are therefore susceptible to recurrent infections with bacteria that form polysaccharide capsules, such as *S pneumoniae* and *H influenzae.* Although the sites of infection tend to be the middle ear and sinuses, pneumonia can also be seen in this group of patients. Later in life, there is also an increased incidence of PCP.

Ataxia-Telangiectasia

Ataxia-telangiectasia (A-T) is a complex multisystem autosomal recessive syndrome with abnormalities of the nervous system, endocrine system, skin, liver, and immune system.[11] Immune dysfunction in A-T is variable and affects both T and B cells. Although A-T is classified as a T cell immunodeficiency, B cell dysfunction due to loss of T cell help is the primary immune problem. Immunoglobulin A and IgG subclass deficiencies are commonly seen in patients with A-T. Pulmonary infections are a common complication in A-T, and a significant cause of mortality. Pneumonia in patients with A-T tends to be caused by bacteria, such as *S pneumoniae, S aureus, H influenzae, Mycoplasma pneumoniae,* and *Pseudomonas aeruginosa.* Respiratory syncytial virus and CMV can also cause lower respiratory tract infection in these patients, but fungi, mycobacteria, and *P jiroveci* rarely are pathogens in this disease.[11] The underlying defect in A-T involves a defect in DNA repair, and patients with A-T are at high risk for the development of malignancy. In some patients with A-T, pulmonary lymphoma has led to cavitary lesions on chest radiographs that were mistaken for pneumonia.[16] It is therefore important to consider the possibility of malignancy when evaluating patients with A-T and pulmonary symptoms and to pursue an appropriate investigation.

Hyper-IgM Syndrome

Hyper-IgM (HIgM) syndrome is characterized by normal or elevated serum IgM levels with decreased or absent levels of IgG, IgA, and IgE.[11] Hyper-IgM syndrome exists in both an X-linked and autosomal recessive form. About 55% to 65% of the patients have the X-linked form that is caused by mutations in the gene for CD40 ligand (CD154), a T cell surface molecule critical for induction of B cell isotype switch. Because of the absence of CD154, B cells from patients with X-linked HIgM can only make IgM, with little or no production of other Ig isotypes. An autosomal recessive form also exists associated with a defect in CD40, the receptor for CD40 ligand. In addition, there are also autosomal recessive forms that are caused by mutations in at least 3 different genes involved directly in B cell isotype switch. Bacterial pneumonia is the most common pulmonary complication in

HIgM syndrome, but PCP and other opportunistic infections are seen in the X-linked form and in CD40 deficiency, indicating that CD154/CD40 interaction also plays a role in T cell-innate immune cell interaction.

Noninfectious Pulmonary Complications of Immunodeficiency

In addition to impaired host defense, patients with immunodeficiency can also develop dysregulated immune responses.[17] Noninfectious pulmonary diseases that have been reported in association with immunodeficiency include interstitial lung disease, bronchiolitis obliterans, and hypersensitivity pneumonitis. The presumed mechanism for these disorders is that defects that result in an impaired ability to generate a protective adaptive immune response may also result in excessive inflammatory responses. Common variable immunodeficiency and A-T are the most common conditions associated with the above disorders,[5,11] although they have been reported in other immunodeficiencies.[18]

Pulmonary Complications Associated With HIV Infection

HIV infection is the most common cause of acquired immunodeficiency.[19] HIV infects CD4 positive Th cells, leading to their loss. As HIV infection progresses, patients have a near total depletion of CD4 T cells. The loss of Th cells impairs both CTL function as well as B cell function.

Infectious Complications of HIV Infection

Pneumocystis jiroveci pneumonia is one of the most common complications of HIV[19,20] and may be the presenting feature in infancy. *Pneumocystis jiroveci* pneumonia infections in patients infected with HIV carry a high degree of morbidity and mortality.[19] Prophylaxis against PCP is an important part of HIV treatment and can be accomplished with either TMP-SMX or inhaled pentamidine.

In endemic areas of developing nations, *Mycobacterium tuberculosis* (TB) has emerged as a major pulmonary complication and cause of death in patients infected with HIV.[19] Tuberculosis infections tend to be more severe and difficult to treat in patients infected with HIV. Non-tuberculous mycobacteria, such as *Mycobacterium avium* complex (MAC) can also cause disseminated disease in adults with HIV. In contrast, the incidence of severe pulmonary MAC disease is less in children infected with HIV.[21]

Respiratory viral infections are another common complication in HIV infection. Respiratory syncytial virus, influenza A and B, and parainfluenza viruses can all cause severe lung disease in infants infected with HIV.[22] Cytomegalovirus can also cause pulmonary disease. However, because CMV is often shed asymptomatically, the diagnosis of true pneumonitis should rest on evidence of systemic dissemination (eg, retinitis or hepatitis) or demonstration of viral inclusion bodies in lung biopsy specimens.

The other major group of respiratory pathogens in individuals infected with HIV is fungi. Histoplasmosis infection is rare, but when present it occurs as disseminated disease that often includes reticulonodular, miliary, or lobar infiltrates. It can often progress to septic shock and death if untreated. *Cryptococcus* and *Coccidioides* species can also cause pulmonary disease. Pulmonary aspergillosis is rare and presents as invasive pulmonary disease rather than as aspergilloma; this can be life-threatening, with poor prognosis despite antifungal therapy.[23]

Although patients with HIV primarily suffer from opportunistic infections as a consequence of their loss of cellular immunity, bacterial infections are also common, especially in children.[20,21,23] These occur despite normal or even elevated Ig levels in patients with HIV, because the loss of CD4 positive Th cells results in a failure to generate effective specific antibody titers. *Streptococcus pneumoniae* is the most common cause of bacterial pneumonia in this patient population. Other common organisms include *S aureus*, group A streptococcus, *Escherichia coli, P aeruginosa, H influenzae,* and *Salmonella.*

Noninfectious Complications of HIV Infection

Dysregulation of the immune system is another consequence of HIV infection, leading to an increased incidence of noninfectious disorders of the lung.[19,20] In children, the most common noninfectious pulmonary complication is lymphocytic interstitial pneumonitis (LIP). The precise pathogenesis of LIP is unknown. It is thought to represent a dysregulated immunologic response to Epstein-Barr virus infection.

Between 30% and 40% of perinatally infected children will have LIP, with an average age of 2.3 years at presentation. Typically, patients with LIP present with gradual onset of cough and dyspnea. Generalized lymphadenopathy and clubbing are associated clinical findings. The chest radiograph demonstrates diffuse reticulonodular densities, frequently with hilar adenopathy. Lymphocytic interstitial pneumonitis is usually quite responsive to systemic corticosteroid therapy, which is the first line of treatment for this condition. The condition may recur, requiring repetitive courses of oral corticosteroids.

In addition to LIP, a nonspecific interstitial pneumonitis can also occur in patients infected with HIV, although this is less common in children. Nonspecific interstitial pneumonitis is thought to result from localized CTL activity against HIV-infected cells in the lung parenchyma. Therefore it is more commonly seen early in HIV infection, when there is still some residual CD4-positive T cell activity present. However, it can occur at any stage of the disease.

Pulmonary Complications Related to HIV Therapy

Highly active antiretroviral therapy (HAART) against HIV infection was introduced in the mid-1990s. Highly active antiretroviral therapy has had a dramatic effect on the prognosis and clinical course of HIV infection.[19] One result of increased survival has been the increased incidence of chronic lung diseases, such as bronchiectasis.[24] The restoration of immune function in patients with previously longstanding immunodeficiency has also led to unexpected complications resulting from either exuberant inflammatory responses or unmasking of latent opportunistic infections.[25,26] As immune function is restored, there is an increased inflammatory response against underlying latent mycobacterial infections, both TB as well as MAC. Highly active antiretroviral therapy may also be associated with reactivation of latent PCP, leading to acute respiratory failure. Noninfectious complications that have been reported with HAART include a sarcoid-like syndrome, hypersensitivity pneumonitis, and pulmonary hypertension.[26,27] Although most published reports have focused on adult patients, it is likely that this same phenomenon will be seen in children as HAART increasingly becomes the standard of care in HIV treatment.

Box 44-1. Evaluation of the Patient With Immunodeficiency

History
- Delayed umbilical cord separation
- History of infections
- Sites and etiologies of infections

Physical Examination
- Head, eyes, ears, nose, throat
  - Presence of tonsils
- Chest
  - Crackles
  - Wheezes
- Extremities
  - Lymphadenopathy
  - Clubbing

Radiographic Imaging
- Chest radiograph
- High-resolution computed tomography
- Evidence of bronchiectasis
- Thymus present?

Pulmonary Function Testing
- Restrictive versus obstructive pattern
- Diffusion defects

Bronchoscopy vs Transthoracic Needle Aspiration/Biopsy

Pulmonary Evaluation of the Patient With Immunodeficiency

The approach to evaluating a patient with immunodeficiency is summarized in Box 44-1. The evaluation begins with a thorough history and physical examination. The history should focus on symptoms of chronic infection or bronchiectasis. The patient or patient's parents should be questioned about the presence of cough and sputum production. However, patients with impaired host responses often do not feel as sick as they are, and are often much less symptomatic than their degree of infection would cause in a normal host. Symptoms of wheezing may suggest an asthma or reactive airways disease component. Elements of the physical examination of particular importance include the patient's height and weight, chest examination, and extremity examination. The height and weight provide important information about the patient's nutritional status, which may be compromised in the setting of chronic pulmonary disease. Auscultation of the chest is important to identify areas of localized crackles or wheezes. The presence of digital clubbing on extremity examination is an indication of underlying bronchiectasis or hypoxemia. Other important aspects of the physical examination include evidence of skin infections, absence of lymphoid tissue (eg, tonsils and lymph nodes), and evidence of chronic or frequently recurring otitis media.

Radiography is an important tool in the evaluation of pulmonary disease in immunodeficient patients. Plain chest radiographs can reveal areas of atelectasis or infiltrate. Although large areas of bronchiectasis can be seen by plain radiographs, high-resolution computed tomography is a more sensitive tool for the detection of early or mild bronchiectasis.[28,29] Computed tomography is also helpful for delineating lesions such as pulmonary abscesses or lymph node pathology.

The results of pulmonary function tests in immunodeficient patients depends on the underlying pulmonary pathology. Patients with bronchiectasis demonstrate an obstructive pattern (see Chapter 6). Patients with interstitial lung processes will have a restrictive pattern, and the diffusion capacity may also be decreased. Pulmonary function tests can be helpful in establishing the severity of disease and in tracking disease progression. Pulmonary function tests can also provide objective assessment of response to medications, such as bronchodilators.

Bronchoscopy can be important both for acute complications as well as for chronic conditions. For patients presenting with acute pulmonary symptoms, bronchoscopy with bronchoalveolar lavage (BAL) can help in the diagnosis of infections such as PCP. For patients with bronchiectasis who cannot expectorate sputum, BAL can provide information about the organisms colonizing the lower respiratory tract. Transbronchial biopsy can also be performed to identify fungal or viral infections. Bronchoscopy can also be helpful in studying the airway anatomy, especially in patients in whom there is concern for compression of the bronchi by enlarged reactive lymph nodes. In most cases, flexible fiberoptic bronchoscopy can be safely performed under moderate or deep sedation on this group of patients. It is important to be aware that BAL may not provide microbiological diagnosis, especially in fungal disease. Percutaneous needle biopsy is another safe alternative and has much higher diagnostic yield in diseases like CGD.

Treating Pulmonary Complications in Immunodeficient Children

Treatment of the underlying immune defect is the best way to prevent pulmonary complications, but since this usually requires bone marrow transplantation, temporizing measures are critical. For patients with SCID or other T cell disorders, bone marrow transplantation can result in complete correction of the immune defect.[11] Antibody deficiency syndromes can be treated with IVIG/SCIG replacement therapy.[5,10] Highly active antiretroviral therapy has had a dramatic effect on survival and the rates of infection in patients with HIV.[19] It is likely that as our understanding of the molecular and cellular basis of congenital and acquired immunodeficiency increases, more therapies aimed at correcting the underlying defect will become available.

Although specific therapy for immunodeficiencies is available, not all patients are candidates for bone marrow transplantation, and other therapies may not lead to complete absence of pulmonary complications. In this situation, antibiotic prophylaxis can be used to reduce the incidence of pulmonary infections. The choice of antibiotic depends on the pathogens most likely to be involved in the underlying disease process. For CGD, prophylaxis with TMP-SMX covers all their bacterial pathogens, whereas for T cell immunodeficiencies and HIV infection, prophylaxis against *P jiroveci* is the major concern. Itraconazole prophylaxis for *Aspergillus* in CGD has been used effectively in many centers.[30]

Many patients with immunodeficiency still develop bronchiectasis, as a result of either delayed diagnosis or continued infection despite treatment. This is especially common in patients with B cell disorders such as XLA and CVID. See Chapter 17 for treatment information.

For patients with irreversible or progressive respiratory failure, lung transplantation is an option. Lung transplantation has been performed on patients with immunodeficiency, but there are limited data on their clinical outcomes.[8,31] Lung transplantation is an arduous process for patients and is associated with numerous short-term and long-term complications. Any decision to proceed with lung transplantation must be made after a careful and thorough consideration of the risks and potential benefits.

When to Refer

Consider referring patients with immunodeficiency to the pulmonologist if they have persistent respiratory symptoms or signs of chronic lung disease (eg, clubbing).

Key Points

- Pulmonary complications are common in patients with immunodeficiency, and pulmonary infections are frequently the initial presenting sign.
- It is important to identify the microbe so that therapy can be directed aggressively to the appropriate organism.
- Defects in different parts of the immune system result in distinctive patterns of infection.
- Although IVIG and antibiotics can help prevent severe infections, bronchiectasis can often still develop in these patients.
- Noninfectious pulmonary diseases, such as interstitial lung disease, can also develop.
- The primary care provider should be aware of the presenting signs of primary immunodeficiency and evaluate patients appropriately.
- The primary care provider should maintain close follow-up of patients with immunodeficiency and evaluate their respiratory status on a regular basis or if signs and symptoms of lung disease develop.

References

1. Lekstrom-Himes JA, Gallin JI. Immunodeficiency diseases caused by defects in phagocytes. *N Engl J Med.* 2000;343(23):1703–1714
2. Goldblatt D, Thrasher AJ. Chronic granulomatous disease. *Clin Exp Immunol.* 2000;122(1):1–9
3. Winkelstein JA, Marino MC, Johnston RB Jr, et al. Chronic granulomatous disease. Report on a national registry of 368 patients. *Medicine (Baltimore).* 2000;79(3):155–169
4. Gallin JI, Alling DW, Malech HL, et al. Itraconazole to prevent fungal infections in chronic granulomatous disease. *N Engl J Med.* 2003;348(24):2416–2422

5. Ballow M. Primary immunodeficiency disorders: antibody deficiency. *J Allergy Clin Immunol.* 2002;109(4):581–591
6. Lederman HM, Winkelstein JA. X-linked agammaglobulinemia: an analysis of 96 patients. *Medicine (Baltimore).* 1985;64(3):145–156
7. Thickett KM, Kumararatne DS, Banerjee AK, Dudley R, Stableforth DE. Common variable immune deficiency: respiratory manifestations, pulmonary function and high-resolution CT scan findings. *QJM.* 2002;95(10):655–662
8. Cunningham-Rundles C, Bodian C. Common variable immunodeficiency: clinical and immunological features of 248 patients. *Clin Immunol.* 1999;92(1):34–48
9. Busse PJ, Razvi S, Cunningham-Rundles C. Efficacy of intravenous immunoglobulin in the prevention of pneumonia in patients with common variable immunodeficiency. *J Allergy Clin Immunol.* 2002;109(6):1001–1004
10. Orange JS, Hossny EM, Weiler CR, et al. Use of intravenous immunoglobulin in human disease: a review of evidence by members of the Primary Immunodeficiency Committee of the American Academy of Allergy, Asthma and Immunology. *J Allergy Clin Immunol.* 2006;117(4 suppl):S525–S553
11. Buckley RH. Primary cellular immunodeficiencies. *J Allergy Clin Immunol.* 2002;109(5):747–757
12. Bacchetta R, Gambineri E, Roncarolo MG. Role of regulatory T cells and FOXP3 in human diseases. *J Allergy Clin Immunol.* 2007;120(2):227–235
13. Chatila TA. Role of regulatory T cells in human diseases. *J Allergy Clin Immunol.* 2005;116(5):949–959
14. Deerojanawong J, Chang AB, Eng PA, Robertson CF, Kemp AS. Pulmonary diseases in children with severe combined immune deficiency and DiGeorge syndrome. *Pediatr Pulmonol.* 1997;24(5):324–330
15. Ochs HD, Thrasher AJ. The Wiskott-Aldrich syndrome. *J Allergy Clin Immunol.* 2006;117(4):725–738
16. Yalcin B, Kutluk MT, Sanal O, et al. Hodgkin's disease and ataxia telangiectasia with pulmonary cavities. *Pediatr Pulmonol.* 2002;33(5):399–403
17. Conces DJ Jr. Noninfectious lung disease in immunocompromised patients. *J Thorac Imaging.* 1999;14(1):9–24
18. Levy J, Espanol-Boren T, Thomas C, et al. Clinical spectrum of X-linked hyper-IgM syndrome. *J Pediatr.* 1997;131(1 pt 1):47–54
19. Moylett EH, Shearer WT. HIV: clinical manifestations. *J Allergy Clin Immunol.* 2002;110(1):3–16
20. Bye MR. Human immunodeficiency virus infections and the respiratory system in children. *Pediatr Pulmonol.* 1995;19(4):231–242
21. Perez MS, Van Dyke RB. Pulmonary infections in children with HIV infection. *Semin Respir Infect.* 2002;17(1):33–46

22. Madhi SA, Schoub B, Simmank K, Blackburn N, Klugman KP. Increased burden of respiratory viral associated severe lower respiratory tract infections in children infected with human immunodeficiency virus type-1. *J Pediatr.* 2000;137(1):78–84
23. Mofenson LM, Yogev R, Korelitz J, et al. Characteristics of acute pneumonia in human immunodeficiency virus-infected children and association with long term mortality risk. National Institute of Child Health and Human Development Intravenous Immunoglobulin Clinical Trial Study Group. *Pediatr Infect Dis J.* 1998;17(10):872–880
24. Sheikh S, Madiraju K, Steiner P, Rao M. Bronchiectasis in pediatric AIDS. *Chest.* 1997;112(5):1202–1207
25. Wolff AJ, O'Donnell AE. Pulmonary manifestations of HIV infection in the era of highly active antiretroviral therapy. *Chest.* 2001;120(6):1888–1893
26. Grubb JR, Moorman AC, Baker RK, Masur H. The changing spectrum of pulmonary disease in patients with HIV infection on antiretroviral therapy. *AIDS.* 2006;20(8):1095–1107
27. Naccache JM, Antoine M, Wislez M, et al. Sarcoid-like pulmonary disorder in human immunodeficiency virus-infected patients receiving antiretroviral therapy. *Am J Respir Crit Care Med.* 1999;159(6):2009–2013
28. Kainulainen L, Varpula M, Liippo K, Svedstrom E, Nikoskelainen J, Ruuskanen O. Pulmonary abnormalities in patients with primary hypogammaglobulinemia. *J Allergy Clin Immunol.* 1999;104(5):1031–1036
29. Barker AF. Bronchiectasis. *N Engl J Med.* 2002;346(18):1383–1393
30. Mouy R, Veber F, Blanche S, et al. Long-term itraconazole prophylaxis against *Aspergillus* infections in thirty-two patients with chronic granulomatous disease. *J Pediatr.* 1994;125(6 pt 1):998–1003
31. Hill AT, Thompson RA, Wallwork J, Stableforth DE. Heart lung transplantation in a patient with end stage lung disease due to common variable immunodeficiency. *Thorax.* 1998;53(7):622–623

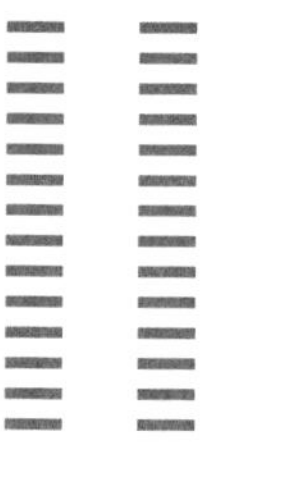

Chapter 45

Pulmonary Complications of Neuromuscular Disorders

Girish D. Sharma, MD

Introduction

Neuromuscular disorders (NMDs) may be associated with a gradual loss of muscle function over time, and children with these disorders are at risk to develop significant respiratory morbidity from recurrent respiratory infections and chronic respiratory insufficiency.[1–4]

Loss of respiratory muscle strength that leads to ineffective cough and decreased ventilation may result in atelectasis, decreased lung volumes, chronic respiratory insufficiency, and respiratory failure.[1] In some children muscle weakness may lead to oropharyngeal incompetence,[5,6] gastroesophageal reflux, feeding problems, and malnutrition[7,8] (Figure 45-1). These complications may be prevented or their onset delayed by careful serial assessment of respiratory function, blood gas monitoring, and investigations to diagnose and treat associated problems, such as obstructive sleep apnea (OSA), oropharyngeal aspiration, gastroesophageal reflux, pneumonia, and asthma.[9–11]

Case Report 45-1

A 7-year-old boy with Duchenne muscular dystrophy was referred to the pulmonary clinic for evaluation and clearance for Achilles tendon release surgery. The muscular dystrophy was diagnosed at age 3 years when he was investigated for delayed motor milestones, frequent falls, and inability to stand. The muscle weakness has been progressive and he has used a wheelchair for the last few weeks. The physical examination was remarkable for weak cough and reduced air exchange on auscultation of chest, and the pulmonary function test showed evidence of mild restrictive defect.

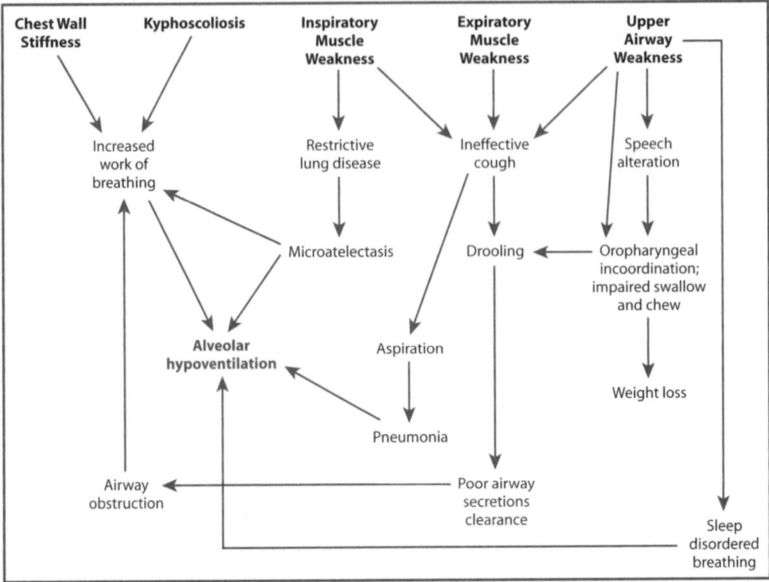

Figure 45-1. Development of severe hypoventilation in neuromuscular disease.

Pathophysiology of Respiratory Impairment in Patients With NMDs

Knowledge of normal respiratory function and control is essential to understand the pathophysiology of respiratory impairment in NMDs.

Three basic components of respiratory control[12] are

1. Sensors, which gather afferent information: central chemoreceptors located in medulla, carotid, and aortic bodies, and the stretch receptors in the lungs
2. Respiratory center in the brain stem, which acts as the central controller by processing afferent impulses and sending out efferent impulses to the periphery
3. Effectors, which are the respiratory muscles that are responsible for ventilation or cough

Respiratory control occurs subconsciously. The cortex can temporarily override the automatic nature of this mechanism if voluntary control is desired. A motor unit comprises an anterior horn cell, its peripheral nerve axon, the neuromuscular junction, and the muscle fibers it innervates. Neuromuscular disease can involve anterior horn cells, peripheral motor nerves, and muscle fibers. Patients with neuromuscular disease often do not report dyspnea until the diaphragm is involved.[13]

Diseases affecting the muscles of respiration or their nerve supply include poliomyelitis, Guillain-Barré syndrome, myasthenia gravis, muscular dystrophies, and spinal muscular atrophy.

Young children with neuromuscular disease have elevated chest wall compliance normalized to body weight.[14] Therefore, the chest wall deforms during tidal breathing resulting in inefficient breathing[15] and predisposes the child to develop atelectasis and chest deformities. A combination of reduced lung compliance due to generalized and widespread atelectasis (increased elastic load on the pump) and chest wall deformity due to reduced chest wall compliance results in increased work of breathing and chronic respiratory insufficiency. Reduced lung stretch because of suboptimal expansion, in conjunction with chest wall deformities, may also result in reduced lung growth.[16]

Respiratory pump function can be assessed by tests of respiratory muscle strength, such as maximum inspiratory pressure (MIP) and maximum expiratory pressure (MEP). Forced vital capacity (FVC) and fractional lung volumes are the result of interplay between respiratory pump and the load and can be used to monitor the progress of the patients with NMD.

Patients with extreme muscle weakness due to NMD may not be able to show the normal response to hypoventilation in the form of increased tidal volume but may have tachypnea. Inspiratory muscle weakness leads to chest wall stiffness and restrictive lung disease and contributes to ineffective cough and microatelectasis. Expiratory muscle weakness results in ineffective cough, inadequate airway clearance, aspiration, pneumonia, and alveolar hypoventilation. Upper airway muscle involvement results in oropharyngeal incompetence, difficulties with swallowing and chewing, speech alteration, and sleep-disordered breathing (SDB). In addition to muscle weakness due to NMD, musculoskeletal deformities, such as kyphoscoliosis, contribute to restrictive lung disease. These consequences are summarized in Box 45-1.

Box 45-1. Consequences of Compromised Respiratory Muscle Function

- Poor clearance of lower airway secretions due to impaired cough
- Hypoventilation during sleep
- Recurrent infections that exacerbate muscle weakness and impair integrity of lung parenchyma
- Chest wall underdevelopment in a growing child

Clinical Manifestations

The consequences of NMDs depend on the stage of the disorder. Most of the disorders are progressive, with resultant pulmonary and nutritional issues. The major findings discovered by history and physical examination are detailed in Box 45-2.

Evaluation and Anticipatory Guidance

Pulmonary Function Testing (PFT)

Indications for PFT include

- Evaluate the respiratory status of patients at the time of diagnosis.
- Monitor the progression and course of pulmonary limitation.
- Evaluate prior to surgical procedure.
- Provide an assessment of prognosis.

Because PFTs require voluntary participation of the patient, they are of limited use in children younger than 6 years. In younger patients, physical examination, clinical observation for work of breathing,

Box 45-2. Pulmonary and Associated Consequences of Neuromuscular Disorders

- Weak and ineffective cough
- History of recurrent respiratory infections and pneumonia
- Respiratory distress, retractions, wheeze, cyanosis
- Speech alteration, weak voice
- Snoring/irregular breathing/apneic episodes during sleep
- Nocturnal awakenings
- Fatigue, daytime somnolence
- Difficulty with chewing and swallowing
- Oropharyngeal incompetence (nasal regurgitation)
- Drooling
- Weight loss

respiratory rate, oxyhemoglobin saturation, end-tidal carbon dioxide measurement, blood gas profile, and chest radiograph may provide useful information. Infant lung function testing, including tidal flow volume loop, partial flow volume curves, raised volume rapid thoracic compression, and infant plethysmography, are available in specialized centers.[17–19]

FVC

During an FVC maneuver, the patient takes a maximum breath and fills lungs to total lung capacity (TLC) and then exhales to the maximum. Total volume of air expelled during forced exhalation after maximum inspiration is FVC. Measurement of vital capacity in sitting, supine, side-lying, and when the patient is wearing a thoracolumber stabilizing device is practiced by some physicians and may give more realistic information. Similarly, vital capacity measured in a recumbent position may be helpful. A greater than 7% fall in vital capacity from sitting to supine position may indicate that diaphragmatic weakness is out of proportion to chest wall muscle weakness.

Peak Flow Rate and Cough Peak Flow (CPF)

Muscle weakness due to NMDs results in reduced values for peak flow.[20] Peak flow rate is effort-dependent. The use of CPF can minimize effort-related variation. Thus, in patients with neuromuscular weakness, CPF is a better and more reliable measurement of expiratory muscle strength. This inexpensive and sturdy device can be used to monitor muscle strength at home.

Assisted CPF

The patient breathes with deep inspiration of successive tidal breaths without expiring (known as air stacking) and abdominal thrust is applied. The CPF is measured by peak flow meter. The difference between assisted and unassisted CPF can be used to measure glottic integrity.

Forced expiratory volume in 1 second (FEV_1) is reduced in proportion to FVC. Thus the FEV_1/FVC ratio remains normal. If the ratio of FEV_1/FVC is below 70% predicted this suggests an obstructive process that may coexist with the restrictive disorder. The percent predicted value for TLC is the best estimate of restriction (Table 45-1).

Table 45-1. Approximate Indicators of Severity of Lung Restriction

Degree of Restriction	Total Lung Capacity	Forced Vital Capacity
Normal	80%–120% predicted	>80% predicted
Mild restriction	70%–79% predicted	60%–79% predicted
Moderate restriction	60%–69% predicted	40%–59% predicted
Severe restriction	<60% predicted	<40% predicted

Respiratory Muscle Strength

Maximum inspiratory pressure and MEP are performed while the patient inhales or exhales maximally against a closed shutter. They are the most sensitive indicators of decreased respiratory muscle strength.

Objective evaluation at each clinic visit should include oxyhemoglobin saturation by pulse oximetry; spirometric measurements of FVC, FEV_1, maximum mid-expiratory flow rate, MIP and MEP; and CPF rate.

Carbon dioxide level should be evaluated when awake at least annually in conjunction with spirometry. When available, capnography is ideal for this purpose. If capnography is not available, a venous or capillary blood sample should be obtained to assess for the presence of alveolar hypoventilation (elevated values for carbon dioxide and bicarbonate).

For younger children, such as patients with spinal muscular dystrophy type 1 or 2, respiratory muscle function tests are indirect measures of cough effectiveness and include CPF, MIP, and MEP. Most children with spinal muscular atrophy who are bedridden may be too weak or too young to perform PFT. Therefore, the most useful evaluation of respiratory muscle function may be observation of cough ability.[2] Older patients and those with relatively mild disease but who are wheelchair bound can do MIP, MEP, and CPF to monitor their respirator muscle function. Older patients and those with still milder disease (able to walk) may be able to perform PFT and respiratory muscle function testing.

Palliative Care

Ventilatory and palliative care options should be discussed early and before complications requiring such intervention occur. Quality of life judgments should be made with the informed participation of the patient and family.[1] All long-term treatment options, including mechanical ventilation, should be discussed even when the treating physician predicts a poor quality of life with long-term ventilation.[21]

Such options must be presented in an open, fair, and balanced manner. End-of-life directives established by the patient, family, and health care team must be clearly documented and must be available in case of an emergency. Patients choosing to forgo long-term ventilation should be provided with palliative care, which may include management of pain, dyspnea, and attending to psychosocial and spiritual needs of the patient and their families.

Nutrition

Patients with NMDs may have feeding and swallowing problems due to bulbar dysfunction and can develop complications such as aspiration pneumonia. Gastrointestinal dysfunction can lead to constipation and delayed gastric emptying, and gastroesophageal reflux.

Ideal body weight percentage and body mass index should be evaluated, and the family should be counseled accordingly. Regular follow-up and evaluation by a nutritionist is recommended. Clinical evaluation for oropharyngeal incompetence and confirmation by studies such as videofluoroscopic swallow study should be considered. Patients should be evaluated for need for supplemental nutrition.

Cardiac Evaluation

Cardiac involvement may be due to cardiomyopathy, such as in patients with Duchenne muscular dystrophy. Chronic respiratory insufficiency may result in pulmonary hypertension or arrhythmia. Therefore, when clinically indicated the child should be evaluated by a cardiologist who may order an electrocardiogram, an echocardiogram, and medications, as well as regular follow-up appointments.

Sleep Evaluation

Patients with NMDs have greater than 40% prevalence of SDB,[22] a 10-fold greater occurrence than the general population.[23] They have a much higher incidence of OSA, gas exchange abnormalities, disrupted sleep architecture, and central apnea.[4,23] Dysfunction of upper airway muscles results in OSA, and dysfunction of diaphragm and intercostal muscles results in hypoventilation. In patients with neuromuscular disease, there may be increased airway resistance during sleep due to weakness of pharyngeal dilator muscles, which is worse during REM stage when these muscles are atonic. In patients with NMD,[24] OSA often precedes hypoventilation. Hypoventilation during sleep as a result of blunting of the response to hypoxia and hypercarbia worsens as muscle weakness progresses. Furthermore, the presence of kyphoscoliosis can contribute to restriction of lung capacity and impaired ventilation.[25]

The nature of SDB in patients with neuromuscular disease reflects the distribution of respiratory muscle involvement.[26] When patients have severe diaphragm dysfunction, suppression of intercostal and accessory muscles during REM sleep leads to hypoventilation. However, if diaphragm strength is intact, but the upper airway or intercostal muscles are weak, then obstructive apneas or hypopneas are more likely to occur. In some forms of neuromuscular disease, such as myotonic dystrophy, primary abnormalities in ventilatory control may also contribute to SDB, often complicated by nocturnal or even diurnal hypoventilation.[27] Arousal response seen with hypoventilation is compensatory as it prevents prolonged hypoxia or hypercarbia, but this is at the expense of adequate sleep and results in daytime fatigue and hypersomnolence. With time and progression of disease the ventilatory, chemosensitivity is reset and the arousal response is blunted, leading to prolongation of REM stage during which alveolar hypoventilation occurs. Eventually respiratory drive is depressed, resulting in severe hypoventilation and ultimate respiratory failure[27] (Figure 45-2).

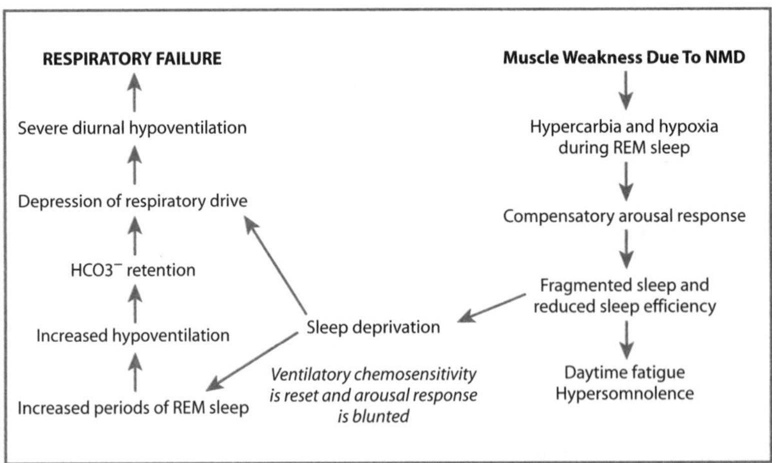

Figure 45-2. Pulmonary pathophysiological consequences of neuromuscular disease.

Nocturnal hypoventilation is not well defined in children. In adults, sleep-induced hypoventilation, according to *International Classification of Sleep Disorders: Diagnostic and Coding Manual* 2007, is defined as a level of arterial carbon dioxide of greater than 45 mm Hg or "disproportionately increased relative to levels during wakefulness."[28] Sleep-induced hypoxemia is defined as oxygen desaturations to less than 90% for at least 5 minutes with a nadir of at least 85% or greater than 30% of total sleep time with oxygen saturation at less than 90%.[29] Quality of sleep and symptoms of SDB should be reviewed at each encounter (see Chapter 36). An annual polysomnogram should be done in each patient with NMD from the time they are wheelchair users or when the clinical situation warrants. If the polysomnogram is not able to be performed, nocturnal pulse oximetry with or without capnography is an alternative.

Management

Multiple approaches to reducing the impact of the progression of neuromuscular weakness are available. The approaches to investigate and treat symptoms will depend on the clinical course and are summarized in Table 45-2.

Airway Clearance

Muscle weakness in patients with NMDs may be associated with weak or ineffective cough leading to pooling of secretions, which may result in airway obstruction. Therefore, airway clearance (either manual chest physiotherapy or using a mechanical device) is very important to prevent respiratory complications, including pneumonia, atelectasis, and respiratory failure. In the initial stages, airway clearance by hand along with postural drainage may be used. As the disease progresses resulting in pooling of secretions, more aggressive methods, such as the use of a mechanical cough-assist device, will help. Use of a high-frequency chest wall oscillation device alone may not help much if the patient has weak/ineffective cough. Use of this device in a patient with significant musculoskeletal deformities (kyphoscoliosis) may be uncomfortable.

Ineffective cough may be clinically suspected when there is a history of lack of secretions while coughing, recurrent pneumonia, and reduced values for CPF. Cough peak flow may be measured in the primary care physician's office, patient's home, or pulmonologist's office by attaching

Table 45-2. Suggested Approach to Investigate and Treat Patients With Progressive Respiratory Muscle Involvement

Clinical Features	Relevant Investigations	Suggested Interventions
No clinical evidence of respiratory muscle involvement	Normal spirometry, normal cough peak flow (>270 L/min)	Regular follow-up in the clinic (6 monthly), monitor spirometry, cough peak flow rate, encourage incentive spirometry
Evidence of respiratory muscle involvement, weak cough, and pooling of secretions	Reduced cough peak flow (<270 L/min), maximum expiratory pressure <60 cm H_2O, restrictive lung disease on spirometry (FVC and FEV_1 <80% predicted)	Initiate airway clearance (cough-assist device)
Snoring, sleep-disordered breathing, nocturnal awakenings due to breathing difficulty, daytime somnolence	Evidence of sleep-disordered breathing on sleep study, evidence of chronic hypoventilation on blood gas (elevated CO_2 and bicarbonate levels), and hypoxia (reduced oxyhemoglobin saturation, Po_2 levels on blood gas), and elevated end-tidal CO_2 levels	Consider noninvasive ventilation during sleep
Hypoventilation, hypercarbia during awake periods	Waking Pco_2 >50 mm of Hg Oxyhemoglobin saturation <92%	Extend noninvasive ventilation during daytime, may be intermittent to begin with
Persistent or worsening hypoventilation, hypercarbia, and hypoxia	As above	Long-term ventilation, may be noninvasive to begin with and if there is contraindication or failure of noninvasive ventilation or patient/family preference, long-term tracheostomy may be considered

Abbreviations: FEV_1, forced expiratory rate in 1 second; FVC, forced vital capacity; Pco_2, partial pressure of carbon dioxide; Po_2, partial pressure of oxygen.

a mask to a peak flow meter and asking the patient to cough in it. This inexpensive, simple device monitors the expiratory muscle strength and the patient can maintain a journal with weekly or monthly readings. Cough peak flows correlate directly to the ability to clear secretions from the respiratory tract,[30] and values below 160 L/min have been associated with ineffective airway clearance.[31] A peak cough expiratory flow rate of 270 L/min has been used to identify patients who would benefit from assisted cough techniques. Similarly, an MEP below 45 cm H_2O has been considered an indication for assisted cough techniques. Various techniques have been developed to overcome ineffective cough in patients with neuromuscular weakness.

Patients or caregivers should be taught strategies to improve airway clearance and how to use those techniques early and aggressively. Patients with clinically weak/ineffective cough and clinical evidence of poor airway clearance should be started on a regular airway clearance regimen. Use assisted cough technologies in patients whose clinical history suggests difficulty in airway clearance, or whose CPF is less than 270 L/min and/or whose maximal expiratory pressures are less than 60 cm H_2O. A mechanical insufflation-exsufflation device (Cough-Assist) is recommended.

Manually Assisted Cough Technique

Manually assisted coughing involves inspiratory assistance followed by augmentation of the forced expiratory effort. An increase in inspiratory capacity can be achieved by the use of glossopharyngeal breathing (in essence forcing air into the lungs using one's mouth), air stacking (taking a series of tidal breaths without exhaling between them), application of positive pressure with self-inflating bag and mask, an intermittent positive pressure breathing device, or a mechanical ventilator. Interfaces for inspiratory assistance include a face mask, mouthpiece, or direct attachment of the assisting device to a tracheostomy tube. Forced exhalation is augmented by pushing on the upper abdomen or chest wall in synchrony with the subject's own cough effort.

Mechanical Techniques

Mechanical insufflator-exsufflators simulate a cough by providing a positive pressure breath followed by a negative pressure exsufflation. This technique has been found to be superior to those generated either by breath stacking or manual cough assistance.[20] In patients with tracheostomies, mechanical insufflation-exsufflation offers a number of advantages over traditional suctioning, including clearance of secretions from peripheral airways, avoidance of mucosal trauma from direct tracheal suction, improved patient comfort,[32] and prevention of atelectasis.

Bronchoscopy has been used in selected patients with Duchenne muscular dystrophy, generally in cases of persistent atelectasis, but has not been of proven benefit and therapy and should be considered only after all noninvasive airway clearance techniques have proven unsuccessful and a mucus plug is suspected.

Respiratory Muscle Training

The rationale for respiratory muscle training in Duchenne muscular dystropy is based on the assumption that improved muscle strength and endurance in patients affected with the condition may lead to improved preservation of lung function over time. Low-intensity inspiratory muscle training at home may improve respiratory muscle endurance in children with Duchenne muscular dystrophy, and the effectiveness of training appears to depend on the quantity of training.[33] Training with an inspiratory threshold load (70%–80% of the maximal inspiratory mouth pressure) provides a stimulus that increases both the pressure- and flow-generating capacities of the respiratory muscles, and therefore may provide a practical approach to inspiratory muscle training in both children and adults with neuromuscular disease.[27]

Noninvasive Nocturnal Ventilation

Onset of moderately severe muscle weakness as evidenced by physical examination, weak/ineffective cough, pooling of secretions, and evidence of hypoventilation or hypoxia during sleep or wakefulness will differ from patient to patient and disease to disease. For example a patient with spinal muscular dystrophy will develop such a weakness much earlier compared with a patient with Duchenne muscular dystrophy. Use of noninvasive ventilatory support may improve quality of life and reduce the high morbidity (SDB, including hypopnea, central and obstructive apnea, and hypoxemia) and early mortality associated with NMDs such as Duchenne muscular dystrophy.[1]

Nocturnal nasal intermittent positive pressure ventilation with a bilevel positive airway pressure (BiPAP) generator or mechanical ventilator has been used successfully in the treatment of SDB, and nocturnal hypoventilation in patients with Duchenne muscular dystrophy and other NMDs.[1] Polysomnography should be done to confirm the presence and extent of SDB, hypoxia, and hypercarbia and for titration to initiate treatment with optimum ventilator settings and to ensure response to treatment. In the absence of polysomnography, overnight pulse oximetry with continuous carbon dioxide monitoring can be used to monitor nighttime gas exchange.[1] Follow-up visits should include monitoring for daytime hypoventilation that may necessitate around-the-clock ventilation.

Daytime ventilation should be considered when measured waking partial pressure of carbon dioxide exceeds 50 mm Hg or when oxygen saturation remains less than 92% while awake. Oxygen supplementation alone should not be used to treat sleep-related hypoventilation without ventilatory assistance due to the potential of exacerbating carbon dioxide retention.

Tracheostomy

Tracheostomy may be considered when contraindications to noninvasive ventilations are present: The patient has an aversion to noninvasive ventilation, the patient lacks sufficient oro-motor or neck control to use a mouthpiece interface during the daytime, or other interfaces are poorly tolerated.[1] However, tracheostomies have many potential complications, including generating more secretions; impairing swallowing and increasing the risk of aspiration; bypassing of airway defenses, likely increasing the risk of infection; and a higher risk of airway occlusion by a mucus plug.[34] Since tracheostomies also impair oral communication, communication may be restored using a relatively small tracheostomy tube, allowing a "leak" around the airway, and a speaking valve (Passey–Muir valve).

Respiratory Management of Patients With NMD Undergoing Sedation or Anesthesia

Preoperative pulmonary evaluation[35] and consultation should be obtained. Pulmonary function testing, including FVC, MIP, MEP, CPF, and oxyhemoglobin saturation measurement in room air should be performed. An FVC value less than 50% is associated with increased risk, and when the values are below 30% preoperative training for noninvasive ventilation should be provided. If indicated the child should be extubated to noninvasive ventilation, such as nasal BiPAP, and appropriate pain management should be provided. Aggressive airway clearance should begin as soon as the patient can tolerate.[35]

When to Refer

Pulmonologist

- Shortly after diagnosis for respiratory care evaluation and discussion of treatment options, including identification of goals for chronic and acute respiratory care. Regular follow-up of pulmonary status should be performed once or twice a year after the patient becomes wheelchair-bound.
- Prior to a proposed surgery for evaluation of pulmonary status and to assess fitness for the proposed anesthesia, sedation, or surgery.
- In case of acute respiratory illness.

Cardiologist

The cardiologist should be consulted to diagnose and manage cardiomyopathy and pulmonary hypertension. Cardiac evaluation for evidence of cardiomyopathy and cardiac dysrhythmias and pulmonary hypertension should be done. Patients with neuromuscular disease are at high risk of developing side effects during the perioperative period due to hypoxemia, anemia, and other causes of impaired oxygen tissue delivery. Intravascular shifts can result in congestive heart failure and impaired ventricular load.[36]

When to Admit

- **At the time of diagnosis**
  Patients with late diagnosis who may have significant pulmonary compromise as evidenced by lung function, or laboratory evidence of respiratory failure or cardiac involvement, may benefit from hospitalization.
- **In case of acute respiratory illness**
  Patients may need aggressive airway clearance; increased respiratory support, such as noninvasive ventilation; management of nutrition; hydration; and initiation of antibiotic therapy. In case of acute respiratory decompensation in a patient already on chronic noninvasive ventilation, endotracheal intubation may be warranted.

- **For elective procedures** such as gastric feeding tube placement, scoliosis surgery, elective tracheostomy and initiation of invasive ventilation, and sleep studies.

Key Points

- History in a patient with NMDs disorder should include questions about strength and efficiency of cough, activity or exercise intolerance, and respiratory distress.
- Sleep-disordered breathing associated with NMDs should be suspected if there is history of snoring, irregular breathing, apneic episodes during sleep, or nocturnal awakenings due to breathing difficulty (not for change of position due to discomfort).
- History of recurrent respiratory infections and pneumonia may suggest chronic aspiration due to oropharyngeal incompetence.
- Videofluoroscopic swallow study may help to confirm oropharyngeal incompetence and associated aspiration.
- Involve the palliative care team to discuss ventilatory and palliative treatment options before they become necessary.

References

1. Finder JD, Birnkrant D, Carl J, et al. Respiratory care of the patient with Duchenne muscular dystrophy: ATS consensus statement. *Am J Respir Crit Care Med.* 2004;170(4):456–465
2. Wang CH, Finkel RS, Bertini ES, et al. Consensus statement for standard of care in spinal muscular atrophy. *J Child Neurol.* 2007;22(8):1027–1049
3. Emery AEH. Fortnightly review: the muscular dystrophies. *BMJ.* 1998;317(7164):991–995
4. Gozal D. Pulmonary manifestations of neuromuscular disease with special reference to Duchenne muscular dystrophy and spinal muscular atrophy. *Pediatr Pulmonol.* 2000;29(2):141–150
5. Willig TN, Paulus J, Lacau Saint Guily J, Beon C, Navarro J. Swallowing problems in neuromuscular disorders. *Arch Phys Med Rehabil.* 1994;75(11):1175–1181
6. Tome FM, Chateau D, Helbling-Leclerc A, Fardeau M. Morphological changes in muscle fibers in oculopharyngeal muscular dystrophy. *Neuromuscul Disord.* 1997;7(suppl 1):S63–S69

7. Pane M, Vasta I, Messina S et al. Feeding problems and weight gain in Duchenne muscular dystrophy. *Eur J Paediatr Neurol.* 2006;10(5-6):231–236
8. Messina S, Pane M, De Rose P, et al. Feeding problems and malnutrition in spinal muscular atrophy type II. *Neuromuscul Disord.* 2008;18(5):389–393
9. Iannaccone ST; American Spinal Muscular Atrophy Randomized Trials (AmSMART) Group. Outcome measures for pediatric spinal atrophy. *Arch Neurol.* 2002;59:1445–1450
10. Oskoui M, Levy G, Garland CJ, et al. The changing natural history of spinal muscular atrophy type 1. *Neurology.* 2007:69:1931–1936
11. Jeppesen J, Green A, Steffensen BF, Rahbek J. The Duchenne muscular dystrophy population in Denmark, 1977–2001: prevalence, incidence and survival in relation to the introduction of ventilator use. *Neuromuscul Disord.* 2003;13(10):804–812
12. West JB. *Respiratory Physiology—The Essentials.* Baltimore, MD: Williams & Wilkins; 1995:117–132
13. West JB. *Pulmonary Pathophysiology—The Essentials.* Baltimore, MD: Williams & Wilkins; 2008:97–132
14. Papastamelos C, Panitch HB, Allen JL. Chest wall compliance in infants and children with neuromuscular disease. *Am J Respir Crit Care Med.* 1996;154(4 pt 1):1045–1048
15. Lissoni A, Aliverti A, Tzeng AC, Bach JR. Kinematic analysis of patients with spinal muscular atrophy during spontaneous breathing and mechanical ventilation. *Am J Phys Med Rehabil.* 1998;77(3):188–192
16. Bach JR, Bianchi C. Prevention of pectus excavatum for children with spinal muscular atrophy type 1. *Am J Phys Med Rehabil.* 2003;82(10):815–819
17. Stocks J, Lum S. Paediatric pulmonary function testing applications and future directions of infant pulmonary function testing. *Prog Respir Res.* 2005;33:78–91
18. Bates JH, Schmalisch G, Filbrun D, et al. Tidal breath analysis for infant pulmonary function testing. ERS/ATS Task Force on Standards for Infant Respiratory Function Testing. European Respiratory Society/American Thoracic Society. *Eur Respir J.* 2000;16:1180–1192
19. Beydon N, Davis SD, Lombardi E, et al. An official American Thoracic Society/European Respiratory Society statement: pulmonary function testing in preschool children. *Am J Respir Crit Care Med.* 2007;175(12):1304–1345
20. Bach JR. Mechanical insufflation-exsufflation: comparison of peak expiratory flows with manually assisted and unassisted coughing techniques. *Chest.* 1993;104:1553–1562
21. Gilgoff I, Prentice W, Baydur A. Patient and family participation in the management of respiratory failure in Duchenne's muscular dystrophy. *Chest.* 1989;95:519–524
22. Labanowski M, Schmidt-Nowara W, Guilleminault C. Sleep and neuromuscular disease: frequency of sleep-disordered breathing in a neuromuscular disease clinic population [see comment]. *Neurology.* 1996;47(5):1173–1180

23. Brunetti L, Rana S, Lospalluti ML, et al. Prevalence of obstructive sleep apnea syndrome in a cohort of 1,207 children of southern Italy. *Chest.* 2001;120(6):1930–1935
24. Suresh S, Wales P, Dakin C, et al. Sleep-related breathing disorder in Duchenne muscular dystrophy: disease spectrum in the paediatric population. *J Paediatr Child Health.* 2005;41(9–10):500–503
25. Panitch HB. Respiratory issues in the management of children with neuromuscular disease. *Respir Care.* 2006;51(8):885–893
26. Piper A. Sleep abnormalities associated with neuromuscular disease: pathophysiology and evaluation. *Semin Respir Crit Care Med.* 2002;23:211–219
27. Perrin C, Unterborn JN, Ambrosio CD, Hill NS. Pulmonary complications of chronic neuromuscular diseases and their management. *Muscle Nerve.* 2004;29 (1):5–27
28. Katz SL. Assessment of sleep-disordered breathing in pediatric neuromuscular disease. *Pediatrics.* 2009;123:S222–S225
29. American Academy of Sleep Medicine. *International Classification of Sleep Disorders: Diagnostic and Coding Manual.* Chicago, IL: American Acaedemy of Sleep Medicine; 2005
30. King M, Brock G, Lundell C. Clearance of mucus by simulated cough. *J Appl Physiol.* 1985;58:1776–1782
31. Bach JR, Saporito LR. Criteria for extubation and tracheostomy tube removal for patients with ventilatory failure: a different approach to weaning. *Chest.* 1996;110:1566–157
32. Garstang SV, Kirshblum SC, Wood KE. Patient preference for in-exsufflation for secretion management with spinal cord injury. *J Spinal Cord Med.* 2000;23:80–85
33. Topin N, Matecki S, Le Bris S, et al. Dose-dependent effect of individualized respiratory muscle training in children with Duchenne muscular dystrophy. *Neuromuscul Disord.* 2002;12:576–583
34. American Thoracic Society. Care of the child with a chronic tracheostomy. *Am J Respir Crit Care Med.* 2000;161:297–308
35. Birnkrant DJ, Panitch HB, Benditt JO, et al. American College of Chest Physicians consensus statement on the respiratory and related management of patients with Duchenne muscular dystrophy undergoing anesthesia or sedation. *Chest.* 2007;132(6):1977–1986
36. American Academy of Pediatrics Section on Cardiology and Cardiac Surgery. Cardiovascular health supervision for individuals affected by Duchenne or Becker muscular dystrophy. *Pediatrics.* 2005;116(6):1569–1573

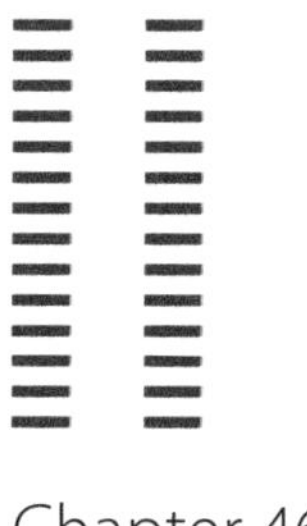

Chapter 46

Airway Clearance Techniques

Karen Hardy, MD

Introduction

Normal Airway Clearance

Typically, the clearance of airway secretions relies on 2 defense mechanisms: the mucociliary escalator and cough clearance. The mucociliary escalator requires normally functioning cilia and a normal airway surface liquid and mucus layer. These components of airway clearance function in the small airways as well as the larger cartilaginous airways (Figure 46-1). Cough clearance function is limited to the larger central airways and requires normal inspiration, vocal cord closure, and expiration, as well as adequate rigidity of the airway.

Abnormal Airway Clearance

Children who lack any factor involved in the 2 main mechanisms of the mucociliary escalator and cough clearance will have difficulty with normal airway clearance. See Table 46-1 for the types of abnormalities that relate to lack of the required components for appropriate airway clearance.

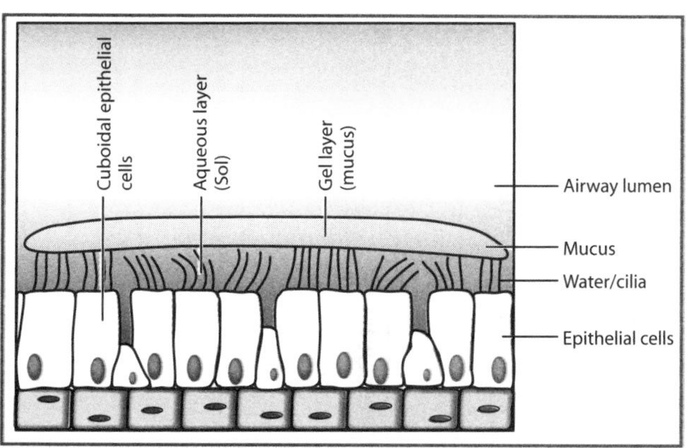

Figure 46-1. Components of normal airway clearance.

Table 46-1. Abnormalities Related to the Lack of Physical Components of Airway Clearance

Anatomical or Functional Abnormality	Diagnostic Category	Pathophysiology
MUCOCILIARY ESCALATOR		
Cilial dysfunction	Primary ciliary dyskinesia (PCD)	Cilia immotile or dyskinetic
Abnormal airway surface liquid/mucus layer	Cystic fibrosis (CF)	Reduced airway surface liquid; thick and viscous mucus layer; increased inflammatory mediators; increased destructive compounds (elastases, proteases)
	Pseudohypoaldosteronism	Increased volume of airway surface liquid; intermittent airway obstruction and infection as young children, typically younger than 6 years
	Asthma	Abnormal and increased mucus Airway edema
COUGH CLEARANCE		
Respiratory muscle dysfunction		
Neuromuscular disease	Duchenne muscular dystrophy (DMD)	Combined respiratory motor defects with abnormal inspiratory pressure generation and/or expiratory pressure generation; bulbar dysfunction with aspiration and/or gastroesophegeal reflux
	Spinal muscular atrophy I	See DMD.
	Spinal muscular atrophy II	Combined respiratory motor defects with abnormal inspiratory pressure generation and/or expiratory pressure generation
	Congenital myopathies	See DMD.

Table 46-1. Abnormalities Related to the Lack of Physical Components of Airway Clearance (continued)

Anatomical or Functional Abnormality	Diagnostic Category	Pathophysiology
COUGH CLEARANCE (continued)		
Neuromotor disease	Cerebral palsy	Inability to sense secretions in the airways or pharynx, bulbar palsies, direct aspiration, severe muscle imbalance causing scoliosis; can be associated with impaired cough, poor nasopharyngeal motor tone with subsequent upper airway obstruction and possible obstructive sleep apnea
	Phrenic nerve injuries	Profound diaphragmatic dysfunction sometimes associated with paradoxical motion
	Traumatic or postoperative head and spinal cord injury	Can damage phrenic nerve and innervation of intercostal muscles and accessory muscles, affecting bellow's function
	Meningomyelocele (spina bifida)	Bellow's dysfunction and progressive scoliosis
Neurologic	Bulbar palsy	Inability to control oral secretions and/or swallow, may include direct aspiration
	Encephalopathy	See bulbar palsy.
Unstable airways	Airway malacia	Airways collapse with dynamic pressure changes during inspiration and/or expiration
	Tracheoesophageal fistula (TEF)	See airway malacia and direct airway damage from aspiration.
	VATER syndrome (TEF)	See TEF.
	Bronchiectasis (bronchiolitis obliterans, CF, immunodeficiency, PCD, postinfections/tuberculosis	See airway malacia.
Obstructed airway	Tracheal stenosis	Inadequate lumen for secretion clearance
	Scoliosis	Airway rotational deformities ("kinking") and muscle imbalance that can be progressive

Considerations Unique to Infants and Children

Children are more susceptible than adults to complications related to compromised airway clearance for several reasons. The mucus of children is more acidic and may have greater viscosity. Infants and children have an overly compliant chest wall and relatively stiff lungs, leading to a lower functional residual capacity. Furthermore, the airways are smaller, have less cartilage support, and tend to collapse more easily than in adults. Finally, the bronchioles and alveoli of children have fewer channels for collateral ventilation than those of adults.[1]

Airway clearance therapy (ACT) is more difficult in infants and children because of difficulties in obtaining cooperation. In addition, gastroesophageal reflux (GER) is common but can be difficult to diagnose and can be aggravated particularly by a head-down drainage position.[2,3] Unfortunately, data regarding the use of ACT in children are limited. Children who require ACT often have rare diseases; adequately powered trials are the exception rather than the rule. Placebo-controlled studies are not possible, and the length of time needed to judge treatment efficacy for chronic conditions can be long, making studies costly and increasing the likelihood of non-adherence and attrition. Much of what is known is based on case reports, small single-center studies, and clinician experience, although a few meta-analyses and Cochrane reviews are available.[4–7]

Airway Clearance Techniques

Airway clearance therapy may be independently performed, relying on the patient's breathing skills, or may depend on other persons or machines. For any patient, the appropriate method is one that is effective, affordable, feasible, and repeatable. Importantly, a patient's ability to choose their method of airway clearance can also improve adherence. Box 46-1 lists the various airway clearance techniques divided into the independent and dependent skills categories with reference to the known physiological effects, costs, and preferences.

Independent Techniques

Huff Cough Maneuver

Coughing clears normal airways quite effectively in healthy people. The components of cough include inspiration, glottic closure, and expulsion via forced exhalation. Coughing causes compression of the airways that

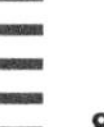

Box 46-1. Airway Clearance Techniques

Independent Methods
- No equipment or assistance needed
- Directed cough huff maneuver
- Active cycle of breathing techniques
- Autogenic drainage

Dependent Methods
- Personnel required
- Chest physical therapy (CPT), also known as postural drainage and percussion and vibration
- Manual cough assist

Handheld Device Required
- Manual percussor for CPT
- Positive expiratory pressure valve
- Flutter valve
- Acapella
- Quake

Large Machine Required
- Vests (high-frequency chest wall compression)
- Cough assist device
- Intrapulmonary percussive ventilator

moves from the smaller to the larger airways and toward the mouth.[8] A cough is less effective if the airways are unstable and collapsible, and a modification of cough (huff cough or forced expiratory maneuver) can help to decrease the compression of these airways. The huff maneuver is performed by inhaling, breath-holding for approximately 3 seconds, and then exhaling with a slightly open glottis. This is easily mimicked by the skill of "fogging a mirror." The force of exhalation is adjusted to avoid wheezing and airway collapse. Maintenance of the open glottis avoids the excessive transmural pressures that cause airway closure and limit secretion clearance. This skill is easy to teach and effective for patients with collapsible airways.

Active Cycle of Breathing Technique (ACBT)

Active cycles of breathing techniques combine the huff maneuver with 2 other skills: diaphragmatic (or relaxed) breathing and thoracic expansions (or deep rib breathing). Relaxed, diaphragmatic breathing occurs during gentle inhalation using the diaphragm and allowing the abdomen to expand.[9] Children often call this "belly breathing." A child may learn this skill by placing a favorite stuffed animal on her abdomen and watching it rise up and down. During exhalation the abdominal muscles are used and with successive breaths, large volumes are moved with improved ventilation of the dependent lung tissue. Thoracic expansions rely more on intercostal muscles with prominent chest expansion that improves upper lung expansion and ventilation. The use of alternating cycles of diaphragmatic breaths with thoracic breaths and huff maneuvers in ACBT can effectively and efficiently mobilize and clear airways.[10,11] This independent skill can be mastered and then used anytime in any position, although it requires attention to be most effective.

Autogenic Drainage

The most advanced and challenging independent skill is autogenic drainage (AD).[12] This technique is applied widely in children with cystic fibrosis (CF), but also is used for adolescents and adults with bronchiectasis from any cause. The skill is difficult to learn and typically requires a series of visits to a skilled teacher. The patient is trained in 3 phases or levels that are serially completed: first breathing at low-lung volumes to dislodge the mucus, then mid-lung volumes to collect the mucus, and then high-lung volumes to expel the mucus[13] (Figure 46-3). Skilled performance of this technique is associated with improved oxygenation and minimization of work to expectorate.[14] It also reduces the likelihood of coughing fits that are so typically caused by forced coughing in those with unstable airways and excessive secretions.

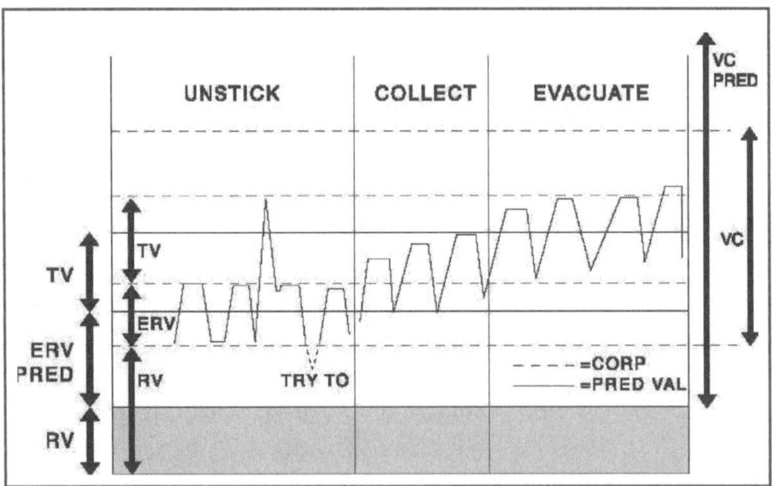

Figure 46-3. The 3 phases or levels of autogenic drainage. (From Basic Bronchial Drainage Course—Autogenic Drainage 2011. Bosschaerts M, Chevaillier J. Copyright 2011, reprinted by permission.)

Dependent Techniques

Chest Physical Therapy

Chest physical therapy (CPT) may include postural drainage, percussion, and vibration. Classically, patients are placed into a position to permit gravity to assist in mucus flow. The chest wall is percussed to loosen the mucus during both inspiration and expiration; intermittently a prolonged exhalation with chest wall vibration is subsequently applied as a final attempt to move mucus. Applying the vibrations is the most difficult component for the respiratory therapist, physical therapist, and families, and as a result is often ignored in many settings. This technique is widely practiced but has a number of drawbacks. Complications have been shown to include desaturations, GER, aspiration, pain, fractured ribs, and headaches.[10,13,15,16] In addition, this is a technique that requires assistance, leading to poor adherence as long-term therapy when patients begin to seek independence.[17,18] Care providers performing CPT can also experience pain or musculoskeletal abnormalities.[19] This can be partially circumvented by the use of mechanical devices. Typical postural drainage positions for children are shown in Figure 46-4.

Augmented cough, also known as manual cough assist, is used for patients with neuromuscular disease who cannot generate an effective cough. This maneuver involves a Heimlich-like procedure where the caregiver uses the heel of the hand to thrust from the abdomen toward the diaphragm in concert with patient efforts to cough. Manual cough assist if most effective if the child is supine.[20]

Positive Expiratory Pressure

Small handheld devices are often used for generating positive expiratory pressure (PEP),[21] which may be constant or oscillatory. In this technique the patient breathes in and out 5 to 20 times through a flow resistor, which creates a positive pressure in the airways during exhalation. After a series of breaths, the patient performs the huff cough maneuver. Positive pressure devices cause motion of air via collateral channels of ventilation (alveolar pores of Kohn and bronchiolar-alveolar channel of Lambert) to equalize alveolar filling and facilitate mucus clearance with the huff cough. Positive expiratory pressure devices can be very inexpensive, ranging from $10 for the valve alone

Self-Percussion—Upper Lobes
Sit upright and reach across the chest to clap self on front of chest over the muscular area between the collarbone and the top of the shoulder blade.

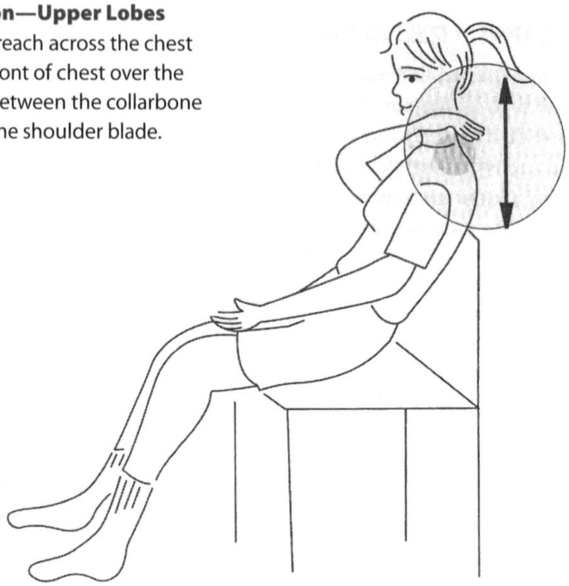

Upper Front Chest—Upper Lobes Sitting
Sit upright. Clap on both sides of upper front chest over the muscular area between the collarbone and the top of the shoulder blade.

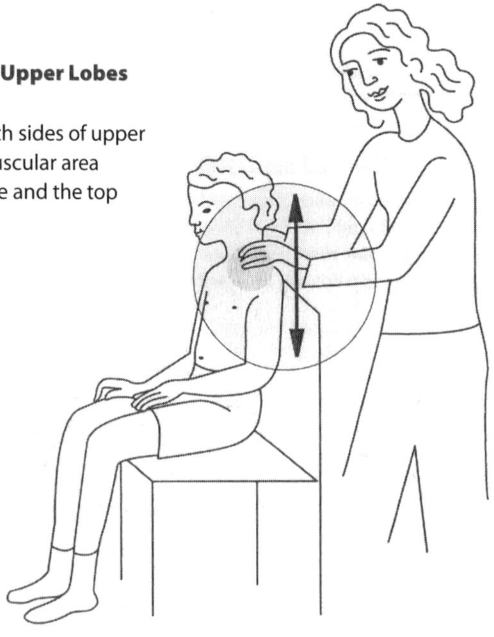

Figure 46-4. Image demonstrates typical chest physical therapy drainage positions for children. (From CF Family Education Program—Baylor College of Medicine, with permission.)

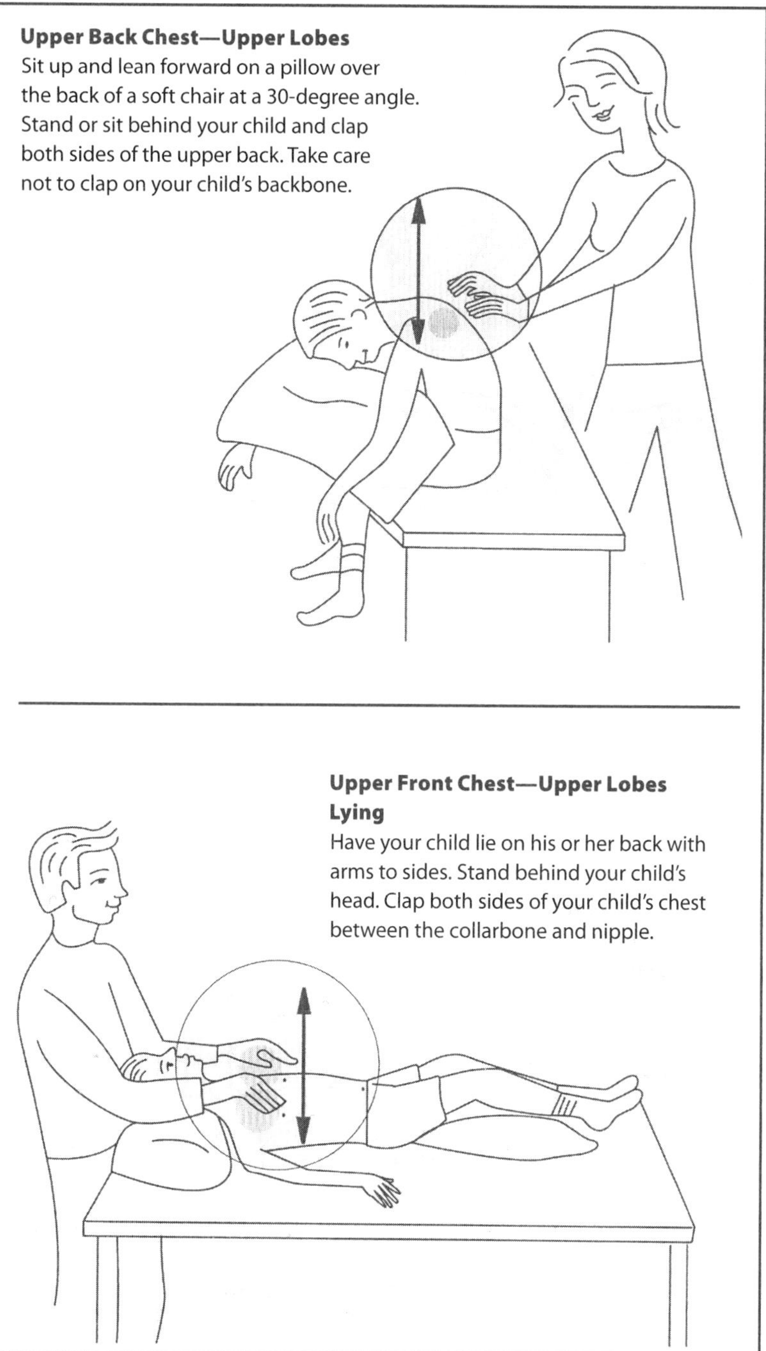
Upper Back Chest—Upper Lobes
Sit up and lean forward on a pillow over the back of a soft chair at a 30-degree angle. Stand or sit behind your child and clap both sides of the upper back. Take care not to clap on your child's backbone.
Upper Front Chest—Upper Lobes Lying
Have your child lie on his or her back with arms to sides. Stand behind your child's head. Clap both sides of your child's chest between the collarbone and nipple.

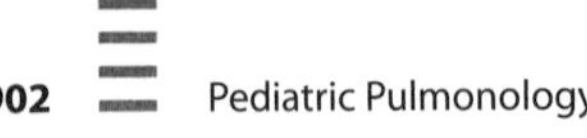

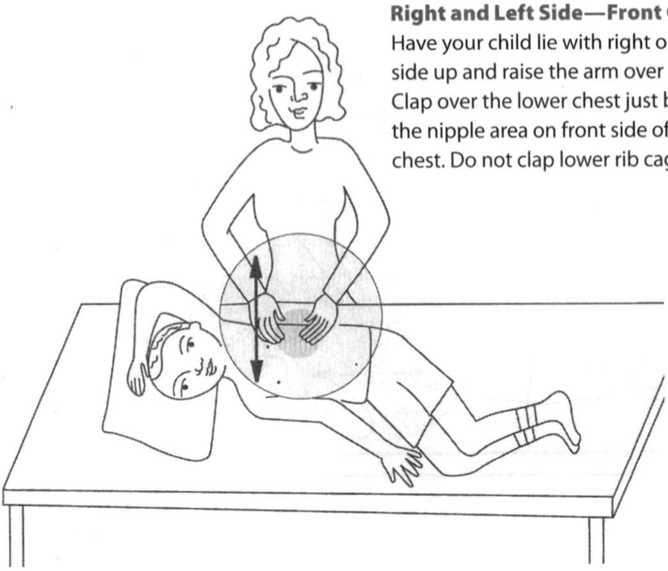

Right and Left Side—Front Chest
Have your child lie with right or left side up and raise the arm over head. Clap over the lower chest just below the nipple area on front side of the chest. Do not clap lower rib cage.

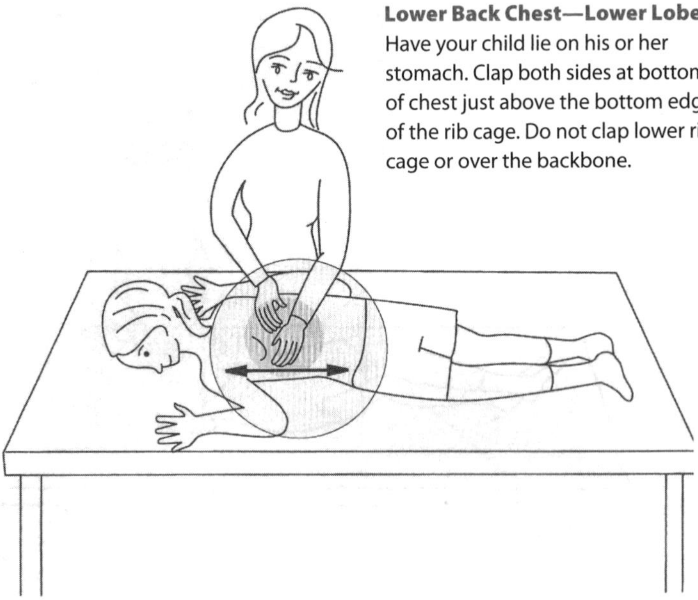

Lower Back Chest—Lower Lobe
Have your child lie on his or her stomach. Clap both sides at bottom of chest just above the bottom edge of the rib cage. Do not clap lower rib cage or over the backbone.

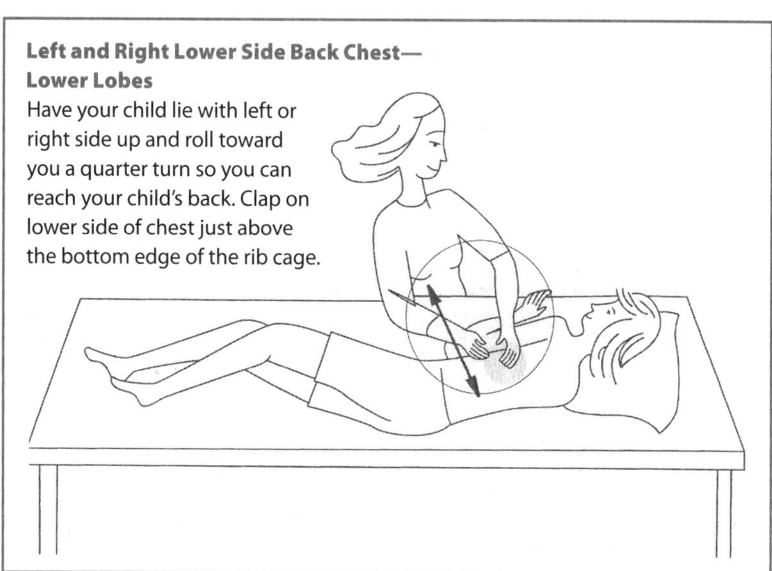
Left and Right Lower Side Back Chest—Lower Lobes
Have your child lie with left or right side up and roll toward you a quarter turn so you can reach your child's back. Clap on lower side of chest just above the bottom edge of the rib cage.

up to $150 for a valve with visual feedback attachments. One example is the TheraPEP valve (Figure 46-5). Multiple studies have documented the efficacy of PEP techniques when compared with CPT and AD.[22]

Oscillating PEP Devices

High-frequency oscillations were added to PEP therapy initially with the advent of the Flutter valve device[23–25] (Figure 46-6), which was then followed by a number of alternative devices, including the Acapella valve and the Quake, that have different mechanisms by which they produce the desired oscillations. As the patient exhales actively into the devices, PEP is initially generated that then rapidly subsides and then recurs. The oscillations produced by the devices and exhalations are passed along the airway walls and loosen mucus. The Flutter valve produces these oscillations with the flutter of a steel ball inside the device that moves during use. The Acapella valve uses magnets adjusted at a specific distance to produce vibrations. Two Acapella

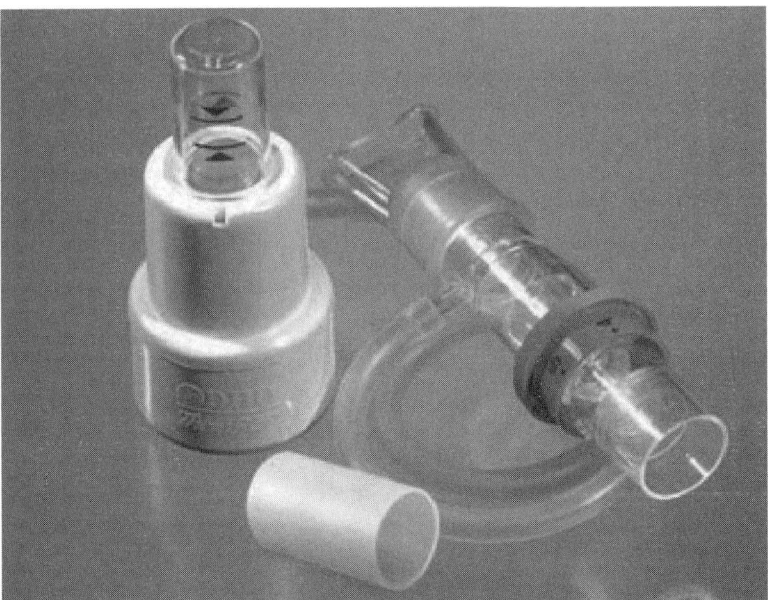

Figure 46-5. Example of TheraPEP, a positive expiratory pressure (PEP) valve. (Image of TheraPEP® PEP Therapy System by Smiths Medical ASD, Inc./Portex from EveryDay Medical Products, LLC http://www.everydaymedical.com/index.asp?PageAction=VIEWPROD&ProdID=3259).

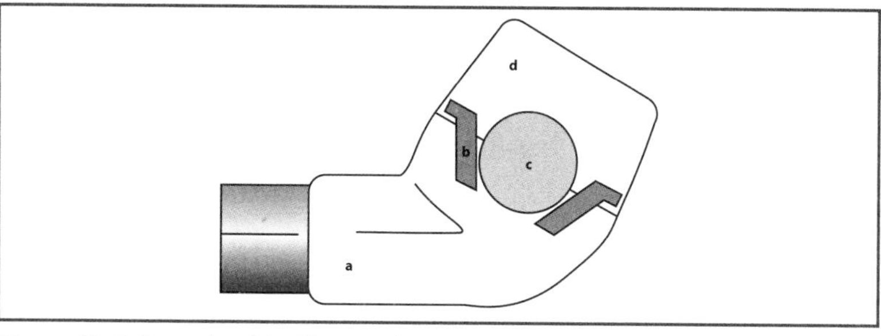

Figure 46-6. Example of the Flutter valve, an oscillating positive expiratory pressure (PEP) valve. The device comprises a mouthpiece **(a)**, a plastic cone **(b)**, a steel ball **(c)**, and a perforated cover **(d)**. During exhalation through the device, the tracheobronchial tree undergoes internal vibrations together with repeated variations of the exhaled airflow against the resistance (PEP) and oscillations of the endobronchial pressure (oscillating pressure). Oscillating PEP is most commonly performed with the Flutter device or the Acapella device. (From Althaus P. Oscillating PEP. In: *Physiotherapy for People with Cystic Fibrosis: From Infant to Adult.* Prague: The International Physiotherapy Group for Cystic Fibrosis; 2009. http://cfww.org/docs/ipg-cf/bluebook/bluebooklet2009.websiteversion.pdf)

colors designate devices designed for younger (blue—low flow) and older (green—high flow) children (Figure 46-7).

The Quake is another handheld device with a crank shaft on the pipe that is turned by the patient; the speed of the rotations determines the frequency of interruption of airflow as small holes in the shaft align to permit airflow or cross to stop airflow (Figure 46-8). These oscillating PEP devices are similar in cost. All require exhalation via a mouthpiece or mask and thus require adequate muscle strength to form a tight seal around the device, since oscillations and pressure can be lost in the oral cavity. Pressure loss can be prevented by tightening the cheek muscles or holding them with thumb and fingers, compressing the cheeks.

High-Frequency Chest-Wall Compression: Vests

A number of manufacturers have devised portable machines that apply variable high-frequency oscillations directly to the chest wall via an inflated jacket. Collectively these machines are called vests. The devices require power sources and tubing to connect the generator to the jacket. The personally fitted jacket is applied to the chest and inflated to avoid frictional loss of energy at the chest wall and to

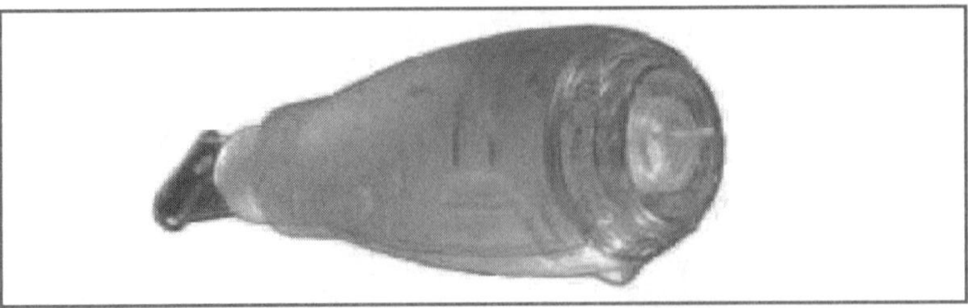

Figure 46-7. Example of the Acapella device, a handheld positive expiratory pressure (PEP) oscillation device designed using magnets; color-coded units (green for high flow, blue for low) help customize treatment for younger and older children. (Image of PEP Therapy | Acapella Vibratory PEP Therapy [Green High Flow and Blue Low Flow w/Mouthpiece] by Smiths Medical ASD, Inc./Portex from EveryDay Medical Products, LLC http://www.everydaymedical.com/index.asp?PageAction=VIEWPROD&ProdID=2095).

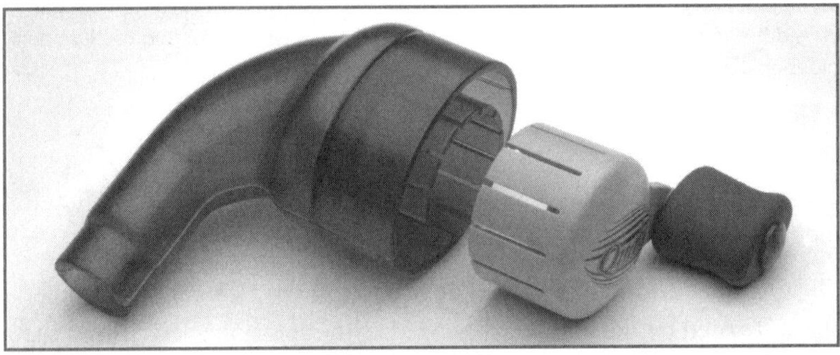

Figure 46-8. Example of the Quake, a handheld oscillating positive expiratory pressure device. (Image of The Quake by Thayer Medical http://www.thayermedical.com/quake.htm).

effectively transmit oscillations simultaneously over the entire chest wall. The inflation pressure can be adjusted, as can the oscillatory frequency. Vest devices move mucus from the periphery to central airways, but actual clearance is required through huff or cough to expectorate mucus (Figure 46-9). Small studies and case series of patients with cerebral palsy and neuromuscular disease suggest that recurrent pneumonia in these patients can be lessened or avoided with routine use.[26]

Cough Assist Device (CAD)

The CAD is used to augment weak and ineffective cough in patients with conditions such as neuromuscular diseases and spinal trauma. Initially called the insufflator-exsufflator, the machine was renamed the cough assist device and has been modified and updated to become truly portable (Figure 46-10). This device generates both positive and negative pressure breaths and can be used in a manual or automatic mode. The interface between the patient and the device can be a mouthpiece, mask, or airway tube (either endotracheal or tracheal). Weaker patients benefit by coughing along with the machine as able or can remain fully passive with glottis open. Even young children and infants can be assisted by using this device. More extensive explanation of teaching and performing these cough assist skills are referenced.[27,28]

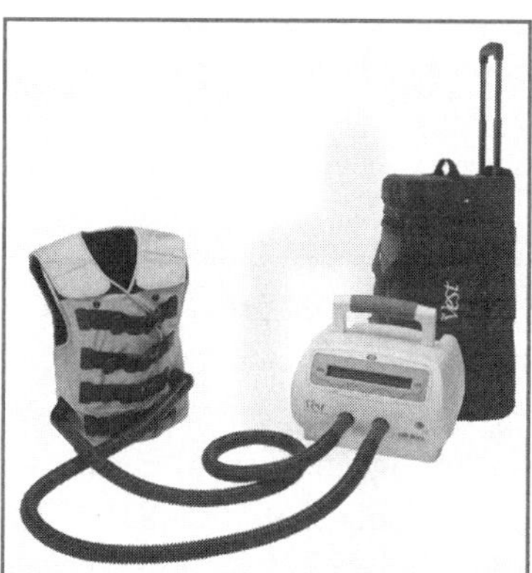

Figure 46-9. Example of the vest. (Image of the Vest airway clearance system. © 2011 Hill Rom Services, Inc. Reprinted with permission. All rights reserved.)

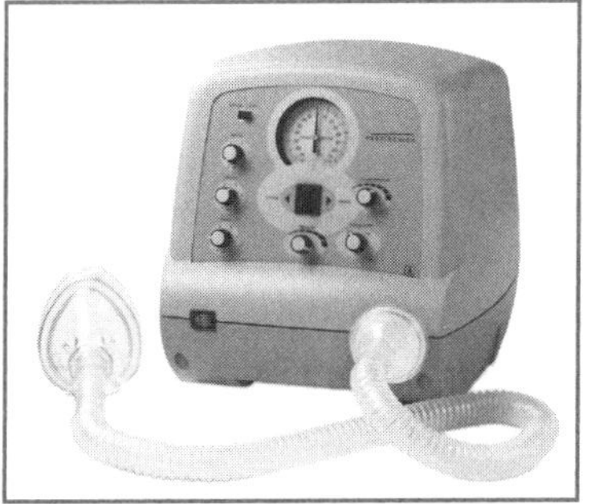

Figure 46-10. Example of a cough assist device. (Image of CoughAssist Mechanical Insufflator-Exsufflator from Phillips Respironics http://www.coughassist.com/).

Intrapulmonary Percussive Ventilator (IPV)

The IPV is another large machine that provides a mouthpiece, mask, or tube interfaces. In this ventilator, positive pressure is generated with jet pulses of air with carefully controlled flow via pistons. The inspiration:expiration ratio is fully controlled so that expiration time always exceeds inspiration time, ensuring that mucus clearance proceeds in the direction of the mouth. Continuous aerosol is required in conjunction with this device because the combination of large airflows and minute volumes is excessively drying to the airways. Epinephrine or selective bronchodilators are recommended for continuous airflow use (Figure 46-11).

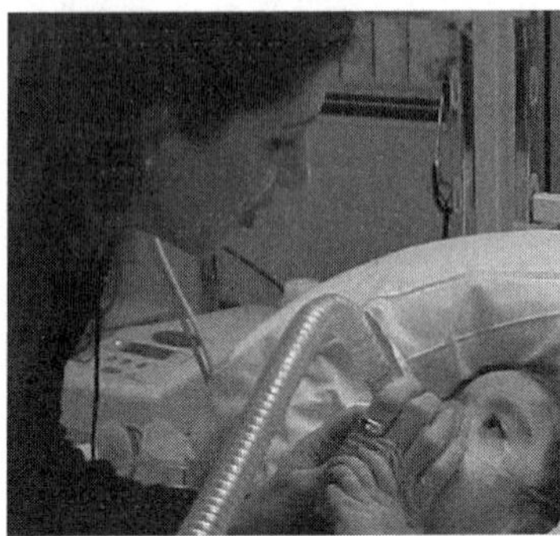

Figure 46-11. Young patient using cough assist device with parental assistance.

Upkeep and Cost Considerations

The devices used require regular cleaning. See Box 46-2 for general care considerations. The prescribing physician should provide detailed information to the family and the primary care physician regarding specific upkeep and maintenance concerns for the specific devices. All the large devices for airway clearance are significantly more costly than handheld devices (Table 46-2). An adherence meter is attached to the vest to generate information regarding usage trends for practitioner review. Disposable vests have also been developed to decrease costliness and are able to function for approximately 1 year before requiring replacement. The standard vest, CAD, and IPV are very durable machines that serve patients for many years. Replacement is most often stimulated by the desire for a newer, more portable device modification rather than a machine failure. These large airway clearance devices can be used passively or combined in the cooperative patient with active respiration strategies as described previously.

Selection of ACT

Infants or very young children typically require assistance and dependent methods of ACT, traditionally using CPT or large machines. Vest jackets have been developed even for infants with a chest size of 19 inches or more. Multiple options are available, and therapies may be modified to suit maturity and lifestyle. Additionally, offering patients input and choice of techniques can increase adherence. Other enhancers of airway clearance can include exercise, playing wind instruments, and vocal training.

Box 46-2. General Care of Airway Clearance Therapy Equipment

Vest

Sponge clean with mild detergent and dry dust machine.
Use germicidal wipes.
Do weekly.

Acapella/Positive Expiratory Pressure (PEP)

Create a water–vinegar solution that has a ratio of 1 part vinegar to 2 parts water.
Place mouthpiece in to soak for 20 minutes.
Let drain and dry on clean towel. Angle Acapella/PEP on towel for best drainage.
Do not immerse TheraPEP.

Table 46-2. Cost Comparisons of Airway Clearance Therapy (ACT) Equipment

ACT Type	Device Cost	Respiratory Therapy Training (approximately 1 hour per session)
Chest physical therapy	$0	1–2 sessions
Huff	$0	1 session
Active cycle of breathing technique	$0	2 sessions
Autogenic drainage	$0	4–6 sessions
Positive expiratory pressure valve	~ $30	1 session
Flutter valve	~ $50	1 session
Acapella	~ $60	1 session
Quake	~ $40	1 session
Vest	~ $9,000–14,000	1 session
Cough assist device	~ $3,500–4,100	2–3 sessions
Intrapulmonary percussive ventilator	~ $5,400–7,000	1 session

Inhaled Medications and ACT

Pharmacologic therapies to aid in airway clearance have primarily been devised for and evaluated in patients with CF. Pulmozyme (recombinant human DNase) enzymatically cleaves DNA that is found in high concentration in the sputum of patients with CF. The DNA is present because of the necrosis of neutrophils that have been drawn into the airway in response to infection. Pulmozyme has a significant impact on mucus viscosity and improves pulmonary function in patients with CF. It is sometimes used in children with other conditions, but there is no evidence of effectiveness outside of CF. Hypertonic saline (7%) has also been shown to be of benefit in patients with CF, presumably by osmotically augmenting airway surface liquid.[29] N-acetyl cysteine (10% solution) is thought to lyse sulfide bonds in mucin and improve the liquidity and ease of removal, but there is little supporting evidence for efficacy. Bronchodilators are helpful to relieve or prevent bronchoconstriction in patients with airway hyperreactivity, but are not universally beneficial and might be detrimental in patients with tracheomalacia or bronchomalacia, who depend on smooth muscle tone to maintain airway patency.[30,31]

Key Points

- A wide selection of independent and dependent techniques is available to improve airway clearance in patients.
- Use CPT for infants and very small children.
- Teach concepts related to breathing at a young age. Children need to learn a vocabulary for these skills. Parents can teach them cough, breathe in, breathe out, blow, etc. Preschool-aged children can learn diaphragmatic breathing and the huff cough.
- Most pulmonary and respiratory specialists and hospital personnel become skilled in the application of these techniques and can assist generalists in decision-making regarding the selection and refinement of ACT skills.
- Weaker patients with poor cough are best managed with manual cough assistance or the CAD.
- The Cystic Fibrosis Foundation has developed comprehensive new guidelines on airway clearance technique, which is a good reference for patients with CF or other diseases causing bronchiectasis and productive cough.

References

1. Schechter MS. Airway clearance applications in infants and children. *Respir Care.* 2007;52(10):1382–1390
2. Button BM, Heine RG, Catto-Smith AG, Phelan PD. Postural drainage in cystic fibrosis: is there a link with gastro-oesophageal reflux? *J Paediatr Child Health.* 1998;34(4):330–334
3. Button BM, Heine RG, Catto-Smith AG, Phelan PD, Olinksy A. Chest physiotherapy, gastro-oesophageal reflux, and arousal in infants with cystic fibrosis. *Arch Dis Child.* 2004;89(5):435–439
4. Thomas J, Cook DJ, Brooks D. Chest physical therapy management of patients with cystic fibrosis: a meta-analysis. *Am J Respir Crit Care Med.* 1995:151(3 pt 1):846–850
5. Bradley JM, Moran RM, Elborn JS. Evidence for physical therapies (airway clearance and physical training) in cystic fibrosis: an overview of five Cochrane systematic reviews. *Respir Med.* 2006;100(2):191–201
6. Main E, Prasad A, Schans C. Conventional chesty physiotherapy compared to other airway clearance techniques for cystic fibrosis. *Conchrane Database Syst Rev.* 2005;(1):CD002011
7. Hough JL, Flenady V, Johnston L, Woodgate PG. Chest physiotherapy for reducing respiratory morbidity in infants requiring ventilatory support. *Cochrane Database Syst Rev.* 2008;(3):CD006445
8. West. J. *Respiratory Physiology: The Essentials.* 7th ed. Philadelphia, PA: Lippincott Williams & Wilkins; 2005:1–12
9. Webber BA, Pryor JA. Physiotherapy techniques. In: Pryor AJ, Webber BA, eds. *Physiotherapy for Respiratory and Cardiac Problems.* 2nd ed. Edinburgh: Churchill Livingstone; 1998;140–155
10. Zapetal A, Stefanova J, Horak J, Vavrova V, Samanek M. Chest physiotherapy and airway obstruction in patients with cystic fibrosis: a negative report. *Eur J Respir Dis.* 1983;64(6):426–433
11. Wilson GE, Baldwin Al, Walshaw MJ. A comparison of traditional chest physiotherapy with the active cycle of breathing in patients with chronic suppurative lung disease. *Euro Resp J.* 1995;8(19):171S
12. Chevaillier J. Autogenic drainage. In: Lawson D, ed. *Cystic Fibrosis: Horizons.* New York, NY: John Wiley & Sons, Inc; 1984:235
13. Pryor JA, Webber VA, Hodson ME. Effect of chest physiotherapy on oxygen saturation in patients with cystic fibrosis. *Thorax.* 1990;45(1):77
14. Giles DR, Wagener JS, Accurso FJ, Butler-Simon N. Short term effects of postural drainage versus autogenic drainage on oxygen saturation and sputum recovery in patients with cystic fibrosis. *Chest.* 1995;108:952–954
15. Murphy MB, Cocannon D, FitzGerald MX. Chest percussion: help or hindrance to postural drainage? *Irish Med J.* 1983;76(4):189–190
16. Selsby DS. Chest physiotherapy. *Br Med J.* 1989;298(6673):541–542

17. Passero MA, Remor, B, Salomon J. Patient-reported compliance with cystic fibrosis therapy. *Clin Pediatr (Phila).* 1981;20:264–268
18. Hardy KA, Elisan I, Johnson C, Sills E, Robles AJ. Novel efficacy score for ACT and medicine delivery in CF patients (abstract). *Pediatr Pulmonol Suppl.* 2008;A601
19. Eid N, Buchheit J, Neuling M, et al. Chest physiotherapy in review. *Respir Care.* 1991;36:270–282
20. Jaeger RJ, Turba RM, Yarkony GM, Roth EJ. Cough in spinal cord injured patients: comparison of three methods to produce cough. *Arch Phys Med Rehabil.* 1993;74(12):1358–1361
21. Falk M, Kelstrup M, Andersen JB, et al. Improving the ketchup bottle method with positive expiratory pressure, PEP, in cystic fibrosis. *Eur J Respir Dis.* 1984;65:423–432
22. Mahlmeister MJ, Fink JB, Hoffman GL, Fifer LF. Positive-expiratory pressure mask therapy: theoretical and practical considerations and a review of the literature. *Respir Care.* 1991;36(6):546–554
23. Althaus P, et al. The bronchial hygiene assisted by the Flutter VRP1 (module regulator of a positive pressure oscillation on expiration). *Eur Respir J.* 1989; 2 (suppl 8):693
24. Hüls G, Lindermann H. Vergleichende Untersuchungen zur Physiotherapie: flutter VRP 1 versus autogene drainage [comparison between two physiotherapeutic methods: the flutter VRP 1 and autogenic drainage]. *Atemw und Lungenkrankheiten.* 1991;17:414
25. Lindemann H. Zum Stellenwert der Physiotherapie mit dem VRP 1-Desitin ("Flutter") [The value of physical therapy with VRP 1 ("Flutter")]. *Pneumologie.* 1992;46(12):626–630
26. Plioplys AV, Lewis S, Kasnicka I. Pulmonary vest therapy in pediatric long-term care. *J Am Med Dir Assoc.* 2002;3(5):318–321
27. Bach JR. Mechanical insufflation-exsufflation. Comparison of peak expiratory flows with manually assisted and unassisted coughing techniques. *Chest.* 1993;104:1553–1562
28. Schwake-Dohna C, Ragette R, Teschler H, Voit T, Mellies U. IPPB-assisted coughing in neuromuscular disorders. *Pediatr Pulmonol.* 2006;41:551–557
29. Elkins MR, Robinson M, Rose BR, et al. A controlled trial of long-term inhaled hypertonic saline in patients with cystic fibrosis. *N Engl J Med.* 2006;354(3):229–240
30. Panitch HB, Keklikian EN, Motley RA, Wolfson MR, Schidlow DV. Effect of altering smooth muscle tone on maximal expiratory flows in patients with tracheomalacia. *Pediatr Pulmonol.* 1990;9(3):1717–1726
31. Panitch HB, Allen JL, Alpert BE, Schidlow DV. Effects of CPAP on lung mechanics in infants with acquired tracheobronchomalacia. *Am J Respir Crit Care Med.* 1994;150(5 pt 1):1341–1346

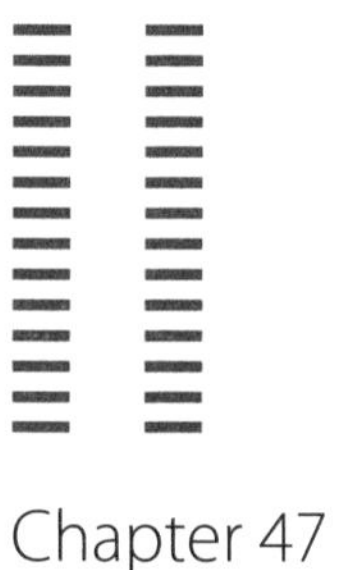

Chapter 47

Aerosol Delivery of Medication

David Geller, MD
Ariel Berlinski, MD

Introduction

Topical application of drugs to the lungs by inhalation is a mainstay of treatment for pulmonary diseases in children. Disease management guidelines stress the importance of inhaled corticosteroids and bronchodilators for controlling asthma, and mucus-active agents and antibiotics for controlling the lung disease in cystic fibrosis (CF).[1,2] There is also interest in using aerosols for systemic delivery of molecules that would otherwise be degraded in the gut or that require injection, although no such drugs are currently approved for children.

As simple as the concept of topical inhalation therapy may seem, the challenges of successful delivery of drugs to the lungs are much greater than those of oral or systemic drug delivery. The respiratory tract has evolved to filter out foreign materials and exclude entry into the lower airways. Aerosol devices and breathing techniques must be able to bypass these defenses to deposit drugs in the lungs. The success of aerosol delivery depends on several complex, interrelated factors. Improper use of aerosol devices is associated with poorer clinical outcomes,[3] so it is crucial that children and their caregivers be familiar with aerosol principles and the correct operation of different aerosol delivery devices.

Aerosol Principles

Advantages of Aerosols

Using inhaled therapy to treat lung diseases is similar to treating skin disorders with topical creams, lotions, and powders in that the goal is to deliver the drug to the site of action (ie, the airways). Inhaled topical therapy potentially provides a high in situ concentration and usually requires lower doses than systemic treatment, thus maximizing the desired effects while reducing systemic effects. In the case of inhaled bronchodilators, the onset of action is far quicker than oral therapy, providing rapid relief of bronchospasm.[4] For corticosteroids, the improved therapeutic index of the inhaled route helps to minimize side effects of adrenal and growth suppression. Antibiotics like tobramycin inhalation solution can achieve 100-fold the concentration in airway secretions versus the intravenous route for children with CF, while reducing the risk of ototoxicity and nephrotoxicity.[5] The gut renders protein-based drugs inactive (eg, dornase alfa for CF), therefore inhalation is the best modality.

Aerosol Drug Delivery

An aerosol is a suspension of solid or liquid particles in a carrier gas. Many patients and clinicians believe that aerosols know how to navigate beyond the upper airway and naturally seek their target receptor in the lung. In fact, there are numerous factors that determine where the particles of an aerosol will deposit, including characteristics of the aerosol itself, as well as variables pertaining to the person inhaling the aerosol[6–9] (Box 47-1).

For inhaled medications, the particle size distribution of the aerosol is one of the important factors that determine the likelihood of drug deposition in the lower airway. The particle size of an aerosol is described by the mass median aerodynamic diameter (MMAD) (ie, the

Box 47-1. Factors Determining Aerosol Deposition

Aerosol Factors	Patient Factors
Particle size	Inspiratory flow rate
Velocity	Age
Hygroscopic properties	Breathing pattern (eg, tidal volume, rate)
Drug viscosity and surface tension	Nasal vs mouth breathing
Suspension vs solution	Upper airway anatomy
	Disease severity
	Physical and cognitive abilities
	Adherence, contrivance

size for which half of the mass of the drug is contained in particles that are larger and half in particles that are smaller). The distribution of particle sizes in an aerosol is described by the geometric standard deviation (GSD). Particles larger than 6 microns tend to impact (be deposited) in the upper airway, which can contribute to local and systemic side effects. Particles under 5 to 6 microns can more easily navigate the upper airway to reach the lower airways and alveoli of the lung. Once aerosol particles pass the first few generations of bronchi, the deposition mechanism switches from impaction to sedimentation (gravity), which is why a breath-hold can be useful with single-breath techniques to allow time for particles to settle. Submicron particles (<1 micron) may be so small that they are exhaled rather than deposited in the lungs in healthy subjects. However, patients with airway obstruction have a greater chance of particle deposition at branch points, so these generalizations do not always apply. Most pharmaceutical aerosols are polydisperse, meaning they contain particles of varying sizes (high GSD). In theory, the larger particles deposit more centrally and the smaller ones more distally in the airways.

Patient Variables Affecting Aerosol Delivery

Patient variables are often more important than aerosol characteristics in determining lung deposition. Particle size and speed are the 2 main factors that determine whether it will impact on an airway (the larger the particle and the faster it travels, the more likely it will crash into an airway and deposit). The speed at which the particle is generated (device-related) as well as the inspiratory flow (patient-related) determines particle velocity. For pressurized metered-dose inhalers (pMDIs) and nebulizers, patients are taught to inhale slowly (ie, <30 L/min) to slow the speed of the particles and avoid upper airway impaction. Conversely, dry-powder inhalers (DPIs) require greater inspiratory force to break the powder apart into small particles.

Patient variables, including tidal volume and respiratory rate, are important for aerosol deposition. In general, the larger the inhaled or tidal volume and the slower the respiratory rate, the higher the lung deposition will be because the aerosol "dwell time" in the lungs is longer. For the same reason, a breath-hold at the end of inspiration improves deposition for pMDIs. For a continuously operating nebulizer a breath-hold may not be beneficial since aerosol will be lost during the breath-hold.

Upper airway anatomy is an often-ignored subject, though it is a crucial determinant of the ability to achieve lung deposition. Nasal breathing can filter half of an aerosol drug before it can reach the lower airways.[10] The upper airways of infants and young children are much smaller than those of an adult, and also filter a considerable amount of drug before it reaches the lungs. Probably for this reason, infants and young children do not require a dose adjustment based on size, since the amount reaching the lung is proportionately smaller.

A lower airway obstruction (as found in asthma, bronchiolitis, and CF) has a profound influence on regional deposition of aerosols in the lung. Aerosol droplets deposit in larger, more central airways and at flow-limiting segments in patients with obstructions. Radiolabeled scintigraphy of aerosol deposition in obstructed patients shows a very patchy, uneven distribution of aerosol.[11] Infants and young children also tend to deposit aerosol more centrally since their lower airways also have a smaller caliber. Therefore, successful aerosol delivery to the peripheral lung in sicker and younger patients is much more challenging.

Case Report 47-1

D.B. is an 18-month-old boy with a history of recurrent wheezing since 2 months of age when he was hospitalized for bronchiolitis. He has atopic dermatitis and wheezes during and between colds. Bronchoscopy ruled out an anatomical reason for wheezing. Chronic inhaled corticosteroids were prescribed, but he has not improved. The parents swear they faithfully give the medication, though most of the time it takes 2 to 3 people to hold him down during the treatment.

Infants and young children are the most challenging group to treat with aerosols, and there are many myths pertaining to this group. None of the factors mentioned in Box 47-1 favor deposition in young children. They tend to be nose-breathers and have smaller upper and lower airway sizes, smaller tidal volumes, and more rapid respiratory rates. They don't have the cognitive ability to follow commands or understand specialized inhalation maneuvers, so they are restricted to devices that only require tidal breathing, and those with a mask as the interface between device and patient. Nebulizers and pMDIs attached to a valved holding chamber (VHC) can have mask attachments, but the masks must be applied close to the child's face with a nebulizer to prevent escape of aerosol, and must be tight-fitting with a VHC to draw the medication out of the chamber. Unfortunately, a high proportion of young children do not tolerate masks, even with repeated use, and become fussy or cry during the treatment.[12]

Some caregivers mistakenly believe that crying will improve aerosol deposition because the child is taking deeper breaths. In fact, the opposite is true. Crying involves a prolonged exhalation, followed by a rapid inhalation. Drug is wasted from the device during the long exhalation, and the rapid inhalation causes the drug to impact on the throat, but very little reaches the lungs.[13]

To optimize aerosol delivery in small children, first choose the delivery device that is best tolerated. This will require some trial and error, and the prescribed drug must be available in the desired delivery devices. Second, distract the child during aerosol administration with toys or videos, and try to make a game out of it with incentives for good performance. They should not regard their treatments as a form of punishment, and they may not comprehend that the medication is to make them feel better. Using the blow-by technique with a nebulizer (holding the mask away from the face) is discouraged, based on in vitro and deposition studies.[13,14] However, there is in vitro evidence that holding a corrugated-tube extension in front of the face instead of using a mask may provide an adequate inhaled dose, although this has not been demonstrated in clinical trials.[15] Finally, there is evidence that providing aerosols with less than 2.5 microns to children younger than 3 years may enhance aerosol delivery to the lungs.[16]

Aerosol Delivery Devices

Systems for delivery of inhaled medications include wet nebulizers, pMDIs, and DPIs. Each of these systems has unique advantages and disadvantages, but most of these technologies are decades old and are relatively inefficient in terms of the proportion of the nominal dose reaching the lower airways (especially in children). Since the dose-response curves for bronchodilators and inhaled corticosteroids are steep at low doses, and since the therapeutic index is high with these drugs, the poor delivery efficiency and high variability of these systems has been tolerated. Novel delivery technologies have been designed to radically improve delivery efficiency for newer therapies that are expensive, have a lower therapeutic index, or require precision targeting to a particular part of the airway (eg, gene therapy in CF).[17]

Nebulizers

Wet Nebulizers

Wet nebulizers are aerosol devices that convert a liquid solution or suspension into an aerosol for inhalation. The 3 main types of nebulizer are the jet nebulizer (sometimes called small-volume nebulizer); ultrasonic nebulizer; and vibrating, perforated-membrane nebulizer. The jet nebulizer is the type most commonly prescribed by pediatricians, probably because of the relatively low cost and availability. Nebulizers are perhaps the most intuitive devices for aerosol delivery in children, because they do not require special breathing techniques and can be used by patients of all ages. Some advantages and disadvantages of jet nebulizers are listed in Box 47-2.

Jet Nebulizers

Jet nebulizers deliver compressed gas (supplied by an electric compressor, hospital air, or oxygen) through a small jet orifice, generating a negative pressure that draws fluid from the nebulizer cup. The fluid is entrained in the stream of gas and sheared into particles. Larger, non-respirable particles impact against a baffle and are recirculated, whereas smaller aerosol particles are directed to the patient. There is some evaporation and cooling that occurs when particles are recycled, causing an increase in drug concentration in the residual volume that remains in the nebulizer cup after the nebulization is complete. In general the residual volume ranges between 0.5 and 1.5 mL, thus wasting a large proportion of the loaded dose. The aerosol charac-

Box 47-2. Advantages and Disadvantages of Jet Nebulizers

Advantages	Disadvantages
Easy technique (tidal breathing)	Bulky, less portable than pressurized metered-dose inhalers or dry-powder inhalers
Can use at any age	Longer treatment times
Can use with any disease severity	Require cleaning and disinfection
Use with artificial airways	Noisy (may disturb infants)
Use with mechanical ventilation	Require power source
High doses possible (eg, antibiotics)	High variability between brands

teristics and efficiencies of many variables. For example, increasing various brands of nebulizer differ by several-fold[18] and depend on the flow rate through a nebulizer may decrease the particle size and reduce delivery time. While this can be accomplished easily in the hospital setting, most electronic compressors (particularly portable, battery-operated models) have low flow rates and longer delivery times. Over time, electronic compressors can lose power and require replacing if the patient experiences long delivery times.

There are 3 different types of jet nebulizer. The most common and least expensive are the so-called t-piece or updraft nebulizers that produce aerosol during both inspiration and expiration. Aerosol is wasted during exhalation. A more efficient nebulizer is the breath-enhanced jet nebulizer (eg, SideStream Plus, Respironics), which incorporates a 1-way valve that entrains inspired air through the drug reservoir, capturing more aerosol during inspiration and wasting less drug during exhalation. This results in improved drug delivery compared with the t-piece nebulizer. Finally, newer types of devices are breath-actuated and only release aerosol on demand during inspiration, with no wasted drug during exhalation. If a unit dose of drug is used, the length of treatment may be longer but delivered dose will be higher. Depending on the drug characteristics (dose-response curve, side-effect profile), dose adjustments may be necessary with a breath-actuated nebulizer.

Nebulizer-Patient Interface

The interface between the nebulizer and patient is very important. Although masks and mouthpieces seem to provide similar clinical benefits,[19] the latter is recommended to avoid drug filtering in the nose and decrease facial deposition and potential side effects.[20] Transition to mouthpiece can usually be done at age 4 or 5 years. Mask design is an important factor in minimizing side effects. Several studies have shown that front-loaded masks lead to less ocular deposition than bottom-loaded masks.[21]

Nebulizing Multiple Drugs

The nebulization of several drugs together is discouraged because of potential changes in particle size characteristics.[22] Albuterol and ipratropium bromide are an exception, though this combination is available commercially. Also, combining unit-dose drugs will significantly increase the delivery time (more fluid to nebulize), so combining drugs in the nebulizer would only be advantageous if one of them is in a concentrated form.

Ultrasonic Nebulizers

Ultrasonic nebulizers operate with piezoelectric crystal that vibrates at a set frequency and transfers energy to the fluid placed in a reservoir to produce a mist.[23] Ultrasonic nebulizers are quieter and faster than jet nebulizers, though they are not commonly prescribed because of their higher cost. Historically they have been large and bulky, though in recent years many models have been introduced that are small, portable, and battery operated. However, ultrasonic nebulizers cannot effectively deliver suspensions like budesonide.[24] They also tend to produce a larger particle size than jet nebulizers, which may reduce the dose reaching the lungs. Finally, some of these devices increase the solution/suspension temperature, which could potentially denature protein drugs like dornase alfa.[25]

Perforated-Membrane Nebulizers

Vibrating, perforated-membrane nebulizers are the most recent addition to the nebulizer menu. These devices use a piezo element to either move a perforated membrane against the solution to "micro-pump" the fluid through the holes (Aeroneb, Aerogen, and eFlow, PARI Pharma), or to move a vibrating horn that shoots the fluid through a mesh to create the aerosol (MicroAir, Omron).[17] Vibrating, perforated membrane nebulizers are small, silent, have small residual volumes, and are faster than most jet nebulizers. The available "open" devices (Aeroneb, Aerogen) were designed to give approximately the same performance efficiency as a breath-enhanced jet nebulizer. To do this, the particle size is larger to compensate for the lower residual volume, thus offering no advantage other than speed. Also, the micron-sized holes in the mesh are easily clogged, so these devices are not recommended for suspensions like budesonide.

The eFlow is a platform that can be customized for specific drugs as a drug-device combination. The eFlow has a higher delivery efficiency than other nebulizers because of a low residual volume, consistent (less heterodisperse) aerosol, and an aerosol chamber that conserves some of the aerosol during exhalation. Though an "open" version is available from a few compounding pharmacies for patients with CF, this device is typically paired with specific drugs, including inhaled antibiotics that are in development for CF and bronchiectasis. Because the eFlow has such a high delivery efficiency, when it is used as an open device, a dose adjustment downward may be necessary to avoid toxicity with some drugs.

Nebulizer Maintenance

Routine maintenance of nebulizers is often ignored. All nebulizers need to be cleaned after each use and disinfected according to manufacturer's instructions. Cleaning can be done by washing with soapy water followed by rinsing and air-drying. Disinfection can be done by several methods, including boiling in water for 5 minutes, or immersion in 70% isopropyl alcohol (5 minutes), 3% hydrogen peroxide (30 minutes), or 1:50 dilution of 5.25% to 6.15% household bleach (3 minutes). Rinsing with sterile or filtered water will be necessary if any of the solutions are used. Other alternatives include microwaving in water (5 minutes) or using a dishwasher (30 minutes), provided water remains hotter than 158°F. Disinfection with a steam sterilizer (like those used for baby bottles) is recommended for vibrating-membrane nebulizers and can be used for jet nebulizers also.

Pressurized Metered-Dose Inhalers

Pressurized metered-dose inhalers are popular as delivery systems because they are small and convenient to use (Box 47-3). The technique for using a pMDI is the most challenging of aerosol devices, with many

Box 47-3. Advantages and Disadvantages of Metered-Dose Inhalers

Advantages	Disadvantages
Compact, portable	Difficult technique to learn/teach
Rapid delivery	Coordination for actuation and inhalation
Multi-dose convenience	High oropharyngeal dose (not with valved holding chamber)
Easy to clean	Dissatisfaction with hydrofluoroalkanes propellant
Any age (when used with a valved holding chamber)	Intolerance of tight face mask (young children)
Dose counters now more common	Limited number of drugs available

errors reported among both patients and caregivers.[26,27] Each pMDI canister contains micronized drug suspended in a propellant. A metering valve holds a few microliters of the suspension, and when the device is actuated, the metering chamber is exposed to the atmosphere and the reduction in chamber pressure causes the rapid boiling of the propellant, releasing the contents at a high velocity. The propellants currently used are hydrofluoroalkanes (HFAs), which replaced chlorofluorocarbons (CFCs, Freon). One advantage of HFAs as propellant is that the plume has a slower velocity with most drugs (except fluticasone), so that the "ballistic" fraction is reduced, with less impaction on the throat. Also, the aerosol is warmer, so there is less risk that the patient will stop inhaling prematurely as the cold aerosol hits the throat (cold Freon effect). On the other hand, some patients accustomed to feeling the cold forceful puff in their throat believe the HFA inhalers don't work as well as the older CFC formulations. These patients will benefit from education regarding the different sensation and taste of the HFA inhalers.

Two of the available inhaled corticosteroids (beclomethasone and ciclesonide) are dissolved in the HFA, forming a stable solution (as opposed to a suspension). This allowed a redesign of the pMDI for those drugs, with a resulting tiny particle size (MMAD 1.1–1.2 microns) that favors improved lung deposition and penetration of the aerosol deep in the lungs,[28] and in theory may be more advantageous for small children than the larger particle devices.[16,29]

Case Report 47-2

B.A. is a 6-year-old with asthma being treated with medium-dose inhaled corticosteroids via pMDI and holding chamber. He takes the medication twice a day as prescribed, but complains of worsening symptoms for the last month. Approximately 3 or 4 weeks prior he lost his holding chamber and he started using the pMDI without it.

Spacers and Valved Holding Chambers

Metered-dose inhalers are often used with add-on devices like spacers and VHCs. Spacers are valveless tubes that work by allowing deceleration of the aerosol and shrinkage of the particles. Conversely, VHCs incorporate a 1-way valve to contain the aerosol in the chamber for a few seconds until the valve is opened by the patient's inspiratory effort.

Both spacers and VHCs reduce the high oropharyngeal deposition (and local side effects) of pMDIs, but only VHCs help overcome the difficulty in coordinating actuation with inhalation, and are therefore favored over simple spacers. In Case Report 47-2, B.A. likely had poor technique without his VHC and wasn't getting adequate medication to his lower airways. However, even the use of a VHC is not foolproof and requires patient education for proper use.

Some of the advantages of pMDIs and VHCs are reviewed in Box 47-3. These delivery systems are portable, noiseless, can be used for children of any age, and can be used with artificial airways (tracheostomies, intubated patients). The biggest attraction is that they are less time-consuming than nebulizers. There are only a few types of drugs available in pMDIs, including bronchodilators and inhaled corticosteroids (asthma medications).

Most VHCs allow insertion of the pMDI mouthpiece into a connector, thus using its own boot (plastic holder). Some VHCs require the pMDI canister to be removed from its own plastic boot and inserted into a universal boot for actuation. However, the universal boots were originally designed for CFC inhalers and may not work well with the newer HFA inhalers.

There are several different brands and designs of VHCs, leading to a high degree of variability in dose delivery between devices.[30] Many early devices are made from polycarbonate, which has a high electrostatic charge and can reduce the drug output. The electrostatic charge can be neutralized by washing the VHC in soapy water and letting it air-dry without rinsing the inside. Some newer VHCs are manufactured with a charge-dissipating material, which increases the "hang time" of the aerosol in the chamber and delivers more of the dose to the patient.[31] Although VHCs overcome the need for precise coordination, the aerosol does not stay suspended for more than a few seconds, so a delay in inhalation will significantly decrease drug output. Patients requiring more than one actuation of medication should shake the canister between actuations and allow a 30-second interval between them. No more than one actuation should be performed at one time into a VHC, since the particles may collide and reduce the total drug output.

Care and Use of Inhalers

The care of HFA inhalers is slightly different from their CFC counterparts in that the actuator orifice can become clogged over time and requires cleaning. Inhalers need to be primed with their first use and each time they are not used for prolonged periods (varies between products but may be as short as 2–3 days).

The VHCs with mask attachments allow infants and young children to use medication via pMDI. It is important to choose a mask with a small dead space made of flexible material that forms a good seal with the face.[32–34] A good seal is necessary for the child to open the valve of the VHC, allowing access to the medication in the chamber. For young children who tolerate a close-fitting face mask, the pMDI with VHC is the preferred method for delivery of inhaled asthma medications. Though the pMDI with VHC and face mask is a quicker way to deliver bronchodilators and inhaled corticosteroids than a nebulizer, more than a third of infants and toddlers do not tolerate the tight-fitting mask and should use the alternate delivery system.[12]

A transition to a VHC with mouthpiece is encouraged at about 3 to 4 years of age to avoid drug filtering by the nose. Young children can use tidal breathing (5–6 breaths) with the VHC until they are old enough to comprehend single-breath technique. When children reach 4 to 6 years of age, they can be taught to exhale first, seal their lips around the mouthpiece, actuate the pMDI, and slowly inhale to full lung capacity, with a 10-second breath-hold to allow particles to settle in the airways. The same technique applies for a pMDI without a VHC, though with corticosteroids the use of a VHC is recommended to reduce topical oropharyngeal effects.

Historically, there were no dose counters on pMDIs, so it was difficult to tell how much drug was left in a canister. The only valid way was to keep track of the number of inhalations taken and subtract from the total starting number in the canister. Placing the canister in water and observing how it submerges is inaccurate and can obstruct the valve. In 2003 the US Food and Drug Administration offered guidance to pharmaceutical companies to incorporate dose counters into pMDIs, and many have done so. This is particularly important for rescue medications. Since their use is not scheduled and there are priming requirements, it is very difficult to keep track of the number of available inhalations.

Finally, there is a breath-actuated pMDI for the rescue drug pirbuterol. This device is activated by the inspiratory flow of the patient, eliminating the need for coordinating actuation and inhalation. It does not eliminate the cold Freon effect. Older children (≥6 years) can be taught how to use this device, which does not require a VHC. More drugs should be available via breath-actuated pMDI in the future.

Dry-Powder Inhalers

Dry-powder inhalers are drug-device combinations that are breath actuated so do not require a coordinated effort as with most pMDIs (Box 47-4). There is a variety of DPI devices, including capsule-based single-dose devices, or multi-dose devices with either a bulk drug reservoir or with individual doses protected by foil. Generally, the drug is milled into very small particles in the respirable size range. However, small micronized drug particles have strong forces of attraction and tend to stick together. The inspiratory energy generated by the patient is responsible for the deagglomeration of the powder into particles that can be inhaled. As the inspiratory force increases, the amount of drug available in small particles also increases and offsets the losses from impaction of the high-velocity particles in the oropharynx.[35] Sometimes, large "carrier" particles of a substance like lactose are used to improve the separation and flow of small drug particles, with the larger carrier particles depositing in the throat and the smaller drug particles passing to the lungs. Novel DPI formulations (antibiotics, insulin) use light, hollow, porous particles to improve particle separation and deliver higher payloads.[36]

Box 47-4. Advantages and Disadvantages of Dry-Powder Inhalers

Advantages	Disadvantages
Compact, portable	Need strong inspiratory effort
Rapid delivery time	High oropharyngeal impaction
Breath-actuated	Vulnerable to humidity
Dose counters in multi-dose devices	Limited to children >5 years
Easier to learn than pressurized metered-dose inhalers	Multiple dry-powder inhaler device types
No need for valved holding chamber, spacer	Technique confusion with other devices

Inspiratory Effort and Dry Delivery

The ideal inspiratory effort is different for various DPI devices depending on their internal resistance. It is a myth that low-resistance devices are better suited for children. Simple physics dictates that with the same inspiratory effort, the flow rate will be higher through a low-resistance device, and vice versa. However, higher resistance devices have internal channels that help the deagglomeration process, and higher resistance may open the glottis to allow more drug to pass the larynx. The belief that asthmatic patients are unable to attain sufficient inspiratory flow to derive clinical benefit from a higher resistance DPI is a misconception.[37] There are too many variables involved to compare DPI devices based on resistance alone.

Case Report 47-3

J.C. is a 4-year-old with asthma. His inhaled steroid was switched 2 months ago from pMDI with VHC to a DPI. The family reports an increase in daytime and nighttime symptoms. He has been requiring more albuterol over the last month.

Use of Dry-Powder Inhalers

The main limiting factors for DPI use in children are that very young children either lack the inspiratory power necessary to power the device, they lack the lung capacity to draw the powder into the lungs, and/or they cannot comprehend the maneuver to operate a DPI. Young children sometimes would rather blow into a device rather than inhale from it, which would moisten the powder and make it impossible to aerosolize. For these reasons it is reasonable to exclude the use of DPIs until about 6 years of age, whether or not they are approved for younger ages.

Though the inhalation technique for a DPI is simpler than a pMDI, there are many types of DPI inhalers that look and operate differently. Each pharmaceutical company has its own proprietary device that has its unique set of instructions. This can be confusing for patients who require more than one device for control of their asthma or other lung disease. For example, in the United States there is no short-acting ß-agonist formulation available as a DPI. Therefore, patients would have to learn to inhale forcefully from their DPI controller medication, and inhale their rescue drug slowly from their pMDI. This can lead to "device delirium" and misuse of one or the other device types.[38] Practitioners need to learn about the specifics for each device they prescribe.

Choosing the Appropriate Delivery Device

The increasing number of device choices can be very confusing and intimidating to patients and clinicians alike. There are hundreds of papers that argue the merits of one device versus another, but a recent comprehensive meta-analysis of this literature provided evidence-based guidelines in a variety of inpatient and outpatient settings,[39] concluding that each of the aerosol devices work equally well in a variety of clinical settings *in patients who can use the devices appropriately.* This work emphasizes the burden that clinicians have to properly educate their patients in the proper techniques for use and maintenance of their devices. Given the high rate of device misuse, reeducation on subsequent clinic visits should repeat until the optimal procedure is followed.

There is a complex relationship between hospitals, suppliers, pharmacies, insurers, caregivers, and patients that can influence the choice of an aerosol device for your patients.[38]

Key Points

- Different medications may require choosing a specific device, for example nebulized budesonide and inhaled antibiotics that have been evaluated in clinical trials.
- The choice of delivery system depends on the age, comprehension, and capability of the child. This will often require a trial in the office to evaluate.
- The third-party payer may dictate which device is covered. Unfortunately this is often state-specific and changes frequently.
- Cost, time savings, and portability should be considered when choosing the device. Decreasing the burden of care enhances adherence to the medical regimen.
- The technique of medication delivery should be reviewed often with the caregiver to ensure that the device is being used correctly. Clinicians need to be familiar with the various devices in order to be able to teach how to use them.
- Acceptability by the child and family is of paramount importance for adherence and clinical outcomes. Sometimes a trial with different delivery systems may be necessary or using 2 types of delivery systems may be appropriate (eg, using a nebulizer at home and a pMDI with VHC at child care for best clinical outcomes).

Current medications for asthma and the devices for which they are formulated are listed in Table 47-1. An updated comprehensive guide on aerosol delivery is available from the American Association for Respiratory Care.[40] This invaluable guide has pictures and detailed instructions for how to use and care for each device (download at http://www.aarc.org/education/aerosol_devices).

Table 47-1. Drug Formulations for Asthma Available in United States

Medication	Nebulizer	pMDI	Breath-actuated pMDI	DPI Single-dose	DPI Multi-dose
Short-acting Bronchodilators					
Albuterol	√	√			
Levalbuterol	√	√			
Pirbuterol[a]			√		
Terbutaline	√	√			
Ipratropium	√	√			
Albuterol + ipratropium[a]	√	√			
Long-acting Bronchodilators					
Salmeterol					√
Formoterol	√			√	
Arformoterol	√				
Tiotropium				√	
Inhaled Corticosteroids					
Budesonide	√				√
Mometasone					√
Fluticasone		√			
Beclomethasone		√			
Ciclesonide		√			
Flunisolide		√			
Combination ICS/LABA					
Budesonide/formoterol		√			
Fluticasone/salmeterol		√			√
Mometasone/formoterol		√			

Abbreviations: DPI, dry-powder inhaler; ICS, inhaled corticosteroid; LABA, long-acting bronchodilator; pMDI, pressurized metered-dose inhaler.
[a]Chlorofluorocarbon formulations will not be available after 12/31/11.

References

1. National Heart, Lung, and Blood Institute, National Asthma Education and Prevention Program. *Expert Panel Report 3: Guidelines for the Diagnosis and Management of Asthma.* Washington, DC: US Department of Health and Human Services, National Institutes of Health; 2007. http://www.nhlbi.nih.gov/guidelines/asthma/asthgdln.htm
2. Flume PA, O'Sullivan BP, Robinson KA, et al. Cystic fibrosis guidelines: chronic medications for maintenance of lung health. *Am J Respir Crit Care Med.* 2007;176:957–969
3. Giraud V, Roche N. Misuse of corticosteroid metered-dose inhaler is associated with decreased asthma stability. *Eur Respir J.* 2002;19:246–251
4. Dulfano MJ, Glass P. The bronchodilator effects of terbutaline: route of administration and patterns of response. *Ann Allergy.* 1976;37(5):357–366
5. Geller DE, Pitlick WH, Nardella PA, Tracewell WG, Ramsey BW. Pharmacokinetics and bioavailability of aerosolized tobramycin (TOBI) in cystic fibrosis. *Chest.* 2002;122(1):219–226
6. Geller DE. The science of aerosol delivery in cystic fibrosis. *Pediatr Pulmonol.* 2008;43(9 suppl A):S5–S17
7. Tiddens HA, Devadason SG. Delivery of therapy to the cystic fibrosis lung. In: Hodson M, Geddes D, Bush A, eds. *Cystic fibrosis.* London: Edward Arnold; 2007:185–198
8. Labiris NR, Dolovich MB. Pulmonary drug delivery. Part I: physiologic factors affecting therapeutic effectiveness of aerosolized medications. *Br J Clin Pharmacol.* 2003;56(6):588–599
9. Zanen P, Laube BL. Targeting the lungs with therapeutic aerosols. In: Bisgaard H, O'Callaghan CO, Smaldone GC, eds. Drug delivery to the lung. New York, NY: Marcel Dekker; 2002:211–268
10. Chua HL, Collis GG, Newbury AM, et al. The influence of age on aerosol deposition in children with cystic fibrosis. *Eur Respir J.* 1994;7:2185–2191
11. Laube BL, Links JM, LaFrance ND, Wagner HN Jr, Rosenstein BJ. Homogeneity of bronchopulmonary distribution of 99mTc aerosol in normal subjects and in cystic fibrosis patients. *Chest.* 1989;95:822–830
12. Marguet C, Couderc L, Le Roux P, Jeannot E, Lefay V, Mallet E. Inhalation treatment: errors in application and difficulties in acceptance of the devices are frequent in wheezy infants and young children. *Pediatr Allergy Immunol.* 2001;12:224–230
13. Erzinger S, Schueepp KG, Brooks-Wildhaber J, Devadason SG, Wildhaber JH. Facemasks and aerosol delivery in vivo. *J Aerosol Med.* 2007;20 (suppl 1):S78–S83
14. Everard ML, Clark AR, Milner AD. Drug delivery from jet nebulisers. *Arch Dis Child.* 1992;67:586–591
15. Restrepo RD, Dickson SK, Rau JL, Gardenhire DS. An investigation of nebulized bronchodilator delivery using a pediatric model of spontaneous breathing. *Respir Care.* 2006;51(1):56–61

16. Schueepp KG, Devadason SG, Roller C, et al. Aerosol delivery of nebulised budesonide in young children with asthma. *Respir Med.* 2009;103(11):1738–1745
17. Kesser KC, Geller DE. New aerosol delivery devices for cystic fibrosis. *Respir Care.* 2009;54(6):754–767
18. Berg EB, Picard RJ. In vitro delivery of budesonide from 30 jet nebulizer/compressor combinations using infant and child breathing patterns. *Respir Care.* 2009;54(12):1671–1678
19. Mellon M, Leflein J, Walton-Bowen K, Cruz-Rivera M, Fitzpatrick S, Smith JA. Comparable efficacy of administration with face mask or mouthpiece of nebulized budesonide inhalation suspension for infants and young children with persistent asthma. *Am J Respir Crit Care Med.* 2000;162:593–598
20. Geller DE. Clinical side effects during aerosol therapy: cutaneous and ocular effects. *J Aerosol Med.* 2007;20(suppl 1):S100–S109
21. Harris KW, Smaldone GC. Facial and ocular deposition of nebulized budesonide: effects of face mask design. *Chest.* 2008;133:482–488
22. Berlinski A, Waldrep JC. Nebulized drug admixtures: effect on aerosol characteristics and nebulized albuterol output. *J Aerosol Med.* 2006;19(4):484–490
23. Hess DR. Aerosol delivery devices in the treatment of asthma. *Respir Care.* 2008;53(6):699–723
24. Berlinski A, Waldrep JC. Effect of aerosol delivery system and formulation on nebulized budesonide output. *J Aerosol Med.* 1997;10(4):307–318
25. Cipolla DC, Clark AR, Chan HK, Gonda I, Shire SJ. Assessment of aerosol delivery systems for recombinant human deoxyribonuclease. *SPT Pharma Sci.* 1994;4:50–62
26. Scarfone RJ, Capraro GA, Zorc JJ, Zhao H. Demonstrated use of metered-dose inhalers and peak flow meters by children and adolescents with acute asthma exacerbations. *Arch Pediatr Adolesc Med.* 2002;156(4):378–383
27. Self TH, Arnold LB, Czosnowski LM, Swanson JM, Swanson H. Inadequate skill of healthcare professionals in using asthma inhalation devices. *J Asthma.* 2007;44:593–598
28. Roller CM, Zhang G, Troedson RG, Leach CL, Le Souef PN, Devadason SG. Spacer inhalation technique and deposition of extrafine aerosol in asthmatic children. *Eur Respir J.* 2007;29:299–306
29. Janssens HM, De Jongste JC, Hop WC, Tiddens HA. Extra-fine particles improve lung delivery of inhaled steroids in infants: a study in an upper airway model. *Chest.* 2003;123(6):2083–2088
30. Asmus MJ, Liang J, Coowanitwong I, Hochhaus G. In vitro performance characteristics of valved holding chamber and spacer devices with a fluticasone metered-dose inhaler. *Pharmacotherapy.* 2004;24(2):159–166
31. Khan Y, Tang Y, Hochhaus G, et al. Lung bioavailability of hydrofluoroalkane fluticasone in young children when delivered by an antistatic chamber/mask. *J Pediatr.* 2006;149(6):793–797

32. Amirav I, Newhouse MT. Dead space variability of face masks for valved holding chambers. *Isr Med Assoc J.* 2008;10(3):224–226
33. Shah S, Berlinski A, Rubin B. Variability in holding chamber mask dead space volume and seal. *Respir Care.* 2006;51(2):140–144
34. Chavez A, McCracken A, Berlinski A. Effect of face mask dead volume, respiratory rate and tidal volume on inhaled albuterol delivery. *Pediatr Pulmonol.* 2010;45:224–229
35. Borgstrom L, Bondesson E, Moren F, Trofast E, Newman SP. Lung deposition of budesonide via Turbuhaler: a comparison with terbutaline sulphate in normal subjects. *Eur Respir J.* 1994;7:69–73
36. Geller DE, Konstan M, Smith J, Noonberg S, Conrad C. A novel tobramycin inhalation powder in cystic fibrosis subjects: pharmacokinetics and safety. *Pediatr Pulmonol.* 2007;42:307–313
37. Borgstrom L. On the use of dry powder inhalers in situations perceived as constrained. *J Aerosol Med.* 2001;14:281–287
38. Geller DE. Comparing clinical features of the nebulizer, metered-dose inhaler, and dry powder inhaler. *Respir Care.* 2005;50(10):1313–1322
39. Dolovich MB, Ahrens RC, Hess DR, et al. Device selection and outcomes of aerosol therapy: evidence-based guidelines. *Chest.* 2005;127:335–371
40. Ari A, Hess D, Myers TR, Rau JL. *A Guide to Aerosol Delivery Devices for Respiratory Therapists.* 2nd ed. Irving, TX: American Association for Respiratory Care; 2009. http://www.aarc.org/education/aerosol_devices

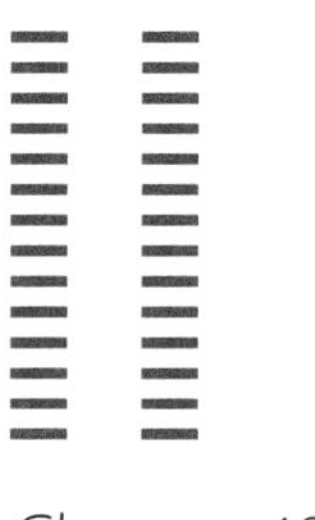

Chapter 48

Bronchodilators

H. William Kelly, PharmD
Leslie Hendeles, PharmD

Introduction

Bronchodilators are used in a number of obstructive respiratory diseases of childhood for the relief of airway smooth muscle contraction (ie, bronchospasm). Although bronchodilators are approved by the US Food and Drug Administration (FDA) only for the treatment of asthma and chronic obstructive pulmonary disease (COPD), they are commonly prescribed for children with cystic fibrosis (CF), bronchiolitis, and bronchopulmonary dysplasia (BPD).

Infants are born with fully functional airway smooth muscle whose mass relative to airway size is fully developed by 25 weeks' gestation.[1] Neonatal bronchial tissue responds similarly to both β_2-agonists and cholinergic stimulation as adult bronchial tissue because neonatal β-adrenergic receptors are in similar density in the airway smooth muscle as in adults.[2,3] Thus differences in response to the various bronchodilators between infants, children, and adults will most likely be due to issues involving mechanisms of airway obstruction, dosing, responsive capacity of the lung, and drug delivery than in pharmacologic responsiveness of the smooth muscle.

Bronchodilator Mechanisms

Three categories of bronchodilators are used clinically. These include β_2-agonists, methylxanthines, and anticholinergic drugs.

β_2-agonists

The β_2-agonists are the most effective bronchodilators used in clinical practice. The β_2-adrenergic receptor is a G-protein coupled transmembrane receptor and exists in a conformational equilibrium between the activated and inactivated states. Agonist binding shifts the equilibrium to the activated state, leading to increased intracellular production of cyclic adenosine monophosphate (cAMP) and a corresponding, proportional decrease in smooth muscle tone. Continued stimulation by an agonist will result in desensitization that occurs within 1 to 2 weeks of regular administration, levels off, and does not then worsen over time.[4] It is a receptor phenomenon and, therefore, cross-tolerance to all of the β_2-agonists occurs.

The small, highly polymorphic gene for the human β_2-adrenergic receptor is located on chromosome 5q31-q32.[5] The most common forms of polymorphisms are single nucleotide substitutions termed single nucleotide polymorphisms (SNPs). The most studied of these are amino acid substitutions at position 16, where the presence of glycine (Gly) versus arginine (Arg) results in functional changes in the receptor in vitro.[5] The Gly/Gly homozygous state is significantly more susceptible to agonist-induced down-regulation of the β_2-adrenergic receptor than the Arg/Arg homozygous state. The heterozygous state at loci 16 (Arg/Gly) shows an intermediate effect. At locus 27 the glutamate (Glu) homozygote (Glu/Glu) protects against β_2-agonist down-regulation when combined with Arg/Arg but not with Gly/Gly. There are racial differences in allele frequency and haplotype structure (paired SNPs) that represent linkage disequilibrium (SNP pairs that occur more frequently together in populations than by chance alone). For example Arg/Arg homozygotes make up 11% to 20% of the white population, 24% to 31% of blacks, and 28% to 35% of Asians, whereas Glu27 homozygotes are found in 19% of whites and only 4% of blacks.[6]

Synthetic β_2-agonists differ in their potency and selectivity for β_2-adrenergic receptors. Naturally occurring epinephrine equally stimulates α-adrenergic receptors (smooth muscle constriction), β_1-adrenergic receptors (cardiac tissue contraction and conductance), and β_2-adrenergic receptors, whereas early synthetic agents such as isoproterenol are equally potent for the β_1-adrenergic and β_2-adrenergic receptors.[4] The currently available short-acting β_2-agonists

(SABAs)—albuterol, pirbuterol, and terbutaline—are equally β_2 selective, whereas the long-acting inhaled β_2-agonists (LABAs)—formoterol and salmeterol—are slightly more β_2 selective.[4] The LABAs have a duration of action of at least 12 hours compared with the 2- to 4-hour duration of SABAs due to their increased lipophilicity, allowing them to be retained in the lung tissue for prolonged periods.[4] Retention in the lung also improves their therapeutic index (bronchodilation:systemic effect ratio) over the SABAs.[6] Although LABAs have a similar duration, the onset of effect for formoterol is similar to that of a SABA.

The synthetic β_2-agonists exist as racemic mixtures of equal amounts of 2 enantiomers (mirror image chemicals) with the exception of levalbuterol and arformoterol, which contain only the most active enantiomers, R-albuterol and R,R-formoterol, respectively. The inactive isomers do not significantly compete for the receptor.[6]

Anticholinergics

The anticholinergics competitively block acetylcholine at the muscarinic receptors in the airways.[7] Unlike the β_2-adrenergic receptors, the distribution of muscarinic receptors in the lung diminishes as the airways become more peripheral as does the cholinergic innervation.[7] Atropine is a tertiary ammonium compound that is readily absorbed across membranes, including the central nervous system, so is of limited clinical utility as an anticholinergic due to adverse effects.[7] The quaternary ammonium compounds, such as ipratropium bromide and tiotropium, are very poorly absorbed across membranes, causing minimal to no systemic effects when applied topically. Tiotropium has a longer duration of action (24 hours) due to its greater lipophilic nature than ipratropium bromide (duration 6 hours).

Methylxanthines

Theophylline is the only methylxanthine that has been used clinically as a bronchodilator. It has modest bronchodilator effects at optimal serum concentrations. In addition, it has modest anti-inflammatory, immunomodulatory, and bronchoprotective effects, which contribute to its efficacy as a controller medication for persistent asthma. It increases intracellular concentrations of cAMP in airway smooth muscle and inflammatory cells by nonspecific phosphodiesterase inhibition.

Theophylline is used infrequently for asthma because of its risk of adverse effects. It may be considered, however, when patients are unable to tolerate first-line therapies. The benefits and risks from theophylline are closely correlated with serum concentrations. The maximum potential benefit with the least risk of adverse effects is achieved at peak concentrations of 10 to 15 mcg/mL. Since concentrations can vary greatly among children receiving the same dose because of variable rates of metabolism, serum concentrations must be measured to adjust dosage.[8]

Pathophysiology and Clinical Features of Airway Obstruction

Airways obstruction of children with asthma is produced by bronchospasm, airway edema, desquamation of airway epithelium, and mucus plugging. In those with acute severe asthma exacerbations, the rapid response to bronchodilators for most patients suggests that much of the obstruction is caused by bronchospasm. The excessive bronchospasm triggered by external stimuli, such as irritants, exercise, chemicals, and allergens, is termed bronchial hyperresponsiveness (BHR) and is a cardinal feature of asthma.[9] While asthma is primarily an inflammatory disease, it is clear that bronchodilators play an important role in treating and preventing ongoing symptoms and reducing the risk of severe exacerbations from asthma.

Bronchospasm plays a less prominent role in the airway obstruction of airway diseases other than asthma, and thus bronchodilators are less likely to be effective. The airway obstruction of children with CF is caused by bacterial infection, inflammation, and increased mucus viscosity that impairs ciliary function.[10] Although some patients with CF also may have asthma, most have a component of reactive airways disease secondary to chronic inflammation. However, infection is the primary cause of acute exacerbations. Bronchopulmonary dysplasia has a component of neutrophilic inflammation as well but is primarily due to a maturational failure of airway development combined with damage from either the high oxygen or barotrauma secondary to mechanical ventilation.[11] Airway edema, increased airway resistance, and BHR are features of BPD.[11] The bronchospasm seems to be primarily induced via cholinergic mechanisms similar to that seen in COPD of adults, where the inflammatory process is also primarily due to neutrophils and not eosinophils.[12] Acute severe bronchiolitis, generally secondary to respiratory syncytial virus and other viruses, induces airway obstruction via inflammation, edema, and mucus plugging.[13] Bronchospasm may play a role in those infants with a family history of asthma or allergy.

Wheezing, hyperinflation, dyspnea, retractions, and cough are all signs of airway obstruction, regardless of mechanism, so the differential diagnosis is broad and includes a number of conditions that are not responsive to the pharmacologic agents generally called bronchodilators.[9] Nonetheless, given the difficulty of establishing a clear diagnosis, many clinicians will give a trial of bronchodilators to assess response.

Clinical Pharmacology and Disease Management

Asthma is the only disease of airway obstruction for which the bronchodilators, β_2–agonists, and theophylline are approved for children by the FDA.[9] The anticholinergics are approved only for COPD in adults. Furthermore, the use of any bronchodilators in children younger than 2 years and the use of metered-dose inhalers (MDIs) in children younger than 4 years is off-label. They have not been evaluated adequately for FDA approval despite extensive clinical experience and use. The dosage recommendations in Table 48-1 are based on clinical trials or clinical use that was not controlled.

Acute Bronchospasm

The β_2-agonists are the most effective bronchodilators for reversing bronchospasm in asthma.[9] As functional antagonists they can reverse bronchospasm secondary to any mediator or neurogenic mechanism.[12] Aerosolized SABAs are the drugs of choice for both the relief of symptoms associated with mild bronchospasm and for the initial treatment for severe asthma exacerbations together with systemic corticosteroids to treat the inflammatory component (see Table 48-2 for dosing).[9] In settings of increased inflammation in the outpatient management of bronchospasm, such as viral-induced exacerbations and nocturnal asthma, the usual dose of SABAs has proven insufficient to reverse the bronchospasm and the doses may be doubled.[9] The short-acting anticholinergic ipratropium bromide provides additive efficacy with SABAs in severe acute exacerbations, but only improves lung function another 10% to 20% (reversing the cholinergic component) over frequent administration of high-dose SABAs.[9] However, the addition of frequent dosing of inhaled ipratropium bromide to SABAs has resulted

Table 48-1. Bronchodilator Medication Dosing Chart for Routine Outpatient Use[a]

	Years of Age		
Medication	**<5**	**5–11**	**≥12**
Inhaled SABAs			
Albuterol MDI 90 mcg/puff, 60 or 200 puffs/canister	2 puffs with VHC/ mask every 4–6 hours as needed for symptoms and 5 minutes prior to exercise	2 puffs as needed every 4–6 hours for symptoms and 5 minutes prior to exercise	2 puffs as needed every 4–6 hours for symptoms and 5 minutes prior to exercise
Nebulizer solutions 0.63 mg/3 mL 1.25 mg/3 mL 2.5 mg/3 mL 5.0 mg/mL (0.5%)	0.63–2.5 mg in 3 cc saline every 4–6 hours as needed 0.1–0.2 mg/kg in 1–2 cc saline every 4–6 hours for bronchopulmonary dysplasia	1.25–5.0 mg in 3 cc saline every 4–8 hours as needed	1.25–5.0 mg in 3 cc saline every 4–8 hours as needed
Levalbuterol MDI[b] 45 mcg/puff, 200 puffs/ canister	2 puffs with VHC/ mask every 4–6 hours as needed for symptoms and 5 minutes prior to exercise	2 puffs as needed every 4–6 hours for symptoms and 5 minutes prior to exercise	2 puffs as needed every 4–6 hours for symptoms and 5 minutes prior to exercise
Nebulizer solutions[c] 0.31 mg/3 mL 0.63 mg/3 mL 1.25 mg/0.5 mL 1.25 mg/3 mL	0.31–1.25 mg in 3 cc saline every 4–8 hours as needed	0.31–0.63 mg every 8 hours as needed	0.63–1.25 mg every 8 hours as needed
Pirbuterol CFC-MDI Autohaler[d] 200 mcg/puff, 400 puffs/ canister	NA	2 puffs as needed every 4–6 hours for symptoms and 5 minutes prior to exercise	2 puffs as needed every 4–6 hours for symptoms and 5 minutes prior to exercise

Table 48-1. Bronchodilator Medication Dosing Chart for Routine Outpatient Use[a]

	Years of Age		
Medication	**<5**	**5–11**	**≥12**
Inhaled LABAs			
Salmeterol DPI 50 mcg/ inhalation, 60 inhalations/ device	NA	1 inhalation every 12 hours and 1 inhalation 30 minutes prior to exercise	1 inhalation every 12 hours and 1 inhalation 30 minutes prior to exercise
Formoterol DPI 12 mcg/single use capsule 12 or 60 capsules/ box	NA	1 capsule inhaled every 12 hours and 1 capsule 15 minutes prior to exercise	1 capsule inhaled every 12 hours and 1 capsule 15 minutes prior to exercise
Anticholinergics			
Ipratropium bromide MDI 17 mcg/puff, 200 puffs/canister	NA	NA	2–3 puffs every 6 hours
Nebulizer solution 0.25 mg/mL (0.025%)	**BPD:** 0.025–0.08 mg/kg in 1.5–2.0 mL saline every 6 hours	NA	0.25 mg every 6 hours
Methylxanthines			
Theophylline liquids, sustained-release capsules, and tablets	Starting dose 10 mg/kg/day usual maximum before serum concentration measurement: <1 year of age: (0.2) (age in weeks) + 5 = mg/kg/day. ≥1 year of age: 16 mg/kg/day	Starting dose 10 mg/kg/day up to maximum of 300 mg then usual maximum before serum concentration monitoring: 16 mg/kg/day, up to maximum of 600 mg/d	Starting dose 10 mg/kg/day up to 300 mg maximum then usual maximum: 16 mg/kg/d up to maximum of 600 mg/day before serum concentration monitoring

Abbreviations: BPD, bronchopulmonary dysplasia; CFC, chlorofluorocarbon; DPI, dry-powder inhaler; LABA, long-acting β_2-agonist; MDI, metered-dose inhaler; NA, not available (either not approved by US Food and Drug Administration and/or insufficient clinical trial data on safety and efficacy in the age group); SABA, short-acting β_2-agonist; VHC, valved holding chamber.

[a] All doses based on studies in asthma unless otherwise indicated. Usual doses for asthma are used for cystic fibrosis.

[b] Not approved for children <12 years.

[c] Not approved for children <6 years.

[d] Likely to be withdrawn from US market in near future because a non-CFC formulation has not been developed.

Table 48-2. Bronchodilator Medication Dosing Chart (Acute Management in Home, Emergency Department, and Hospital)[a,b]

	Years of Age		
Medication	**<5**	**5–11**	**≥12**
Inhaled SABA[s]			
Albuterol MDI 90 mcg/puff, 200 puffs/canister	**Home:** 2–4 puffs with VHC + face mask up to every 20 minutes for 3 doses then every 2–4 hours as needed **ED:** 4–8 puffs with VHC + face mask every 20 minutes for 3 doses then every 1–4 hours as needed **Hosp:** 4–8 puffs with VHC + face mask every 1–4 hours as needed	**Home:** 2–4 puffs up to every 20 minutes up to 3 doses then every 2–4 hours as needed **ED:** 4–8 puffs with VHC every 20 minutes for 3 doses then every 1–4 hours as needed **Hosp:** 4–8 puffs with VHC every 1–4 hours as needed	**Home:** 2–4 puffs up to every 20 minutes up to 3 doses then every 2–4 hours as needed **ED:** 4–8 puffs every 20 minutes for 3 doses then every 1–4 hours as needed **Hosp:** 4–8 puffs every 1–4 hours as needed
Nebulizer solutions 0.63 mg/3 mL 1.25 mg/3 mL 2.5 mg/3 mL 5.0 mg/mL (0.5% diluted with 2–3 mL of normal saline)	**Home:** 1.25–2.5 mg up to every 20 minutes by face mask for up to 3 doses then every 2–4 hours as needed **ED:** 0.15 mg/kg (minimum 2.5 mg) every 20 minutes for 3 doses then 0.15–0.3 mg/kg up to 10 mg every 1–4 hours as needed or 0.5 mg/kg/hour by continuous nebulization **Hosp:** 0.15–0.3 mg/kg up to 10 mg every 1–4 hours as needed or 0.5 mg/kg/hour by continuous nebulization **Bronchiolitis:** 0.15 mg/kg up to 5 mg every 30 minutes for 3 doses then every 2 hours if patient responds	**Home:** 1.25–2.5 mg up to every 20 minutes for up to 3 doses then every 2–4 hours as needed **ED:** 0.15 mg/kg (minimum 2.5 mg) every 20 minutes for 3 doses then 0.15–0.3 mg/kg up to 10 mg every 1–4 hours as needed or 0.5 mg/kg/hour by continuous nebulization **Hosp:** 0.15–0.3 mg/kg up to 10 mg every 1–4 hours as needed or 0.5 mg/kg/hour by continuous nebulization	**Home:** 2.5–5 mg up to every 20 minutes for up to 3 doses then every 2–4 hours as needed **ED:** 2.5–5.0 mg every 20 minutes for 3 doses then 2.5–10 mg every 1–4 hours as needed or 10–15 mg/hour by continuous nebulization **Hosp:** 2.5–10 mg every 1–4 hours as needed or 10–15 mg/hour by continuous nebulization

Table 48-2. Bronchodilator Medication Dosing Chart (Acute Management in Home, Emergency Department, and Hospital)[a,b]

	Years of Age		
Medication	**<5**	**5–11**	**≥12**
Levalbuterol MDI[c] 45 mcg/puff, 200 puffs/canister	See albuterol MDI doses above.	See albuterol MDI doses above.	See albuterol MDI doses above.
Nebulizer solutions 0.31 mg/3 mL 0.63 mg/3 mL 1.25 mg/0.5 mL 1.25 mg/3 mL	**Home:** 0.63–1.25 mg up to every 20 minutes by face mask for up to 3 doses then every 2–4 hours as needed **ED:** 0.075 mg/kg (minimum 1.25 mg) every 20 minutes for 3 doses then 0.075–0.15 mg/kg up to 5 mg every 1–4 hours as needed or 0.25 mg/kg/hour by continuous nebulization **Hosp:** 0.075–0.15 mg/kg up to 5 mg every 1–4 hours as needed or 0.25 mg/kg/hour by continuous nebulization	**Home:** 0.63–1.25 mg up to every 20 minutes for up to 3 doses then every 2–4 hours as needed **ED:** 0.075 mg/kg (minimum 1.25 mg) every 20 minutes for 3 doses then 0.075–0.15 mg/kg up to 5 mg every 1–4 hours as needed or 0.25 mg/kg/hour by continuous nebulization **Hosp:** 0.075–0.15 mg/kg up to 5 mg every 1–4 hours as needed or 0.25 mg/kg/hour by continuous nebulization	**Home:** 1.25–2.5 mg up to every 20 minutes for up to 3 doses then every 2–4 hours as needed **ED:** 1.25–2.5 mg every 20 minutes for 3 doses then 1.25–5 mg every 1–4 hours as needed or 5–7.5 mg/hour by continuous nebulization **Hosp:** 1.25–5 mg every 1–4 hours as needed or 5–7.5 mg/hour by continuous nebulization
Injectable epinephrine 1:1,000 (1 mg/ mL)	**ED:** 0.01 mg/kg up to 0.3–0.5 mg sq every 20 minutes for 3 doses sq	**ED:** 0.01 mg/kg up to 0.3–0.5 mg sq every 20 minutes for 3 doses sq	**ED:** 0.3–0.5 mg sq every 20 minutes for 3 doses
Injectable terbutaline (1 mg/mL)	**ED:** 0.01 mg/kg up to 0.3–0.5 mg sq every 20 minutes for 3 doses sq then every 2–6 hours as needed	**ED:** 0.01 mg/kg up to 0.3–0.5 mg sq every 20 minutes for 3 doses sq then every 2–6 hours as needed	**ED:** 0.25 mg sq every 20 minutes for 3 doses
Intravenous terbutaline		**ED, PICU** 0.01 mg/kg IV over 1–2 minutes Continuous infusion starting at 0.001 mg/kg/min titrated to effect and heart rate	**ED, PICU** 0.01 mg/kg IV over 1–2 minutes Continuous infusion starting at 0.001 mg/kg/min titrated to effect and heart rate

Table 48-2. Bronchodilator Medication Dosing Chart (Acute Management in Home, Emergency Department, and Hospital)[a,b] (continued)

	Years of Age		
Medication	**<5**	**5–11**	**≥12**
Anticholinergics			
Ipratropium bromide MDI 17 mcg/puff, 200 puffs/canister	**ED:** 4 puffs with VHC + face mask every 20 minutes times 3 doses then every 1 hour up to 3 hours	**ED:** 4–8 puffs with VHC every 20 minutes times 3 doses then every 1 hour up to 3 hours	**ED:** 8 puffs every 20 minutes as needed up to 3 hours
Nebulizer solution 0.25 mg/mL (0.025%)	**ED:** 0.25-0.5 mg every 20 minutes then as needed (May mix with albuterol nebulizer solution.)	**ED:** 0.25–0.5 mg every 20 minutes then as needed (May mix with albuterol nebulizer solution.)	**ED:** 0.5 mg every 20 minutes then as needed (May mix with albuterol nebulizer solution.)
Ipratropium/albuterol nebulizer solution 0.5mg/2.5mg per 3 mL	**ED:** 1.5 mL every 20 minutes for 3 doses then as needed	**ED:** 1.5–3 mL every 20 minutes for 3 doses then as needed	**ED:** 3 mL every 20 minutes for 3 doses then as needed

Table 48-2. Bronchodilator Medication Dosing Chart (Acute Management in Home, Emergency Department, and Hospital)[a,b] (continued)

	Years of Age		
Medication	**<5**	**5–11**	**≥12**
Methylxanthines			
Aminophylline	**PICU:** Loading dose 6 mg/kg IV over 20 minutes Initial continuous infusion: Neonate: 1.5 mg/kg every 12 hours 6 weeks–6 months: mg/kg/hour = (0.01) (age in weeks) + 0.26 6 months–1 year: 0.6 mg/kg/hour 1–4 years: 1 mg/kg/hour Monitor serum concentrations to adjust infusion rate	**PICU:** Loading dose 6 mg/kg IV over 20 minutes Initial continuous infusion: 4–11 years: 1.0 mg/kg/hour Monitor serum concentrations to adjust infusion rate	**PICU:** Loading dose 6 mg/kg IV over 20 minutes Initial continuous infusion: 12–16 years: 0.7 mg/kg/hour Monitor serum concentrations to adjust infusion rate

Abbreviations: ED, emergency department; Hosp, hospitalized patient; IV, intravenously; MDI, metered-dose inhaler; PICU, pediatric intensive care unit; SABA, short-acting β_2-agonist; sq, subcutaneously; pediatric intensive care unit; VHC, valved-holding chamber.

[a] Table derived from reference 10 the NHLBI, NAEPP EPR-3.

[b] All doses for asthma unless otherwise indicated.

[c] At equimolar doses levalbuterol is neither more effective nor does it have fewer systemic effects than racemic albuterol.

in a significant reduction in hospitalizations of children presenting to the emergency department (ED) with severe obstruction.[13] It has not been shown to be beneficial in any other clinical scenario in childhood, either at home or in the hospital. Theophylline and intravenous aminophylline have not demonstrated additive benefit to optimal aerosolized β_2-agonists in the ED.[14]

Intravenous magnesium sulfate has been recommended for adults and children with severe asthma that is unresponsive to the usual doses of SABAs in the ED.[15] Magnesium sulfate is a moderately potent smooth muscle relaxant and some studies, but not all, have demonstrated improved bronchodilation and reduced hospitalizations in children when added to usual SABA therapy in the ED.[9,15] There are no studies comparing magnesium sulfate with other treatment strategies in patients with severe, unresponsive asthma, including the addition of frequent doses of ipratropium bromide or providing continuous nebulization of SABA, both of which improve lung function and reduce the risk of hospitalization.[9] Thus the National Heart, Lung, and Blood Institute's National Asthma Education and Prevention Program's Expert Panel Report 3 (EPR-3) Guidelines for the Diagnosis and Management of Asthma states that magnesium sulfate can be considered but falls short of recommending its use.[9]

During hospitalization the doses of SABAs are based on the severity of the asthma and the patient's response to therapy.[9] As the patients improve, lowering the dose and spreading out the dosing interval may proceed quickly. Once the child is hospitalized, the addition of ipratropium bromide to SABAs does not improve outcomes and is not recommended.[9] For the patient who does not respond and requires intensive care unit (ICU) admission, continuous nebulization of albuterol has been shown to reduce ICU stay.[16] Two studies have shown marginal benefit (improved symptom score and lung function) from addition of theophylline at the cost of more adverse effects (vomiting and tachycardia) in patients admitted to the ICU, but there was no effect on ICU admission or length of stay.[9]

Administration of aerosolized SABAs is more effective and produces fewer adverse effects than oral or parenteral administration.[9] Aerosolized SABAs can be administered by either jet nebulization or MDI with equivalent results. A nebulizer or valved holding chamber fitted with appropriately sized face masks may be used for delivery to infants and children younger than 5 years (see Chapter 47).[9] In addition to requiring higher doses in severe asthma exacerbations, the duration of significant bronchodilation is decreased so more frequent administration (every 20 minutes initially) and even continuous nebulization can improve outcomes over administration on an hourly basis in the patients with more severe asthma.[16]

Administering high doses of SABAs can lead to β_2-agonist mediated systemic side effects, including tachycardia, hypokalemia, hyperglycemia, and prolonged QTc interval, so these should be monitored.[9] Although QTc interval is prolonged by all β_2–agonists, reports of significant cardiac arrhythmias, such as torsades de pointes, are exceedingly rare.[6] Metabolic acidosis is a common finding in those who are quite ill with asthma and who are on β_2-agonist therapy. Due to vascular dilatation, SABAs can also slightly worsen the ventilation/perfusion mismatching seen in severe exacerbations, so low-flow oxygen should always be administered during severe exacerbations and transcutaneous partial pressure of oxygen should be monitored.[9] Tachycardia from hypoxemia and stimulation of irritant receptors is common in severe asthma exacerbations and is not a contraindication for high doses of SABAs. Indeed the heart rate often decreases in patients receiving high-dose aerosolized SABAs as the airway obstruction improves.[9] There is no advantage among any of the β_2-selective SABAs (albuterol, levalbuterol, pirbuterol, or terbutaline) when given in equipotent doses.[6,9] They all produce a similar degree of bronchodilation and amount of β_2-adrenergic–mediated side effects. Isoproterenol and epinephrine have the potential to produce significantly greater cardiac toxicity, and the outdated practice of using intravenous isoproterenol in children with severe asthma resulted in myocardial ischemia and is no longer recommended.[9]

Chronic Persistent Asthma

The SABAs are indicated for as-needed treatment for symptoms associated with bronchospasm (cough, wheezing, and dyspnea) in the outpatient management of asthma.[9] They constitute the primary treatment for intermittent asthma and the primary prevention of exercise-induced bronchospasm (EIB).[9,17] They are not indicated for regular maintenance administration. Patients who require as-needed SABA therapy for more than 2 days per week, not counting prevention of EIB, should generally not be considered well controlled and should either be placed on regular anti-inflammatory controller therapy or have their regular controller therapy increased if their compliance is adequate. The use of 2 or more canisters per month of SABAs has been associated with a significant increase in the risk of severe asthma exacerbations, including death, and the use of 4 or more canisters per year indicates poor asthma control and an increased risk of ED use.[9]

The inhaled β_2-agonists are the most effective preventive therapy for EIB.[10] The SABAs have a duration of protection of 2 to 4 hours, whereas the LABAs protect for up to 12 hours after a single dose. However, the duration of protection against EIB from LABAs when taken regularly decreases to 4 to 6 hours due to tolerance.[6,12] Despite the tolerance from regular administration of a β_2-agonist, most patients are fully protected against EIB in the 1 to 2 hours following SABA administration.[6] Theophylline requires serum concentrations greater than 10 mcg/mL to block EIB, and ipratropium is ineffective. Leukotriene receptor antagonists are only partially effective for prevention of EIB, and they are ineffective in up to 40% to 50% of children.[18]

Because of their lack of clinically significant anti-inflammatory effects, LABAs are currently only indicated as adjunct therapy in patients incompletely controlled on low to medium doses of inhaled corticosteroids.[9] They improve baseline lung function and decrease symptoms and as-needed SABA use when added to inhaled corticosteroid therapy. Early studies in which monotherapy with a LABA was added to the usual therapy in children showed an increased risk of serious asthma exacerbations (hospitalization for asthma).[9,19] This same finding did not occur in studies of combination LABA and inhaled corticosteroids.[20,21] Currently LABAs are not approved for use in children younger than 4 years, and there are no clinical trials evaluating them in that age group. Thus the EPR-3 recommends combination therapy in only those toddlers and infants not responding to medium-dose inhaled corticosteroids.[9]

A mechanism for the increase in serious asthma exacerbations from monotherapy with LABAs has not been elucidated. Although tolerance in patients receiving LABAs is measurable, it primarily affects duration of bronchoprotection against induced bronchospasm and does not affect response to the usual doses of SABAs administered in the ED.[6] Clinical trials examining tolerance to exogenous β_2-agonists have not consistently demonstrated a genotypic response. The reason for the difference between regular administration of SABAs and LABAs is unclear, but early trials consistently reported increased BHR following regular use of SABAs but not LABAs.[6]

The LABA formoterol is less lipophilic than salmeterol, which allows for a more rapid onset of bronchodilation similar to the SABAs albuterol and terbutaline.[4,12] As a result of this property it has been investigated for as-needed use similar to SABAs.[9] Preliminary studies have reported improved outcomes compared with SABAs as measured by fewer exacerbations requiring oral corticosteroids or ED visits.[6] In addition, the combination inhaler containing both budesonide and formoterol has received a maintenance plus relief indication in numerous countries outside the United States, including the United Kingdom, Australia, and Canada, because clinical trials in children and adults have demonstrated fewer exacerbations with lower overall corticosteroid dosing compared with standard dosing of combination or higher-dose inhaled corticosteroids plus SABAs as reliever.[21] The FDA-approved labeling for combination budesonide/formoterol states the drug is only for maintenance therapy and the recommended daily doses are not to be exceeded and not to be used for acute exacerbations, and all patients must be prescribed a SABA for treatment of exacerbations. Thus the use of budesonide/formoterol for maintenance and relief is still considered experimental in the United States.[9]

Sustained-release theophylline is still considered an alternative, not preferred, maintenance and adjunctive therapy to the inhaled corticosteroids in children 5 to 11 years of age but not in children 0 to 4 years of age.[9] It is no longer recommended in 0- to 4-year-olds because of a lack of clinical trial data on efficacy and the potential for serious adverse effects in young children and infants.[22] When using theophylline in 5- to 11-year-old children, serum drug concentration monitoring is required to prevent serious toxicity.

The anticholinergics do not have an FDA-approved indication in children with asthma and have not been shown to improve outcomes in clinical trials.[23] Some have advocated that ipratropium bromide could be used as a reliever in patients unable to tolerate SABAs. It has been used successfully as a reliever in clinical trials involving patients with mild asthma but has a slower onset of action and is not as effective as SABAs.[9]

Bronchiolitis

The use of bronchodilators in the treatment of acute viral bronchiolitis has been controversial for years. Systematic reviews of SABA use indicate a modest short-term improvement in clinical scores but no improvement in hospitalization rates or duration of hospitalization.[24] However, some of the studies may have included infants with recurrent wheezing and family histories of asthma. Some experts have advocated aerosolized epinephrine for its α-agonist effect producing pulmonary vascular constriction, thus decreasing airway edema.[25] Studies show no benefit of epinephrine in hospitalized infants but show a slightly greater benefit compared with albuterol in outpatient treatment.[25] However, the studies comparing epinephrine either as a single isomer or racemic mixture often used doses of epinephrine that were higher than that of albuterol in terms of β_2-adrenergic potency, so it is unclear whether the slight difference was due to an α-agonist effect or just greater β_2-agonist dose. A large study giving equivalent β_2-agonist doses found no difference between epinephrine and albuterol.[26] Epinephrine may be more effective when given in combination with oral dexamethasone.[27] The current recommendation is that if SABAs are to be used in acute bronchiolitis, response should be carefully assessed and the drugs discontinued if a beneficial clinical response is not observed.

Bronchopulmonary Dysplasia

Aerosolized bronchodilators, both SABAs and ipratropium bromide, reduce airway resistance and improve dynamic compliance in infants with BPD.[11] Use of bronchodilators does not prevent the development or change the natural history of BPD and are therefore indicated for symptomatic control of increased airway resistance. Continuous treatment without evidence of symptomatic improvement is not indicated. Albuterol and ipratropium last 4 to 6 hours and in some patients produce an additive effect when used together.[11]

Cystic Fibrosis

Some patients with CF have a component of BHR and will respond to bronchodilators. Recurrent wheezing or dyspnea that responds to a SABA is an indication for the use of bronchodilators. In patients older than 5 years an objective bronchodilator response of greater then 12% in forced expiratory volume in 1 second or positive BHR should be documented.[10] Albuterol is often given before hypertonic sodium chloride, chest physiotherapy, and inhaled tobramycin[28] to prevent reflex bronchospasm, but has not been assessed in controlled trials. The LABAs also improve lung function in the short term but have produced inconsistent long-term effects. Anticholinergics have not demonstrated beneficial responses in patients with CF.[10]

Key Points

- The SABAs are the most effective bronchodilators for all clinical situations involving bronchoconstriction because they are functional antagonists.
- Although desensitization occurs with regular β_2-agonist use, it is not progressive and is easily overcome with 1 or 2 extra doses of a SABA.
- The LABAs should only be used as adjunctive therapy to inhaled corticosteroids.
- Anticholinergics are second-line agents that should only be used in specific indications (acute severe asthma in the ED, and BPD).
- Numerous pulmonary diseases other than asthma (ie, CF, BPD, bronchiolitis) are associated with wheezing that may or may not be secondary to bronchospasm. Bronchodilators should only be used if there is a documented positive response.

References

1. Sward-Comunelli SL, Mabry SM, Truog WE, Thibeault DW. Airway muscle in preterm infants: changes during development. *J Pediatr.* 1997;130(4):570–576
2. Sparrow MP, Weichselbaum M, McCray PB. Development of the innervation and airway smooth muscle in human fetal lung. *Am J Respir Cell Mol Biol.* 1999;20(4):550–560
3. McCray PB Jr. Spontaneous contractility of human fetal airway smooth muscle. *Am J Respir Cell Mol Biol.* 1993;8(5):573–580
4. Anderson GP. Interactions between corticosteroids and β-adrenergic agonists in asthma disease induction, progression, and exacerbation. *Am J Respir Crit Care Med.* 2000;61(3 pt 2):S188–S196
5. Small KM, McGraw DW, Liggett SB. Pharmacology and physiology of adrenergic receptor polymorphisms. *Annu Rev Pharmacol Toxicol.* 2003;43:381–411

6. Kelly HW. What is new with the β2 agonists: issues in the management of asthma. *Ann Pharmacother.* 2005;39(5):931–938
7. Barnes PJ. Distribution of receptor targets in the lung. *Proc Am Thorac Soc.* 2004;1:345–351
8. Hendeles L, Weinberger M. Theophylline use in asthma. In: Rose BD, ed. *UpToDate* [CD-Rom]. Waltham, MA: UpToDate Inc; 2008
9. National Heart, Lung, and Blood Institute, National Asthma Education and Prevention Program. *Full Report of the Expert Panel: Guidelines for the Diagnosis and Management of Asthma (EPR-3).* Washington, DC: US Department of Health and Human Services, National Institutes of Health; 2007. http://www.nhlbi.nih.gov/guidelines/asthma
10. Halfhide C, Evans HJ, Couriel J. Inhaled bronchodilators for cystic fibrosis. *Cochrane Database Syst Rev.* 2005;(4):CD003428
11. Pantalitschka T, Poets CF. Inhaled drugs for the prevention and treatment of bronchopulmonary dysplasia. *Pediatr Pulmonol.* 2006;41(8):703–708
12. Anderson GP. Current issues with β2-adrenergic agonists: pharmacology and molecular and cellular mechanisms. *Clin Rev Allergy Immunol.* 2006;31(2–3):119–130
13. Plotnick L, Ducharme F. Combined inhaled anticholinergics and beta2-agonists for initial treatment of acute asthma in children. *Cochrane Database Syst Rev.* 2000;(3):CD000060
14. Mitra AAD, Bassler D, Watts K, Lasserson TJ, Ducharme F. Intravenous aminophylline for acute severe asthma in children over two years receiving inhaled bronchodilators. *Cochrane Database Syst Rev.* 2005;(2):CD001276
15. Rowe BH, Bretzlaff JA, Bourdon C, Bota GW, Camargo CA Jr. Magnesium sulfate for treating exacerbations of acute asthma in the emergency department. *Cochrane Database Syst Rev.* 2000;(2):CD001490
16. Camargo CA, Spooner C, Rowe BH. Continuous versus intermittent beta-agonists for acute asthma. *Cochrane Database Syst Rev.* 2003;(4):CD001115
17. Spooner C, Spooner GR, Rowe BH. Mast-cell stabilising agents to prevent exercise-induced bronchoconstriction. *Cochrane Database Syst Rev.* 2003;(4):CD002307
18. Raissy HH, Kelly F, Harkins M, Kelly HW. Pretreatment with albuterol vs. montelukast in exercise induced bronchospasm in children. *Pharmacotherapy.* 2008;28(3):287–294
19. Cates CJ, Cates MJ, Lasserson TJ. Regular treatment with formoterol for chronic asthma: serious adverse events. *Cochrane Database Syst Rev.* 2008;(4):CD006923
20. Sorkness CA, Lemanske RF, Mauger DT, et al. Long-term comparison of 3 controller regimens for mild-moderate persistent childhood asthma: the Pediatric Asthma Controller Trial. *J Allergy Clin Immunol.* 2007;119(1):64–72

21. Bisgaard H, Le Roux P, Bjamer D, Dymek A, Vermeulen JH, Hultquist C. Budesonide/formoterol maintenance plus reliever therapy: a new strategy in pediatric asthma. *Chest.* 2006;130(6):1733–1743
22. Seddon P, Bara A, Ducharme FM, Lasserson TJ. Oral xanthines as maintenance treatment for asthma in children. *Cochrane Database Syst Rev.* 2006;(1):CD002885
23. McDonald N, Bara A, McKean MC. Anticholinergic therapy for chronic asthma in children over two years of age. *Cochrane Database Syst Rev.* 2003;(1):CD003535
24. Gadomski AM, Bhasale AL. Bronchodilators for bronchiolitis. *Cochrane Database Syst Rev.* 2006;(3):CD001266
25. Hartling L, Wiebe N, Russell KF, Patel H, Klassen TP. Epinephrine for bronchiolitis. *Cochrane Database Syst Rev.* 2004;(1):CD003123
26. Ralston S, Hartenberger C, Anaya T, Qualls C, Kelly HW. Randomized, placebo-controlled trial of albuterol and epinephrine at equipotent beta-2 agonist doses in acute bronchiolitis. *Pediatr Pulmonol.* 2005;40(4):292–299
27. Plint AC, Johnson DW, Patel H, et al. Epinephrine and dexamethasone in children with bronchiolitis. *N Engl J Med.* 2009;360(20):2079–2089
28. Nikolaizik WH, Trociewicz K, Ratjen F. Bronchial reactions to the inhalation of high-dose tobramycin in cystic fibrosis. *Eur Respir J.* 2002;20:122–126

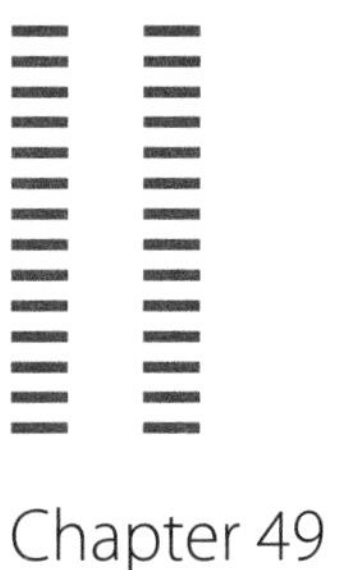

Chapter 49

Antibiotics for Pulmonary Conditions

Michael J. Light, MD
John S. Bradley, MD

Introduction

Here is presented antibiotics that may be prescribed for pulmonary disorders of children, with the major focus on the ambulatory patient. Parenteral antibiotics are included because increasingly children with illnesses or diseases requiring these antibiotics are managed outside the hospital environment.

There are many considerations for the choice of antibiotic, as there are with any prescription. The product label (package insert) provides the indications that have been approved by the US Food and Drug Administration (FDA). The FDA-approved indication means that adequate and controlled clinical trials have been conducted and reviewed by the FDA. Accepted medical practice often includes drug use that is not reflected in approved drug labeling. Lack of approval for an indication does not necessarily mean lack of effectiveness, but indicates that appropriate studies have not been performed or that data have not been submitted to the FDA for approval for that indication. The decision to prescribe a drug is deemed in the best interest of the patient, taking into account the reasonable medical evidence. The physician who prescribes the drug must weigh the benefits and risks of using the drug, regardless of whether the drug has received approval from the FDA for the specific indication and age of the patient. Consultation with infectious disease and pulmonology specialists is often indicated.

Choice of Antibiotic and Dosage

There are multiple factors that guide the choice of antibiotic and are included in Box 49-1. Dosages that are listed in this chapter are for the "usual" patient and should be considered as guidance for care and individualized for the patient that is being treated (Table 49-1). The dosage recommendations are for patients who are adequately hydrated and have normal renal and hepatic function. The duration of treatment should be individualized. The recommendations are based on the literature, common practice, and experience.

Box 49-1. Considerations for the Choice of Antibiotic

- Condition to be treated
- Specific illness suspected or proven
- Proven efficacy in clinical trials
- Degree of potency for a particular pathogen
- Age of the child
- Immune status of the child
- Weight of the child
- Tolerance
- Degree of hydration
- Renal function
- Liver function
- Cost

Table 49-1. Antibiotic Choices

UPPER AIRWAY INFECTIONS		
Clinical Diagnosis	**Therapy**	**Comments**
Epiglottitis (aryepiglottitis, supraglottitis; *H influenzae* type b in an unimmunized child); rarely pneumococcus, *S aureus*	Ceftriaxone 50 mg/kg/day IV, IM q24h OR cefotaxime 150 mg/kg/day IV div q8h x 7–10 d	Emergency: provide airway For *S aureus* (causes only 5% of epiglottitis), consider adding clindamycin 40 mg/kg/day IV div q8h
Tracheitis, bacterial (*S aureus,* including CA-MRSA; group A streptococcus; pneumococcus; *H influenzae* type b)	Vancomycin 40–60 mg/kg/day IV div q8h or clindamycin 40 mg/kg/ day IV div q8h AND ceftriaxone 50 mg/kg/day q24h or cefotaxime 150 mg/kg/day div q8h	For susceptible *S aureus,* oxacillin or cefazolin May represent bacterial superinfection of viral laryngotracheobronchitis
LOWER RESPIRATORY TRACT INFECTIONS		
Clinical Diagnosis	**Therapy**	**Comments**
Abscess, lung		
– Primary (severe, necrotizing community-acquired pneumonia caused by pneumococcus, *S aureus,* including CA-MRSA, group A streptococcus)	Empiric therapy with ceftriaxone 50–75 mg/kg/day q24h or cefotaxime 150 mg/kg/day div q8h For severe disease (presumed *S aureus),* ADD clindamycin 40 mg/kg/day div q8h; x 14–21 d or longer	Bronchoscopy necessary if abscess fails to drain; surgical excision rarely necessary for pneumococcus, but more important for CA-MRSA and MSSA For susceptible staph: oxacillin or cefazolin
– Primary, putrid (ie, foul-smelling; polymicrobial infection with oral aerobes and anaerobes)	Clindamycin 40 mg/kg/day IV div q8h OR meropenem 60 mg/kg/day IV div q8h x 10 d or longer	Alternatives: imipenem IV, or pip/tazo IV, or ticar/clav IV

Table 49-1. Antibiotic Choices (continued)

LOWER RESPIRATORY TRACT INFECTIONS		
Clinical Diagnosis	**Therapy**	**Comments**
Allergic bronchopulmonary Aspergillosis (ABPA)	See Chapter 9.	
Aspiration pneumonia (polymicrobial infection with oral aerobes and anaerobes)	Clindamycin 40 mg/kg/day IV div q8h OR meropenem 60 mg/kg/day IV div q8h if additional gram-negative aerobic coverage is needed; x 10 d or longer	Alternatives: imipenem IV or pip/tazo IV or ticar/clav IV
Atypical pneumonia (see *Mycoplasma*, Legionnaire's disease)		
Bronchitis, acute	No antibiotic needed for most cases, as disease is usually viral	If bacterial infection suspected, treat with antibiotics
Cystic fibrosis, acute exacerbation (*P aeruginosa* primarily; and other gram negatives)	Ceftazidime 150–200 mg/kg/day IV divided q6–8h Older children (maximum dose) 2 grams q8h or 3 g q12h OR piperacillin 300–400 mg/kg/day IV div q4h AND tobramycin 8–10 mg/kg/day IV once a day, or divided q8h for younger children Alternatives: meropenem, imipenem, or cefepime AND aminoglycosides; OR ciprofloxacin 30 mg/kg/day PO, IV bid (maximum 500 mg or 750 mg per dose)	Larger than normal dosages of antibiotics required in most patients with CF; monitor trough serum concentrations of aminoglycosides after 3 doses and weekly Cultures with susceptibility testing and synergy testing may help select antibiotics If dominant organism gram-negative may also need gram-positive coverage (see below) Combination therapy may provide synergistic killing and delay the emergence of resistance Inhaled tobramycin 300 mg twice daily, cycling 28 days on therapy, 28 days off therapy, is effective adjunctive therapy between exacerbation

Table 49-1. Antibiotic Choices (continued)

LOWER RESPIRATORY TRACT INFECTIONS		
Clinical Diagnosis	**Therapy**	**Comments**
Cystic fibrosis, acute exacerbation due to MSSA or MRSA	MSSA Oxacillin 100–200 mg/kg/day IM/IV div q4–6h; Maximum (adult) dose Mild to moderate infections 250–500 mg IV q4–6h Severe infection 1 g IV q4–6h MRSA Vancomycin 40–60 mg/kg/day IV divided into 2 or 3 doses Maximum (adult) dose daily 2 g divided either as 500 mg every 6 hours or 1 g every 12 hours If intolerant to vancomycin Linezolid 30 mg/kg/day IV, PO div q8h (follow platelets and WBC weekly) Older children (maximum dose) 600 mg q12h	Treatment of exacerbation of CF patients who only have gram-positive organisms If dominant organism gram-negative may also need gram-positive coverage IV vancomycin should be administered at no more than 10 mg/min or over a period of at least 60 minutes Check vancomycin peak and trough levels

Table 49-1. Antibiotic Choices (continued)

LOWER RESPIRATORY TRACT INFECTIONS		
Clinical Diagnosis	**Therapy**	**Comments**
Pertussis	Azithromycin (10 mg/kg/day x 5 d) or clarithromycin (15 mg/kg/day div bid x 7 d) or erythromycin (estolate preferable) 40 mg/kg/day PO div qid; x 14 d Alternative: TMP/SMX (8 mg/kg/day TMP) div bid x 14 d	Azithromycin and clarithromycin are better tolerated than erythromycin. Azithromycin is preferred in young infants to reduce pyloric stenosis risk. The azithromycin dosage that is recommended for infants <1 month of age, but this dosage is well tolerated and safe for older children (12 mg/kg/ day X 5 d is actually FDA approved for other indications). Alternatively, 10 mg/kg on day 1, followed by 5 mg/kg on days 2–5 should also be effective. Isolate for the first 5 days of therapy. Provide prophylaxis to family members.

Table 49-1. Antibiotic Choices (continued)

LOWER RESPIRATORY TRACT INFECTIONS		
Clinical Diagnosis	**Therapy**	**Comments**
Pneumonia: Community-acquired, bronchopneumonia		
– Mild to moderate illness (overwhelmingly viral, especially in preschool children)	No antibiotic therapy unless epidemiological, clinical, or laboratory reasons to suspect bacteria or *Mycoplasma*	Broad-spectrum antibiotics may increase risk of subsequent infection with antibiotic-resistant pathogens
– Moderate to severe illness (pneumococcus; group A streptococcus; *S aureus,* including CA-MRSA; or *Mycoplasma pneumoniae)*	Empiric therapy: ceftriaxone 50–75 mg/kg/day q24h or cefotaxime 150 mg/kg/day div q8h For suspected CA-MRSA, use vancomycin 40–60 mg/kg/day Alternative for MSSA or CA-MRSA is clindamycin, if organisms susceptible For suspect *Mycoplasma*/atypical pneumonia agents, particularly in school-aged children, ADD azithromycin 10 mg/kg IV, PO x 1, then decrease dose to 5 mg/kg once daily for days 2–5 of treatment	Tracheal aspirate or bronchoalveolar lavage for Gram stain/culture when indicated Daptomycin should NOT be used for treatment of pneumonia caused by any pathogen. Check vancomycin serum concentrations and renal function, particularly at the higher dosage for CA-MRSA. Alternatives to azithromycin for atypical pneumonia include erythromycin IV, PO, or clarithromycin PO, or doxycycline IV, PO for children >7 years of age, or levofloxacin for postpubertal older children.

Table 49-1. Antibiotic Choices (continued)

LOWER RESPIRATORY TRACT INFECTIONS		
Clinical Diagnosis	**Therapy**	**Comments**
Pneumonia: Community-acquired, lobar consolidation		
Pneumococcus (even if immunized), *S aureus,* including CA-MRSA (can cause necrotizing pneumonia) and group A streptococcus. Consider *H influenzae* type b in the unimmunized child. *M pneumoniae* may cause lobar pneumonia.	Empiric therapy: ceftriaxone 50–75 mg/kg/day q24h or cefotaxime 150 mg/kg/day div q8h; for more severe disease ADD clindamycin 40 mg/kg/day div q8h or vancomycin 40–60 mg/kg/day div q8h for *S aureus* For suspect *Mycoplasma/*atypical pneumonia agents, particularly in school-aged children, ADD azithromycin 10 mg/kg IV, PO x 1, then decrease dose to 5 mg/kg once daily for days 2–5 of treatment Empiric oral outpatient therapy for less severe illness: high dosage amoxicillin 80–100 mg/kg/day PO div q8h (NOT q12h); for *Mycoplasma,* ADD a macrolide as above	If clindamycin is used, verify that organisms are susceptible. Daptomycin should NOT be used for treatment of pneumonia caused by any pathogen. Change to PO after improvement (decreased fever, no oxygen needed); treat until clinically asymptomatic and chest radiography significantly improved (7–21 days) No reported failures of ceftriaxone/cefotaxime for pen-R pneumococcus: no need to add empiric vancomycin for this reason Oral therapy for pneumococcus and *Haemophilus* may also be successful with amox/clav, cefdinir, cefpodoxime, or cefuroxime Levofloxacin is an alternative but due to cartilage toxicity concerns, should not be first-line therapy.
– Pneumococcal, pen-S	Penicillin G 250,000–400,000 U/kg/day IV div q4–6h x 10 d	After improvement, change to PO amoxicillin 50–75 mg/kg/day PO div tid, or penicillin V 50–75 mg/kg/day div qid–tid

Table 49-1. Antibiotic Choices (continued)

LOWER RESPIRATORY TRACT INFECTIONS		
Clinical Diagnosis	**Therapy**	**Comments**
– Pneumococcal, pen-R	Ceftriaxone 75 mg/kg/day q24h, or cefotaxime 150 mg/kg/day div q8h for 10–14 d	Addition of vancomycin has not been required for eradication of pen-R strains For oral convalescent therapy, clindamycin (if organism susceptible) (30 mg/kg/day PO div tid), or linezolid (30 mg/kg/day PO div tid), or high-dosage amoxicillin (100–150 mg/kg/day PO div tid)
– *S aureus* (including CA-MRSA)	For MSSA: oxacillin or cefazolin For CA-MRSA: vancomycin 60 mg/kg/day; alternatives for CA-MRSA are clindamycin or linezolid, if organisms susceptible. For life-threatening infection caused by CA-MRSA, some experts recommend combination therapy although no prospectively collected data exist to support or refute better outcomes.	Alternative for MSSA or CA-MRSA is clindamycin, if organisms susceptible. Daptomycin should NOT be used for treatment of pneumonia caused by any pathogen. Check vancomycin serum concentrations and renal function, particularly at the higher dosage needed for invasive CA-MRSA disease. Linezolid 30 mg/kg/day IV, PO div q8h is another option (follow platelets and WBC weekly) Older children 600 mg q12h

Table 49-1. Antibiotic Choices (continued)

LOWER RESPIRATORY TRACT INFECTIONS		
Clinical Diagnosis	**Therapy**	**Comments**
Pneumonia: with empyema (same pathogens as for community-associated bronchopneumonia)	Empiric therapy: ceftriaxone 50–75 mg/kg/day q24h or cefotaxime 150 mg/kg/day div q8h AND vancomycin 40–60 mg/kg/day IV div q8h	Initial therapy based on Gram stain of empyema fluid; typically clinical improvement is slow, with persisting but decreasing "spiking" fever for 2–3 wks
– Group A streptococcal	Penicillin G 250,000 U/kg/day IV div q4–6h x 10 d	Change to PO amoxicillin 75 mg/kg/day div tid or penicillin V 50–75 mg/kg/day, div qid to tid after clinical improvement
– *S aureus* (including CA-MRSA)	For MSSA: oxacillin or cefazolin For CA-MRSA: use vancomycin 60 mg/kg/day (follow serum concentrations and renal function); may need additional antibiotics	For life-threatening disease, optimal therapy of CA-MRSA is not defined: add gentamicin and/or rifampin Oral convalescent therapy for MSSA: cephalexin PO; for CA-MRSA: clindamycin (if organism susceptible) PO at 30–40 mg/kg/day div tid Total course x 21 d or longer Linezolid 30 mg/kg/day IV, PO div q8h is another option (follow platelets and WBC weekly) Older child (maximum dose 600 mg q12h)

Table 49-1. Antibiotic Choices (continued)

LOWER RESPIRATORY TRACT INFECTIONS		
Clinical Diagnosis	**Therapy**	**Comments**
Pneumonia: Immuno-suppressed, neutropenic host *P aeruginosa,* other community-associated or nosocomial gram-negative bacilli, *S aureus,* fungi, AFB, *Pneumocystis,* viral (adenovirus, CMV, EBV, influenza, RSV, others)	Ceftazidime 150 mg/kg/day IV div q8h and tobramycin 6.0–7.5 mg/kg/day IM, IV div q8h, OR cefepime 150 mg/kg/day div q8h, or meropenem 60 mg/kg/day div q8h ± tobramycin; AND if *S aureus* suspected clinically, ADD vancomycin 40–60 mg/kg/day IV div q8h Biopsy or bronchoalveolar lavage may be needed to determine need for antifungal, antiviral, antimycobacterial treatment	Amikacin 15–22.5 mg/kg/day is alternative aminoglycoside. Use 2 active agents for improved efficacy and decreased risk of emergence of resistance.
– **Pneumonia: Interstitial pneumonia syndrome of early infancy**	If *Chlamydia trachomatis* suspected, azithromycin 10 mg/kg on day 1, followed by 5 mg/kg/day once daily days 2–5 OR erythromycin 40 mg/kg/day PO div qid; x 14 d	Most often respiratory viral pathogens, CMV, or chlamydial; role of *Ureaplasma* uncertain

Table 49-1. Antibiotic Choices (continued)

LOWER RESPIRATORY TRACT INFECTIONS		
Clinical Diagnosis	**Therapy**	**Comments**
– **Pneumonia, Nosocomial (HAP/VAP)** *P aeruginosa*, gram-negative enteric bacilli *(Enterobacter, Klebsiella, Serratia, Escherichia coli), Acinetobacter, Stenotrophomonas,* and gram-positive organisms including CA-MRSA and *Enterococcus*	Commonly used regimens: Meropenem 60 mg/kg/day div q8h, OR pip/tazo 240–300 mg/kg/day div q6–8h, OR cefepime 150 mg/kg/day div q8h; ± gentamicin 6.0–7.5 mg/kg/day div q8h; ADD vancomycin 40–60 mg/kg/day div q8h for suspect CA-MRSA	For multidrug-resistant gram-negative bacilli, colistin may be required. Should be institution-specific, based on your hospital's nosocomial pathogens and susceptibilities. Pathogens that cause nosocomial pneumonia often have multidrug resistance. Cultures are critical. Empiric therapy also based on child's prior colonization/infection.
Pneumonias of other established etiologies		
– *Chlamydia* (now *Chlamydophila) pneumoniae, C psittaci,* or *C trachomatis*	Azithromycin 10 mg/kg on day 1, followed by 5 mg/kg/day once daily days 2–5 or erythromycin 40 mg/kg/day PO div qid; x 14 d	Doxycycline (patients >7 yrs) 100 mg oral twice daily
– CMV (immune-compromised host)	Ganciclovir IV 10 mg/kg/day IV div q12h for 2 weeks; if needed, continue at 5 mg/kg/day q24h to complete 4–6 weeks total	Add IVIG or CMV immune globulin to provide a small incremental benefit. For older children, oral valganciclovir may be used for convalescent therapy.

Table 49-1. Antibiotic Choices (continued)

LOWER RESPIRATORY TRACT INFECTIONS		
Clinical Diagnosis	**Therapy**	**Comments**
– *E coli*	Ceftriaxone 50–75 mg/kg/day q24h or cefotaxime 150 mg/kg/day div q8h	For resistant strains (ESBL-producers), use meropenem, imipenem, or ertapenem
– *Enterobacter* spp	Cefepime 100 mg/kg/day div q12h or meropenem 60 mg/kg/day div q8h; OR ceftriaxone 50–75 mg/kg/day q24h or cefotaxime 150 mg/kg/day div q8h AND gentamicin 6.0–7.5 mg/kg/day IM, IV div q8h	Addition of aminoglycoside to 3rd generation cephalosporins may retard the emergence of resistance; not needed with cefepime, meropenem, or imipenem
– *Francisella tularensis*	Gentamicin 6.0–7.5 mg/kg/day IM, IV div q8h x 10 d or longer for more severe disease; for less severe disease, doxycycline PO	Alternatives for oral therapy of mild disease: ciprofloxacin or *levofloxacin* The rate of relapse seems to be higher with tetracycline.
– Fungi – Community-associated pathogens vary by region (eg, coccidioides, histoplasma) – *Aspergillus*, mucor, others in immune-compromised hosts	For suspected deep fungi in immune-compromised host, treat empirically with a lipid amphotericin B AND voriconazole and/or an echinocandin; biopsy needed to guide therapy	For normal hosts, triazoles (fluconazole for coccidioidomycosis, and itraconazole for histoplamosis) are better tolerated than amphotericin and equally effective for mild to moderate disease. For severe disease in normal hosts, empiric therapy with AmB provides the broadest coverage.

Table 49-1. Antibiotic Choices (continued)

LOWER RESPIRATORY TRACT INFECTIONS		
Clinical Diagnosis	**Therapy**	**Comments**
– Influenza virus For 2010–11, circulating strains of influenza A and B identified as of December 2010 are virtually all susceptible to the neuraminidase inhibitors (oseltamivir and zanamivir) and resistant to the adamantanes (amantadine and rimantadine). The CDC Web site contains current information about susceptibility of circulating influenza virus strains.	Empiric therapy for influenza A or B: 1 yr to ≤7 years old: oseltamivir; for >7 years old: zanamivir inhaled alone OR oseltamivir Oseltamivir dose by body weight: ≤15 kg: 30 mg twice daily ≥15 kg to 23 kg: 45 mg twice daily ≥23 kg to 40 kg: 60 mg twice daily ≥40 kg: 75 mg twice daily Zanamivir inhalation for children >7 years of age: 10 mg (two 5-mg inhalations) twice daily	For empiric therapy of infants younger than 1 year, oseltamivir can be prescribed at 3 mg/kg/dose twice daily as was recommended during the swine flu pandemic.
– *Klebsiella pneumoniae*	Ceftriaxone 50–75 mg/kg/day IV, IM q24h OR cefotaxime 150 mg/kg/day IV, IM div q8h; for ceftriaxone-resistant strains (ESBL strains), use meropenem 60 mg/kg/day IV div q8h	For *K pneumoniae* carbapenemase-producing strains: alternatives include fluoroquinolones or colistin
– Legionnaire's disease *(Legionella pneumophila)*	Azithromycin 10 mg/kg IV, PO q24h x 5 d	Alternatives: clarithromycin, erythromycin, ciprofloxacin, levofloxacin, doxycycline

Table 49-1. Antibiotic Choices (continued)

LOWER RESPIRATORY TRACT INFECTIONS		
Clinical Diagnosis	**Therapy**	**Comments**
– *Mycobacteria,* nontuberculous (*M avium* complex most common)	In a normal host: azithromycin PO or clarithromycin PO x 6–12 wks if susceptible For more extensive disease: a macrolide AND rifampin AND ethambutol; ± amikacin or streptomycin	Highly variable susceptibilities of different nontuberculous mycobacterial species Check for immune-compromise: HIV or γ-interferon receptor deficiency
– *Mycobacterium tuberculosis* (see Tuberculosis)		
– *M pneumoniae*[1]	Azithromycin 10 mg/kg on day 1, followed by 5 mg/kg/day once daily days 2–5, or clarithromycin 15 mg/kg/day div bid x 7–14 d, or erythromycin 40 mg/kg/day PO div qid x 14 d	*Mycoplasma* often cause self-limited infection and does not require treatment. For children older than 7 years, doxycycline 100 mg bid is an alternative.
– *Pneumocystis jiroveci* (previously *Pneumocystis carinii)*	Mild-moderate disease: TMP/SMX 20 mg of TMP/kg/day PO div qid x 14–21 d Moderate-severe disease: same dosage of TMP/SMX given IV, each dose over 1 h Use steroid adjunctive treatment for more severe disease	Alternatives: pentamidine 3–4 mg IV once daily, infused over 60–90 minutes; TMP AND dapsone; OR primaquine AND clindamycin; OR atovaquone Prophylaxis: TMP/SMX 5 mg TMP/kg/day PO daily or 3x/wk; OR dapsone 1 mg/ kg PO once daily
– *P aeruginosa*	Ceftazidime 150 mg/kg/day IV div q8h AND tobramycin 6.0–7.5 mg/kg/day IM, IV div q8h. Alternatives: cefepime 150 mg/kg/day div q8h or meropenem 60 mg/kg/day div q8h ± tobramycin	Ciprofloxacin for short-term oral convalescent therapy of a few weeks (less safety data in children for long-term therapy)

Table 49-1. Antibiotic Choices (continued)

LOWER RESPIRATORY TRACT INFECTIONS		
Clinical Diagnosis	**Therapy**	**Comments**
– RSV infection (bronchiolitis, pneumonia)	For immune-compromised hosts: ribavirin aerosol: 6-g vial (20 mg/mL in sterile water), by SPAG-2, over 18–20 h daily x 3–5 d	Treat only for severe disease, immune-compromise, severe underlying cardiopulmonary disease Ribavirin may also be given systemically (no data on efficacy) Palivizumab is not effective for treatment, only prevention
Tuberculosis		
– Primary pulmonary disease	INH 10–15 mg/kg/day (max 300 mg) PO qd x 6 mos AND rifampin 10–20 mg/kg/day (max 600 mg) PO qd x 6 mos AND PZA 20–40 mg/kg/day PO qd x first 2 mos therapy only If risk factors present for multidrug resistance, add ethambutol 20 mg/kg/day PO qd OR streptomycin 30 mg/kg/day IV, IM div q12h initially	Contact TB specialist for therapy of drug-resistant TB. Fluoroquinolones may play a role. Directly observed therapy preferred; after 2 wks of daily therapy, can change to twice weekly dosing (double dosage of INH (max 900 mg), PZA (max 2 g) and ethambutol (max 2.5 g); rifampin remains same dosage (10–20 mg/kg/day, max 600 mg) LP ± computed tomography of head for children ≤2 years old to rule out occult, concurrent CNS infection; consider test for HIV infection
– Skin test conversion (latent TB infection)	INH 10–15 mg/kg/day (max 300 mg) PO daily x 9 mos (12 mos for immune-compromised patients); treatment with INH at 20–30 mg twice weekly x 9 mos is also effective	Single drug therapy if no clinical or radiographic evidence of active disease. For exposure to known INH-R but rifampin-S strains, use rifampin 6 mos

Table 49-1. Antibiotic Choices (continued)

LOWER RESPIRATORY TRACT INFECTIONS		
Clinical Diagnosis	**Therapy**	**Comments**
– Exposed infant <4 yrs, or immune-compromised patient (high risk of dissemination)	INH 10–15 mg/kg PO daily x 2–3 mos after last exposure with repeat skin test or interferon-γ release assay test negative	If PPD remains negative at 2–3 mos and child well, consider stopping empiric therapy. PPD may not be reliable in immune-compromised patients.

Abbreviations: AFB, acid-fact bacilli; Amb, amphotericin B; amox/clav, amoxicillin/clavulanate; bid, twice a day; CA-MRSA, community-associated methicillin-resistant *Staphylococcus aureus;* CDC, Centers for Disease Control and Prevention; CF, cystic fibrosis; CMV, cytomegalovirus; CNS, central nervous system; div, divided; EBV, Epstein-Barr virus; ESBL, extended spectrum ß-lactamase; FDA, US Food and Drug Administration; HAP, hospital-acquired pneumonia; IM, intramuscular; INH, isoniazid; IV, intravenous; IVIG, intravenous immune globulin; LP, lumbar puncture; MRSA, methicillin-resistant *Staphylococcus aureus;* MSSA, methicillin-susceptible *Staphylococcus aureus;* pip/tazo, piperacillin/tazobactam; PO, orally; PPD, purified protein derivative; PZA, pyrazinamide; q, every; qid, 4 times daily; RSV, respiratory syncytial virus; SPAG-2, small particle aerosol generator-2; TB, tuberculosis; ticar/clav, ticarcillin/clavulanate; tid, 3 times daily; tmp/smx, trimethoprim/sulfamethoxazole; VAP, ventilator-acquired pneumonia; WBC, white blood cell.

[a] Adapted from Bradley JS, Nelson JD, eds. *2010–2011 Nelson's Pocket Book of Pediatric Antimicrobial Therapy.* Elk Grove Village, IL: American Academy of Pediatrics; 2010.

Classes of Antibiotics

Oral Cephalosporins

The oral cephalosporins (Box 49-2) have an advantage over the oral penicillins of a somewhat greater safety profile and greater palatability of the suspension. The serum half lives of cefpodoxime, ceftibuten, and cefixime are greater than 2 hours. This allows for twice-daily dosing. There is varying activity against *Haemophilus influenzae* and *Streptococcus pneumoniae.*

Box 49-2. Oral Cephalosporins

- Cephalexin
- Cefadroxil
- Cefaclor
- Cefprozil
- Cefuroxime
- Cefixime
- Cefdinir
- Cefditoren (≥12 years)
- Ceftibutin

Box 49-3. Parenteral Cephalosporins

First Generation
- Cefazolin

Second Generation
- Cefamandole
- Cefuroxime
- Cephamycins
  - Cefoxitin
  - Cefotetan

Third Generation
- Cefotaxime
- Ceftrizxone
- Ceftozoxime
- Ceftazidime
- Cefoperazone

Fourth Generation
- Cefipime

First generation cephalosporins (Box 49-3) are mainly used for gram-positive infections. Cefazolin is well tolerated by intramuscular or intravenous injection.

Second generation cephalosporins (Box 49-3) provide increased activity against many gram-negative organisms. Cefoxitin has increased activity against approximately 80% of strains of *Bacteroides fragilis* and can be considered for use in place of metronidazole, clindamycin, and carbapenems when that organism is implicated in non–life-threatening disease. Cefotetan has a spectrum similar to cefoxitin with a longer half-life, so it can be given every 12 hours. Cefuroxime has been given as a single injection in many countries for pneumonia that is caused by gram-positive cocci or *Haemophilus.*

Third generation cephalosporins (Box 49-3) all have enhanced potency against gram-negative bacilli, but lack activity against the newly emergent extended-spectrum ß-lactamases (ESBLs). They are inactive against enterococci and *Listeria* and have variable activity against *Pseudomonas* and *Bacteroides.*

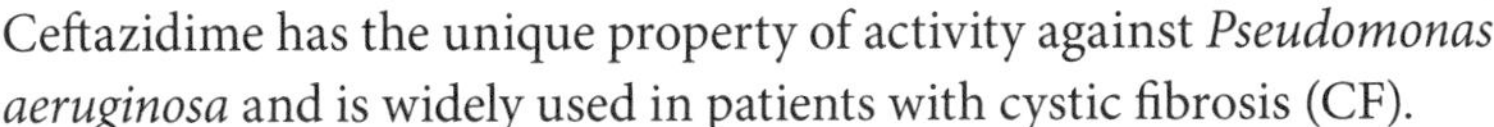

Ceftazidime has the unique property of activity against *Pseudomonas aeruginosa* and is widely used in patients with cystic fibrosis (CF).

The fourth generation cephalosporin cefepime has antipseudomonal activity as well as activity against gram-positive organisms and gram-negative bacilli, such as *Enterobacter* and *Serratia.*

The fifth generation cephalosporin ceftaroline is the first of the ß-lactam antibiotics to demonstrate activity against methicillin-resistant *Staphylococcus aureus* (MRSA). In addition, it provides activity against the gram-negative enteric bacilli similar to the third generation cephalosporins and lacks activity against ESBL-producing pathogens.

Penicillinase-Resistant Penicillins

The penicillinase-resistant penicillins (Box 49-4) were specifically formulated to address stability against the ß-lactamase produced by *Staphylococcus aureus.* These compounds are not stable to the ß-lactamases produced by gram-negative bacteria. They are active against methicillin-sensitive *Staphylococcus aureus* (MSSA) but not MRSA. Nafcillin is excreted primarily by the liver rather than the kidneys, compared with the others in this group, and may be preferred over methicillin except in neonates and patients with hepatic disease. Methicillin causes nephrotoxicity or hemorrhagic cystitis in 5% of children.

Box 49-4. Penicillinase-Resistant Penicillins

- Cloxacillin
- Dicloxacillin
- Methicillin
- Nafcillin
- Oxacillin

The oral antibiotics cloxacillin, dicloxacillin, and oxacillin are equivalent in activity but they are virtually unpalatable.

Antipseudomonal ß-Lactams

Timentin (ticarcillin/clavulanate [TC]) (Box 49-5) and Zosyn (piperacillin/tazobactam [PT]) represent combinations of 2 ß-lactam drugs. The antibiotic binds effectively to the target site in the bacteria, resulting in death of the organism whereas the second ß-lactamase inhibitor binds irreversibly to and neutralizes the ß-lactamase enzyme the organism produced to degrade the original antibiotic. The antipseudomonal activity of the combination is no different than the original ticarcillin and piperacillin, but there is increased activity to other ß-lactamase–positive bacteria, including *S aureus* (MSSA strains only) and *B fragilis.*

Box 49-5. Antipseudomonal ß-lactams

- Ticarcillin
- Piperacillin
- Aztreonam
- Ceftazidime
- Cefipime
- Meropenem
- Imipenem

Ticarcillin/clavulanate
Piperacillin/tazobactam

Pseudomonas has an intrinsic capacity to develop resistance to ceftazidime, ticarcillin (and TC), or piperacillin (and PT). Single therapy with these antibiotics commonly results in resistance, so combination with an aminoglycoside is recommended with these antibiotics. Cefepime, meropenem, and imipenem are less likely to develop resistance and can be used as single therapy. However, in CF, immunocompromised hosts, and life-threatening infections, these antibiotics should be used in combination with an aminoglycoside.

Aminopenicillins

Ampicillin, an aminopenicillin (Box 49-6), is more likely than the others to cause diarrhea and to cause overgrowth of *Candida.* Amoxicillin is well absorbed, good tasting, and has few side effects. Augmentin is available in the United States in oral form, and for parenteral use in many other countries. Augmentin is the combination of amoxicillin and clavulanic acid and has activity against many ß-lactamase–producing bacteria, including *H influenzae* and *S aureus* (MSSA strains only).

Box 49-6. Aminopenicillins

- Amoxicillin
- Amoxicillin/clavulanate
- Ampicillin
- Ampicillin/sulbactam

Box 49-7. Carbapenems

- Meropenem
- Imipenem
- Dorapenem (not approved in children)
- Ertapenem

Carbapenems

Carbapenems (Box 49-7) have a broader spectrum of activity than any other ß-lactams currently available. They are active against streptococci and *S aureus* (MSSA strains only); *Pseudomonas;* most coliform bacilli, including cefotaxime-resistant strains; and anaerobes, including *B fragilis.*

Macrolides

Erythromycin is the prototype of macrolide antibiotics, and the 3 shown in Box 49-8 are the only commercial macrolide antibiotics available in the United States. Azithromycin is more accurately called an azalide but is structurally very similar to macrolides. Azithromycin and clarithromycin have activity against certain nontuberculous mycobacteria but should not be used as monotherapy if possible, because of the potential to develop resistance.

Box 49-8. Macrolides

- Erythromycin
- Azithromycin
- Clarithromycin

Aminoglycosides

The first 3 aminoglycosides listed in Box 49-9 are in widespread use for systemic therapy of aerobic gram-negative infections and for synergy in the treatment of certain gram-positive infections. It is advisable to monitor levels early in the course of treatment because of potential toxicity to the kidneys and eighth cranial nerve. With amikacin, the desired peak concentrations are 25 to 30 mcg/mL and trough concentration less than 10 mcg/mL; for gentamicin and tobramycin peak concentrations should be 5 to 10 mcg/mL and trough concentrations less than 2 mcg/mL. Children with CF will require significantly higher dosages. Aminoglycosides demonstrate concentration-dependent killing of organisms, and the peak serum concentrations are greater than those achieved with dosing 3 times daily. Once-daily dosing of tobramycin is increasingly being prescribed, with doses of 5 to 7.5 mg/kg and, in patients with CF, doses of 9 to 10 mg/kg. The peak levels are often not measured, but it is important that the trough level is less than 1.0 mcg/mL in order to avoid renal toxicity and ototoxicity. There are insufficient prospectively collected comparative data to recommend once-daily treatment, compared with hourly dosing in young children, but based on retrospective data and present experience it is likely that once-daily treatment will become the standard.

Box 49-9. Aminoglycosides

- Amikacin
- Gentamycin
- Tobramycin
- Streptomycin[a]
- Spectinomycin[a]
- Kanamycin[a]

[a]Not commonly used

Fluoroquinolones

Ciprofloxacin has excellent gram-negative coverage against enteric bacteria *(Escherichia coli, Klebsiella, Enterobacter, Salmonella,* and *Shigella* as well as coverage against *P aeruginosa).* Ciprofloxacin has minimal coverage for gram-positive organisms, so if *S aureus,* streptococcus or pneumococcus is suspected alternate coverage should be added. The newer quinolones—levofloxacin and gatifloxacin—have improved coverage against these organisms, but should not be considered optimal therapy for staphylococcal infections.

Box 49-10. Fluoroquinolones

- Ciprofloxacin
- Gatifloxacin
- Moxifloxacin

There are concerns regarding toxicity of fluoroquinolones to cartilaginous weight-bearing joints, so the fluoroquinolones (Box 49-10) should not be considered a first choice treatment of infections in children.

Antifungal Agents

Amphotericin B

Amphotericin is a polyene antifungal antibiotic that has been available since 1960 for the treatment of invasive fungal infections. It remains the most broad-spectrum antifungal available for clinical use, with a mechanism of action against the fungal cell membrane in which pores are created, compromising the integrity of the membrane and creating a fungicidal effect. The toxicity of the original formulation, amphotericin B deoxycholate (AmB-D), is substantial from the standpoints of both systemic reactions (fever and chills) and renal toxicity. Premedication with acetaminophen, diphenhydramine, and meperidine is often required to prevent systemic reactions during infusion. Renal dysfunction manifests primarily as decreased glomerular filtration with a rising serum creatinine concentration, but substantial tubular nephropathy is associated with potassium wasting, requiring supplemental potassium for virtually all neonates and children, regardless of clinical symptoms associated with infusion. Newer lipid preparations decrease toxicity with no apparent decrease in clinical efficacy. The lipid formulations should be used despite their increased cost, as they are far better tolerated than AmB-D.

Azoles

A new class of systemic agents for the treatment of fungal infections was first approved in 1981: an imidazole, ketoconazole. All of the azoles work by inhibition of ergosterol synthesis (fungal cytochrome P450 sterol 14-demethylation), required for fungal cell membrane integrity. In general, the azoles are fungistatic in vivo, in contrast to polyenes like AmB, which are fungicidal. Primarily active against *Candida* species, ketoconazole is available for systemic treatment in an oral formulation.

Fluconazole is active against a broader range of fungi than ketoconazole, and includes clinically relevant activity against *Cryptococcus, Coccidioides,* and *Histoplasma.* Fluconazole remains one of the most active, and so far the safest, systemic antifungal agent for the treatment of most *Candida* infections, although some resistance is present in many non-*albicans Candida* species as well as in *C albicans* in children repeatedly exposed to fluconazole. Available in both oral and parenteral formulations, clinical data have been generated in pediatrics, including premature neonates. Toxicity is unusual, but when it occurs is primarily hepatic.

Itraconazole is active against an even broader range of fungi and molds, including *Aspergillus.* Pediatric clinical data are limited. Voriconazole was approved for adults in 2002 and at present is only FDA-approved for those older than 12 years. It is now the treatment of choice for *Aspergillus* infections. Voriconazole is active against *Candida* species, including some that are fluconazole resistant, but fluconazole is preferred if the *Candida* is susceptible. Voriconazole may produce transient visual disturbances early in the course of therapy, but no long-term visual or ocular toxicity has been documented. Hepatotoxicity is uncommon, occurring in 2% to 5% of patients. Voriconazole is cytochrome P450 metabolized, interacts with any similarly metabolized drugs, and may produce profound changes in serum concentrations of many concurrently administered drugs.

Posaconazole is the most recently FDA-approved triazole for adults and is not approved for children younger than 13 years. It has activity against *Candida* and *Aspergillus,* but importantly it has substantial activity against *Rhizopus* species and *Mucor* species, as well as *Coccidioides, Histoplasma,* and *Blastomyces.*

Echinocandins

This new class of antifungals was approved in 2001. The echinocandins prevent cell wall formation by inhibiting glucan synthesis. Caspofungin was the first to be approved. Active in vitro against most *Candida* and *Aspergillus* species, published data suggest that the echinocandins produce equivalent outcomes in the therapy of invasive *Candida* infections compared with AmB, but with fewer side effects. Caspofungin has received FDA approval for children 3 months to 17 years of age for

- Empiric therapy of presumed fungal infections in febrile neutropenic children
- Treatment of candidemia (including esophagitis, peritonitis, and empyema)
- Salvage treatment of invasive *Aspergillus*

Micafungin and anidulafungin are similar echinocandin agents and are approved for adults; both are under investigation for use in children. The echinocandins are highly protein-bound (>95%) but unlike some of the triazole antifungals, they are not metabolized by the P450 system.

Adverse Reactions to Antibiotics

Adverse drug reaction to antibiotics should be considered whenever there is a symptom that is associated with the side-effect profile of the drug and when unexpected symptoms and signs arise. The most common of these is a rash, often with itching, but more severe reactions can occur, including anaphylaxis. The child who has a reaction may require discontinuation of the drug or further supportive treatment.

Drug Interactions

Infectious disease consultants and pharmacists should be consulted whenever there is a potential for drug interaction. There are sources on the Internet that also are able to provide extensive information concerning drug interactions.

Acknowledgment

Chapter adapted from Bradley JS, Nelson JD, eds. *2010–2011 Nelson's Pocket Book of Pediatric Antimicrobial Therapy.* Elk Grove Village, IL: American Academy of Pediatrics; 2010.

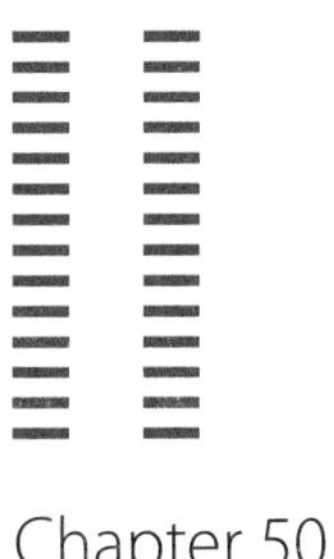

Chapter 50

Nutritional Aspects of Pulmonary Conditions

Ellen K. Bowser, MS, RD, LD/N, RN
Mary H. Wagner, MD

Pulmonary disorders such as cystic fibrosis (CF), bronchopulmonary dysplasia, and asthma may compromise a child's growth and acquisition of specific nutrients, and nutritional deficiencies might worsen the overall course of children with these conditions. On the other hand, overnutrition plays a role in the development or severity of pulmonary disorders, such as obstructive sleep apnea (OSA) or hypercapnic response in persons with Prader Willi syndrome.[1] Thus understanding nutritional issues is important in the care of children with pulmonary disorders.

General Nutritional Evaluation

Nutritional assessment of children with pulmonary conditions can be accomplished using the ABCDEF method (Table 50-1). Anthropometry determines the child's growth and body composition in comparison to their peers. Biochemical indices assist the pediatrician in determining hematologic, protein, and vitamin and mineral status. Clinical examination helps in the determination of nutritional status, and dietary, elimination, and feeding information assists in the formulation of a diagnosis.

Anthropometric Evaluation

Anthropometric data include growth plotted on standard growth charts. Genetics plays a major role in each child's growth potential. Evaluation of the parent's height (mid-parental height calculation) provides an estimate of the child's potential for height. Well-nourished

Table 50-1. ABCDEF Method of Nutritional Assessment in Children With Pulmonary Conditions

Components of Interest for Specific Conditions				
Assessment	**All Children**	**CF**	**Asthma/OSA**	**BPD**
Anthropometry	Weight percentile Height percentile Weight/height percentile (<3 years) BMI percentile (>3 years) Head circumference (<3 years)	Skinfold measurements (TSF, subscapular) Mid-upper arm circumference	Neck size	Correction for prematurity
Biochemical indices	Albumin Prealbumin Hemoglobin Hematocrit	Vitamins A, D, E, K (PT/INR) Zinc Essential fatty acids		
Clinical examination	Appearance Skin turgor Wasting or excess weight	Increased work of breathing	Acanthosis, striae	Increased work of breathing, pulse oximetry
Dietary information	24-hour dietary recall	3-day diet record	3-day diet record	Formula preparation, solid foods
Elimination patterns	Bladder, bowel habits Emesis	Detailed stooling history, constipation or DIOS?		
Feeding history	Location and timing of meals and snacks	Enzyme dosing		Oral-motor feedings/skills

Abbreviations: BPD, bronchopulmonary dysplasia; CF, cystic fibrosis; DIOS, distal intestinal obstruction syndrome; INR, international normalized ratio; OSA, obstructive sleep apnea; PT, prothrombin time; TSF, triceps skinfold.

children with CF and asthma are able to meet their genetic potential for growth.[2] Children with bronchopulmonary dysplasia (BPD) who were premature infants are often shorter and weigh less than their peers.

Body mass index (BMI, weight in kg/[height in m^2]) is an overall assessment of the child's weight for their height. Because children are growing, their actual BMI value changes as they get older. Body mass index percentiles provide a better assessment of the child's level of overweight and underweight. Normal or healthy BMI percentiles for children are between the fifth and less than the 85th percentiles (children with CF have different BMI goals as described on page 981).

Skinfold measurements are often used to assess nutritional status in children and adolescents with pulmonary diseases. Percentile standards[3] are available for ages 2 to 21, and the most commonly used measurements are triceps skinfolds, subscapular skinfolds, and mid-upper arm circumference. These values are most useful when assessing changes (ie, response to nutrition intervention) on a longitudinal basis. Skinfold measurements should always be taken by a trained anthropometrist. Calipers such as the Lange or Harpenden models are the most widely used in clinical settings.

Biochemical Evaluation

Biochemical indices that are most commonly used for nutritional assessment include albumin and prealbumin, hemoglobin and hematocrit, and vitamin levels. Albumin and prealbumin are serum proteins synthesized by the liver. Serum albumin levels are indicators of protein status. However, albumin reflects the protein status of the preceding 21 days. Prealbumin is a more immediate indicator of current nutritional status and reflects the protein status of the preceding 2 to 3 days. Prealbumin can be decreased in various circumstances, including liver disease and acute illness.

Hemoglobin and hematocrit are indicators of anemia. Anemia in children with lung conditions can be caused by poor dietary intake of iron, folate, vitamin B_{12}, or vitamin E. Malabsorption can also contribute to anemia in children with CF. Anemia of chronic disease also may be found in children with CF.

Serum fat-soluble vitamin levels are routinely measured in children with CF with exocrine pancreatic insufficiency. Low essential fatty acid levels and zinc levels may also contribute to poor weight gain in children with CF.

Clinical Evaluation

Clinical examination of the child with a pulmonary condition includes evaluation of overall appearance, skin turgor, and evidence of wasting or excess weight. Acanthosis or striae may be found in obese children, and it may be of interest to measure neck size in children with OSA, as neck size is associated with OSA in adults.[4]

Dietary Evaluation

Dietary information is essential in assessing the nutritional status of a child with a pulmonary condition. A 24-hour dietary recall is useful in obtaining a general indicator of a child's caloric and protein intake. However, these are often inaccurate and may not reflect usual intake. A 3-day diet record is the most accurate means to assess intake, but these are difficult and should be done in consultation with a registered dietitian. Specific instructions need to be given to the caregivers and child on estimating portion size and providing details, such as product brands and restaurant names. Dietary information can be entered into the US Department of Agriculture Web site (www.mypyramid.gov) for an assessment.

Elimination Evaluation

Elimination patterns include bladder and bowel habits as well as emesis. In addition to determining current patterns, it is important to assess if there are any recent changes. The number and consistency of stool should be established. In patients with CF, pancreatic insufficiency (PI) is associated with steatorrhea with malodorous, greasy stools.

Feeding Evaluation

Feeding information should include location and timing of meals and snacks. Length of meals and oral-motor and feeding skills are also important to assess. Children with BPD often have a delay in the normal oral-motor skill development due to their prematurity and length of time on a ventilator. The calorie intake should be assessed and, as recall is often poor, a prospective 3-day dietary record of intake is useful.

Nutritional Management of Respiratory Conditions Associated With Undernutrition

Cystic Fibrosis

Nutrition plays a key role in the management of persons with CF. Adequate nutrition is important in maintaining health, fighting infection, and avoiding deficiencies that may accompany the disorder. Assessment of nutritional parameters is an important part of routine care of persons with CF (see Chapter 37). A decline in growth may herald worsening pulmonary status, onset of diabetes, or increased involvement of the liver. The Cystic Fibrosis Foundation (CFF) recommends that children with CF maintain normal weight and height for age, as normal growth has been associated with better lung function and survival.[5] The CFF suggests that children (those >2 years, including adolescents) should achieve energy intake at levels of 110% to 200% above the usual requirements in healthy children to achieve age-appropriate weight gain.[6] This may require a combination of approaches, including calorie boosting, nutritional supplements, and behavioral interventions.

Nutritional intervention begins when a diagnosis of CF is made. Approximately 85% to 90% of persons with CF will have exocrine PI. This most often presents at birth or shortly thereafter, but in some children it develops after the first year. The diagnosis of PI may be confirmed by finding a low level of fecal elastase. Persons with PI have malabsorption of fat, protein, and other nutrients, including the fat-soluble vitamins (A, D, E, and K).

Anthropometric measurements, including height, weight, and BMI, should be obtained at each clinic visit. A target of maintaining BMI at the 50th percentile or greater is suggested because this level of growth is associated with a forced expiratory volume in 1 second near 80% of predicted.[5] Those with BMI less than the 25th percentile are considered nutritionally at risk, and a child with a BMI less than the 10th percentile is considered in nutritional failure.[6] All persons with CF should have additional monitoring of their nutritional status by yearly laboratory evaluation, including complete blood cell count, differential, liver function tests, clotting studies, and vitamin levels (A, E, and D 25-OH).

Enzyme Replacement Therapy

Patients with PI should be given pancreatic enzyme replacement therapy, with all meals and snacks, including human milk and pre-digested formulas. The microsphere tablet preparations are enteric coated to avoid degradation in the acidic gastric environment, so the enzymes are released in the proximal small intestine to optimize nutrient absorption. Some patients may benefit from the addition of a histamine-2 receptor blocker or proton pump inhibitor because gastric acid passing into the duodenum, unbuffered by pancreatic bicarbonate secretion, may decrease the effectiveness of pancreatic enzymes.

Pancreatic enzyme products were not approved by the US Food and Drug Administration (FDA) for many years. In April 2004 the FDA mandated that all makers of pancreatic enzymes submit their products for FDA approval based on safety, efficacy, and product quality by April 28, 2010. As of June 1, 2010, 3 pancreatic enzyme products have received FDA approval: Zenpep (Eurand Pharmaceuticals), Creon (Abbott Products, Inc), and Pancreaze (Johnson & Johnson). Other products are in the process of gaining FDA approval.[7]

Enzymes should be taken before every meal or snack unless the snack is pure carbohydrate, such as fruit. Patients usually take half of the typical meal dose before a snack. The dose of enzymes for a meal may need to be distributed throughout the meal for patients who take an extended period to eat or who are snacking throughout the day. The family and patient need to learn how to adjust the enzyme dose depending on the size, content, and duration of the meal. All caregivers, including child care and school environments, need to be educated about the need for enzymes with all snacks and meals.

Enzyme doses should be in the range of 1,500 to 2,500 units of lipase per kilogram of body weight per meal, with a ceiling of 10,000 units of lipase per kilogram per day.[5] These dose ranges are formulated to avoid risk of fibrosing colonopathy. Patients with persistent malabsorption need further evaluation for other conditions, such as small bowel bacterial overgrowth, celiac disease, or lactase deficiency.

Infants With Cystic Fibrosis

Infants with CF may be identified by clinical history or by newborn screening for CF. For most infants, the major form of nutrition in the first year of life should be human milk. Formulas with a caloric density greater than 20 kcal/oz or human milk are often necessary to maintain the desirable level of weight gain. The caloric density of formula or human milk can be augmented by concentrating the formula or adding fat or carbohydrate. Solid foods can be added at age 4 to 6 months as per recommendations of the American Academy of Pediatrics (AAP). However, the primary source of caloric intake should remain formula or human milk, especially if adequate growth is an issue. Infant cereal should be mixed with formula or human milk rather than juice or water. Whole milk can be used after 1 year of age for infants who are growing well.

For patients with PI, enzymes should be administered in a small amount of formula or baby food. Infants should receive vitamin supplementation, including vitamins A, D, E, and K. The adequacy of dietary iron and fluoride should be evaluated and supplements added if necessary. Those infants with suboptimal growth may need supplementation of their caloric intake by addition of carbohydrate polymers (Polycose, Ross Laboratories Division, Abbott Labs, or Moducal, Mead Johnson) and/or fats such as Microlipid (Mead Johnson) or vegetable oil to solids or formulas.

Because of extra salt loss in their sweat, infants with CF should be supplemented with one-eighth teaspoon daily for infants up to 6 months and one-quarter teaspoon of salt daily for infants older than 6 months.[5] This can be given in 1 or 2 doses mixed with formula or expressed human milk or given in the applesauce and enzyme mixture for nursing babies.

Toddlers and Preschool-aged Children With CF

Families with toddlers and preschool children with CF have more mealtime difficulties (ie, more feeding resistance, longer mealtimes) than families who do not have children with CF.[8] This can lead to mealtime battles and dysfunctional eating behaviors. Clinical or behavioral psychology services can be useful to enhance positive feeding behaviors and consistent weight gain.

School-aged Children With CF

Children with CF who are of school age may experience decreased growth[9] because of the number of activities that limit time for meals and snacks. Disease progression may also affect growth velocity.

Diets high in protein and fat should be encouraged, with continued vitamin supplementation. Behavioral interventions may be required if mealtime problems are identified. Children of this age with PI should have an understanding of why they need enzyme supplementation.

Ingesting enzymes at school or child care may be problematic. The staff may not understand that enzymes should be given just before eating. It may be difficult for the student to obtain the enzymes in a timely manner so that they have time to consume their food. School personnel may benefit from instruction on the importance of the child with CF having rapid access to enzymes before snacks and meals to facilitate their ability to eat and digest what they have eaten. There are educational materials available for caregivers, teachers, and coaches who work with children with CF.

Adolescents With CF

Calorie and nutrient requirements increase in adolescents for several reasons, including pubertal growth spurt, increased activity, and disease progression in some children. Girls are at greater risk of nutritional failure[10] primarily because of gender-specific social norms and expectations regarding weight. Some patients may develop CF-related diabetes. Decreased growth or delayed sexual maturation may occur in those with severe disease.[6] Additional issues that may be encountered with adolescents with CF include loss of parental control over medication administration and intentional weight loss. The adolescent should understand the link between good nutrition, good lung health, and avoiding hospitalization. Adolescents experiencing weight loss should be questioned about their perspective on their body image and whether or not the loss was intentional. Patients with CF can develop eating disorders with potentially severe consequences. Adolescents should be involved with their own treatment plan to improve adherence and results.

Nutritional Supplements and Calorie Boosters

Children and adolescents with chronic pulmonary conditions benefit from strategies to increase the caloric density of their usual diet. This can be accomplished using milk shakes or calorie boosters with their daily foods (Box 50-1). Other children and adolescents with suboptimal growth may benefit from the use of commercial formulas. These preparations can be useful and convenient but entail additional

Box 50-1. Tips to Help Your Child Gain Weight[a]

Feeding Suggestions

Stick to a regular meal schedule (for example, 3 meals and 3 snacks each day).
Offer solid foods first and then liquids.
Limit juice to 4 oz per day.
Praise for good behavior and ignore bad behavior.
Do not force your child to eat. Forcing a child to eat may actually cause him or her to eat less.
Avoid the TV and other distractions during mealtimes.
Limit meals and snacks to 20–30 minutes.

Calorie Boosters

Adding extra calories to your child's diet will help him or her to gain weight. There are many ways to add extra calories to common foods. Below are some examples.

Sour cream

Put on baked potatoes.
Add to burritos and tacos.
Stir into cream soups.

Cheese dip

Eat with pretzels.
Eat on apples or celery.
Melt over broccoli or cauliflower.

Nut butters

Spread on breads, crackers, apples, bananas, and celery.

Cream cheese

Spread on bagels.
Use flavored cream cheese as a dip for fruits.

Vegetable oil

Drizzle over noodles and vegetables.
Use in salad dressings.
Use to make scrambled eggs.
Use as dipping oil for breads and rolls.

Salad dressings

Serve with salads.
Use as dip for vegetables.
Use as spread with sandwiches.

Box 50-1. Tips to Help Your Child Gain Weight[a] (continued)

Healthy High-Calorie Foods

Cereal with whole milk: Kellogg's Frosted Mini Wheats, Post Banana Nut Crunch, Granola, General Mills Honey Nut Clusters, Raisin Bran, Post Blueberry Morning

Hot cereal: 1 packet of flavored instant oatmeal made with ½ cup heavy cream

Dairy: Dannon La Crème with Chocolate, Stonyfield Farms organic whole milk yogurt, Yoplait custard style yogurt (any flavor), Yoplait Nouriche Drink, Dannon Frusion Drink

Nuts: Trail mix (nuts, seeds, dried fruit, pretzels, chocolate chips—buy or make your own), sunflower seeds, oil roasted mixed nuts

Recipes

Power milk: 1 cup whole milk, 2 tbsp heavy whipping cream, 2 tbsp chocolate syrup

Nachos: 15 tortilla chips, ¼ cup cheese, 2 tbsp sour cream, 2 tbsp black olives, 2 tbsp guacamole or avocado dip

Chocolate peanut butter shake: ½ cup heavy whipping cream, 3 tbsp creamy peanut butter, 3 tbsp chocolate syrup, 1½ cups chocolate ice cream. Mix in blender and top with crushed Oreos.

Apple pie a la mode shake: 1 cup apple pie filling, ½ cup whole milk, 1 cup vanilla ice cream, dash of cinnamon. Mix in blender and top with caramel and crushed graham crackers.

French toast sandwich: spread 2 tbsp of peanut butter and 1 tbsp of jelly between 2 slices of French toast.

No bake chocolate cookies: mix ¼ cup softened margarine, ¼ cup peanut butter, ½ cup instant sweet cocoa mix, 1 cup oatmeal. Form into 1-inch balls and chill in refrigerator for 10 minutes.

Cooked carrots: 2 tbsp apricot preserves and brown sugar, or 2 tbsp honey added to buttered, cooked carrots.

Chocolate pudding: use 1 can (12–14 oz) sweetened condensed milk instead of regular milk when making pudding and sprinkle white chocolate chips on top

[a]Pediatric Pulmonary Center—University of Florida, 2007.

expense and may be difficult for the families to obtain. Dietary intake should be monitored so that these preparations are used to supplement rather than replace meals. They can be delivered orally or enterally if a feeding tube is present. Nutritional supplements of the patient's choice are the best. Most patients will benefit from a rotation of different supplements because they may tire of the same one if used repeatedly. Patients and families should be questioned about what over-the-counter supplements they may be using to avoid excess intake of specific nutrients.

Medications used to stimulate appetite, such as cyproheptadine (an antihistamine) have been used in school-aged and older children with CF with some success.[11]

Tube Feedings

Children who are unable to consume adequate calories during their daily intake may benefit from tube feedings. This approach should be considered in those whose anthropometric parameters put them in the category of nutritional failure.[6] Feedings can be administered via tubes place nasally (nasogastric [NG]) or percutaneously (gastrostomy [G-tubes]). Some children who are unable to consume adequate calories will appreciate the option of being able to supplement their intake with NG feedings delivered during sleep. Others will benefit from G-tube placement. Pancreatic enzymes are usually given prior to the start of the feeding and again in the morning. Some children require additional enzyme administration during the midpoint of the feeding period. Patient response to these feedings should be carefully monitored, including weight gain, symptoms of malabsorption, and daytime appetite. Other strategies include using predigested formulas with and without enzymes. These formulas incur additional expense and have not been shown to be better absorbed, but may be preferred in those who have had small intestine resection.[12] Tube feedings should stop at least 2 hours prior to the usual wake-up time in order for the child to be able to feel hungry for breakfast.

Vitamins

Persons with CF are at risk for deficiencies of fat-soluble vitamins, including A, D, E, and K. The CF Consensus Conference for pediatric nutrition has made specific recommendations for supplementation of fat-soluble vitamins.[6] Several vitamin formulations are available containing water-soluble forms of the fat-soluble vitamins (A, D, E, and K). These include AquADEK, ADEK (Scandipharm), SourceCF (SourceCF), and Vitamax (CF Pharmacy Services). These preparations are available in a variety of forms (soft gels, chewable tablets, and drops). These preparations have variable vitamin content, so each patient's vitamin levels should be monitored yearly and followed by a registered dietitian specializing in CF care.

All patients should receive the Dietary Reference Intake (DRI) suggested for calcium based on age. Calcium supplementation may be required for those on steroids, with decreased dietary calcium intake, or decreased bone density. Suboptimal serum levels of vitamin D (<30 ng/mL of 25 hydroxyvitamin D) are seen commonly in children with CF. This is thought to be a combination of inadequate intake, decreased storage, and decreased synthesis. Osteopenia and osteoporosis are frequent findings.[13]

Salt

Patients with CF experience increased losses of sodium and chloride through their sweat. Infants with CF should be supplemented with 3 to 4 Meq/kg body weight per day of sodium even when not exposed to heat stress.[6] Salt requirements in older children and adolescents can be met with liberal use of high-salt foods or the salt shaker. They may require additional salt supplementation at times of increased salt losses, such as with fever, hot weather exposure, vigorous physical activity, or diarrhea.

Bronchopulmonary Dysplasia

Infants with BPD are often of extremely low or very low birth weight due to their prematurity. Weight gain in the neonatal intensive care unit (NICU) early in their disease process is often poor, and these infants tend to remain small for their gestational age. On discharge from the NICU they may continue to experience growth failure. Adequate nutrition to allow normal growth and development is key to the resolution of BPD. Growth of new lung tissue can occur in humans up to 8 years of age, therefore it is important to continue to encourage good nutrition.

Numerous factors need to be considered in evaluating and managing the nutritional needs of children with BPD. These include increased metabolic rate, increased work of breathing, need for catch-up growth, volume intolerance, feeding issues, frequent respiratory infections, and fluid restrictions.

The effects of increased metabolic rate and increased work of breathing increase energy expenditure by 25% for infants with BPD.[14] Human milk is considered the optimal form of nutrition for all infants because exclusive breastfeeding until age 4 months and partial breastfeeding thereafter is associated with significant reduction of respiratory and gastrointestinal morbidity rates in infants up to 1 year of age. For infants with BPD, the increase in caloric expenditure, along with the need for catch-up growth, often mandate the use of human milk fortifiers or the addition of concentrated formula to human milk. Human milk can be enhanced by one of these methods to reach a caloric density of 24 to 30 kcal/oz. If human milk is not available, special infant formulas designed for the premature or low birth weight infant are recommended. These formulas have higher caloric and nutrient density. The AAP Committee on Nutrition recommends formulas designed for preterm infants after discharge from the NICU be given up to 9 months postnatal age.[15] Recommendations have been made to continue to use these formulas up to 12 months postnatal age in the infant with BPD.[16] When using high caloric density formulas caution should be taken due to the dilution of protein, vitamins, and minerals, and the need for free water. A registered dietitian familiar with the nutritional care of the child with BPD should be consulted if an increased caloric density formula is required. Infants with BPD are often fluid restricted and given diuretics to improve lung function and prevent pulmonary edema.[14]

Volume intolerance can be caused by hyperinflation of the lungs and compression of the diaphragm and stomach. This can lead to limited intake of the nutrient-enriched formula. Gastroesophageal reflux (GER), which commonly occurs in premature infants,[14] can make feeding the infant with BPD more challenging. Evaluation for GER may be appropriate, as medical or even surgical treatment may be necessary to ensure adequate oral intake and prevent aspiration. Feeding issues for the infant or toddler with BPD may include uncoordinated suck, swallow, and breathing; oral-motor dysfunction; and adverse feeding behaviors. If these are suspected, a feeding evaluation should be done by a speech-language or occupational therapist to determine if these are present. Ongoing therapy may be required to allow the child with BPD to achieve adequate oral intake for growth.

Feeding Disorders

Most children with pulmonary conditions such as CF and asthma will have normal oral-motor skill development. However, children with a history of prematurity are at increased risk for delayed development of oral-motor skills. Children who were premature are at increased risk for impairments in swallowing and feeding disruptions.[17] Periods of non-oral feedings, aspiration events, and the need for alternative feeding methods are more likely to occur in children who were premature compared with term infants.

Chronic lung disease is associated with uncoordinated suck, swallow, and breathing patterns, which increase the risk of aspiration. Infants who were mechanically ventilated for an extended period may develop oral-motor defensiveness. Those who remain on supplemental oxygen may experience fatigue with feeding and tolerate only small volumes of formula. Infants and children with neuromuscular, genetic, and craniofacial disorders may also experience feeding difficulties. Infants and older children with feeding issues should receive treatment from a speech-language pathologist or occupational therapist.

Children with tracheostomies can feed orally once it is ascertained that the child is not aspirating. Children who receive exclusive tube feedings should receive oral-motor stimulation during feedings to help associate the sensations of fullness with oral involvement. Failure to cough or clear the throat in response to aspiration is common in children with complex medical conditions.

Parental feeding behaviors and the feeding environment are also vital to appropriate feeding skills. A calm, non-stimulating setting (TV and other distractions turned off) is important. Scheduled meals and snacks, parental role modeling, and the use of positive reinforcement should be encouraged.[18]

Gastrostomy tube feedings are often used when a child with a pulmonary disorder is unable to maintain adequate oral intake over time. These feedings may be either bolus or continuous feedings. Gastrostomy tube feedings may be used to supplement inadequate oral intake or as a substitute for oral intake in children who may be at significant risk for aspiration. Oral-motor stimulation should be encouraged if the child is receiving exclusive tube feedings.

Nutritional Aspects of Respiratory Conditions Associated With Obesity

The overall prevalence of obesity in the US population is 17.1%, and its prevalence has been increasing in all age groups over recent years, especially in racial and ethnic minority groups.[19] Obesity is associated with a variety of pulmonary disorders including OSA, asthma, and restrictive lung disease (see Chapter 34).

A meta-analysis examining 12 articles from 1966 to 2004 noted that children with high body weight were at increased risk of future asthma.[20] Obesity has been shown to be a risk factor for OSA in both adults and children. Many children seen with OSA will require a multi-modal approach, which often includes weight management. Children with extreme obesity may have restricted chest wall movement and a restrictive pattern on their lung disease, and if obesity is severe they may suffer from obesity hypoventilation syndrome with impaired response to carbon dioxide.

Recently published clinical practice guidelines for the prevention and treatment of pediatric obesity[21] recommend that treatment for overweight and obesity includes appropriate lifestyle changes, including diet, physical activity, and behavioral counseling for the patient and the family. Dietary recommendations include (1) avoidance of high-calorie, low-nutrient foods, including fast foods, sweetened beverages, fruit drinks, juices, and sports drinks; (2) control of caloric intake via portion control as recommended by the AAP; (3) decrease in the amount of saturated fat in the diet for children older than 2 years of age; (4) increased dietary intake of fruits, vegetables, and fiber; and (5) meals at regular intervals, including breakfast with limited "grazing." This panel recommended physical activity, including moderate to vigorous exercise for 60 minutes per day, and restriction of sedentary activities, including TV viewing, video gaming, and use of computers. They suggested families be educated about the importance of parents modeling good dietary and exercise behaviors. Many of these recommendations are mirrored by the American Dietetic Association, suggesting multi-component programs including diet, physical activity, nutritional counseling, and parent participation for the intervention to be successful.[22]

Asthma

An association between overweight and asthma has been reported in the literature, but a cause and effect relationship has not been clear.[23] A recent meta-analysis examined the effect on high body weight in childhood on the future risk of asthma[20] and concluded that school-aged children with BMI at the 85th percentile or greater had a 50% higher risk of developing asthma than their normal weight peers. They also found infants with a birth weight of 3.8 kg or higher had a 20% higher risk of future asthma than their peers. Weight loss has been shown to improve asthma outcomes (symptoms, use of medications, or hospitalizations) in overweight adults.[24] However, there is little information on the effects of weight loss in overweight children with asthma.

Children and adolescents with asthma are often discouraged from drinking milk or other calcium-rich dairy products due to the ongoing myth that milk or dairy consumption increases mucus production. Although this theory has been disproved,[25] the milk-mucus connection remains widespread. Parents of children with asthma often report avoiding dairy in their asthmatic children's diets.[26,27] This is important because a recent study found that children with asthma, regardless of steroid intake, had decreased bone density.[28] Children with asthma should be encouraged to consume adequate amounts of calcium and vitamin D for bone growth and mineralization. Pediatricians should inquire about calcium and vitamin D intakes when working with children with asthma. Parents who remain hesitant to give their children dairy products should be encouraged to give their children calcium and vitamin D supplements to meet the Institute of Medicine Food and Nutrition Board's DRI levels.

Several dietary interventions have been proposed for reducing the severity of asthma, including supplementation with fish oils, antioxidants, vitamin C and E, and beta carotene, and reduction in dietary sodium. However, recent analyses do not support these interventions.[29]

Obstructive Sleep Apnea

Obstructive sleep apnea is estimated to occur in 1% to 3% of the general pediatric population.[30] Obesity is a risk factor for the development of OSA.[31] However, some children will present with failure to thrive. Many children will have no growth issues. Several studies have shown improvements in growth percentiles after adenotonsillectomy for OSA in children with normal, decreased, and increased growth at baseline.[32] Weight loss has been shown to result in an improvement in sleep-related breathing disorders,[33] thus assessment of nutritional status is important in children with OSA. Nutritional intervention may be an important component of the multifaceted management plan in these children (Box 50-2).

Prader-Willi Syndrome

Prader-Willi syndrome (PWS) has an estimated prevalence of 1/10,000 to 1/25,000 live births[34] and initial nutritional symptoms that include poor suck, hypotonia, and poor growth. Patients with PWS evolve to a pattern of food-seeking behavior, and insatiable appetite with subsequent development of obesity.[35] Pulmonary manifestations can include restrictive lung disease and sleep-related breathing disorders, including OSA, central apnea, and excessive daytime sleepiness. Dietary management is very important to deal with the different nutritional phases these patients experience and should be under the direction of a registered dietitian experienced in the care of these patients.[35] Strategies for dietary management include environmental management of food intake, a low-calorie diet, and constant supervision.

Box 50-2. Tips to Help Your Child Lose Weight or Slow Weight Gain

Feeding Suggestions

- Limit fast-food intake to 1 time/week.
- Avoid soft drinks, soda, or drinks with added sugar.
- Drink water or sugar-free drinks.
- Sit down and have meals as a family.
- Encourage fruits and vegetables as snacks.
- Exercise as a family 30–60 minutes daily.
- Limit TV or screen time to 1 hour daily.
- Switch to low-fat or skim milk.
- Switch to baking or broiling rather than frying.
- Be aware of appropriate portion sizes for children.

Key Points

- A progressive approach to weight gain for children with CF includes calorie boosters, oral nutritional supplements, and tube feedings.
- The Cystic Fibrosis section contains specific strategies and recommendations that can be used for children with other conditions.
- The general approach to weight loss depends on the child's age, BMI percentile, and medical condition. See the American Dietetic Association's guidelines.[22]
- See Boxes 50-1 and 50-2 for tips to increase or decrease weight gain.
- The ABCDEF method of assessment provides a comprehensive evaluation of a child's nutritional status.
- Nutritional status is linked to pulmonary status and outcomes in CF.
- Patients with CF and PI should take pancreatic enzymes before all meals and snacks and be supplemented with fat-soluble vitamins.
- Obesity is on the rise, and successful weight loss programs incorporate the family; lifestyle changes, including exercise; and moderation in caloric intake.
- Overnutrition in infancy and early childhood has been linked with the subsequent development of asthma.
- Obstructive sleep apnea can be found in children with normal, overnutrition, or undernutrition.
- A registered dietitian should be consulted to manage the nutritional aspects of CF, BPD, and PWS.

References

1. Arens R, Gozal D, Omlin KJ, et al. Hypoxic and hypercapnic ventilatory responses in Prader Willi syndrome. *J Appl Physiol.* 1994;77:2224–2230
2. Wooldridge N. Pulmonary diseases. In: Samour PQ, King K, eds. *Handbook of Pediatric Nutrition.* 3rd ed. Sudbury, MA: Jones and Bartlett; 2005:307–349
3. Frisancho AR. New norms of upper arm limb and fat and muscle areas for assessment of nutritional status. *Am J Clin Nutr.* 1981;34:2540–2545
4. Davies RJ, Stradling JR. The relationship between neck circumference, radiographic pharyngeal anatomy, and the obstructive sleep apnea syndrome. *Eur Respir J.* 1990;3:509–514

5. Stallings VA, Stark LJ, Robinson KA, et al. Evidence-based practice recommendations for nutrition-related managements of children and adults with cystic fibrosis and pancreatic insufficiency: results of a systematic review. *J Am Diet Assoc.* 2008;108:832–839
6. Borowitz D, Baker RD, Stallings VA. Consensus report on nutrition for pediatric patients with cystic fibrosis. *J Pediatr Gastroenterol Nutr.* 2002;35(3):246–259
7. FDA Approves Pancreatic Enzyme Product, Pancreaze. Press Release. http://www.fda.gov/newsevents/newsroom/pressannouncements/ucm208135.htm. Accessed October 28, 2010
8. Powers SW, Mitchell MJ, Patton SR, et al. Mealtime behaviors in families of infants and toddlers with cystic fibrosis. *J Cystic Fibrosis.* 2005;4(3):175–182
9. Lai HC, Corey M, FitzSimmons S, et al. Comparison of growth status in patients with cystic fibrosis between United States and Canada. *Am J Clin Nutr.* 1999;69:531–538
10. Lai HC, Kasorok MR, Sondel SA, et al. Growth status of children with cystic fibrosis based on the National Cystic Fibrosis Patient Registry: evaluation of various criteria used to identify malnutrition. *J Pediatr.* 1998;132:478–485
11. Homnick DN, Homnick BD, Reeves AJ, Marks JH, Pimental RS, Bonnema SK. Cyproheptakine is an effective appetite stimulant in cystic fibrosis. *Pedatr Pulmonol.* 2004;38(2):129–134
12. Erskine JM, Lingard CD, Sontag MK, et al. Enteral nutrition for patients with cystic fibrosis: comparison of a semi-elemental and non-elemental formula. *J Pediatr.* 1998;132:265–269
13. Hall WB, Sparks AA, Aris RA. Vitamin D deficiency in cystic fibrosis. *Int J Endocrinol.* 2010;2010:218691
14. Kelly MM. The medically complex premature infant in primary care. *J Pediatr Health Care.* 2006:20:367–373
15. American Academy of Pediatrics Committee on Nutrition. *Pediatric Nutrition Handbook.* 5th ed. Elk Grove Village, IL: American Academy of Pediatrics; 2004
16. Atkinson SA. Special nutritional needs of infants for prevention of and recovery from bronchopulmonary dysplasia. *J Nutr.* 2001;131:942s–946s
17. Lefton-Greif MA, Arvedson JC. Schoolchildren with dysphagia associated with medically complex conditions. *Lang Speech Hear Serv Sch.* 2008:39:237–248
18. Tobin SP, Cheng V, Schumacher C, et al. The role of the interdisciplinary feeding team in the assessment and treatment of feeding problems. *Building Block for Life.* 28(3):1–17. www.pnpg.org/bb
19. Wofford LG. Systematic review of childhood obesity prevention. *J Ped Nurs.* 2008;23(1):5–19
20. Flaherman V, Rutherford GW. A meta-analysis of the effect of high weight on asthma. *Arch Dis Child.* 2006;91:334–339

21. August GP, Caprio S, Fennoy I, et al. Prevention and treatment of pediatric obesity: an endocrine society clinical practice guideline based on expert opinion. *J Clin Endocrin Metab.* 2008;93(12):4576–4599
22. Pediatric Weight Management Evidence-Based Nutrition Practice Guideline. Executive summary of recommendations. http://www.adaevidencelibary.com/topic.cfm?cat=3013
23. Eneli IU, Skybo T, Camargo CA Jr. Weight loss and asthma: a systematic review. *Thorax.* 2008;63:671–676
24. Stenius-Aarniala B, Poussa T, Kvarnstrom J, Gronlund EL, Ulikarhi M, Mustajoki P. Immediate and long term effects of weight reduction in obese people with asthma: randomized controlled study. *BMJ.* 2000;320:827–832
25. Wuthrich B, Schmid A, Walther B, Seiber R. Milk consumption does not lead to mucus production or occurrence of asthma. *J Am Coll Nutr.* 2005;24(6 suppl):547S–555S
26. Dawson KP, Ford RPK, Mogridge N. Childhood asthma: what do parents add or avoid in their children's diets? *N Z Med J.* 1990;103:239–240
27. Lee C, Dozor AJ. Do you believe milk makes mucus? *Arch Pediatr Adolesc Med.* 2004;158:601–602
28. Ducharme FM, Chabot G, Polychronakos C, Glorieux F, Mazer B. Safety profile of frequent short courses of oral glucocorticoids in acute pediatric asthma: impact on bone metabolism, bone density, and adrenal function. *Pediatrics.* 2003;111:376–383
29. Gao J, Gao X, Li W, Zhu Y, Thompson PJ. Observational studies on the effect of dietary antioxidants on asthma: a meta-analysis. *Respirology.* 2008;13:528–536
30. Redline S, Tishler PV, Schluchter M, et al. Risk factors for sleep-disordered breathing in children: associations with obesity, race, and respiratory problems. *Am J Respir Crit Care Med.* 1999;159:1527–1532
31. Marcus CL, Curtis S, Koerner CB, et al. Evaluation of pulmonary function and polysomnography in obese children and adolescents. *Pediatr Pulmonol.* 1996;21:176–183
32. Lind MG, Lundell BP. Tonsillar hyperplasia in children: a cause of obstructive sleep apneas, CO2 retention, and retarded growth. *Arch Otolaryngol.* 1982;108:650–654
33. Kudoh F, Sanai A. Effect of tonsillectomy and adenoidectomy on obese children with sleep associated breathing disorders. *Acta Otolaryngol Suppl (Stockh).* 1996;523:216–218
34. Keens TG, Davidson Ward SL. Syndromes affecting respiratory control during sleep. In: Loughlin GM, Carroll JL, Marcus CL, eds. *Sleep and Breathing in Children: A Developmental Approach.* New York, NY: Marcel Dekker; 2000:535–537
35. Chen C, Visootsak J, Dills S, et al. Prader-Willi syndrome: an update and review for the primary pediatrician. *Clin Pediatr.* 2007;46(7):580–591

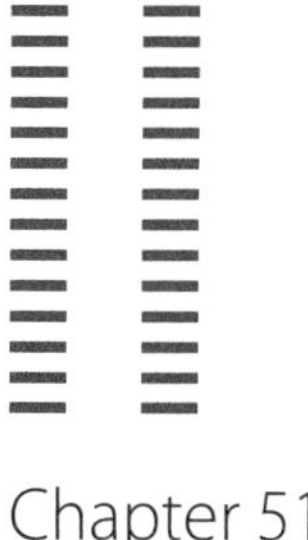

Chapter 51

Oxygen Therapy

Patricia M. Quigley, MD
Elizabeth K. Fiorino, MD

Pathophysiology

Oxygen Content and the Oxyhemoglobin Dissociation Curve

Oxygen is both dissolved in blood (a small portion) and bound to hemoglobin. The oxyhemoglobin dissociation curve (Figure 51-1) depicts how the percent saturation of hemoglobin corresponds to the partial pressure of oxygen. When hemoglobin is 90% saturated, the

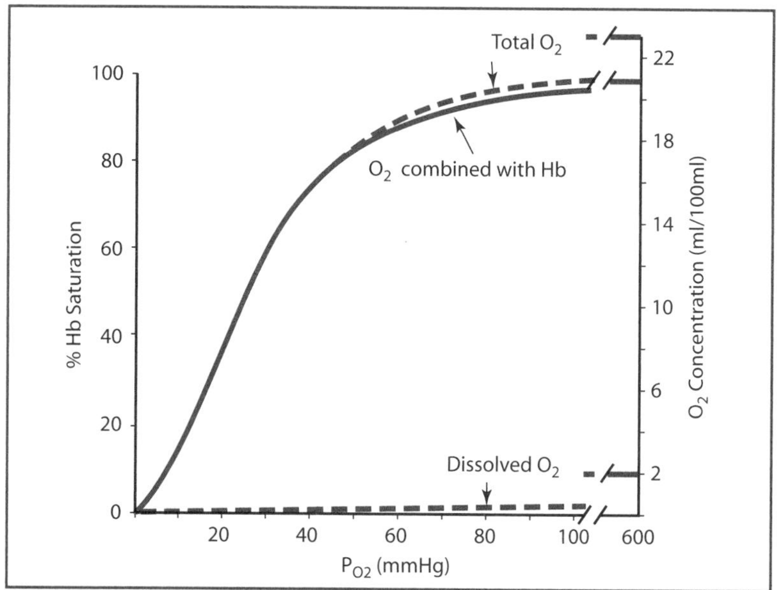

Figure 51-1. The oxygen dissociation curve. (From West JB. *Respiratory Physiology: The Essentials.* Philadelphia, PA: Lippincott, Williams and Wilkins; 2005, with permission.)

arterial partial pressure of oxygen (Pao_2) is 60 mm Hg. Above this value, though Pao_2 changes, oxyhemoglobin saturation (Spo_2) will not change appreciably. Below 60 mm Hg, however, Spo_2 changes significantly with small changes in Pao_2. Certain conditions, such as elevated partial pressure of carbon dioxide (Pco_2), increased temperature, and acidosis, decrease hemoglobin's affinity for oxygen and encourage increased unloading of oxygen at the tissue level, shifting the curve rightward. In contrast, lower Pco_2, decreased temperature, and alkalosis increase hemoglobin's affinity for oxygen, and facilitate oxygen uptake by red blood cells, shifting the curve leftward.[1]

Causes of Hypoxemia

There are 5 major causes of hypoxemia: ventilation/perfusion ($\dot{V}/\dot{Q}$) mismatch, hypoventilation, diffusion defect, ascent to high altitude, and shunt. In pediatrics, the most common cause of hypoxemia is $\dot{V}/\dot{Q}$ mismatch, followed by hypoventilation. A true shunt is most commonly observed in cyanotic congenital heart disease, and a physiologically significant diffusion impairment is rare.

$\dot{V}/\dot{Q}$ Mismatch

This term refers to an imbalance between ventilation, or gas flow into, and blood flow through different parts of the lung. Both blood flow and ventilation vary according to region of the lung and the patient's position. In healthy individuals, pulmonary blood vessels are regulated such that if a particular gas exchange unit is not receiving adequate ventilation, the vascular supply to that area will constrict. This compensation, however, does not always occur in an ideal fashion. In a patient with a $\dot{V}/\dot{Q}$ mismatch, a lung unit is perfused but not ventilated. This is most commonly seen with atelectasis, which may be found in association with pneumonia, pulmonary edema, asthma, and acute lung injury/acute respiratory distress syndrome.

Hypoventilation

Hypoventilation is insufficient ventilation to adequately remove carbon dioxide. This results in hypoxemia via simple displacement: If additional carbon dioxide remains in the alveolus, there is simply not enough space for the oxygen to enter and diffuse.

Multiple conditions may lead to hypoventilation. Sedation with its attendant cardiorespiratory depression, obstructive sleep apnea, and neuromuscular weakness are among the most common causes in children, and hypoventilation may be an important component of impending respiratory failure in children with severe conditions such as pneumonia or asthma, or neonatal respiratory disease. It is important to consider hypoventilation as a cause for hypoxemia in any child who is given supplemental oxygen. The application of supplemental oxygen may correct the Spo_2 in a child with hypoventilation but it does not remedy the root cause of the problem, and may even place the patient at greater risk because of blunting of the hypoxic drive. Patients who have hypoventilation may require ventilatory support, rather than supplemental oxygen alone.

Use of the modified alveolar gas equation (Box 51-1) allows for determination of the alveolar-arterial oxygen gradient, or difference (A-a gradient), which can be useful in circumstances when the cause of hypoxemia is not readily apparent. Solving the equation, using arterial partial pressure of carbon dioxide ($Paco_2$), determined via arterial blood gas, and fraction of inspired oxygen (FIO_2), yields the alveolar partial pressure of oxygen (PAO_2); from this value subtract the Pao_2 (from arterial blood gas). If the A-a oxygen gradient is normal (4–10 mm Hg), then hypoventilation is the only explanation for the patient's hypoxemia.

Box 51-1. The Alveolar Gas Equation[a]

PAO_2	=	**PIO_2 - $PACO_2$/R**
Abbreviations		
PAO_2	=	partial pressure of oxygen in the alveolus, mm Hg
FIO_2	=	fraction of inspired oxygen, percent
PIO_2	=	partial pressure of inspired oxygen
	=	(Barometric pressure – water vapor pressure) x FIO_2
	=	in room air: (760 – 47) x 0.21 = 150, mm Hg
$PACO_2$	=	partial pressure of carbon dioxide in the alveolus, mmHg
R	=	respiratory exchange ratio (CO_2 produced/O_2 absorbed, usually 0.8), no dimensions

[a] Valid if inspired air contains no carbon dioxide. We assume that arterial Pco_2 is equivalent to alveolar Pco_2.

Diffusion Defect

A diffusion defect usually occurs when there is a thickening or disruption of the normal surface area available for gas exchange in the lung. The space across which oxygenation of the blood occurs is less than a micron thick, ideal for gas exchange. At baseline, the red blood cells have plenty of time in which to traverse the pulmonary capillary and receive oxygen from the alveolus. In the healthy individual, this arrangement accommodates states of increased demand, such as exercise, during which the cardiac output increases up to 5-fold and the capillary transit time decreases. In children, true diffusion defects are rare, occurring in conditions such as surfactant dysfunction disorders and pulmonary hemosiderosis. Interstitial lung diseases may also demonstrate diffusion defects, which are often temporary, improving when the underlying disease process resolves.

Shunts

Intrapulmonary shunts result in hypoxemia that can be corrected to an extent by administering oxygen. Hypoxia caused by $\dot{V}/\dot{Q}$ mismatch is corrected by breathing 100% oxygen, whereas true intrapulmonary shunts only partially correct. Oxygen saturation in patients with intracardiac right-to-left shunts does not improve when 100% oxygen is administered.

Changes in Oxygenation at High Altitude

A less frequent cause of hypoxemia is inspiration of a lower concentration of ambient oxygen, which occurs at high altitude or during air travel. (See Chapter 3.) The body's normal compensatory response in the setting of hypoxemia is to increase ventilatory drive. A child with neuromuscular weakness, for example, may not have the strength necessary to initiate and sustain the necessary response successfully. Similarly, individuals who use supplemental oxygen at baseline to maintain a normal saturation may require an increase during air travel. The high altitude simulation test involves the patient breathing air with a known, decreased F_{IO_2} (usually 0.15, which simulates 8,000 feet), calibrated to approximate a pressurized airline cabin. This is accomplished with the patient breathing via a mask, with continual monitoring of Sp_{O_2}, respiratory rate, and heart rate. The body's normal response is to increase minute ventilation to maintain adequate oxygenation. Once it is established that the patient is unfit for air travel on room air, the testing session may be used to calibrate the flow needed by the patient.[2] The cutoff value for initiating supplemental oxygen with flight is controversial.[3]

New Federal Aviation Administration regulations specify that only certain portable oxygen devices may be brought on board for flight. Some of these include conserving devices, which are flow triggered and deliver oxygen only in response to a patient's inhalation. These are sufficient for older children and adults; however, the young child, infant, or child with neuromuscular weakness may not be able to actively trigger this delivery. Therefore, for these children, it is best to procure a portable concentrator with continuous flow. Insurance payment is often a problem with portable concentrators, and families often must pay a short-term rental fee out of pocket.

Clinical Features of Hypoxemia

Signs on Physical Examination

The hypoxic patient may demonstrate cyanosis of the mucous membranes. If a patient is acutely hypoxemic, they will manifest signs of respiratory distress, such as tachypnea, tachycardia, and use of accessory muscles of respiration. One may observe supraclavicular, suprasternal, intercostal, and subcostal retractions, as well as thoracoabdominal asynchrony and nasal flaring. If the patient has been chronically hypoxemic, one may observe digital clubbing.

Evaluation of Hypoxemia

Pulse oximetry is a quick way to assess a patient's degree of hypoxemia. The technology is based on detection of hemoglobin's absorbance of light at 2 wavelengths. Absorbance changes, depending on hemoglobin's percent saturation with oxygen. The oximeter can detect oxygenated and deoxygenated hemoglobin. Of note, standard spectra were developed and assessed using hemoglobin A, complicating somewhat the use of pulse oximetry in individuals with hemoglobinopathies.

Arterial blood gas is an accurate tool assessing oxygenation. It provides direct measurement of Pao_2 and $Paco_2$, as well as pH. Venous blood gas is less useful, because the values obtained may be variable and inconsistent. Capillary gas is somewhat more useful. Mixed venous saturation, obtained directly from a central line or during cardiac catheterization, can provide a measure of oxygen extraction at the tissue level. Because of the potential for error in blood gas measurement, proper collection of the specimen is paramount. The sample should be of sufficient quantity and collected directly into a heparinized syringe that is quickly placed on ice. The quantity of heparin may adversely affect the pH measurement. Care must also be taken not to introduce air into the syringe; an air bubble may falsely elevate the Pao_2 or depress the $Paco_2$.

Cooximetry is useful in determining the cause of a discrepancy between percent saturation and partial pressure of oxygen, as may be seen in carbon monoxide poisoning or methemoglobinemia. Cooximetry uses technology that is similar to pulse oximetry, but evaluates absorbance using multiple wavelengths; thus, the cooximeter determines not only the percent saturation of hemoglobin by oxygen (oxyhemoglobin), but also carboxyhemoglobin and methemoglobin. An individual with carbon monoxide poisoning will often present with bright or cherry red mucous membranes; the blood similarly is bright red. The pulse oximeter will display a normal Spo_2 in the face of a low Pao_2. In contrast, those with methemoglobinemia will appear cyanotic, and the blood specimen will appear chocolate brown; Pao_2 can be normal, but the Spo_2 is low. Anemic patients will often not appear cyanotic, despite a low Pao_2, whereas patients with polycythemia will appear cyanotic at more mild levels of desaturation. Pulse oximetry results are not completely accurate in patients with hemoglobinopathies.

Uses of Oxygen Therapy

In general, the clinical goals of home oxygen therapy include maintaining saturation within a safe range (>92%; possibly higher in children with pulmonary hypertension and lower for children with congenital heart disease), limiting potential complications of hypoxemia, improving symptoms associated with hypoxemia, and promoting sustained adequate growth.[4,5] Optimal somatic growth is crucial for children with lung disease because there is a finite window, usually up to 6 to 8 years of age, in which to grow new alveoli.

The most important consequences of chronic hypoxemia are due to reflex increases in pulmonary vascular resistance leading to pulmonary hypertension and cor pulmonale, increased right-to-left shunting through a patent foramen ovale, and poor growth.[6]

Chronic Oxygen Therapy

Neonatal Chronic Lung Disease

Bronchopulmonary dysplasia (BPD) is defined by the need for supplemental oxygen at 36 weeks' postmenstrual age in the premature infant. Some studies suggest that the incidence of supplemental oxygen dependence in infants with BPD is decreasing,[7] but this may reflect changed practices and new definitions of BPD.[8] In general, prescribing supplemental oxygen in the infant with BPD results in a quicker discharge, improvement in growth, and reduced episodes of desaturation. In addition, prevention of hypoxemia reduces the risk of development of pulmonary hypertension.

Optimal target oxyhemoglobin saturations are still being determined in BPD. Saturation targets of 90% to 92% are well tolerated in the nursery setting and are associated with similar rates of infant growth and development over time. To promote adequate growth and help prevent pulmonary hypertension, American Thoracic Society (ATS) guidelines recommend that in-home oxygen saturation levels be 95% to 99% for children no longer at risk for oxygen-induced retinopathy. These saturations should be maintained while the child is awake and asleep.[5]

Home oxygen is often prescribed for infants with other lung diseases and malformations, such as congenital diaphragmatic hernia.[9] These infants may experience a component of BPD as well because of exposure to high pressures and oxygen concentration while receiving mechanical ventilation.

Cyanotic Heart Disease

Children with cyanotic congenital heart disease usually do not require supplemental oxygen. An exception is the child with cyanotic congenital heart disease and pulmonary hypertension. Supplemental oxygen therapy is used as a palliative measure, to alleviate symptoms, and to promote good growth. (See Chapter 39.)

Pulmonary Hypertension

Pulmonary hypertension may develop secondary to persistent hypoxemia in the context of lung disease, may be idiopathic in nature, or may develop in those with long-standing congenital heart disease. In individuals with lung disease, hypoxemia leads to smooth muscle contraction in pulmonary arteries, with likely endothelial remodeling. Hypoxic crises may be episodic, and the severity of hypoxemia often worsens with stressors such as illness or exercise.

Interstitial Lung Disease

Interstitial lung disease in infants has undergone reclassification over the last several years, and may be referred to as diffuse lung disease of childhood. The conditions that cause diffuse lung disease of childhood are heterogeneous, with a variable age of onset and prognosis, and are quite different from the conditions causing interstitial lung disease in older children and adults. Children with these conditions often require long-term oxygen supplementation throughout infancy, and sometimes through childhood. The goals are similar to oxygen supplementation in infants with BPD: good growth, decreasing the risk of pulmonary hypertension, and alleviating the dyspnea and increased respiratory work associated with hypoxemia.

Obstructive Sleep Apnea

Supplemental oxygen is generally not indicated in obstructive sleep apnea, in which hypoxemia, when it occurs, is due to hypoventilation. Supplemental oxygen may depress the respiratory drive, especially in those children who have hypoventilation as a component of their disease. Positive pressure is more physiologically appropriate in these patients, but some children may not tolerate the interface necessary for delivery of positive pressure. In those cases, it is therefore necessary to weigh the risks of worsened hypoventilation with the benefits of normalizing oxygenation, such as augmented growth and decreased likelihood of developing pulmonary hypertension. Careful titration of optimal supplemental oxygen and monitoring for induced hypoventilation by polysomnogram is necessary.[10]

Short-term Oxygen Therapy

Patients without preexisting pulmonary disease may require short-term oxygen supplementation following an acute illness. In small

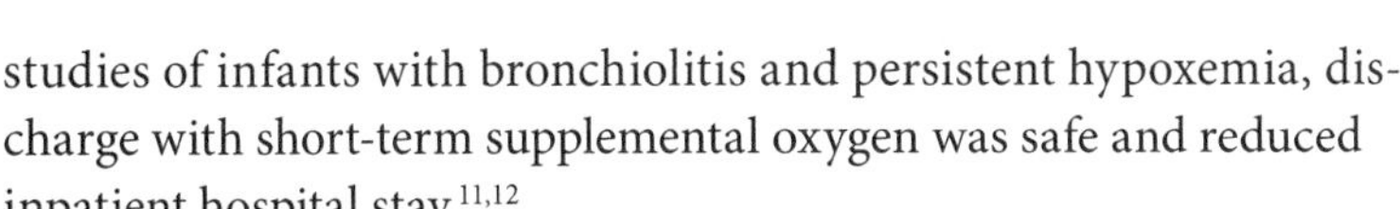

studies of infants with bronchiolitis and persistent hypoxemia, discharge with short-term supplemental oxygen was safe and reduced inpatient hospital stay.[11,12]

Criteria for Discharge With Supplemental Oxygen

Before going home with supplemental oxygen, the child must both maintain stable oxygen levels within his targeted saturation goal and demonstrate sustained adequate growth on a fixed amount of low-flow oxygen. The child's family must be familiar and comfortable with the care plan and have suitable resources in place (eg, for reliable access to electrical sources). Family members should receive training in the care of a child receiving supplemental oxygen, and they must feel secure in providing this care.[5,13] Table 51-1 outlines further concerns and planning for the child discharged on home oxygen.

A pulse oximeter or cardiorespiratory monitor should be used to monitor the child on oxygen at home, during awake and sleeping states, as well as with feeding and activity. A pulse oximeter provides immediate heart rate and oxygen saturation data, but can be fraught with difficulty in the home, as movement artifact causes frequent false alarms and falsely low oxygen saturation readings. The ATS recommends home monitoring for infants with BPD because the children may develop apnea or bradycardia should the flow of oxygen become disrupted and hypoxemia ensue. Parameters for heart rate, respiratory rate, apnea delay, or saturation for the monitoring equipment should be determined based on the needs of the child, in conjunction with the pulmonary specialist. Caregivers should be proficient in the use of this equipment, and they should be aware that most alarms are false alarms, resulting from poor lead placement, shallow respirations or, in the case of pulse oximetry, movement artifact. Should an alarm occur, caregivers first should assess the child, looking for clinical signs of hypoxia.

Successful discharge planning requires a team approach. Often, this begins with a multidisciplinary meeting, including the durable medical equipment company, social work, the child's physician, and the family. The child's family (and the child, if developmentally appropriate) should be educated regarding use and maintenance of all equipment.

Table 51-1. Considerations for Discharge of the Child Requiring Oxygen Therapy[a]

Topic	Teaching Component
Reason for supplemental oxygen need	Disease process, sequelae, management
Assessment	Vital signs (temperature, pulse, respirations) Evaluation of color Breathing pattern Lung auscultation Fluid balance, skin turgor Neurologic status Changes in appetite, behavior Use of pulse oximeter—technique and interpretation
Safety issues	Home safety Smoke-free environment Adequate and safe electrical system Car safety
Nutrition	Feeding schedule Importance of weight gain
Oxygen	Purpose, flow rate Method of administration Reading the flow meter Maintenance and cleaning of equipment Weaning plan and procedure Safety considerations
Emergency management	Who and when to call for symptoms Procedure for emergency assistance CPR technique Telephone numbers posted near phone
Anticipatory guidance	Emotional, social, and financial needs of family Sibling rivalry Rehospitalization
Travel	Transport bag with emergency supplies Air travel with supplemental oxygen

[a] Adapted from Allen J, Zwerdling R, Ehrenkranz R, et al. Statement on the care of the child with chronic lung disease of infancy and childhood. *Am J Respir Crit Care Med.* 2003;168:356–396. Copyright © American Thoracic Society. Reprinted by permission.

The family should be comfortable troubleshooting the cause of equipment alarms. In addition, caregivers should be able to recognize the signs and symptoms of hypoxia and any worsening of the child's baseline pulmonary status. There should be a written care plan to follow, should this occur. Education should occur repeatedly, until caregivers feel comfortable with the child's needs and can demonstrate competency in managing both the child's disease and her accompanying technology.

Special attention should be paid to precautions and safety measures. There should be no smoke exposure in the home. The electrical system should be functional, safe, and able to provide the power necessary to maintain equipment; this assessment may be performed, at least in part, by personnel from the medical equipment company.

Equipment for Oxygen Therapy

Delivery interface and oxygen source must be considered in light of patient size, disease process, and patient and family preference when selecting equipment for an individual patient, both in the inpatient and ambulatory settings.[14] Box 51-2 is a list of equipment typically necessary for home oxygen delivery.

Box 51-2. Typical Equipment for Delivery of Supplemental Oxygen at Home

- For portable use: concentrator, small liquid portable unit, or lightweight compressed gas cylinder
- For home: concentrator, liquid oxygen reservoir, or large compressed gas tank
- Low-flow meter
- Humidification system, if needed
- Appropriately sized cannulae/mask/tubing
- Adhesive to keep cannula in place (tape, "tender grips")
- Stroller with necessary structure to transport concentrator or cylinders
- Pulse oximeter with extra probes

Delivery Interfaces

When prescribing oxygen therapy, the patient's actual FIO_2 is important. Fraction of inspired oxygen is determined by individual patient characteristics, such as size, tidal volume, and breathing pattern (slow or fast, rapid or shallow) and by characteristics of the delivery device (flow, oxygen concentration, amount of room air entrained). Nasal cannulae, for example, entrain, or include, a certain proportion of room air with each breath, lowering the inspired concentration of oxygen. This, however, depends on the patient's tidal volume and flow generated with inspiration. For example, though one cannot practically measure an infant's FIO_2 while receiving 0.25 L/minute of 100% oxygen via nasal cannula, the FIO_2 will be greater than a 2-year-old child receiving the same amount as, proportionally, the 0.25 L/minute comprises a greater proportion of the infant's tidal volume and inspiratory flow.

Low-Flow Devices

Nasal prongs, or cannulae, sit directly in the anterior nares. They are made in several sizes appropriate for infants, children, and adults. Typically, infants can tolerate flows up to 2 L/minute, whereas an older child or adult can tolerate higher flows, up to 4 L/minute. In the hospital setting, these and higher flows may be used; if the air is dry, it will be irritating to the nares, so the air should be humidified. In the home setting, flows are generally lower, so humidification may not be as critical. The prongs must be held in place in infants and young children, typically by using an adhesive to affix tubing to the cheeks. For short-term administration, tape is often sufficient, but for long-term home use, this is often irritating, especially to infant skin. There are tapes made especially for sensitive skin and several different types of gentle adhesives that are applied to the skin that may remain in place for several days. Parents should be cautioned to be especially careful during sleep because prongs may dislodge and infants may become entangled in long cords.

Transtracheal oxygen administration, though better studied in adults, has been used in children successfully, although it is rarely prescribed.[15] For the older child with chronic supplemental oxygen need, the device is more cosmetically appealing, as there is no tubing over the face. Because the oxygen is delivered immediately into the lower airway, a certain amount of dead space is overcome, often allowing for decreased flow rates and overall oxygen usage, but necessitating constant humidification. Risks associated with transtracheal oxygen catheters include infection, mucus plugging and, rarely, frank airway obstruction, in addition to intraoperative risks. The likelihood of mucus plugging decreases with adequate humidification.

High-Flow and Reservoir Devices

There are several mask interfaces that may be used to deliver oxygen therapy, mostly in the inpatient setting. Standard masks have a hole on either side to allow for exhalation and room air entrainment. Oxygen is delivered through a tube at the bottom of the mask and, similar to a nasal cannula, actual FIO_2 depends on patient factors. Venturi masks allow for oxygen to be administered at a set concentration, at high flows. Oxygen is delivered to the mask under high pressure, via high flows. The high flows create a shearing effect, entraining a specific proportion of room air; because the flow often exceeds an individual's peak inspiratory flow, the FIO_2 is more predictable. A non-rebreathing mask administers 100% oxygen using 2 one-way valves, to prevent mixing of delivered supplemental oxygen with both expired gas and entrained room air. This mask achieves the highest FIO_2 (though not 1.0) in an unintubated patient.

Oxygen Sources

Oxygen may be stored and delivered in several ways: compressed gas, in tanks of several sizes; liquid oxygen, contained in a large central reservoir to distribute to smaller tanks for portability; and concentrating devices, which capture oxygen from the air. Each of these systems has its own advantages and disadvantages, and a patient's prescription may include more than one modality, accounting for cost, convenience, and portability.

Compressed gas comes in large and small tanks and is readily available. The family must maintain close contact with their medical equipment company to keep track of when deliveries are needed (Table 51-2 and Table 51-3). A consistent source of power is not a requirement, which makes this a good option in parts of the country where power outages are frequent. If compressed gas is used in the home, it is from a large cylinder, or an "H" cylinder, weighing 200 pounds; it is quite large, and must be secured properly. Portable tanks include the "E" tank, which weighs 22 pounds with a carrier, and the "M" tank, which

Table 51-2. E Cylinder Oxygen Supply Time Guide

	Approximate Time Remaining				
Pressure Gauge Reading	**1 L/min**	**2 L/min**	**3 L/min**	**4 L/min**	**5 L/min**
2000 psi	8 h	4 h	2.5 h	2 h	1.5 h
1500 psi	6.5 h	3 h	2 h	1.5 h	1 h
1000 psi	4 h	2 h	1.25 h	1 h	30 min
500 psi	2 h	1 h	25 min	15 min	5 min

Table 51-3 Approximate Oxygen Tank Duration Times[a]

Flow rate (L/min)	**Use Times (Hours)**							
	1	1.5	2	2.5	3	4	5	6
M4								
Pulse dose	5.7	3.8	2.9	2.3	1.9	1.4	1.1	.9
Continuous flow	1.9	1.3	.9	.7	.6	.5	.4	.3
M6								
Pulse dose	8.3	5.5	4.1	3.3	2.8	2.1	1.7	1.4
Continuous flow	2.7	1.8	1.4	1.1	.9	.7	.6	.4
ML6								
Pulse dose	8.6	5.7	4.3	3.4	2.9	2.1	1.7	1.4
Continuous flow	2.8	1.9	1.4	1.1	.9	.7	.6	.4
C								
Pulse dose	12.1	8.1	6.1	4.9	4.0	3.0	2.4	2.0
Continuous flow	4.0	2.7	2.0	1.6	1.3	1.0	.8	.7
D								
Pulse dose	21.0	14.0	10.5	8.4	7.0	5.2	4.2	3.5
Continuous flow	6.9	4.6	3.5	2.8	2.3	1.7	1.4	1.2
E								
Pulse dose	34.4	23.0	17.2	13.8	11.5	8.6	6.9	5.8
Continuous flow	11.4	7.6	5.7	4.6	3.8	2.8	2.3	1.9

[a] Ranges are calculated assuming 20 breaths per minute and a full tank.

is much lighter, at 4 pounds. The tanks must be secured and kept from potential fire sources. Another option is a filling system, which uses a concentrator to maintain a reservoir of gas, which may be transferred into a compressed gas cylinder; the availability of this system is more limited and requires electrical power.

Liquid oxygen is based on a reservoir system, with a large device maintained in the home, which must be refilled periodically. Parents fill smaller tanks for travel purposes. Similar to compressed gas, parents must be alert to when they will need replenishment. Liquid oxygen requires no electricity for maintenance.

Concentrators are the most economical of oxygen delivery devices, because they do not require deliveries or refilling. They function by taking oxygen from the ambient air; however, they do require electricity to function, a cost that must be absorbed by the patient. One must use caution in prescribing these devices to small or weak patients, as the delivery of oxygen may not be constant, but flow-triggered. Small infants, especially, often cannot generate the inspiratory force necessary for oxygen to be delivered. If patients are to travel by air, they likely will need to use a concentrator. Patients should be observed using these devices prior to travel.

Monitoring

A pulse oximeter is a useful tool for families to use to become familiar with a child's normal baseline, heart rate, and oxygen saturation. Often, tachycardia may be the first sign of distress. Tracking the child's normal values, especially resting heart and respiratory rates, in conjunction with oxygen saturation, provides trends that may be used to begin the weaning process. This information, though useful, is not always necessary. In conjunction with the child's medical equipment company, downloads of pulse oximeter data over a night of sleep can provide accurate oxygen saturation and heart rate. The quality of data is variable, however, and must be interpreted with caution. In special situations, polysomnography, in a laboratory familiar with pediatric patients, may provide a more accurate record of overnight oxygenation, and provides a full picture of the child's respiratory status with sleep, including variation in heart and respiratory rates, end-tidal carbon dioxide levels, and differences with sleep stages.

Oxygen Weaning

There are no evidence-based guidelines for the weaning process, though ATS guidelines provide a useful approach and algorithm (Figure 51-2). There is significant variability in practice, monitoring, and assessment.[16] Oxygen needs during wakefulness are often less than that during sleep. Thus, as a first step in the weaning process, a trial of supplemental oxygen may be performed with the child awake in a monitored setting, such as during a prolonged visit to a physician's office, with the child monitored both clinically and with pulse oximetry. Once the child has been weaned to room air while awake, and has tolerated this well for a period at home, demonstrating continued good growth and acceptable oxygen saturation, then oxygen weaning during sleep can be attempted. It should be remembered that oxygen levels while awake do not accurately reflect oxygen levels during sleep. Nighttime weaning requires at least a review of downloadable readings from overnight pulse oximeter monitoring, and is done most accurately in a pediatric sleep laboratory.

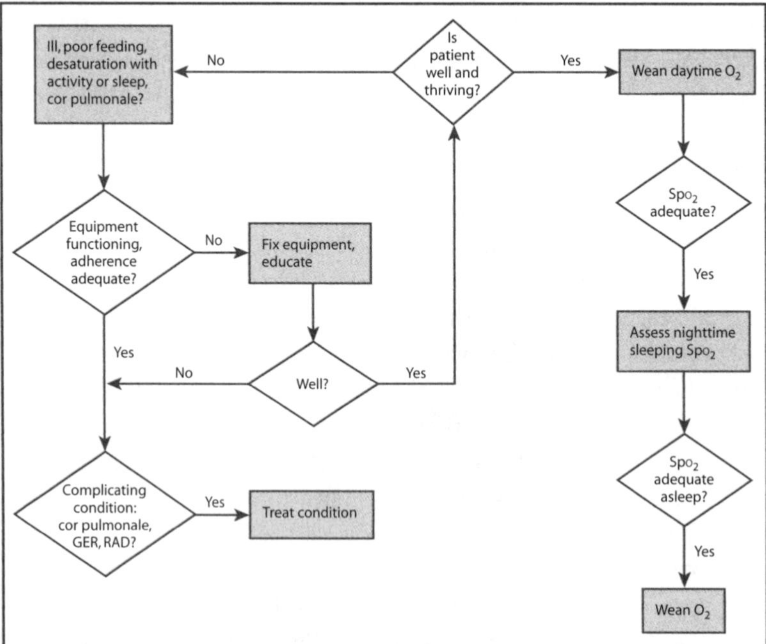

Figure 51-2. An approach to weaning supplemental oxygen in the child with chronic lung disease. GER, gastroesophageal reflux; RAD, reactive airway disease; Spo_2, oxyhemoglobin saturation. (Adapted from Allen J, [a]Adapted from Allen J, Zwerdling R, Ehrenkranz R, et al. Statement on the care of the child with chronic lung disease of infancy and childhood. *Am J Respir Crit Care Med.* 2003;168:356–396. Copyright © American Thoracic Society. Reprinted by permission.)

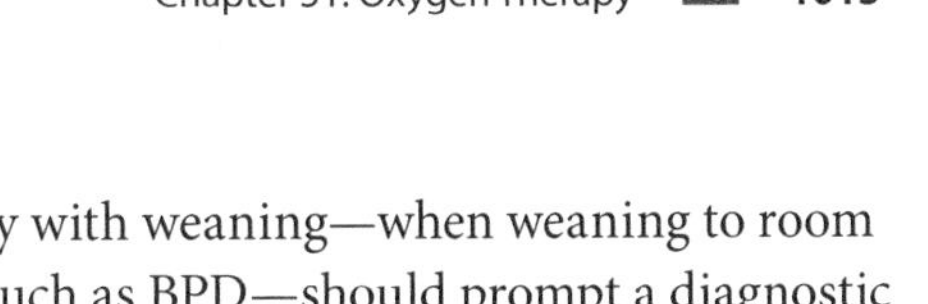

Failure to progress successfully with weaning—when weaning to room air is expected, in conditions such as BPD—should prompt a diagnostic workup for other conditions, including aspiration of gastric or oral contents, gastroesophageal reflux, airway malformations, pulmonary hypertension, and congenital heart disease.

When to Refer

- Documented persistent hypoxemia or frequent episodes of subnormal oxyhemoglobin saturation
- Any child requiring chronic supplemental oxygen
- Intermittent desaturation during pneumogram or polysomnogram
- Poor growth despite adequate caloric intake

When to Admit

- Documented persistent significant increase in supplemental oxygen requirement, despite additional airway clearance and other measures
- Significant signs and symptoms of respiratory distress, such as accessory muscle use
- For children receiving supplemental oxygen at home, the threshold for hospitalization may be individualized. In certain circumstances, particularly if the patient has only a mild illness, and if there is significant nursing support in the home, then pulmonary care, including increased oxygen administration and airway clearance, may escalate safely without hospitalization. In these cases, there must be close communication between the child's home care provider and pulmonary specialist or pediatrician. For example, some children will require supplemental oxygen only with sleep when in usual health; with an intercurrent viral illness, the child may require supplemental oxygen during the day as well. If there is adequate monitoring in the home, and if adequate communication occurs between family, home care providers, and physicians, this works quite well. Should this occur, the child should be evaluated by her physician on an ambulatory basis. If there is any concern about the patient's stability, then it is best to err on the side of caution and hospitalize the patient for closer evaluation.

Key Points

- The number of children with complex respiratory care provided in the home setting is increasing, so the general pediatrician must be familiar with equipment such as supplemental oxygen and attendant home monitoring requirements.
- The 5 causes of hypoxemia are $\dot{V}/\dot{Q}$ mismatch, hypoventilation, diffusion defect, ascent to high altitude, and shunt; of these, $\dot{V}/\dot{Q}$ mismatch is the most common.
- Administering supplemental oxygen without also investigating the root cause may mask hypoventilation; the alveolar gas equation helps to differentiate hypoventilation from other causes of hypoxemia.
- A patient's required F_{IO_2} is determined by her size, tidal volume, underlying lung disease, and mode of supplemental oxygen delivery. An infant, for example, receiving 2 L/minute of oxygen via nasal cannula has a significantly higher F_{IO_2} than an adult receiving the same.
- Family education is vital.
- Open lines of communication between primary care provider, medical equipment company, nursing agency, pulmonary specialist, and families are essential for the success of home supplemental oxygen therapy.

Related AAP Policy Statements

American Academy of Pediatrics Committee on Child Health Financing, Section on Home Care. Financing of pediatric home health care. *Pediatrics.* 2006;118(2):834–838

American Academy of Pediatrics Committee on Fetus and Newborn. Apnea, sudden infant death syndrome, and home monitoring. *Pediatrics.* 2003;111(4):914–917

American Academy of Pediatrics Committee on Fetus and Newborn. Hospital discharge of the high-risk neonate—proposed guidelines. *Pediatrics.* 1998;102(2):411–417

Higgins RD, Bancalari E, Willinger M, Raju TNK. Executive summary of the Workshop on Oxygen in Neonatal Therapies: controversies and opportunities for research. *Pediatrics.* 2007;119(4):790–796

Useful Web Resources

http://www.portableoxygen.org/

http://www.thoracic.org/sections/education/patient-education/patient-education-materials/patient-information-series/oxygen-therapy.html

http://www.thoracic.org/sections/copd/for-health-professionals/management-of-stable-copd/long-term-oxygen-therapy/oxygen-sources-and-delivery-devices.html

References

1. West JB. *Respiratory Physiology: The Essentials.* Philadelphia, PA: Lippincott, Williams and Wilkins; 2005
2. Dine CJ, Kreider ME. Hypoxia altitude simulation test. *Chest.* 2008;133(4):1002–1005
3. Martin AC, Verheggen M, Stick SM, et al. Definition of cutoff values for the hypoxia test used for preflight testing in young children with neonatal chronic lung disease. *Chest.* 2008;133(4)914–919
4. Moyer-Mileur LJ, Nielson DW, Pfeffer KD, et al. Eliminating sleep-associated hypoxemia improves growth in infants with bronchopulmonary dysplasia. *Pediatrics.* 1996;98:779–783
5. Allen J, Zwerdling R, Ehrenkranz R, et al. Statement on the care of the child with chronic lung disease of infancy and childhood. *Am J Respir Crit Care Med.* 2003;168:356–396
6. Poets CF. When do infants need additional inspired oxygen? A review of the current literature. *Pediatr Pulmonol.* 1998;26:424–428
7. Geary C, Caskey M, Fonseca R, Malloy M. Decreased incidence of broncho-pulmonary dysplasia after early management changes, including surfactant and nasal continuous positive airway pressure treatment at delivery, lowered oxygen saturation goals, and early amino acid administration: a historical cohort study. *Pediatrics.* 2008;121(1):89–96
8. Davis PG, Thorpe K, Roberts R, et al. Evaluating "old" definitions for the "new" bronchopulmonary dysplasia. *J Pediatr.* 2002;140:555–560
9. American Academy of Pediatrics Section on Surgery, Committee on Fetus and Newborn. Postdischarge follow-up of infants with congenital diaphragmatic hernia. *Pediatrics.* 2008;121(3):627–632
10. Marcus CL, Carroll JL, Bamford O, et al. Supplemental oxygen during sleep in children with sleep-disordered breathing. *Am J Respir Crit Care Med.* 1995;152:1297–1301
11. Joseph L, Goldberg S, Picard E. A randomized trial of home oxygen therapy from the emergency department for acute bronchiolitis. *Pediatrics.* 2006;118(3):1319–1320

12. Tie SW, Hall GL, Peter S, et al. Home oxygen for children with acute bronchiolitis. *Arch Dis Child.* 2009;94(8):641–643
13. Gracey K, Talbot D, Lankford R, et al. The changing face of bronchopulmonary dysplasia: part 2. Discharging an infant home on oxygen. *Adv Neonatal Care.* 2003;3:88–98
14. Myers TR; American Association for Respiratory Care. AARC clinical practice guideline: selection of an oxygen delivery device for neonatal and pediatric patients—2002 revision and update. *Respir Care.* 2002;47(6):707–716
15. Preciado DA, Pantich HB, Thatcher G, Rimell FL. Transtracheal oxygen catheters in a pediatric population. *Ann Otlo Rhinol Laryngol.* 2002;111:310–314
16. Solis A, Harrison G, Shaw BN. Assessing oxygen requirement after discharge in chronic lung disease: a survey of current practice. *Eur J Pediatr.* 2002;161:428–430

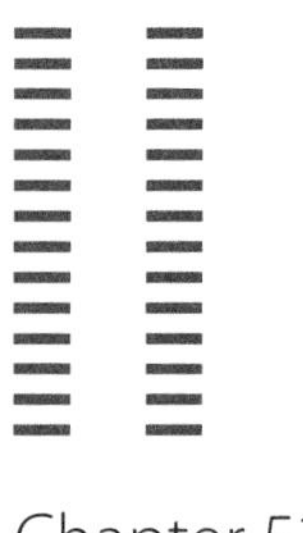

Chapter 52

Secondhand Tobacco Smoke Exposure and Active Smoking in Childhood and Adolescence

Marianna Sockrider, MD, DrPH, FAAP
Harold J. Farber, MD, MSPH, FAAP

Introduction

The United States Surgeon General's Report finds, "Massive and conclusive scientific evidence documents adverse effects of involuntary smoking on children and adults, including cancer and cardiovascular diseases in adults, and adverse respiratory effects in both children and adults."[1] Tobacco smoke is a complex air pollutant that is made up of more than 4,000 substances, including respiratory irritants, toxins, and carcinogens.[1] While the rate of adult tobacco smoking has declined in the United States in recent years, children's secondhand smoke (SHS) exposure remains common.

The American Academy of Pediatrics recommends that pediatricians ask about and document tobacco use and SHS exposure at all clinical encounters, know the harms of tobacco use and SHS exposure and educate patients and their families about those harms, and routinely offer help and referral to those who use tobacco—even if the person is not your patient.[2] Pediatric health care providers also have important responsibilities to advocate for public policies to decrease and eliminate children's SHS exposure and risk for becoming tobacco dependent. These recommendations are summarized in Table 52-1.[3]

Table 52-1. Pediatric Health Care Provider Actions to Prevent Tobacco Exposure[a]

Clinical Practice	Public Policy
Ask about and document tobacco use and secondhand smoke exposure at all clinical encounters.	Advocate for tobacco-free indoor and outdoor public places, particularly for environments in which children learn, live, and play, such as schools, multiunit housing, public parks, child care settings, public beaches, sidewalks, restaurants, and sporting arenas.
Discuss the dangers of second-hand smoke exposure with parents and encourage parents to stop smoking.	Advocate for health care and educational facilities to be completely tobacco-free, inside and outside, at all times.
Routinely offer help with nicotine dependence and referral to those who use tobacco—even if the person is not your patient.	Advocate for all public and private health insurance to provide coverage for comprehensive tobacco cessation treatment.
Encourage families to establish smoking bans in their homes and cars.	Advocate for local, state, and federal authorities to promote programs that contribute to the prevention and decrease of tobacco use by youth, including programs that discourage tobacco use, support antitobacco advertising, and teach skills to resist peer and advertising influences.
Provide anticipatory guidance to children about the dangers of smoking and smoke exposure, starting by age 5 years.	Support tobacco prevention programs in schools.
Maintain a smoke-free office. Eliminate tobacco advertising from all materials associated with your clinical practice, including magazines and other media in patient care and waiting areas.	• Marketing of tobacco products should be banned from all media, events, and venues, including the Internet. • Sales of candy cigarettes, cigars, and other products that imitate tobacco products or smoking should be banned. • Exposure to and depiction of tobacco use should be reduced in films, videos, DVDs, and television programs. A film that shows or implies tobacco use should be given a Motion Picture Association of America rating of R or greater.

[a] Adapted from American Academy of Pediatrics Committee on Environmental Health, Committee on Substance Abuse, Committee on Adolescence, and Committee On Native American Child Health.[3]

Prenatal Effects of Maternal Active and SHS Exposure

Involuntary exposure to tobacco can begin in the womb. Nicotine, carbon monoxide, and other tobacco smoke toxins readily cross the placenta. Given the developmental processes in progress, fetuses as well as young children are considered to be at greater risk of adverse effects of SHS exposure than adults.[1] Maternal smoking increases risk for premature birth and decreases birth weight, with clear dose-response effects demonstrated.[1]

Secondhand maternal smoke exposure also impacts the fetus. Increased risk for preterm birth and lower birth weight have been documented.[1,4] A study of pregnant African-American women exposed to SHS reduced rates of very low birth weight and prematurity using a cognitive-behavioral intervention to reduce SHS exposure.[6]

Maternal smoking increases a child's risk for wheezing illnesses, including bronchiolitis and asthma.[7,8] How much of the risk is from in-utero versus postnatal smoke exposure is difficult to sort out as maternal smoking is often the largest contributor to a child's smoke exposure both in utero and subsequently.[9] Active maternal smoking during pregnancy increases the risk for asthma in infants and preschool children.[10,11] In-utero exposures from maternal smoking may affect lung development. In-utero exposure to maternal smoking is associated with decreased lung function in childhood.[12–14]

Active maternal smoking is associated with increased risk for orofacial clefts and has possible associations with congenital heart defects, particularly septal and right-sided obstructive defects.[1] Adverse effects of in-utero or postnatal exposure to SHS on neuropsychological development have also been postulated. Numerous components of SHS, including nicotine and carbon monoxide, may produce these effects. A review of 16 longitudinal studies showed that most found cognitive deficits among children whose mothers smoked during pregnancy.[15] However, the sizes of the effects were small, and the long-term consequences remain unclear.

Sudden Infant Death Syndrome and SHS Exposure

Risk for sudden infant death syndrome (SIDS) is increased by both active and secondhand maternal smoking during pregnancy,[1,16,17] with reduced arousal responses[18] and reduced recovery from hypoxic challenge[19] as likely mechanisms to account for this risk. An estimated

25% to 40% of SIDS cases are related to smoking during pregnancy. The relationship between smoking during pregnancy and SIDS was studied prospectively in 24,986 Danish infants.[17] Compared with the children of nonsmokers, the children of smokers had more than 3 times the risk of SIDS; the risk of SIDS increased with the number of cigarettes smoked per day.

Lower Respiratory Problems and SHS Exposure

Lung Function

Secondhand smoke exposure is associated with reduced lung function (as assessed by reduced forced expiratory flows) from birth forward.[1,12–14,20,21] Studies on rodents show that in-utero smoke exposure reduces alveolar numbers and simplifies alveolar structure.[22] These children will enter adulthood with less pulmonary reserve. Children of smokers are more likely to become smokers and thus face risk of further impairment from active smoking.[1]

Respiratory Infections

Infants with parents who smoke have an increased risk of lower respiratory tract illness, including bronchiolitis, bronchitis, and pneumonia.[1,7,23,24] The finding of an association between parental smoking and lower respiratory infections is consistent across diverse study populations, study designs, and diagnostic groupings.[1] Most studies have shown that maternal smoking rather than paternal smoking contributes the predominant component of the increased risk associated with parental smoking, as maternal and caregiver smoking are the greatest contributors to a child's tobacco smoke exposure.[1,9] Nonetheless, studies from countries such as Vietnam and Hong Kong, where women rarely smoke, show that paternal smoking alone can increase the incidence of lower respiratory illness.[25,26] The mechanisms for these risks are complex and likely reflect both prenatal effects on lung development as well as postnatal injury from SHS exposure. These mechanisms operate to make respiratory infections more severe or to possibly increase the likelihood of infection.[1]

Respiratory Symptoms

Numerous surveys demonstrate a greater frequency of the most common respiratory symptoms—cough, phlegm, and wheeze—in the children of smokers.[1,11,27,28] The highest risks for these symptoms occurred in children with 2 parents who smoked. The less prominent effects compared with infant risks may reflect lower exposures to SHS by older children who spend less time with their parents. However, there is sufficient evidence to support this association even in school-aged children.[1]

Asthma and Other Lung Diseases

Exposure to SHS is associated with increased asthma prevalence and severity. Although the underlying mechanisms remain to be fully identified, the epidemiologic evidence linking SHS exposure and childhood asthma is substantial.[1,7,11,12,29,30–32] A significant excess of childhood asthma occurs if both parents or the mother smoke. A dose-response relationship exists between SHS and childhood asthma, and no defined threshold level of exposure is without risk.[32] A study in Germany suggests this excess occurs primarily in children with allergic predisposition.[33] Exposure to SHS during childhood is also associated with increased prevalence of asthma in adults.[34]

Exposure to SHS worsens the status of children with asthma. Population studies also have shown increased airway responsiveness for SHS-exposed children with asthma.[1] Exposure to smoking in the home increases the number of emergency department visits made by children with asthma. Inhaled and oral corticosteroid responsiveness is decreased for exposed children with asthma.[35]

Reducing parental smoking can result in reduced asthma morbidity and decreased airway hyperreactivity.[36,37] Parents frequently misperceive a child's level of smoke exposure and may not recognize tobacco smoke as a trigger if the child does not have immediate symptoms.[25] Children with pulmonary problems such as cystic fibrosis may experience greater adverse effects on lung function from regular SHS exposure.[38] Parents may underreport exposure in children with respiratory diseases.[39]

Otitis Media and SHS Exposure

Secondhand smoke exposure is associated with increased risk for otitis media, with the strongest effects demonstrated for recurrent otitis media and maternal smoking.[1] Risk of acute infections remained even after tympanostomy surgery in infants with SHS exposure.[40]

Resolution of severe chronic otitis media with effusion (glue ear) was prolonged by parental smoking, irrespective of adenoidectomy or ventilation tube insertion.[41]

Dental Caries and SHS exposure

Exposure to SHS may be associated with an increased risk of dental caries in children. A cross-sectional study in 3,531 children ages 4 to 11 found that elevated serum cotinine levels were associated with caries in deciduous but not permanent teeth in a multivariate model.[42]

Cancer Risk and SHS Exposure

There is limited evidence suggesting a causal relationship between prenatal and postnatal exposure to SHS and childhood cancers.[1,43,44] Studies of leukemia, the most common cancer in children, and SHS exposure are mixed, and further research is needed to determine if a significant association exists.[44] The consequences of SHS exposure in childhood may not be realized until later in life. Numerous studies have concluded that SHS exposure in any location, including workplace or home, is a cause of lung cancer among lifetime nonsmoker adults.[1] The pooled evidence indicates a 20% to 30% increased risk of lung cancer associated with living with a smoker.[1] There has been some evidence to suggest that childhood exposure increases risk of cancer in adulthood; however, the studies are limited in part by potential recall misclassification of childhood exposure and additional SHS exposure during adulthood.[1,45]

Cardiovascular Risk and SHS Exposure

Causal associations between active smoking and coronary heart disease (CHD) outcomes have long been demonstrated.[1] The risk of CHD in active smokers increases with the amount and duration of cigarette smoking and decreases quickly with cessation. Although the strength of SHS exposure on a child's future risk of cardiovascular disease requires further study, growing evidence suggests it is a risk. Evidence is also growing regarding the mechanisms through which SHS exposure may contribute to cardiovascular disease. For example, exposure to SHS has been found to be associated with subtle changes in endothelial function, which are in turn associated with atherogenesis, as well as decreased high-density lipoprotein cholesterol.[46] Parental health behaviors such as tobacco smoking can influence their children's adverse health behaviors that increase risk of cardiovascular disease.[47]

Thirdhand Smoke Exposure

Thirdhand smoke exposure is the exposure that a child gets from contact with surfaces that have absorbed smoke exposure. Residual nicotine and other substances can also form other carcinogenic substances. The persistence of these substances represents an unappreciated health hazard through dermal exposure, dust inhalation, and ingestion. Discussion of this exposure risk may be a further incentive for families to adopt home nonsmoking policies.[47,48]

Screening for SHS Exposure

Screening questions to identify children with SHS exposure should be used routinely in clinical practice (Box 52-1). Ask whether a child is regularly exposed to smoke. Screen for any adults who smoke living in the child's home. If there are smokers or the child is exposed, make time to discuss individualized risks and control measures that can be undertaken. Assess readiness to quit and offer help to the parent who smokes. See Chapter 53 for more about tobacco dependence treatment for parents.

Exposure to SHS can be estimated by measuring the biomarker cotinine. Cotinine is a sensitive and specific biomarker of tobacco product exposure and reflects the prior 4 days of exposure.[49] It can be measured

Box 52-1. Screening for Secondhand Smoke Exposure in Pediatric Practice[a]

Questions to Ask

1. Does anyone who lives with (name of child) use tobacco?
2. Does anyone who provides care for (name of child) use tobacco?
3. Does (name of child) visit places where people use tobacco?

Charting Stamp

Tobacco use exposure from

___ Person(s) who lives in the home

___ Person(s) who provides child care

___ Places the child visits

[a] Adapted from Sachs DPL; 2010. Reprinted with permission.

in urine, saliva, and blood and other tissues. When using a urine cotinine assay to assess for SHS exposure, it is important that the assay used detects cotinine levels as low as 2 ng/mL.[49] The clinical benefit of routine urine cotinine measurement is not well established. There have been few studies incorporating feedback about child cotinine levels; however, feedback without smoking cessation behavioral counseling showed no benefit.[37,50,51]

Anticipatory Guidance and SHS Exposure

Anticipatory guidance is a key part of well-child care and has been incorporated with the National Cancer Institute's algorithm for tobacco control, now the "5 As"[51] (Box 52-2). This is a useful mnemonic for pediatric health care providers in smoking counseling.

Reducing SHS exposure in the home and car is critical since the home and car are major locations of children's exposure. Pediatricians should encourage parents to maintain a smoke-free home and car. Smoking should be kept well away from doors, windows, and any area where children are playing. Children who grow up in a smoke-free home will be less likely to start smoking as adolescents.[53] Household smoking bans can be helpful even when parents are smokers. A smoke-free home is also associated with increased smoking cessation and decreased cigarette consumption in adult smokers.[54] A smoking ban must be strictly enforced in order for it to be effective. Pediatric health care providers can access resources to help promote smoke-free homes at the Environmental Protection Agency Web site (www.epa.gov).[55]

Box 52-2. The 5 As of Tobacco Use Prevention[a]

- Anticipatory guidance—address tobacco use and exposure as a part of well-child care.
- Ask about smoking activity and secondhand smoke exposure.
- Advise nonsmoking, avoidance of exposure, and smoking cessation.
- Assist in eliminating tobacco use exposure and smoking cessation efforts.
- Arrange follow-up to provide reinforcement and support.

[a] Adapted from Epps and Manley.[51]

Tobacco Smoking Behavior in Children and Teens

Childhood is the time when most people who will become regular smokers first start. More than 80% of current adult tobacco users started smoking cigarettes before age 18 years.[3] While smoking rates have declined in adolescents, the best opportunity to prevent future morbidity and mortality from tobacco is to prevent smoking initiation. Risk factors for acquisition of tobacco dependence include previous smoking experimentation and lack of a firm decision not to smoke. Pediatric health care providers should work with parents early to engage them in actions that will help prevent smoking behavior in their children.

In addition to smoking cigarettes, many teens use other forms of tobacco, including chewing tobacco (dip), snuff, bidis, kreteks, snus, hookahs, and electronic cigarettes (e-cigarettes). Some teens may be misinformed about the dangers of smokeless tobacco. It is important to screen for all forms of tobacco use, as teens and parents may fail to mention other forms of tobacco when asked about smoking.

Peers

Peers' attitudes and behavior with regard to smoking are a strong influence on smoking experimentation and development of tobacco dependence. Teens with friends who smoke are more likely to experiment with smoking and become regular smokers.[56]

Parents

Parental smoking behavior is a strong predictor of teen smoking behavior. Children whose parents smoke are more likely to smoke, particularly if both parents smoke. Parents can also be positive role models. Parents who quit smoking are less likely to have their children become smokers. The earlier in the child's life the parent quits, the less likely the child will smoke. Adolescents who perceive strong parental disapproval of smoking are less likely to smoke and more resistant to the influence of peer smoking.[57] Parental use of positive family management can also reduce teen smoking.[56]

Low Socioeconomic Status and Education

Lower socioeconomic status is associated with higher rates of smoking in teens. It has been observed that students living in ZIP codes with a low mean education level were more likely to smoke. Poor school performance, skipping school, and higher rates of school absence are associated with higher risk of adolescent smoking.[56,57]

Emotional/Mental Health and Expectations

Teens with depressive or anxiety symptoms are more likely to become smokers.[58,59] Teens can have expectations regarding the benefits of smoking that influence smoking initiation, such as relaxation and stress reduction or weight control and appetite suppression, which may vary by gender.[60]

Other Behaviors

Youth antisocial behavior is a risk factor for progression to daily smoking.[56] Teens' use of alcohol and/or marijuana is associated with tobacco smoking. Engaging in unprotected intercourse has also been shown to be correlated with early smoking initiation among females.[61] In contrast, teens who attend religious activities[57] and those who feel it is important to contribute to their community are less likely to smoke.[61]

Marketing and Media Influences

The role of the media on smoking experimentation and regular smoking among teens has been described in a growing number of studies and is a reflection of the aggressive marketing efforts of the tobacco industry.[62] Owning or willingness to own tobacco promotional items and having a favorite cigarette advertisement are risk factors for regular teen smoking.[57] The Smoking Prevention and Tobacco Control Act of 2009 has expanded the US Food and Drug Administration's ability to regulate tobacco products and the advertising and promotion of such products.[63] This is a significant advancement in smoking prevention, and pediatric health care providers should continue to support legislative efforts and enforcement at state and local levels.

Anticipatory Guidance and Smoking Prevention

Pediatric health care providers should screen for active tobacco use at every opportunity. Smoking can start as young as 8 years. Health risk behavior screening should be done with the teen separately from the parents. Confidentiality should be established early in the discussion, outlining what information must be shared with a parent and offering to help the teen talk with the parent if needed.

Some of the reasons teens cite as motivation to quit can also be used to help dissuade teens from becoming smokers. Tobacco smoking is a costly habit—helping teens calculate the costs of current and future smoking may provide an incentive to quit or not start. Teens can have concerns about current health and cosmetic effects, such as bad breath and reduced athletic performance. Discussing a teen's goals with respect to sports may be valuable. Recreational sports activity has been associated with greater success in smoking cessation. Provide guidance in healthy ways to concerns such as stress management and weight control.

Teen Smoking Cessation and Nicotine Dependence

Many teens who smoke indicate an interest in quitting, though only a small percentage stop smoking without help. Just as peers influence smoking behavior, friends may also have a role in supporting smoking cessation, particularly if they are nonsmokers themselves. Talk with the teen about friends' behavior and willingness to help. School-based multi-session behaviorally based programs for tobacco-dependent teenagers, such as American Lung Association's Not-On-Tobacco program, have shown some benefit in facilitating smoking cessation, although brief interventions can be useful, particularly with adolescents who use fewer cigarettes.[64,65]

Nicotine dependence can develop early, even before the onset of regular smoking. Teens can have withdrawal symptoms with attempts at smoking cessation. Research on tobacco dependence treatment of adolescents is limited. Studies of nicotine patch combined with cognitive behavioral counseling for tobacco-dependent teens who wanted to quit did show effectiveness.[66] While further research in treating adolescent tobacco dependence is needed, it is reasonable to apply treatment strategies demonstrated to be effective in adults to teens. Close follow-up is essential. Effective tobacco dependence treatment prevents a lifetime of tobacco-related morbidity and premature mortality. See Chapter 53 for a discussion of tobacco dependence treatment.

Key Points

- Active smoking and secondhand tobacco smoke exposure (prenatal and postnatal) have substantial adverse health effects on children from conception through adolescence and beyond.
- Pediatric health care providers should take an active role in addressing tobacco smoke exposure and smoking prevention through clinical practice and advocacy efforts. These actions are outlined in Table 52-1.
- Screening for exposure and tobacco use should be done at every clinic visit. Pediatric health care providers should follow the "5 As" approach (Box 51-2) in counseling patients and families. Pediatric health care providers can assist smokers in quitting and guide children to healthy behaviors.
- Providers need to be advocates for legislation and community action to reduce the incidence of tobacco dependence and reduce the risk for involuntary tobacco smoke exposure, both locally and worldwide.

Related American Academy of Pediatrics Policy Statements

American Academy of Pediatrics Committee on Environmental Health, Committee on Substance Abuse, Committee on Adolescence, Committee on Native American Child Health. Tobacco use: a pediatric disease. *Pediatrics.* 2009;124:1474–1487

Best D; American Academy of Pediatrics Committee on Environmental Health, Committee on Native American Child Health, Committee on Adolescence. Secondhand and prenatal tobacco smoke exposure. *Pediatrics.* 2009;124(5):e1017–e1044. http://aappolicy.aappublications.org/cgi/content/abstract/pediatrics;124/5/e1017. Accessed November 8, 2010

Sims TH; American Academy of Pediatrics Committee on Substance Abuse. Tobacco as a substance of abuse. *Pediatrics.* 2009;124(5):e1045–e1053. http://aappolicy.aappublications.org/cgi/content/abstract/pediatrics;124/5/e1045. Accessed November 8, 2010

References

1. US Department of Health and Human Services. *The Health Consequences of Involuntary Exposure to Tobacco Smoke: A Report of the Surgeon General.* Atlanta, GA: US Department of Health and Human Services, Centers for Disease Control and Prevention, Coordinating Center for Health Promotion, National Center for Chronic Disease Prevention and Health Promotion, Office on Smoking and Health; 2006
2. World Health Organization International Agency for Research on Cancer. *Tobacco Smoke and Involuntary Smoking.* Geneva, Switzerland: IARC Press; 2004. *IARC Monographs on the Evaluation of Carcinogenic Risks to Humans;* vol 83. http://monographs.iarc.fr/ENG/Monographs/vol83/mono83.pdf. Accessed April 24, 2010
3. American Academy of Pediatrics Committee on Environmental Health, Committee on Substance Abuse, Committee on Adolescence, Committee on Native American Child Health. Tobacco use: a pediatric disease. *Pediatrics.* 2009;124:1474–1487
4. Jaakkola JJ, Jaakkola N, Zahlsen K. Fetal growth and length of gestation in relation to prenatal exposure to environmental tobacco smoke assessed by hair nicotine concentration. *Environ Health Perspect.* 2001;109(6):557–561
5. El-Mohandes AA, Kiely M, Blake SM, et al. An intervention to reduce environmental tobacco smoke exposure improves pregnancy outcomes. *Pediatrics.* 2010;125(4):721–728
6. Bradley JP, Bacharier LB, Bonfiglio J, et al. Severity of respiratory syncytial virus bronchiolitis is affected by cigarette smoke exposure and atopy. *Pediatrics.* 2005;115(1):e7–e14
7. Farber HJ, Wattigney W, Berenson G. Trends in asthma prevalence: the Bogalusa Heart Study. *Ann Allergy Asthma Immunol.* 1997;78(3):265–269
8. Farber HJ, Knowles SB, Brown NL, et al. Secondhand tobacco smoke in children with asthma: sources of and parental perceptions about exposure in children and parental readiness to change. *Chest.* 2008;133(6):1367–1374
9. Young S, Le Souef PN, Geelhoed GC, et al. The influence of a family history of asthma and parental smoking on airway responsiveness in early infancy. *N Engl J Med.* 1991;324:1168
10. Xepapadaki P, Manios Y, Liarigkovinos T, et al. Association of passive exposure of pregnant women to environmental tobacco smoke with asthma symptoms in children. *Pediatr Allergy Immunol.* 2009;20(5):423–429
11. Wang L, Pinkerton KE. Detrimental effects of tobacco smoke exposure during development on postnatal lung function and asthma. *Birth Defects Res C Embryo Today.* 2008;84(1):54–60
12. Young S, Sherrill DL, Arnott J, et al. Parental factors affecting respiratory function during the first year of life. *Pediatr Pulmonol.* 2000;29(5):331–340
13. Gilliland FD, Berhane K, McConnell R, et al. Maternal smoking during pregnancy, environmental tobacco smoke exposure and childhood lung function. *Thorax.* 2000;55:271

14. Lassen K, Oei, TP. Effects of maternal cigarette smoking during pregnancy on long-term physical and cognitive parameters of child development. *Addict Behav.* 1998;23:635
15. Pollack HA. Sudden infant death syndrome, maternal smoking during pregnancy, and the cost-effectiveness of smoking cessation intervention. *Am J Public Health.* 2001;91:432
16. Wisborg K, Kesmodel U, Henriksen TB, et al. A prospective study of smoking during pregnancy and SIDS. *Arch Dis Child.* 2000;83:203
17. Sawnani H, Jackson T, Murphy T, et al. The effect of maternal smoking on respiratory and arousal patterns in preterm infants during sleep. *Am J Respir Crit Care Med.* 2004;169(6):733–738
18. Schneider J, Mitchell I, Singhal N, et al. Prenatal cigarette smoke exposure attenuates recovery from hypoxemic challenge in preterm infants. *Am J Respir Crit Care Med.* 2008;178(5):520–526
19. Landau LI. Tobacco smoke exposure and tracking of lung function into adult life. *Paediatr Respir Rev.* 2008;9(1):39–43
20. Tager IB. The effects of second-hand and direct exposure to tobacco smoke on asthma and lung function in adolescence. *Paediatr Respir Rev.* 2008; 9(1):29–37
21. Collins MH, Moessinger AC, Kleinerman J, et al. Fetal lung hypoplasia associated with maternal smoking: a morphometric analysis. *Pediatr Res.* 1985;19(4):408–412
22. Haberg SE, Stigum H, Nystad W, Nafstad P. Effects of pre- and postnatal exposure to parental smoking on early childhood respiratory health. *Am J Epidemiol.* 2007;166(6):679–686
23. Li JS, Peat JK, Xuan W, et al. Meta-analysis on the association between environmental tobacco smoke (ETS) exposure and the prevalence of lower respiratory tract infection in early childhood. *Pediatr Pulmonol.* 1999;27(1):5–13
24. Suzuki M, Thiem VD, Yanai H, et al. Association of environmental tobacco smoking exposure with an increased risk of hospital admissions for pneumonia in children under 5 years of age in Vietnam. *Thorax.* 2009;64(6):484–489
25. Kwok MK, Schooling CM, Ho LM, et al. Early life second-hand smoke exposure and serious infectious morbidity during the first 8 years: evidence from Hong Kong's "Children of 1997" birth cohort. *Tob Control.* 2008;17(4):263–270
26. Cook DG, Strachan DP. Health effects of passive smoking. 3. Parental smoking and prevalence of respiratory symptoms and asthma in school age children. *Thorax.* 1997;52:1081
27. Jaakkola JJ, Jaakkola MS. Effects of environmental tobacco smoke on the respiratory health of children. *Scand J Work Environ Health.* 2002;28 (suppl 2):71–83

28. Goksor E, Amark M, Alm B, et al. The impact of pre- and post-natal smoke exposure on future asthma and bronchial hyper-responsiveness. *Acta Paediatr.* 2007;96:1030
29. Vork KL, Broadwin RL, Blaisdell RJ. Developing asthma in childhood from exposure to secondhand tobacco smoke: insights from a meta-regression. *Environ Health Perspect.* 2007;115(10):1394–1400
30. Mannino DM, Homa DM, Redd SC. Involuntary smoking and asthma severity in children: data from the Third National Health and Nutrition Examination Survey. *Chest.* 2002;122(2):409–415
31. Committee on the Assessment of Asthma and Indoor Air. Exposure to environmental tobacco smoke. In: Institute of Medicine. *Clearing the Air: Asthma and Indoor Air Exposures.* Washington, DC: National Academy Press; 2000:263–297
32. Keil T, Lau S, Roll S, et al. Maternal smoking increases risk of allergic sensitization and wheezing only in children with allergic predisposition: longitudinal analysis from birth to 10 years. *Allergy.* 2009;64(3):445–451
33. Larsson ML, Frisk M, Hallstrom J, et al. Environmental tobacco smoke exposure during childhood is associated with increased prevalence of asthma in adults. *Chest.* 2001;120:711
34. Farber HJ. Optimizing maintenance therapy in pediatric asthma. *Curr Opin Pulm Med.* 2010;16(1):25–30
35. Gerald LB, Gerald JK, Gibson L, et al. Changes in environmental tobacco smoke exposure and asthma morbidity among urban school children. *Chest.* 2009;135(4):911–916
36. Wilson SR, Yamada EG, Sudhakar R, et al. A controlled trial of an environmental tobacco smoke reduction intervention in low-income children with asthma. *Chest.* 2001;120(5):1709–1722
37. Collaco JM, Vanscoy L, Bremer L, et al. Interactions between secondhand smoke and genes that affect cystic fibrosis lung disease. *JAMA.* 2008;299:417
38. Köhler E, Sollich V, Schuster R, et al. Passive smoke exposure in infants and children with respiratory tract diseases. *Hum Exp Toxicol.* 1999; 18(4):212–217
39. Hammarén-Malmi S, Saxen H, Tarkkanen J, et al. Passive smoking after tympanostomy and risk of recurrent acute otitis media. *Int J Pediatr Otorhinolaryngol.* 2007;71(8):1305–1310
40. Maw R, Bawden R. Spontaneous resolution of severe chronic glue ear in children and the effect of adenoidectomy, tonsillectomy, and insertion of ventilation tubes (grommets). *BMJ.* 1993;306(6880):756–760
41. Aligne CA, Moss ME, Auinger P, et al. Association of pediatric dental caries with passive smoking. *JAMA.* 2003;289:1258
42. Pang D, McNally R, Birch JM. Parental smoking and childhood cancer: results from the United Kingdom Childhood Cancer Study. *Br J Cancer.* 2003;88:373

43. Chang JS. Parental smoking and childhood leukemia. *Methods Mol Biol.* 2009;472:103–137
44. Olivo-Marston SE, Yang P, Mechanic LE, et al. Childhood exposure to secondhand smoke and functional mannose binding lectin polymorphisms are associated with increased lung cancer risk. *Cancer Epidemiol Biomarkers Prev.* 2009;18(12):3375–3383
45. Kallio K, Jokinen E, Raitakari OT, et al. Tobacco smoke exposure is associated with attenuated endothelial function in 11-year-old healthy children. *Circulation.* 2007;115:3205
46. Burke V, Gracey MP, Milligan RA, et al. Parental smoking and risk factors for cardiovascular disease in 10- to 12-year-old children. *J Pediatr.* 1998;133:206
47. Winickoff JP, Friebely J, Tanski SE, et al. Beliefs about the health effects of "thirdhand" smoke and home smoking bans. *Pediatrics.* 2009;123(1):e74–e79
48. Benowitz NL, Hukkanen J, Jacob P III. Nicotine chemistry, metabolism, kinetics and biomarkers. *Handb Exp Pharmacol.* 2009;192:29–60
49. Wakefield M, Banham D, McCaul K, et al. Effect of feedback regarding urinary cotinine and brief tailored advice on home smoking restrictions among low-income parents of children with asthma: a controlled trial. *Prev Med.* 2002;34:58–65
50. Woodruff SI, Conway TL, Elder JP, et al. Pilot study using hair nicotine feedback to reduce Latino children's environmental tobacco smoke exposure. *Am J Health Promot.* 2007;22(2):93–97
51. Epps RP, Manley MW. A physicians' guide to preventing tobacco use during childhood and adolescence. *Pediatrics.* 1991;88(1):140–144
52. Farkas AJ, Gilpin EA, White MM, et al. Association between household and workplace smoking restrictions and adolescent smoking. *JAMA.* 2000;284:717
53. Mills AL, Messer K, Gilpin EA, et al. The effect of smoke-free homes on adult smoking behavior: a review. *Nicotine Tob Res.* 2009;11(10):1131–1141
54. US Environmental Protection Agency. Indoor air quality: smoke-free homes and cars program. http://www.epa.gov/smokefree/. Accessed May 1, 2010
55. Kim MJ, Fleming CB, Catalano RF. Individual and social influences on progression to daily smoking during adolescence. *Pediatrics.* 2009;124:895–1092
56. Sargent JD, Dalton M. Does parental disapproval of smoking prevent adolescents from becoming established smokers? *Pediatrics.* 2001;108:1256
57. Kaufman NJ, Castrucci BC, Mowery PD, et al. Predictors of change on the smoking uptake continuum among adolescents. *Arch Pediatr Adolesc Med.* 2002;156(6):581–587
58. Bush T, Richardson L, Katon, W, et al. Anxiety and depressive disorders are associated with smoking in adolescents with asthma. *J Adolesc Health.* 2007;40:425

59. Lotrean LM, Mesters I, Ionut C, et al. Smoking among Romanian adolescents: do the gender differences exist? *Pneumologia.* 2009;58(4):240–246
60. DiNapoli PP. Early initiation of tobacco use in adolescent girls: key sociostructural influences. *Appl Nurs Res.* 2009;22(2):126–132
61. DiFranza JR, Wellman RJ, Sargent JD, et al. Tobacco promotion and the initiation of tobacco use: assessing the evidence for causality. *Pediatrics.* 2006;117:e1237
62. US Food and Drug Administration. Tobacco Products: Guidance, Compliance and Regulatory Information. US Food and Drug Administration Web site. http://www.fda.gov/TobaccoProducts/GuidanceComplianceRegulatoryInformation/default.htm. Accessed May 1, 2010
63. Sussman S, Sun P, Dent CW. A meta-analysis of teen cigarette smoking cessation. *Health Psychol.* 2006;25(5):549–557
64. Horn K, Fernandes A, Dino G, et al. Adolescent nicotine dependence and smoking cessation outcomes. *Addict Behav.* 2003;28:769–776
65. Moolchan ET, Robinson ML, Ernst M, et al. Safety and efficacy of the nicotine patch and gum for the treatment of adolescent tobacco addiction. *Pediatrics.* 2005;115;407–414
66. Sachs DPL, Leone F, Farber HJ, et al. *Tobacco Dependence Treatment ToolKit.* 3rd ed. Northbrook, IL: American College of Chest Physicians; 2010. http://tobaccodependence.chestnet.org/

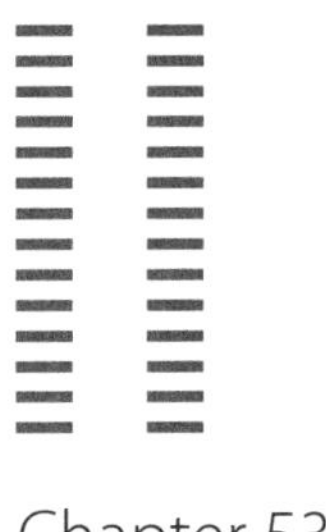

Chapter 53

Treating Tobacco Dependence

Harold J. Farber, MD, MSPH, FAAP
Marianna Sockrider, MD, DrPH, FAAP
David P. L. Sachs, MD

Importance of Tobacco Dependence Treatment

Tobacco dependence is one of the most important preventable causes of premature death and disability.[1] Tobacco dependence most commonly starts in adolescence.[2] Tobacco dependence is not simply a bad habit; it is a chronic illness with serious consequences for the smoker and individuals close to him or her.[3] Nicotine addiction is a severe addiction. Tobacco use causes changes in brain nicotinic receptors,[4] making exogenous nicotine required for normal functioning. Withdrawal symptoms (Box 53-1) can lead to mood disturbances of similar intensity to that seen in psychiatric outpatients, including irritability, depression, restlessness, anxiety, and anhedonia.[5,6]

Secondhand (SHS) smoke exposure is either a cause or an exacerbating factor for most childhood respiratory illnesses[3] (see Chapter 52). Although having a smoke-free home and car may reduce a child's smoke exposure, this rarely eliminates it. The greatest contribution to the SHS exposure of children is from their parents and caregivers.[7] Providing tobacco-dependent patients, parents, and other caregivers with effective treatment is important for achieving and maintaining respiratory health—of not just the smoker, but also the smoker's children. The American Academy of Pediatrics advises that pediatric health care providers "Routinely offer help and referral to those who use tobacco—even if the person is not your patient."[8]

Box 53-1. Nicotine Withdrawal Symptoms

- Cravings
- Irritability, frustration, anger
- Anxiety, restlessness
- Difficulty concentrating, slowed cognitive performance
- Insomnia
- Increased appetite
- Constipation
- Tremors
- Dysphoric or depressed mood
- Anhedonia—inability to feel pleasure

Pediatric health care providers should seize available opportunities to (1) prevent initiation of tobacco use in children and adolescents and (2) assist their tobacco-dependent patients and parents/caregivers to obtain effective treatment.

Box 53-2. Counseling Approaches

Counseling to Facilitate Smoking Cessation: 6 As	Not Ready to Stop Smoking: 5 Rs	Facilitate Behavior Change: ASK NOW
Anticipate risk of tobacco use	**Relevance** of smoking cessation	**Assess** the health behavior
Ask about tobacco use and exposure history	**Risks** of tobacco use	Determine the **Stage** of change
Advise about the harm of active smoking and secondhand exposure	**Rewards** of smoking cessation	Keep in mind **Key** facts
Assess readiness to change and severity of nicotine dependence	**Roadblocks** to smoking cessation	Jointly **Negotiate** an action plan
Assist in developing a tobacco dependence treatment plan	**Repetition** at every office visit follow-up	**Observe** outcome in follow-up
Arrange follow-up		**Work** toward the next stage

Tobacco dependence often requires repeated interventions to effectively treat.[9] Most parents who are tobacco dependent would accept treatment or referral from their child's health care provider.[10,11] Pediatricians may be the only health care provider that parents interact with. Routinely offering tobacco dependence treatment to parents as part of their child's health care can confer profound benefits to children and their families.[8,12]

Counseling to Facilitate Smoking Cessation

The "6 As" is a systematic method for counseling about tobacco (Box 53-2).

1. **Anticipate** risk of tobacco use: Routinely ask parents and patients about smoking and tobacco exposure. Make parents aware of age of smoking onset and risk factors. Discuss the many adverse health effects of tobacco use. Use individualized messages that are personally relevant. Be aware of populations at increased risk of tobacco initiation.

2. **Ask:** Obtain a tobacco use and smoke exposure history. Ask about smokers in child care settings and homes visited by the child.

   Useful questions to ask about tobacco use and tobacco smoke exposure include
   - Does anyone who lives with (child's name) smoke?
   - Does anyone who provides care for (child's name) smoke?
   - Does (child's name) visit places where people smoke?
   - Does (child's name) have any regular exposure to tobacco smoke?

   Useful questions to ask about active smoking in an adolescent include
   - How many of your friends smoke?
   - Have you ever tried (name of tobacco product)?
   - How many times have you tried (name of tobacco product)?
   - When was the last time you used (name of tobacco product)?

3. **Advise:** Provide strong messages about the harm of active smoking and SHS exposure. Use messages that are individualized and personally relevant. Discuss the benefit of effective tobacco dependence pharmacotherapy.

4. **Assess:** Determine readiness to stop smoking. Determine barriers to smoking cessation. Determine the level of tobacco (nicotine) dependence (as discussed in later in this chapter).

5. **Assist:** For the patient interested in stopping smoking, develop an individualized tobacco dependence treatment plan (as discussed in later in this chapter) and/or refer for counseling or additional treatment.

6. **Arrange follow-up:** For the patient willing to initiate tobacco dependence treatment, arrange for follow-up contacts, beginning within the first week after the target stop smoking date. For patients unwilling to initiate tobacco dependence treatment, address tobaccodependence during the next clinic visit.

If a smoker does not want to stop, the "5 Rs" is a counseling method to overcome resistance (Box 53-2).

1. **Relevance:** Encourage the patient/parent to consider the personal relevance of stopping smoking, being as specific as possible. Personalize the benefits of quitting to their individual situation.

2. **Risks:** Ask the patient/parent to identify potential negative consequences of tobacco use. The clinician may suggest and highlight those that seem most relevant. Ask the person to list pros and cons of smoking.

3. **Rewards:** Ask the patient/parent to identify potential benefits of stopping tobacco use. The clinician may suggest and highlight those that seem most relevant.

4. **Roadblocks:** Ask the parent/patient to identify barriers or impediments to quitting and provide treatment (problem-solving counseling, medication) that could address barriers.

   Common barriers include withdrawal symptoms, fear of failure, fear of weight gain, enjoyment of tobacco, stress management, psychiatric comorbidities, and ignorance of effective treatment options.

5. **Repetition:** Repeat the message every time parents/patients who use tobacco visit the office.

   Make notes regarding previous counseling to help guide future contacts. Tobacco-dependent persons commonly make multiple attempts before smoking cessation is sustained.

A theory-based approach to counseling to facilitate health behavior change for tobacco dependence can be described using the acronym

ASK NOW (Box 53-2). This approach incorporates use of the 6 As and 5 Rs.

A: **A**ssess the health behavior of concern.

S: Determine the patient's **S**tage of Change. Stages of change include pre-contemplation (no intention to make the behavior change), contemplation (intends to make the change within the next 6 months, but not now), preparation (intends to make the change within the next month), action (has recently made the change, within the past 6 months), and maintenance (usually considered 6 months to 5 years after the change is made).[13]

K: Keep in mind **K**ey facts, such as previous experience with making the change, social stresses, barriers, areas of resistance, etc.

N: Jointly **N**egotiate an action plan. The action plan should be based on both the smoker's stage of change and key facts. For example, in pre-contemplation the plan might be to consider how to minimize harm from the continued behavior (such as adopting smoke-free home and car policies). In contemplation one would develop a set of steps to get ready to stop smoking and/or accept tobacco dependence treatment. In preparation one would develop a concrete action plan and ask the smoker to set a stop smoking date (see section on tobacco dependence treatment below). In action and maintenance the risk of relapse should be assessed and strategies to handle difficult situations discussed.[14] Keep in mind that change is not a linear process. Sometimes stages are skipped. Sometimes patients regress. Asking the person to weigh the pros and cons of the behavior and its change can aid in advancing to the next stage.

O: **O**bserve outcome in follow-up. How has their stage of change progressed or regressed? How did the action plan work? What barriers were encountered? Does the action plan need to be updated or modified? Learn from slips and lapses. Provide follow-up.

W: **W**ork toward the next stage. Acknowledge and reinforce any progress. Jointly negotiate a plan to consolidate gains and move forward.

Principles of Tobacco Dependence Treatment

The principles of effective tobacco dependence treatment are similar to those of asthma treatment. Both are chronic diseases with exacerbations and remissions. In asthma, the goal is to minimize symptoms and normalize lung function. Similarly, in tobacco dependence the goal is to feel normal or near normal without use of tobacco products.

ARMR is an acronym for a systemic approach to tobacco dependence treatment.

- **A**ssess severity of tobacco dependence, experience with prior quit attempts, and relevant comorbidities.
- **R**ecommend effective tobacco dependence therapy and negotiate a tobacco dependence treatment plan. Encourage efforts to mobilize a personal support system.
- **M**onitor for treatment effectiveness and for side effects.
- **R**evise the treatment plan as needed to improve treatment effectiveness and minimize side effects.

Assess Tobacco Dependence Severity

The Fagerström Test of Nicotine Dependence measures nicotine dependence severity,[15] the modified Fagerström Tolerance Questionnaire can be used for adolescents.[16] Asking about the number of cigarettes smoked per day and time to first cigarette provides a rough estimate of nicotine dependence. Risk factors such as starting tobacco use at a young age (≤17 years old), multiple previous quit attempts, another smoker in the household, psychiatric comorbidities, and current other substance abuse indicate a need for more intensive treatment. Assess experience with prior quit attempts, triggers for smoking, readiness to change, and therapies they would be willing to accept. Most smokers make multiple stop smoking attempts prior to complete cessation of smoking. Incorporating the experience of these attempts helps in negotiation of a better tobacco dependence treatment plan.

Table 53-1 provides a classification of tobacco dependence severity. This classification is used to help determine intensity of initial tobacco dependence treatment.

Recommend Tobacco Dependence Treatment

For tobacco dependence, the best available treatment includes the use of pharmacotherapy in combination with education and behavioral counseling. Medications can be characterized as long-acting controllers (nicotine transdermal patch, bupropion, varenicline) and shorter-acting relievers (nicotine gum, lozenge, inhaler, and nasal spray). Relievers can also be used to pre-medicate for situations at risk for

Table 53-1. Classification of Tobacco Dependence Severity: Clinical Features Before Treatment[a,b]

Step	Cigarette Use	Nicotine Withdrawal Symptoms	Fagerström Test of Nicotine Dependence
Step 4 Very severe	>40/day Time to first cigarette 0–5 min	Constant	8–10
Step 3 Severe	20–40/day Time to first cigarette: 6–30 min	Constant	6–7
Step 2 Moderate	6–19/day Time to first cigarette 31–60 min	Frequent	4–5
Step 1 Mild	1–5/day Time to first cigarette >60 min	Intermittent	2–3
Step 0 Non-daily/ social	Non-daily Social settings only Time to first cigarette >60 min	None	0–1 Healthy
Note: If chronic medical or psychiatric disease is present in the smoker, more intensive treatment is needed. Escalate severity assessment by 1 to 2 steps.			

[a] Adapted with permission from Sachs DPL, Leone FT, Farber HJ, et al. *American College of Chest Physicians Tobacco-Dependence Treatment Tool Kit.* 3rd ed. Northbrook, IL: American College of Chest Physicians; 2010. http://tobaccodependence.chestnet.org.
[b] The presence of one feature of severity is sufficient to place patient in that category.

smoking at any step. At all steps, individualized behavioral counseling should be provided. Match the intensity of pharmacotherapy to the severity of tobacco dependence (Figure 53-1).

For example, with Step 1 (mild) tobacco dependence, start either one *controller* medication or the regular use of a *reliever* medication. If the individual is tobacco dependent and has a moderate to severe chronic medical or psychiatric illness, more intensive therapy would be needed; escalate by 1 to 2 steps.

Create a written tobacco independence action plan. Like some asthma action plans, a green, yellow, red zone plan can be used.

- In the green zone, nicotine withdrawal symptoms are well controlled.

Step 0 Non-daily/social	Step 1 Mild	Step 2 Moderate	Step 3 Severe	Step 4 Very Severe	Step Down and Maintenance
Controller: None **Reliever:** As needed reliever use may be considered	**Controller:** Nicotine patch *or* bupropion SR *or* varenicline **OR** **Reliever** as needed	**Controller:** Nicotine patch or bupropion SR **Plus *reliever as needed*** **OR** Varenicline alone	**Controllers:** Varenicline + bupropion SR **OR** Nicotine patch + bupropion SR **AND** **Reliever** as needed	**Controllers:** Varenicline and/or bupropion-SR **and/or** High-dose nicotine patch **AND** **Multiple reliever** medications as needed	When tobacco dependence is controlled • Gradually reduce medications, one at a time • Monitor, to maintain good control of nicotine withdrawal symptoms

Figure 53-1. Pharmacologic management of tobacco dependence. (Adapted with permission from Sachs DPL, Leone FT, Farber HJ, et al. *American College of Chest Physicians Tobacco-Dependence Treatment Tool Kit.* 3rd ed. Northbrook, IL: American College of Chest Physicians; 2010. http://tobaccodependence.chestnet.org.)

- The yellow zone is for mild withdrawal symptoms, indicating the need for reliever medicine.
- The red zone is for moderate to severe nicotine withdrawal and indicates the need for intensified reliever medication and physician contact.

A sample action plan form can be found in the American College of Chest Physicians *Tobacco Dependence Treatment Toolkit* (available free of charge at http://tobaccodependence.chestnet.org/).[17] Give the number for the National Cancer Institute toll-free telephone quitline (1-800-QUIT NOW), it provides free access to a cessation counselor. Consider referral to a local counseling or cessation support group. Be sure that the support group endorses up-to-date tobacco dependence treatment approaches, including pharmacotherapy.

When prescribing smoking cessation pharmacotherapy for a parent or caregiver, document the assessment, counseling, and plan (including follow-up) in the medical record. If the pediatrician is not comfortable with prescribing medication for adults, counseling about treatment needed and treatment resources available can still be of great value. Instructions on proper use of over-the-counter (OTC) nicotine replacement products can also help tobacco-dependent individuals.

It is important to provide support and follow-up. Make a plan to check on the patient/parent's progress by phone or a clinic visit. Ask the person to identify a person or persons in their family or social network to serve as a support person, coach, or smoking cessation buddy. Encourage the person to share the smoking cessation plan and talk about how to communicate needs to others when facing possible triggers to relapse. Be available to escalate pharmacotherapy, if needed, for nicotine withdrawal symptoms that are not well controlled.

Monitor

Monitor to assess adequacy of nicotine withdrawal control (use the Nicotine Withdrawal Symptom Scale[17,18]), adherence to medications, side effects of treatment, presence/risk of relapse, and plans to handle potentially difficult situations. Lapses and relapses are common, particularly if pharmacotherapy is inadequate to control withdrawal symptoms. A lapse is a sign that treatment needs to be intensified. Psychiatric conditions may be unmasked by stopping smoking; in such cases referral to a psychiatrist may be needed.

Revise

Revise the treatment plan as necessary to achieve goals of therapy. If nicotine withdrawal is not well controlled, explore medication adherence, side effects, delivery technique, dose, and triggers to smoking. Some triggers may not have been recognized or considered important before stopping smoking. Consider stepping up pharmacotherapy (Figure 53-1). Significant or bothersome side effects may require either a change in medication or modification of technique for use.

If nicotine withdrawal symptoms have been well controlled without tobacco use for 3 to 6 months or more, consider stepping down medications.

Medications

Long-Acting Controller Medications

Long-acting controller medications help to control nicotine withdrawal; they do not give quick relief of acute withdrawal symptoms.

Nicotine Patch

The OTC nicotine transdermal patch gives a constant low dose of nicotine. The nicotine patch produces peak nicotine levels after 4 to 12 hours (depending on the patch brand).

Standard patch doses alone may not be sufficient to control nicotine withdrawal for those with severe tobacco dependence (Figure 53-1). The nicotine patch comes in 3 strengths: 21 mg, 14 mg, and 7 mg. Do not step down the dose on a fixed schedule; step down when good control of nicotine withdrawal symptoms has been achieved and maintained.

Side Effects: The most common side effects from nicotine patch use are sleep disturbance and bizarre or vivid, unpleasant dreams. These can usually be managed by removal of the patch before bedtime. Skin irritation usually responds to the use of topical hydrocortisone and is minimized by rotating patch sites. Nausea can be a sign that the dose of nicotine is too high for the patient.

Special Precautions: Be sure to keep patches—whether used or not—well out of reach of children. A used patch still has enough nicotine to be dangerous to a child.

Bupropion

Bupropion is an antidepressant that, independent of its antidepressant properties, is effective for the treatment of tobacco dependence. Bupropion is available by prescription as sustained release (SR—dosed twice daily) and extended release (dosed once a day, in the morning). Adherence is usually best with once-daily dosing. Although all bupropion formulations share the same pharmacologic activity, only the SR preparation has been approved by the US Food and Drug Administration (FDA) for tobacco dependence treatment.

Side Effects: Bupropion may cause agitation and sleeplessness. Other potential side effects include weight loss, dry mouth, nausea or vomiting, or headaches. These side effects tend to improve over time, even with continued use.

Special Precautions: Bupropion may lower seizure threshold. Seizure risk is lower when the dose is divided twice daily. Presence of a seizure disorder, head injury, anorexia, bulimia, and alcohol abuse are considered relative contraindications to its use. Do not administer to patients receiving a monoamine oxidase inhibitor. See Black Box Warnings below.

Varenicline

Varenicline is a central nervous system $\alpha_4 \beta_2$ nicotinic receptor partial agonist. This receptor is primarily responsible for the reinforcing effects of nicotine on smoking behavior. Varenicline use results in both reduced nicotine withdrawal symptoms and decreased reinforcing effect of nicotine. It is available by prescription only.

Side Effects: Possible side effects include nausea, vomiting, flatulence, vivid or unusual dreams, constipation, and dry mouth. Nausea is common (30%) with varenicline use; it usually improves or resolves with continued use.[19]

Black Box Warnings

Treatment-emergent depression and suicidality have been reported with use of bupropion and varenicline,[20] although the causal role of the medication remains to be demonstrated.[21–23] Inadequate control of nicotine withdrawal may also lead to depression, anger, or suicidality.[22,23] Psychiatric conditions and suicide are more common among smokers than the general population,[24–27] especially in adolescents.[28–30]

Regardless of therapy, it is important to monitor patients for treatment-emergent psychiatric symptoms.

Rapidly Acting Reliever Medications

Rapidly acting reliever, or rescue, medications provide quick relief of acute or breakthrough nicotine withdrawal symptoms.

Nicotine Polacrilex Gum and Lozenge

Absorption of nicotine from Polacrilex gum and lozenges is through the oral mucosa, leading to peak nicotine levels in about 20 minutes. Although onset is much faster than the nicotine patch, this is still much slower than a cigarette.

Proper technique is key to best effect. Nicotine gum is chewed until a tingling or peppery nicotine taste appears, then the gum is parked until the taste disappears, then repeat chew and park cycles. The nicotine lozenge is placed between the cheek and gum and allowed to slowly dissolve. Too rapid release of nicotine (such as from too rapid chewing of the nicotine gum, or placing the nicotine lozenge under the tongue) can lead to swallowed nicotine, which can cause nausea and hiccups. The liver rapidly inactivates swallowed nicotine.

In these products, nicotine is bound to a resin; release is pH-dependent. Eating or drinking anything that lowers mouth pH (such as tea, coffee, soft drinks) will reduce the therapeutic effect. Advise the patient to wait 15 minutes after eating any acidic food or beverage before using the nicotine gum or lozenge.[31] This pH-dependent release is not an issue with nicotine nasal spray or nicotine oral inhaler.

Nicotine Nasal Spray

Nicotine nasal spray, available by prescription, delivers peak levels of nicotine to the brain within 6 minutes after use. Nasal irritation is a common side effect.

Nicotine Oral Inhaler

The nicotine oral inhaler, available by prescription, delivers a nicotine vapor that is absorbed through the oral mucosa (not the lungs).[32] Its pharmacokinetics are similar to nicotine gum. The nicotine inhaler has the benefit of providing oral sensory feedback. Mild throat irritation is common. Inhaled nicotine may cause bronchospasm, hence this is not as good a choice for people with asthma.

Other Cessation Pharmacotherapy Tips

- Cigarettes produce peak nicotine levels in 5 to 7 *seconds,* faster than that provided by any of the rapidly acting reliever medications. Nicotine replacement medications are best used early, BEFORE there are strong cravings or severe withdrawal symptoms.
- Combinations of first-line tobacco dependence pharmacotherapies are more effective than single-agent therapies.[9] Combination of pharmacotherapy with counseling and/or cognitive-behavioral therapy is more effective than pharmacotherapy alone.[9]
- If the individual is not yet ready to stop smoking, use of the nicotine patch can aid in reduction of smoking in preparation for cessation.[33]

Treating Tobacco Dependence in Adolescents

Adolescent smoking is driven by many factors, including family and peer relations, activities, positive and negative emotions, social ramifications, cultural images, and role models. In adolescents, smoking can rapidly progress from intermittent to daily use and full-blown tobacco dependence. Loss of autonomy over smoking has been documented within 2 days of first cigarette use.[34] Many tobacco-dependent teens are interested in quitting,[35] yet without treatment, only 3% of adolescents who want to quit report sustained smoking cessation.[36] In contrast to the large amount of research on treatment of tobacco dependence in adults, the literature in adolescents is limited. Reliance on self-report of cessation in adolescents (without biochemical confirmation) can overestimate cessation rates and bias study results.[37] Clinical trials of motivational interviewing versus brief advice interventions for tobacco-dependent adolescents have not demonstrated significant differences in biochemically confirmed tobacco cessation rates.[38,39]

Multi-session, school-based group interventions, including Project EX[40] and Not On Tobacco,[41] have shown positive benefit. Cessation rates in these programs were substantially greater for those with the minimal to no nicotine dependence compared with those who were highly addicted.[40,42]

Research on the use of smoking cessation pharmacotherapy of tobacco-dependent adolescents is limited. Among moderate to severely tobacco-dependent adolescents motivated to quit smoking there is some evidence to support benefit of regular use of nicotine patches combined with cognitive behavioral therapy[43] and bupropion[44] when used in combination with standardized individual cessation counseling. A 12-week randomized controlled clinical trial comparing the addition of nicotine patches versus placebo to cognitive behavioral therapy showed benefit of the patch at 1 week post-target quit date (26.5% vs 5%, $P = 0.02$) and at 3 months after the 12-week intervention concluded (20.6% vs 5%, $P = 0.06$).[43] A study of bupropion 150 mg twice a day given for 6 weeks demonstrated benefit only during the active treatment period (29% vs 16% abstinence at 6 weeks, $P = 0.02$); it was not sustained after medication discontinuation.[44] Randomized clinical trials using as-needed therapy with nicotine gum or nicotine nasal spray for strong cravings failed to demonstrate a benefit due to non-adherence.[43,45] The instruction to wait for strong cravings may have been too little, too late. Poorly controlled nicotine withdrawal has been associated with lapses of smoking in adolescents on tobacco dependence treatment.[46]

Although not currently FDA approved, the approach outlined above for tobacco dependence in adults may be applied to adolescents who are moderately to highly tobacco dependent and want to stop smoking.[17] Combining pharmacotherapy with behavioral counseling and maintaining close physician follow-up is essential for adolescents. The goal of pharmacotherapy should be to control nicotine withdrawal symptoms and to allow the adolescent to feel normal. Medications should be gradually reduced as control of nicotine withdrawal is achieved and maintained. It is important to screen adolescents for other substance abuse and psychiatric comorbidities and address those as well.

For teens who are not ready to quit, focus on the "5 Rs": **R**elevance, **R**isks, **R**ewards, **R**oadblocks, **R**epetition.[9,47] Give messages that are age appropriate and personally relevant. Risks of bad breath, yellowed fingers, smelly clothes, and rewards of better performance in sports and money saved may be more relevant to a teen than risk of future lung disease, cancer, or premature death. Contact information for local tobacco cessation resources and/or quitlines (1-800-QUIT NOW) should be provided.

"E-Cigarettes": Unapproved and Inappropriate for Tobacco Dependence Treatment

The "e-cigarette" is a battery-powered device that delivers a vaporized propylene glycol/nicotine mixture. There have been no safety or efficacy studies of these devices. An FDA analysis found carcinogenic and toxic substances in its vapor, including tobacco-specific nitrosoamines and antifreeze (diethylene glycol).[48] Use of flavorings (such as chocolate, strawberry, and mint) is designed to appeal to young people[49] to recruit them to a life of nicotine dependence. *This product is potentially harmful and should not be recommended.*

Prevention

The most important and most effective approach to tobacco dependence is primary prevention. Physicians should encourage parents to model nonsmoking behavior. Pediatricians should support or advocate for public policies to de-normalize smoking behavior. Smoking bans in public areas, schools, and workplaces need to be expanded and enforced. Depictions of smoking behavior in media that either target or are accessible to young people should be restricted. Raising tobacco prices decreases tobacco use.[50] Laws prohibiting purchase of tobacco products by minors need to be enforced. Box 53-3 provides a summary of tobacco control policy recommendations for pediatricians and the public.[8]

Box 53-3. Summary of Tobacco Control Recommendations From the American Academy of Pediatrics Policy Statement—Tobacco Use: A Pediatric Disease (2009)[8]

Pediatricians Have Important Roles in Efforts to Reduce Family Tobacco Use and Secondhand Smoke Exposure

Recommendations for Pediatricians

1. Maintain a tobacco-free environment. Do not wear or display tobacco products, advertisements, or promotional items. Eliminate tobacco advertising and depictions of tobacco use from all materials associated with your clinical practice, including magazines, videos, and other media in patient care and waiting areas.
2. Ask about and document tobacco use and secondhand smoke exposure at all clinical encounters. Advise all families to make their homes and cars smoke-free, and urge all tobacco users to stop using tobacco.
3. Provide counseling to expectant parents to quit using tobacco products and avoid secondhand smoke exposure during and after pregnancy. Assist new parents in their efforts to continue their tobacco use abstinence or cessation efforts after delivery.
4. Counsel preadolescents and adolescents to prevent initiation of tobacco use.
5. Encourage tobacco-dependent persons to include appropriate pharmacotherapy in their smoking cessation plans.
   a. Pediatricians may either prescribe this medication to the child's caregivers themselves (with appropriate documentation), recommend use of over-the-counter tobacco dependence treatment products, or may choose to refer to cessation services and recommend that parents discuss appropriate pharmacotherapy with their health care providers.
   b. Memorize the national quitline telephone number (1-800-QUIT NOW), prominently post it, and provide it to all tobacco users.
6. Advocate for tobacco-free homes, cars, schools, child care programs, playgrounds, and other venues.

Box 53-3. Summary of Tobacco Control Recommendations From the American Academy of Pediatrics Policy Statement—Tobacco Use: A Pediatric Disease (2009)[8] (continued)

Pediatricians Have Important Roles in Efforts to Reduce Family Tobacco Use and Secondhand Smoke Exposure

Recommendations for Public Policy

1. The use of tobacco products in all indoor and outdoor public places should be prohibited.
2. Health care and educational facilities should be completely tobacco-free, inside and outside, at all times.
3. Treatment of tobacco use and dependence should be available to patients and their families in both inpatient and outpatient settings.
4. Public and private employers should develop or provide access to tobacco use cessation programs for their employees.
5. All public and private health insurance should provide coverage for comprehensive tobacco dependence treatment.
6. Sales and distribution of tobacco to youth should be strictly prohibited. The sale of tobacco products on the same premises as pharmacies should be eliminated.
7. Advertising of tobacco products should be banned from all media, events, and venues, including the Internet. All forms of advertising and media, especially advertising and media aimed at children, adolescents, and young adults, should not contain messages that promote tobacco use or images of tobacco or tobacco use.
8. Exposure to and depiction of tobacco use should be reduced in films, videos, DVDs, and television programs. Definitive and unambiguous antismoking ads (not produced or funded by a tobacco company) should be required to preview before any film with any tobacco presence.
9. The evidence-based recommendations of *Best Practices for Comprehensive Tobacco Control Programs*[a] should be funded and implemented.
10. Pediatric tobacco-control research should be considered a high priority and funded accordingly. Funding should not be accepted from the tobacco industry.

[a]Centers for Disease Control and Prevention. *Best Practices for Comprehensive Tobacco Control Programs: 2007*. Atlanta, GA: US Department of Health and Human Services, Centers for Disease Control and Prevention, National Center for Chronic Disease Prevention and Health Promotion, Office on Smoking and Health; 2007

Key Points

- The pediatric health care provider needs to be knowledgeable about tobacco dependence treatment and ROUTINELY offer help and referral to those who are tobacco dependent—both among patients and parents or caregivers.
- Counseling starts with the "6 As": **A**nticipate, **A**sk, **A**dvise, **A**ssess, **A**ssist, and **A**rrange follow-up.
- If not yet ready to stop smoking, focus on the "5 Rs": **R**elevance, **R**isks, **R**ewards, **R**oadblocks, and **R**epetition.
- Use ASK NOW to facilitate behavior change: **A**ssess behavior of concern, determine **S**tage of change, keep in mind **K**ey facts, jointly **N**egotiate an action plan, **O**bserve the outcome, **W**ork toward the next stage.
- ARMR approach to tobacco dependence treatment
  - **A**ssess the severity of tobacco dependence. Based on that assessment,
  - **R**ecommend effective tobacco-dependence therapy. Encourage efforts to mobilize a personal support system.
  - **M**onitor for treatment effectiveness and for side effects.
  - **R**evise the treatment plan as needed to improve treatment effectiveness and reduce side effects.
- Principles of tobacco dependence treatment are similar to asthma treatment.
  - The goal of tobacco dependence treatment is for the patient to feel normal or near normal without use of tobacco products.
  - Medications include long-acting controllers (nicotine patch, bupropion, varenicline) and rapidly acting relievers (nicotine gum, lozenge, inhaler, and nasal spray).
  - Intensity of therapy should be based on severity of tobacco dependence.
  - Therapy is stepped up or down based on adequacy of control of nicotine withdrawal—not on a fixed timetable.
  - Nicotine replacement therapy can be started in the smoker not yet ready to stop to allow them to gain greater control over their smoking, gain experience with treatment, and prepare for cessation.

Key Points

- Smoking in adolescents
  - Smoking can rapidly progress from intermittent to daily use.
  - School-based multi-session group tobacco cessation programs are useful, especially for those with minimal to mild levels of tobacco dependence.
  - Approaches to tobacco dependence treatment that have been shown to be effective in tobacco-dependent adults can be applied to moderately to severely tobacco-dependent adolescents, although such pharmacotherapy is not currently FDA approved for use in minors.
- Pediatricians should encourage public policies to de-normalize smoking behavior and reduce initiation of smoking by young people.

Acknowledgment

The principles of treatment described here are adapted from those of the American College of Chest Physicians *Tobacco Dependence Treatment Toolkit,* 3rd Edition, (tobaccodependence.chestnet.org). Dr Farber is a coauthor of the toolkit. Dr Sachs is lead author of the toolkit.

Key Resources

- National Cancer Institute Quit Line for free telephone counseling on tobacco cessation (connects caller to their state quitline): **1-800-QUIT NOW.**
- American College of Chest Physician's *Tobacco Dependence Treatment Toolkit,* 3rd Edition: http://tobaccodependence.chestnet.org.
- Campaign for Tobacco Free Kids advocates for public policies to decrease smoking initiation and secondhand smoke exposure. http://www.tobaccofreekids.org/index.php
- American Academy of Pediatrics Policy Statement
  - Committee on Environmental Health, Committee on Substance Abuse, Committee on Adolescence, Committee on Native American Child Health. Tobacco use: a pediatric disease. *Pediatrics.* 2009;124(5):1474–1487. http://aappolicy.aappublications.org/cgi/content/full/pediatrics;124/5/1474

- American Academy of Pediatrics Technical Reports
  - Committee on Environmental Health, Committee on Native American Child Health, Committee on Adolescence. Secondhand and prenatal tobacco smoke exposure. *Pediatrics.* 2009;124(5):e1017–e1044. http://aappolicy.aappublications.org/cgi/content/full/pediatrics;124/5/e1017
  - Committee on Substance Abuse. Tobacco as a substance of abuse. *Pediatrics.* 2009;124(5):e1045–e1053. http://aappolicy.aappublications.org/cgi/content/full/pediatrics;124/5/e1045 Fagerström Tolerance Questionnaire, modified version: http://dccps.nci.nih.gov/TCRB/mftq.html.

References

1. Centers for Disease Control and Prevention. Smoking-attributable mortality, years of potential life lost, and productivity losses—United States, 2000–2004. *MMWR Morb Mortal Wkly Rep.* 2008;57(45):1226–1228
2. Elders MJ, Perry CL, Eriksen MP, Giovino GA. The report of the Surgeon General: preventing tobacco use among young people. *Am J Public Health.* 1994;84(4):543–547
3. US Department of Health and Human Services. *The Health Consequences of Involuntary Exposure to Tobacco Smoke: A Report of the Surgeon General.* Atlanta, GA: US Department of Health and Human Services, Centers for Disease Control and Prevention, Coordinating Center for Health Promotion, National Center for Chronic Disease Prevention and Health Promotion, Office on Smoking and Health; 2006
4. Breese CR, Marks MJ, Logel J, et al. Effect of smoking history on [3H] nicotine binding in human postmortem brain. *J Pharmacol Exp Ther.* 1997;282(1):7–13
5. Hughes JR. Clinical significance of tobacco withdrawal. *Nicotine Tob Res.* 2006;8(2):153–156
6. Benowitz NL. Nicotine addiction. *N Engl J Med.* 2010;362(24):2295–2303
7. Farber HJ, Knowles SB, Brown NL, et al. Secondhand tobacco smoke in children with asthma: sources of and parental perceptions about exposure in children and parental readiness to change. *Chest.* 2008;133(6):1367–1374
8. American Academy of Pediatrics Committee on Environmental Health, Committee on Substance Abuse, Committee on Adolescence, Committee on Native American Child Health. Tobacco use: a pediatric disease. *Pediatrics.* 2009;124:1474–1487
9. Fiore MC, Jaén CR, Baker TB, et al. *Treating Tobacco Use and Dependence: 2008 Update. Clinical Practice Guideline.* Rockville, MD: US Department of Health and Human Services, Public Health Service; 2008

10. Winickoff JP, Tanski SE, McMillen RC, Klein JD, Rigotti NA, Weitzman M. Child health care clinicians' use of medications to help parents quit smoking: a national parent survey. *Pediatrics.* 2005;115(4):1013–1017
11. Winickoff JP, Tanski SE, McMillen RC, Hipple BJ, Friebely J, Healey EA. A national survey of the acceptability of quitlines to help parents quit smoking. *Pediatrics.* 2006;117(4):e695–e700
12. Winickoff JP, Berkowitz AB, Brooks K, et al. State-of-the-art interventions for office-based parental tobacco control. *Pediatrics.* 2005;115(3):750–760
13. Prochaska JO, Velicer WF. The transtheoretical model of health behavior change. *Am J Health Promot.* 1997;12(1):38–48
14. Farber HJ. High-quality asthma care: it's not just about drugs. *Permanente J.* 2005;9(3):32–36
15. Heatherton TF, Kozlowski LT, Frecker RC, et al. The Fagerström Test for nicotine dependence: a revision of the Fagerström Tolerance Questionnaire. *Br J Addict.* 1991;86:1119–1127
16. Prokhorov AV, De Moor C, Pallonen UE, Hudmon KS, Koehly L, Hu S. Validation of the modified Fagerström Tolerance Questionnaire with salivary cotinine among adolescents. *Addict Behav.* 2000;25(3):429–433
17. Sachs DPL, Leone FT, Farber HJ, et al. *American College of Chest Physicians Tobacco-Dependence Treatment Tool Kit.* 3rd ed. Northbrook, IL: American College of Chest Physicians; 2010. http://tobaccodependence.chestnet.org
18. Hughes JR, Hatsukami DK, Pickens RW, Krahn D, Malin S, Luknic A. Effect of nicotine on the tobacco withdrawal syndrome. *Psychopharmacology (Berl).* 1984;83(1):82–87
19. Gonzales D, Rennard SI, Nides M, et al. Varenicline, an alpha4beta2 nicotinic acetylcholine receptor partial agonist vs sustained-release bupropion and placebo for smoking cessation: a randomized controlled trial. *JAMA.* 2006;296(1):47–55
20. Pollock M, Lee JH. Postmarket reviews: the smoking cessation aids varenicline (marketed as Chantix) and bupropion (marketed as Zyban and generics)—suicidal ideation and behavior. *FDA Drug Safety Newsletter.* 2009;2(1):1–4
21. Hughes JR. Smoking and suicide: a brief overview. *Drug Alcohol Depend.* 2008;98(3):169–178
22. Medical Letter. Safety of smoking cessation drugs. *Med Lett Drugs Ther.* 2009;51(1319):65
23. Drugs for tobacco dependence. *Treat Guide Med Lett.* 2008;6(73):61–66
24. Miller M, Hemenway D, Bell NS, Yore MM, Amoroso PJ. Cigarette smoking and suicide: a prospective study of 300,000 male active-duty Army soldiers. *Am J Epidemiol.* 2000;151(11):1060–1063
25. Miller M, Hemenway D, Rimm E. Cigarettes and suicide: a prospective study of 50,000 men. *Am J Public Health.* 2000;90(5):768–773
26. Boden JM, Fergusson DM, Horwood LJ. Cigarette smoking and suicidal behaviour: results from a 25-year longitudinal study. *Psychol Med.* 2008;38(3):433–439

27. Grant BF, Hasin DS, Chou SP, Stinson FS, Dawson DA. Nicotine dependence and psychiatric disorders in the United States: results from the national epidemiologic survey on alcohol and related conditions. *Arch Gen Psychiatry.* 2004;61(11):1107–1115
28. Escobedo LG, Reddy M, Giovino GA. The relationship between depressive symptoms and cigarette smoking in US adolescents. *Addiction.* 1998;93(3):433–440
29. Alvarado GF, Breslau N. Smoking and young people's mental health. *Curr Opin Psychiatry.* 2005;18(4):397–400
30. Patten CA, Choi WS, Vickers KS, Pierce JP. Persistence of depressive symptoms in adolescents. *Neuropsychopharmacology.* 2001;25(5 suppl):S89–S91
31. Henningfield JE, Radzius A, Cooper TM, Clayton RR. Drinking coffee and carbonated beverages blocks absorption of nicotine from nicotine Polacrilex gum. *JAMA.* 1990;264:1560–1564
32. Lunell E, Bergstrom M, Antoni G, Langstrom B, Nordberg A. Nicotine deposition and body distribution from a nicotine inhaler and a cigarette studied with positron emission tomography. *Clin Pharmacol Ther.* 1996;59(5):593–594
33. Rose JE, Behm FM, Westman EC, et al. Precessation treatment with nicotine skin patch facilitates smoking cessation. *Nicotine Tob Res.* 2006;8:89–101
34. DiFranza JR, Savageau JA, Fletcher K, et al. Symptoms of tobacco dependence after brief intermittent use: the Development and Assessment of Nicotine Dependence in Youth-2 study. *Arch Pediatr Adolesc Med.* 2007;161(7):704–710
35. Centers for Disease Control and Prevention. Youth tobacco surveillance United States, 2000. *MMWR Surveill Summ.* 2001;50(no. SS-4)
36. Burt RD, Peterson AV Jr. Smoking cessation among high school seniors. *Prev Med.* 1998;27(3):319–327
37. Robinson LA, Vander Weg MW, Riedel BW, Klesges RC, McLain-Allen B. "Start to stop": results of a randomised controlled trial of a smoking cessation programme for teens. *Tob Control.* 2003;12 suppl 4:IV26–33
38. Colby SM, Monti PM, O'Leary Tevyaw T, et al. Brief motivational intervention for adolescent smokers in medical settings. *Addict Behav.* 2005;30(5):865–874
39. Horn K, Dino G, Hamilton C, Noerachmanto N. Efficacy of an emergency department-based motivational teenage smoking intervention. *Prev Chronic Dis.* 2007;4(1):A08
40. Sussman S, Dent CW, Lichtman KL. Project EX: outcomes of a teen smoking cessation program. *Addict Behav.* 2001;26(3):425–438
41. Grimshaw GM, Stanton A. Tobacco cessation interventions for young people. *Cochrane Database Syst Rev.* 2006;(4):CD003289
42. Horn K, Fernandes A, Dino G, Massey CJ, Kalsekar I. Adolescent nicotine dependence and smoking cessation outcomes. *Addict Behav.* 2003;28(4):769–776

43. Moolchan ET, Robinson ML, Ernst M, et al. Safety and efficacy of the nicotine patch and gum for the treatment of adolescent tobacco addiction. *Pediatrics.* 2005;115;407–414
44. Muramoto ML, Leischow SJ, Sherrill D, et al. Randomized, double-blind, placebo-controlled trial of 2 dosages of sustained-release bupropion for adolescent smoking cessation. *Arch Pediatr Adolesc Med.* 2007;161:1068–1074
45. Rubinstein ML, Benowitz NL, Auerback GM, Moscicki AB. A randomized trial of nicotine nasal spray in adolescent smokers. *Pediatrics.* 2008;122(3):e595–e600
46. Bagot KS, Heishman SJ, Moolchan ET. Tobacco craving predicts lapse to smoking among adolescent smokers in cessation treatment. *Nicotine Tob Res.* 2007;9(6):647–652
47. Sims TH; American Academy of Pediatrics Committee on Substance Abuse. Tobacco as a substance of abuse. *Pediatrics.* 2009;124(5):1045–1053
48. Westenberger BJ. Evaluation of e-cigarettes. Food and Drug Administration Center for Drug Evaluation and Research, Division of Pharmaceutical Analysis. May 4, 2009. http://www.fda.gov/downloads/Drugs/ScienceResearch/UCM173250.pdf. Accessed November 16, 2009
49. FDA Warns of Health Risks Posed by E-Cigarettes. FDA Consumer Health Information, July 2009. http://www.fda.gov/downloads/ForConsumers/ConsumerUpdates/UCM173430.pdf Accessed November 16, 2009
50. Roeseler A, Burns D. The quarter that changed the world. *Tob Control.* 2010;19 suppl 1:i3–15

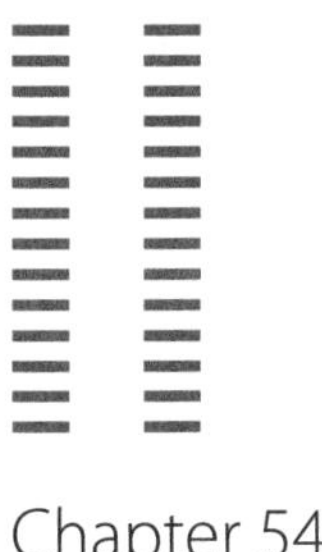

Chapter 54

Home Apnea Monitoring

Suzanne E. Beck, MD
Lee J. Brooks, MD

Introduction

Cardiorespiratory monitors were originally designed and used in clinical care in the 1960s for the management of apnea of prematurity in the hospital setting.[1] Currently home cardiorespiratory monitoring (HCRM) supports the care of infants with a variety of acute and chronic disorders.[2,3]

Continuous cardiorespiratory monitors at home were intended to prevent sudden infant death syndrome (SIDS), centering on the hypothesis that prolonged apnea caused or preceded SIDS.[4] Despite independent research spanning several decades, however, the apnea theory has never been proven.[5–9] There have been no randomized, controlled studies demonstrating the effectiveness of home apnea monitoring devices, or that SIDS is prevented in infants receiving cardiorespiratory monitoring at home. Epidemiological studies have shown that the death rate attributable to SIDS did not decline as a result of widespread home monitor usage and in fact did not decline until public education, such as the Back to Sleep campaign, focused on reducing modifiable SIDS risk factors.[10–14] However, this lack of data may, at least in part, be due to the infrequency of SIDS deaths and hence the enormous numbers of subjects required for study. Despite the lack of data, home apnea monitoring became popular and commonplace in high-risk infants, based on the hypothesis that by identifying episodes of central apnea or bradycardia, and alerting caregivers to a pathologic event, an intervention could be performed to prevent a terminal cardiorespiratory event.[4,15,16]

Collaborative Home Infant Monitoring Evaluation (CHIME) Study

Analysis of data from longitudinal multi-channel home cardiorespiratory recordings of infants, available from the CHIME Study Group[17] has given insight into the range and variability of cardiorespiratory physiology in healthy term infants compared with infants thought to be at risk for SIDS. The study monitored 1,079 infants and included 718,000 hours of monitoring time. These infants were divided into the following subgroups: those who had had an idiopathic apparent life-threatening event (ALTE) (n=152), a sibling who died of SIDS (n=178), asymptomatic healthy preterm (≤34 weeks' gestation, weighing <1,750 g at birth) (n=443), and asymptomatic healthy term (n=306) infants. The study defined extreme apnea as 30 seconds or longer for all ages and extreme bradycardia as a heart rate less than 60 beats per minute (bpm) and lasting more than 10 seconds for infants younger than 44 weeks' postmenstrual age (PMA*) and less than 50 bpm and lasting more than 10 seconds for infants at least 44 weeks' PMA. Conventional events, including 20 seconds of apnea and bradycardia ranging from 50 to 80 bpm depending on PMA were also recorded. Events exceeding the conventional thresholds occurred in 41% of infants. Extreme events occurred in 10% of all infants, including 2.3% of healthy term infants.

The study demonstrated that preterm infants, up to approximately 43 weeks' PMA, were the only group that had a higher risk of "extreme events" compared with healthy term infants. The study demonstrated that many infants experienced apnea and bradycardia exceeding conventional alarm thresholds without serious sequelae, and by 41 weeks' PMA the "at-risk" groups were indistinguishable from healthy controls.[17]

The CHIME study characterized cardiorespiratory events only in infants in whom the cause of the event was unknown and excluded any infant with known problems, such as those on concurrent treatment with supplemental oxygen, diuretics, steroids, and medications for gastroesophageal reflux or seizures; those with abnormal chest radiographs, congenital heart disease (except asymptomatic patent

*Please note that in the CHIME reports the term *postconceptional age (PCA)* was used in place of *postmenstrual age (PMA)*. PMA is the actual age and correct terminology when referring to these data. (Personal communication with Carl E. Hunt, MD, and Michael J. Corwin, MD)

ductus arteriosis, muscular wall ventricular septal defect), ventricular-peritoneal shunt, congenital brain anomalies, chromosomal abnormalities, facial anomalies, and metabolic anomalies; or infants whose caregiver used illicit drugs or was not able to communicate (language barrier or had no telephone). Only 16% of the mothers of the healthy control group smoked cigarettes during pregnancy, while up to 43% of the mothers of the "at-risk" groups smoked.[17] Therefore, what is considered normal based on data in the CHIME study might not pertain to medically ill infants or the population of patients being monitored for other reasons.

Indications for Home Cardiorespiratory Monitoring

With the above background in mind, there may be a group of infants at risk for sudden death because of factors other than SIDS, in whom use of a HCRM may be warranted. This group is different from SIDS because the definition of SIDS implies that the death is not associated with such risk factors, for example chronic lung disease (bronchopulmonary dysplasia). The American Academy of Pediatrics (AAP) does not recommend home apnea monitoring to prevent SIDS; however, the AAP has published guidelines for the appropriate use of HCRM in certain groups of infants who are at risk of sudden death or of extreme events.[2,18] The AAP states: "HCRM may be justified to allow rapid recognition of apnea, airway obstruction or respiratory failure, interruption of supplemental oxygen supply, or failure of mechanical respiratory support[2] and may be useful in some infants who have had an apparent life-threatening event (ALTE)"[18] (Box 54-1). For a full discussion on ALTE, please see Chapter 32.

Pediatricians should continue to promote proven practices that decrease the risk of SIDS: supine sleep position, safe sleeping environments, elimination of prenatal and postnatal tobacco smoke exposure, etc (refer to references 20 and 21 for a more in depth discussion of SIDS prevention).

Home Cardiorespiratory Monitoring

The monitor at home will not prevent apneas or other cardiorespiratory events. It merely alerts the caretakers that the child needs attention. Parents and other caretakers must be trained in how to respond to monitor alarms and the steps to take in properly caring for the child.

Box 54-1. Recommendations for Home Monitoring With Clinical Rationale[a]

1. Home cardiorespiratory monitoring (HCRM) should not be used to prevent sudden infant death syndrome (SIDS). Rationale: The data do not support the use of monitors to prevent SIDS.
2. HCRM may be warranted for premature infants who are at high risk of recurrent episodes of apnea, bradycardia, and hypoxia. Use should be limited to 43 weeks' postmenstrual age (PMA) or after the cessation of extreme events. Rationale: Preterm infants are at greater risk of extreme apnea episodes than term infants; risk decreases with time, ceasing at approximately 43 weeks' PMA.[17]
3. HCRM may be warranted for infants who are technologically dependent (tracheostomy, continuous positive airway pressure, mechanical ventilation) or who have unstable airways, have rare medical conditions affecting the regulation of breathing (such as central hypoventilation syndrome, metabolic disorders, central nervous system disorders), or who have symptomatic chronic lung disease (especially those requiring supplemental oxygen) or who have experienced an unexplained apparent life-threatening event. Rationale: Monitoring of these infants may alert the caregiver to extreme events that may have been due to apnea, airway obstruction, respiratory failure, interruption of supplemental oxygen supply, or failure of mechanical respiratory support, allowing rapid intervention and prevention of hypoxia due to or resulting in bradycardia or prolonged apnea.
4. If a home monitor is prescribed it should be equipped with an event recorder. Rationale: Event recorders allow the physician to review cardiorespiratory events and determine their clinical significance.
5. Parents should be advised that HCRM has not been proven to prevent sudden unexpected events in infants (see Family Education section). Indeed, there have been reports of infants dying suddenly and unexpectedly at home despite using a monitor.[19] Parents should be taught proper use of the monitor, placement of leads, troubleshooting of frequent alarms, proper response to alarms and clinical scenarios, and cardiopulmonary resuscitation, as well as safe infant sleeping practices.

[a]Based on the 2003 American Academy of Pediatrics policy statement "Apnea, Sudden Infant Death and Home Monitoring."[2]

Impedance Monitors

A standard home monitor is designed to detect breathing effort and heart rate with a 2-channel signal via 2 electrodes placed on the anterior chest or via a belt around the chest. These types of monitors will detect central apnea (ie, lack of chest wall movement) and heart rate. A transthoracic impedance signal from the chest detects chest wall movement (or lack thereof) and is calculated into a respiratory rate.

A QRS electrocardiogram signal is calculated into a heart rate. The heart rate and respiratory rate parameters vary by age. Limits for recording and alarming should be specifically ordered by the prescribing clinician and adjusted, if necessary, as the child grows and matures (Table 54-1). The parameters communicated to and set by the home care or equipment company are (1) duration of apnea for recording and alarming; (2) heart rate minimum (bradycardia limit), usually set with a 5-second delay to account for beat-to-beat variability, and maximum (tachycardia limit). Since most tachycardia alarms are false, due to movement artifacts while awake, and take up valuable memory space, the tachycardia limit may be turned off depending on the indications for monitoring. However, tachycardia may also be a sign of respiratory distress and one of the first signs of distress in children with neuromuscular weakness.

Standard monitors are designed to detect extremes of heart rate, namely bradycardia and central apnea, and specifically do not detect obstructive apnea or hypoxemia. This is problematic because the initial pathophysiological event causing central apnea or bradycardia may have been obstructive apnea or hypoxemia. In any case, the apnea monitors can be a useful tool to look for central apnea or bradycardia, and once detected, the infant can be appropriately evaluated for a specific cause. Home cardiorespiratory monitoring may be a useful tool to monitor an infant who suffered from a severe, unexplained ALTE to provide information on the physiological consequences of subsequent events, and similarly to monitor for physiological aberrations after specific therapy has been initiated or weaned.

Table 54-1. Suggested Home Cardiorespiratory Parameters

Parameter	Postmenstrual Age			
	<40 weeks	40–44 weeks	44 weeks–2 months	>2 months
Apnea alarm (seconds)	20	20	20	20
Apnea record (seconds)	16–19	16–19	16–19	16–19
Bradycardia (seconds)	80	80	70	60
Bradycardia delay (seconds)	5	5	5	5
Tachycardia	off	off	off	off

A standard monitor has a memory capable of storing data from individual events and is often referred to as an event recorder. The device will indicate when the memory is nearly full so it can be downloaded in a timely manner without loss of data. Once the memory is full, the device will either not record any further events or erase earlier events until it is downloaded and refreshed. The memory function does not have to be used if the device is used for an alerting instrument only (eg, in a patient with an established pattern of events). Event recorders allow the physician to review cardiorespiratory events and determine their clinical significance. Alarms may be false because of motion on the part of the infant or improper lead placement, which may result in a low amplitude signal that is misinterpreted by the monitor as apnea. The monitor should be downloaded periodically for review of events and interpreted by a qualified physician. If the clinician ordering the monitor does not feel comfortable in the review or interpretation of monitor downloads, the child should be referred to an appropriate specialist, usually a pulmonologist or a neonatologist, who can be expected to follow the child and assist in managing the child on a monitor.

A standard monitor is usually prescribed for use when the child is asleep or unattended. Event recording monitors are able to record and tabulate when the monitor is being used. This is important to ensure patient safety, and to confirm that parental reports of "no alarms" are not due to underutilization of the equipment. If a family is using the monitor around the clock, there may be many false alarms due to motion or lead detachment. Too many false alarms may result in parental desensitization, perhaps resulting in their failure to respond to an alarm that may herald a true, significant event. The cost benefit of continued monitoring must be reevaluated in the patient who is poorly compliant, and it may be necessary to contact local child welfare authorities.

Oximetry Monitor

Oxyhemoglobin saturation (Spo_2) can be monitored via a pulse oximeter. The unit monitors Spo_2, heart rate derived from the pulse signal, and strength of the signal displayed as the pulse waveform. Oxyhemoglobin saturation and a calculated heart rate are displayed on the monitor screen. The strength of signal may also be displayed in some models.

Continuous pulse oximetry monitoring is notoriously difficult in the home and can lead to inaccurate readings and many false alarms due to movement, poor perfusion, or loose connections. Some newer pulse oximeters monitor the quality of the signal to minimize artifacts due to movements and limit false alarms.

Continuous pulse oximetry monitoring in the home setting can be useful in patients at risk for subtle or intermittent hypoxemia whether or not supplemental oxygen is required. This includes patients with severe chronic lung disease, patients with profound respiratory muscle weakness, young patients with tracheostomies, or patients requiring ventilatory support. Intermittent pulse oximetry monitoring in the home setting may be recommended in otherwise stable patients, during certain periods when the risk of oxyhemoglobin desaturation is more likely. Some patients may require oximetry monitoring only during sleep or during periods of respiratory illnesses. Patients on supplemental oxygen at home do not necessarily require continuous pulse oximetry but may need monitoring during periods of illness.

The pulse oximetry device is usually used as an alerting instrument only and the memory function is often not used, as the memory can fill within several hours or days. It may be used diagnostically to detect suspected or unsuspected oxyhemoglobin desaturation related to chronic lung disease or apnea in an infant or child, and is the preferred study to evaluate the child who is being weaned from supplemental oxygen.

Oximetry monitoring in the home requires education for the caretakers to recognize false readings and to troubleshoot abnormal signals or measurements. Whether the device is used as an alerting instrument alone or whether it is being used to record, alarm parameters are prescribed by the clinician and communicated to and set by the home care or nursing company (if applicable). These parameters include (1) low saturation and length of time below that level for alarming and or recording and (2) heart rate minimum (bradycardia limit), usually set with a 5-second delay to account for beat-to-beat variability, and maximum for alarming and recording. It is important to specify and note the averaging time for the oximeter. Beat-to-beat recording will lead to many false alarms due to motion or other artifact, while too long an averaging time will result in smoothing of the data and clinically important events may be missed. The prescription should also specifically include when to use the monitor. For recording devices, the prescription should include how often to download and who is interpreting the downloads. The caretakers should have a clear understanding of the limitations of the monitor and what to do if the readings are low.

Interpretation of Home Cardiorespiratory Monitor Downloads

A typical cardiorespiratory monitor will store about 50 seconds of data from each event according to the set parameters, including some time before and after the event. In addition the monitor will store adherence data, recording and graphing all of the time the monitor is in actual use (Figure 54-1). With appropriate software, data can be downloaded and analyzed for review of each event. The download may be reviewed by the patient's primary care provider or a specialist (usually a pulmonologist or neonatologist) who may or may not be involved in the care of the patient. Typically, the specialist prepares a report that includes the name and date of birth of the patient, gestational age and reason for monitoring if known, and the dates of monitoring reviewed. A diary of usage and events is also desirable. The report should include the date range of monitor usage, number of events (ie, number of alarms), number of alarms available for review (which may be less if the

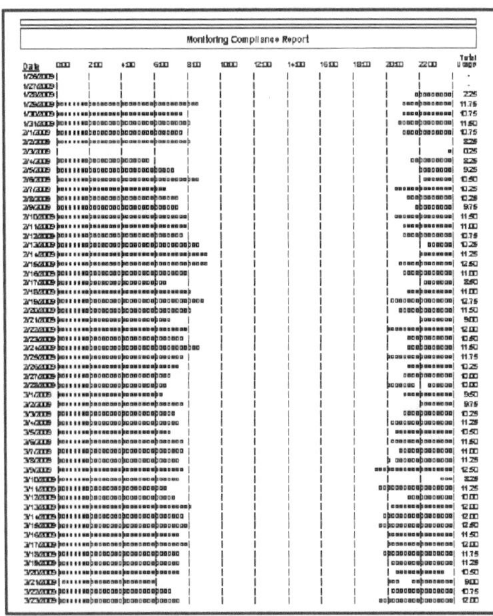

Figure 54-1. Examples of compliance reports from 3 individual typical home cardiorespiratory monitor downloads showing 3 different scenarios of usage: **(A)** consistent and uniform use from bedtime (approximately 8–9 pm) to wake time (approximately 7–8 am), **(B)** continuous usage almost 24 hours/day, and **(C)** intermittent usage.

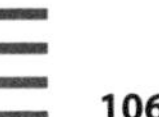

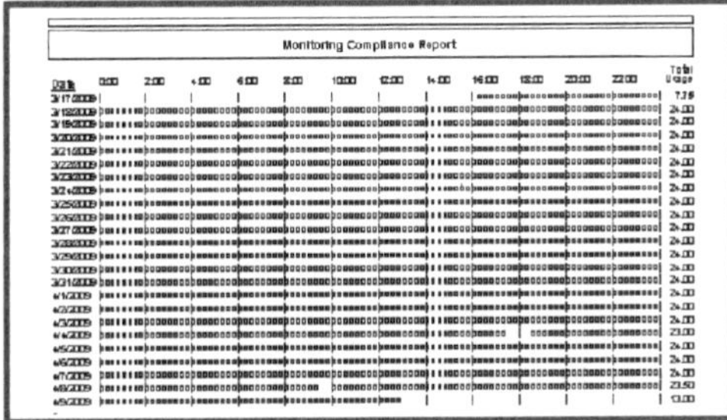

B

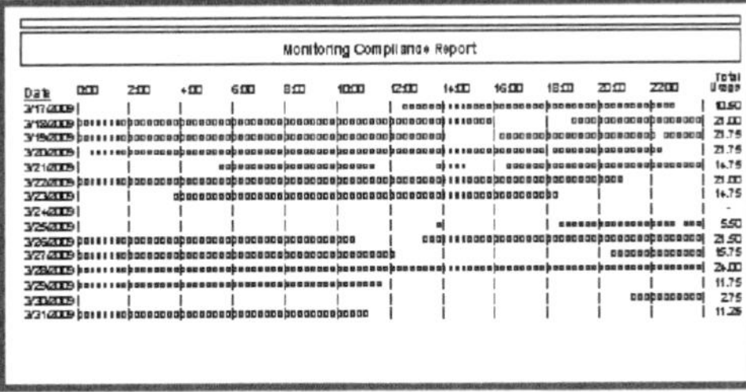

C

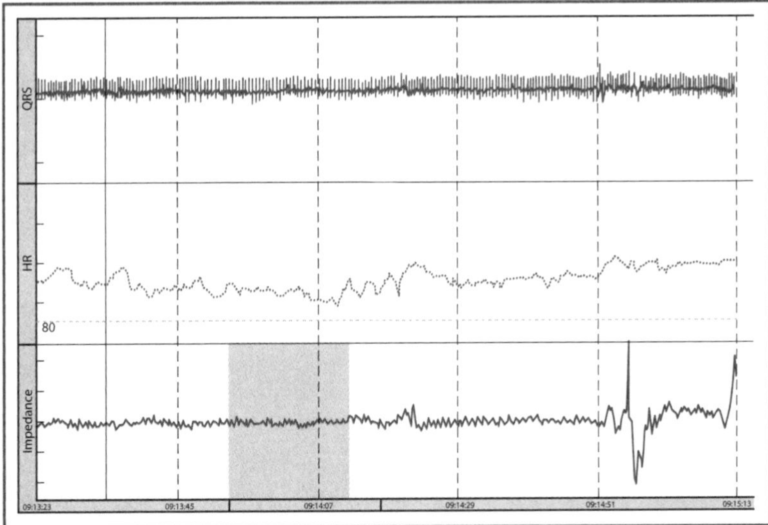

Figure 54-2. 150-second epoch of a home apnea monitor recording showing a false apnea alarm. Note top panels showing QRS complex; middle panels showing heart rate, above 80 beats per minute in this case; and in the lower panels chest wall impedence showing continued chest wall movement. The shaded area indicates a 26-second apneic event as detected by the monitor, but it is in fact a false apnea due to low amplitude of the signal.

memory exceeded capacity and deleted events), the number and type of true alarms by reviewing each individual event to determine if each event is real or false, and the days and hours used. Figures 54-2 through 54-4 show typical monitor events.

The significance of events will be based on number, length, and association with each other in relation to the patient's age and underlying medical problems. Prompt communication via a report from the interpreting physician to the primary care provider is essential. However, it is unwise to make clinical decisions based solely on monitor downloads. Decisions to alter therapy, change monitoring parameters, or stop the monitor should be made by the clinician caring for the child, taking into account monitoring data, underlying conditions, and clinical progress.

Ordering Home Cardiorespiratory Monitors

A prescription for a home monitor should include the indication for monitoring and age-appropriate alarm and recording parameters (see Table 54-1), which is then communicated to a durable medical equipment (DME) company. The company will deliver the equipment to the hospital or to the home and teach the family how to keep a log of events, use the equipment, and order supplies. If the monitor is started on an inpatient, the bedside nurse should review all teaching prior to discharge.

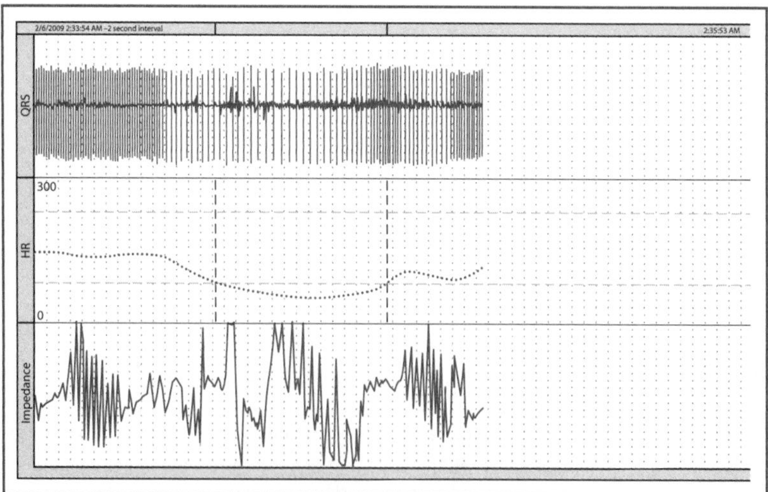

Figure 54-3. 120-second epoch of a home apnea monitor recording showing a true bradycardia alarm. Note top panels showing electrocardiogram, with a heart rate dipping below 80 beats per minute for 30 seconds (middle panels); and impedance showing continued chest wall movement (lower panels). This is an example of a true bradycardia.

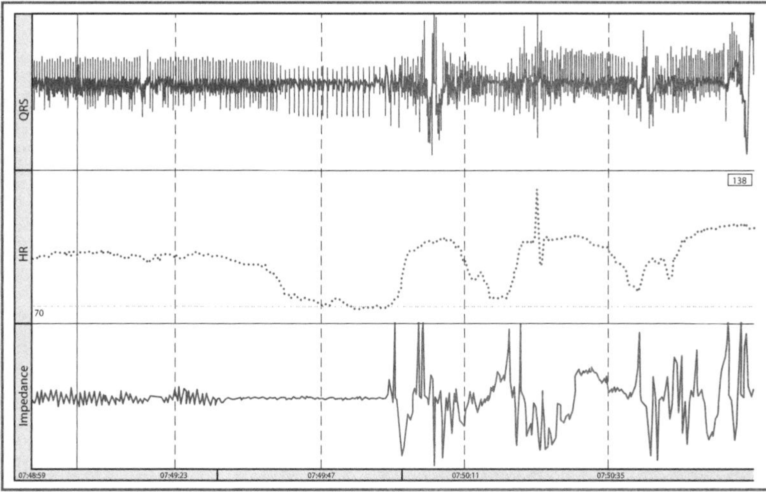

Figure 54-4. 150-second epoch of a home apnea monitor recording showing a true central apnea followed by bradycardia with quick recovery. Note top panels with electrocardiogram showing intact waveforms in the first half of the event with heart rate decelerations from 140 to 68 beats per minute (middle panels) and chest wall impedence showing lack of chest wall movement with a true 25-second apnea (lower panels) follow by a period of erratic chest wall movement associated with poor QRS waveforms typical of movement artifact (top panels). This is an example of a 25-second central apnea associated with physiological heart rate deceleration followed bymovement. An accompanying diary of events would help determine whether the movement after the apnea alarm was spontaneous or caused by a caretaker intervention.

Family Education

Family education is vital to adherence and proper use of home monitors. Safe infant sleep practices, including sleeping place and position, and avoidance of tobacco exposure, should be emphasized. The family requires instruction on proper use of the monitor and basic safety measures. This includes how to turn the monitor on and off and proper placement of the belt or leads. The monitor should be kept away from other children in the home who might have access to the child's bedroom. Skin care is an important topic to discuss, as skin irritation from the belt or leads is common, as is artifact from topical creams and lotions. In addition, the power company needs to be notified should an outage occur or failure to pay a bill on time results in discontinuation of service. It should be clear in the discharge orders to the caregivers and to the DME company when and how often the child should be placed on the monitor (24 hours a day vs only when asleep or unobserved). The family should know how often the monitor is to be downloaded. One possibility is to have the data in the monitor downloaded for interpretation every 1 to 3 months, depending on the indication for monitoring, to reassess continuing need for the monitoring (see Discontinuing Home Cardiorespiratory Monitoring). The recorded data should also be downloaded when the memory is nearly full. The memory may fill quickly with false alarms if inappropriate parameters are set, if there is poor lead placement, or with overuse. Once the memory is full, future events may record over the existing recordings. The data may also need to be downloaded after consulting with their practitioners should the family notice frequent or unusual cardiorespiratory events.

The family should have a clear understanding of what to do and whom to call should an alarm or an event occur. They need to understand that the monitor does not stop a cardiorespiratory event, it simply alerts caretakers that the baby needs attention. All caregivers of home-monitored patients should be instructed in proper assessment of the infant's breathing as well as CPR.

If the monitor alarms, the parent (or caretaker) should assess the child and particularly note the baby's color, and whether he or she is in distress. This may involve turning on the light to properly assess the child. They should note the presence and quality of breathing, central color, tone, position, and sounds. If the child is pink and breathing, no intervention may be needed. If the child is comfortable but apneic, mild stimulation may be required, moving to vigorous stimulation, and finally CPR, if necessary. If the child is not breathing, is cyanotic, has a change in tone, or is lethargic, CPR should be initiated and emergency protocols, such as calling 911, activated. A log or diary of events can be helpful during retrospective review of events.

Discontinuing Home Cardiorespiratory Monitoring

The physician who is taking care of the patient determines when the monitor should be discontinued. The home monitor is generally discontinued when the

1. Infant is older than 43 weeks' PMA
2. Reasons for starting it have resolved
3. Patient has weaned off therapy that was treating the events (eg, caffeine)
4. Patient is no longer exhibiting significant cardiorespiratory events

Many clinicians consider 3 months without an event requiring intervention and 2 months without a real event documented on monitor downloads to be adequate periods of observation to consider discontinuation.[22]

When to Refer

The primary care physician should be comfortable with caring for an infant on a cardiorespiratory monitor. If not, they should seek consultation and follow up with an experienced specialist, such as a neonatologist or pulmonologist. The role of the specialist may simply be to receive and evaluate monitor downloads, or they may provide consultative services and regular follow-up, adjusting monitor parameters as the child matures, and making the decision when monitoring is no longer needed. Communication from the specialist to the patient's primary outpatient physician is essential. The DME company should have a clear plan as to where the monitor downloads will be sent for interpretation. Some examples of abnormal findings and recommendations are included in Table 54-2.

Key Points

- Home cardiorespiratory monitors are useful tools to monitor preterm infants or other high-risk infants for central apnea or bradycardia.
- Home cardiorespiratory monitors have not been demonstrated to prevent SIDS.
- Heart rate and apnea alarm limits should be adjusted for age (Box 54-1).
- Children at risk for hypoxemia should be monitored with a pulse oximeter, understanding the limitations of home pulse oximetry.
- Family education, including CPR, is vital for proper adherence and usage of home apnea monitors.
- Communication among DME company, ordering physician, interpreting physician, and outpatient primary care providers is vital.
- Children at risk for obstructive sleep apnea should be evaluated with polysomnography and appropriate treatment initiated; a home monitor is not appropriate treatment for obstructive sleep apnea.

Table 54-2. Abnormal Monitor Recordings, Causes, and Actions

Monitor Result	Further Description	Common Cause	What to Do
False bradycardia alarms	Monitor alarms because EKG signal was lost due to movement	Movement	Communicate to family to limit monitor use while awake (if appropriate); check positioning of leads.
False bradycardia alarms	Beat-to-beat variability without true bradycardia detected because bradycardia delay was too short	Bradycardia delay was not set to 5 seconds.	Communicate to DME to reset bradycardia delay to 5 seconds.
Real but physiological bradycardia alarms	HR alarms for bradycardia, but low HR is within the normal range for age	HR alarm or record was not set according to age-appropriate parameters.	1. Validate with caretakers' observations of infant (no color change, baby doing well, etc). 2. Reassure caretakers. 3. Communicate to DME to reset HR alarm and record to age-appropriate parameters (see Box 54-1).
Real bradycardia alarms	HR alarms for bradycardia because HR is below what is expected for age	1. Gastroesophageal reflux[a] 2. Apnea, obstructive[a] or central[b] 3. Hypoxia[a]	Evaluate the child. Consider referral to a pediatric pulmonologist for further evaluation. (May need to expedite the referral.) If bradycardia alarms are frequent, prolonged, or severe, urgent inpatient evaluation is recommended.
Frequent short apnea alarms	Apnea alarms for apneas of <20 seconds	Alarm was inappropriately set to alarm at <20 seconds' duration.	1. Validate with caretakers' observations of infant (no color change, baby doing well, etc). 2. Reassure caretakers. 3. Communicate to DME to reset apnea alarm to 20 seconds.

Table 54-2. Abnormal Monitor Recordings, Causes, and Actions

Monitor Result	Further Description	Common Cause	What to Do
False apnea alarms	Apnea alarms because monitor did not detect respiratory effort due to low amplitude respiratory signal or shallow breathing	1. Poor connection (eg, lotion on skin) 2. Shallow breathing 3. Improper lead placement	1. Validate with caretakers' observations of infant (no color change, baby doing well, etc). 2. Reassure/educate caretakers. 3. Communicate to DME to reeducate caretakers on proper lead placement. 4. Consider changing to EKG leads ("patches") if an impedance belt is currently used.
Real apnea alarms	Apnea alarms for apneas of ≥20 seconds	1. Pathologic 2. Central apnea 3. Apnea of prematurity 4. Central causes 5. Infection 6. Metabolic 7. Other	Validate with caretakers' observations of the child. If stable, refer to pediatric pulmonologist. If unstable, admit for further evaluation.
Loose connections	Loose connections	Loose connections (Note: Loose connections can cause parental desensitization to real alarms or undue anxiety.)	1. Reassure and educate caretakers. 2. Limit monitor use to periods of sleep or when unobserved, if appropriate. 3. Communicate to DME to reeducate caretakers on proper lead placement.

Table 54-2. Abnormal Monitor Recordings, Causes, and Actions (continued)

Monitor Result	Further Description	Common Cause	What to Do
Tachycardia	HR alarms for tachycardia, usually due to movement. These are usually physiological.	High HR alarm was inappropriately set. (Note: Tachycardia alarms are often physiological and may cause desensitization to real alarms or undue anxiety.)[c]	1. Reassure/educate caretakers. 2. Limit monitor use to periods of sleep or when unobserved, if appropriate. 3. Communicate to DME to increase the tachycardia alarm parameter or turn tachycardia alarm off.
Poor compliance	Monitor is not being used regularly	Many	Validate with caretakers. May need to reeducate why monitor is being used.

Abbreviations: DME, durable medical equipment; EKG, electrocardiogram; HR, heart rate.

[a] These causes are not detected by the monitor.

[b] This cause might be present and detected but shorter events might not be detected.

[c] Tachycardia alarm may be useful in a few clinical scenarios; however, trends in heart rate rather than alarms may be more useful because of the frequency of false alarms caused by movement.

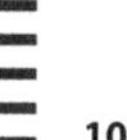

References

1. Daily WJ, Klaus M, Mayer HB. Apnea in premature infants: monitoring, incidence, heart rate changes, and effect on environmental temperature. *Pediatrics.* 1969;43:510–518
2. American Academy of Pediatrics Committee on Fetus and Newborn. Apnea, sudden death syndrome, and home monitoring. *Pediatrics.* 2003;111 (4 pt 1):914–917
3. National Institutes of Health. National Institutes of Health Consensus Development Conference on Infantile Apnea and Home Monitoring. Sept 29 to Oct 1, 1986. *Pediatrics.* 1987;79:292–299
4. Steinschneider A. Prolonged apnea and the sudden infant death syndrome: clinical and laboratory observations. *Pediatrics.* 1972;50:646–654
5. Franks CI, Watson JB, Brown BH, Foster EF. Respiratory patterns and risk of sudden unexpected death in infancy. *Arch Dis Child.* 1980;55:595–599
6. Southall DP, Richards JM, Rhoden KJ, et al. Prolonged apnea and units: failure to predict an increased risk for sudden infant death syndrome. *Pediatrics.* 1982;70:844–851
7. Rosen CL, Frost JD Jr, Harrison GM. Infant apnea: polygraphic studies and follow-up monitoring. *Pediatrics.* 1983;71:731–736
8. Southall DP, Richards JM, Stebbens V, et al. Cardiorespiratory function in 16 full-term infants with sudden infant death syndrome. *Pediatrics.* 1986;78:787–796
9. Schwartz PJ, Southall DP, Valdes-Dapena M. The sudden infant death syndrome: cardiac and respiratory mechanisms and interventions. Proceedings. May 24–27, 1987, Como, Italy. *Ann N Y Acad Sci.* 1988;533:1–474
10. Leach CE, Blair PS, Fleming PJ, et al. Epidemiology of SIDS and explained sudden infant deaths: CESDI SUDI Research Group. *Pediatrics.* 1999;104:e43
11. Carpenter RG, Irgens LM, Blair PS, et al. Sudden unexplained infant death in 20 regions in Europe: case control study. *Lancet.* 2004;363:185–191
12. Wennergren G, Alm B, Oyen N, et al. The decline in the incidence of SIDS in Scandinavia and its relation to risk intervention campaigns: Nordic Epidemiologic SIDS Study. *Acta Paediatr.* 1997;86;963–968
13. MacKay M, Abreu e Silva FA, MacFadyen UM, Williams A, Simpson H. Home monitoring for central apnoea. *Arch Dis Child.* 1984;59:136–142
14. Ward SL, Keens TG, Chan LS, et al. Sudden infant death syndrome in infants evaluated by apnea programs in California. *Pediatrics.* 1986;77:451–458
15. Hunt CE, Brouillette RT. Sudden infant death syndrome: 1987 perspective. *J Pediatr.* 1987;110:669–678
16. Daniels H, Naulaers G, Deroost F, et al. Polysomnography and home documented monitoring of cardiorespiratory patterns. *Arch Dis Child.* 1999;81:434–436
17. Ramanathan R, Corwin MJ, Hunt CE, et al. Cardiorespiratory event recorded on home monitors: comparison of healthy infants with those at increased risk for SIDS. *JAMA.* 2001;285:2199–2207

18. American Academy of Pediatrics Task Force on Sudden Infant Death Syndrome. The changing concept of sudden infant death syndrome: diagnosing coding shifts, controversies regarding the sleeping environment, and new variables to consider in reducing risk. *Pediatrics.* 2005;116;5:1245–1255
19. Meny RG, Carroll JL, Carbone MT, Kelly DH. Cardiorespiratory recordings from infants dying suddenly and unexpectedly at home. *Pediatrics.* 1994;93:44–49
20. Hunt CE, Corwin MJ, Lister G, et al. Precursors of cardiorespiratory events in infants detected by home memory monitor. *Pediatr Pulmonol.* 2008;43:87–98
21. American Academy of Pediatrics Task Force on Infant Sleep Position and Sudden Infant Death Syndrome. Changing concepts of sudden infant death syndrome: implications for infant sleeping environment and sleep position. *Pediatrics.* 2000;105:650–656
22. Pohl CA, Spitzer AR. Infant apnea. In: Dozor AJ, ed. *Primary Pediatric Pulmonology.* Armonk NY: Futura; 2001:43–62

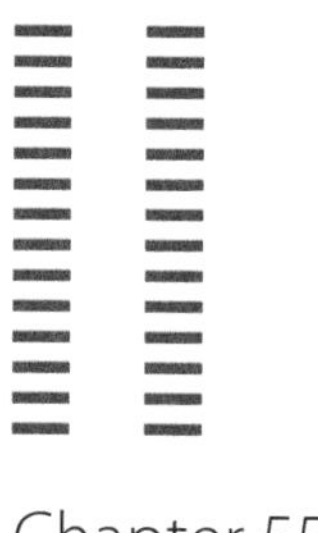

Chapter 55

Tracheostomies

Renée C. Benson, MD
Manisha Newaskar, MBBS

Introduction

Increasingly, general pediatricians care for children with long-term tracheostomies in the outpatient setting. Optimal care for the child with a long-term tracheostomy requires an interdisciplinary team. In addition to the primary care physician, the team usually includes an otolaryngologist or surgeon to place the tracheostomy and coordinate equipment and supplies, a pulmonologist to monitor the patient and coordinate care with the otolaryngologist, a speech therapist, home nursing care, and family members well trained in tracheostomy care. The general pediatrician should understand indications for tracheostomy placement, changes in normal physiology following tracheostomy, the patient's respiratory equipment, home care procedures, common complications of tracheostomy, and indications for decannulation.

Indications for Tracheostomy

With the advent of vaccines against *Corynebacterium diphtheriae* and *Haemophilus influenzae,* the most common indications for tracheostomy have shifted away from acute inflammatory airway compromise to anatomical upper airway obstruction caused by underlying chronic conditions.[1] Of pediatric tracheotomies, 40% to 70% are now performed on children younger than 1 year.[2–4] Indications for tracheostomy fall into 2 main categories delineated in Box 55-1.

Most commonly tracheostomy is indicated for congenital or acquired anatomical abnormalities leading to critical upper airway obstruction,

Case Report 55-1

A.N. is an 8-year-old girl with mucopolysaccharidosis (MPS) type VI who emigrated from Mexico to the United States for treatment of her MPS. She has a history of obstructive sleep apnea after her adenotonsillectomy at 3 years of age, but continues to snore and obstruct, requiring frequent position changes during sleep. Two months after her arrival in the United States she was found to have papilledema during a routine ophthalmology examination. Computed tomography scan revealed moderately severe hydrocephalus, and she was admitted for placement of a ventriculoperitoneal shunt. The anesthesiologist was unable to intubate her through either direct or fiberoptic laryngoscopy because laryngeal landmarks could not be visualized due to significant redundant tissue. She underwent emergency tracheostomy due to severe upper airway obstruction (Figures 55-1 and 55-2).

such as subglottic stenosis following prolonged intubation in the neonatal intensive care unit period. Children who require prolonged mechanical ventilation for longer than 2 to 3 weeks for acute or chronic respiratory failure may need a tracheostomy for more comfortable long-term ventilation. Finally, children with neuromuscular conditions leading to weak cough, aspiration, and difficulty clearing secretions may benefit from tracheostomy for improved control of secretions and pulmonary toilet.

Box 55-1. Indicators for Tracheostomy

Upper Airway Obstruction

- Foreign body
- Laryngeal or pharyngeal cysts/neoplasms
- Craniofacial disorders, such as macroglossia/micrognathia
- Epiglottitis
- Severe laryngotracheomalacia
- Bilateral true vocal cord paralysis
- Subglottic stenosis
- Facial or laryngeal trauma
- Laryngeal edema after burns

Prolonged Ventilatory Support

- Chronic respiratory failure
- Neuromuscular diseases
- Bronchopulmonary dysplasia
- Guillain-Barré syndrome
- Coma with respiratory dysfunction

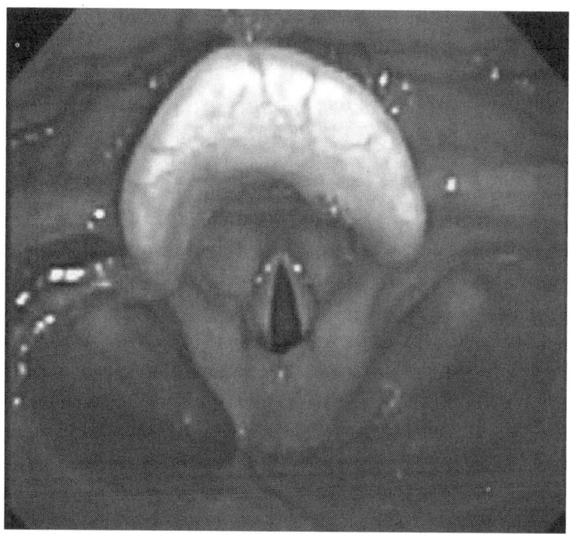

Figure 55-1. Normal larynx.

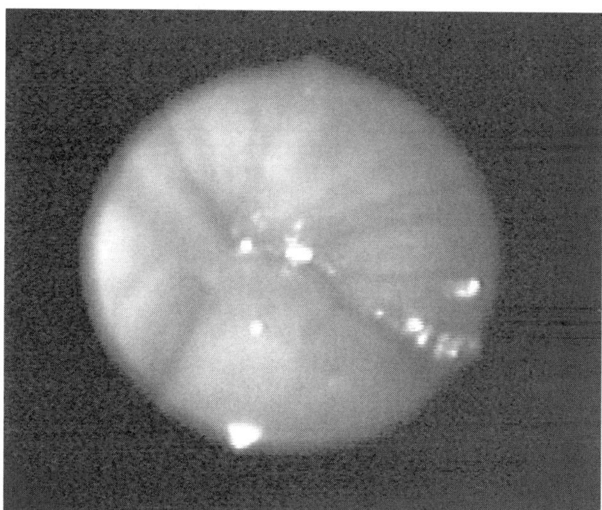

Figure 55-2. Mucopolysaccharidosis type VI with no visible laryngeal landmarks due to redundant tissue.

Surgical Methods

Surgical methods for tracheostomy include vertical incision (most common), circular window, inferior flap, or superior flap (Figure 55-3). The x-shaped starplasty incision is a newer technique that creates a tracheocutaneous fistula at the stoma leading to persistent fistula after decannulation, and as such should only be considered for conditions that are not expected to resolve. With any technique there is a risk of tracheal stenosis at the tracheostomy site and collapse of the anterior tracheal wall superior to the stoma.[5]

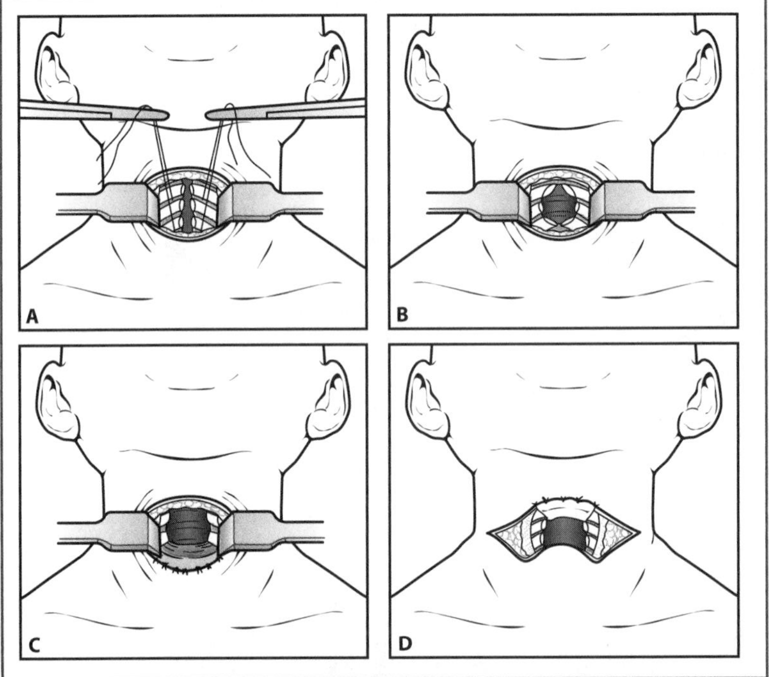

Figure 55-3. A. Standard pediatric tracheostomy with a vertical tracheal incision and silk retention sutures on either side of the tracheostomy opening. **B.** A circular shield of anterior tracheal wall cartilage has been removed to fenestrate the trachea and facilitate placement of the tracheostomy tube. **C.** An inferiorly based anterior tracheal wall flap, designed by Bjork, is sewn to the inferior edge of the horizontal tracheostomy skin incision. **D.** The Eliachar technique for a permanent stoma using an omega-shaped skin incision and a superiorly based tracheal flap, the construction of which results in a circumferential mucocutaneous suture line.

Altered Physiology After Tracheostomy

Once tracheostomy is performed, there are multiple physiological effects on normal tracheal function that may be altered. Airway clearance may become impaired because scar tissue can develop in the anterior trachea at the tracheostomy site, and normal ciliary function will be disrupted in that location leading to mucus stasis. In addition, cough clearance is less effective because the compressive phase of glottic closure before forced expiration is bypassed with the tracheostomy in place.[6] As a result, the patient is at increased risk for recurrent tracheitis and pneumonia. A normal sense of smell requires airflow through the nose, and if upper airway obstruction is significant airflow will be directed through the tracheostomy tube, thereby decreasing subjective sense of smell. Similarly, speech requires adequate airflow past the vocal cords, which depends on the severity of upper airway obstruction and tolerance of tracheostomy tube capping with a speaking valve. In order to achieve speech without augmentative communication devices, the tracheostomy tube must not exceed two-thirds of the tracheal lumen.[7] Development of normal speech requires early speaking valve assessment and speech therapy. The humidification of inspired air is another important function of the nasopharynx that is bypassed with a tracheostomy. The lack of humidity can lead to dessication of secretions, damage to mucus glands, mucus plugging, and impaired ciliary function unless external humidification is provided.[8] This in turn can cause increased infection risk and reduction of lung function. Finally, swallowing function can be affected by the presence of the tracheostomy tube because it limits superior excursion of the larynx with deglutition, may inhibit the normal laryngeal reflex that prevents aspiration, and may contribute to mass effect on the esophagus posteriorly.[1,9] Dysphagic symptoms are extremely common in infants with tracheostomies.[10]

Choice of Tube

Tracheostomy tubes are available in neonatal, pediatric, and adult sizes, which vary by length and radius or curvature (Figure 55-4). Customized tubes can be manufactured if standard tubes do not conform well to the child's anatomy. Choice of tube size depends on the initial indication for tracheostomy, keeping in mind the patient's lung function, tracheal size and shape, upper airway resistance, and allowance for air leak to achieve vocalization. Tubes can be made out of silicone,

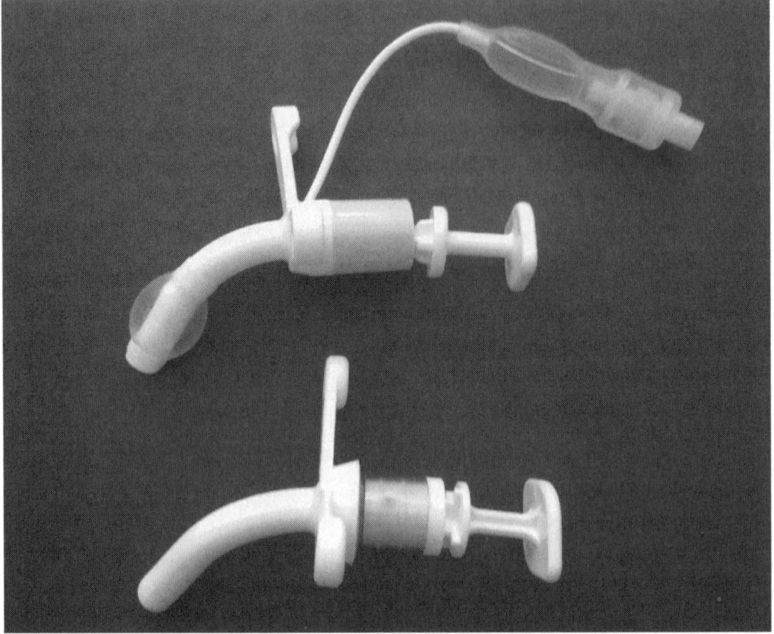

Figure 55-4. Bivona TTS cuffed tracheostomy tube, Shiley uncuffed tracheostomy tube. (From http://www.smiths-medical.com/catalog/bivona-tracheostomy-tubes/neonatal-pediatric/neo-tts/bivona-tts-cuffed-neonatal.html, http://www.shopmedrx.com/mp_images/MAL45PED.jpg.)

polyvinyl chloride and, uncommonly, metal. Bivona silicone tracheostomy tubes manufactured before 2007 are not compatible with magnetic resonance imaging, but subsequently manufactured tubes are compatible. Cuffed tubes are used for patients requiring mechanical ventilation with high pressures, or who are at risk for aspiration. Cuff pressures are kept below 20 cm H_2O to prevent necrosis injury to airway epithelium. In general, uncuffed tubes are preferred for children to allow for vocalization. Fenestrated tubes may be used by adults to promote translaryngeal airflow, but are not commonly used for children and may be associated with increased propensity to form granulomas.[7]

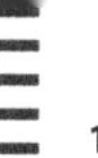

Home Care

Caregiver education is an important step in successful transition from hospital to home care. The benefits and risks of tracheostomy as well as its associated care should be discussed with the caregivers before the child receives a tracheostomy. As soon as the tracheostomy is placed, hands-on teaching starts at the bedside. Education should include decision-making as well as technical skills. It should also include stoma care, tracheostomy tube and tie changes, appropriate suctioning techniques, CPR training, recognizing signs and symptoms of respiratory problems, and troubleshooting any problems. This teaching should be individualized to the child and family, taking into account the cultural and language needs. Audiovisual aids may be used in addition to written materials. If appropriate, older siblings should be included in this process. Some institutions require at least 2 adult caregivers, who will provide consistent care to the child. They must receive training in tracheostomy care and demonstrate proficiency in skills and decision-making. A child with a tracheostomy must have constant supervision from an adult trained in tracheostomy care. If at any time after discharge a trained adult caregiver is not available, the child should be readmitted until a trained adult caregiver is available. All children should receive skilled home nursing care during a transitional adjustment time after discharge.

Every child with a tracheostomy should have adequate supplies at home (Box 55-2). These include spare tracheostomy tubes (including one size smaller for emergencies), cleaning supplies, tracheostomy ties, suctioning equipment and catheters, humidification equipment, etc. Before a child goes home, it is important to make sure all the essential supplies are available from the durable medical equipment company. All home care equipment, including portable equipment, should be used in the hospital before discharge.

Tracheostomy tubes should be changed on a regular basis. Different sources recommend tube change frequency, ranging from daily to monthly.[11,12] However, no objective data are available to support these practices. Weekly changes at baseline are usual and more frequent when the child is sick and has increased secretions. The advantages of frequent tube changes include keeping caregivers well practiced in tube changing to decrease airway infection or granuloma formation, and to reduce the risk of tube occlusion by thick secretions.[7]

Box 55-2. Tracheostomy Home Care Supplies

- Extra trach tube, same size
- Extra trach tube, 0.5 size smaller
- Suction machine and tubing
- Suction catheters and olive tip
- Ambu-bag with trach adapter and face mask
- Scissors
- External humidification (nebulizer/compressor or heat and moisture exchanger)
- Trach ties
- Clean jar of water
- Normal saline for suctioning
- Cotton swabs and gauze
- Oxygen with tubing (if ordered)
- Breathing monitor, such as pulse oximeter (if ordered)

Tracheostomy tubes made of polyvinyl chloride (PVC) can become rigid or stiff with repeated use and may develop splits or cracks. All tubes should be inspected for any cracks or splits before insertion. Clinical experience suggests that individual tracheostomy tubes made of PVC, when changed routinely, are appropriate for 6 months to 1 year before stiffening. Used tracheostomy tubes are best cleaned using a mild liquid detergent and water. After rinsing thoroughly, the tube should be allowed to air-dry completely and then stored in a plastic bag. Tracheostomy ties should be replaced during tracheostomy tube changes or when soiled. Soft Velcro material helps to minimize irritation of the skin. The ties should be tight enough to minimize movement of the tube, but still allow a finger to be inserted underneath the tie. If tracheostomy ties are too tight skin breakdown can occur.

Suctioning is a vital component to the management of a child with a chronic tracheostomy because occlusion of the tube by secretions or mucus plugs can be life-threatening. Attention to clean technique is important.[13] Caregivers should thoroughly wash their hands before and after each suctioning procedure. After suctioning, the catheter should be flushed with tap water until secretions are cleared from lumen. The catheter should then be wiped with alcohol and allowed to air-dry, and then stored in a clean, dry area.

Ensuring adequate humidification is important because the tracheostomy bypasses the upper airway and the inspired air may have significantly lower humidity than normal. External humidification can be delivered with a heated humidifier, jet nebulizer, or heat and moisture exchanger ("artificial nose"). The latter is a passive humidification device that collects moisture from the patient's exhaled gas and delivers it during inspiration. These devices also contribute to resistance and dead space and, as such, each patient must undergo evaluation with the device before using routinely.[7]

Speech can be facilitated with the use of a speaking valve, although not all patients are suitable candidates. To use the speaking valve, the patient must be awake, interactive, and medically stable. The child should also be able to tolerate deflation of the tracheostomy tube cuff, and must not have excessive thick secretions or high tracheal pressures. A speech-language pathologist plays an important role in speech development, and should be consulted as soon as possible to assist with the care of every child with a tracheostomy.[7,14]

A well-trained, vigilant, and properly equipped caregiver should be able to provide excellent monitoring. For young children or those unable to provide self-care of the tracheostomy, an awake caregiver should be available for monitoring for airway obstruction, which means many children require 8 to 12 hours of overnight nursing. Monitoring devices like a pulse oximeter should be considered for children who are at high risk of airway complications. Home apnea monitors may not be appropriate to monitor tracheostomy patients because they do not diagnose airway obstruction. For high-risk tracheostomy patients (ie, those patients who are tracheostomy dependent secondary to a critically narrow airway), 24-hour nursing may be necessary.

Routine Evaluation

Regular follow-up with a primary care physician, otolaryngologist, and pulmonologist is indicated for children with chronic tracheostomies. During the follow-up visit, the child should be assessed for the ongoing need for the tracheostomy tube and for complications. Routine evaluation with rigid or flexible bronchoscopy is usually performed every 6 to 12 months. The purpose of this evaluation is to assess the underlying airway pathology, detect and treat complications, assess tube size and position, and determine the readiness for decannulation. Decannulation should be considered if the original condition or need for the tracheostomy is no longer present and the patient is able to maintain a safe and adequate airway.

Complications

Between 25% to 50% of children will develop complications following tracheostomy, and each child should be routinely evaluated to minimize morbidity. Complications are more common in younger children and those with long-term tracheostomies (Box 55-3).[7] Tracheal lesions, such as granulomas, fistulas, and erosions, can develop as a result of rubbing of the tracheostomy tube against the tracheal wall. The suprastomal region is particularly vulnerable to collapse and granuloma formation. Suction catheters can also contribute to traumatic injury to the trachea and subsequent granuloma formation. Routine bronchoscopic evaluation can identify granulomas, which can then be excised.[1] Infection, particularly tracheitis, can develop as a result of direct communication with the external environment and inhibition of the normal defense mechanisms of mucociliary transport, cough, and upper airway filtration. Most patients with tracheostomies quickly become colonized with bacteria such as *Pseudomonas aeruginosa*. Erythema and drainage of the stoma site are usually managed with more frequent tube changes and topical antibiotics. Clinical signs of tracheitis or pneumonia, including increased cough and change in quality and color of secretions, accompanied by leukocytes and organisms

Box 55-3. Late Postoperative Complications of Pediatric Tracheostomy[a]

- Suprastomal collapse
- Tracheal wall granuloma
- Tracheoesophageal fistula
- Depressed scar
- Laryngotracheal stenosis
- Tracheal wall erosion
- Catastrophic hemorrhage
- Tracheomalacia
- Tube obstruction or displacement
- Decannulation failure
- Recurrent tracheitis/bronchitis/pneumonia
- Death

[a] From Sherman JM. American Thoracic Society statement: care of the child with a chronic tracheostomy. *Am J Respir Crit Care Med.* 2000;161:297–308. Copyright © American Thoracic Society. Reprinted by permission.

identified by Gram stain indicate acute infection. Cultures aspirated from the tracheostomy tube should guide antibiotic therapy.[15] Catastrophic bleeding as a result of erosion of the tracheostomy tube into a major vessel is rare, but any recurrent or significant bleeding should be promptly evaluated by the pulmonologist or otolaryngologist.[7] Lastly, obstruction or displacement of the tube can lead to life-threatening airway obstruction and even death; therefore, the family should be comfortable with suctioning, replacing the tube, and providing positive pressure resuscitation through the tube or upper airway with a mask should such an event take place.[16]

Decannulation

Decannulation should only be performed once the initial indication for tracheostomy placement has resolved and the patient has demonstrated the ability to maintain a patent airway and adequate respiratory physiology independent of the tracheostomy tube. Decannulation is ultimately achieved in 50% to 70% of patients; the average time to decannulation ranges from 4 to 21 months and varies based on original indication.[3,17,18] The patient should first undergo laryngoscopy and bronchoscopy to evaluate the airway for feasibility of decannulation, including the presence or absence of granulomas, suprastomal collapse,

Case Report 55-2

E.C. is a 4-year-old girl with a history of congenital hydrocephalus status. She has a ventriculoperitoneal shunt and pervasive developmental delay. She developed vomiting initially thought to be due to gastroenteritis, but later became lethargic and was found to have bilateral medial temporal, occipital, and midbrain ischemic infarcts due to shunt failure. She underwent tracheostomy for inability to protect her airway due to compromised neurologic function. She was admitted to the rehabilitation service and made significant improvements in her functional status, recovering her ability to speak and use her upper and lower extremities. She was successfully weaned to room air, and she began evaluation for decannulation. She did well with downsizing her tracheostomy tube and with capping trials during the daytime. Polysomnography demonstrated increased work of breathing, snoring, and arousals when the tracheostomy tube was capped. Flexible bronchoscopy revealed enlarged tonsils and adenoids and the presence of suprastomal granulation tissue obstructing 50% of the tracheal lumen (Figure 55-5). She was referred to a pediatric otolaryngologist for adenotonsillectomy and excision of the granuloma. Following surgery her snoring resolved, she was able to tolerate overnight capping, and she was successfully decannulated.

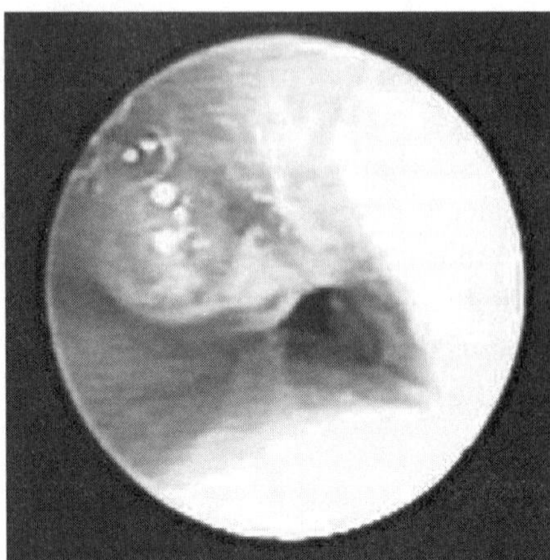

Figure 55-5. Suprastomal granulation tissue proximal to tracheostomy tube obstructing approximately 50% of airway lumen.

hypopharyngeal collapse, or tracheomalacia. Capping trials are first evaluated in the office of the specialist. If tolerated, the specialist will provide instruction on short capping trials to be initiated at home with supervision to determine how well the patient tolerates occlusion of the tube for extended periods. The tube can also be progressively downsized, although this approach is limited in very small children due to the proportionately larger increase in airway resistance and mucus plugging of the smaller tube. Finally, polysomnogram can be performed to assess the adequacy of gas exchange with a capped tracheostomy tube prior to decannulation. Decannulation should be attempted as an inpatient if the patient passes the aforementioned evaluations and tolerates capping for a minimum of 24 hours. The patient should be monitored in the hospital for 24 to 48 hours following decannulation to observe for any obstructive symptoms.[1,7,19]

Key Points

- Caring for a child with a chronic tracheostomy requires a multidisciplinary team.
- Indications for tracheostomy placement include causes of critical upper airway obstruction and conditions requiring prolonged mechanical ventilation.
- Changes in airway clearance, sense of smell, speech, humidification, and swallowing function can be expected following tracheostomy.
- Tracheostomy tubes are made in neonatal, pediatric, and adult sizes and are most commonly made of silicone or polyvinyl chloride.
- Uncuffed tubes are generally preferred to allow for vocalization, but cuffed tubes can be used for patients who are on ventilators or at risk for aspiration.
- Parents and other caregivers should be trained in suctioning, positive pressure resuscitation, stoma and skin care, tie and tube changes, cleaning tubes, troubleshooting, and CPR prior to discharge from the hospital.
- Patients with chronic tracheostomies should undergo semi-annual to annual bronchoscopic evaluations to assess size and fit, complications, and readiness for decannulation.
- Long-term complications of tracheostomy include granulomas, fistulae, erosions, infection, bleeding, and life-threatening obstruction of the tube.
- Decannulation can be considered in patients once initial indication for tracheostomy placement has resolved.
- Evaluation for decannulation includes flexible bronchoscopy, capping trials, downsizing of the tube, and polysomnogram.

References

1. Wetmore RF. Tracheotomy. In: Bluestone CD, Stool SE, et al, eds. *Pediatric Otolaryngology.* 4th ed. Philadelphia, PA: Saunders; 2003:1583–1598
2. Lewis CW. Tracheotomy in pediatric patients: a national perspective. *Arch Otolaryngol Head Neck Surg.* 2003;129:523–529
3. Shinkwin C. Tracheostomy in children. *J R Soc Med.* 1996;89:188–192
4. Corbett H. Tracheostomy—a 10-year experience from a UK pediatric surgical center. *J Pediatr Surg.* 2007;42(7):1251–1254
5. Koltai PJ. Starplasty: a new technique of pediatric tracheotomy. *Arch Otolaryngol Head Neck Surg.* 1998;124:1105–1111
6. McCool FD. Global physiology and pathophysiology of cough: ACCP evidence-based clinical practice guidelines. *Chest.* 2006;129(1 suppl):48S–53S
7. Sherman JM. American Thoracic Society statement: care of the child with a chronic tracheostomy. *Am J Respir Crit Care Med.* 2000;161:297–308
8. Van Oostdam JC, Walker DC, Knudson K, Dirks P, Dahlby RW, Hogg JC. Effect of breathing dry air on structure and function of airways. *J Appl Physiol.* 1986;61:312–317
9. Abraham SS, Wolf EL. Swallowing physiology of toddlers with long-term tracheostomies: a preliminary study. *Dysphagia.* 2000;15(4):206–212
10. Norman V. Incidence and description of dysphagia in infants and toddlers with tracheostomies: a retrospective review. *Int J Pediatr Otorhinolaryngol.* 2007;71(7):1087–1092
11. Hazinski M. Pediatric home tracheostomy care: a parent's guide. *Pediatr Nurs.* 1986;12:41–48, 69
12. Fitton C. Nursing management of the child with a tracheostomy. *Pediatr Clin North Am.* 1984;41:515
13. Fitton C, Myers C. Home care of the child with a tracheostomy. In: Myer C, Cotton R, Shott S, eds. *The Pediatric Airway: An Interdisciplinary Approach.* Philadelphia, PA: JB Lippincott; 1995
14. Hess D. Facilitating speech in the patient with a tracheostomy. *Respir Care.* 2005;50(4):519–525
15. Rusakow L. Suspected respiratory tract infection in the tracheostomized child: the pediatric pulmonologist's approach. *Chest.* 1998;113(6):1549–1554
16. Toder DS, McBride JT. Consultation with the specialist: home care of children dependent on respiratory technology. *Pediatr Rev.* 1997;18:273–281
17. Zenk J, Fyrmpas G, Zimmerman T, Koch M, Constantindis J, Iro H. Tracheostomy in young patients: indications and long-term outcome. *Eur Arch Otorhinolaryngol.* 2009;266:705–711
18. Leung R, Berkowitz RG. Decannulation and outcome following pediatric tracheostomy. *Ann Otol Rhinol Laryngol.* 2005;114(10):743–748
19. Clark K. Tracheotomy. In: Hilman BC, ed. *Pediatric Respiratory Disease: Diagnosis and Treatment.* Philadelphia, PA: WB Saunders; 1993

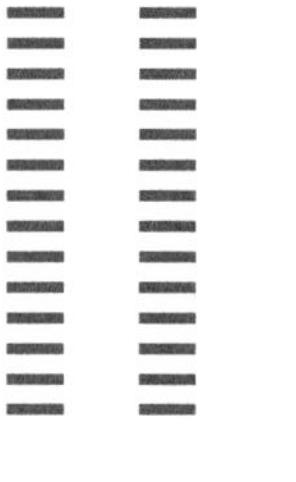

Chapter 56

Home Ventilation

Howard B. Panitch, MD

Case Report 56-1

A 6-month-old male was born at 24 weeks' gestation weighing 570 g. He developed respiratory distress, requiring endotracheal intubation and mechanical ventilation. Following stabilization, repeated efforts to wean ventilatory support resulted in episodes of respiratory distress and weight loss. At 5 months of age, he underwent elective tracheostomy placement to facilitate long-term mechanical ventilation. Following an interdisciplinary team meeting with the child's family where options for his ongoing care were discussed, the family expressed a desire to bring him home while he was still being supported by mechanical ventilation. Over the ensuing 8 weeks, his parents learned all aspects of their child's medical care, including how to suction and change his tracheostomy tube, how to assess his respiratory status, and how to ventilate him manually in the event of a ventilator failure. The necessary equipment and skilled nursing services were arranged, and the child was successfully discharged from the hospital at 8 months of age. With assisted ventilation, he demonstrated both somatic and developmental catch-up, and his respiratory status improved. He weaned completely off mechanical ventilation by 17 months, and had his trachea decannulated by 20 months.

History and Epidemiology of Pediatric Home Mechanical Ventilation

Chronic respiratory failure (CRF) can be defined as the need for mechanical ventilatory support for at least 4 hours per day for a month or longer.[1] The concept of supporting patients with CRF at home arose during the polio epidemics of the late 1940s and early 1950s, both because of the numbers of patients versus the number of available acute care beds and the desire of families to have their loved ones home.

The medical indications for chronic ventilatory support have shifted over time. In the 1970s and 1980s, the group of children with CRF comprised infants with chronic respiratory disease, those with anoxic encephalopathy, and infants surviving formerly fatal congenital anomalies.[2] Infants chronically dependent on ventilatory support were identified as having a new form of disability, and were considered "a creature of our new technology."[3] Over the last 2 decades, the population most likely to require chronic ventilatory support at home has shifted again, from survivors of neonatal disease to those children with underlying neuromuscular or central nervous system (CNS) diseases.[4,5]

As the types of patients receiving mechanical ventilation at home has changed over the years, the number of children receiving such care has continued to increase. In 1987 there were an estimated 600 to 2,000 ventilator-dependent children in the United States.[6] In 2004 the estimated number of children receiving home mechanical ventilation via tracheostomy grew to 4,100.[5] In Massachusetts, a 2005 survey of children supported by mechanical ventilation outside of an acute care hospital showed an almost 3-fold increase in number when compared with numbers derived from a similar survey conducted 15 years earlier. A similar shift was seen in the reasons for mechanical ventilation from children born prematurely with chronic lung disease to those with neuromuscular and CNS conditions.[4]

Goals of Home Mechanical Ventilation

No matter the diagnosis, growing up in an acute care hospital is considered detrimental to a child's overall health. Children who receive their respiratory support in hospitals for prolonged periods are at risk for nosocomial infection, in part because resistant bacteria are selected for in hospital environments and also because other children with communicable diseases from the community are admitted into the hospital and so increase the risk of exposure. Growth and development are slowed by prolonged hospitalization, because therapies and play activities must fit into regimented days with caregivers who are responsible for the care of several other children as well. In addition to the drawbacks for the child, caring for children in acute care hospitals is expensive, and excellent quality care can typically be accomplished for less in the home environment.[1,7]

The goals of home mechanical ventilation are listed in Box 56-1.

Box 56-1. Goals of Home Mechanical Ventilation[a]

- Extend life and enhance its quality.
- Reduce morbidity.
- Improve physiological function.
- Achieve normal growth and development whenever possible.
- Reduce health care costs.

[a]Adapted from O'Donohue WJ Jr, Giovannoni RM, Goldberg AI, et al. Long-term mechanical ventilation. Guidelines for management in the home and at alternate community sites. Report of the Ad Hoc Committee, Respiratory Care Section, American College of Chest Physicians. *Chest.* 1986;90:1S–37S.

Assisted ventilation for the hospitalized child represents an impediment to advancing to the next step of rehabilitation and eventual discharge; thus the focus is on withdrawing support even at the expense of increasing the patient's own breathing effort. Since the home ventilation patient is no longer taking up the limited resources of a hospital, weaning can proceed as the natural outcome of growth, development, and rehabilitation; as a child's underlying disease improves and growth and developmental milestones are acquired, mechanical ventilatory support becomes less needed and finally unnecessary. This philosophy is the key to understanding many of the factors that are considered in the weaning process of children with CRF, as discussed below.

Causes of Chronic Respiratory Failure

Conditions that cause respiratory failure in children can be broadly considered within the context of disorders of the respiratory pump (the chest wall, ventral abdominal wall, and muscles of respiration), abnormalities in the respiratory control center, lung parenchymal abnormalities, and airway anomalies. One way to categorize these conditions is listed in Box 56-2. In general, the suitability for home mechanical ventilation has less to do with the underlying diagnosis than with the degree of medical stability and the extent of support available for home care.

Clinical Features of Chronic Respiratory Failure

Often CRF follows an acute illness from which the child does not recover completely. In such situations, it is not possible to reduce ventilatory support because respiratory distress or signs of respiratory

Box 56-2. Conditions for Which Home Mechanical Ventilation Might Be Considered

Thoracic/Intrathoracic

- Obstructive lung disease
  - Chronic lung disease of infancy (bronchopulmonary dysplasia)
  - Tracheomalacia
  - Cystic fibrosis
- Restrictive lung disease
  - Neuromuscular diseases
  - Chest wall disorders
  - Spinal cord injury
  - Lung hypoplasia
  - Recurrent aspiration syndromes

Extrathoracic

- Craniofacial malformations
- Obstructive sleep apnea

Central Control

- Congenital central hypoventilation syndrome
- Brain/brain stem injury
- Central nervous system tumors

insufficiency quickly ensue. In other situations, the effects of respiratory failure are more insidious. Children with progressive neuromuscular diseases, for example, develop sleep-disordered breathing and will complain of frequent awakenings and morning headaches when nocturnal hypoventilation is present.[8] As respiratory muscle weakness progresses, daytime fatigue, poor school functioning, and weight loss will ensue. Older children and adolescents with respiratory muscle weakness who chronically breathe at low tidal volumes eventually develop reduced chest wall compliance as ligaments and tendons stiffen and ankylosis of the costovertebral joints develops,[9] adding to the load against which respiratory muscles have to work.

Respiratory load can also increase because of airway obstruction from uncontrolled bronchospasm or during acute viral illnesses, with atelectasis or pneumonia, or when mechanical ventilator support is weaned too aggressively. When the respiratory load increases, the work of the respiratory pump must also increase to avoid failure. This work of increasing respiratory pump expenditure to attain near-normal gas exchange often comes at the expense of growth,[10] or energy for play or acquisition of developmental milestones. Inadequate ventilatory support can also be associated with hypoxemia, and even intermittent hypoxemia can lead to pulmonary hypertension, cor pulmonale, and right heart failure.

Mechanical ventilation can be used to provide sigh breaths to maintain chest wall flexibility and reverse areas of microatelectasis that occur after prolonged low tidal volume breathing. By shifting inspiratory work from the muscles of ventilation to the mechanical ventilator, calories can be conserved and redistributed for somatic growth and other physical (developmental) activities. Ventilatory support improves sleep quality in patients who have sleep-related hypoventilation,[8] and restoration of normal gas exchange can often help reverse pulmonary hypertension and cor pulmonale.

Patient Selection for Home Ventilation

There are several criteria that must be fulfilled to consider a child eligible for home ventilation, independent of the cause of CRF. These include medical, social, and economic factors. If a child with a life-threatening condition or irreversible, progressive respiratory failure does not meet the usual criteria but would be better managed in the home environment, the approach and assessment must be individualized.

Medical Stability

The child must fulfill both physiological and clinical requirements for safe care outside of the intensive care unit (ICU) (Box 56-3). Physiological criteria refer to the child's airway and gas exchange capabilities. The child's airway must be stable, whether it is the natural airway or an artificial one. A stable airway means that under usual circumstances; there is a patent passage from atmosphere to alveoli; that any artificial airway will remain in place despite movement of the child; and tube repositioning, if it occurs, does not require routine radiographic confirmation. Children with parenchymal lung disease should be able to maintain a partial pressure of oxygen in arterial blood (Pa_{O_2}) above 60 mm Hg in an fraction of inspired oxygen (F_{IO_2}) less than 0.40. This is not only a practical consideration (it is technically difficult to maintain a supply of home oxygen when demands are >0.50), but it is also somewhat of a pragmatic one; it suggests that the child has some degree of reserve so that in the event of a mild illness, the child's

Case Report 56-2

A female neonate was discovered during her first examination to have a congenital diaphragmatic hernia and severe pulmonary hypoplasia. She required support with extracorporeal membrane oxygenation therapy for 19 days, and underwent patch repair of her defect at 9 days of age. She developed persistent pulmonary hypertension that was managed with chlorothiazide and sildenafil. She underwent tracheostomy placement to facilitate chronic mechanical ventilation at 3 months of age. Her parents discussed home care issues with the care team and learned all aspects of their daughter's medical care. At the same time, a home equipment company and nursing agency were identified. The home was assessed for adequacy of supporting the child, and the care team and insurance case managers agreed on the amount of nursing care and types of durable and disposable equipment that would be covered by the insurance company. Episodically, however, the infant experienced severe spells of respiratory distress, with oxyhemoglobin desaturation, diaphoresis, and poor air entry on chest auscultation. Treatment of the spells typically required sedation rescues, a temporary increase in positive end-expiratory pressure, and increased F_{IO_2}. The planned discharge was suspended. Evaluation disclosed severe gastroesophageal reflux despite the use of acid blockers and motility agents. The child underwent fundoplication and placement of a gastrostomy tube at 4 months. Following recovery from her surgery, she experienced a 2-week period without spells. Over the same time, no changes were made to any of her medications or ventilator settings. At 5 months of age she was considered to be safe for home care and was successfully discharged home on continuous mechanical ventilation and medications for the treatment of her pulmonary hypertension.

condition is unlikely to deteriorate precipitously, and the child might be able to be cared for through the acute illness at home. The child's partial pressure of carbon dioxide in arterial blood ($Paco_2$) should be less than 50 mm Hg on the current level of ventilatory support. In the case of children with respiratory failure from causes other than parenchymal lung disease, the Pao_2 and $Paco_2$ should both be normal on ventilatory support without the need for supplemental oxygen. Frequent changes in ventilator settings should not be required to maintain adequate gas exchange.

Clinical criteria that must be satisfied include a positive trend on the growth curve for infants and young children or weight maintenance for older children, stamina for periods of play or participation in therapy sessions, freedom from infection or frequent fevers, and resolution of any outstanding diagnostic considerations. Once a decision has been made to send a child home on mechanical ventilatory support,

Box 56-3. Determinants of Medical Stability for Ventilator-Dependent Children Outside of the Intensive Care Unit

Physiological Criteria

- Stable airway
- Parenchymal lung disease
  - Pao_2 >60 mm Hg in Fio_2 <0.40
  - $Paco_2$ <50 mm Hg
- Chest wall/neuromuscular disease
  - Pao_2 >60 mm Hg in room air
  - $Paco_2$ <45 mm Hg
- No need for frequent ventilator changes to maintain adequate gas exchange

Clinical Criteria

- Positive trend on growth curve
- Stamina for periods of play or therapies
- No frequent fevers or infections
- Resolution of any outstanding medical issues requiring evaluation

Abbreviations: Fio_2, fraction of inspired oxygen; $Paco_2$, partial pressure of arterial carbon dioxide; Pao_2, partial pressure of arterial oxygen.

there must be a predefined period, which can range from 1 to 4 weeks before the planned discharge, where no changes are made to any aspect of the medical regimen. In this way, the treating team gains understanding of how the patient is tolerating the current level of support. Furthermore, the care team is better able to smooth the transition to home, which often is a tumultuous time, and unexpected medical issues resulting from a change in support are avoided.

Caregiver Training

Early in the process of identifying a child as a candidate for home ventilation, the family must agree to the concept and be willing and able to learn all aspects of the child's medical care. A brief checklist of the issues that need to be addressed before a child can be safely discharged on assisted ventilation is presented in Box 56-4. There should be at least 2 adults available to learn the care, although additional family members should be encouraged to learn as well, to provide support to the primary caregivers. This will require family caregivers to understand the ventilator or bi-level pressure generator and its circuit, issues related to the patient/machine interface (eg, tracheostomy care or skin care for noninvasive ventilation), a general respiratory assessment and what to do in emergency situations, and all aspects of the child's medical regimen.

Box 56-4. Checklist of Items Required for Safe Home Ventilation Discharge

Caregiver training (2 people)
- Ventilator and monitors
- Tracheostomy or noninvasive interface
- Airway clearance equipment
- General respiratory assessment
- Medications
- CPR

Identification of home care providers
- Primary care provider
- Skilled nursing agency
- Durable medical equipment company
- Local ambulance service/emergency care facility

Written agreement with insurance company of what and how much will be covered
- Durable and disposable equipment
- Hours of skilled nursing
- Therapies

Home assessment and any necessary modifications
- Electrical, water, heat
- Generator if frequent power outages expected
- Telephone
- Ramps

Notification to community services
- Electrical company
- Local ambulance service/emergency department

Prescriptions filled

All necessary equipment and supplies delivered to home before discharge

Child adequately supported on home equipment in the hospital 1–7 days

The family should also have some understanding of the child's underlying condition that has caused the CRF. The primary caregivers need not necessarily be the child's biological parents; in single-parent homes, a grandparent, close friend, or neighbor can be the backup caregiver. Depending on insurance plans, the family may also be responsible for the selection of professional caregivers (home durable medical equipment [DME] company and nurses). Given the plethora of information and skills that family members must acquire, the family can expect the process to take 6 to 8 weeks between the time that they commit to taking the child home and being prepared to do so.

Preparing the Home

The home environment must also be adequate to support a ventilator-dependent child. There must be sufficient space for the equipment and additional personnel who will be caring for the child, as well as adequate heat, electricity, and water supply. A working telephone is critical, as the telephone becomes the lifeline between the family and the child's medical caregivers. Those children confined to a wheelchair will require alterations to the home for access and egress. If the child lives in a remote area, or in an area where power outages are frequent, it is prudent for the family to have a backup generator. When the child lives at a distance from the discharging tertiary care center, community resources like the local hospital's emergency department and local ambulance service must be identified, so that the child can be stabilized and transported in the event of an acute illness.

Skilled Nursing Care

Care of a child with CRF at home is stressful for parents, and parental stress has been shown to increase with duration of time at home.[7] Skilled nursing care is often prescribed to help parents cope with the extraordinary demands of caring for these children. Any child who would experience life-threatening respiratory embarrassment if the ventilator interface were to become inadvertently disconnected or obstructed, and who would be unable physically to correct the problem, should receive a minimum of 8 hours of skilled nursing care. In this way, parents can be assured that a trained adult is available to assess and intervene on their child's behalf while they sleep. The nurse provides care as directed by a written medical plan and provides ongoing assessments and documentation of the child's medical status as well as the family's level of functioning. The nurse can also teach and reinforce procedures and assessment skills that were introduced to the family during the initial hospitalization of the child. The home care nurse must be knowledgeable and proficient in all aspects of high-technology home care, including function of home ventilators, assessment of respiratory and cardiac status, care of long-term tracheostomies or nasal interfaces, and use of airway clearance techniques and devices.

Depending on the medical needs of the child, up to 24 hours per day of nursing care may be necessary for the safety and well-being of the child.[11] Nursing care represents the most expensive aspect of home mechanical ventilation.[1] Nevertheless, there are no uniform criteria to determine the quantity or duration of nursing care that the ventilator-dependent child should receive. The period following the initial discharge of a ventilator-dependent child is perhaps the most tenuous with regard to achieving a successful transition from hospital to home care. For this reason, many advocate that families receive around-the-clock nursing care for 1 to 2 weeks until the child's home regimen is well established, after which a reduction in the number of nursing hours provided can occur based on the child's status and level of the family's functioning.[11] The number of nursing hours funded by third-party payers may require temporary increases during periods of acute illness of the child or family caregivers. In addition, the well-being of caregivers demands a rational approach for providing funded periods of respite care for families.[12] The need for respite care services, to allow families some time off from the highly stressful duties of caring for a ventilator-dependent child, has been repeatedly identified both by parents and experts in the field as essential, and a mechanism to help avoid a care crisis or family breakdown.[11–13]

Economic and Payment Issues

Home mechanical ventilation is purported to be cost-saving when compared with caring for children in ICUs.[1] Nevertheless, it is still expensive and beyond the capabilities of most families to pay for. Thus funding for DME, nursing services, disposable supplies, medications, and specialized formulas all must be established and guaranteed. This is typically accomplished through third-party payers, state Medicaid programs, or model waiver programs. The items and services that these programs will cover must be established before the child is discharged from the hospital to avoid unexpected catastrophic financial burdens for the family. Some expenses that are bundled into a hospital stay will become out-of-pocket costs for families, such as medications or formula. The home electric, water, and telephone bills are also likely to increase. Each family must consider this in their decision to bring the child home. Families must also try to anticipate the effect of lost income related to the child's unexpected illnesses and there is no nurse available. By discussing these issues early in the discharge process, the family can often make contingency plans, seek additional funding from other community resources, or devise alternate strategies to make up any shortfalls.

Organizational Issues

Successful discharge of a ventilator-dependent child requires the efforts and input of a multidisciplinary team that includes appropriate medical subspecialists; case managers; nurse coordinators; social workers; nutritionists; respiratory, speech, physical, and occupational therapists from the discharging institution; a case manager from the insurance company; and the primary care physician and home nursing and DME company personnel in the community.[11,14–16]

Any child who receives skilled nursing care at home must also have a set of written medical orders. These encompass everything from the recommended ventilator settings and routine medication regimen to frequency of vital signs, types of monitoring to be used, the amount of skilled nursing the child should receive, the type and frequency of airway clearance to provide, and the nutritional plan. Actions to take in case of a change in the child's medical status, such as the range of supplemental oxygen permissible, frequency of extra bronchodilator aerosol treatments to be given, or other changes in support, are documented as well. The initial plan is written by the discharging team before the child first leaves the hospital, but it must be reviewed periodically. This review can be the responsibility of the primary care physician or the subspecialist (usually a pulmonologist or critical care medicine physician) who monitors the child's ventilator care.

The role and responsibilities of the primary care physician will vary depending on the level of comfort of the physician regarding the care of ventilator-dependent children, prior training, proximity of the patient to the tertiary care center, regional customs of care delivery, and established relationships with the family.[17] In general, the primary care physician is the person responsible for general pediatric care but, as noted previously, he or she may also want to be responsible for care plan review and even ventilator management. In some programs, a multidisciplinary team of pulmonologists, advanced practice nurses, social worker, nutritionist, and therapists provide ongoing care through telephone contact and scheduled outpatient visits, and work in concert with the primary care physician to ensure continued success of the child and family at home. Ventilator-dependent patients are seen for routine visits at intervals from 1 to 6 months, depending on their underlying disease, expected trajectory with regard to weaning, and degree of illness. In many programs in the United States, when children require rehospitalization, they return to the discharging institution. In contrast, in other systems like that found in the United Kingdom, when a child is discharged home with ventilatory support, the care of the child is also transferred from the tertiary care center to a community health care team.[14]

Modes of Mechanical Ventilation

Most types of mechanical ventilation provided at home involve the application of positive pressure to the airway, although negative pressure and positive pressure body ventilators are occasionally used. Whether a child receives positive pressure noninvasively or invasively depends on several factors, as listed in Box 56-5. In general, if a child cannot control his secretions, requires support for more than 16 hours per day, has facial features that make a standard nasal interface difficult to use, or is not (or his caregivers are not) committed to a noninvasive approach, then tracheostomy placement should be considered to facilitate assisted ventilation. At times, supporting a young child with noninvasive ventilation can increase the complexity of care for families who must also manage airway clearance and provide physical and other therapies. In these situations, placement of a tracheostomy can actually simplify care, even though the caregivers must learn additional skills related to tracheostomy management. Thus the decision to manage a child with invasive or noninvasive ventilation is a highly individualized one.

The mode of ventilation, whether pressure or volume controlled, is also a choice that is individualized. There are no data that generally support one style over the other, and several newer portable mechanical ventilators designed for home use can provide either method of support. Occasionally, one style is preferred over the other. In cases of large leaks around tracheostomies, for example, ventilation in a volume control mode will be unreliable and can lead to significant episodes of hypoventilation.[18] In this situation, pressure

Box 56-5. Factors to Consider for Noninvasive Versus Tracheostomy Positive Pressure Ventilation

- Level of consciousness
- Ability to control oral secretions
- Duration of daily support
- Adequacy of available interfaces
- Willingness of patient and family
- Caregiver skills and aptitude

control ventilation can help overcome the leak, and avoid the need for a cuffed tracheostomy tube.

Equipment and Monitoring

There is no single home mechanical ventilator that is the most appropriate for all situations. Newer, smaller models provide continuous flow and are capable of giving pressure support during spontaneous efforts. This is ideal for infants and young children, but may not be necessary for patients who do not breathe spontaneously or who are supported in an assist/control mode of ventilation. The model of ventilator or bi-level pressure generator chosen should be based on whether it can deliver the mode of support prescribed, adequate trigger and cycle sensitivity, and portability (for those who require support for most of the day). Accompanying equipment for the ventilator will vary, depending on whether the child receives support via tracheostomy or noninvasively.[2,11]

Children who cannot be independent of mechanical ventilation for at least 4 hours of the day, or who live more than 1 hour from their DME company or health care facility, should have a second complete ventilator and circuit in the event that the primary unit fails,[15] although this is uncommon.[19]

While all portable ventilators have alarms to detect obstruction, accidental disconnection, or decannulation, these are not adequate to be used as the sole means of monitoring patients. This is especially true for children with tracheostomy tubes that have inside diameters smaller than 4.5 mm, where high tube resistance can mask an inadvertent tracheal decannulation.[20]

There is, however, no consensus regarding the type and extent of monitoring to be used beyond that supplied by the ventilator. Pulse oximetry can be used both as a routine monitoring device and as an aid in adjusting ventilator settings during acute illnesses, or as a monitoring device during weaning of the patient if appropriate. Cardiorespiratory monitors are advocated by some,[2] but considered redundant by others.[21] Continuous capnometry is not indicated for patients at home, but intermittent determinations of end-tidal carbon dioxide can be useful to assess adequacy of ventilation, especially during weaning trials or during acute illnesses.

Long-term Outcomes of Home Mechanical Ventilation

Outcomes of ventilator-dependent children can be gauged in terms of survival, ability to wean from support, quality of life of the child, and quality of life of the caregivers. In general, survival is considered quite good, although it differs by diagnostic groups. Factors to consider regarding survival include the natural history of the underlying disease (ie, is the child's underlying condition expected to improve over time, remain static, or worsen), and whether the child is supported noninvasively or via tracheostomy.

The average 5-year cumulative survival from published reports of 265 children treated with home mechanical ventilation between 1983 and 1998 was approximately 85%.[22] Of 137 patients with neuromuscular diseases who were receiving home mechanical ventilation, the 5-year cumulative survival estimate was slightly lower (75%). In most series abstracted, death was most commonly a result of progression of the underlying disease.

Chronic mechanical ventilation does not reverse the respiratory failure associated with a progressive parenchymal disease like cystic fibrosis,[23] but it does contribute to a longer survival of patients with neuromuscular disease after the onset of respiratory failure.[24] Reported differences in survival by disease groups might not be apparent when the follow-up period is short.

The presence of a tracheostomy adds a small but significant survival risk because of the possibility of inadvertent decannulation, tube obstruction and, less commonly, serious bleeding from erosion of the tube into a major vessel. Furthermore, life-threatening tracheostomy-related accidents are more likely to occur in the home than in the hospital. In one review, life-threatening airway accidents in children receiving chronic mechanical ventilation by tracheostomy occurred among hospitalized children at a rate of 0.9/10,000 patient days, whereas the rate at home was almost 3 times greater, or 2.3/10,000 patient days.[25] In a review of 101 children with CRF cared for over 18 years, 30 children died, of whom one-third had already been liberated completely from mechanical ventilation but had not yet undergone tracheal decannulation.[26] Six of the deaths (20%) were attributable to airway accidents, and all but one occurred at home. Three of the 5 children at home had already been liberated from mechanical ventilation, but had a tracheostomy in place because of subglottic stenosis.

Other outcomes frequently measured in children receiving mechanical ventilatory support outside of the ICU are reduction of mechanical ventilator support to fewer than 12 hours per day and complete liberation from mechanical ventilation.[27] The likelihood that a child with CRF will wean from mechanical ventilation is greatly influenced by the underlying cause of respiratory failure. Children with chronic lung disease after prematurity or a central airway problem like tracheomalacia are less likely to require long-term mechanical ventilation compared with children who have underlying neurologic or neuromuscular conditions.[27–29] In the home setting, 30% to 56% of children with CRF can be liberated from mechanical ventilation, most of whom are infants with a history of chronic lung disease or a central airway disorder.[28,29]

In general, home mechanical ventilation is positively viewed by the patients supported by it. Its use is associated with improved physiological function and sleep quality, and fewer rehospitalizations.[8,24,30] Home ventilation of 23 males with Duchenne muscular dystrophy not only resulted in 1- and 5-year survival of 85% and 73%, respectively, but nocturnal ventilatory support also normalized daytime unassisted oxygen and carbon dioxide values.[24] Among 15 children with neuromuscular diseases receiving noninvasive mechanical ventilation at home, there was an 85% reduction in the number of hospital days after initiation of mechanical ventilation compared with the pre-ventilation period.[8] In another retrospective series, patients experienced an average of only 0.7 rehospitalizations per year over the 20-year observation period.[31]

Home ventilation is also psychologically acceptable to the children who use it. Interviews with 38 ventilator-dependent children showed that 79% were satisfied with their quality of life.[32] Most (77%) were also considered to be well adjusted. Adolescents were, in general, less content with their daily activities than were younger children, but greater satisfaction trended with greater activity levels. Notably, quality of life did not correlate with whether the child had been ventilator-dependent from birth or acquired respiratory failure later in life, with duration of ventilation at home, or if the child's disease was static or progressive.

Although ventilator-dependent children have expressed concern about their health and being a burden to their families,[13] in general their outlook toward mechanical ventilation is a positive one, and mechanical ventilation is considered a minor aspect of their lives.[33,34] Furthermore, older ventilator-dependent patients express overall satisfaction with their lives.[35] Gilgoff and Gilgoff[31] noted that 83% of their subjects left home each day to attend school, and many reported traveling for vacations. Perhaps paramount in the discussion is that health care providers routinely underestimate the quality of life of ventilator-dependent patients, and so might not consider chronic mechanical ventilation as a reasonable choice for some patients.[36]

While ventilator-dependent children generally express satisfaction with their general condition, the feelings of their family caregivers are more complicated. Parents (or other family caregivers) commonly express that having their ventilator-dependent child at home is both good and desirable, but they also speak about the stresses of caring for their ventilator-dependent children.[7,13,37–39] Parents frequently voice a fear of having the child die at home.[13] In contrast, neither the severity of respiratory insufficiency, amount of ventilator support, nor long-term prognosis predicts caregiver stress.[37] Several studies cite a lack of privacy associated with home nursing care, as well as a concern for the quality of professional care provided as sources of family stress.[37,39] Financial concerns result not only from increased expenses (utility bills, special formulas, medications), but also from the loss of income that occurs when one spouse must remain home to care for the child. Parents often feel isolated, since it is difficult or impossible to find a babysitter who is trained to care for a ventilator-dependent child, and some public facilities restrict access to people with tracheostomies or mechanical ventilators.[13,37] Parents also experience frequent sleep disruption to answer alarms or to provide care when nighttime nursing is not available.[40] The stresses related to caring for a ventilator-dependent child at home increase over time.[7] Despite these hardships, parents who have cared for their ventilator-dependent children at home would choose to do so again if given the choice.[38] In general, both medical professionals and family members have a sense that having a ventilator-dependent child at home improves both growth and developmental outcomes.

When to Admit

The general goal of chronic mechanical ventilation is to support the child's growth and development. These, therefore, must be monitored routinely either by the primary care provider or the team managing the child's ventilator care. Adjustments to routine care, including a change in ventilator settings, can be achieved without the need for hospitalization. If ventilator support is being gradually weaned, weekly status updates with the caregivers should be arranged by phone. Acute illnesses often can be cared for without the need for emergency department or hospital visits. Tracheal samples and even appropriate blood work can be obtained at home and sent for analysis with advanced planning. Antibiotic therapy can be instituted, and bronchodilator administration can be started or increased based on reports and observations of home nurses or family caregivers. Ventilatory support can also be adjusted based on reports of physical examination, pulse oximetry, and capnography evaluations.

Hospitalization for acute illnesses or deterioration in the patient's status is recommended any time anyone on the family–health care team feels uncomfortable with the child's situation. That means if the parent or home nurse is uneasy keeping the child home under current conditions, or if members of the health care team do not feel that they have an adequate understanding of the child's status, hospitalization or a visit to the emergency department should be recommended. Practical limitations of care delivery also will dictate hospitalization. This could include a need for supplemental oxygen beyond what is deliverable in the home environment (eg, FIO_2 >0.50), or exhaustion of caregivers, especially if skilled nursing care is not available. Return to the hospital must never be seen as a hurdle for families, because this undermines the relationship with the health care team. Rarely, children will be hospitalized electively for a comprehensive evaluation. Hospitalization, however, is disruptive for the patient and the family; thus this should occur only when the tests deemed necessary cannot be performed on an outpatient basis.

Key Points

- The indications for chronic home mechanical ventilation, and the number of children so supported, continue to grow.
- Successful discharge of a ventilator-dependent child requires careful planning and intense training of family caregivers.
- Maintaining a ventilator-dependent child at home successfully requires a hospital-based multidisciplinary team of health care professionals, the primary care provider, community health care professionals, and family working together with defined roles.
- Outcomes of ventilator-dependent children generally are good, and are determined primarily by the prognosis of the underlying disease.
- While the practice of caring for a child with CRF at home on mechanical ventilatory support has become more commonplace, such care must be considered an extraordinary commitment on the part of the health care team, and especially on the part of the family who agrees to undertake this care.
- The remarkable efforts and needs of families and ventilator-dependent patients must be recognized and supported by health care and societal systems so that they may achieve their best outcomes.

References

1. Downes JJ, Parra MM. Costs and reimbursement issues in long-term mechanical ventilation of patients at home. In: Hill NS, ed. *Long-Term Mechanical Ventilation.* Vol. 152. New York, NY: Marcel Dekker, Inc.; 2001:353–374
2. Schreiner MS, Donar ME, Kettrick RG. Pediatric home mechanical ventilation. *Pediatr Clin North Am.* 1987;34:47–60
3. Koop CE. Keynote Address: Report of the Surgeon General's Workshop on Children with Handicaps and Their Families. Philadelphia, PA; 1982
4. Graham RJ, Fleegler EW, Robinson WM. Chronic ventilator need in the community: a 2005 pediatric census of Massachusetts. *Pediatrics.* 2007;119:e1280–e1287
5. Gowans M, Keenan HT, Bratton SL. The population prevalence of children receiving invasive home ventilation in Utah. *Pediatr Pulmonol.* 2007;42:231–236

6. US Congress, Office of Technology Assessment. *Technology-Dependent Children: Hospital v. Home Care—A Technical Memorandum.* Washington, DC: US Government Printing Office; 1987
7. Quint RD, Chesterman E, Crain LS, Winkleby M, Boyce WT. Home care for ventilator-dependent children. Psychosocial impact on the family. *Am J Dis Child.* 1990;144:1238–1241
8. Katz S, Selvadurai H, Keilty K, Mitchell M, MacLusky I. Outcome of non-invasive positive pressure ventilation in paediatric neuromuscular disease. *Arch Dis Child.* 2004;89:121–124
9. Estenne M, De Troyer A. The effects of tetraplegia on chest wall statics. *Am Rev Respir Dis.* 1986;134:121–124
10. Loui A, Tsalikaki E, Maier K, Walch E, Kamarianakis Y, Obladen M. Growth in high risk infants <1500 g birthweight during the first 5 weeks. *Early Hum Dev.* 2008;84:645–650
11. Panitch HB, Downes JJ, Kennedy JS, et al. Guidelines for home care of children with chronic respiratory insufficiency. *Pediatr Pulmonol.* 1996;21:52–56
12. Parra MM. Nursing and respite care services for ventilator-assisted children. *Caring.* 2003;22:6–9
13. Carnevale FA, Alexander E, Davis M, Rennick J, Troini R. Daily living with distress and enrichment: the moral experience of families with ventilator-assisted children at home. *Pediatrics.* 2006;117:e48–e60
14. Jardine E, Wallis C. Core guidelines for the discharge home of the child on long-term assisted ventilation in the United Kingdom. UK Working Party on Paediatric Long Term Ventilation. *Thorax.* 1998;53:762–767
15. Make BJ, Hill NS, Goldberg AI, et al. Mechanical ventilation beyond the intensive care unit. Report of a consensus conference of the American College of Chest Physicians. *Chest.* 1998;113:289S–344S
16. Plummer AL, O'Donohue WJ Jr, Petty TL. Consensus conference on problems in home mechanical ventilation. *Am Rev Respir Dis.* 1989;140:555–560
17. Goldberg AI, Monahan CA. Home health care for children assisted by mechanical ventilation: the physician's perspective. *J Pediatr.* 1989;114:378–383
18. Gilgoff IS, Peng RC, Keens TG. Hypoventilation and apnea in children during mechanically assisted ventilation. *Chest.* 1992;101:1500–1506
19. Srinivasan S, Doty SM, White TR, et al. Frequency, causes, and outcome of home ventilator failure. *Chest.* 1998;114:1363–1367
20. Kun SS, Nakamura CT, Ripka JF, Davidson Ward SL, Keens TG. Home ventilator low-pressure alarms fail to detect accidental decannulation with pediatric tracheostomy tubes. *Chest.* 2001;119:562–564
21. Kacmarek RM. Home mechanical ventilatory assistance for infants. *Respir Care.* 1994;39:550–561

22. Teague WG. Long-term mechanical ventilation in infants and children. In: Hill NS, ed. *Long-Term Mechanical Ventilation.* Vol. 152. New York, NY: Marcel Dekker, Inc.; 2001:177–213
23. Young AC, Wilson JW, Kotsimbos TC, Naughton MT. Randomised placebo controlled trial of non-invasive ventilation for hypercapnia in cystic fibrosis. *Thorax.* 2008;63:72–77
24. Simonds AK, Muntoni F, Heather S, Fielding S. Impact of nasal ventilation on survival in hypercapnic Duchenne muscular dystrophy. *Thorax.* 1998;53:949–952
25. Downes JJ, Pilmer SL. Chronic respiratory failure—controversies in management. *Crit Care Med.* 1993;21:S363–S364
26. Schreiner MS, Downes JJ, Kettrick RG, Ise C, Voit R. Chronic respiratory failure in infants with prolonged ventilator dependency. *JAMA.* 1987;258:3398–3404
27. Kharasch VS, Haley SM, Dumas HM, Ludlow LH, O'Brien JE. Oxygen and ventilator weaning during inpatient pediatric pulmonary rehabilitation. *Pediatr Pulmonol.* 2003;35:280–287
28. Wheeler WB, Maguire EL, Kurachek SC, Lobas JG, Fugate JH, McNamara JJ. Chronic respiratory failure of infancy and childhood: clinical outcomes based on underlying etiology. *Pediatr Pulmonol.* 1994; 17:1–5
29. Edwards EA, O'Toole M, Wallis C. Sending children home on tracheostomy dependent ventilation: pitfalls and outcomes. *Arch Dis Child.* 2004;89:251–255
30. Khan Y, Heckmatt JZ, Dubowitz V. Sleep studies and supportive ventilatory treatment in patients with congenital muscle disorders. *Arch Dis Child.* 1996;74:195–200
31. Gilgoff RL, Gilgoff IS. Long-term follow-up of home mechanical ventilation in young children with spinal cord injury and neuromuscular conditions. *J Pediatr.* 2003;142:476–480
32. Lumeng JC, Warschausky SA, Nelson VS, Augenstein K. The quality of life of ventilator-assisted children. *Pediatr Rehabil.* 2001;4:21–27
33. Earle RJ, Rennick JE, Carnevale FA, Davis GM. 'It's okay, it helps me to breathe': the experience of home ventilation from a child's perspective. *J Child Health Care.* 2006;10:270–282
34. Noyes J. Health and quality of life of ventilator-dependent children. *J Adv Nurs.* 2006;56:392–403
35. Bach JR, Campagnolo DI, Hoeman S. Life satisfaction of individuals with Duchenne muscular dystrophy using long-term mechanical ventilatory support. *Am J Phys Med Rehabil.* 1991;70:129–135
36. Gibson B. Long-term ventilation for patients with Duchenne muscular dystrophy: physicians' beliefs and practices. *Chest.* 2001;119:940–946
37. Aday LA, Wegener DH. Home care for ventilator-assisted children: implications for the children, their families, and health policy. *Child Health Care.* 1988;17:112–120

38. Allen NL, Simone JA, Wingenbach GF. Families with a ventilator-assisted child: transitional issues. *J Perinatol.* 1994;14:48–55
39. Hazlett DE. A study of pediatric home ventilator management: medical, psychosocial, and financial aspects. *J Pediatr Nurs.* 1989;4:284–294
40. Meltzer LJ, Mindell JA. Impact of a child's chronic illness on maternal sleep and daytime functioning. *Arch Intern Med.* 2006;166:1749–1755

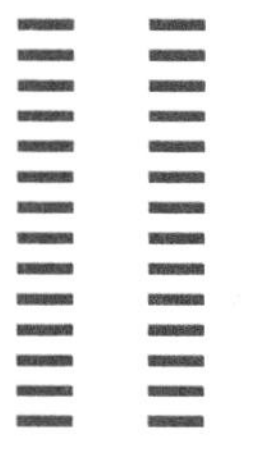

Index

C

E

F

G

H

I

M

N

Q

R

T

U

V

W

X

Y

Z